P9-CQA-821

THE WASHINGTON MANUAL OF OUTPATIENT INTERNAL MEDICINE

First Edition

Department of Medicine
Washington University
School of Medicine
St. Louis, Missouri

Executive Editor

Thomas M. De Fer, MD
Associate Professor of Internal Medicine

Editors

Meredith A. Brisco, MD
Instructor in Medicine

Rashmi S. Mullur, MD
Chief Resident

Wolters Kluwer | Lippincott Williams & Wilkins
Health
Philadelphia · Baltimore · New York · London
Buenos Aires · Hong Kong · Sydney · Tokyo

Acquisitions Editor: Avé McCracken
Product Manager: Michelle M. LaPlante
Marketing Manager: Kimberly Schonberger
Vendor Manager: Bridgett Dougherty
Manufacturing Manager: Ben Rivera
Design Coordinator: Teresa Mallon
Compositor: Aptara, Inc.

First Edition

Library of Congress Cataloging-in-Publication Data

The Washington manual of outpatient internal medicine / Dept. of
Medicine, Washington University School of Medicine ; executive editor,
Thomas M. De Fer ; editors, Meredith A. Brisco, Rashmi S. Mullur.—1st ed.
    p. ; cm.
  Includes bibliographical references and index.
  ISBN 978-0-7817-8977-6 (alk. paper)
  1. Ambulatory medical care—Handbooks, manuals, etc. I. De Fer,
Thomas M. II. Brisco, Meredith A. III. Mullur, Rashmi S. IV. Washington
University (Saint Louis, Mo.). Dept. of Medicine. V. Title: Manual of outpatient internal medicine.
  [DNLM: 1. Ambulatory Care—Handbooks. 2. Internal
Medicine—methods—Handbooks. WB 39 W3196 2010]
  RC55.W375 2010
  362.12—dc22
                                                                    2009052705

DISCLAIMER
Care has been taken to confirm the accuracy of the information present and to describe generally accepted practices. However, the authors, editors, and publisher are not responsible for errors or omissions or for any consequences from application of the information in this book and make no warranty, expressed or implied, with respect to the currency, completeness, or accuracy of the contents of the publication. Application of this information in a particular situation remains the professional responsibility of the practitioner; the clinical treatments described and recommended may not be considered absolute and universal recommendations.

  The authors, editors, and publisher have exerted every effort to ensure that drug selection and dosage set forth in this text are in accordance with the current recommendations and practice at the time of publication. However, in view of ongoing research, changes in government regulations, and the constant flow of information relating to drug therapy and drug reactions, the reader is urged to check the package insert for each drug for any change in indications and dosage and for added warnings and precautions. This is particularly important when the recommended agent is a new or infrequently employed drug.

  Some drugs and medical devices presented in this publication have Food and Drug Administration (FDA) clearance for limited use in restricted research settings. It is the responsibility of the health care provider to ascertain the FDA status of each drug or device planned for use in their clinical practice.

To purchase additional copies of this book, call our customer service department at (800) 638-3030 or fax orders to (301) 223-2320. International customers should call (301) 223-2300.

Visit Lippincott Williams & Wilkins on the Internet: http://www.lww.com. Lippincott Williams & Wilkins customer service representatives are available from 8:30 am to 6:00 pm, EST.

Contributors

Maria Q. Baggstrom, MD
Assistant Professor of Medicine
Division of Oncology

Thomas C. Bailey, MD
Professor of Medicine
Division of Infectious Diseases

Benico Barzilai, MD
Professor of Medicine
Division of Cardiology

Ernesto Bernal-Mizrachi, MD
Assistant Professor of Medicine, Cell Biology
and Physiology
Division of Endocrinology, Metabolism,
and Lipid Research

Melvin Blanchard, MD
Associate Professor of Medicine
Chief, Division of Medical Education

Morey A. Blinder, MD
Associate Professor of Medicine
Assistant Professor of Pathology and
Immunology
Division of Hematology

Debaroti M. Borschel, MD
Assistant Professor of Medicine
Director, Internal Medicine House
Staff Clinic
Division of Medical Education

Richard D. Brasington, MD
Professor of Medicine
Division of Rheumatology

Meredith A. Brisco, MD
Instructor in Medicine
Division of Medical Education

J. Chad Byrd, MD
Fellow
Division of Rheumatology
Former Chief Resident

Michelle C.L. Cabellon, MD
Assistant Professor of Medicine
Division of Renal Diseases

Amanda Camp, MD
Senior Assistant Resident
Internal Medicine Residency

David B. Carr, MD
Associate Professor of Medicine and
Neurology
Division of Geriatrics and Nutritional
Sciences

Murali M. Chakinala, MD
Associate Professor of Medicine
Division of Pulmonary and Critical
Care Medicine

Jinny E. Chang, MD
Instructor in Medicine
Division of Hospitalist Medicine

Ying Chen, MD
Fellow
Division of Renal Diseases

Steven Cheng, MD
Assistant Professor of Medicine
Division of Renal Diseases

Matthew A. Ciorba, MD
Instructor in Medicine
Division of Gastroenterology

William E. Clutter, MD
Associate Professor of Medicine
Division of Endocrinology, Metabolism,
and Lipid Research

Maria C. Dans, MD
Assistant Professor of Medicine
Division of Hospitalist Medicine
Clinical Director, Palliative Care Services

Thomas M. De Fer, MD
Associate Professor of Medicine
Division of Medical Education

Kathryn M. Diemer, MD
Assistant Professor of Medicine
Assistant Dean for Career Counseling

Dayna S. Early, MD
Associate Professor of Medicine
Division of Gastroenterology

Charles S. Eby, MD
*Associate Professor of Medicine and
Pathology and Immunology
Division of Hematology*

Brian F. Gage, MD
*Associate Professor of Medicine
Division of General Medical Sciences*

Prateek C. Gandiga, MD
*Instructor in Medicine
Division of Hospitalist Medicine*

Anne C. Goldberg, MD
*Associate Professor of Medicine
Division of Endocrinology, Metabolism,
and Lipid Research*

C. Prakash Gyawali, MD
*Associate Professor of Medicine
Division of Gastroenterology*

Christina Ha, MD
*Fellow
Division of Gastroenterology*

Katherine E. Henderson, MD
*Assistant Professor of Medicine
Division of Medical Education*

Warren Isakow, MD
*Assistant Professor of Medicine
Division of Pulmonary and Critical
Care Medicine*

Raksha Jain, MD
*Fellow
Division of Pulmonary and Critical
Care Medicine*

Omar Jassim, MD, PhD
*Resident
Division of Dermatology*

Mariko K. Johnson, MD
*Fellow
Division of Endocrinology, Metabolism,
and Lipid Research*

Shirley D. Joo, MD
*Assistant Professor of Medicine
Division of Allergy and
Immunology*

Stephen A. Kamenetzky, MD
*Resident
Department of Ophthalmology and
Visual Sciences*

Syed Khalid, MD
*Fellow
Division of Geriatrics and Nutritional
Sciences*

Nadia Khoury, MD
*Senior Assistant Resident
Internal Medicine Residency*

Eric C. Klawiter, MD
*Fellow
Department of Neurology*

Kevin M. Korenblat, MD
*Associate Professor of Medicine
Division of Gastroenterology*

F. Matthew Kuhlmann, MD
*Fellow
Division of Infectious Diseases*

Brendan Lloyd, MD
*Resident
Division of Dermatology*

Vinay Madan, MD
*Senior Assistant Resident
Internal Medicine Residency*

Scott B. Marrus, MD, PhD
*Fellow
Division of Cardiology*

Martin L. Mayse, MD
*Assistant Professor of Medicine
Division of Pulmonary and Critical
Care Medicine*

Rashmi S. Mullur, MD
*Chief Resident
Internal Medicine Residency*

Jawad Munir, MD
*Fellow
Division of Renal Diseases*

Mohsen Nasir, MD
*Senior Assistant Resident
Internal Medicine Residency*

E. Turner Overton, MD
Assistant Professor of Medicine
Division of Infectious Diseases

Vikrant Rachakonda, MD
Senior Assistant Resident
Internal Medicine Residency

Reshma Rangwala, MD, PhD
Instructor in Medicine
Division of Hospitalist Medicine

Hilary E.L. Reno, MD, PhD
Instructor in Medicine
Division of Infectious Diseases

Michael W. Rich, MD
Professor of Medicine
Division of Cardiology

Ilana Rosman, MD
Resident
Division of Dermatology

Tonya D. Russell, MD, BS
Associate Professor of Medicine
Division of Pulmonary and Critical
Care Medicine

Joel D. Schilling, MD, PhD
Instructor in Medicine
Division of Cardiology

Todd J. Schwedt, MD
Assistant Professor of Neurology

Amy Sheldahl, MD
Instructor in Medicine
Division of Hospitalist Medicine

Devin P. Sherman, MD
Fellow
Division of Pulmonary and Critical
Care Medicine

Timothy W. Smith, DPhil, MD
Associate Professor of Medicine
Division of Cardiology

Joshua M. Stolker, MD
Assistant Professor of Medicine
Division of Cardiology

Michael D. Straiko, MD
Resident
Department of Ophthalmology and Visual
Sciences

Shelby A. Sullivan, MD
Instructor in Medicine
Division of Endocrinology, Metabolism,
and Lipid Research

R. Brian Sommerville, MD
Fellow
Department of Neurology

Linda M. Tsai, MD
Associate Professor of Ophthalmology and
Visual Sciences

Peter G. Tuteur, MD
Associate Professor of Medicine
Division of Pulmonary and Critical Care
Medicine

Babac Vahabzadeh, MD
Senior Assistant Resident
Internal Medicine Residency

Leo Wang, MD
Fellow
Department of Neurology

Karen S. Winters, MD
Assistant Professor of Medicine
Director, Student and Employee Health
Services

Megan E. Wren, MD
Associate Professor of Medicine
Division of Medical Education

Roger D. Yusen, MD, MPH
Associate Professor of Medicine
Division of Pulmonary and Critical Care
Medicine

Preface

Welcome to the first edition of *The Washington Manual of Outpatient Internal Medicine.* This book is intended to be a companion to the 33rd edition of *The Washington Manual of Medical Therapeutics* and focuses almost entirely on the practice of internal medicine in the ambulatory setting. It is an outgrowth of *The Washington Manual of Ambulatory Therapeutics* published in 2002. We are, of course, indebted to the original editors (Tammy L. Lin and Scott W. Rypkema) and authors.

The continued focus is to provide a reference that covers common ambulatory medical problems encountered in each medical subspecialty. Recognizing that the approach to each may be handled differently, most of the subspecialties have separate symptom- and disease-based chapters. Many problems seen in the ambulatory setting fall outside traditional internal medicine subspecialties; therefore, we have included chapters on topics such as dermatology, neurology, ophthalmology, otolaryngology, and psychiatry. Following the tradition of our other publications, all chapters are authored by house staff and faculty at Barnes-Jewish Hospital and Washington University School of Medicine.

We have, however, departed from tradition in an important way—readers will find the format rather different from the preceding publication. We have purposely chosen to move away from the strictly outline format to a standard chapter template with a more bulleted style and more tables and figures. We are confident that the reader will find this more appealing and easier to navigate. These changes greatly facilitate future sharing with electronic media. Also, for the first time, two-color printing has been used.

The time from inception to completion has been considerable (longer than ever imagined) and the editors are enormously grateful for the patience shown by all involved. We especially thank the staff at Wolters Kluwer/Lippincott Williams & Wilkins for their superior guidance, assistance, encouragement, and forbearance, particularly Avé McCracken, Michelle LaPlante, and Kimberly Schonberger.

Finally, we have received tremendous support from the Department of Medicine. There are multiple people without whom this manual would not have been possible, including the Chief of the Division of Medical Education, Melvin Blanchard, and the department Chairman, Kenneth Polonsky. Both have been unwavering in the belief that the project could and should come to fruition.

Thomas M. De Fer, MD
Meredith A. Brisco, MD
Rashmi S. Mullur, MD

December 2009

Contents

1 Approach to the Ambulatory Patient

Debaroti M. Borschel and Thomas M. De Fer

Ambulatory care is any medical care delivered on an outpatient basis. The goals of the ambulatory visit are many and will vary from visit to visit. Not every issue can or needs to be addressed at each visit. The primary aims are management of current medical issues and prevention of future health problems.

Current Disease Management

- Diagnosis and treatment of disease are key elements of each visit.
- The clinician should evaluate the status of chronic diseases and any new problems.
- Because of time constraints, **not every problem can be analyzed exhaustively at each visit.**
- **Prioritization must occur** and is usually based on what the clinician feels is the most serious or active problem or problems and also what the patient feels is the most pressing matter, often the chief complaint.
- Explanation and relief of symptoms are key to the patient's satisfaction. Relief of symptoms does not always necessitate drug therapy but may include lifestyle changes.
- Some patients may only be seeking reassurance that a symptom is not indicative of a more serious illness.

Prevention of Future Health Problems

Screening may involve primary, secondary, or tertiary prevention.
- The four major types of clinical preventive care are as follows:
  - Immunizations (discussed in detail in Chapter 43).
  - Screening (discussed in detail in Chapter 43).
  - Behavioral counseling (lifestyle changes).
  - Chemoprevention.
- All four apply throughout the life span.
- **Primary prevention** keeps disease from occurring at all, by removing the cause, for example, with immunizations. Also, much of primary prevention is done at the community level with efforts such as fluorination of water, iodination of salt, and laws to require seatbelt and car seat usage.
- **Secondary prevention** entails screening for asymptomatic disease while in an early treatable phase. This includes screening for common cancers, as with Papanicolaou (Pap) smears or screening colonoscopy or mammograms. It can also include screening for common disease processes such as osteoporosis or hypertension.
- **Tertiary prevention** refers to those activities that prevent worsening of a disease or further complications, for example, using β-blockers or statins in patients with known coronary disease.

- **The periodic health examination,** formerly known as the "annual examination," is often used to address these preventive issues.

The Periodic Health Examination

- It is not often possible to cover all the issues that need to be covered during a periodic health examination at one visit and **many insurance companies may not cover a "routine visit."** It is generally better policy to have continuous health maintenance and address these issues in an ongoing manner.
- Preventive medicine requires an **individualized assessment** tailored to each patient's age, sex, risk factors, and existing illnesses.
- **Counseling** about a healthy lifestyle is a critical component of health care at any age. Refer to the individual sections for further details on cancer screening, immunizations, geriatrics, and so forth.

Adolescents and Young Adults

- Adolescents and young adults are at risk for serious morbidity and even mortality related to the **risky behaviors** that are common in this age group.
- The clinician should maintain an **open and nonjudgmental attitude** to encourage the adolescent to speak frankly.
- **Confidentiality** should be assured.
- **Important topics to discuss** include the avoidance of smoking, drinking, and illicit drug use; the use of bike helmets and car seat belts; firearm safety; depression and suicide; the potential consequences of sexual activity and how to avoid them; healthy dietary habits and eating disorders; and appropriate exercise.
- The physical examination should include height, weight, blood pressure (BP), testicular or breast and pelvic examinations, and possibly patient instruction on self-examination of the breasts or testes.
- Laboratory tests should include Pap smear, screening for *Chlamydia trachomatis* and *Neisseria gonorrhoeae*, and targeted screening for syphilis, hepatitis B, and HIV.
- Preventive measures include updating immunizations, especially rubella in women.
- Women of childbearing age should take a daily vitamin with 0.4 mg folic acid to reduce the risk of neural tube defects in their offspring.

Midlife Adults

- **Important topics to discuss** include continued reinforcement of the importance of healthy habits, especially diet, exercise, avoidance of tobacco, and moderation in alcohol consumption.
- Physical and laboratory examinations should include height, weight, BP, and screening for hyperlipidemia and common treatable cancers.
- In most women, annual mammography should begin at age 40 (see Chapter 43).
- Men can be offered screening for prostate cancer beginning at age 50 (see Chapter 38).
- All patients should be screened for colorectal cancer beginning at age 50. Patients with high-risk factors, including a family history of disease, need more aggressive screening (see Chapter 43).
- Preventive measures at age 50 include starting annual influenza vaccination and assessing the need for a tetanus booster or pneumococcal vaccination.
- Perimenopausal women should be counseled and should be offered screening for osteoporosis (see Chapter 37).

Older Adults

- **Important topics to discuss** include continued reinforcement of the importance of healthy habits, especially diet, exercise, avoidance of tobacco, and moderation in alcohol.
- As patients age, it is important to review medication lists for avoidance of polypharmacy and surveillance for side effects, drug interactions, and the need for dose adjustments due to changes in age, weight, and renal or hepatic function (see Chapter 34).
- Physical and laboratory examinations generally continue as for younger adults.
- Cessation of cancer screening is an individualized decision with no definite age end point and is based on patient preferences, age, comorbidities, functional status, and estimated life expectancy.
- Ongoing attention should be paid to minimizing the impact of deficits in vision, hearing, and mobility.
- Patients should be monitored for their ability to perform activities of daily living, including the ability to take medications accurately.
- Preventive measures include offering one-time pneumococcal and annual influenza vaccinations.
- Many elderly patients would benefit from a daily multivitamin to prevent micronutrient deficiencies as the daily caloric intake wanes with aging.
- Discussion of home safety may reduce the risk of falls (see Chapter 34).
- One should enlist family and community resources, which can provide essential support to enable the aging patient to remain as independent and active as possible.
- End-of-life care should be discussed on an ongoing basis with patients and their families.

Screening for Disease

- The benefit of screening depends on the prevalence of the disease, the sensitivity and specificity of the screening test, the ability to change the natural course of disease with treatment, and the acceptability of the test to the patient.
- Various professional organizations have made recommendations regarding screening for disease; these guidelines apply only to **asymptomatic patients at average risk,** and they must be individualized.
  - United States Preventive Services Task Force (USPSTF) usually takes a less-is-more standpoint and does not recommend screening without relatively clear evidence for a meaningful change in outcome (www.ahrq.gov/CLINIC/uspstfix.htm). Table 1 lists screening activities currently recommended by the USPSTF specifically for asymptomatic patients at average risk.
  - Disease-specific and subspecialty groups often advocate for more rather than less screening.
  - More general groups, for example, the American College of Physicians, have a tendency to take the middle ground.
- **Many areas of controversy exist,** including ages to start and stop screening, which tests to use, or whether to screen at all.
- For many diseases, there is a lack of definitive research evidence regarding the effect of screening on morbidity and mortality.

Hypertension

- **All patients should have their BP measured every 1 to 2 years but the optimum screening interval is unknown.**

TABLE 1	Screening and Preventive Measures Recommended by the USPSTF for *Asymptomatic Average Risk* Individuals

Breast cancer screening
Mammography
Colorectal cancer screening
  Fecal occult blood testing or
  Flexible sigmoidoscopy or
  Colonoscopy
Cervical cancer screening
  Pap smear
Hypertension screening
Dyslipidemia screening
Diabetes screening
  Only in those with BP >135/80 mm Hg
Osteoporosis
  Dual-energy x-ray absorptiometry
Abdominal aortic aneurysm screening
  Ultrasound once for men only for those aged between 65 and 75 years who
    have ever smoked
Chlamydia screening
  Nonpregnant, sexually active females <24 years
Syphilis screening
  All pregnant females
Hepatitis B screening
  All pregnant females
Obesity screening
Depression screening
Alcohol misuse screening
Tobacco use screening

BP, blood pressure; USPSTF, United States Preventive Services Task Force.

- Optimal/normal BP is <120/80 mm Hg.[1]
- A diastolic BP of >90 mm Hg or a systolic BP of >140 mm Hg (measured on more than one reading) is considered hypertension.
- Prehypertension is defined by a systolic BP of 120 to 139 mm Hg and/or a diastolic BP of 80 to 89 mm Hg. Prehypertensives are at high risk of developing hypertension, and early intervention can decrease the rate of BP progression with age but this does not denote a disease category.
- Initial therapy includes counseling on weight loss, aerobic exercise, limiting alcohol intake, and reduction in sodium intake. The decision to start drug therapy should depend on the severity of hypertension, the presence of other disease, and evidence of end-organ damage (see Chapter 3).

Dyslipidemia
- **Cholesterol screening is recommended every 5 years for all adults >20 years of age.**[2,3]
- Screening is best performed with a lipid profile (total cholesterol, low-density lipoprotein cholesterol, high-density lipoprotein cholesterol, and triglycerides) obtained after a 12-hour fast.

- Initial therapy for patients with elevated cholesterol levels includes counseling to decrease consumption of fats and to promote weight loss in overweight patients (see Chapter 8).

Diabetes Mellitus

- The USPSTF recommendations for diabetes mellitus (DM) screening are as follows:
  - **In asymptomatic adults with sustained BP of >130/85 mm Hg, screen for DM.**
  - In asymptomatic adults with sustained BP of <130/85 mm Hg, do NOT screen for DM (insufficient evidence).
  - Also consider screening those with other major coronary heart disease risk factors.
  - The optimal screening interval is unknown.
- The American Diabetes Association standards of care are as follows[4]:
  - Appropriate screening test is fasting plasma glucose or a 2-hour oral glucose tolerance test.
  - Fasting plasma glucose of ≥126 mg/dL on two separate occasions is diagnostic of DM. A casual plasma glucose of ≥200 mg/dL **with** symptoms of hyperglycemia (e.g., polyuria, polydipsia, and unexplained weight loss) is also diagnostic.
  - Recently an international expert committee has recommended the adoption of hemoglobin A_{1c} (the assay standardized and aligned with the Diabetes Control and Complications trial/UK Prospective Diabetes Study assay) as the diagnostic test of choice, ≥6.5% being diagnostic. Those with an A_{1c} level of ≥6% but <6.5% are at highest risk for progression to DM.[5] The American Diabetes Association has not officially accepted these recommendations, but it may do so in the future.
  - Based on expert opinion, screen overweight (body mass index [BMI] ≥25 kg/m^2) adults and those who have additional risk factors (presented in Table 2).
  - In those without risk factors, begin screening at age 45.
  - If screening is normal, repeat at 3-year intervals.
- Also refer to Chapter 16.

TABLE 2	Risk Factors for Diabetes Mellitus

BMI ≥ 25 kg/m^2
Are habitually physically inactive
Have a first-degree relative with diabetes
Are members of a high-risk ethnic group (e.g., African American, Latino, Native American, Pacific Islander)
Have delivered a baby weighing >9 lb or have been diagnosed with gestational diabetes
Are hypertensive (BP ≥140/90 mm Hg)
Have an HDL cholesterol level of <35 mg/dL and/or a triglyceride level of >250 mg/dL
Have polycystic ovary syndrome
On previous testing had impaired glucose tolerance or impaired fasting glucose
Have other clinical conditions associated with insulin resistance (e.g., severe obesity, acanthosis nigricans)
Have a history of vascular disease

BMI, body mass index; BP, blood pressure; HDL, high-density lipoprotein.
Modified from American Diabetes Association. Standards of Medical Care in Diabetes—2009. *Diabetes Care* 2009;32:S13–S61.

Thyroid Disease

- **According to the USPSTF, there is insufficient evidence to recommend for or against routine screening for thyroid disease in asymptomatic adults.** It does, however, note that some persons are at increased risk (e.g., elderly, postpartum, radiation exposure, and Down syndrome).
- The American Thyroid Association recommends that adults should be screened for thyroid dysfunction with TSH beginning at age 35 and every 5 years thereafter.[6]
- The American College of Physicians recommends screening women >50 years.
- Screening in pregnancy is controversial, with various organizations making rather different recommendations.
- Also refer to Chapter 17.

Obesity

- Periodic height and weight measurements are recommended for all patients.
- The BMI is calculated by dividing the body weight in kilograms by the square of the height in meters.
  - A person with a BMI of ≥25 kg/m^2 is considered overweight.
  - A person with a BMI of ≥30 kg/m^2 is considered obese.
  - A person with a BMI of ≥40 kg/m^2 is considered severely obese.
- Morbid obesity is obesity accompanied by medical complications (see Chapter 18).

Osteoporosis

- **The USPSTF and the National Osteoporosis Foundation recommend that all women >65 years be screened for osteoporosis with bone mineral density testing** (i.e., dual-energy x-ray absorptiometry).[7]
- The National Osteoporosis Foundation also recommends screening all men >70 years.
- Premenopausal women and men aged 50 to 69 years may be screened earlier if they have clinical risk factors.
- Risk factors for osteoporosis are listed in Table 3.[8]

TABLE 3	Risk Factors for Osteoporosis

Age
Female gender
Prior osteoporotic fracture (including morphometrics vertebral fractures)
Low body mass index
Oral steroids (equivalent to prednisone ≥5 mg/day for ≥3 months)
Rheumatoid arthritis
Parental history of hip fracture, current smoking
Three or more alcoholic drinks per day
Conditions associated with secondary osteoporosis (e.g., hyperthyroidism, hyperparathyroidism, hypogonadal states, Cushing syndrome, inflammatory bowel disease)

Modified from Kanis JA on behalf of the World Health Organization Scientific Group. Assessment of Osteoporosis at the Primary Health Care Level. 2008 Technical Report. University of Sheffield, UK: WHO Collaborating Center, 2008.

- All women should receive counseling regarding dietary calcium, vitamin D, weight-bearing exercise, and smoking cessation.
- Also see Chapter 37.

Depression

- **Screening all adults for depression is recommended by the USPSTF.**
- There is insufficient data to strongly recommend one screening method over another.
- Asking two simple questions about mood and anhedonia, "Over the past two weeks have you felt down, depressed, or hopeless" and "Over the past two weeks have you felt little interest or pleasure in doing things?" may be as effective as longer screening instruments.[9]
- Also refer to Chapter 40.

Sexually Transmitted Infections

- **Syphilis** serologic testing is recommended by the USPSTF for **all pregnant women and for all patients at increased risk for infection** (i.e., men who have sex with men and engage in high-risk sexual behavior, commercial sex workers, persons who exchange sex for drugs, and those in adult correctional facilities). The optimal screening interval is unknown.
- **Chlamydia** screening (with a nucleic acid amplification test) is recommended by the USPSTF **for all sexually active/pregnant young women aged 24 or younger and for older sexually active/pregnant women who are at increased risk** (e.g., <25 years of age, previous chlamydial infection or other sexually transmitted infections [STIs], new or multiple sexual partners, inconsistent condom use, sex work, African American, Hispanic). The optimum screening interval is unclear, but the Centers for Disease Control and Prevention recommends annual screening for those at increased risk.[10]
- **Gonorrhea** screening (with culture, nucleic acid amplification, or hybridization testing) is recommended by the UPSTF for **all sexually active women, including those who are pregnant, for gonorrhea infection if they are at increased risk for infection** (i.e., <25 years of age, previous gonorrhea infection or other STIs, new or multiple sexual partners, inconsistent condom use, sex work, and drug use). Routine screening of those not at increased risk is not recommended. The optimal screening interval is unknown.

HIV

- **HIV screening is recommended by the UPSTF for all pregnant women and all adolescents and adults with risk factors** (Table 4).

TABLE 4	Risk Factors for HIV

Men who have had sex with men after 1975
Men and women having unprotected sex with multiple partners
Past or present injection-drug users
Men and women who exchange sex for money or drugs or have sex partners who do
Individuals whose past or present sex partners were HIV infected, bisexual, or injection-drug users
Persons being treated for sexually transmitted diseases
Persons with a history of blood transfusion between 1978 and 1985

Modified from www.ahrq.gov/clinic/uspstfix.htm.

TABLE 5	Risk Factors for Hepatitis B

Persons born in regions of high and intermediate HBV endemicity, HBsAg
   positivity ≥ 2% U.S.-born persons not vaccinated as infants whose parents
   were born in regions with high HBV endemicity (≥8%)
Injection-drug users
Men who have sex with men
Persons needing immunosuppressive therapy
Persons with elevated ALT/AST levels of unknown etiology
Donors of blood, plasma, organs, tissues, semen
Hemodialysis
Pregnant women
Infants born to HBsAg-positive mothers

ALT, alanine aminotransferase; AST, aspartate aminotransferase; HBsAg, hepatitis B
surface antigen; HBV, hepatitis B virus.
Modified from Weinbaum CM, Williams I, Mast EE, et al. Recommendations for identification and public health management of persons with chronic hepatitis B infection.
MMWR Recomm Rep 2008;57:1–20.

- The Centers for Disease Control and Prevention recommends screening all individuals 13 to 64 years of age regardless of recognized risk factors in any health care
  setting. This recommendation presupposes that patients are notified that such testing will be done and they do not decline. They further recommend annual screening for those at high risk.[10]

Hepatitis B
- The USPSTF strongly recommends that **pregnant women be screened** for hepatitis B
  at their first prenatal visit. It recommends against broad screening of the general
  asymptomatic population.
- The Centers for Disease Control and Prevention advises screening for those who are
  at increased risk (Table 5).[11]

Alcohol Abuse
- **Screening for alcohol abuse and dependence is an important part of the routine checkup.**
- The UPSTF recommends screening and behavioral counseling intervention to
  reduce alcohol misuse.
- The "CAGE" questions are a useful screening tool.[12] If a patient has one or more
  positive responses that occurred in the last year, she or he may be at risk for alcohol-
  related problems:
  - Have you ever felt that you should **C**ut down on drinking?
  - Have you ever been **A**nnoyed with people's criticism about your drinking?
  - Have you ever felt **G**uilty about drinking?
  - Have you ever needed an **E**ye-opener in the morning to relieve the shakes?
- Alcohol Use Disorder Identification Test (AUDIT) is another screening test that
  may be more sensitive in populations with lower alcohol use.[13]
- A single-question screen may be just as effective, "How many times in the past year have
  you had four/five or more drinks in one day?" (four for women, five for men).[14,15]
- A detailed discussion of alcohol misuse is presented in Chapter 45.

Cancer Screening

- Cancer screening recommendations have been issued by many organizations, including the American Cancer Society (ACS; http://www.cancer.org), the National Cancer Institute (http://www.nci.nih.gov), the American College of Physicians (ACP; http://www.acponline.org), the USPSTF (http://www.ahrq.gov/clinic), and many specialty societies.
- As with other screening for other conditions, the approach much be individualized.
- Recommendations are discussed in detail in Chapter 43.

Tobacco Use and Cessation

- Nearly one-fourth of American adults smoke, but an estimated 70% want to quit.
- Although only approximately 7% of patients are able to quit long-term on their own, it is estimated that counseling and appropriate pharmacotherapy can increase the quit rate to 15% to 30%.
- A widely accepted approach to brief office-based counseling and pharmacotherapy was published as a U.S. Public Health Service Report.[16]
- Brief counseling should be provided to all smokers at every visit. Interventions as short as 3 minutes can increase the quit rate significantly.
- A detailed discussion of tobacco cessation is presented in Chapter 44.

Lifestyle Counseling

- The most important interventions for promoting good health center on changing personal health behaviors and habits rather than specific clinical interventions.
- Tobacco users should receive brief counseling at every visit (see Chapter 44).
- Regular **physical activity** is important at all ages. Patients should be encouraged to stay physically active, either through formal vigorous exercise (30 minutes three to four times per week) or by incorporating physical activity into the daily routine, with a goal of accumulating 30 minutes of moderate-to-vigorous activity on most or all days of the week. Activities may include walking, stair-climbing, gardening, and other "lifestyle exercise."
- All patients should be counseled regarding a prudent low-fat **diet** with abundant fruits, vegetables, and whole grains. Some patients may benefit from decreased sodium intake. Women, particularly those at risk for osteoporosis, should be counseled to consume between 1,000 and 1,500 mg calcium each day, and women of childbearing age should consume at least 0.4 mg folic acid daily by diet or supplements.
- Patients should be advised to use **lap/shoulder belts** for themselves and their passengers, to use **safety helmets** when riding motorcycles or bicycles, and to avoid alcohol or sedating drugs when driving.
- Elderly patients should be advised regarding home safety (see Chapter 34).
- Other areas for counseling and screening include alcohol use, dental health, domestic violence, unintended pregnancy, and sexually transmitted diseases.
- Use of alternative health care practices, including herbal medicine, chiropractic care, acupuncture, or hypnosis, should be inquired about in a nonjudgmental manner.

Patient Safety

- Patient safety and medical errors are pertinent topics in the ambulatory setting, where pharmaceutical drugs are frequently prescribed. Adverse drug events can account for hospital admissions and significantly contribute to increased morbidity and mortality. Some simple actions can be easily incorporated into routine clinical practice to reduce the number of errors.

- **Involve your patients and make them active participants in their care.**
  - This helps avoid misinterpretations of diagnostic or therapeutic plans and problems with compliance or follow-up. Involving other members of the health care team, including nurses, dietitians, and therapists, is vital.
  - Ensure that the patient leaves with clear comprehensible written directions for whom to contact and how to do so if he or she has any questions.
- **Know what medications your patients are taking.**
  - Ask them (or a family member) to bring all of the medicines and supplements (nutritional and alternative) they are currently taking to each visit. Keep an accurate ongoing list of all medications the patient is on.
  - Always review and inquire about any new allergies or adverse reactions.
  - Errors due to illegible handwriting are easily preventable and ensuring that your patients know their medications is essential in case there is a mistake.
- **Educating patients about their medications helps ensure their safety.**
  - Ask them to check with their pharmacist that the medication they receive is the one you meant to prescribe.
  - Make sure that they know what the medication is prescribed for, the dosing schedule, how long they should take it, what to do about a missed dose, interactions with other medications and alcohol, any monitoring or screening that may be necessary, and the importance of compliance with the medication to their overall health.
- To minimize and prevent errors, use computerized order entry, a reminder or alert system when available, and attempt to identify and minimize systemic errors in your practice.

Adherence

- Assessment of adherence requires a nonjudgmental attitude and acknowledgment of the many challenges to compliance.
  - Open-ended questions are more productive.
  - Pill counts may occasionally be useful but may be insulting to the patient.
  - The patient's pharmacist can provide information on the frequency of refills.
  - Low serum drug levels may represent failure to take the medication, poor absorption, rapid metabolism, and/or large volume of distribution.
- Noncompliance must be distinguished from ineffectiveness of treatment. Presumed nonadherence should be approached as any other clinical symptom by forming a differential diagnosis of possible etiologies.

Strategies to Enhance Adherence

- **Educate** the patient about the medical condition, the risks and benefits of therapy, and alternatives, using understandable language.
- **Collaborate** on the treatment plan; involve the patient in decision making to establish reasonable goals. Clarify expectations, and address fears and concerns.
- **Consider the patient's perspective and keep an open nonjudgmental attitude.** The patient's health belief model includes acceptance of diagnosis, perceived seriousness of condition, perceived benefits of the treatment, perceived barriers, readiness for change, and the level of confidence in the ability to carry out the plan.

- **Maintain contact** by follow-up visits and telephone calls.
- **Keep care simple and inexpensive** by using generic drugs, once-daily or combination formulations, and drugs that are not affected by meals.
- **Give written instructions.** Have the patient repeat the instructions to assess understanding.
- **Encourage self-monitoring** so that the patient feels a sense of control over his/her own health (e.g., home BP, blood sugar, peak flows, exercise log).
- **Identify and address barriers,** which can include limitations of time, money, transportation, functional illiteracy, social isolation or conflict, depression, mental illness, substance abuse, or cognitive dysfunction.
- **Focus on the positive benefits** of treatment and reinforce the patient's efforts. Set small specific goals that are achievable by breaking large projects into smaller steps. A relapse is not a failure: take a problem-solving approach to analyze causes and work out alternative strategies.
- **Ask about side effects.**
- **Discuss adherence strategies,** such as the use of medication log sheets, calendars, or daily pillboxes.
  - A wristwatch alarm can provide reminders, or medication taking can be tied to well-established daily routines such as meals or toothbrushing.
  - Help with lifestyle changes can include substitution of other activities to cope with cravings or stress and avoidance of situations that tempt old habits.
  - Achievement of new behaviors should be celebrated with small frequent rewards, such as a new book, a movie, or an outing.
  - Family and friends should encourage healthy new habits by joining smoking cessation attempts or new diet and exercise plans.

Difficult Doctor-Patient Interactions

- One great advantage of an ongoing physician-patient relationship is that it allows an opportunity to become familiar with all of a patient's problems and understand them in the context of the patient's personality and life circumstances. Hopefully, for most patients, mutual understanding and trust will grow as a therapeutic relationship develops.
- Sometimes issues can arise with physician's perception of a "difficult patient" or other issues with differences in styles of communication. This is a fairly common occurrence, about 15% of visits.[17–20]
- A full discussion of this subject is beyond the scope of this book but a brief overview will be provided.
- It is important to point out that improved physician communication skills can result in better patient outcomes, improved satisfaction (of the patient and the doctor), decreased litigation, and less physician burnout.
- At the most basic level, the "difficult patient" refers to those patients with whom a physician has trouble forming a normal therapeutic relationship.[21]
- **It is important not to lose sight of the contributions the clinician makes to the doctor-patient relationship, even when it is difficult.**
- In general, it is far more productive to consider the interaction itself "difficult" rather than the actual patient.
- **Patient-related characteristics** that appear to be associated with difficult doctor-patient interactions include the following[17–20,22–29]:

- Emotional.
- Psychosocial problems/distress.
- Mental disorders (e.g., multisomatoform disorder, dysthymia, generalized anxiety disorder, major depressive disorder, and alcohol abuse/dependence).
- Functional impairment/disability.
- High health care utilization.
- Multiple somatic complaints (vague, difficult to describe, undifferentiated, unexplained).
- More severe complaints/distress.
- Bring up new symptoms at the last moment.
- Does not take responsibility for their own health care; perceived lack of control over illness; nonadherence.
- Demanding/controlling.
- Unmet expectations/expects a "cure."
- Lower satisfaction with care.
- Abrasive personality style/personality disorder.
- Physicians may not be aware of **their own negative reactions** to these characteristics and are encouraged to be generally more mindful/self-aware in their practice.[13,23,30] Such negative responses can be the actual genesis of a difficult encounter and/or make an already difficult situation worse.
- **Potentially contributory physician factors** include the following[17,28,31]:
  - Less experienced.
  - Younger.
  - Poorer psychosocial attitudes.
  - Work more hours.
  - Have higher stress.
  - More patients with psychosocial problems or substance abuse.
- Given the fiduciary nature of the doctor-patient relationship, it is generally accepted that the physician has a much greater responsibility to resolve relationship issues and to ensure that the interactions are as therapeutic and productive as possible.
- Potentially helpful recommendations include the following[32,33]:
  - Recognize when an interaction is not going as well as it could be—acknowledge this to yourself and to the patient. Ask yourself what the problem might be.
  - It is fine to start over if you get off on the wrong foot.
  - Keep in mind that you are not required to solve every problem in a single visit.
  - **Carefully consider how your own responses to certain patient characteristics are contributing to the interaction.** Be cognizant of your own "hot-button issues" and biases. Are you tired? Frazzled? Threatened? Frustrated? Uncomfortable? Inadequate?
  - Try to understand the patient's perspective but do not make assumptions about what that might be.
  - Consider if there are any cross-cultural issues.
  - Be willing to accommodate, within reason, different personality types.
  - Be empathetic regarding displays of sadness and fear. Acknowledge anger.
  - Always **keep in mind your fundamental responsibilities to the patient.** Make sure you have taken care of the basics, for example, take a **patient-centered** history,[34] perform an examination, make an assessment, and offer your best medical advice in clear, nonjudgmental terms.
  - Remember that it is a two-way street and negotiation may be very appropriate.

- Set clear expectations/limits and maintain boundaries particularly with sometimes very challenging patients such as those with personality disorders (e.g., borderline, antisocial, histrionic, narcissistic) or ongoing substance abuse.
- After a difficult interaction, reflect and deconstruct it. Talk to your colleagues about it. What seemed to work? What did not work? What will you do differently next time?

REFERENCES

1. Chobanian AV, Bakris GL, Black HR, et al. National High Blood Pressure Education Program Coordinating Committee on Prevention, Detection, Evaluation, and Treatment of High Blood Pressure: the JNC 7 report. *JAMA* 2003;289:2560–2572.
2. Expert Panel on Detection, Evaluation, and Treatment of High Blood Cholesterol in Adults. Executive summary of the third report of the National Cholesterol Education Program (NCEP) Expert Panel on Detection, Evaluation, and Treatment of High Blood Cholesterol in Adults (Adult Treatment Panel III). *JAMA* 2001;285:2486–2497.
3. Grundy SM, Cleeman C, Merz NB, et al. Implications of recent clinical trials for the National Cholesterol Education Program Adult Treatment Panel III Guidelines. *Circulation* 2004;110:227–239.
4. American Diabetes Association. Standards of medical care in diabetes—2009. *Diabetes Care* 2009;32:S13–S61.
5. Internal Expert Committee. International Expert Committee report on the role of the A_{1c} assay in the diagnosis of diabetes. *Diabetes Care* 2009;32:1327–1334.
6. Ladenson PW, Singer PA, Ain KB, et al. American Thyroid Association guidelines for detection of thyroid dysfunction. *Arch Intern Med* 2000;160:1573–1575.
7. National Osteoporosis Foundation. Clinician's Guide to Prevention and Treatment of Osteoporosis. Washington, DC: National Osteoporosis Foundation, 2008.
8. Kanis JA on behalf of the World Health Organization Scientific Group. Assessment of osteoporosis at the primary health care level. 2008 Technical Report. University of Sheffield, UK: WHO Collaborating Center, 2008.
9. Whooley MA, Avins AL, Miranda J, Browner, WS. Case-finding instruments for depression. Two questions are as good as many. *J Gen Intern Med* 1997;12:439–445.
10. Centers for Disease Control and Prevention. Sexually transmitted diseases treatment guidelines, 2006. *MMWR Recomm Rep* 2006;55:1–94.
11. Weinbaum CM, Williams I, Mast EE, et al. Recommendations for identification and public health management of persons with chronic hepatitis B infection. *MMWR Recomm Rep* 2008;57:1–20.
12. Mayfield D, McLeod G, Hall P. *Am J Psychiatry* 1974;131:1121–1123.
13. Buchsbaum DG, Buchanan RG, Centor RM, et al. Screening for alcohol abuse using CAGE scores and likelihood ratios. *Ann Intern Med* 1991;115:774–777.
14. National Institute of Alcohol Abuse and Alcoholism. Helping Patients Who Drink Too Much: A Clinician's Guide. 2005 Ed. Bethesda, MD: National Institute of Alcohol Abuse and Alcoholism, 2007.
15. Smith PC, Schmidt SM, Allensworth-Davies D, Saitz R. Primary care validation of a single-question alcohol screening test. *J Gen Intern Med* 2009;24:783–788.
16. Fiore MC, Jaen CR, Baker TB, et al. Treating Tobacco Use and Dependence: 2008 Update. Clinical Practice Guideline. Washington, DC: Public Health Service, U.S. Department of Health and Human Services, 2008.
17. Crutcher JE, Bass MJ. The difficult patient and the troubled physician. *J Fam Pract* 1980; 11:933–938.
18. Hahn SR, Thompson KS, Wills TA, et al. The difficult doctor-patient relationship: somatization, personality and psychopathology. *J Clin Epidemiol* 1994;47:647–657.
19. Hahn SR, Kroenke K, Spitzer RL, et al. The difficult patient: prevalence, psychopathology and functional impairment. *J Gen Intern Med* 1996;11:1–8.

20. Jackson JL, Kroenke K. Difficult patient encounters in the ambulatory clinic: clinical predictors and outcomes. *Arch Intern Med* 1999;159:1069–1075.
21. Simon JR, Dwyer J, Goldfrank LR. The difficult patient. *Emerg Med Clin North Am* 1999;17:353–370.
22. John C, Schwenk TL, Roi LD, Cohen M. Medical care and demographic characteristics of "difficult" patients. *J Fam Pract* 1987;24:607–610.
23. Schwenk TL, Marquez JT, Lefever RD, Cohen M. Physician and patient determinants of difficult physician-patient relationships. *J Fam Pract* 1989;28:59–63.
24. Lin EH, Katon W, Von Korff M, et al. Frustrating patients: physician and patient perspectives among distressed high users of medical services. *J Gen Intern Med* 1991;6:241–246.
25. Levinson W, Stiles WB, Inui TS, Engle R. Physician frustration in communicating with patients. *Med Care* 1993;31:285–295.
26. Katz RC. "Difficult patients" as family physicians perceive them. *Psychol Rep* 1996;79:539–544.
27. Walker EA, Katon WJ, Keegan D, et al. Predictors of physician frustration in the care of patients with rheumatological complaints. *Gen Hosp Psychiatry* 1997;19:315–323.
28. Steinmetz D, Tabenkin H. The "difficult patient" as perceived by family physicians. *Fam Pract* 2001;18:495–500.
29. Hahn SR. Physical symptoms and physician-experienced difficulty in the physician-patient relationship. *Ann Intern Med* 2001;134:897–904.
30. Epstein RM. Mindful practice. *JAMA* 1999;282:833–839.
31. Krebs EE, Garrett JM, Konrad TR. The difficult doctor? Characteristics of physicians who report frustration with patients: an analysis of survey data. *BMC Health Serv Res* 2006;6:128.
32. Platt FE, Gordon GH. Filed Guide to the Difficult Patient Interview. 2nd Ed. Philadelphia, PA: Lippincott Williams & Wilkins, 2004.
33. Coulehan JL, Block MR. The Medical Interview: Mastering Skills for Clinical Practice. 5th Ed. Philadelphia, PA: F.A. Davis Company, 2006.
34. Smith RC. Patient-Centered Interviewing: An Evidence-Based Method. 2nd Ed. Philadelphia, PA: Lippincott Williams & Wilkins, 2002.

Care of the Surgical Patient

Meredith A. Brisco, Rashmi S. Mullur, and Thomas M. De Fer

General Considerations

- The role of the primary physician is to risk stratify patients, determine the need for further evaluation, and prescribe possible interventions to mitigate risk.
- Although preoperative evaluation often focuses on cardiac risk, it is essential to remember that poor outcomes can result from significant disease in other organ systems. Evaluation of the entire patient is necessary to provide optimal perioperative care.
- It is important to remember that no patient is ever truly "cleared for surgery," as there will always be some risk of adverse outcome and only approximations of risk can be offered.

Elective versus Emergent

- Elective surgery carries less risk of perioperative complications, allowing time for optimization of a patient's general medical condition and treatment of cardiovascular and pulmonary disease.
- **Emergent surgeries are often associated with serious medical comorbidities,** but the disadvantages of delaying surgery may outweigh the benefits in stabilizing the patient.

Routine Preoperative Laboratory Testing

- **The frequency of unanticipated abnormalities or abnormalities that ultimately change management is too low to justify "routine labs" for all patients.**[1–4]
- A large randomized study of preoperative medical testing before cataract surgery failed to show a significant difference in the rates of intraoperative and postoperative events between the testing group and the nontesting group.[5]

Complete Blood Cell Count

- Depending on the patient's age, gender, and current medical conditions, the prevalence of preoperative anemia can range from 0% to 30%.[6]
- In older men, mild preoperative anemia or polycythemia is associated with increased 30-day postoperative mortality and cardiac events; whether treatment decreases postoperative mortality in this and other populations remains unknown.[7]
- **Therefore, preoperative** complete blood cell counts **(CBCs) are usually not warranted unless more than minimal blood loss is expected or the history or physical examination indicates them.**

Serum Electrolytes

- A significant number of patients may have abnormalities but only a small percentage of results affect management.
- Hypokalemia specifically is not associated with adverse events or incidence of perioperative arrhythmias.[8]

Renal Function Tests
- Renal insufficiency is a risk factor for postoperative complications in cardiac and noncardiac surgery and is a clinical risk predictor in the 2007 ACC/AHA guidelines and one of six predictors of risk in the Revised Cardiac Risk Index.[9,10]
- Unlike other clinical conditions, moderate renal insufficiency may not always be clinically apparent, such that some experts advocate preoperative renal function testing in patients with the following factors[3]:
  - Age >50.
  - Diabetes.
  - Hypertension.
  - Cardiac disease.
  - Taking medications that affect renal function (angiotensin-converting enzyme [ACE] inhibitors).
  - Undergoing major surgical procedures.

Coagulation Studies
- Testing should be performed only in those patients currently anticoagulated or whose history and physical examination suggest prior bleeding problems.
- The prothrombin time and activated partial thromboplastin time are not predictive of perioperative hemorrhage.[3]

Anesthesia Modality: General versus Regional
- The modality of anesthesia is an often-debated aspect of preoperative assessment for which **there is no absolute consensus.**
- Multiple individual studies and meta-analyses have produced conflicting results, and most data specifically relate only to hip-fracture repair and total hip/knee replacement.[11–16]
- Whether or not epidural or spinal anesthesia reduces postoperative morbidity and mortality compared with general anesthesia is still unclear. However, a reduced risk of deep venous thrombosis does seem to be a fairly consistent finding.

PREOPERATIVE CARDIOVASCULAR RISK ASSESSMENT

General Principles

Epidemiology
- Of the millions of patients undergoing noncardiac surgery annually, 1% to 6% (depending on the population studied and diagnostic criteria used) will suffer a major cardiac event.
- Overall, an estimated 50,000 perioperative myocardial infarctions (MIs) and 1 million other cardiovascular complications occur annually.[17]
- Of those who have a perioperative MI, the risk of in-hospital mortality is estimated at 10% to 15%.[18]
- Patients who have noncardiac complications are more likely to develop cardiac complications and vice versa.[19]

Pathophysiology
- The exact mechanism of perioperative MIs is not clear.

- Based on the autopsy studies and angiographic evidence, it is likely that plaque rupture plays an integral role in a large number of these events, just as in nonperioperative infarcts.
- However, an undetermined number may be due to supply/demand mismatch engendered by the stresses of surgery.

Diagnosis

Clinical Presentation

History

- The focus of the history is to identify factors/comorbid conditions that will affect perioperative risk.
- Different classification schemas have identified somewhat different risk factors.
- **The most current guidelines** are those of the American College of Cardiology (ACC) and the American Heart Association (AHA), and they focus on the identification of active cardiovascular conditions and known risks factors.[9]
- **Active cardiovascular conditions** that should be investigated in the history are presented in Table 1.
- The history should also seek to elucidate validated independent predictors of postoperative complications (MI, pulmonary edema, cardiac arrest, and cardiac death) using the **Revised Cardiac Risk Index** (Table 2).[10] Further validation of the index suggests that the class-associated risks may be less than originally derived/validated and that the index may also be predictive of late mortality and impaired health status.[20,21]

TABLE 1	Active Cardiac Conditions

Unstable coronary syndromes
Unstable angina
Severe angina (CCS Class III or IV)
Recent myocardial infarction (>7 days but ≤30 days)
Decompensated heart failure
NYHA Class IV
New-onset heart failure
Worsening heart failure
Significant arrhythmias
Symptomatic bradycardia
High-grade AV block (third degree, Mobitz II)
Symptomatic ventricular arrhythmias (>100)
SVT with uncontrolled ventricular rate
Newly recognized VT
Severe valvular disease
Severe aortic stenosis (valve area < 1.0 cm^2 or mean gradient > 40 mm Hg)
Symptomatic mitral stenosis (dyspnea on exertion, exertional presyncope, heart failure)

AV, atrioventricular; CSS, Canadian Cardiovascular Society; NYHA, New York Heart Association; SVT, supraventricular tachycardia; VT, ventricular tachycardia.
Modified from Fleisher LA, Beckman JA, Brown KA, et al. ACC/AHA 2007 guidelines on perioperative cardiovascular evaluation and care for noncardiac surgery: a report of the American College of Cardiology/American Heart Association Task Force on Practice Guidelines (Writing Committee to Revise the 2002 Guidelines on Perioperative Cardiovascular Evaluation for Noncardiac Surgery). *Circulation* 2007;116:e418–e499.

TABLE 2	Revised Cardiac Risk Index

High-risk surgery[a]
   Intraperitoneal
   Intrathoracic
   Suprainguinal vascular procedures
History of ischemic heart disease
   History of MI (not acute or recent)
   ECG with pathological Q waves
   History of a positive exercise stress test
   Stable angina
   Nitrate therapy
History of compensated or prior CHF
   History of CHF
   History of pulmonary edema
   History of paroxysmal nocturnal dyspnea
   Bilateral rales
   S3 gallop
   Chest radiograph showing pulmonary vascular redistribution
   History of cerebrovascular disease
Stroke
   TIA
   Insulin therapy for diabetes
   Preoperative serum creatinine > 2.0 mg/dL

Associated major cardiac complication rate

No risk factor/Class I, 0.4%–0.5%
One risk factor/Class II, 0.9%–1.3%
Two risk factors/Class III, 3.6%–6.6%
Three or more risk factors/Class IV, 9.1%–11%

CHF, congestive heart failure; ECG, electrocardiogram; MI, myocardial infarction;
TIA, transient ischemic attack.
[a]Considered separately in the ACC/AHA 2007 Guidelines.
Modified from Lee TH, Marcantonio ER, Mangione CM, et al. Derivation and prospective
validation of a simple index for prediction of cardiac risk of major noncardiac surgery.
Circulation 1999;100:1043–1049.

- Prior iterations of the ACC/AHA guidelines have included **minor predictors** (e.g., age >70 years, certain abnormal echocardiograms [ECG] [left ventricular hypertrophy, left bundle-branch block, ST-T abnormalities], rhythm other than sinus, and uncontrolled hypertension); however, these have not been conclusively shown to independently increase perioperative risk. Although potentially suggestive of a higher risk of coronary artery disease (CAD), they are no longer a part of the most recent guidelines.
- Similarly, **known independent CAD risk factors** (e.g., age, smoking, increased low-density lipoprotein [LDL], decreased high-density lipoprotein [HDL], hypertension, diabetes, and family history), though clinically very important, are not specifically used to assess perioperative cardiovascular risk.
- It is worth noting that one study from Brazil did identify increasing age as an independent predictor for perioperative complications and in-hospital mortality but also that the mortality rate is still relatively low even in those >80.[22]

- Older patients, particularly those with dementia, are at increased risk for postoperative agitation and delirium.
- A preoperative mental status examination may identify patients with developing dementia, potentially identify those at risk for delirium, and serve as a useful comparison if there is a question of altered mental status postoperatively.
- Careful attention should be paid to the medical factors that may be contributory (e.g., sedative/alcohol abuse, other medications, and infection).
- The history should also focus on an assessment of the patient's functional status, which has been shown to be independently associated with perioperative risk and can be assessed by the patient's report (Table 3).[23] **In general, those with a good functional status (>4 METs) without symptoms are at relatively low risk.**

Physical Examination

- A complete physical examination is essential.
- Specific attention should be paid to the following:
  - Vital signs, especially blood pressure. Systolic blood pressure (SBP) of <180 mm Hg and diastolic blood pressure (DBP) of <110 mm Hg are generally considered acceptable. The management of SBP >180 mm Hg or DBP >110 mm Hg is controversial. Postponing elective surgery to allow adequate BP control in this setting is acceptable, but this is poorly studied and how long to wait after treatment is instituted is unclear.
  - Murmurs suggestive of significant valvular lesions such as aortic stenosis and mitral stenosis.
  - Evidence of congestive heart failure (CHF) (jugular vein distension, crackles, S3, etc.).

TABLE 3	Estimated Metabolic Equivalents (METs) of Various Activities		
1 MET	Can you take care of yourself?	4 METs	Climb a flight of stairs or walk up a hill?
			Walk on level ground briskly?
	Eat, dress, use the toilet?		Run a short distance?
			Do heavy housework (e.g., scrubbing floors, lifting/ moving heavy furniture)?
	Walk indoors around the house?		
			Participate in moderate recreational activity (e.g., bowling, dancing, doubles tennis, golf, throwing a baseball/football)?
	Walk 1–2 level blocks slowly?		
			Participate in strenuous sports (e.g., basketball, football, singles tennis, skiing, swimming)?
	Do light housework (e.g., dusting,		
4 METs	washing dishes)?	>10 METs	

Modified from Fleisher LA, Beckman JA, Brown KA, et al. ACC/AHA 2007 guidelines on perioperative cardiovascular evaluation and care for noncardiac surgery: a report of the American College of Cardiology/American Heart Association Task Force on Practice Guidelines (Writing Committee to Revise the 2002 Guidelines on Perioperative Cardiovascular Evaluation for Noncardiac Surgery). *Circulation* 2007;116:e418–e499.

Diagnostic Criteria

Figure 1 presents an overview of the ACC/AHA 2007 guidelines for the cardiovascular risk assessment of patients undergoing noncardiac surgery.[9]

Step 1:
- **Establish the need for emergency surgery.**
- For truly emergent surgery, proceed to surgery.

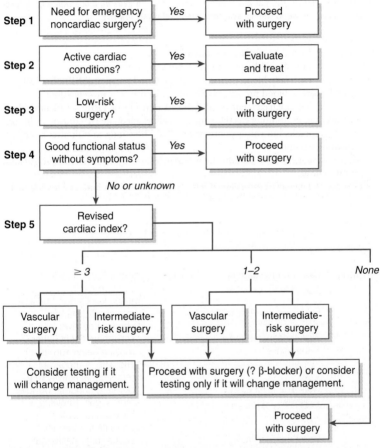

Figure 1. ACC/AHA 2007 cardiovascular risk assessment algorithm. (Modified from Fleisher LA, Beckman JA, Brown KA, et al. ACC/AHA 2007 guidelines on perioperative cardiovascular evaluation and care for noncardiac surgery: a report of the American College of Cardiology/American Heart Association Task Force on Practice Guidelines (Writing Committee to Revise the 2002 Guidelines on Perioperative Cardiovascular Evaluation for Noncardiac Surgery). *Circulation* 2007;116:e418–e499.)

TABLE 4	Cardiac Risk of Noncardiac Surgeries	
Risk Group	Risk of Cardiac Death and Nonfatal Myocardial Infarction (MI)	Examples
Vascular	≥5%	Aortic and other major vascular surgery Peripheral vascular surgery
Intermediate	1%–5%	Intraperitoneal surgery Intrathoracic surgery Carotid endarterectomy Head and neck surgery Orthopedic surgery Prostate surgery
Low	<1%	Endoscopic procedures Superficial procedures Cataract surgery Breast surgery Ambulatory surgery

Modified from Fleisher LA, Beckman JA, Brown KA, et al. ACC/AHA 2007 guidelines on perioperative cardiovascular evaluation and care for noncardiac surgery: a report of the American College of Cardiology/American Heart Association Task Force on Practice Guidelines (Writing Committee to Revise the 2002 Guidelines on Perioperative Cardiovascular Evaluation for Noncardiac Surgery). *Circulation* 2007;116:e418–e499.

Step 2:
- **Determine if active cardiac conditions are present** (Table 1).
- If active cardiac conditions are present, postpone surgery, evaluate, and treat.

Step 3:
- **Determine the risk of the specific surgery** (Table 4).
- **Patients undergoing low-risk surgery can generally proceed to the procedure without any further evaluation.**
- Superficial procedures in the ambulatory setting have a particularly low rate of MI, well below 0.1%.[24,25]

Step 4:
- **Assess the patient's functional capacity** (Table 3).
- Low functional capacity (<4 METs) is associated with increased risk of perioperative cardiovascular complications.[23]
- **Patients with a functional capacity of >4 METs without symptoms can proceed to surgery with relatively low risk.**

Step 5:
- **Assess clinical risk factors** (Table 2).
- **Patients with no clinical risk factors are inherently low risk** (<1% risk of cardiac events) and are unlikely to benefit from further intervention. **They may proceed to surgery.**

- Patients with one or two clinical risk factors undergoing intermediate risk or vascular procedures can typically proceed to surgery.
  - Stress testing should be considered only if it will change management, but recent data regarding preoperative percutaneous coronary interventions (PCIs) have called this somewhat into question (see the "Treatment" section).
  - The use of β-blockers in this group has become controversial (see the "Treatment" section).

Diagnostic Testing

12-Lead Electrocardiogram

- The current ACC/AHA guidelines recommend an ECG for the following patients[9]:
  - Patients with one or more risk factors (Table 2) undergoing vascular surgery and patients with known peripheral vascular disease, CAD, or cerebrovascular disease undergoing intermediate risk surgery (Class I recommendation).
  - Patients without risk factors undergoing vascular surgery and patients with other clinical risk factors undergoing intermediate risk surgery (Class II recommendation).
- The primary utility of a preoperative ECG in most patients will be for comparison with ECGs that may be obtained postoperatively.

Resting Echocardiogram

- Indications for echocardiography are no different than in the nonoperative setting and is **not routinely recommended.**[9]
- Murmurs found on physical exam suggestive of significant underlying valvular disease should be evaluated by echo just as they should be in a nonperioperative setting.
- An assessment of left ventricular function should be considered when there is concern for CHF not previously diagnosed or deterioration since the last examination. Again, this would be done without regard to impending surgery.

Noninvasive Stress Testing

- The decision to pursue a stress evaluation should be guided by an assessment of preoperative risk as detailed above.
- **Routine stress testing of all patients undergoing surgery is not warranted.**
- Stress testing should not generally be pursued unless subsequent clearly indicated treatments would be undertaken without regard to noncardiac surgery (see the "Treatment" section).
- Recent data suggest that noninvasive stress testing in intermediate-risk patients does not significantly change outcome.[26–28]
- However, such data do not preclude potential benefit in certain patient groups where the outcome of noninvasive testing would change management.[29] The ACC/AHA guidelines recommend the following[9]:
  - Noninvasive stress testing is reasonable for patients with three or more risk factors and poor functional capacity (<4 METs) undergoing vascular surgery, only if it will change management.
  - Consider noninvasive stress testing for patients with one to two or more risk factors and poor functional status (<4 METs) undergoing intermediate-risk surgery, if it will change management.
  - Consider noninvasive stress testing for patients with one to two or more risk factors and good functional capacity (>4 METs) undergoing vascular surgery.

- Recommendations regarding noninvasive stress testing must also be considered in the light of newer data regarding β-blockers and revascularization (see the "Treatment" section).

Coronary Angiography

- Some patients will have a clear indication for angiography on clinical grounds apart from perioperative risk stratification, and standard guidelines for the nonperioperative setting should guide the management of these patients.
- Indications for preoperative coronary angiography in the majority of patients are in flux because of concerns that revascularization of lesions identified at angiography may not improve outcomes (see the "Treatment" section).
- It is reasonable to pursue angiography in patients with high-risk results on noninvasive testing to further define their level of perioperative risk and to determine if they have disease that would generally mandate consideration of revascularization.
- **Routine use of coronary angiography as a method of risk stratification cannot be recommended.**

Treatment

Medications

β-Blockers

- Multiple, earlier, smaller studies suggested that perioperative β-blockade improved mortality and cardiovascular outcome.[30-34]
- More recent data, however, have questioned the utility of perioperative β-blockade.[35-38]
  - In particular, the large POISE trial, while confirming the decrease in cardiac events with aggressive perioperative β-blockade, showed increase in overall mortality and stroke risk.[37]
  - An important difference between the studies showing benefit and the POISE trial was the β-blocker regimen used. The POISE trial employed a relatively high dose of extended-release metoprolol beginning on the day of surgery. The others started a long-acting β-blocker days to weeks prior to the surgery and titrated the dose preoperatively.
- The most recent ACC/AHA guidelines regarding perioperative β-blocker use were released prior to the POISE trial.[9,39] For now, the most prudent recommendations are as follows:
  - β-Blockers should be continued in those taking them for clear indications.
  - Suddenly withdrawing β-blockers in the immediate preoperative period is not recommended.
  - Instituting β-blockade for patients at high risk for perioperative myocardial injury (three or more risk factors and/or a positive stress evaluation) seems reasonable, particularly for those undergoing vascular surgery. β-Blockade should begin two or more weeks prior to surgery.
  - The utility of β-blockade in intermediate-risk patients is, at present, questionable.
  - β-Blockade is not indicated for low-risk patients.

α_2-Agonists

- Data suggest that α_2-agonists reduce perioperative risk of myocardial ischemia and death.[40-42]
- α_2-Agonists may be an option when β-blockers are otherwise contraindicated.

Statins
- Statins show promise in reducing perioperative events, particularly in those undergoing vascular surgery.[43–45]
- Statin therapy should be continued in those currently taking statins.
- Statin therapy should be started in all with otherwise appropriate indications (see Chapter 8).
- Statin therapy is reasonable for anyone undergoing vascular surgery.[9]

Revascularization
- The utility of preoperative revascularization has been very much called into question with the result of recent trials.[46–48]
  - In the CARP trial, patients with angiographically significant CAD were randomized to revascularization (coronary artery bypass grafting [CABG] or PCI) or nonrevascularization.[46]
    - No difference between the groups in occurrence of postoperative MI or long-term survival was demonstrated.
    - Notable exclusions from the study were patients found to have significant left main disease, severe LV dysfunction, severe aortic stenosis, and the presence of severe coexisting illnesses.
  - In the DECRASE-V trial, preoperative coronary revascularization in high-risk patients undergoing vascular surgery was not associated with short- or long-term improved outcome.[47,48]
- Given the results above, data from the COURAGE trial,[49] and issues of stent thrombosis (see below), **a strategy of routinely pursuing coronary revascularization as a method of decreasing perioperative cardiac risk cannot be recommended at this time.**
  - Careful screening of patients is essential to identify those high-risk subsets excluded from the above study and to identify patients who may obtain a survival benefit from revascularization **independent of their need for noncardiac surgery.**

Preoperative PCI: ACC/AHA Advisory
- If a bare-metal intracoronary stent is utilized, the risk of adverse cardiac outcomes perioperatively is greatly increased in the first few weeks following the PCI.[50,51] This is thought largely to be due to in-stent restenosis related to the cessation of antiplatelet therapy in the perioperative period. **Any subsequent surgery needs to be delayed for a minimum of 2 weeks, though 6 weeks is preferred.**
- The ACC/AHA recommends dual antiplatelet therapy with aspirin 325 mg daily and clopidogrel 75 mg daily for a minimum duration of[52]
  - **one month** in patients receiving **bare-metal stents and**
  - **twelve months** in patients receiving **drug-eluting stents.**
- In patients likely to have surgery within the next 12 months, consideration should be given to a bare-metal stent or balloon angioplasty alone.
- **Elective procedures with significant risk of bleeding should be postponed until patients have completed the minimum duration of antiplatelet therapy.**
- For patients who have received a drug-eluting stent who are undergoing surgery that cannot be postponed, and that mandate discontinuation of thienopyridine therapy with clopidogrel or ticlopidine, aspirin should be continued if possible and thienopyridine therapy restarted as soon as possible postprocedure.
- Antiplatelet therapy should not be discontinued without consulting the patient's cardiologist.

- For angioplasty alone, 2 to 4 weeks delay is recommended, though the event rates appear to be considerably lower.[53,54]

PERIOPERATIVE CONSIDERATIONS FOR SPECIFIC CARDIOVASCULAR CONDITIONS

Hypertension

- Hypertension <180/110 mm Hg is not an independent predictor of perioperative complications.
- However, severe hypertension >180/110 mm Hg may be associated with intraoperative BP fluctuations and myocardial ischemia.[9]
- Antihypertensive agents that patients are taking prior to admission for surgery may have an impact on the perioperative period:
  - Patients on β-blockers or clonidine chronically should continue therapy to avoid tachycardia and rebound hypertension.
  - Consideration can be given to holding ACE inhibitors and angiotensin receptor blockers on the day of surgery and not resuming until the patient is euvolemic because of the potential for hypotensive episodes.[55–57]

Valvular Heart Disease

- Symptomatic stenotic lesions such as mitral stenosis and aortic stenosis are associated with perioperative CHF and shock, and preoperative valvotomy or replacement is often needed.
- Severe aortic stenosis is associated with a very high incidence of perioperative MI and mortality.[58]
- Symptomatic regurgitant lesions are generally better tolerated perioperatively and can generally be managed medically so long as the patient is well compensated preoperatively.
- If surgery is emergent, elective valvular repair needs to be deferred.
- If surgery can be delayed for a short period, preoperative valvotomy can be considered.
- Endocarditis prophylaxis should be considered.
- Cardiology consultation should be considered when severe disease is present.

Pacemakers and Implantable Cardioverter Defibrillators

- Electrocautery intraoperatively can have adverse effects on the function of implanted cardiac devices.
- Various errors may occur from resetting of the device to inadvertent discharge of an implantable cardioverter defibrillator.
- Optimally the device should be interrogated pre- and postoperatively to ensure proper function.
- Rate-responsive pacemakers should have this mode deactivated intraoperatively.
- Implantable cardioverter defibrillators should be deactivated immediately preoperatively and reactivated postoperatively to avoid accidental discharge.

Congestive Heart Failure

- Active, decompensated heart failure is a contraindication to surgery.
- The study by Lee et al. defined heart failure as indicated in Table 2.[10]
- The history and physical examination should seek out symptoms and signs of CHF.
- Medical treatment for CHF should be carefully optimized prior to elective noncardiac surgery (see Chapter 5).

PREOPERATIVE PULMONARY EVALUATION

General Principles

- Postoperative pulmonary complications are as common and as morbid and mortal as cardiac complications.[59,60]
- Occurrence of one complication probably increases the chance of others occurring.[19]
- The most significant complications include atelectasis, pneumonia, respiratory failure, and exacerbation of underlying lung disease.
- The American College of Physicians practice guideline recognizes the following patient-related factors that increase the risk of postoperative pulmonary complications[59,60]:
  - History of chronic obstructive pulmonary disease (COPD).
  - Age >60.
  - American Society of Anesthesiology Class >II (a patient with a severe but not incapacitating systemic disease).
  - CHF.
  - Functional dependence.
- Other data also support the following as additional patient-related risk factors: smoking, weight loss/malnutrition, impaired sensorium, alcohol use, obstructive sleep apnea, and pulmonary hypertension.[61–63]
- Procedure-related risk factors include the following[59–63]:
  - Aortic aneurysm repair.
  - Thoracic surgery.
  - Abdominal surgery.
  - Neurosurgery.
  - Prolonged surgery.
  - Head and neck surgery.
  - Emergency surgery.
  - Vascular surgery.
  - General anesthesia.

Diagnosis

Clinical Presentation

History
- Focus should be placed on identifying the presence of patient-related risk factors.
- A complete respiratory history should be obtained.
- Any symptoms of current upper respiratory infection should be ascertained but is not an absolute contraindication to surgery.
- A full smoking history should be obtained.
- Patients should be questioned about their general functional status.

Physical Examination

- Attention should be paid to evidence of chronic lung disease such as increased anteroposterior dimensions of the chest, hyperresonance, diminished breath sounds, and the presence of adventitious lung sounds such as wheezing.
- Signs of CHF should also be sought, including rales, increased jugular venous pressure, and peripheral edema.
- Body habitus may suggest the possibility of obstructive sleep apnea and obesity hypoventilation syndrome.

Diagnostic Criteria

- Unlike the relatively well-defined risk assessment strategy for cardiovascular complications described above, there is no single, evidence-based algorithmic approach for the assessment of pulmonary risk.
- The postoperative pneumonia risk index is presented in Table 5.[61]

TABLE 5		Postoperative Pneumonia Risk Index	
Risk Factor	**Point Value**	**Risk Factor**	**Point Value**
Type of surgery		Weight loss >10% in past 6 months	7
AAA repair	15		
Thoracic	14	History of COPD	5
Upper abdominal	10	General anesthesia	4
Neck	8	Impaired sensorium	4
Neurosurgical	8	History of CVA	4
Vascular	3	BUN, mg/dL	
Age, y		<8	4
≥80	17	22–30	2
70–79	13	≥30	3
60–69	9	Transfusion >4 units	3
50–59	4	Emergency surgery	3
Functional status		Steroid use for chronic condition	3
Totally dependent	10	Current smoker with 1 y	3
Partially dependent	6	Alcohol intake >2 drinks/d in past 2 wk	2

Risk Class	**Risk of Pneumonia**
1 (0–15 points)	0.2%
2 (16–25 points)	1.2%
3 (26–40 points)	4.0%
4 (41–55 points)	9.4%
5 (>55 points)	15.3%

AAA, abdominal aortic aneurysm; COPD, chronic obstructive pulmonary disease; CVA, cerebrovascular accident; d, day; m, month; wk, weeks; y, year.
Modified from Arozullah AM, Khuri SF, Henderson WG, Daley J; Participants in the National Veterans Affairs Surgical Quality Improvement Program. Development and validation of a multifactorial risk index for predicting postoperative pneumonia after major noncardiac surgery. *Ann Intern Med* 2001;135:847–857.

- A model, the respiratory failure risk index, has also been developed that can predict the rate of postoperative respiratory failure.[62] This index is fairly complex and not likely to be used frequently in routine clinical practice.

Diagnostic Testing

Laboratories
- A decreased **serum albumin level** is a potent predictor of pulmonary risk.[59,60]
  - A level <3.5 mg/dL appears to be indicative of increased risk.
  - Measure albumin in all patients who are clinically suspected of having hypoalbuminemia and in patients with one or more risk factors for perioperative pulmonary complications.
  - There is at present, however, no conclusive evidence that enteral or parenteral nutritional supplementation decreases the risk.
- **Arterial blood gases** (ABG).
  - It is unclear that ABG results add to the estimate of preoperative pulmonary risk beyond other clinically derived variables.
  - There are no proven abnormal levels beyond which surgery is contraindicated.
  - An ABG should be obtained when otherwise clinically necessary.
  - Its primary purpose in most patients will be to serve as a baseline comparison for ABGs that may be obtained in the immediate postoperative period.

Imaging
- Many chest radiography findings deemed abnormal are chronic and rarely affect management.[3,59,60,64]
- **Routine preoperative chest radiography in all patients is not recommended.**
- Limited evidence suggests that preoperative chest radiography may be beneficial in those with known cardiopulmonary disease and in those >50 years undergoing upper abdominal, thoracic, or abdominal aortic aneurysm surgery.[59]

Diagnostic Procedures
- General consensus exists on the value of **pulmonary function testing** before lung resection and determining candidacy for CABG.[59,60]
- Otherwise, spirometry may identify patients at higher risk for pulmonary complications but the data are mixed.
- Spirometry has not been shown superior to history and physical examination.
- No prohibitive spirometric threshold has been identified below which the risk of surgery is unacceptable.
- Pulmonary function testing is indicated for those patients with a suspected but undiagnosed pulmonary condition, for which they would otherwise be indicated outside of the context of surgery.

Treatment

Smoking Cessation
- Benefit has been shown if patients stop smoking at least 6 to 8 weeks before surgery.[63,65,66]
- All patients should be counseled to stop even if < 8 weeks from surgery as previous concerns about paradoxical increase in complications appear unwarranted.[66]

COPD Therapy

- Therapy should be optimized and elective surgery postponed in the setting of an acute exacerbation.
- COPD exacerbations should be treated in the usual manner (see Chapter 11).

Postoperative Interventions

- **Lung expansion maneuvers** (i.e., incentive spirometry, deep breathing exercises, and continuous positive airway pressure) reduce the risk of postoperative pulmonary complications.[59,63,65]
- A strategy of selective nasogastric tube placement after abdominal surgery rather than routine use has also been shown to decrease the risk of pulmonary complications.[59,65]

PERIOPERATIVE CONSIDERATIONS IN OTHER DISEASE STATES

Liver Disease

General Principles

- Patients with hepatic dysfunction suffer from an increased risk of morbid outcomes when undergoing surgery.
- Probably because of decreased hepatic perfusion during anesthesia, patients with underlying liver disease are at substantial risk for acute hepatic decompensation postoperatively.[67]
- The systemic effects of liver dysfunction result in an increased frequency of other complications as well, such as bleeding and renal failure.

Diagnosis

- Because of the low prevalence and because significant disease is usually clinically suspected, **routine laboratory screening for hepatic dysfunction in patients presenting for surgery who are without clinically suspected or known liver disease is not recommended.**[68]
- Patients with known or suspected liver disease should undergo a thorough evaluation of liver function including hepatic enzyme levels, albumin and bilirubin measurements, and evaluation for coagulopathy.
- In patients with cirrhosis, increasing **Child-Pugh score** correlates with greater degrees of hepatic dysfunction and increasing perioperative morbidity and mortality[69] (refer to Chapter 26, Table 2).
- Studies indicate that the **Model of End-Stage Liver Disease (MELD) score** may also be a reliable indicator of postoperative mortality. The MELD score is discussed in detail in Chapter 26.
- Recent data suggest that MELD scores of > 14 more accurately predict poor outcomes than does a Child's class C.[70]

Treatment

- Patients with acute viral or alcoholic hepatitis tolerate surgery poorly, and delaying surgery until recovery is recommended if possible. Patients with chronic hepatitis without evidence of hepatic decompensation generally tolerate surgery well.

- With regard to postoperative mortality after 7 days, the AGA Institute suggests the following management of patients with cirrhosis undergoing surgery[70]:
  - For patients with a MELD score of <11, the postoperative mortality is low enough that the risks of surgery are generally acceptable.
  - Patients with a MELD score of 12 to 19 should have evaluation for liver transplantation completed prior to any elective surgeries so that they may proceed to urgent liver transplantation if necessary.
  - Patients with a MELD score of ≥20 should have most elective procedures postponed until after liver transplantation.
- Based on the high perioperative mortality rates in patients with advanced cirrhosis, nonoperative alternatives should be strongly considered.
- For patients who require surgery, steps should be taken to optimize the preoperative status including coagulopathy, thrombocytopenia, renal and electrolyte abnormalities, volume status, ascites, and encephalopathy. These subjects are discussed in detail in Chapter 26.

CHRONIC KIDNEY DISEASE

General Principles

- Chronic kidney disease is an independent risk factor for perioperative cardiac complications, so all patients with renal disease need appropriate cardiac risk stratification.[9]
- Patients with end stage renal disease have a substantial mortality risk when undergoing surgery.[71]
- Most general anesthetic agents have no appreciable nephrotoxicity or effect on renal function other than that mediated through hemodynamic changes.[72]

Treatment

- Every effort should be made to achieve euvolemia preoperatively to reduce the incidence of volume-related complications intra- and postoperatively.[73]
  - Although this typically entails removing volume, some patients may be hypovolemic and require hydration.
  - Patients with chronic renal insufficiency not receiving hemodialysis may require treatment with loop diuretics.
  - Patients being treated with hemodialysis should undergo dialysis preoperatively.
  - This is commonly performed on the day prior to surgery.
  - Hemodialysis can be performed on the day of surgery as well, but the possibility that transient electrolyte abnormalities and hemodynamic changes postdialysis can occur should be considered.
- Hyperkalemia in the preoperative setting should be treated, particularly as tissue breakdown associated with surgery may elevate the potassium level further postoperatively (see Chapter 20).
- Platelet dysfunction has long been associated with uremia.
  - The value of a preoperative bleeding time in predicting postoperative bleeding has been questioned.[74]
  - A preoperative bleeding time is, therefore, not recommended.
  - Patients who evidence perioperative bleeding should, however, be treated (see Chapter 9).

DIABETES MELLITUS

GENERAL PRINCIPLES

- **Hospitalized patients with diabetes and hyperglycemia are at increased risk for poor outcomes.**[75–77]
- Data concerning glycemic control in critically ill/intensive care unit (ICU) patients initially suggested improved outcome. However, more recent trials with very stringent targets (e.g., 80 to 110 mg/dL) have failed to demonstrate this outcome because of the difficulty in achieving the goal without increasing the risk of severe hyperglycemia.[77,78]
- It is unclear if improving glucose control in the non-ICU setting improves mortality, but given the association between hyperglycemia and poor outcomes in the general inpatient setting, this is suggested.[77]
- **Significant hypoglycemia is independently associated with in-hospital mortality and should be scrupulously avoided.**

Treatment

- **Elective surgery in patients with uncontrolled diabetes mellitus should preferably be scheduled after acceptable glycemic control has been achieved.**
- If possible, the operation should be scheduled for early morning to minimize prolonged fasting.
- **Frequent monitoring of blood glucose levels is required in all situations.**
- **Significant hypoglycemia must be avoided with the same vigilance as hyperglycemia** (>180 mg/dL).
- **Traditional "sliding scale insulin" alone is usually ineffective and should not be used as monotherapy.**

Target Glucose Levels

- The most current American Diabetes Association recommended goals for inpatients take into account the most recent trial data regarding very tight glycemic control and the risk of hypoglycemia.[77]
- For critically ill patients, therapy should be initiated for persistent hyperglycemia (starting at a threshold no >180 mg/dL) and a target glucose range of 140 to 180 mg/dL.
- For noncritically ill patients, the preprandial goal is <140 mg/dL and random levels <180 mg/dL.

Type 1 Diabetes

- **Some form of basal insulin is required at all times.**
- On the evening prior to surgery, the regularly scheduled basal insulin should be continued. If taken in the morning, it is still recommended to give the regularly scheduled basal insulin without dose adjustment.
- Intravenous (IV) glucose (i.e., D5-containing fluids) can be administered to avoid hypoglycemia while the patient is NPO and until tolerance of oral intake postoperatively is established.
- For complex procedures and procedures requiring a prolonged NPO status, a continuous insulin infusion will likely be necessary.

- Caution should be exercised with the use of subcutaneous insulin in the intraoperative and critical care settings, as alterations in tissue perfusion may result in variable absorption.

Type 2 Diabetes

Diet-Controlled Diabetes

- These patients can generally be managed without insulin therapy.
- Glucose values should be checked regularly and elevated levels (>180 mg/dL) can be treated with intermittent doses of short-acting insulin.

Type 2 Diabetes Managed with Oral Therapy

- Short-acting sulfonylureas and other oral agents should be **held on the operative day.**
- Metformin and long-acting sulfonylureas (e.g., chlorpropamide) should be withheld 1 day before planned surgical procedures.
- Metformin is generally held for 48 hours postoperatively. **Renal function should be normal prior to resuming metformin.**
- **Other oral agents can be resumed when patients are tolerating their preprocedure diet.** This recommendation assumes that such patients will be rapidly discharged to home; otherwise, **oral hypoglycemic agents are generally inappropriate for most hospitalized patients.**
- Glucose values should be checked regularly and elevated levels (>180 mg/dL) can be treated with intermittent doses of short-acting insulin.
- Most patients can be managed without an insulin infusion.

Type 2 Diabetes Managed with Insulin

- **Traditional "sliding scale insulin" alone is usually ineffective and should generally not be used as monotherapy.**
- If it is anticipated that the patient will be able to eat postoperatively, basal insulin is still given on the morning of surgery.
- If given as long-acting insulin (e.g., glargine insulin) and the patient usually takes the dose in the morning, 80% to 90% of the usual dose can be given.
- If the patient utilizes intermediate-acting insulin (e.g., NPH), half to two-thirds of the usual morning dose is given to avoid periprocedural hyperglycemia.
- Glucose-containing IV fluids may be required to avoid hypoglycemia.
- Patients undergoing major procedures will typically require an insulin drip perioperatively.
- Glucose and potassium will need to be administered concomitantly to avoid hypoglycemia and hypokalemia, respectively.
- The usual insulin treatment can be resumed once oral intake is established postoperatively.

PERIOPERATIVE ANTIPLATELET AND ANTICOAGULATION MANAGEMENT

Antiplatelet Agents

- Some controversy exists over the use of aspirin in the perioperative period.
- Traditionally, aspirin is withheld for approximately 1 week prior to invasive procedures to minimize bleeding risk.

- However, some evidence suggests that withdrawal of aspirin may be associated with an increased risk of cardiac events.[79]
- Also, early use of aspirin postoperatively appears to improve outcomes in coronary artery bypass surgery.[80]
- For patients **not at high risk** for cardiac events undergoing noncardiac surgery, the 2008 American College of Chest Physicians (ACCP) guideline[81] recommends stopping antiplatelet agents 7 to 10 days before surgery.
- For patients **at high risk** for cardiac events, the recommendation is to continue aspirin but to withhold clopidogrel 5 to 10 days before surgery.
- For patients having a **PCI**, aspirin should be continued without interruption.
- For patients having **CABG**, aspirin should be continued up to and after surgery but clopidogrel should be held 5 to 10 days before surgery.
- Regarding an existing PCI scheduled for noncardiac surgery, refer to the "Revascularization" section.

Warfarin

- Anticoagulation strategy should always be discussed with the surgeon and precise recommendations depend on the exact patient situation.
- The benefit of treatment should be weighed against the risk of hemorrhage for each patient.
- Surgery is generally felt to be safe with an INR of ≤1.5.
- Some procedures may be safely done even with an INR of 2.0 to 3.0 (e.g., endoscopy without biopsy, dental procedures, and skin biopsies).
- If interruption of warfarin therapy is necessary, it should be discontinued 4 to 5 days before the procedure, allowing the INR to drift below 1.5.[82]
- If a temporary interruption of anticoagulation is unacceptable (e.g., mechanical heart valve, atrial fibrillation, or VTE at high/moderate risk), parenteral **bridging anticoagulation** (i.e., low-molecular-weight heparin [LMWH] or unfractionated heparin [UFH]) should be initiated approximately 3 days after the last warfarin dose and discontinued 4 to 24 hours prior to the procedure, depending on the half-life of the drug. **LMWH will be simpler and more cost-effective for most patients and does not routinely require monitoring of antifactor Xa levels.**
- Bridging anticoagulation after **minor surgery** or invasive procedures can be resumed in approximately 24 hours.
- After **major surgery** (e.g., open abdominal surgery) or **surgery with a high bleeding risk** (e.g., cardiac, neurosurgical, urologic, or major orthopedic surgeries), bridging anticoagulation can be resumed in approximately 48 to 72 hours.
- After the procedure, warfarin (at the previous dose) and/or parenteral anticoagulation are resumed as soon as adequate hemostasis and low bleeding risk have been achieved, typically within 24 hours.

PERIOPERATIVE CORTICOSTEROID MANAGEMENT

General Principles

- Surgery is a potent activator of the hypothalamic-pituitary axis (HPA).
- Patients with adrenal insufficiency may lack the ability to respond appropriately to surgical stress.

- Furthermore, patients receiving corticosteroids as medical therapy for indications other than adrenal dysfunction may develop adrenal insufficiency.

Etiology/Pathophysiology

- The subtype of adrenal insufficiency has implications on management.
  - **Tertiary adrenal insufficiency** due to exogenous corticosteroid administration is the most common adrenal problem encountered. These patients should have intact mineralocorticoid function and therefore require only glucocorticoid supplementation.
  - Likewise, **secondary adrenal insufficiency** should not result in mineralocorticoid deficiency. The possibility of deficits in other hormones due to pituitary disease should be considered.
  - **Primary adrenal insufficiency** requires replacement of both mineralocorticoids and glucocorticoids.
- The dose and duration of exogenous corticosteroids required to produce clinically significant tertiary adrenal insufficiency is highly variable, but general principles can be outlined[83]:
  - **Daily therapy with ≤5 mg of prednisone (or equivalent), alternate day corticosteroid therapy, and any dose given for <3 weeks should not result in clinically significant adrenal suppression.**
  - Patients receiving >20 mg/day of prednisone (or equivalent) for >3 weeks and patients who are clinically cushingoid in appearance can be expected to have significant suppression of adrenal responsiveness.
  - The function of the HPA cannot be readily predicted in patients receiving prednisone doses of 5 to 20 mg for >3 weeks and patients receiving doses of >5 mg for >3 weeks within the prior year.

Diagnosis

- For patients in whom clinical prediction of adrenal function is difficult, a cosyntropin stimulation test can be performed.
- The diagnosis of adrenal failure is discussed in detail in Chapter 17.

Treatment

- It is generally agreed that patients with known or expected adrenal insufficiency should be treated with perioperative glucocorticoids.
- In patients whose HPA axis status is uncertain and there is inadequate time to perform a cosyntropin stimulation test, corticosteroids can be administered preoperatively.
- The following guidelines are based on extrapolation from small studies in the literature, expert opinion, and clinical experience[83]:
  - **Minor surgical stress** (e.g., colonoscopy, cataract surgery, and inguinal hernia repair): Give 25 mg hydrocortisone or 5 mg methylprednisolone IV on the day of the procedure only.
  - **Moderate surgical stress** (e.g., cholecystectomy and hemicolectomy): Give 50 to 75 mg hydrocortisone or 10 to 15 mg methylprednisolone IV on the day of the procedure and taper quickly over 1 to 2 days to the usual dose.
  - **Major surgical stress** (e.g., major cardiothoracic surgery, Whipple procedure, and liver resection): Give 100 to 150 mg hydrocortisone or 20 to 30 mg methylprednisolone IV on the day of the procedure and taper to the usual dose over the next 1 to 2 days.
  - **Critically ill patients undergoing emergent surgery** (e.g., sepsis and hypotension): Give 50 to 100 mg hydrocortisone IV every 6 to 8 hours or 0.18 mg/kg/hour as a continuous

infusion plus 0.05 mg/day of fludrocortisone until the shock has resolved. Then gradually taper the dose, monitoring vital signs and serum sodium closely.

- Additional mineralocorticoid supplementation for patients with primary adrenal insufficiency may or may not be necessary, depending on the dose and mineralocorticoid potency of the corticosteroid given.
- A recent systematic review suggests that stress dose steroids are not routinely required for patients receiving therapeutic doses who undergo a surgical procedure, as long as they continue to receive their usually daily dose.[84]

OTHER MEDICATION ADJUSTMENTS IN PERIOPERATIVE PERIOD

Thyroid Hormone Replacement

- Patients with hypothyroidism who are clinically euthyroid receiving thyroxine treatment can safely skip this medication for several days due to its long half-life.
- Patients may resume therapy once they can take PO.
- In patients who cannot resume oral intake in 5 to 7 days, IV thyroxine should be given at approximately 80% of the oral dose.

Anticonvulsants

- **Patients with poorly controlled seizures should not undergo elective surgery.**
- Anticonvulsants for generalized seizures should be continued parenterally if needed.
- Phenytoin has a fairly long half-life and a single dose may be withheld safely.
- When IV or IM preparations are not available, phenytoin or phenobarbital should be substituted.

Psychiatric Medications

- **Benzodiazepines** should be continued postoperatively in those who take them chronically.
- **Selective serotonin reuptake inhibitors** can be given safely in the perioperative period.
- **Antipsychotics** can generally be continued without adverse effects.
- **Tricyclic antidepressants** can have significant anticholinergic and α-adrenergic blocking properties and there is a high potential for drug interactions. Tricyclic antidepressants **should preferably be stopped several days before elective surgery.**
- **Monoamine oxidase inhibitors** (MAOIs) have the potential for severe drug interactions and **must be stopped at least 2 weeks prior to elective surgery.**
- Lithium has a narrow margin of safety and serious side effects when overdosed.
  - Lithium can cause fluid and electrolyte abnormalities and prolong the effects of anesthetic and neuromuscular blocking agents.
  - Lithium should usually be stopped 1 to 2 days preoperatively and can be resumed once the patient is reliably taking PO.

Herbal Medications

- Be sure to ask the patient specifically about the use of alternative or herbal preparations, as many patients may not report this when asked for a medication list.

TABLE 6	Venous Thromboembolism Risk Factors
Surgery	Erythropoiesis-stimulating agents
Trauma (major or lower extremity)	Acute medical illnesses
Prolonged immobility/paralysis	Inflammatory bowel disease
Cancer or cancer therapy	Nephrotic syndrome
Venous compression (e.g., tumor, hematoma, arterial abnormality)	Myeloproliferative disorders
Prior DVT or PE	Paroxysmal nocturnal hemoglobinuria
Age > 40 years	Obesity
Pregnancy/postpartum	Varicose veins
Estrogen use (e.g., OCPs or HRT)	Central venous catheterization
Selective estrogen receptor modulators	Inherited or acquired thrombophilia

DVT, deep vein thrombosis; HRT, hormone replacement therapy; OCP, oral contraceptive pill; PE, pulmonary embolism.
Modified from Geerts WH, Bergqvist D, Pineo GF, et al. American College of Chest Physicians. Prevention of venous thromboembolism: American College of Chest Physicians Evidence-Based Clinical Practice Guidelines (8th Edition). *Chest* 2008; 133:381S–453S.

- All of the following herbal remedies should probably be stopped before surgery[85–87]:
  - **Feverfew, ginger, and gingko** may potentially increase the risk of bleeding.
  - **Valerian root** can potentiate the effects of sedatives and anxiolytics.
  - **St. John's wort** may have MAOI-like activity.
  - Toxic effects of **ma huang** include hypertension, arrhythmias, and myocardial ischemia.

Prophylactic Measures

Venous Thromboembolism Prophylaxis

- Venous thromboembolism (VTE) prophylaxis is generally relevant only in the inpatient setting. However, because of its importance, the topic will be briefly covered here.
- VTE encompasses deep vein thrombosis (DVT) and pulmonary embolism (PE). Prophylaxis is of paramount importance as DVT/PE continues to be a leading cause of in-hospital mortality.
- Risk factors for VTE are listed in Table 6.[88]
- The 2008 ACCP thromboprophylaxis recommendations are presented in Table 7.[88]

ENDOCARDITIS PROPHYLAXIS

General Principles

- In 2007, the AHA released its most recent guideline regarding infective endocarditis (IE) prophylaxis; it contains major changes compared with prior guidelines.[89]
- There is a notable lack of data supporting the use of antibiotic prophylaxis in the setting of dental, gastrointestinal, and genitourinary (GU) procedures and evidence of causation is circumstantial.

TABLE 7	Level of Risk and Thromboprophylaxis	
Level of Risk	DVT Risk Without Prophylaxis	Thromboprophylaxis
Low risk	<10%	
Minor surgery in mobile patients		No specific thromboprophylaxis
Fully ambulatory medical patients		Early and aggressive ambulation
Moderate risk	10%–40%	
Most general, open gynecologic, or urologic surgery patients		LMWH, LDUH bid or tid, fondaparinux
Medical patients, bed rest, or sick		
Moderate VTE risk plus high bleeding risk		Mechanical thromboprophylaxis
High risk	40%–80%	
Hip or knee arthroplasty, hip fracture surgery		LMWH, fondaparinux, warfarin
Major trauma, spinal cord injury (presuming there is no major contraindication)		
High VTE risk plus high bleeding risk		Mechanical thromboprophylaxis

DVT, deep vein thrombosis; LDUH, low-dose unfractionated heparin; LMWH, low-molecular-weight heparin; VTE, venous thromboembolism.
Modified from Geerts WH, Bergqvist D, Pineo GF, et al. American College of Chest Physicians. Prevention of venous thromboembolism: American College of Chest Physicians Evidence-Based Clinical Practice Guidelines (8th Edition). *Chest* 2008;133: 381S–453S.

- There has been no prospective, placebo-controlled, multicenter, randomized, double-blind study of the efficacy of IE antibiotic prophylaxis.
- Based on a synthesis of available data, it is likely that **most cases of IE are not directly caused by dental or other procedures** and that even if antibiotic prophylaxis were completely effective, a very large number of prophylactic doses would be needed to prevent a very small number of cases or IE.
- **The cumulative risk for IE is much greater with ordinary daily activities** (e.g., chewing, brushing, and flossing).
- On the other hand, the risks of single-dose antibiotic prophylaxis are quite low but they do exist (e.g., increased antibiotic resistance and rare cases of anaphylaxis).
- The AHA suggests that there be greater emphasis on oral health in individuals with high-risk cardiac conditions.
- The guidelines conclude that **antibiotic prophylaxis is reasonable in very few clinical situations.**

Treatment

- Prophylaxis is now recommended (despite the lack of conclusive evidence) **only** for patients undergoing certain dental procedures with cardiac conditions associated with the highest risk of adverse outcome (Table 8). This does **not** include patients with mitral valve prolapse.
- Only those dental procedures that involve manipulation of the gingival tissue or the periapical region (i.e., near the roots) of teeth or perforation of the oral mucosa warrant prophylaxis. Tooth extractions and cleanings are included. In these instances, prophylactic antibiotics should be directed against viridans streptococci. Despite known resistance patterns, the recommended regimens for dental procedures are as follows:
  - **Amoxicillin 2 g PO 30 to 60 minutes before the procedure.**
  - **If unable to take PO,** ampicillin 2 g IM/IV **OR** cefazolin 1 g IM/IV **OR** ceftriaxone 1 g IM/IV 30 to 60 minutes before the procedure.
  - **If allergic to penicillins,** cephalexin 2 g PO (do not use if there is a history of anaphylactoid reactions) **OR** clindamycin 600 mg PO **OR** azithromycin/clarithromycin 500 mg PO 30 to 60 minutes before the procedure. Another first- or second-generation cephalosporin may be used in doses equivalent to cephalexin.
  - For patients who are **penicillin allergic AND cannot take PO,** cefazolin/ceftriaxone 1 g IM/IV (do not use if there is a history of anaphylactoid reactions) **OR** clindamycin 600 mg IM/IV 30 to 60 minutes before the procedure.
- IE prophylaxis may also be reasonable for high-risk patients (see Table 3 of Chapter 28) having **procedures on the respiratory tract involving incision or biopsy of the respiratory mucosa.** The same regimens recommended above for dental procedures should be used.
- For **procedures on infected skin, skin structures, or musculoskeletal tissue,** it is reasonable that treatment for the infection itself should be active against staphylococci and β-hemolytic streptococci, that is, an antistaphylococcal penicillin or cephalosporin. For patients unable to tolerate penicillins or who are suspected or known to have an oxacillin-resistant *Staphylococcus aureus* infection, vancomycin or clindamycin may be used.
- **Antibiotics solely for the purpose of IE prophylaxis are no longer recommended for gastrointestinal (including endoscopy) or genitourinary procedures on any patient.**

TABLE 8	Cardiac Conditions with the Highest Risk of Adverse Outcome from Infective Endocarditis

Prosthetic valve or prosthetic material used for valve repair
Previous infective endocarditis
Congenital heart disease (CHD)
Unrepaired cyanotic CHD, including palliative shunts and conduits
Completely repaired CHD with prosthetic material or device, whether placed by surgery or by catheter intervention, during the first 6 months after the procedure
Repaired CHD with residual defects at the site or adjacent to the site of a prosthetic patch or prosthetic device (which inhibit endothelialization)
Cardiac transplantation recipients who develop cardiac valvulopathy

Modified from Wilson W, Taubert KA, Gewitz M, et al. Prevention of infective endocarditis: guidelines from the American Heart Association. *Circulation* 2007;116:1736–1754.

REFERENCES

1. Macpherson DS. Preoperative laboratory testing: should any tests be "routine" before surgery? *Med Clin North America* 1993;77:289–308.
2. Johnson RK, Mortimer AJ. Routine pre-operative blood testing: is it necessary? *Anaesthesia* 2002;57:914–917.
3. Smetana GW, Macpherson DS. The case against routine preoperative laboratory testing. *Med Clin N Am* 2003;87:7–40.
4. Dzankic S, Pastor D, Gonzalez C, Leung JM. The prevalence and predictive value of abnormal preoperative laboratory tests in elderly surgical patients. *Anesth Analg* 2001;93:301–308.
5. Schein OD, Katz J, Bass EB, et al. The value of routine preoperative medical testing before cataract surgery. *New Engl J Med* 2000;342:168–175.
6. Marcello PW, Roberts PL. "Routine" preoperative studies. Which studies, which patients? *Surg Clin North Am* 1996;76:11–23.
7. Wu WC, Schifftner TL, Henderson WG, et al. Preoperative hematocrit levels and postoperative outcomes in older patients undergoing noncardiac surgery. *JAMA* 2007;297:2481–2488.
8. Hirsch IA, Tomlinson DL, Slogoff S, et al. The overstated risk of preoperative hypokalemia. *Anesth Analg* 1988;67:131–136.
9. Fleisher LA, Beckman JA, Brown KA, et al. ACC/AHA 2007 guidelines on perioperative cardiovascular evaluation and care for noncardiac surgery: a report of the American College of Cardiology/American Heart Association Task Force on Practice Guidelines (Writing Committee to Revise the 2002 Guidelines on Perioperative Cardiovascular Evaluation for Noncardiac Surgery). *Circulation* 2007;116:e418–e499.
10. Lee TH, Marcantonio ER, Mangione CM, et al. Derivation and prospective validation of a simple index for prediction of cardiac risk of major noncardiac surgery. *Circulation* 1999;100:1043–1049.
11. Sorenson RM, Pace NL. Anesthetic techniques during surgical repair of femoral neck fractures. A meta-analysis. *Anesthesiology* 1992;77:1095.
12. Urwin SC, Parker MJ, Griffiths R. General versus regional anaesthesia for hip fracture surgery: a meta-analysis of randomized trials. *Br J Anaesth* 2000;84:450–455.
13. Rodgers A. Walker N, Schug S, et al. Reduction of postoperative mortality and morbidity with epidural or spinal anesthesia: results from overview of randomized trials. *BMJ* 2000; 321:1493–1497.
14. Parker MJ, Handoll HH, Griffiths R. Anaesthesia for hip fracture surgery in adults. *Cochrane Database Syst Rev* 2004 Oct 18;(4):CD000521.
15. Mauermann WJ, Shilling AM, Zuo Z. A comparison of neuraxial block versus general anesthesia for elective total hip replacement: a meta-analysis. *Anesth Analg* 2006;103:1018–1025.
16. Hu S, Zhang ZY, Hua YQ, et al. A comparison of regional and general anaesthesia for total replacement of the hip or knee: a meta-analysis. *J Bone Joint Surg Br* 2009;91:935–942.
17. Fleisher LA, Eagle KA. Clinical practice. Lowering cardiac risk in noncardiac surgery. *N Engl J Med* 2001;345:1677–1682.
18. Adesanya AO, de Lemos JA, Greilich NB, Whitten CW. Management of perioperative myocardial infarction in noncardiac surgical patients. *Chest* 2006;130:584–596.
19. Fleischmann KE, Goldman L, Young B, Lee TH. Association between cardiac and noncardiac complications in patients undergoing noncardiac surgery: outcomes and effects on length of stay. *Am J Med* 2003;115:515–520.
20. Boersma E, Kertai MD, Schouten O, et al. Perioperative cardiovascular mortality in noncardiac surgery: validation of the Lee cardiac risk index. *Am J Med* 2005;118:1134–1141.
21. Hoeks SE, op Reimer WJ, van Gestel YR, et al. Preoperative cardiac risk index predicts long-term mortality and health status. *Am J Med* 2009;122:559–565.
22. Polanczyk CA, Marcantonio E, Goldman L, et al. Impact of age on perioperative complications and length of stay in patients undergoing noncardiac surgery. *Ann Intern Med* 2001; 134:637–643.
23. Reilly DF, McNeely MJ, Doerner D, et al. Self reported exercise tolerance and the risk of serious perioperative complications. *Arch Intern Med* 1999;159:2185–2192.

24. Backer CL, Tinker JH, Robertson DM, Vlietstra RE. Myocardial reinfarction following local anesthesia for ophthalmic surgery. *Anesth Analg* 1980;59:257–262.

25. Warner MA, Shields SE, Chute CG. Major morbidity and mortality within 1 month of ambulatory surgery and anesthesia. *JAMA* 1993;270:1437–1441.

26. Falcone RA, Nass C, Jermyn R, et al. The value of preoperative pharmacologic stress testing before vascular surgery using ACC/AHA guidelines: a prospective, randomized trial. *J Cardiothorac Vasc Anesth* 2003;17:694–698.

27. Poldermans D, Bax JJ, Schouten O, et al. Dutch Echocardiographic Cardiac Risk Evaluation Applying Stress Echo Study Group. Should major vascular surgery be delayed because of preoperative cardiac testing in intermediate-risk patients receiving beta-blocker therapy with tight heart rate control? *J Am Coll Cardiol* 2006;48:964–969.

28. Brett AS. Coronary assessment before noncardiac surgery: current strategies are flawed. *Circulation* 2008;117:3145–3151.

29. Gregoratos G. Current guideline-based preoperative evaluation provides the best management of patients undergoing noncardiac surgery. *Circulation* 2008;117:3134–3144.

30. Mangano DT, Layug EL, Wallace A, et al. Effect of atenolol on mortality and cardiovascular morbidity after noncardiac surgery. *N Engl J Med* 1996;335: 1713–1720.

31. Poldermans D, Boersma E, Bax JJ, et al. The effect of bisoprolol on perioperative mortality and myocardial infarction in high-risk patients undergoing vascular surgery. Dutch Echocardiographic Cardiac Risk Evaluation Applying Stress Echocardiography Study Group. *N Engl J Med* 1999;341:1789–1794.

32. Wallace A, Layug B, Tateo I, et al. Prophylactic atenolol reduces postoperative myocardial ischemia. McSPI Research Group. *Anesthesiology* 1998;88:7–17.

33. Stevens RD, Burri H, Tramèr MR. Pharmacologic myocardial protection in patients undergoing noncardiac surgery: a quantitative systematic review. *Anesth Analg* 2003;97:623–633.

34. McGory ML, Maggard MA, Ko CY. A meta-analysis of perioperative beta blockade: what is the actual risk reduction? *Surgery* 2005;138:171–179.

35. Juul AB, Wetterslev J, Bluud C, et al. Effect of perioperative beta blockade in patients with diabetes undergoing major non-cardiac surgery: randomized placebo controlled, blinded multicenter trial. *BMJ* 2006;332:1482–1488.

36. Yang H, Raymer K, Butler R, et al. The effects of perioperative beta-blockade: results of the Metoprolol after Vascular Surgery (MaVS) study, a randomized controlled trial. *Am Heart J* 2006;152:983–990.

37. POISE Study Group, Devereaux PJ, Yang H, Yusuf S, et al. Effects of extended-release metoprolol succinate in patients undergoing non-cardiac surgery (POISE trial): a randomised controlled trial. *Lancet* 2008;371:1839–1847.

38. Bangalore S, Wetterslev J, Pranesh S, et al. Perioperative beta blockers in patients having non-cardiac surgery: a meta-analysis. *Lancet* 2008;372:1962–1976.

39. Fleisher LA, Beckman JA, Brown KA, et al. ACC/AHA 2006 guideline update on perioperative cardiovascular evaluation for noncardiac surgery: focused update on perioperative beta-blocker therapy: a report of the American College of Cardiology/American Heart Association Task Force on Practice Guidelines. *J Am Coll Cardiol* 2006;47:2343–2355.

40. Nishina K, Mikawa K, Uesugi T, et al. Efficacy of clonidine for prevention of perioperative myocardial ischemia: a critical appraisal and meta-analysis of the literature. *Anesthesiology* 2002;96:323–329.

41. Wijeysundera DN, Naik JS, Beattie WS. Alpha-2 adrenergic agonists to prevent perioperative cardiovascular complications: a meta-analysis. *Am J Med* 2003;114:742–752.

42. Wallace AW, Galindez D, Salahieh A, et al. Effect of clonidine on cardiovascular morbidity and mortality after noncardiac surgery. *Anesthesiology* 2004;101:284–293.

43. Poldermans D, Bax JJ, Kertai MD, et al. Statins are associated with a reduced incidence of perioperative mortality in patients undergoing major noncardiac vascular surgery. *Circulation* 2003;107:1848–1851.

44. Lindenauer PK, Pekow P, Wang K, et al. Lipid-lowering therapy and in-hospital mortality following major noncardiac surgery. *JAMA* 2004;291:2092–2099.

45. Durazzo AE, Machado FS, Ikeoka DT, et al. Reduction in cardiovascular events after vascular surgery with atorvastatin: a randomized trial. *J Vasc Surg* 2004;39:967–976.

46. McFalls EO, Ward HB, Moritz TE, et al. Coronary-artery revascularization before elective major vascular surgery. *N Engl J Med* 2004;351:2795–2804.

47. Poldermans D, Schouten O, Vidakovic R, et al. DECREASE Study Group. A clinical randomized trial to evaluate the safety of a noninvasive approach in high-risk patients undergoing major vascular surgery: the DECREASE-V Pilot Study. *J Am Coll Cardiol* 2007;49: 1763–1769.

48. Schouten O, van Kuijk JP, Flu WJ, et al. DECREASE Study Group. Long-term outcome of prophylactic coronary revascularization in cardiac high-risk patients undergoing major vascular surgery (from the randomized DECREASE-V Pilot Study). *Am J Cardiol* 2009; 103:897–901.

49. Boden WE, O'Rourke RA, Teo KK, et al. COURAGE Trial Research Group. Optimal medical therapy with or without PCI for stable coronary disease. *N Engl J Med* 2007;356: 1503–1516.

50. Kaluza GL, Joseph J, Lee Jr, et al. Catastrophic outcomes of noncardiac surgery soon after coronary stenting. *J Am Coll Cardiol* 2000;35:1288–1294.

51. Wilson SH, Fasseas P, Orford JL, et al. Clinical outcome of patients undergoing noncardiac surgery in the two months following coronary stenting. *J Am Coll Cardiol* 2003;42:234–240.

52. Grines CL, Bonow RO, Casey DE, et al. Prevention of premature discontinuation of dual antiplatelet therapy in patients with coronary artery stents. *J Am Coll Cardiol* 2007;49: 734–739.

53. Brilakis ES, Orford JL, Fasseas P, et al. Outcome of patients undergoing balloon angioplasty in the two months prior to noncardiac surgery. *Am J Cardiol* 2005;96:512–514.

54. Leibowitz D, Cohen M, Planer D, et al. Comparison of cardiovascular risk of noncardiac surgery following coronary angioplasty with versus without stenting. *Am J Cardiol* 2006; 97:1188–1191.

55. Coriat P, Richer C, Douraki T, et al. Influence of chronic angiotensin-converting enzyme inhibition on anesthetic induction. *Anesthesiology* 1994;81:299–307.

56. Pigott DW, Nagle C, Allman K, et al. Effect of omitting regular ACE inhibitor medication before cardiac surgery on hemodynamic variables and vasoactive drug requirements. *Br J Anaesth* 1999;83:715–720.

57. Brabant SM, Bertrand M, Eyraud D, et al. The hemodynamic effects of anesthetic induction in vascular surgical patients chronically treated with angiotensin II receptor antagonists. *Anesth Analg* 1999;89:1388–1392.

58. Kertai MD, Bountioukos M, Boersma E, et al. Aortic stenosis: an underestimated risk factor for perioperative complications in patients undergoing noncardiac surgery. *Am J Med* 2004;116:8–13.

59. Qaseem A, Snow V, Fitterman N, et al. Risk assessment for and strategies to reduce perioperative pulmonary complications for patients undergoing noncardiothoracic surgery: a guideline from the American College of Physicians. *Ann Intern Med* 2006;144:575–580.

60. Smetana GW, Lawrence VA, Cornell JE. American College of Physicians. Preoperative pulmonary risk stratification for noncardiothoracic surgery: systematic review for the American College of Physicians. *Ann Intern Med* 2006;144:581–595.

61. Arozullah AM, Khuri SF, Henderson WG, Daley J. Participants in the National Veterans Affairs Surgical Quality Improvement Program. Development and validation of a multifactorial risk index for predicting postoperative pneumonia after major noncardiac surgery. *Ann Intern Med* 2001;135:847–857.

62. Johnson RG, Arozullah AM, Neumayer L, et al. Multivariable predictors of postoperative respiratory failure after general and vascular surgery: results from the patient safety in surgery study. *J Am Coll Surg* 2007;204:1188–1198.

63. Bapoje SR, Whitaker JF, Schulz T, et al. Preoperative evaluation of the patient with pulmonary disease. *Chest* 2007;132:1637–1645.

64. Archer C, Levy AR, McGregor M. Value of routine preoperative chest x-rays: a meta-analysis. *Can J Anaesth* 1993;40:1022–1027.

65. Lawrence VA, Cornell JE, Smetana GW. American College of Physicians. Strategies to reduce postoperative pulmonary complications after noncardiothoracic surgery: systematic review for the American College of Physicians. *Ann Intern Med* 2006;144:596–608.

66. Barrera R, Shi W, Amar D, et al. Smoking and timing of cessation: impact on pulmonary complications after thoracotomy. *Chest* 2005;127:1977–1983.

67. Wiklund RA. Preoperative preparation of patients with advanced liver disease. *Crit Care Med* 2004;32:S106–S115.

68. Rizvon MK, Chou CL. Surgery in the patient with liver disease. *Med Clin N Am* 2003;87: 211–227.

69. Mansour A, Watson W, Shayani V, et al. Abdominal operations in patients with cirrhosis: still a major surgical challenge. *Surgery* 1997;122:730–735.

70. Teh SH, Nagorney DM, Stevens SR, et al. Risk factors for mortality after surgery in patients with cirrhosis. *Gastroenterology* 2007;132:1261–1269.

71. Kellerman PS. Perioperative care of the renal patient. *Arch Intern Med* 1994;154:1674–1688.

72. Wagener G, Brentjens TE. Renal disease: the anesthesiologist's perspective. *Anesthesiol Clin* 2006;24:523–547.

73. Joseph AJ, Cohn SL. Perioperative care of the patient with renal failure. *Med Clin North Am* 2003;87:193–210.

74. Lind SE. The bleeding time does not predict surgical bleeding. *Blood* 1991;77:2547–2552.

75. Umpierrez GE, Isaacs SD, Bazargan N, et al. Hyperglycemia: an independent marker of in-hospital mortality in patients with undiagnosed diabetes. *J Clin Endocrinol Metab* 2002; 87:978–982.

76. ACE/ADA Task Force on Inpatient Diabetes. American College of Endocrinology and American Diabetes Association Consensus statement on inpatient diabetes and glycemic control. *Diabetes Care* 2006;29:1955–1962.

77. Moghissi ES, Korytkowski MT, DiNardo M, et al. American Association of Clinical Endocrinologists; American Diabetes Association. American Association of Clinical Endocrinologists and American Diabetes Association consensus statement on inpatient glycemic control. *Diabetes Care* 2009;32:1119–1131.

78. Finfer S, Chittock DR, Su SY, et al. NICE-SUGAR Study Investigators. Intensive versus conventional glucose control in critically ill patients. *N Engl J Med* 2009;360:1283–1297.

79. Ferrari E, Benhamou M, Cerboni P, et al. Coronary syndromes following aspirin with-drawal: a special risk for late stent thrombosis. *J Am Coll Cardiol* 2005;45:456–459.

80. Mangano DT. Aspirin and mortality from coronary bypass surgery. *N Engl J Med* 2002; 347:1309–1317.

81. Douketis JD, Berger PB, Dunn AS, et al. American College of Chest Physicians. The peri-operative management of antithrombotic therapy: American College of Chest Physicians Evidence-Based Clinical Practice Guidelines (8th Edition). *Chest* 2008;133:299S–339S.

82. White RH, McKittrick T, Hutchinson R, Twitchell J. Temporary discontinuation of warfarin therapy: changes in the international normalized ratio. *Ann Intern Med* 1995;122:40–42.

83. Coursin DB, Wood KE. Corticosteroid supplementation for adrenal insufficiency. *JAMA* 2002;287:236–240.

84. Marik PE, Varon J. Requirement of perioperative stress doses of corticosteroids: a system-atic review of the literature. *Arch Surg* 2008;143:1222–1226.

85. Winslow LC, Kroll DJ. Herbs as medicines. *Arch Intern Med* 1998;158:2192–2199.

86. Miller LG. Herbal medicinals: selected clinical considerations focusing on known or poten-tial drug-herb interactions. *Arch Intern Med* 1998;158:2200–2211.

87. Lee A, Chui PT, Aun CST, et al. Incidence and risk of adverse perioperative events among surgical patients taking traditional Chinese herbal medicines. *Anesthesiology* 2006;105: 454–461.

88. Geerts WH, Bergqvist D, Pineo GF, et al. American College of Chest Physicians. Preven-tion of venous thromboembolism: American College of Chest Physicians Evidence-Based Clinical Practice Guidelines (8th Edition). *Chest* 2008;133:381S–453S.

89. Wilson W, Taubert KA, Gewitz M, et al. Prevention of infective endocarditis: guidelines from the American Heart Association. *Circulation* 2007;116:1736–1754.

3

Hypertension
Vinay Madan and Thomas M. De Fer

General Principles

Introduction/Background

- Hypertension (HTN) is one of the most commonly encountered diseases in the outpatient setting with an **estimated prevalence rate of 30%.**
- Starting from as low as 115/75 mm Hg, the mortality from cardiovascular disease doubles for every increase by 20 mm Hg systolic or 10 mm Hg diastolic, highlighting the tremendous burden that elevated blood pressure (BP) places on society as well as the importance of prompt recognition and treatment.[1]
- Although considerable progress has been made in raising awareness of HTN over the last few decades, current recognition of those affected is far from adequate. **Approximately one-third of adults are unaware of their HTN and nearly two-thirds of those who are aware fall short of their treatment goals.**[2]
- As a physician in the outpatient setting, achieving better control of HTN is of paramount importance.

Definition

- For epidemiologic and practical reasons, HTN is currently defined as a systolic pressure of ≥140 mm Hg and/or a diastolic pressure of ≥90 mm Hg. This is based upon the **average of two or more properly measured readings** at each of two or more visits following an initial screen.[2]
- However, BP is a continuously distributed trait with a correspondingly variable risk of cardiovascular disease, so defining HTN in terms of numbers is somewhat arbitrary.
- HTN can perhaps be better described as a progressive cardiovascular syndrome characterized by the presence of BP elevation to a level that places patients at increased risk for target organ damage in multiple vascular beds.

Classification

- HTN is further stratified into stages of severity based on both systolic and diastolic pressure. Table 1 provides the classification scheme for adults aged 18 and older from the Seventh Report of the Joint National Committee on Prevention, Detection, Evaluation, and Treatment of High Blood Pressure (JNC 7).[2]
- The term "prehypertension" was adopted to identify those at high risk of developing HTN in whom early intervention can decrease the rate of BP progression with age but does not denote a disease category.[2,3]

Epidemiology

- An estimated 65 million people with on **overall prevalence rate of approximately 30%** have HTN based on 1999–2000 National Health and Nutrition Examination Survey (NHANES) data, a substantial increase from earlier estimates of 50 million only a decade before.[4]

TABLE 1	Classification of Blood Pressure for Adults	
BP Classification	SBP (mm Hg)	DBP (mm Hg)
Normal	<120	And <80
Prehypertension	120–139	Or 80–89
Stage 1 hypertension	140–159	Or 90–99
Stage 2 hypertension	≥160	Or ≥100

BP, blood pressure; DBP, diastolic blood pressure; SBP, systolic blood pressure.
Modified from Chobanian AV, Bakris GL, Black HR, et al. National High Blood Pressure Education Program Coordinating Committee on Prevention, Detection, Evaluation, and Treatment of High Blood Pressure: the JNC 7 report. *JAMA* 2003;289:2560–2572.

- This growing prevalence is directly related to an **aging population and a higher rate of obesity.** HTN affects >50% of those aged 60 to 69 and approximately 75% of those 70 or older.[5]
- HTN is more common in African-Americans and those with a positive family history. The prevalence is higher in men than in women until the age of 60, after which women are affected in greater numbers.
- HTN is a major risk factor for the development of cardiovascular disease, chronic kidney disease, and dementia, with most affected patients dying from ischemic heart disease.
- **Reversible risk factors** include prehypertension, being overweight or obese, metabolic syndrome, tobacco use, excessive alcohol intake, a high-sodium low-potassium diet, and a sedentary lifestyle.

Etiology

Essential Hypertension
- Most common cause of HTN affecting approximately 95% of patients.
- Because of a complex interplay of multiple factors including genetics, increased sympathetic and angiotensin II activity, insulin resistance, salt sensitivity, and environmental influences.

Secondary Hypertension
- Affects a smaller minority (about 5%) of patients.
- Secondary to a disease process with a specific identifiable structural, biochemical, or genetic defect resulting in elevated BP.
- Some of the more common examples include renovascular disease, renal parenchymal disease, endocrinopathies, side effect of other drugs, and obstructive sleep apnea. These entities are described further in the "Special Considerations" section.

Diagnosis

Screening

- Elevated BP is usually discovered in asymptomatic patients during routine office visits and should therefore be checked as part of every health care encounter.
- **The optimal screening interval for HTN is unknown.** Current recommendations call for checking BP at least every 2 years in those with normal BP (<120/80 mm Hg) and

TABLE 2	Recommendations for Follow-Up Based on Initial Blood Pressure Measurements for Adults without Acute End-Organ Damage

Initial Blood Pressure (mm Hg)	Follow-up Recommended
Normal	Recheck in 2 years
Prehypertension	Recheck in 1 year
Stage 1 hypertension	Confirm within 2 months
Stage 2 hypertension	Evaluate within 1 month
	For those with higher pressures (>180/110 mm Hg), evaluate and treat immediately or within 1 week depending on clinical situation and complications

Modified from Chobanian AV, Bakris GL, Black HR, et al. National High Blood Pressure Education Program Coordinating Committee on Prevention, Detection, Evaluation, and Treatment of High Blood Pressure: the JNC 7 report. *JAMA* 2003;289:2560–2572.

annually for persons with prehypertension. Table 2 presents a suggested time frame for follow-up evaluations based on BP measurements.[2]
- If systolic and diastolic categories are different, follow recommendations for the shorter follow-up.
- The schedule may be modified based on reliable information about past BP measurements, other cardiovascular risk factors, and target organ damage.

Measuring Blood Pressure/Technique
- Optimal detection of HTN depends on proper technique.[6]
- BP should be measured while the patient is in the **seated position** with the arm supported at the heart level.
- The patient should have avoided caffeine, exercise, and smoking for at least 30 minutes prior to measurement.
- An **appropriately sized cuff** with the bladder encircling at least 80% of the arm circumference should be used to ensure accuracy.
- The cuff should be inflated at a rate of 20 to 30 mm Hg past the level where the radial pulse is no longer felt and then deflated at a rate of 2 mm Hg/sec.
- The stethoscope should be placed lightly over the brachial artery.
- Systolic blood pressure (SBP) should be noted at the sound of the brachial pulse (Korotkov phase I) and diastolic blood pressure (DBP) at the disappearance of the pulse (Korotkov phase V).
- Two readings should be taken, ideally separated by at least 2 minutes.
- Elevated values should be confirmed in both arms. If there is a disparity due to a unilateral arterial lesion, the reading from the arm with higher pressure should be used.

Ambulatory Blood Pressure Monitoring
- In some situations, **ambulatory blood pressure monitoring** (ABPM) can be used to provide further information.[2]
- With ABPM, patients wear automated, lightweight devices that obtain multiple BP measurements at specific intervals throughout a 24- to 48-hour period.

- More effectively reflects a patient's true diurnal variation in BP with lower values during sleep and higher values during wakefulness or activity.
- Studies have suggested that values obtained with ABPM more closely correlate with end-organ complications than do values obtained in the physician's office.[7]
- Particularly useful in suspected cases of "white coat HTN" in which the anxiety of the physician encounter may falsely elevate BP while values outside of the office are often normal.[2]
- Also helpful in guiding treatment decisions in patients with borderline HTN, resistant HTN, or symptoms suggestive of hypotension on treatment.[2]
- In general, self-recorded measurements are less reliable but may serve as a practical alternative in patients whose values are consistently <130/80 mm Hg despite an elevated office value.

Making the Diagnosis

- The diagnosis is established by documenting SBP of ≥140 mm Hg and/or DBP of ≥90 mm Hg, based on the average of two or more readings obtained on each of two or more office visits.
- A patient may be diagnosed on the basis of an elevated SBP alone even if the DBP is normal (i.e., isolated systolic HTN).
- With extreme elevations of BP (>210/120 mm Hg), the diagnosis can usually be safely made without the need for serial evaluations. **In these circumstances, one should focus on the evaluation of end-organ damage and treatment of hypertensive crises as indicated.**
- After the diagnosis of HTN has been made, there are three major objectives:
  - Assess lifestyle or other cardiovascular risk factors that may affect prognosis and guide treatment.
  - Reveal a cause of secondary HTN (most often NOT present).
  - Assess the presence or absence of target organ damage.
- The history, physical examination, and further diagnostic testing are the primary tools to achieve these objectives.

History

- Seek evidence of **target organ damage** that may be either known or suggested by characteristic symptoms:
  - Coronary artery disease (CAD) or prior myocardial infarction (MI) (angina or exertional dyspnea).
  - Heart failure (symptoms of volume overload and/or dyspnea).
  - Prior transient ischemic attack or stroke (dementia or focal deficits).
  - Peripheral artery disease (claudication).
  - Renal disease.
- Determine additional **risk factors** that increase the risk for a cardiovascular event. Modifiable risk factors should be treated.
  - Increased age (men >55, women >65).
  - Cigarette smoking.
  - Obesity (body mass index [BMI] >30 kg/m^2).
  - Physical inactivity.
  - Dyslipidemia.
  - Diabetes mellitus (DM).
  - Microalbuminuria or estimated glomerular filtration rate of <60 mL/min.
  - Family history of premature cardiovascular disease (for men, age <55, for women, age <65).

- **Secondary HTN** should be considered when BP becomes severely elevated acutely in a previously normotensive individual, at extremes of age (<20 or >50), or if refractory to treatment with multiple medications. Other symptoms that may be helpful include muscle weakness, palpitations, diaphoresis, skin thinning, flank pain, snoring, or daytime somnolence.
- Conduct a thorough evaluation of the patient's **medications,** as many agents have side effects of elevated BP. Common examples include oral contraceptives, nonsteroidal anti-inflammatory drugs (NSAIDs), and tricyclic antidepressants. Recent alcohol consumption or illicit substances such as cocaine can also raise BP.
  - Oral contraceptives induce sodium retention and potentiate the action of catecholamines.
  - NSAIDs block the formation of vasodilating, natriuretic prostaglandins and interfere with the effectiveness of many antihypertensives.
  - Tricyclic antidepressants inhibit the action of centrally acting agents (e.g., clonidine).

Physical Examination

- After obtaining accurate BP measurements, the physical examination should be tailored to evaluate the presence and severity of target end-organ damage and any features that may suggest secondary HTN.
- **Cardiopulmonary exam:** S4 gallop suggesting left ventricular hypertrophy (LVH), murmurs, or rales suggesting heart failure.
- **Funduscopic exam:** papilledema, arteriolar narrowing, cotton wool spots, and microaneurysms.
- **Vascular exam:** bruits of major arterial vessels (carotids, femorals, and aorta), asymmetric or diminished distal pulses.
- **Neurologic exam:** altered mental status or focal findings suggestive of prior stroke.
- **Endocrine:** elevated BMI, thyroid enlargement, and Cushingoid features (e.g., buffalo hump, striae, and skin thinning).

Diagnostic Testing

- Routine laboratory tests recommended before initiating therapy include serum electrolytes, blood urea nitrogen (BUN), creatinine, blood glucose, hematocrit, lipoprotein profile, thyroid-stimulating hormone, and urinalysis.
- Measurement of microalbuminuria is recommended in those with DM or renal disease but is otherwise elective and may add to the overall assessment of cardiovascular risk.
- An electrocardiogram (ECG) should be obtained in all patients to look for LVH and/or signs of previous infarct. Although ECG is more sensitive at diagnosing LVH, it is not recommended in all patients.
- A more detailed workup can be pursued for features highly suggestive of a secondary cause of HTN. Some of these are described in Table 3.[2]

Treatment

Principles of Therapy

- The goal of therapy is to eliminate the morbidity and mortality of cardiovascular disease attributable to HTN by decreasing BP to <140/90 mm Hg. A lower target of <130/80 mm Hg is recommended for those with DM or chronic kidney disease.[2]

TABLE 3	Secondary Causes of Hypertension	
Disease	**History and Exam Findings**	**Further Studies**
Renal parenchymal disease	History of DM, polycystic kidney disease, glomerulonephritis	Creatinine clearance Renal ultrasound
Renovascular disease	Abdominal bruit (50%), hypokalemia, proteinuria, episode of AKI induced by ACE inhibitor/ARB, recurrent pulmonary edema	Duplex ultrasonography MRA Spiral CT angiography
Cushing syndrome	Central obesity, buffalo hump, bruising, moon faces, wasting of extremities, hypokalemia	Dexamethasone suppression test Urinary free cortisol, serum ACTH Pituitary or adrenal imaging as indicated
Primary hyperaldo-steronism and other mineralocorticoid excess states	Hypokalemia, metabolic alkalosis, muscle weakness	Screen: plasma aldo-sterone (>15 ng/dL), aldosterone: renin ratio (>20) Confirm: salt suppression test CT or MRI to evaluate adrenals
Pheochromocytoma	Paroxysms of headaches, palpitations, diaphoresis	Serum and/or urine metanephrines
Coarctation of the aorta	Asymptomatic, BP greater in upper than in lower extremities, cold feet, claudication, dyspnea, fatigue	Chest radiograph Echocardiogram MRI
Obstructive sleep apnea	Obesity, frequent awakening with daytime somnolence, loud snoring, morning headache	Nocturnal polysomnography

ACE inhibitor, angiotensin-converting enzyme inhibitor; ACTH, adrenocorticotropic hormone; AKI, acute kidney injury; ARB, angiotensin-receptor blocker; BP, blood pressure; CT, computed tomography; DM, diabetes mellitus; MRI, magnetic resonance imaging. Modified from Chobanian AV, Bakris GL, Black HR, et al. National High Blood Pressure Education Program Coordinating Committee on Prevention, Detection, Evaluation, and Treatment of High Blood Pressure: the JNC 7 report. *JAMA* 2003;289:2560–2572.

- Patient education is an essential component of the treatment plan and promotes better adherence. Physicians should stress the following:
  - Lifelong treatment is often required.
  - **Symptoms are an unreliable gauge of severity** (despite many patients' claims that they can "feel" when their BP is high).

TABLE 4	Lifestyle Modifications to Prevent and Manage Hypertension

Modification	Recommendation	SBP Reduction (Range)
Weight reduction	Maintain normal body weight (body mass index 18.5–24.9 kg/m²)	5–20 mm Hg/10 kg
DASH diet	Consume a diet rich in fruits, vegetables, and low-fat dairy products with a reduced content of saturated and total fat	8–14 mm Hg
Sodium reduction	Reduce dietary sodium intake to no >100 mmol/day (2.4 g sodium or 6 g sodium chloride)	2–8 mm Hg
Exercise	Engage in regular aerobic physical activity such as brisk walking (at least 30 minutes/day, most days of the week)	4–9 mm Hg
Moderation of alcohol consumption	Limit consumption to no more than two drinks (e.g., 24 oz beer, 10 oz wine, or 3 oz 80-proof whiskey) per day in most men and to no more than one drink per day in women and lighter-weight persons	2–4 mm Hg

DASH, Dietary Approaches to Stop Hypertension.
Modified from Chobanian AV, Bakris GL, Black HR, et al. National High Blood Pressure Education Program Coordinating Committee on Prevention, Detection, Evaluation, and Treatment of High Blood Pressure: the JNC 7 report. *JAMA* 2003;289:2560–2572.

- Prognosis improves with effective management.
- Adherence to therapy is critically important.

Nonpharmacologic Therapy

- **Therapeutic lifestyle changes** described in Table 4 should be instituted in all patients with HTN and prehypertension.[2,8] These represent a critical component of both prevention and management of those on drug therapy.
- Therapeutic lifestyle changes may be employed as sole therapy for 6 to 12 months to manage stage 1 HTN in the absence of DM, target organ damage, evidence of cardiovascular disease, or multiple other risk factors.[2]
- **Weight loss:** Although achieving ideal body weight should be the goal, weight loss as little as 10 lb reduces both SBP and DBP.
- **Exercise:** Moderate- and high-intensity aerobic activity reduces BP independent of weight loss.
- **Diet:**
  - Reducing sodium levels decreases BP in some individuals but often enhances the antihypertensive effects of medications.

- **The DASH (Dietary Approaches to Stop Hypertension) diet** has been shown in studies to lower BP within 2 weeks.[9]
- **Alcohol and Tobacco:**
  - Cessation of smoking is advised for overall cardiovascular health.
  - Alcohol intake should be limited to one to two drinks per day at most. Those who drink more have a higher incidence of HTN, most notably when intake exceeds five drinks per day.
- **Stress:** Although relieving stress may improve one's overall health, no studies have successfully demonstrated a link between stress reduction and a sustained reduction in BP.

Pharmacologic Therapy

General Considerations/Introduction
- Many factors should be taken into consideration when initiating drug therapy including the following:
  - Evidence of improved clinical outcomes with certain drug classes.
  - Comorbid diseases and other cardiovascular risk factors.
  - Demographic differences in response.
  - Affordability.
  - Lifestyle issues.
  - Likelihood of adherence.
- **There is a high interpatient variability in response, with many patients responding well to one drug class but not to another.**
- The amount of BP reduction rather than the specific antihypertensive drug is the major determinant in reducing cardiovascular risk in hypertensive patients.

Who Should Be Treated?
- Drug therapy is indicated in patients if the systolic pressure is persistently ≥140 mm Hg and/or the diastolic pressure is persistently ≥90 mm Hg despite a 6- to 12-month trial of lifestyle modification and can be considered earlier if multiple risk factors for cardiovascular disease are present.[2]
- Drug therapy should be started initially in addition to lifestyle modifications in those with stage 2 HTN or stage 1 HTN and known DM, cardiovascular disease, or end-organ damage.[2]

Initial Monotherapy
- Figure 1 presents JNC 7's basic HTN treatment algorithm.[2]
- First-line antihypertensive drug classes include thiazide diuretics, angiotensin-converting enzyme (ACE) inhibitors, angiotensin-receptor blockers (ARBs), and calcium channel blockers (CCBs).[2,10]
- **Thiazide diuretics** are recommended as the initial choice in most patients. Multiple trials have shown them to be as effective as other agents in lowering BP and preventing the cardiovascular complications of HTN.
- **ACE inhibitors, ARBs,** and **CCBs** have all been shown to be effective as first-line agents and are acceptable alternatives to thiazides in many cases.
- Although appropriate in many circumstances, **β-blockers have fallen out of favor as first-line agents due to the lack of consistent data supporting an independent positive effect on cardiovascular morbidity and mortality.**[11]
- Many patients have **compelling indications** for specific antihypertensive agents based on other comorbidities. Table 5 lists some common clinical conditions for which certain drug classes have been shown to be particularly effective.[2]

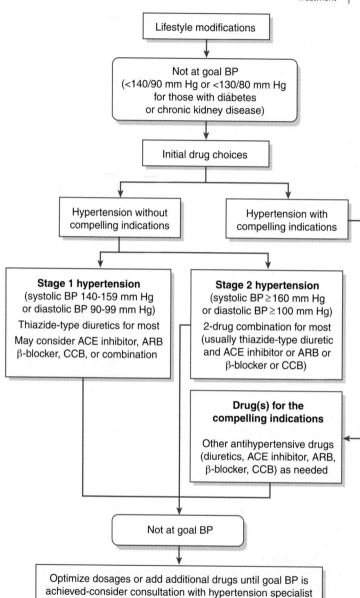

Figure 1. JNC 7 basic hypertension treatment algorithm. JNC, The Seventh Report of Joint National Committee on Prevention, Detection, Evaluation, and Treatment of High Blood Pressure. Modified from: Chobanian AV, Bakris GL, Black HR, et al. National High Blood Pressure Education Program Coordinating Committee on Prevention, Detection, Evaluation, and Treatment of High Blood Pressure: the JNC 7 report. *JAMA* 2003;289:2560–2572.

TABLE 5	Compelling Indications for Individual Drug Classes					
Compelling Indication	**Recommended Drugs**					
	Diuretic	BB	ACE-I	ARB	CCB	Aldo ANT
Heart failure[12–21]	X	X	X	X		X
Postmyocardial infarction[22–26]		X	X			X
High coronary disease risk[10,27–32]	X	X	X		X	
DM[10,28–35]	X	X	X	X	X	
Chronic kidney disease[34,36–40]			X	X		
Recurrent stroke prevention[41]	X				X	

ACE-I, angiotensin converting enzyme inhibitor; Aldo ANT, aldosterone antagonist; ARB, angiotensin-receptor blocker; BB, β-blocker; CCB, calcium channel blocker. Modified from Chobanian AV, Bakris GL, Black HR, et al. National High Blood Pressure Education Program Coordinating Committee on Prevention, Detection, Evaluation, and Treatment of High Blood Pressure: the JNC 7 report. *JAMA* 2003;289:2560–2572.

- A patient with mild HTN who is relatively unresponsive to one drug has an almost 50% likelihood of responding to a second drug, so trials of different agents are warranted before moving to combination therapy.[42]

Combination Therapy
- More than two-thirds of hypertensive patients will not reach treatment goal BP on one drug and will require two or more drugs.[2]
- The typical decrease in BP with a single agent is approximately 8 to 15 mm Hg systolic and 7 to 12 mm Hg diastolic.[43–46] Most patients with HTN, however, will eventually require two or more medications.[2]
- Combination therapy is appropriate if BP cannot be controlled with a single agent, in patients with stage 2 HTN, and in patients with compelling indications for multiple agents described above.
- **A diuretic should be considered as part of a two-drug combination due to the enhanced benefit with multiple other drug classes.**[2]
- Fixed-dose combination pills offer the advantage of convenience that may improve adherence but sometimes at a higher cost to the patient and with less flexibility in adjusting doses.

Specific Populations
Ischemic Heart Disease
- **β-Blockers are first-line therapy both in patients with stable angina and a history of acute coronary syndrome.** They have powerful anti-ischemic effects and proven mortality benefits in these patients.[11]
- CCBs may be used if β-blockers are contraindicated or if additional BP of angina control is necessary. **A long-acting dihydropyridine is recommended** to limit the risk of heart block and bradycardia.
- ACE inhibitors also have mortality benefit in patients following an MI, **especially those with impaired LV function.**[17,18]

Heart Failure

- ACE inhibitors, β-blockers, aldosterone antagonists, and the combination of hydralazine and nitrates have all been shown to have mortality benefit in this population depending on disease severity.[13–16,19–21]
- Diuretics constitute an important aspect of fluid management and are typically an essential part of the patient's regimen.
- While CCBs may cause adverse effects due to their negative inotropic properties, long-acting dihydropyridines can provide additional BP control with less potential for myocardial depression than with verapamil and diltiazem.

Diabetes

- HTN occurs twice as frequently in diabetics compared with nondiabetics.[47] These two conditions together significantly increase a patient's risk of developing both major cardiovascular events and microvascular disease.
- Lower treatment goals (<130/80 mm Hg) have been established by the American Diabetes Association, reflected in the JNC 7 recommendations.[2]
- The United Kingdom Prospective Diabetes Study (UKPDS) demonstrated a reduction in mortality (15%), MI (11%), and retinopathy/nephropathy (13%) for every 10 mm Hg reduction in SBP.[35]
- Diuretics, ACE inhibitors, ARBs, β-blockers, and CCBs have all been shown to have benefit in diabetics. **ACE inhibitors should be considered first-line therapy,** given their ability to retard loss of renal function and proteinuria independent of antihypertensive effects.[33–38]

Chronic Kidney Disease

- HTN can accelerate the loss of renal function up to fourfold if uncontrolled, leading to end-stage renal disease (ESRD) and the need for renal replacement therapy.[48]
- Similar to DM, a lower treatment goal of <130/80 mm Hg has been recommended to slow down the progression to ESRD.[2]
- **An ACE inhibitor or ARB is commonly combined with a diuretic** (many will require a loop diuretic rather than a thiazide diuretic) to achieve this goal.[39,40]

Elderly

- Isolated systolic HTN becomes much more common with advancing age. SBP should be the primary target in this group.
- The elderly often have other medical conditions that may make a particular drug class more appropriate. Diuretics decrease the incidence of stroke, fatal MI, and overall mortality in this group when used as initial therapy.[49,50] CCBs are also very effective and well tolerated.
- Care should be taken when titrating medications to avoid causing orthostatic hypotension. Following the standing BP may be helpful.

African-Americans

- HTN is more common, is more severe, and has a higher morbidity compared with non-Hispanic whites.
- African-Americans have lower plasma renin levels, increased plasma volume, and higher peripheral vascular resistance (PVR) compared with Caucasian patients.
- Dietary sodium reduction may be more effective in this population with a greater decrease in BP compared with other demographic groups.[51]
- On the basis of ALLHAT, African-Americans appear to respond better to thiazide diuretics and CCBs compared with ACE inhibitors.[10] **ACE inhibitors and ARBs can still be very effective (particularly when combined with a diuretic).**[2,52]

Drug Classes

Diuretics

- **Thiazides** (hydrochlorothiazide, chlorthalidone, metolazone, and indapamide):
  - **Mechanism:** Block sodium reabsorption at the distal convoluted tubule by inhibition of Na/Cl cotransporter.
  - Recommended as the initial choice in most patients in the absence of compelling indications.
  - Multiple trials have shown thiazides to be effective in lowering BP, preventing initial and subsequent strokes, and reducing cardiovascular mortality.[10,41,49]
  - They are particularly effective in African-Americans and the elderly who have a greater tendency to be sodium sensitive but less effective in patients with renal insufficiency (CrCl <30 mL/min). In the latter case, a loop diuretic may be more appropriate.
  - Generally well tolerated and affordable.
  - **Side effects** include electrolyte abnormalities (hypokalemia, hypomagnesemia, hypercalcemia, and hyperuricemia), muscle cramps, dyslipidemia, and glucose intolerance.
- **Loop diuretics** (furosemide, bumetanide, torsemide, and ethacrynic acid):
  - **Mechanism:** Block Na reabsorption at the ascending loop of Henle.
  - Appropriate for patients with HTN and renal insufficiency (CrCl <30 mL/min).
  - **Side effects** include electrolyte abnormalities (hypokalemia, hypomagnesemia, hypocalcemia, and hyperuricemia), ototoxicity (less common with oral rather than intravenous), and glucose intolerance.
- **Potassium-sparing agents** (spironolactone, eplerenone, amiloride, and triamterene):
  - **Mechanism:** Spironolactone and eplerenone inhibit the action of aldosterone on the kidney and have benefit on improving mortality in patients with heart failure.[20] Amiloride and triamterene inhibit the reabsorption of Na and secretion of K in the distal nephron.
  - Appropriate for patients with primary or secondary hyperaldosteronism, including severe heart failure.
  - May be added to thiazides to limit hypokalemia.
  - **Side effects** include hyperkalemia, renal calculi, and gynecomastia (spironolactone).

Renin-Angiotensin System Inhibitors

- **ACE inhibitors** (benazepril, captopril, enalapril, fosinopril, lisinopril, moexipril, perindopril, quinapril, ramipril, and trandolapril):
  - **Mechanism:** Inhibit ACE leading to a decreased conversion of angiotensin I to angiotensin II, which reduces vasoconstriction, reduces aldosterone secretion, promotes natriuresis, and increases vasodilatory bradykinins.
  - Appropriate as initial therapy in most patients.
  - Works well in combination with other agents, particularly diuretics.
  - Considered first-line therapy in patients with heart failure or asymptomatic left ventricular dysfunction, prior MI or high risk for coronary disease, and DM or chronic kidney disease.[16–18,24,27,32,35,36,39]
  - **Contraindicated in pregnancy.**
  - **Side effects** include hyperkalemia, orthostatic hypotension, cough, angioedema, and worsening renal function. However, an increase in serum creatinine is expected in most patients and up to 30% is acceptable and not a reason to discontinue therapy.

- **ARBs** (candesartan, eprosartan, irbesartan, losartan, olmesartan, telmisartan, and valsartan):
  - **Mechanism:** Limit the pressor effects of angiotensin II by blocking its interaction with cell surface receptors.
  - Appropriate as initial therapy in most patients and generally effective in the same clinical settings as an alternative to ACE inhibitors.
  - **May be specifically beneficial in patients with LVH.**[29]
  - Additive to ACE inhibitors in reducing proteinuria but may worsen outcome.[53]
  - May be better tolerated than an ACE because of a lack of increase in bradykinin levels, which is responsible for cough in up to 33% of patients.
  - **Contraindicated in pregnancy.**
  - **Side effects** are similar to those of ACE inhibitors with a smaller incidence of cough.
- **Direct renin inhibitors** (aliskiren):
  - **Mechanism:** Directly inhibit plasma renin, thus dramatically decreasing levels of angiotensin I, II, and aldosterone.
  - First new class of drugs introduced to treat HTN since ARBs in 1994.
  - Trials have demonstrated comparable efficacy in lower BP compared with thiazides, ACE inhibitors, and ARBs. Aliskiren may be used alone or in combination with other agents. Most experience is with diuretics (hydrochlorothiazide) or ARBs (valsartan).[54]
  - Because long-term outcome data are not available, the role of direct renin inhibitors continues to evolve.
  - **Side effects** include diarrhea, dyspepsia, edema, and cough.

Calcium Channel Blockers

- **Mechanism:** Selectively block the slow inward calcium channels in vascular smooth muscle causing arteriolar vasodilation.
- Appropriate as an initial treatment of HTN in most patients.
- Should be considered first-line therapy in patients with ischemic heart disease, coronary vasospasm or Raynaud phenomenon, and supraventricular arrhythmias.
- Particularly effective in older patients with isolated systolic HTN and African-Americans.[2,10,52]
- As a class, have no significant effect on glucose tolerance, electrolytes, or lipid profiles and are not adversely affected by NSAIDs.
- Benzothiazepines (diltiazem) and phenylalkylamines (verapamil):
  - Have negative cardiac inotropic and chronotropic effects and thus should be used with caution in patients with heart failure or conduction system disease.
  - **Side effects** include nausea, headache, constipation, esophageal reflux, and heart block (especially in combination with β-blockers).
- Dihydropyridines (nifedipine, amlodipine, felodipine, isradipine, and nicardipine):
  - Have less effect on cardiac conduction and contractility and thus may be used cautiously in patients with impaired ventricular function.
  - **Side effects** include flushing, headache, dependent edema, gingival hyperplasia, and esophageal reflux.

Adrenergic Blockers

- **β-Blockers:**
  - **Mechanism:** Competitively inhibit the effects of catecholamines at β-receptors to decrease heart rate and cardiac output. They also decrease plasma renin and release vasodilatory prostaglandins.

- **β-Blockers have fallen out of favor as first-line agents** in the absence of compelling indications because of the lack of data supporting an independent positive effect on morbidity and mortality.[11]
- Appropriate for patients with ischemic heart disease, heart failure, or as rate control agents in patients with supraventricular tachycardias. May also be beneficial in patients with glaucoma, essential tremor, or migraines.
- Organized based on selectivity for β-receptors and the presence of intrinsic sympathomimetic activity (ISA).
  - **Nonselective** (nadolol, propranolol, and timolol):
    - Acts on both β_1- and β_2-receptors.
    - Risk of hypoglycemia in diabetics and bronchospasm in patients with chronic obstructive pulmonary disease (COPD) or reactive airway disease.
  - **Cardioselective** (acebutolol, atenolol, betaxolol, bisoprolol, celiprolol, esmolol, metoprolol, and nebivolol):
    - Primarily acting on β_1-receptors in the heart at low doses but with less selectivity at higher doses.
    - May be used cautiously in patients with COPD or diabetics with less risk of bronchospasm and masking hypoglycemia, respectively.
  - **β-Blockers with ISA** (acebutolol, pindolol, carteolol, penbutolol, and celiprolol):
    - Exert low-level agonist activity at β-receptors while simultaneously antagonizing the site.
    - May be useful in patients with excessive bradycardia.
    - Have not demonstrated benefit in patients post-MI and are less effective in managing tachyarrhythmias.
- Cardioselective β-blockers act preferentially on β_1-receptors of the heart and may therefore be used cautiously in patients with COPD or diabetics with less risk of bronchospasm and masking hypoglycemia, respectively. Drugs with ISA cause less bradycardia because of their partial agonist activity at the receptor.
- **Side effects** include fatigue, nausea, dizziness, heart block (especially when used with CCBs), worsening of heart failure, dyslipidemia, erectile dysfunction, and bronchospasm. Abrupt withdrawal can precipitate angina or a dramatic elevation of BP because of the increase in adrenergic tone with chronic β-blocker use.
- **α-Blockers** (prazosin, terazosin, and doxazosin):
  - **Mechanism:** Block α_1-receptors on vascular smooth muscle cells, impairing catecholamine-induced vasoconstriction.
  - **Less efficacious** than thiazides, CCBs, and ACE inhibitors as monotherapy based on the ALLHAT and are **not recommended as first-line therapy.**[10]
  - Characterized by a "first-dose effect" with a larger decrease in BP than subsequent doses making use before bedtime more appropriate than the morning.
  - May decrease urinary symptoms in patients with prostate enlargement.
  - **Side effects** include orthostatic hypotension, GI distress, and drowsiness.
- **Mixed α- and β-blockers** (labetalol and carvedilol):
  - These drugs exert activity against both β- and α-receptors.
  - Preferential to conventional nonselective β-blockers based on the latter being associated with inferior outcomes, an increased rate of stroke, and an increased risk of developing DM.
  - **Labetalol** acts on postsynaptic α-receptors to decrease PVR and is useful in hypertensive crises.
  - **Carvedilol** has proven efficacy in decreasing the morbidity and mortality of heart failure patients.[14]

- **Side effects** are similar to those of other β-blockers. In addition, labetalol has been associated with hepatocellular damage and a lupus-like syndrome characterized by positive antinuclear antibody titers.
- **Centrally acting adrenergic agents** (clonidine):
  - **Mechanism:** Stimulate α_2-receptors in the central nervous system leading to decreased peripheral sympathetic tone, PVR, heart rate, and cardiac output.
  - Abrupt cessation can precipitate acute withdrawal syndrome characterized by tachycardia, diaphoresis, and severe elevations in BP.
  - **Side effects** include bradycardia, sedations, orthostatic hypotension, and sexual dysfunction.
- **Other sympatholytics** (reserpine, guanethidine, and guanadrel):
  - **Mechanism:** Inhibit the release of norepinephrine from peripheral neurons.
  - These agents are **no longer considered first- or second-line therapy** because of their significant side-effect profile and the availability of more effective and better-tolerated drugs.
  - **Side effects** include severe depression, sedation, nasal congestion, severe orthostatic hypotension, and lower extremity edema.

Direct Vasodilators (Hydralazine and Minoxidil)

- **Mechanism:** Hyperpolarize arteriolar smooth muscle to produce direct relaxation.
- Potent agents typically used in cases of refractory HTN in addition to multiple other drug classes.
- Hydralazine is particularly useful in addition to nitrates in providing afterload reduction in patients with heart failure.[55]
- Both agents lead to reflex sympathetic hyperactivity and fluid retention that makes concomitant treatment with a diuretic and/or β-blocker desirable.
- **Side effects** of hydralazine include headache, tachycardia, orthostatic hypotension, GI distress, and a lupus-like syndrome. Minoxidil can lead to weight gain, hirsutism, hypertrichosis, ECG abnormalities, and pericardial effusions.

Resistant Hypertension

- Defined as the persistent elevation of BP above goal despite the concurrent use of antihypertensive agents from three different classes. This includes BP that is adequately controlled on a four-drug regimen.[56]
- The exact prevalence is unknown, but clinical trials and surveys suggest that it is a common phenomenon occurring in an estimated 20% to 30% of the population.
- Characteristics associated with resistant HTN include high baseline BP, older age, obesity, excessive dietary salt intake, chronic kidney disease, diabetes, LVH, female gender, African-American race, and residence in the Southeast Unite States.
- Resistant HTN should be distinguished from **"pseudoresistance,"** which may be due to poor medication adherence, poor BP measurement technique, or white coat HTN.
- Careful evaluation of the patient's medication profile may reveal agents that commonly contribute to this condition, including NSAIDs, sympathomimetic compounds, glucocorticoids, oral contraceptives, cyclosporine, erythropoietin, and herbal compounds.
- **Secondary causes** of HTN are more common in patients with resistant HTN, particularly obstructive sleep apnea, renal parenchymal disease, primary hyperaldosteronism, and renovascular disease. Screening should be based on clinical suspicion.
- Treatment strategies should focus on **maximizing medication adherence,** lifestyle modification (e.g., weight loss, daily exercise, reduced dietary salt intake, and reduced alcohol consumption), and treatment of secondary causes of HTN when present.

- Drug therapy should combine agents with different mechanisms of action. Specifically, one should **maximize the use of diuretics** and consider the addition of a mineralocorticoid antagonist and/or loop diuretics.
- Referral to a specialist is recommended if BP cannot be controlled after 6 months of treatment or for specific secondary etiologies that may require assistance.

Special Considerations

Secondary Hypertension

Renal Parenchymal Disease
- HTN is a major contributor to the development of chronic kidney disease, but impaired renal function can also elevate BP resulting in a vicious cycle.
- Approximately 80% of patients with chronic kidney disease have HTN characterized by a combination of sodium retention, activation of the renin-angiotensin system, enhanced sympathetic activity, and impaired endothelium-mediated vasodilation.
- Treatment should stress sodium restriction, use of diuretics, and the use of ACE inhibitors to reduce proteinuria and intraglomerular pressure.

Renovascular Disease
- Important correctable cause of HTN responsible for up to 10% of patients with severe HTN resistant to multiple medications.
- Because of both fibromuscular disease (more common in the young and in women) and atheromatous disease (more common in the elderly with other cardiovascular risk factors).
- Critical stenosis of the renal artery leads to increased renin release from the ischemic kidney, which causes both volume expansion and increased PVR.
- Bilateral disease may present as a sudden decline in renal function after use of anACE or ARB. These agents should be avoided if bilateral disease is known.
- Should be considered in young patients without family history.
- Commonly evaluated with duplex ultrasonography, magnetic resonance angiography, or computed tomography angiography.
- Angioplasty with or without stent placement may be a treatment option that offers improvement rates of up to 85% in fibromuscular dysplasia and 70% in atherosclerotic disease.[57]

Primary Hyperaldosteronism
- Prevalence ranges from 5% to 10% of the hypertensive population.[58]
- Caused by a unilateral adrenal adenoma in most cases with the remainder (20% to 30%) due to bilateral adrenal hyperplasia.[59]
- Difficult to distinguish based on clinical symptoms but should be considered in the presence of unexplained hypokalemia and metabolic alkalosis, especially if also on an ACE or ARB.
- **Diagnostic studies:**
  - *Initial screen:* Serum aldosterone of >15 and the aldosterone/renin ratio of >20 both suggest the diagnosis.
  - *Confirmation:* A salt suppression test (oral salt load × 3 days, followed by measurement of 24-hour urinary aldosterone) should follow. All drugs that interfere with the renin-angiotensin-aldosterone axis should be discontinued first for at least 6 weeks. Inappropriately high aldosterone excretion (>12 mcg/day) with Na >200 mEq/day confirms the diagnosis.

- CT or magnetic resonance imaging (MRI) of the adrenal glands can help distinguish between the subtypes when the disease is confirmed.
- **Treatment** includes surgical resection of a single adenoma or use of **potassium-sparing diuretics** as part of the regimen.

Cushing Syndrome

- Cortisol excess is **not a common cause of HTN overall** but when present, it leads to HTN in approximately 80% of patients.
- Treatment should focus on determining the source of glucocorticoid excess and removing it if possible.

Pheochromocytoma

- **Rare** cause of HTN with incidence of five cases per million persons per year.
- Characterized by tumors that release catecholamines into the bloodstream leading to paroxysms of headaches, palpitations, or diaphoresis.
- BP is paroxysmal in <50% of patients and sustained in the majority. A few patients have interspersed episodes of hypotension.
- Patients with highly suggestive symptoms may be screened with plasma metanephrines (more sensitive) or urinary metanephrines and catecholamines (more specific).

Other Endocrine Disorders

- Hypothyroidism is associated with elevated diastolic pressure and an increased PVR to offset the decreased cardiac output.
- Hyperthyroidism is associated with elevated systolic pressure due to an increased cardiac output.
- Hypercalcemia may increase BP directly by increasing PVR and indirectly by increasing sensitivity to catecholamines.

Obstructive Sleep Apnea

- Episodes of apnea lead to increased sympathetic activity, which directly raises BP.
- Should be considered in patients with the appropriate clinical picture: overweight with a history of snoring, daytime somnolence, and morning headache.
- Beyond weight loss, treatment with continuous positive airway pressure (CPAP) has been shown to and improve overall cardiac performance.[60]

Coarctation of the Aorta

- Major cause of HTN in **young children.**
- Caused by constriction of the aorta just beyond the takeoff of the left subclavian, which leads to increased renin secretion and volume retention.
- Classically associated with increased BP in the upper extremities and lower BP in the lower extremities. Patients may have headache, cold feet, or claudication.
- Diagnosed with ECG or MRI.
- May be treated surgically or with angioplasty.

Pregnancy

General

- HTN is the most common medical problem encountered during pregnancy and can pose a threat to both the mother and the fetus depending on the specific clinical situation.
- Some common antihypertensives are teratogenic and should be avoided in pregnancy.

Classification[2]

- **Chronic HTN** is defined by a BP of >140/90 mm Hg before the 20th week of pregnancy and persisting for >12-week postpartum.
- **Preeclampsia** occurs in approximately 5% of pregnancies after 20 weeks gestation and is characterized by BP of >140/90 mm Hg and proteinuria, typically accompanied by other abnormalities such as liver function abnormalities or thrombocytopenia. **Eclampsia** denotes the addition of generalized seizures. Patients suspected of having these conditions should be referred to an obstetrician urgently.
- **Preeclampsia superimposed on chronic HTN** denotes the new onset or sudden increase in proteinuria in patients with preexisting HTN.
- **Gestational HTN** results in transient increases in BP occurring after 20 weeks' gestation without features of preeclampsia and often returns to normal within 2 weeks of delivery.

Treatment

- Typical nonpharmacologic measures such as weight reduction and exercise should NOT be advised during pregnancy.
- Patients should be strongly encouraged to abstain from alcohol and tobacco.
- Drug therapy is recommended for SBP of >160 mm Hg or DBP of >100 mm Hg and may be provided selectively at lower values but without demonstrable benefit of short-term maternal and fetal outcomes.
- **Methyldopa** has proven safety and effectiveness and is considered first-line therapy.
- Other common and safe options include β-blockers (labetalol and metoprolol), **CCBs** (nifedipine), and **hydralazine.**
- ACE inhibitors have been associated with fetal renal dysgenesis or death and should be avoided in pregnancy. ARBs should be avoided due to a similar mechanism.

Hypertensive Crisis

- Hypertensive crises are often result from the rebound effects of withdrawal and noncompliance but can be a manifestation of many causes of secondary HTN.
- **Hypertensive emergencies** are characterized by severe elevations in BP (>180/120 mm Hg) complicated by evidence of target organ damage (hypertensive encephalopathy, intracranial hemorrhage, papilledema, acute coronary syndrome, aortic dissection, acute pulmonary edema, acute renal failure, microangiopathic hemolytic anemia, and preeclampsia).
  - IV agents should be used to decrease mean arterial pressure by 25% urgently (within the hour) to arrest the progression of damage.
  - Commonly used drugs for this purpose include nitroprusside, nitroglycerine, labetalol, and hydralazine.
- **Hypertensive urgencies** are characterized by similarly severe elevations but without any of the above clinical manifestations of organ damage.
  - Rapid-acting oral agents (captopril, labetalol, clonidine, and hydralazine) can be used to reduce BP over several hours in cases of hypertensive urgency. Once BP is <180/110 mm Hg, a longer-acting drug may be given.

REFERENCES

1. Lewington S, Clarke R, Qizilibash N, et al. Age-specific relevance of usual blood pressure to vascular mortality: a meta-analysis of individual data for one million adults in 61 prospective studies. *Lancet* 2002;360:1903–1913.

2. Chobanian AV, Bakris GL, Black HR, et al. National High Blood Pressure Education Program Coordinating Committee on Prevention, Detection, Evaluation, and Treatment of High Blood Pressure: the JNC 7 report. *JAMA* 2003;289:2560–2672.

3. Julius S, Nesbitt SD, Egan BM, et al. Trial of Preventing Hypertension Study Investigators. Feasibility of treating prehypertension with an angiotensin-receptor blocker. *N Engl J Med* 2006;354:1685–1697.

4. Fields LE, Burt VL, Cutler JA, et al. The burden of adult hypertension in the United States 1999 to 2000: a rising tide. *Hypertension* 2004;44:398–404.

5. Burt VL, Whelton P, Roccella EJ, et al. Prevalence of hypertension in the US adult population. Results from the Third National Health and Nutrition Examination Survey, 1988–1991. *Hypertension* 1995;25:305–313.

6. Reeves RA. The rational clinical examinations. Does this patient have hypertension? How to measure blood pressure. *JAMA* 1995;273:1211–1218.

7. Dolan E, Stanton A, Hisjs L, et al. Superiority of ambulatory over clinic blood pressure measurement in predicting mortality: the Dublin outcome study. *Hypertension* 2005;46:156–161.

8. Elmer PJ, Obarzanek E, Vollmer WM, et al. Effects of comprehensive lifestyle modification on diet, weight, physical fitness, and blood pressure control: 18-month results of a randomized trial. *Ann Intern Med* 2006;144:485–495.

9. Appel LJ, Moore TJ, Obarzanek E, et al. A clinical trial of the effects of dietary patterns on blood pressure. DASH Collaborative Research Group. *N Engl J Med* 1997;336:1117–1124.

10. The ALLHAT Officers and Coordinators for the ALLHAT Collaborative Research Group. Major outcomes in high-risk hypertensive patients randomized to angiotensin-converting enzyme inhibitor or calcium channel blocker vs diuretic: The Antihypertensive and Lipid-Lowering Treatment to Prevent Heart Attack Trial (ALLHAT). *JAMA* 2002;288:2981–2997.

11. Wiysonge CS, Bradley H, Mayosi BM, et al. Beta-blockers for hypertension. *Cochrane Database Syst Rev* 2007;(1):CD002003.

12. Hunt SA. American College of Cardiology; American Heart Association Task Force on Practice Guidelines (Writing Committee to Update the 2001 Guidelines for the Evaluation and Management of Heart Failure). ACC/AHA 2005 guideline update for the diagnosis and management of chronic heart failure in the adult: a report of the American College of Cardiology/American Heart Association Task Force on Practice Guidelines (Writing Committee to Update the 2001 Guidelines for the Evaluation and Management of Heart Failure). *J Am Coll Cardiol* 2005 Sep 20;46:e1–e82.

13. Tepper D. Frontiers in congestive heart failure: effect of metoprolol CR/XL in chronic heart failure: Metoprolol CR/XL Randomised Intervention Trial in Congestive Heart Failure (MERIT-HF). MERIT-HF Study Group. *Congest Heart Fail* 1999;5:184–185.

14. Packer M, Coats AJ, Fowler MB, et al. Effect of carvedilol on survival in severe chronic heart failure. *N Engl J Med* 2001;344:1651–1658.

15. CIBIS Investigators and Committees. A randomized trial of beta-blockade in heart failure. The Cardiac Insufficiency Bisoprolol Study (CIBIS). *Circulation* 1994;90:1765–1773.

16. The SOLVD Investigators. Effect of enalapril on survival in patients with reduced left ventricular ejection fractions and congestive heart failure. *N Engl J Med* 1991;325:293–302.

17. The Acute Infarction Ramipril Efficacy (AIRE) Study Investigators. Effect of ramipril on mortality and morbidity of survivors of acute myocardial infarction with clinical evidence of heart failure. *Lancet* 1993;342:821–828.

18. Kober L, Torp-Pedersen C, Carlsen JE, et al. A clinical trial of the angiotensin-converting-enzyme inhibitor trandolapril in patients with left ventricular dysfunction after myocardial infarction. Trandolapril Cardiac Evaluation (TRACE) Study Group. *N Engl J Med* 1995; 333:1670–1676.

19. Cohn JN, Tognoni G. A randomized trial of the angiotensin-receptor blocker valsartan in chronic heart failure. The Valsartan Heart Failure Trial Investigators. *N Engl J Med* 2001;345:1667–1675.

20. Pitt B, Zannad F, Remme WJ, et al. The effect of spironolactone on morbidity and mortality in patients with severe heart failure. Randomized Aldactone Evaluation Study Investigators. *N Engl J Med* 1999;341:709–717.

21. McMurray J, Ostergren J, Pfeffer M, et al. Clinical features and contemporary management of patients with low and preserved ejection fraction heart failure: baseline characteristics of patients in the Candesartan in Heart Failure—Assessment of Reduction in Mortality and Morbidity (CHARM) programme. *Eur J Heart Fail* 2003;5:261–270.

22. Fraker TD Jr, Fihn SD. 2002 Chronic Stable Angina Writing Committee; American College of Cardiology; American Heart Association. 2007 chronic angina focused update of the ACC/AHA 2002 guidelines for the management of patients with chronic stable angina: a report of the American College of Cardiology/American Heart Association Task Force on Practice Guidelines Writing Group to develop the focused update of the 2002 guidelines for the management of patients with chronic stable angina. *J Am Coll Cardiol.* 2007;50: 2264–2274.

23. β-Blocker Heart Attack Trial Research Group. A randomized trial of propranolol in patients with acute myocardial infarction. I. Mortality results. *JAMA* 1982;247:1707–1714.

24. Pfeffer MA, Braunwald E, Moye LA, et al. Effect of captopril on mortality and morbidity in patients with left ventricular dysfunction after myocardial infarction. Results of the Survival and Ventricular Enlargement Trial. The SAVE Investigators. *N Engl J Med* 1992;327:669–677.

25. The Capricorn Investigators. Effect of carvedilol on outcome after myocardial infarction in patients with left-ventricular dysfunction: The CAPRICORN randomised trial. *Lancet* 2001;357:1385–1390.

26. Pitt B, Remme W, Zannad F, et al. Eplerenone, a selective aldosterone blocker, in patients with left ventricular dysfunction after myocardial infarction. *N Engl J Med* 2003;348: 1309–1321.

27. Heart Outcomes Prevention Evaluation Study Investigators. Effects of an angiotensin-converting enzyme inhibitor, ramipril, on cardiovascular events in high-risk patients. *N Engl J Med* 2000;342:145–153.

28. Wing LM, Reid CM, Ryan P, et al. A comparison of outcomes with angiotensin-converting enzyme inhibitors and diuretics for hypertension in the elderly. *N Engl J Med* 2003;348: 583–592.

29. Dahlof B, Devereux RB, Kjeldsen SE, et al. Cardiovascular morbidity and mortality in the Losartan Intervention For Endpoint Reduction in Hypertension Sudy (LIFE): A randomised trial against atenolol. *Lancet* 2002;359:995–1003.

30. Black HR, Elliott WJ, Grandits G, et al. Principal results of the Controlled Onset Verapamil Investigation of Cardiovascular End Points (CONVINCE) Trial. *JAMA* 2003;289: 2073–2082.

31. The European Trial on Reduction of Cardiac Events with Perindopril in Stable Coronary Artery Disease Investigators. Efficacy of perindopril in reduction of cardiovascular events among patients with stable coronary artery disease: randomised, double-blind, placebo-controlled, multicentre trial (the EUROPA Study). *Lancet* 2003;362:782–788.

32. Pepine C, Handberg E, Cooper-DeHoff R, et al. for the INVEST Investigators. A calcium antagonist vs a noncalcium antagonist hypertension treatment strategy for patients with coronary artery disease. The International Verapamil-Trandolapril Study (INVEST): a randomized controlled trial. *JAMA* 2003;290:2805–2816.

33. American Diabetes Association. Treatment of hypertension in adults with diabetes. *Diabetes Care* 2003;26:S80–S82.

34. National Kidney Foundation Guideline. K/DOQI clinical practice guidelines for chronic kidney disease: evaluation, classification, and stratification. Kidney Disease Outcome Quality Initiative. *Am J Kidney Dis* 2002;39:S1–S246.

35. UKPDS 39. Efficacy of atenolol and captopril in reducing risk of macrovascular and microvascular complications in type 2 diabetes: UKPDS 39. UK Prospective Diabetes Study Group. *BMJ* 1998;317:713–720.

36. Lewis EJ, Hunsicker LG, Bain RP, Rohde RD. The effect of angiotensin-converting enzyme inhibition on diabetic nephropathy. The Collaborative Study Group. *N Engl J Med* 1993;329:1456–1462.

37. Brenner BM, Cooper ME, de Zeeuw, et al. Effects of losartan on renal and cardiovascular outcomes in patients with type 2 diabetes and nephropathy. *N Engl J Med* 2001;345: 861–869.
38. Lewis EJ, Hunsicker LG, Clarke WR, et al. Renoprotective effect of the angiotensin-receptor antagonist irbesartan in patients with nephropathy due to type 2 diabetes. *N Engl J Med* 2001;345:851–860.
39. The GISEN Group (Gruppo Italiano di Studi Epidemiologici in Nefrologia). Randomised placebo-controlled trial of effect of ramipril on decline in glomerular filtration rate and risk of terminal renal failure in proteinuric, non-diabetic nephropathy. *Lancet* 1997;349:1857–1863.
40. Wright JT Jr, Agodoa L, Contreras G, et al. Successful blood pressure control in the African American Study of Kidney Disease and Hypertension. *Arch Intern Med* 2002;162:1636–1643.
41. PROGRESS Collaborative Group. Randomised trial of a perindopril-based blood-pressure-lowering regimen among 6,105 individuals with previous stroke or transient ischaemic attack. *Lancet* 2001;358:1033–1041.
42. Materson BJ, Reda DJ, Preston RA, et al. Response to a second single antihypertensive agent used as monotherapy for hypertension after failure of the initial drug. Department of Veterans Affairs Cooperative Study Group on Antihypertensive Agents. *Arch Intern Med* 1995;155:1757–1762.
43. Materson BJ, Reda DJ, Cushman WC, et al. Single-drug therapy for hypertension in men. A comparison of six antihypertensive agents with placebo. The Department of Veterans Affairs Cooperative Study Group on Antihypertensive Agents. *N Engl J Med* 1993;328:914–921.
44. Neaton JD, Grimm RH Jr, Prineas RJ, et al. Treatment of Mild Hypertension Study. Final results. Treatment of Mild Hypertension Study Research Group. *JAMA* 1993;270:713–724.
45. Staessen JA, Wang JG, Thijs L. Cardiovascular prevention and blood pressure reduction: a quantitative overview updated until 1 March 2003. *J Hypertens* 2003;21:1055–1076.
46. Wald DS, Law M, Morris JK, et al. Combination therapy versus monotherapy in reducing blood pressure: meta-analysis on 11,000 participants from 42 trials. *Am J Med* 2009;122: 290–300.
47. Sowers JR, Epstein M, Frohlich ED. Diabetes, hypertension, and cardiovascular disease: an update. *Hypertension* 2001;37:1053–1059.
48. Bakris GL, Williams M, Dworkin L, et al. Preserving renal function in adults with hypertension and diabetes: a consensus approach. National Kidney Foundation Hypertension and Diabetes Executive Committees Working Group. *Am J Kidney Dis* 2000;36:646–661.
49. Prevention of stroke by antihypertensive drug treatment in older persons with isolated systolic hypertension. Final results of the Systolic Hypertension in the Elderly Program (SHEP). SHEP Cooperative Research Group. *JAMA* 1991;265:3255–3264.
50. Perry HM Jr, Davis BR, Price TR, et al. Effect of treating isolated systolic hypertension on the risk of developing various types and subtypes of stroke: the Systolic Hypertension in the Elderly Program (SHEP). *JAMA* 2000;284:465–471.
51. Sacks FM, Svetkey LP, Vollmer WM, et al. Effects on blood pressure of reduced dietary sodium and the Dietary Approaches to Stop Hypertension (DASH) diet. DASH-Sodium Collaborative Research Group. *N Engl J Med* 2001;344:3–10.
52. Douglas JG, Bakris GL, Epstein M, et al. Hypertension in African Americans Working Group of the International Society on Hypertension in Blacks. Management of high blood pressure in African Americans: consensus statement of the Hypertension in African Americans Working Group of the International Society on Hypertension in Blacks. *Arch Intern Med* 2003;163:525–541.
53. Mann JF, Schmieder RE, McQueen M, et al. ONTARGET investigators. *Lancet* 2008;372: 547–553.
54. Sepehradad R, Frishman WH, Stier CT, et al. Direct inhibition of renin as cardiovascular pharmacotherapy: focus on aliskiren. *Cardiol Rev* 2007;15:242–256.
55. Cohn JN, Archibald DG, Ziesche S, et al. Effect of vasodilator therapy on mortality in chronic congestive heart failure. Results of a Veterans Administration Cooperative Study. *N Engl J Med* 1986;314:1547–1552.

56. Calhoun DA, Jones D, Textor S, et al. Resistant hypertension: diagnosis, evaluation, and treatment. A Scientific Statement from the American Heart Association Professional Education Committee of the Council for High Blood Pressure Research. *Hypertension* 2008;51:1403–1419.

57. Ramsay LE, Waller PC. Blood pressure response to percutaneous transluminal angioplasty for renovascular hypertension: an overview of published series. *BMJ* 1990;300:569–572.

58. Mosso L, Carvajal C, Gonzalez A, et al. Primary aldosteronism and hypertensive disease. *Hypertension* 2003;42:161–165.

59. Ganguly A. Primary aldosteronism. *N Engl J Med* 1998;339:1828–1834.

60. Shivalkar B, Van De Heyning C, Kerremans M, et al. Obstructive sleep apnea syndrome: more insights on structural and functional cardiac alterations, and the effects of treatment with continuous positive airway pressure. *J Am Coll Cardiol* 2006:47;1433–1439.

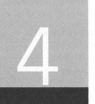

4

Ischemic Heart Disease
Joshua M. Stolker

General Principles

Epidemiology

- Ischemic heart disease (IHD) is the leading cause of mortality in adults in most developed countries.
- >1 million Americans experience a myocardial infarction (MI) each year.
- Lifetime risk of developing significant atherosclerotic coronary artery disease (CAD) after age 40 is nearly 50% for men and 33% for women,[1] with a new coronary event occurring about every 26 seconds.
- About 90% of patients experiencing an ischemic coronary event will have prior exposure to at least one major CAD risk factor.

Risk Factors

- Traditionally, major cardiovascular risk factors[2] have been defined by the National Cholesterol Education Program (NCEP) and other organizations as the following:
  - Increasing age.
  - Elevated low-density lipoprotein (LDL) cholesterol.
  - Low high-density lipoprotein (HDL) cholesterol.
  - Hypertension (HTN).
  - Cigarette smoking.
  - Family history of premature CAD.
- **Note that diabetes mellitus (DM)—a traditional risk factor in the past—is now considered a CAD risk equivalent.**
  - A diabetic without known CAD has approximately the same risk (~20%) of experiencing an MI over a 7-year period as a nondiabetic with prior MI.[3]
  - Diabetic patients who develop CAD have significantly higher rates of reinfarction and death, so aggressive risk factor modification and maintenance of hemoglobin A_{1c} level at <7% is particularly important in these individuals.
- **Peripheral arterial disease (PAD) is also considered a CAD risk equivalent,** and like DM, therapeutic targets with lifestyle modifications should be geared toward levels appropriate for patients with known CAD.[4]
- Also note that traditional NCEP risk factors do not include measures of physical activity, obesity, psychosocial stress, diet, alcohol use, other lipid parameters, etc. despite clear contributions to cardiovascular risk from these additional variables.[5]
- Newer quantitative measures such as C-reactive protein (CRP) and other serum biomarkers, coronary calcium scores on computed tomography (CT), carotid artery intima-media thickness, ankle-brachial indices, creatinine clearance, left ventricular hypertrophy (LVH), etc. are also underrepresented in traditional clinical prediction models.
- Estimating an individual's approximate risk of experiencing an initial cardiovascular event (utilizing risk assessment algorithms such as the one from the NCEP,

| TABLE 1 | Ten-Year Risk for Developing Coronary Artery Disease[a] |

A.

| | Points | | | Points | |
Age (Years)	Men	Women	Age (Years)	Men	Women
20–34	–9	–7	55–59	8	8
35–39	–4	–3	60–64	10	10
40–44	0	0	65–69	11	12
45–49	3	3	70–74	12	14
50–54	6	6	75–79	13	16

| Points | | Points | | | | |
| HDL Cholesterol (mg/dL) | (Either Gender) | Systolic BP (mm Hg) | Untreated | | On Medications | |
			Men	Women	Men	Women
≥60	–1	<120	0	0	0	0
50–59	0	120–129	0	1	1	3
40–49	1	130–139	1	2	2	4
<40	2	140–159	1	3	2	5
		≥160	2	4	3	6

| | Points | | | | | | | | |
| Total Cholesterol (mg/dL) | Age 20–39 Years | | Age 40–49 Years | | Age 50–59 Years | | Age 60–69 Years | | Age 70–79 Years | |
	Men	Women	Men	Women	Men	Women	Men	Women	Men	Women
<160	0	0	0	0	0	0	0	0	0	0
160–199	4	4	3	3	2	2	1	1	0	1
200–239	7	8	5	6	3	4	1	2	0	1
240–279	9	11	6	8	4	5	2	3	1	2
≥280	11	13	8	10	5	7	3	4	1	2

| | Points | | | | | | | | |
| Cigarette Smoking Status | Age 20–39 Years | | Age 40–49 Years | | Age 50–59 Years | | Age 60–69 Years | | Age 70–79 Years | |
	Men	Women	Men	Women	Men	Women	Men	Women	Men	Women
Nonsmoker	0	0	0	0	0	0	0	0	0	0
Smoker	8	9	5	7	3	4	1	2	1	1

[a]Add points in each category (age, HDL cholesterol, total cholesterol, systolic blood pressure, smoking status) to determine point total and then refer to Table 1B.

(*continued*)

TABLE 1	Ten-Year Risk for Developing Coronary Artery Disease[a] *(Continued)*

B.

Point Total (Men)	10-Year Risk (%)	Point Total (Women)	10-Year Risk (%)
<0	<1	<9	<1
0–4	1	9–12	1
5	2	13	2
6	2	14	2
7	3	15	3
8	4	16	4
9	5	17	5
10	6	18	6
11	8	19	8
12	10	20	11
13	12	21	14
14	16	22	17
15	20	23	22
16	25	24	27
≥17	≥30	≥25	≥30

Modified from Executive Summary of the Third Report of The National Cholesterol Education Program (NCEP) Expert Panel on Detection, Evaluation, and Treatment of High Blood Cholesterol in Adults (Adult Treatment Panel III). *JAMA* 2001;285:2486–2497.

which is shown in Table 1) provides clinicians with guidance and targets for therapeutic intervention.

Increasing Age
- This vital risk factor is frequently underappreciated during risk assessment, as traditional algorithms suggest that increased age is "present" when men are >45 and women are >55 (or postmenopausal).
  - In reality, the incidence of acute MI increases continuously with age (Fig. 1), and >83% of people who die from CAD are geriatric in age.[6]

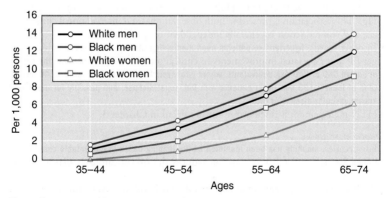

Figure 1. Annual rate of first heart attacks by age, gender, and race in the Atherosclerosis Risk in Communities (ARIC) study, 1987–2000. (From www.americanheart.org.)

• Note the prominent point total associated with age in Table 1, plus the increasing weight assigned to lipid parameters as patient age increases.

Lipids
• Cholesterol is a necessary ingredient in the atherosclerotic process, and as a result its components are important targets for therapeutic intervention.
• **Lipids should be evaluated in adults every ≥5 years, frequently in subjects with additional risk factors.**[2]
• Clinical and epidemiologic trial data are based on venous blood samples drawn after fasting for 12 hours.
• Total cholesterol, HDL, and triglyceride levels are measured directly, whereas very low-density lipoprotein (VLDL) cholesterol level is usually estimated by dividing the triglyceride concentration by 5.
  • This method is accurate only when triglyceride levels are below 400 mg/dL, so that LDL may be calculated from the following formula:

Total cholesterol = HDL + LDL + VLDL

• Since LDL traditionally has been identified as the primary therapeutic target, some laboratories have developed direct measurements of LDL.
• HDL is the only nonatherogenic subtype of cholesterol, so many authorities (including the NCEP) have recommended additional emphasis on lowering all forms of non-HDL rather than LDL alone (therapeutic targets illustrated in Table 2).[2,7]
• Lipid management is discussed in further detail in Chapter 8.

Hypertension
• Guidelines from the Seventh Joint National Committee on Prevention, Detection, Evaluation, and Treatment of Hypertension (JNC 7) have emphasized the classification of blood pressure (BP) into categories designed to affect patient management.[8]
• **Prehypertension signals the need to intensify lifestyle modifications**[9] (with possible medical therapy in select patients), **whereas Stage I and Stage II HTN generally require initiation of one and two BP medications, respectively, if lifestyle modifications have proven inadequate.**
• Of paramount importance is the consistent linear risk of cardiovascular events with increasing BP—particularly in adults >50—starting from systolic BP of 115 mm Hg.[8] This association is present in both observational and interventional clinical trials, and risk reduction is generally independent of specific drugs.
• In other words, **hypertensive patients need medication titration over time** to achieve target BP and associated improvements in clinical outcomes—**particularly in the setting of known CAD or CAD risk equivalents, where goal systolic BP (SBP) is at least <140 mm Hg (and at least <130 mm Hg in patients with DM, renal disease, and possibly for those with known vascular disease or CAD).**
• HTN management is discussed in further detail in Chapter 3.

Cigarette Smoking
• For decades, **smoking has been identified as the leading cause of preventable death in the United States,**[10] and tobacco cessation reduces the risk of cardiovascular events by 25% to 50%.
• Within 3 years of quitting smoking, an individual's risk of CAD returns to normal. Tobacco cessation also results in improved lipid parameters, BP, inflammatory biomarkers, and multiple measures of endothelial and plaque stability.

TABLE 2	Therapeutic Lipid Targets, Depending on Underlying Degree of Cardiovascular Risk

0–1 Major Risk Factors[a] or 10-Year CAD Risk <10%	Two or More Risk Factors[a] or 10-Year CAD Risk 10%–20%	Established CAD, or CAD Risk Equivalent[b] or 10-Year CAD Risk >20%
LDL <160 mg/dL	LDL <130 mg/dL (optional <100 mg/dL)	LDL <100 mg/dL (optional <70 mg/dL)
Non-HDL <190 mg/dL	Non-HDL <160 mg/dL (optional <130 mg/dL)	Non-HDL <130 mg/dL (optional <100 mg/dL)

All groups: HDL goal >40–50 mg/dL when possible, triglyceride goal <150 mg/dL

All groups: Weight loss to <125% ideal weight, regular cardiovascular exercise, low-cholesterol diet, tobacco cessation

CAD, coronary artery disease; HDL, high-density lipoprotein; LDL, low-density lipoprotein.
[a]Major CAD risk factors: increasing age, high LDL, low HDL, hypertension, cigarette smoking, family history of premature CAD.
[b]CAD risk equivalents: significant peripheral arterial disease, diabetes mellitus, or 10-year CAD risk > 20% by standard NCEP risk.
Modified from Executive Summary of the Third Report of The National Cholesterol Education Program (NCEP) Expert Panel on Detection, Evaluation, and Treatment of High Blood Cholesterol in Adults (Adult Treatment Panel III). *JAMA* 2001;285:2486–2497 and Grundy SM, Cleeman JI, Merz CN, et al. Implications of recent clinical trials for the National Cholesterol Education Program Adult Treatment Panel III guidelines. *J Am Coll Cardiol* 2004;44:720–732.

- Clinical studies have demonstrated the key role of physician counseling in facilitating an individual's interest and motivation for quitting.
- Nicotine replacement may be helpful for some patients, but oral medications such as bupropion or varenicline may improve cessation rates.
- Secondhand smoke also increases the risk of cardiovascular events and mortality.
- Smoking cessation is discussed in Chapter 44.

Family History
- Genetic testing and other markers of atherosclerosis may contribute to future models of risk assessment, but epidemiologic data suggest that a simple assessment for family history of premature CAD contributes to an individual's cardiovascular risk.[2]
- In particular, a first-degree relative with CAD at a relatively young age **(men <55 years, women <65 years)** is considered a major risk factor by the NCEP.

Lifestyle Factors
Although variables such as physical activity, diet, obesity, stress levels, etc. are not formally quantified by most traditional risk prediction models, multiple observational and interventional trials demonstrate the utility of modifying high-risk lifestyle behaviors for preventing CAD.

Aerobic Exercise
- **Aerobic exercise** for at least 30 minutes per day, with more vigorous exercise for 2 to 3 days per week, has been associated with reductions in cardiovascular events and is

recommended by national guidelines for both primary and secondary prevention of heart disease.[11]

- Selected patients at higher risk for CAD—particularly diabetics or patients with known CAD—should undergo stress testing prior to beginning a strenuous exercise regimen.[12]
- In general, patients should start by achieving ~50% of maximal predicted heart rate (MPHR = 220 − age) and gradually increase over several months to ~70% to 80% of MPHR.

Diet

- **Dietary modifications** include avoidance of saturated fat when possible, plus increased intake of fish and other sources of polyunsaturated fats to reduce CAD and cardiovascular mortality.[13]
  - Step I and Step II diets from the NCEP both recommend that <30% of daily caloric intake should come from dietary fat, with 50% to 60% of calories from carbohydrates and 10% to 20% from protein.[14]
  - The more restrictive Step II diet is designed for patients with established CAD; recommendations include <7% caloric intake from saturated fatty acids and <200 mg of cholesterol intake per day, versus <10% and <300 mg for the Step I diet.
  - Interestingly, a large multinational study identified low daily fruit and vegetable consumption as a risk factor for CAD,[5] although the utility of higher dose or supplemental fruit and vegetables above standard dietary recommendations remains unclear.
- **Stress management** and **moderation of alcohol consumption** (among those who drink) are also recommended for reduction of cardiovascular event rates.

Obesity

- **Obesity** has become increasingly important in the United States, as approximately one-fourth of all U.S. adults meet criteria for the **metabolic syndrome,** and the prevalence is increasing—particularly in the geriatric population.[15]
  - The diagnosis of metabolic syndrome requires three of the components listed in Table 3.[16]
  - Population studies suggest that subjects with metabolic syndrome have a twofold increase in cardiovascular risk, and in patients without DM, approximately a fivefold increased risk for developing overt DM.
  - Although the utility of diagnosing metabolic syndrome remains controversial, aggressive lifestyle modifications such as weight loss and exercise are of paramount importance given the clustering of risk factors and associated magnified risk in these individuals (Fig. 2).[17,18]

Newer Methods of Risk Assessment

- Current risk prediction algorithms suffer significant limitations when applied to individual patients.
- In 2001, the NCEP acknowledged the emergence of additional risk factors or markers which may help better refine estimates of CAD risk.[2]
- Inflammatory biomarkers and imaging studies in particular have been addressed in scientific statements by national organizations.[19,20]

C-Reactive Protein

- **CRP** exhibits the best combination of assay stability, epidemiologic data, and cost-effectiveness when compared to other inflammatory markers.

TABLE 3	American Heart Association Criteria for Metabolic Syndrome (≥31 in for women)	

Criteria (Any Three for Diagnosis)	Men	Women
Elevated waist circumference[a]	≥102 cm (40 in)	≥88 cm (35 in)
Reduced high-density lipoprotein cholesterol	<40 mg/dL	<50 mg/dL
Elevated triglycerides	≥150 mg/dL or drug treatment for triglycerides	
Elevated blood pressure	Systolic ≥130 mm Hg or diastolic ≥85 mm Hg	
Elevated fasting glucose	≥100 mg/dL or drug treatment for glucose	

[a]Waist circumference measured horizontally at the iliac crest, at the end of normal expiration; lower cutoffs may be appropriate in Asian Americans (≥90 cm or ≥35 in for men, ≥80 cm or ≥31 in for women).
Modified from Grundy SM, Cleeman JI, Daniels SR, et al. Diagnosis and management of the metabolic syndrome. *Curr Opin Cardiol* 2006;21:1–6.

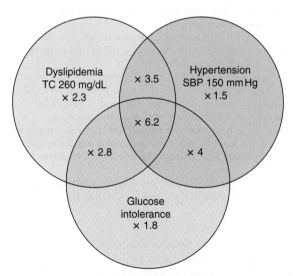

Figure 2. Elevated cardiovascular risk with multiple components of the metabolic syndrome. Risk ratios listed are compared to a 40-year-old male nonsmoker with total cholesterol (TC) of 185 mg/dL, systolic blood pressure (SBP) of 120 mm Hg, no glucose intolerance, no left ventricular hypertrophy on electrocardiogram, and whose probability of developing coronary artery disease is around 1.5% in 8 years. (Modified from Wilson PW, Kannel WB, Silbershatz H, D'Agostino RB. Clustering of metabolic factors and coronary heart disease. *Arch Intern Med* 1999;159:1104–1109 and Poulter N. Coronary heart disease is a multifactorial disease. *Am J Hypertens* 1999;12(Suppl 1):92S–95S.

TABLE 4	Variables Associated with CRP Concentration

Increased Levels of CRP	Decreased Levels of CRP
Elevated blood pressure	Moderate alcohol consumption
Elevated body mass index	Increased activity/endurance exercise
Cigarette smoking	Weight loss
Metabolic syndrome/diabetes mellitus	Statin drug therapy
Low HDL/high triglycerides	Fibrate drug therapy
Estrogen/progesterone use	Niacin drug therapy
Chronic infections (gingivitis, bronchitis)	
Chronic inflammation (e.g., rheumatoid arthritis)	

CRP, C-reactive protein; HDL, high-density lipoprotein cholesterol.
Modified from Pearson TA, Mensah GA, Alexander RW, et al. Markers of inflammation and cardiovascular disease: application to clinical and public health practice. *Circulation* 2003;107:499–511.

- For primary prevention of CAD, meta-analyses suggest that CRP levels >3.0 mg/L are associated with approximately twice the relative risk of cardiovascular events, although some of this risk is attenuated after adjustment for traditional risk factors and patient characteristics (Table 4).[19]
- Given the rise in CRP with acute inflammation or infection, multiple assessments may be necessary, and higher cutoffs may be appropriate in patients with known atherosclerotic disease or heart failure (HF).
- Although subjects with low levels of both CRP and LDL have demonstrated lower rates of CAD and cardiovascular events in some observational[21] and clinical interventional trials,[22,23] several other large-scale studies have failed to demonstrate incremental utility of CRP or many other inflammatory markers.[24,25]
- At the present time, **most authorities consider CRP to be a marker with moderate prognostic utility, which may help direct risk assessment and therapeutic approaches in patients at intermediate risk, although the benefits of CRP-guided treatment remain unproven.**[19]
- Applying secondary prevention therapies should not depend on CRP levels, and the role of intensified pharmacologic therapy to achieve lower CRP levels remains unclear.

Other Biomarkers
- **Other biomarkers**[26] are generally measured only in select patients, including several in commercially available assays for clinical use:
  - Homocysteine (often evaluated in young patients with premature vascular disease)
  - Lipoprotein(a) (genetically determined and probably not modifiable)
  - Fibrinogen (stronger predictor for peripheral arterial disease than for CAD)
  - LDL particle size (small/dense pattern is more atherogenic, but inconsistent risk prediction)
  - B-type natriuretic peptide (more useful in HF or for diagnosing left ventricular [LV] dysfunction)

- Of note, the field of cardiac biomarkers tends to change rapidly, and the utility of additional markers will likely change as more data and clinical assays become available.

Coronary Calcium Scores

- **Coronary calcium scores** by CT have generated considerable controversy, as much of the initial experience was generated through industry and propagated outside of clinical medicine (i.e., direct-to-consumer advertising).
- Small studies suggested that aggressive lipid management may slow down the progression of vascular calcification, although larger prospective trials failed to demonstrate reduction in calcium deposition or improved clinical outcomes independent of therapy directed at standard CAD risk factors.[27]
- Nevertheless, guidelines from the American Heart Association confirm **incremental prognostic utility of CT calcium scores for refining risk stratification in intermediate-risk patients by standard NCEP assessment, but more data are needed prior to recommending treatment options or intensification of therapy.**[28]
- Coronary calcium assessment should not be performed in low-risk patients.[29]
- Although data are very limited, stress testing is reasonable in patients with severe coronary calcification on CT.

Peripheral Arterial Studies

- Measurement of carotid intima-media thickness, assessment of endothelial function using brachial artery reactivity, and other imaging modalities often require specialized centers for accurate and reproducible measurements.
- Ankle-brachial index (also called ankle-arm index) is readily available as a screening test for peripheral arterial disease, and its prognostic utility has been demonstrated most consistently in the geriatric population.

Other Medical Conditions Contributing to Risk

Autoimmune Disease

- A growing body of literature has suggested that autoimmune conditions such as rheumatoid arthritis or lupus also are associated with higher rates of MI and other cardiovascular events.[30–32]
- This risk appears to be independent of hypercoagulable states that frequently accompany these disease processes, although chronic inflammation (i.e., with elevated CRP levels) may play a pathogenic role.
- Paradoxically, however, chronic steroids and other immune-suppressive drugs may also increase the risk of CAD.

Human Immunodeficiency Virus

Infection with human immunodeficiency virus (HIV) may be associated with accelerated atherosclerosis, particularly when treatment includes medications such as **protease inhibitors,** which promote atherogenic dyslipidemia and glucose intolerance.[33]

Cocaine Abuse

Cocaine abuse may dramatically accelerate atherosclerosis in certain individuals, particularly with chronic abuse, and both angina and MI may be precipitated acutely by cocaine-induced vasospasm, thrombosis, and increased myocardial demand from hyperadrenergic tone.[34]

Diagnosis

Clinical Presentation

History

- **The most common manifestation of CAD is angina,** which is generally described as a crushing, squeezing, pressure-like deep visceral pain.
  - Symptoms may radiate into the arm, jaw, neck, or back and are frequently associated with a profound sense of discomfort or uneasiness.
  - Typical angina may be difficult for many patients to describe, and the discomfort tends to be more generalized than focal.
  - Some individuals experience nausea, diaphoresis, epigastric discomfort, or dyspnea; symptoms are often precipitated by emotional or physical stress or a medical illness.
- Of note, **diabetics may not experience chest discomfort** despite having significant CAD, and because of chronic underrepresentation in most clinical studies of CAD, **women and elderly patients often experience more "atypical" forms of chest discomfort** than "classic" anginal symptoms described historically in the medical literature.
  - Geriatric patients may not describe chest pain at all, and frequently an acute coronary syndrome (ACS) is discovered in an elderly subject with generalized malaise, confusion, dyspnea, fatigue, etc.
- Since *quality* of angina varies significantly among individuals, the Canadian Cardiovascular Society has classified the *amount* of angina in terms of symptomatic limitations to performing daily activities (Table 5). This allows clinicians to titrate medical or surgical therapy geared toward the reduction of angina severity.[35]

Physical Examination

- **Physical examination is notoriously unreliable for the diagnosis of CAD,** although angina and discomfort may lead to HTN, tachycardia, and diaphoresis in some subjects.
- Exam findings concerning for acute MI often relate to evolving complications such as significant bradycardia, hypotension, rales, new heart murmurs, pericardial rub, muffled heart sounds, new S3 gallop, or end-organ hypoperfusion (altered mental status, pallor, etc.).
- Evidence of undiagnosed cardiac risk factors may be noted on examination (e.g., tendon xanthomas in hypercholesterolemia and abnormalities of pulse suggestive of PAD).
- Severe HTN alone may provoke coronary ischemia (hypertensive emergency), so rapid reduction of systolic BP by approximately one-third—generally in a monitored

TABLE 5	Classification of Angina
Class	**Onset of Angina**[a]
I	With strenuous activity
II	With moderate activity such as brisk walking or climbing stairs
III	With mild activity such as walking on level ground
IV	With minimal activity or at rest

[a]Unstable angina is generally considered Class IV angina, or progression of Classes II–III angina over the preceding 2 months.
Modified from Campeau L. Grading of angina pectoris. *Circulation* 1976;54:522–523.

setting such as an emergency department—with gradual reduction over the subsequent 48 hours is imperative in patients with chest discomfort and high BP.[36]

Differential Diagnosis

The differential diagnosis of chest pain is broad (Table 6), so the diagnosis of obstructive CAD relies heavily on the history and electrocardiogram (ECG).

Ischemia from Etiologies Other than Atherosclerotic CAD
- **Subendocardial ischemia** related to myocardial strain requires management of the underlying cause of strain (i.e., BP control, β-blockers or calcium channel blockers [CCBs] for hypertrophic cardiomyopathy, valve replacement for aortic stenosis).
- **Coronary vasospasm** is an uncommon cause of angina, usually associated with ST-segment elevation on the ECG.
  - Treatment of spasm using CCBs and/or nitrates should be combined with interventions aimed at endothelial stabilization (e.g., tobacco cessation, aspirin therapy, weight loss and exercise, possibly angiotensin-converting enzyme [ACE] inhibitors).

TABLE 6	Differential Diagnosis of Chest Pain
Cardiac	**Noncardiac**
Potentially dangerous	**Potentially dangerous**
Atherosclerotic coronary artery disease	Aortic dissection
Coronary stent thrombosis or in-stent restenosis	Pulmonary embolus
Hypertrophic cardiomyopathy	Esophageal rupture, Mallory-Weiss tear
Severe aortic stenosis	Peptic ulcer, cholecystitis, pancreatitis
Severe hypertension with subendocardial ischemia	Pneumonia
Arrhythmias	Pulmonary hypertension (usually with right ventricular strain)
Coronary vasospasm	Pneumothorax
Coronary artery aneurysm, dissection, fistula, embolus	Mediastinitis
Myocardial bridging	Supply-demand mismatch (e.g., tachycardia, severe anemia, hypoxia, thyrotoxicosis)
Anomalous coronary artery	
Usually not life threatening	**Usually not life threatening**
Mitral valve prolapse	Reflux, esophagitis, gastritis, esophageal spasm, biliary colic
Pericarditis	Costochondritis, chest wall trauma, musculoskeletal abnormality
Cardiac syndrome X (believed to represent microvascular dysfunction with widely patent coronaries)	Cervical or thoracic spine disease
	Pleurisy, pleuritis, bronchitis
	Herpes zoster

- Provocation in the catheterization laboratory, or 24-hour ECG monitoring to diagnose ST elevations, may be necessary for definitive diagnosis.
- Rarely, **myocardial bridging** (or certain congenital coronary artery anomalies) may also cause angina, which is best relieved by reducing inotropy and improving diastolic flow with β-blockers and possibly CCBs.
- **Cocaine** or other stimulants may provoke ischemia via tachycardia, HTN, and vasoconstriction.[34]
  - Atherosclerosis and thrombosis are accelerated, so inpatient evaluation is usually necessary to rule out MI.
  - Other than cessation of cocaine usage, management is similar to vasospasm and β-blockers are generally avoided because of the risk of unopposed α-adrenergic stimulation with repeated cocaine exposure.

Diagnostic Testing

Laboratories

To correct precipitating causes of chest pain and to assess the patient's degree of risk, **initial tests should include hemoglobin, white blood cell count, renal function and electrolytes, and fasting glucose.** Lipids are often measured if not recently assessed.

Imaging

- **Chest radiography** is indicated if there is evidence of HF, pericardial or aortic disease, or other noncardiac etiologies potentially causing the discomfort (e.g., pulmonary disease, rib or musculoskeletal abnormalities).
- **Echocardiography** is indicated when chest symptoms or examination findings are potentially related to significant valvular heart disease, undiagnosed LV dysfunction, or hypertrophic cardiomyopathy.[37]

Diagnostic Procedures

Stress Testing

- **In patients whose chest pain has an intermediate probability of being caused by CAD, stress testing provides both diagnostic and prognostic information.**[12]
  - High-risk angina (>80% to 85% likelihood of severe or obstructive CAD) should proceed to cardiac catheterization, while stress testing for low-risk chest pain (<10% to 15% likelihood) will result in more false-positive tests than true-positive tests for prevalent CAD.
- Other situations where stress testing may help evaluate for CAD include the following[12,37]:
  - For sedentary or asymptomatic diabetic patients interested in starting a vigorous exercise program.
  - To assess adequacy of medical therapy for CAD.
  - Prior to cardiac rehabilitation, and to assess ischemic burden and prognosis after MI.
  - In certain high-risk occupations (e.g., pilots, firefighters) as screening for CAD.
  - Preoperatively in very specific situations (see Chapter 2).
- **Interpretation of stress testing should include symptomatic response, exercise capacity, hemodynamic response, and ECG/imaging response.**
  - Significant HTN during exercise may require treatment to avoid exertional angina from subendocardial ischemia.
  - Exercise-induced hypotension or sustained ventricular arrhythmias signify poor prognosis (i.e., multivessel CAD or very large ischemic burden), and these patients should be referred for coronary angiography.

TABLE 7	Contraindications to Exercise Testing

Absolute Contraindications	Relative Contraindications
Acute myocardial infarction within 2 days	Known left main coronary stenosis (not bypassed)
High-risk unstable angina	Moderate stenotic valvular heart disease
Uncontrolled symptomatic cardiac arrhythmias	Severe arterial hypertension (e.g., systolic blood pressure >200 mm Hg at rest)
Symptomatic severe aortic stenosis	Significant electrolyte abnormalities
Uncontrolled symptomatic heart failure	Uncontrolled tachyarrhythmia or bradyarrhythmia
Acute pulmonary embolus or pulmonary infarction	Significant obstruction of left ventricular outflow tract
Acute myocarditis or pericarditis	Mental or physical impairment precluding adequate exercise
Acute aortic dissection	High-degree atrioventricular block
Severe comorbidity limiting life expectancy and/or candidacy for revascularization	

Modified from Gibbons RJ, Balady GJ, Bricker JT, et al. ACC/AHA 2002 guideline update for exercise testing: summary article. *Circulation* 2002;106:1883–1892.

- Contraindications to exercise stress testing[12] are listed in Table 7.
- Depending on patient characteristics and stability, **β-blockers and nondihydropyridine CCBs may need to be held prior to exercise or dobutamine stress testing to permit an adequate heart rate response.**
- Screening for silent ischemia in the absence of symptoms is indicated only in specific patient subsets such as high-risk patients undergoing surgery (see Chapter 2), longstanding DM (especially with neuropathy), certain high-risk occupations such as pilots and firefighters, etc.
  - **In asymptomatic patients, risk stratification and prognosis are more important considerations at stress testing than diagnosis (as treatment is geared toward reduction of MI and mortality—not symptom relief), and incident event rates are low regardless of whether interventions are performed.**

Stress ECG
- Sensitivity and specificity of exercise ECG are generally 70% to 75% in clinical studies, but sensitivity is closer to 50% in general medical practice.
  - **ST elevation during stress testing localizes myocardial injury and suggests high-grade obstruction of an epicardial coronary artery;** these patients are usually referred urgently for cardiac catheterization.
  - Upsloping ST depression or inadequate heart rate response (<85% of the MPHR) renders the stress test nondiagnostic.
  - **Downsloping or horizontal ST-segment depression is more closely associated with CAD** than upsloping ST depression, although **the leads with ST depression do not correlate with stenosis location** at catheterization.[38]
  - A positive test is defined as ≥1 mm of ST depression in two contiguous ECG leads, 60 to 80 ms after the J-point, when compared with the PR segment.[39]

TABLE 8	Duke Treadmill Score[a] for Exercise Stress Testing

High-risk findings
Duke Treadmill Score −11 or lower (suggests 5.25% annual CAD mortality)
Systolic blood pressure reduction ≥10 mm Hg during exercise
Persistent ST-segment changes >5 minutes into recovery
Poor functional capacity (e.g., unable to progress beyond Stage I of Bruce
    protocol, or <4 METs)
New ST depression >2 mm
New ST elevation >1 mm
Sustained ventricular tachycardia

Intermediate-risk findings
Duke Treadmill Score −10 to 4 (suggests 1.25% annual CAD mortality)

Low-risk findings
Duke Treadmill Score ≥5 (suggests 0.25% annual CAD mortality)
High exercise tolerance (i.e., >10 METs)

CAD, coronary artery disease; MET, metabolic equivalent.
[a]Duke Treadmill Score = minutes of exercise on Bruce protocol − (5 × ST deviation
in mm) − (4 × exercise angina score). Here exercise angina score: 0 = no angina,
1 = angina during the test, 2 = angina causing test termination.
Modified from Mark DB, Shaw L, Harrell FE, et al. Prognostic value of a treadmill exercise score in outpatients with suspected coronary artery disease. *N Engl J Med* 1991;
325:849–853.

- **Prognosis at exercise stress testing is directly related to functional capacity, plus magnitude and number of leads with ST-segment deviation.**
  - Patients undergoing exercise testing have better outcomes than patients unable to exercise.
  - The **Duke Treadmill Score**[40] incorporates several factors from exercise testing into a simple formula (see Table 8).
  - **High-risk patients should be referred for coronary angiography,** whereas intermediate-risk patients may be further stratified by either angiography or a repeat stress test with echocardiographic or nuclear imaging to better assess ischemic burden and LV systolic function.
- Pharmacologic stress tests involve redistribution of myocardial blood flow (adenosine or dipyridamole) or adrenergic stimulation (dobutamine).
  - **Adenosine and dipyridamole** may provoke bronchospasm in patients with reactive airway disease, and balanced ischemia from multivessel CAD may be missed because of the reliance of these agents on comparative blood flow relative to contralateral myocardial territories.
  - **Dobutamine** may provoke arrhythmias or hypotension, and should be avoided in patients with paroxysmal atrial fibrillation, high risk of ventricular tachycardia, or other high-risk clinical features rendering adrenergic stimulation dangerous (e.g., ACS within the past 24 to 48 hours).

Stress Tests with Imaging
- **Echocardiographic or nuclear imaging is recommended if the baseline ECG is abnormal** (LV hypertrophy with secondary ST-segment changes, resting ST depression >1 mm,

digoxin effects, left bundle branch block [LBBB], ventricular pacemaker beats, pre-excitation) **or if prior revascularization (percutaneous or surgical) has been performed.**[12]

- **When baseline LBBB or electronic ventricular pacing is present, avoidance of tachycardia during stress testing helps maximize accuracy of imaging results** (i.e., adenosine or dipyridamole nuclear perfusion studies should be performed rather than exercise or dobutamine tests in these individuals).
- Sensitivity and specificity of imaging stress tests vary between studies but generally are improved compared with stress ECG alone.
- **Choice of echocardiography versus nuclear imaging generally depends on the level of expertise at a given center, although each modality has unique advantages.**
  - Stress echocardiography is more versatile (allowing evaluation of valvular disease, diastolic function, pericardial abnormalities, and pulmonary artery pressures) with higher specificity and lower cost, but acquisition and interpretation of stress images may be technically more demanding.
  - Thallium and technetium nuclear studies have extensive prognostic utility in the published literature with higher technical success rates, higher sensitivity, and higher overall accuracy in patients with multivessel CAD or prior MI—but handling of nuclear isotopes is significantly more expensive and requires specialized handling.
- **High-risk findings during stress testing (Table 9) should prompt coronary angiography for prognostic assessment and potential revascularization in appropriate candidates.**[37]

TABLE 9	Risk Markers from Stress Testing

High risk (>3% annual mortality)
Severe resting left ventricular systolic dysfunction (ejection fraction <35%)
Poor Duke Treadmill Score (≤ -11)
Severe exercise-induced left ventricular systolic dysfunction
Large or multiple stress-induced nuclear perfusion defects (especially if anterior location)
Significant nuclear perfusion abnormality with stress-induced left ventricular dilation or lung uptake (thallium-201 isotope)
Stress-induced wall motion abnormality on echocardiogram at low heart rate (≤ 120 beats/min) or low dobutamine dose (≤ 10 mg/kg/min)
Extensive or multiple wall motion abnormalities on stress echocardiogram

Intermediate risk (1%–3% annual mortality)
Mild-to-moderate left ventricular systolic dysfunction (ejection fraction 35%–49%)
Intermediate Duke Treadmill Score (-11 to 5)
Moderate stress-induced nuclear perfusion defect
Stress-induced echocardiographic wall motion abnormality at higher dobutamine doses

Low risk (<1% annual mortality)
Low-risk Duke Treadmill Score (≥ 5)
Normal or small nuclear perfusion abnormality (in the absence of other high-risk features)

Modified from Gibbons RJ, Abrams J, Chatterjee K, et al. ACC/AHA 2002 guideline update for the management of patients with chronic stable angina—summary article. *J Am Coll Cardiol* 2003;41:159–168.

Other Imaging Modalities

- With improved gating techniques and spatial resolution, **CT angiography** may provide noninvasive imaging options for specific subsets of patients with chest pain.
  - Unfortunately, CT angiography requires a bolus of intravenous dye (generally equivalent or greater volume than diagnostic catheterization), radiation exposure is greater, and spatial resolution is significantly lower compared with diagnostic angiography.
  - Adequate imaging requires relatively low heart rate, regular heart rhythm, and low levels of "scatter" from coronary calcifications and metallic artifact from stents or surgical clips.
  - Despite these limitations, **CT angiography is improving rapidly and is considered a reasonable option for the assessment of obstructive disease in symptomatic patients with a low or intermediate pretest probability for CAD.**[28,41]
  - **Current guidelines do not recommend CT angiography following stent placement, for tracking atherosclerosis progression, or for screening asymptomatic patients to diagnose occult CAD.**
  - Estimates of LV size and systolic function may also be obtained from cardiac CT.
- **Magnetic resonance angiography (MRA)** is another noninvasive imaging option, although prolonged breath holding and slow heart rates in regular heart rhythms are necessary during image acquisition, so coronary arterial resolution remains highly variable.
- Limited experience with combined structural-functional imaging (e.g., CT angiography plus nuclear imaging or positron emission tomography) suggests a potential role for this noninvasive approach in the future.
- Ambulatory ECG monitoring for ischemia is rarely indicated, and ischemia usually needs to be confirmed with exercise stress testing if abnormal.[37]

Coronary Angiography

- **Diagnostic left heart catheterization is the gold standard for assessing coronary anatomy, plus severity and location of atherosclerotic narrowing,** in conjunction with additional data including LV systolic and diastolic function, atherosclerotic burden, and left-sided valvular function.
  - Despite providing direct visualization of CAD, angiography does not reliably identify plaque stability, intracoronary thrombus, or functional significance of coronary lesions.
  - Nevertheless, interventional techniques such as pressure- and flow-wire assessments or intravascular ultrasound help quantify the significance of intermediate coronary stenoses, and **the extent and severity of CAD and LV dysfunction are powerful predictors of long-term outcome.**[42–45]
    - The prognosis of medically managed patients with varying degrees of CAD is detailed in Table 10.[42]
    - Although these data from a large observational registry are compelling, risk assessment should combine angiographic CAD severity with clinical factors and LV function when estimating a particular individual's degree of risk.
    - For example, a 65-year-old man with stable angina and 3-vessel CAD has a 5-year survival rate of 93%, versus only 58% if the same patient also has HF and LV ejection fraction of 30%.[37]
  - Complication rates from diagnostic catheterization are generally <1% to 2%, although higher risks are associated with increasing age, PAD, renal dysfunction,

TABLE 10	Prognosis of Medically Managed Patients with Significant Coronary Disease at Angiography	

Extent of Coronary Disease	Prognostic Weight (0–100)[a]	5-Year Survival Rate (%)
1 vessel, 75% stenosis	23	93
>1 vessel, 50%–74% stenosis	23	93
1 vessel, ≥95%	32	91
2 vessels	37	88
2 vessels, both ≥95%	42	86
1 vessel, ≥95% proximal LAD	48	83
2 vessels, including ≥95% LAD	48	83
2 vessels, including ≥95% proximal LAD	56	79
3 vessels	56	79
3 vessels, ≥95% in at least one location	63	73
3 vessels, 75% proximal LAD	67	67
3 vessels, ≥95% proximal LAD	74	59

LAD, left anterior descending artery.
[a]Prognostic weight compared with the prognosis for ≥95% left main stenosis, which is given a value of 100, whereas patients with no angiographic coronary disease are given a value of zero.
Modified from Califf RM, Armstrong PW, Carver JR, et al. Task Force 5: stratification of patients into high, medium, and low risk subgroups for purposes of risk factor management. *J Am Coll Cardiol* 1996;27:1007–1019.

coagulopathy, and extremes of body weight. Mortality risk is approximately 0.1%.
- **In suitable candidates for revascularization, and without limited life expectancy or severe comorbidities which markedly increase procedural risk, coronary angiography is recommended for the following scenarios**[37]:
  - Angina with high-risk criteria by clinical assessment.
  - Disabling angina despite medical therapy.
  - Angina with intermediate-risk stress test findings.
  - High-risk stress test findings, with or without angina.
  - Nondiagnostic stress test results despite intermediate-to-high pretest probability of obstructive CAD.
  - Inadequate prognostic information obtained from stress testing.
  - Angina with HF or significant LV systolic dysfunction.
  - Sustained ventricular arrhythmias or sudden cardiac death without other clear etiology.
  - Intermediate or high pretest probability for CAD and planned heart valve or other cardiac surgery.
  - Selected at-risk individuals unable to undergo noninvasive stress testing, or with specific occupational requirements (e.g., airline pilots or firefighters in certain states).

TREATMENT

General Principles

- **Hospitalization should be arranged urgently for high-risk features concerning for MI,**[37] such as the following:
  - Class IV or unstable angina, particularly if prolonged (i.e., >20 minutes) or nocturnal.
  - New HF, rales, or hypotension.
  - ST-segment deviations on ECG.
  - New LBBB with angina.
  - Significant new T-wave inversions.
  - Elevated cardiac biomarkers.
  - Known atherosclerosis at risk of progressing.
- More aggressive testing and/or hospitalization should be considered in patients with recent MI (<30 days) or recent percutaneous or surgical revascularization procedure (<6 months).
- Treatment of IHD is intended to reduce the risks of cardiovascular mortality and MI, while also reducing symptoms and improving quality of life.
- Outpatient therapies are directed toward increasing coronary blood flow, reducing myocardial oxygen demand, reducing thrombosis, lowering sympathetic tone, preventing adverse remodeling of ischemic or infarcted myocardium, and correcting any illness which may precipitate ischemia.

Medications

Primary Prevention

- **Primary prevention of CAD can be best achieved by identifying and treating the risk factors discussed above.**
- **Aspirin** has been extensively studied in multiple populations and is recommended for patients with established vascular disease including CAD.
  - The benefits of aspirin in primary prevention are less clear, as therapy reduces the incidence of MI but the modest benefit is counteracted by bleeding risk.
  - The U.S. Preventative Services Task Force "strongly recommends that clinicians discuss aspirin chemoprevention with adults who are at increased risk" for CAD, especially when risk is >3% in the upcoming 5 years.[46]
    - Data are most compelling for primary prevention in men >40 years, postmenopausal women, and younger people with risk factors—although therapy should be individualized after weighing the risks of MI versus bleeding, peptic ulcer formation, etc.
    - Many clinicians recommend lower doses (75 to 81 mg daily) to avoid these potential side effects in primary prevention.
- Despite promising pathophysiologic and small-scale clinical studies suggesting benefit, multiple large clinical trials have shown that **prophylactic hormone replacement, supplemental vitamins, or antioxidant therapies do not prevent CAD** in their current formulations.[37,47]
- **Omega-3 fatty acids may play a role in reducing cardiovascular risk,** but diets rich in polyunsaturated fats (in conjunction with weight management and physical exercise) likely improve clinical outcomes more effectively than do adjunctive supplements.[13]
- **Moderate alcohol consumption** (one to two drinks per day) has been associated with lower BP and lower rates of cardiovascular events in observational trials, but higher

intake appears detrimental, and alcohol as a therapeutic measure has not been studied in randomized controlled trials.[48]

Antiplatelet Therapy for Established CAD

- **In patients with known CAD, aspirin 81 to 325 mg orally reduces the risk of MI and reduces mortality by approximately one-third.**
  - Clopidogrel is an adequate substitute for patients with true aspirin allergy (i.e., anaphylaxis).
- When added to aspirin, **clopidogrel 75 mg daily for at least 1 month and as long as 1 year** (generally after a 300 to 600 mg load in the hospital) **improves cardiovascular outcomes after ACS or after percutaneous coronary intervention (PCI)** (see the section "Revascularization").[49,50]
  - Cost and hemorrhagic risk often limit clopidogrel usage, particularly in patients at lower risk or without prior ACS,[51] and the utility of clopidogrel is unclear for patients >75.
  - Clopidogrel significantly increases bleeding complications during surgery, so therapy should be withheld for 5 days beforehand whenever possible (see Chapter 2).
  - Ticlopidine may be substituted for subjects with rash or other significant allergy to clopidogrel, although higher rates of blood dyscrasias (i.e., severe thrombocytopenia, neutropenia, anemia) require ongoing periodic monitoring of blood counts during treatment.

Anti-ischemic Therapy
β-Blockers

- **β-Blockers** (Table 11) reduce ischemic complications by lowering myocardial oxygen demand, and **should be given to all patients with prior MI or LV systolic dysfunction**[52] **in the absence of contraindications** (hypotension, severe bradycardia or heart block, decompensated HF, and bronchospasm).
  - Goal heart rate is generally 55 to 60 beats per minute; slow titration may be necessary in HF or with advanced age.
  - Agents more selective for β_1-receptors at low doses may cause fewer side effects related to β_2 antagonism (i.e., bronchospasm, worsening leg claudication, and differential pancreatic cell function in DM).
  - Hydrophilic β-blockers may theoretically cause less sedation, depression, or other central nervous system effects because of reduced crossing of the blood-brain barrier.
  - Some nonselective β-blockers may have benefits in treating other medical problems (i.e., improved antihypertensive effects from concurrent α-receptor antagonism, migraine therapy with propranolol, HF therapy with metoprolol succinate or carvedilol, and possible improved therapy of esophageal varices with nadolol).
  - Antianginal effects are somewhat less effective in Classes III to IV angina when β-blockers with intrinsic sympathomimetic activity are used.

Calcium Channel Blockers

- CCBs may reduce angina by causing arteriolar vasodilation and reductions in myocardial oxygen demand (Table 12), and **CCBs may be added to β-blockers for patients with continued symptoms, or used as alternatives for individuals with contraindications to β-blockers.**[37]
  - CCBs, in conjunction with nitrates, are preferable when treating coronary vasospasm.
  - Short-acting dihydropyridines (e.g., nifedipine) are contraindicated in patients with CAD, but longer-acting CCBs are considered relatively safe in CAD.

TABLE 11 — Commonly Used β-Blockers

Medication	Usual Dosing Regimen	Elimination Half-Life (Hours)	Characteristics
Acebutolol	200–1,200 mg qd or divided bid	3–4 (metabolite 8–15)	B_1 selective, ISA
Atenolol	25–100 mg qd	6–9	B_1 selective, hydrophilic
Bisoprolol	2.5–20 mg qd	9–12	B_1 selective
Carvedilol	3.125–50 mg bid	7–10	Combined α- and β-receptor antagonism
Carvedilol CR	10–80 mg qd	11	Combined α- and β-receptor antagonism
Labetalol	200–2,400 mg bid	6–8	Combined α- and β-receptor antagonism
Metoprolol tartrate	50–200 mg bid	3–4	B_1 selective, lipophilic
Metoprolol succinate	25–200 mg qd	4–7	B_1 selective, lipophilic
Nadolol	40–240 mg qd	14–24	Hydrophilic
Pindolol	5–20 mg bid or tid	3–4	ISA
Propranolol	10–80 mg qid	4–6	Lipophilic
Propranolol LA	60–320 qd	10	Lipophilic
Timolol	10–30 mg bid	3–4	Hydrophilic

ISA, intrinsic sympathomimetic activity.

TABLE 12 — Calcium Channel Blockers

	Usual Dosing Regimen	Elimination Half-Life (Hours)
Nondihydropyridines		
Diltiazem	30–120 mg tid or qid	3–5
Diltiazem CD	120–480 mg qd	5–8
Diltiazem LA	120–480 mg qd	6–9
Verapamil	80–120 mg tid or qid	3–7
Verapamil SR	120–480 mg qd	5–12
Dihydropyridines		
Amlodipine	2.5–10 mg qd	30–50
Felodipine	5–10 mg qd	9
Isradipine	2.5–5 mg bid	8
Isradipine SR	5–10 mg qd	8
Nicardipine	20–30 mg bid or tid	2–8
Nifedipine	10–30 mg tid or qid	2
Nifedipine SR	30–90 mg qd	7
Nisoldipine	10–40 mg qd or bid	7–12

CD, continuous duration; LA, long-acting; SR, sustained-release.

- Nondihydropyridines may be useful for suppressing atrial arrhythmias or atrioventricular conduction, but given their negative chronotropic and inotropic effects, these agents should be used with caution in patients with LV systolic dysfunction.
- Nifedipine may cause reflex tachycardia, and any CCB may cause peripheral edema, constipation, headaches, or flushing.

Nitrates

- **Nitroglycerin** reduces preload (venodilation) and afterload (arterial dilation) in patients with angina, and therefore improves both myocardial supply and demand.
- Headaches are common but benign and often treatable with acetaminophen.
- Hypotension may be precipitated in patients with intravascular depletion, severe aortic stenosis, hypertrophic cardiomyopathy, or concomitant therapy with sildenafil or similar agents (vardenafil, tadalafil) within the preceding 24 to 48 hours.
- **Sublingual nitroglycerin spray or tablets provide rapid relief for many individuals with stable angina, but prolonged discomfort after 2 to 3 doses should prompt immediate evaluation in an emergency department.**
- Longer-acting nitrates (isosorbide dinitrate and mononitrate, transdermal nitroglycerin patch) may help avoid angina in chronic symptomatic CAD, but all forms require an 8 to 12-hour nitrate-free period to avoid tachyphylaxis.
- These agents have never been demonstrated to improve long-term outcomes, so **nitrates should be prescribed for symptom relief in patients with inadequate responses or contraindications to β-blockers or CCBs.**[37]
- As with CCBs, nitrates may help prevent or minimize angina from coronary vasospasm.

Ranolazine

Ranolazine is an anti-ischemic agent with unclear mechanism which has been shown to reduce angina severity and frequency when added to traditional therapy for chronic CAD,[53,54] although reductions in clinical events have not been demonstrated conclusively to date.[55]

Disease-Modifying Therapy

Statins

- **Statin therapy should be administered to all patients with CAD or CAD risk equivalents** (i.e., PAD, DM), with clinical trials demonstrating improved cardiovascular outcomes with lower LDL levels (at least <100 mg/dL, and <70 mg/dL in high-risk individuals).[7,56]
  - **Patients with myalgias or other adverse effects to one statin should be tried on other statins and/or lower doses of the initial statin, as patients able to tolerate these agents demonstrate consistent reductions in cardiovascular events—particularly in the setting of known CAD or prior ACS.**
  - Aside from event reduction, higher-potency statins appear to modify plaque composition over time, with reductions in atherosclerotic progression demonstrated in several studies.[57]
  - Niacin, fibrates, and fish oil tablets may also be administered as add-on or second-line therapies, but clinical outcomes and mortality benefits are significantly more established and consistent in clinical trials of statins. The effects of ezetimibe, cholestyramine, and colesevelam on clinical outcomes remain inadequately defined.

Angiotensin-Converting Enzyme Inhibitors

- **ACE inhibitors** should be added for patients with prior MI, known CAD, or other vascular disease.[37,52]

- Benefits are most pronounced for CAD patients with DM, HF, LV systolic dysfunction, or mild-to-moderate renal dysfunction.
- Angiotensin receptor blockers (ARBs) may be reasonable alternatives for patients with intolerance to ACE inhibitors (e.g., significant cough, angioedema).

Aldosterone Antagonists
- **Eplerenone,** an aldosterone antagonist related to spironolactone, improves short- and long-term mortality and cardiovascular outcomes when given to patients with acute MI, LV systolic dysfunction (ejection fraction <40%), clinical HF or DM, and no other contraindication to aldosterone blockade (i.e., creatinine >2.5 mg/dL, hyperkalemia >5.0 mmol/L).[58]
- Therapy should be continued for 2 years after the MI.

Other Medication Therapies
- **Intensive DM management** is imperative, with goal hemoglobin A_{1c} <7% if possible.
- Empiric intravenous magnesium, prophylactic antiarrhythmic therapy, long-term systemic anticoagulation, dipyridamole, vitamin or garlic or chelation therapy, hormone replacement therapy, acupuncture, or glucose-insulin-potassium infusions are **not indicated** unless targeting a specific indication such as sustained ventricular arrhythmias, atrial fibrillation, LV thrombus, severe menopausal symptoms, etc.
- Folate therapy for hyperhomocysteinemia, stress reduction techniques, and pharmacotherapy for depression (particularly in patients with new depression after ACS) may have some benefits in select patients but clinical outcome data are variable.[37,59]

Other Nonoperative Therapies
- **Tobacco cessation counseling, and pharmacologic therapy if needed, is imperative to reduce the risk of MI** in patients at risk of CAD or with known CAD (see Chapter 44).
- **Cardiac rehabilitation,** including both structured and nonstructured approaches to increasing cardiovascular exercise, has been demonstrated to reduce recurrent events in patients with known CAD.
- **Weight reduction** to <125% of ideal body mass—particularly in patients with the metabolic syndrome—also is associated with improved cardiovascular outcomes for patients with CAD.
- **Influenza vaccine** is recommended annually for patients with known cardiovascular disease.[52]
- **Enhanced external counterpulsation (EECP)** involves sequential inflations and deflations of cuffs on a subject's limbs, and for patients with refractory angina despite maximal medical and interventional therapy, symptoms may be improved after several weeks of daily therapy.[60]

Revascularization

- **In general, patients with acute MI or high-risk symptomatic CAD identified at diagnostic coronary angiography should undergo revascularization when feasible** from a technical and clinical standpoint.[41]
  - These individuals are usually hospitalized, and details of management are beyond the scope of this book.
  - Long-term management should include the antiplatelet, anti-ischemic, and disease-modifying therapies described above in conjunction with aggressive lifestyle modification and targets appropriate for patients with known CAD.
- **Indications for revascularization in ambulatory patients with IHD, or for those with chronic stable angina, are listed in Table 13.**[37]

TABLE 13	Indications and Levels of Evidence[a] for Revascularization in Chronic Stable Angina

Clinical and Angiographic Findings[b]	PCI[c]	CABG
Left main coronary stenosis ≥50%	No (Class III)[d]	Yes (Class I)
Obstructive CAD in three major arteries		
Normal LVSF	Yes (Class I)	Yes (Class I)
Abnormal LVSF	Yes (Class IIb)	Yes (Class I)
Concomitant diabetes mellitus	Yes (Class IIb)	Yes (Class I)
Obstructive CAD in two major arteries which include the proximal LAD		
Normal LVSF	Yes (Class I)	Yes (Class I)
Abnormal LVSF	Yes (Class IIb)	Yes (Class I)
Concomitant diabetes mellitus	Yes (Class IIb)	Yes (Class I)
Demonstrable ischemia on noninvasive stress testing	Yes (Class I)	Yes (Class I)
Obstructive CAD in proximal LAD alone	Yes (Class IIa)	Yes (Class IIa)
Obstructive CAD in one to two major arteries, not including the proximal LAD		
Large area of viable myocardium and high-risk criteria on noninvasive stress testing	Yes (Class I)	Yes (Class I)
Mild symptoms/unlikely to be caused by CAD	No (Class III)	No (Class III)
Inadequate trial of medical therapy and low-risk noninvasive findings (small area of viable myocardium, no ischemia on stress testing, etc.)	No (Class III)	No (Class III)
Recurrent obstruction despite prior PCI, with large area of viable myocardium and/or high-risk criteria on noninvasive stress testing	Yes (Class I)	Yes (Class I)
Obstructive CAD in patients who have not been successfully treated by medical therapy and who can undergo revascularization with acceptable risk	Yes (Class I)	Yes (Class I)
Obstruction of bypass grafts		
Multiple, especially if graft to LAD involved	Unclear	Yes (Class IIa)
Single/focal stenosis, or multiple in poor candidate for repeat heart surgery	Yes (Class IIa)	N/A
Borderline (e.g., 50%–60%) obstruction outside of left main and no ischemia on stress testing	No (Class III)	No (Class III)
Insignificant stenosis (<50% narrowing)	No (Class III)	No (Class III)

[a]Class I recommendation = evidence and/or general agreement that treatment is useful and effective; Class II recommendation = conflicting evidence and/or divergence of opinion; IIa implies weight of evidence is in favor of usefulness/efficacy; IIb implies usefulness/efficacy is less well established by available evidence/opinion; Class III recommendation = evidence and/or general agreement that treatment is NOT useful and effective, and may be harmful.
[b]Obstructive CAD is defined as stenosis ≥50% of the left main, stenosis ≥70% of other arteries or bypass grafts, or evidence of impaired flow by other invasive methods (e.g., intracoronary Doppler or flow wire assessment).
[c]Eligibility for PCI implies coronary anatomy suitable for catheter-based therapy.
[d]Unless very severe CAD with high-risk features and ineligibility for CABG.
CABG, coronary artery bypass surgery; CAD, coronary artery disease; LAD, left anterior descending coronary artery; LVSF, left ventricular systolic function; PCI, percutaneous coronary intervention.
Modified from Gibbons RJ, Abrams J, Chatterjee K, et al. ACC/AHA 2002 guideline update for the management of patients with chronic stable angina—summary article. *J Am Coll Cardiol* 2003;41:159–168.

Coronary Artery Bypass Surgery

- **Coronary artery bypass surgery (CABG)** is recommended for appropriate subjects with ≥50% stenosis of the left main coronary artery, or with ≥70% stenosis of other major vessels as described in Table 13.
  - Internal mammary artery grafts to the left anterior descending (LAD) artery have >90% patency rates at 10 years, versus vein graft patency rates of around 40% to 60% in older studies but approaching 75% on modern and more aggressive lipid therapies.[61–63]
  - Radial artery grafts have slightly lower short-term success rates in observational studies, but in radial grafts remaining patent after 1 year, long-term success is similar to that with internal mammary grafts.
  - Few studies have addressed medical therapy after CABG, but statins and aspirin appear to prevent recurrent cardiovascular events and reduce mortality rates in these patients.[64,65]

Percutaneous Coronary Intervention

- PCI using balloon angioplasty may clear the obstruction of a coronary artery, but most PCI procedures require concomitant placement of an intracoronary stent for maximal vessel patency and durability.
  - **In addition to lifelong aspirin, patients generally require at least one month of clopidogrel therapy after PCI with angioplasty or bare-metal stents, and at least 12 months of clopidogrel therapy after placement of a drug-eluting stent.**[66]
  - Longer duration of clopidogrel therapy is recommended (i.e., 12 to 24 months) in patients at higher risk of stent thrombosis (hypercoagulability, very long regions of stent placement, bifurcation stents, prior thrombosis).
  - In the absence of bleeding or upcoming surgery or other confounding issues, **clopidogrel should be prescribed for at least 12 months after acute MI—with or without concomitant PCI.**[41,67]
  - As described previously, ticlopidine may be substituted for subjects with significant allergy to clopidogrel, but monitoring of blood counts is imperative during treatment.

Stress Testing Postrevascularization

- **Routine stress testing or angiography is NOT indicated after revascularization.**[37]
  - However, repeat ischemic assessment or catheterization could be considered in the setting of specific patient subsets with unique elevations in risk for recurrent ischemic events, including subjects with
    - recurrent symptoms (especially within the first 6 months after PCI or CABG),
    - other changes in clinical status such as sustained ventricular arrhythmias or significant new LV systolic dysfunction,
    - specific high-risk features for restenosis and undergoing PCI (e.g., longstanding or labile DM—especially with neuropathy—which could mask anginal symptoms, end-stage renal disease, suboptimal angiographic results after PCI, bifurcation stents, multivessel PCI, or PCI to the proximal LAD).
- If symptoms recur or persist, **nuclear stress tests are relatively inaccurate for the first 2 months after PCI** because of perfusion abnormalities resulting in high rates of false-positive studies.[12]
- Most clinical trials demonstrate symptomatic improvement after PCI, but in general mortality benefits are seen only in patients undergoing PCI for acute MI.[41,67]

- Above all, **modification of underlying risk factors is imperative because revascularization does not modify the progression of atherosclerosis.**
  - Future angina prevalence and ischemic burden is associated more with progression of native CAD than with the type of revascularization performed.[68]

Treatment after Acute MI

- **Recurrent symptoms, hemodynamic instability or HF, or sustained ventricular arrhythmias after MI should prompt coronary angiography.[41,67]**
- **All eligible individuals should be treated with aspirin, β-blockers, statins, and ACE inhibitors after MI. Clopidogrel for 1 year is recommended if hemorrhagic risk is low.** Certain patient subsets may benefit from additional nitrate or anticoagulation therapy.
- Most patients may resume driving, sexual activity, commercial air travel, and return to work approximately 1 to 2 weeks after MI, although occupations involving strenuous physical activity may require a stress test prior to returning to full duty.

Risk Modification
- Diet and weight loss to <125% of ideal body weight when possible.
- Tobacco cessation to reduce reinfarction risk (see Chapter 44).
- LDL cholesterol should be lowered to at least <100 mg/dL, and to <70 mg/dL when possible.[69,70]
- In a large national registry, early statin initiation (i.e., prior to hospital discharge) was associated with improved 1-year survival after MI (Fig. 3).[71]
- Systolic BP should be targeted to be <130 mm Hg at all times.
- Hemoglobin A_{1c} level should be managed to <7%.

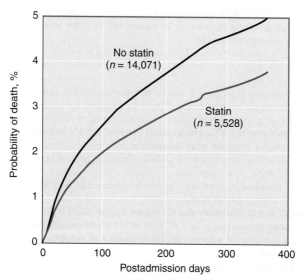

Figure 3. Predischarge statin therapy and survival after hospitalization for myocardial infarction. (From Stenestrand U, Wallentin L, for the Swedish Register of Cardiac Intensive Care (RIKS-HIA). Early statin treatment following acute myocardial infarction and 1-year survival. *JAMA* 2001;285:430–436, with permission.)

Cardiac Rehabilitation

- Cardiac rehabilitation in a structured format has been shown to reduce long-term mortality after MI or coronary revascularization procedures by approximately 25%.[11]
  - Initial goal is 50% to 60% of MPHR (estimated as 220 −age) for 10 to 30 minutes, at least three times per week.
  - Gradual escalation of exercise duration and heart rate to 75% to 85% of maximal predicted.
  - Supervision and hemodynamic surveillance is recommended initially, particularly in the elderly.
  - Warm-up and cool-down periods of 5 to 15 minutes are recommended.

Assessment of Cardiac Function

Stress Testing

- **If angiography was not performed during the MI, symptom-limited inpatient stress testing (or maximal stress testing 3 to 6 weeks later on medical therapy) is recommended to identify patients with high-risk features warranting late angiography.**[67]
  - Pharmacologic testing is considered safe after 48 to 72 hours for adenosine/dipyridamole, and after 72 to 96 hours for dobutamine.
  - High-risk findings include the following:
    - Anterior ischemia or large ischemic burden.
    - Stress-induced ventricular arrhythmias.
    - Significant LV systolic dysfunction or dilation during stress.
    - Hypotension or fall in systolic BP after exercise.
    - Recurrent symptoms concerning for ischemia.

Echocardiography

- **All patients surviving acute MI should undergo assessment of LV systolic function prior to hospital discharge, or shortly afterward, as LV ejection fraction is the benchmark predictor of long-term clinical outcome after MI.**
  - Survival at 1 year is >95% if LV systolic function is normal, whereas observational studies suggest that survival is closer to 50% with severe LV systolic dysfunction after MI.[72]
  - Ventriculography is frequently performed during cardiac catheterization, but patients managed noninvasively should be assessed by echocardiography or nuclear imaging (especially if concurrent stress testing is performed).
  - **If LV ejection fraction is <40%, patients should be treated with ACE inhibitors plus β-blockers (plus aldosterone blockade when appropriate)** to prevent adverse remodeling of ischemic/infarcted myocardium, and doses should be titrated upward as tolerated over several weeks as an outpatient.
  - Medically managed patients with LV systolic dysfunction after MI should be considered for angiography if feasible.
  - **Persistent LV systolic dysfunction after MI (ejection fraction <30% to 40%), despite aggressive medication titration over at least 40 days, should prompt evaluation for an implantable defibrillator in appropriate subjects with mild-to-moderate HF symptoms and otherwise good long-term prognosis.**[73]
  - Therapy for post-MI depression does not improve outcomes,[59] although subsets of clinical trials suggest greater benefits in patients treated for with new incident depression after MI, when compared with patients with prior history of depression.

REFERENCES

1. Rosamand W, Flegal K, Friday G, et al. Heart disease and stroke statistics—2007 update. *Circulation* 2007;115:e69–e171.
2. Expert Panel on Detection, Evaluation, and Treatment of High Blood Cholesterol in Adults. Executive summary of the third report of the National Cholesterol Education Program. *JAMA* 2001;285:2486–2497.
3. Haffner SM, Lehto S, Ronnemaa T, et al. Mortality from coronary heart disease in subjects with type 2 diabetes and in nondiabetic subjects with and without prior myocardial infarction. *N Engl J Med* 1998;339:229–234.
4. Hirsch AT, Haskal ZJ, Hertzer NR, et al. ACC/AHA 2005 guidelines for the management of patients with peripheral arterial disease: executive summary. *J Am Coll Cardiol* 2006;47: 1239–1312.
5. Yusuf S, Hawken S, Ôunpuu S, et al. Effect of potentially modifiable risk factors associated with myocardial infarction in 52 countries (the INTERHEART study): case-control study. *Lancet* 2004;364:937–952.
6. American Heart Association. Heart disease and stroke statistics—2006 update. *Circulation* 2006;113:85–151.
7. Grundy SM, Cleeman JI, Merz CN, et al. Implications of recent clinical trials for the National Cholesterol Education Program Adult Treatment Panel III guidelines. *J Am Coll Cardiol* 2004;44:720–732.
8. JNC-VII Executive Committee. The seventh report of the Joint National Committee on Prevention, Detection, Evaluation, and Treatment of High Blood Pressure. Bethesda, MD: National Heart, Lung, and Blood Institute, 2003. NIH publication 03-5233. Available at: http://www.nhlbi.nih.gov/guidelines.
9. Appel LJ, Brands MW, Daniels SR, et al. AHA scientific statement: dietary approaches to prevent and treat hypertension. *Hypertension* 2006;47:296–308.
10. U.S. Department of Health and Human Services. The health consequences of smoking: a report of the Surgeon General. Atlanta, GA: U.S. Department of Health and Human Services, Centers for Disease Control and Prevention, National Center for Chronic Disease Prevention and Health Promotion, Office on Smoking and Health, 2004. Also see www.cdc.gov/tobacco/data_statistics.
11. Haskell WL, Lee I, Pate RR, et al. Physical activity and public health: updated recommendation for adults from the American College of Sports Medicine and the American Heart Association. *Circulation* 2007;116:1081–1093.
12. Gibbons RJ, Balady GJ, Bricker JT, et al. ACC/AHA 2002 guideline update for exercise testing: summary article: a report of the American College of Cardiology/ American Heart Association Task Force on Practice Guidelines. *Circulation* 2002;106:1883–1892.
13. Kris-Etherton PM, Harris WS, Appel LJ, for the Nutrition Committee. AHA scientific statement: fish consumption, fish oil, omega-3 fatty acids, and cardiovascular disease. *Circulation* 2002;106:2747–2757.
14. Lichtenstein AH, Appel LJ, Brands M, et al. Diet and lifestyle recommendations revision 2006: a scientific statement from the American Heart Association Nutrition Committee. *Circulation* 2006;114:82–96.
15. Ford ES, Giles WH, Dietz WH. Prevalence of the metabolic syndrome among US adults: findings from the third National Health and Nutrition Examination Survey. *JAMA* 2002; 287:356–359.
16. Grundy SM, Cleeman JI, Daniels SR, et al. Diagnosis and management of the metabolic syndrome: an American Heart Association/National Heart, Lung, and Blood Institute scientific statement. *Curr Opin Cardiol* 2006;21:1–6.
17. Wilson PWF, Kannel WB, Silbershatz H, D'Agostino RB. Clustering of metabolic factors and coronary heart disease. *Arch Intern Med* 1999;159:1104–1109.
18. Poulter N. Coronary heart disease is a multifactorial disease. *Am J Hypertens* 1999;12(Suppl 1): 92–95.

19. Pearson TA, Mensah GA, Alexander RW, et al. Markers of inflammation and cardiovascular disease: application to clinical and public health practice: a statement for healthcare professionals from the Centers for Disease Control and Prevention and the American Heart Association. *Circulation* 2003;107:499–511.

20. Naghavi M, Falk E, Hecht HS, et al. From vulnerable plaque to vulnerable patient—part III: executive summary of the Screening for Heart Attack Prevention and Education (SHAPE) Task Force report. *Am J Cardiol* 2006;98(Suppl 1):2–15.

21. Ridker PM, Rifai N, Rose L, et al. Comparison of C-reactive protein and low-density lipoprotein cholesterol levels in the prediction of first cardiovascular events. *N Engl J Med* 2002;347:1557–1565.

22. Ridker PM, Cannon CP, Morrow D, et al. C-reactive protein levels and outcomes after statin therapy. *N Engl J Med* 2005;352:20–28.

23. Nissen SE, Tuzcu EM, Schoenhagen P, et al. Statin therapy, LDL cholesterol, C-reactive protein, and coronary artery disease. *N Engl J Med* 2005;352:29–38.

24. Folsom AR, Chambless LE, Ballantyne CM, et al. An assessment of incremental coronary risk prediction using C-reactive protein and other novel risk markers: the Atherosclerosis Risk in Communities study. *Arch Intern Med* 2006;166:1368–1373.

25. Miller M, Zhan M, Havas S. High attributable risk of elevated C-reactive protein level to conventional coronary heart disease risk factors: the third National Health and Nutrition Examination Survey. *Arch Intern Med* 2005;165:2063–2068.

26. Kullo IJ, Ballantyne CM. Conditional risk factors for atherosclerosis. *Mayo Clin Proc* 2005;80:219–230.

27. Arad Y, Spadaro LA, Roth M, et al. Treatment of asymptomatic adults with elevated coronary calcium scores with atorvastatin, vitamin C, and vitamin E: the St. Francis Heart Study Randomized Clinical Trial. *J Am Coll Cardiol* 2005;46:166–172.

28. Budoff MJ, Achenbach S, Blumenthal RS, et al. Assessment of coronary artery disease by cardiac computed tomography: a scientific statement from the American Heart Association Committee on Cardiovascular Imaging and Intervention, Council on Cardiovascular Radiology and Intervention, and Committee on Cardiac Imaging, Council on Clinical Cardiology. *Circulation* 2006;114:1761–1791.

29. U.S. Preventive Services Task Force. Screening for coronary heart disease: recommendation statement. *Ann Intern Med* 2004;140:569–572.

30. Maradit-Kremers H, Gabriel SE. Epidemiology. In: St. Clair EW, Pisetsky DS, Haynes BF, eds. Rheumatoid Arthritis. Philadelphia, PA: Lippincott Williams & Wilkins, 2004:1–10.

31. Solomon DH, Karlson EW, Rimm EB, et al. Cardiovascular morbidity and mortality in women diagnosed with rheumatoid arthritis. *Circulation* 2003;107:1303–1307.

32. Urowitz MB, Ibañez D, Gladman DD. Atherosclerotic vascular events in a single large lupus cohort: prevalence and risk factors. *J Rheumatol* 2007;34:70–75.

33. Lai S, Lai H, Celentano DD, et al. Factors associated with accelerated atherosclerosis in HIV-1-infected persons treated with protease inhibitors. *AIDS Patient Care & Stds* 2003; 17:211–219.

34. Lange RA, Hillis LD. Cardiovascular complications of cocaine use. *N Engl J Med* 2001;345: 351–358.

35. Campeau L. Grading of angina pectoris. *Circulation* 1976;54:522–523.

36. Fisher NDL, Williams GH. Hypertensive vascular disease. In: Kasper DL, Braunwald E, Fauci AS, et al., eds. Harrison's Principles of Internal Medicine. Chicago: McGraw-Hill, Inc., 2005:1463–1481.

37. Gibbons RJ, Abrams J, Chatterjee K, et al. ACC/AHA 2002 guideline update for the management of patients with chronic stable angina—summary article: a report of the American College of Cardiology/American Heart Association Task Force on practice guidelines, Committee on the Management of Patients With Chronic Stable Angina. *J Am Coll Cardiol* 2003;41:159–168.

38. Mark DB, Hlatky MA, Lee KL, et al. Localizing coronary artery obstructions with the exercise treadmill test. *Ann Intern Med* 1987;106:53–55.

39. Chaitman BR. Exercise stress testing. In: Zipes DP, Libby P, Bonow RO, eds. Braunwald's Heart Disease: A Textbook of Cardiovascular Medicine. Philadelphia: Elsevier Saunders, 2005:153–178.

40. Mark DB, Shaw L, Harrell FE, et al. Prognostic value of a treadmill exercise score in outpatients with suspected coronary artery disease. *N Engl J Med* 1991;325:849–853.

41. Anderson JL, Adams CD, Antman EM, et al. ACC/AHA 2007 guidelines for the management of patients with unstable angina/non-ST-elevation myocardial infarction—executive summary. *J Am Coll Cardiol* 2007;50:652–726.

42. Califf RM, Armstrong PW, Carver JR, et al. Task Force 5: stratification of patients into high, medium, and low risk subgroups for purposes of risk factor management. *J Am Coll Cardiol* 1996;27:1007–1019.

43. Ringqvist I, Fisher LD, Mock M, et al. Prognostic value of angiographic indices of coronary artery disease from the Coronary Artery Surgery Study (CASS). *J Clin Invest* 1983;71: 1854–1866.

44. Emond M, Mock MB, Davis KB, et al. Long-term survival of medically treated patients in the Coronary Artery Surgery Study (CASS) Registry. *Circulation* 1994;90:2645–2657.

45. The Veterans Administration Coronary Artery Bypass Cooperative Study Group. Eleven year survival in the Veterans Administration randomized trial of coronary bypass surgery for stable angina. *N Engl J Med* 1984;311:1333–1339.

46. U.S. Preventive Services Task Force. Aspirin for the primary prevention of cardiovascular events: recommendation and rationale. *Ann Intern Med* 2002;136:157–160.

47. Kris-Etherton PM, Lichtenstein AH, Howard BV, et al. Antioxidant vitamin supplements and cardiovascular disease. *Circulation* 2004;110:637–641.

48. Pearson TA, Blair SN, Daniels SR, et al. AHA guidelines for primary prevention of cardiovascular disease and stroke: 2002 update: consensus panel guide to comprehensive risk reduction for adult patients without coronary or other atherosclerotic vascular diseases. *Circulation* 2002;106:388–391.

49. Yusuf S, Zhao F, Mehta SR, et al. The Clopidogrel in Unstable Angina to Prevent Recurrent Events (CURE) Trial Investigators. *N Engl J Med* 2001;345:494–502.

50. Smith SC, Feldman TE, Hirshfeld JW, et al. ACC/AHA/SCAI 2005 guideline update for percutaneous coronary intervention—summary article. *Circulation* 2006;113:156–175.

51. Bhatt DL, Fox FAA, Hacke W, et al. Clopidogrel and aspirin versus aspirin alone for the prevention of atherothrombotic events. *N Engl J Med* 2006;354:1706–1717.

52. Smith SC, Allen J, Blair SN, et al. AHA/ACC guidelines for secondary prevention for patients with coronary and other atherosclerotic vascular disease: 2006 update. *Circulation* 2006;113:2363–2372.

53. Stone PH, Gratsiansky NA, Blokhin A, et al., for the ERICA Investigators. Antianginal efficacy of ranolazine when added to treatment with amlodipine: the ERICA (Efficacy of Ranolazine in Chronic Angina) trial. *J Am Coll Cardiol* 2006;48:566–575.

54. Chaitman BR, Pepine CJ, Parker JO, et al., for the Combination Assessment of Ranolazine In Stable Angina (CARISA) Investigators. Effects of ranolazine with atenolol, amlodipine, or diltiazem on exercise tolerance and angina frequency in patients with severe chronic angina: a randomized controlled trial. *JAMA* 2004;291:309–316.

55. Morrow DA, Scirica BM, Karwatowska-Prokopczuk E, et al., for the MERLIN-TIMI 36 Trial Investigators. Effects of ranolazine on recurrent cardiovascular events in patients with non-ST-elevation acute coronary syndromes. *JAMA* 2007;297:1775–1783.

56. LaRosa JC, Grundy SM, Waters DD, et al., for the Treating to New Targets (TNT) Investigators. Intensive lipid lowering with atorvastatin in patients with stable coronary disease. *N Engl J Med* 2005;352:1425–1435.

57. Crestor (rosuvastatin calcium) [package insert]. Wilmington, DE: AstraZeneca Pharmaceuticals LP, 2007. Also see FDA website: http://www.fda.gov/cder/rdmt/ESCY07AP.htm for summary of 2007 medication updates.

58. Pitt B, Remme W, Zannad F, et al., for the Eplerenone Post-Acute Myocardial Infarction Heart Failure Efficacy and Survival Study (EPHESUS) Investigators. Eplerenone, a selective

aldosterone blocker, in patients with left ventricular dysfunction after myocardial infarction. *N Engl J Med* 2003;348:1309–1321.

59. Carney RM, Jaffe AS. Treatment of depression following acute myocardial infarction [editorial]. *JAMA* 2002;288:750–751.

60. Shea ML, Conti CR, Arora RR. An update on enhanced external counterpulsation. *Clin Cardiol* 2005;28:115–118.

61. Lytle BW, Cosgrove DM. Coronary artery bypass surgery. *Curr Prob Surg* 1992;29: 743–807.

62. Bourassa MG, Fisher LD, Campeau L, et al. Long-term fate of bypass grafts: the Coronary Artery Surgery Study (CASS) and Montreal Heart Institute experiences. *Circulation* 1985;72(Suppl IV):V71–V78.

63. The Post-Coronary Artery Bypass Graft Trial Investigators. The effect of aggressive lowering of low-density lipoprotein cholesterol levels and low-dose anticoagulation on obstructive changes in saphenous-vein coronary-artery bypass grafts. *N Engl J Med* 1997; 336:153–162.

64. Okrainec K, Platt R, Pilote L, Eisenberg MJ. Cardiac medical therapy in patients after undergoing coronary artery bypass graft surgery: a review of randomized controlled trials. *J Am Coll Cardiol* 2005;45:177–184.

65. Pan W, Pintar T, Anton J, et al. Statins are associated with a reduced incidence of perioperative mortality after coronary artery bypass graft surgery. *Circulation* 2004;110(Suppl II):II45–II49.

66. Grines CL, Bonow RO, Casey DE Jr, et al. Prevention of premature discontinuation of dual antiplatelet therapy in patients with coronary artery stents: a science advisory from the American Heart Association, American College of Cardiology, Society for Cardiovascular Angiography and Interventions, American College of Surgeons, and American Dental Association, with representation from the American College of Physicians. *J Am Coll Cardiol* 2007;49:734–739.

67. Antman EM, Anbe DT, Armstrong PW, et al. ACC/AHA guidelines for the management of patients with ST-elevation myocardial infarction—executive summary. *J Am Coll Cardiol* 2004;44:671–719.

68. Alderman EL, Kip KE, Whitlow PL, et al. Native coronary disease progression exceeds failed revascularization as cause of angina after five years in the Bypass Angioplasty Revascularization Investigation (BARI). *J Am Coll Cardiol* 2004;44:766–774.

69. Cannon CP, Braunwald E, McCabe CH, et al., for the Pravastatin or Atorvastatin Evaluation and Infection Therapy-Thrombolysis in Myocardial Infarction 22 (PROVE-IT-TIMI-22) Investigators. Intensive versus moderate lipid lowering with statins after acute coronary syndromes. *N Engl J Med* 2004;350:1495–1504.

70. Schwartz GG, Olsson AG, Ezekowitz MD, et al., for the Myocardial Ischemia Reduction with Aggressive Cholesterol Lowering (MIRACL) Study Investigators. Effects of atorvastatin on early recurrent ischemic events in acute coronary syndromes. *JAMA* 2001;285: 1711–1718.

71. Stenestrand U, Wallentin L, for the Swedish Register of Cardiac Intensive Care (RIKS-HIA). Early statin treatment following acute myocardial infarction and 1-year survival. *JAMA* 2001;285:430–436.

72. Deedwania PC, Amsterdam EA, Vagelos RH. Evidence-based, cost-effective risk stratification and management after myocardial infarction. *Arch Intern Med* 1997;157:273–280.

73. Zipes DP, Camm AJ, Borggrefe M, et al., for the Writing Committee to Develop Guidelines for Management of Patients With Ventricular Arrhythmias and the Prevention of Sudden Cardiac Death. ACC/AHA/ESC 2006 guidelines for management of patients with ventricular arrhythmias and the prevention of sudden cardiac death—executive summary. *J Am Coll Cardiol* 2006;48:e247–346.

5 Heart Failure and Cardiomyopathy

Joel D. Schilling and Michael W. Rich

HEART FAILURE

General Principles

- The primary goals of heart failure (HF) management in the outpatient setting are to improve patient symptoms, reduce mortality and hospitalizations, and delay disease progression.
- The role of the primary physician is to appropriately diagnose HF in at-risk or symptomatic individuals and to initiate management. Early referral to a cardiologist may also be appropriate in selected patients.

Definition

- HF is a clinical syndrome characterized by the inability of the heart to support the metabolic needs of the body while maintaining normal intracardiac filling pressures.
- The primary clinical manifestations of HF are symptoms and signs of increased fluid retention (e.g., pulmonary/peripheral edema, pleural effusions, ascites) and/or reduced cardiac output (e.g., fatigue, oliguria, hypotension).

Classification

The classification of HF into disease stage and symptom class can help direct optimal patient management and assist in assessing prognosis.

American College of Cardiology Staging

- **Stage 1:** Patients at risk for developing HF (hypertension [HTN], diabetes mellitus [DM], coronary artery disease [CAD], family history, exposures to cardiotoxins) but with no structural heart disease.
- **Stage 2:** Patients with evidence of structural heart disease (left ventricular hypertrophy [LVH], decreased ejection fraction [EF], valvular disease) but without clinical evidence of HF.
- **Stage 3:** Patients with clinically evident HF.
- **Stage 4:** Patients with end stage HF.

New York Heart Association Functional Class

New York Heart Association (NYHA) functional class is a standard tool for assessing the severity of patient symptoms:

- **Class I:** No limitations of activity; no symptoms during ordinary activity.
- **Class II:** Mild limitation of activity; comfortable at rest and with mild exertion.
- **Class III:** Marked limitation of activity; comfortable at rest, but ordinary activity causes dyspnea and fatigue.

- **Class IV:** Unable to carry out any physical activity without discomfort; HF symptoms at rest.

Epidemiology

- HF is a very common disorder. >5 million people in the United States have a diagnosis of HF and there are upwards of 550,000 new diagnoses each year.[1]
- There are >1 million hospitalizations for HF annually, and it is the number one admitting diagnosis for patients >65.[2]
- Up to 30% of patients hospitalized with an HF exacerbation will be rehospitalized within the subsequent 3 months.[3]
- Mortality from HF ranges from 10% to 50% within 1 year following diagnosis depending on disease severity.[3]
- Up to 50% of patients who present with clinical HF have preserved left ventricular (LV) systolic function (EF ≥40%). Three-month mortality is similar in patients with preserved or reduced LV systolic function (Fig. 1).[4]

Etiology

- The potential causes of HF are diverse. In the United States, CAD, HTN, and DM are the most common disorders leading to cardiac dysfunction.

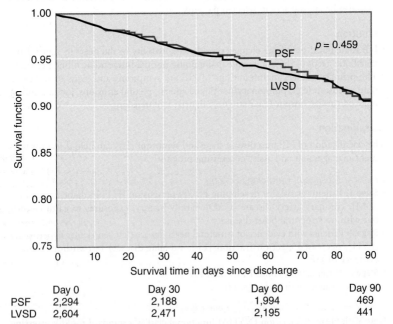

	Day 0	Day 30	Day 60	Day 90
PSF	2,294	2,188	1,994	469
LVSD	2,604	2,471	2,195	441

Figure 1. Mortality following hospitalization in heart failure patients with systolic dysfunction (LVSD) or preserved systolic function (PSF). (From Yancy CW, Lopatin M, Stevenson LW, et al. Clinical presentation, management, and in-hospital outcomes of patients admitted with acute decompensated heart failure with preserved systolic function: a report from the Acute Decompensated Heart Failure National Registry (ADHERE) database. *J Am Coll Cardiol* 2006;47:76–84, with permission.)

TABLE 1	Causes of Heart Failure (HF)
HF with Systolic Dysfunction	**HF with Preserved Systolic Function**
Coronary artery disease	Hypertension
Hypertension	Diabetic cardiomyopathy (early)
Myocarditis	Coronary artery disease
Viral	Restrictive cardiomyopathy
Autoimmune	Amyloidosis
Giant cell	Hemochromatosis
Diabetic cardiomyopathy (late)	Sarcoidosis
Familial/genetic cardiomyopathy	Genetic
Toxin induced	Constrictive pericarditis
Chemotherapy (anthracyclines, trastuzumab)	Right HF (in the absence of left HF)
Cocaine	Pulmonary hypertension
Alcohol	High-output HF
Postpartum cardiomyopathy	Hyperthyroidism
Valvular cardiomyopathy	Arteriovenous malformations
Tachycardia-induced cardiomyopathy	Anemia
Idiopathic	

- The differential diagnosis for HF according to LV systolic function is shown in Table 1.

Risk Factors

- Recognition of patients at risk for HF is important. The early initiation of behavioral interventions and HF therapies can significantly improve patient outcomes and delay or prevent the onset of clinical disease.
- The primary modifiable risk factors associated with HF are HTN, DM, and CAD; therefore, identification and treatment of these diseases and their risk factors (e.g., smoking, obesity, physical inactivity, dyslipidemia) is critical.
- Other factors associated with increased risk of HF include a family history of cardiomyopathy and exposure to cardiotoxins such as chemotherapy drugs (especially anthracyclines and trastuzumab), alcohol, or illicit drugs (especially cocaine).

Pathophysiology

- HF is the consequence of an acute or chronic injury to one or more cardiac structures that leads to impaired cardiac function and diminished cardiac reserve.
- Early in the course of HF, the renin-angiotensin-aldosterone system (RAAS), the sympathetic nervous system, and the vasopressin system are activated to maintain normal cardiac output and tissue perfusion. However, these initially adaptive neurohumoral pathways ultimately lead to further cardiac injury. This process is known as **adverse myocardial remodeling.**

Diagnosis

- HF is a clinical diagnosis based on patient symptoms and physical findings consistent with cardiac dysfunction.

- Laboratory testing and echocardiography are also important tools to aid in the diagnosis and characterization of patients presenting with HF syndromes.

Clinical Presentation

History
- In patients with **new-onset HF,** the history should probe for potential causes:
  - **Ischemic heart disease:** chest pain, history of myocardial infarction (MI), presence of CAD risk factors.
  - **Myocarditis:** recent viral illness, rheumatologic symptoms.
  - **Genetic cardiomyopathy:** family history of HF or sudden death.
  - **Toxic cardiomyopathy:** history of chemotherapy, alcohol or drug abuse.
  - **Hypertensive cardiomyopathy:** history of HTN and intensity of HTN treatment.
  - **Diabetic cardiomyopathy:** known history or family history of DM, polyuria.
  - **Peripartum cardiomyopathy:** recent pregnancy.
  - **Constrictive pericarditis:** history of trastuzumab, chest irradiation, or pericarditis.
  - **Valvular heart disease:** history of a heart murmur, rheumatic fever.
  - **Infectious endocarditis:** fever, chills, recent dental work or other procedures.
- In patients with **established HF,** there are three primary objectives of the history:
  - **Define current patient functional status:**
    - How far can the patient walk before becoming short of breath?
    - How many flights of stairs can the patient climb?
    - Can the patient perform activities of daily living?
    - Compare with previous visits to assess rate of decline.
    - Determine the patient's NYHA functional class.
  - **Assess patient volume status:**
    - Determine presence of paroxysmal nocturnal dyspnea (PND), orthopnea, lower extremity (LE) edema, increased abdominal girth, and increased weight.
  - **Determine adherence to diet and medications.**

Physical Examination
- At each visit, heart rate, respiratory rate, blood pressure, and body weight should be reviewed to direct therapeutic changes.
- Another important function of the physical exam in an initial evaluation is to identify possible causes of HF (e.g., valvular disease, pericardial disease).

Assessment of Volume Status
- **Jugular venous distention (JVD):** Defined as jugular venous pulse >3 to 4 cm above the sternal notch with the patient at 45 degrees. JVD usually correlates with elevated left-sided intracardiac filling pressures unless pulmonary HTN, pericardial constriction, or severe tricuspid regurgitation is present.
- **S3:** A low-frequency heart sound present following S2 that signifies impaired rapid, early diastolic filling of the LV. This finding is specific but not sensitive for determining the presence of LV diastolic volume overload.
- **Pulmonary crackles:** A sign of fluid accumulation in the alveolar air spaces. Present only in ~50% to 60% of HF patients with elevated intracardiac filling pressures due to pulmonary lymphatic compensation. Crackles can also be present in other forms of lung disease (e.g., pneumonia, pulmonary fibrosis).
- **Hepatomegaly/ascites:** Reflects elevated central venous pressure (CVP) from right heart volume overload.
- **LE pitting edema:** A late sign of fluid overload that is ~30% sensitive for diagnosing hypervolumia in HF patients; not a specific sign of HF as many other diseases can produce LE edema.

- **Narrow pulse pressure and pulsus alternans:** Markers of significantly reduced cardiac stroke volume.

Diagnostic Testing

Laboratories
- Laboratory testing in HF can help in determining etiology but is more important for defining disease-modifying comorbidities such as DM, renal insufficiency, and anemia.
- The initial lab evaluation for all patients with newly diagnosed HF should include a **complete blood cell count (CBC), basic metabolic panel (BMP), liver function tests, fasting lipid panel, fasting blood glucose, urinalysis (UA), and thyroid-stimulating hormone (TSH).**
- In select patients with HF of unknown etiology, serum iron studies and tests for HIV and hepatitis C should also be considered.

B-Type Natriuretic Peptide
- **B-type natriuretic peptide (BNP)** is released from myocytes in response to wall stress. A level >400 pg/mL is diagnostic of HF (in the absence of chronic kidney disease), whereas a level <100 pg/mL has a high negative predictive value for active HF.
- BNP levels have also been shown to correlate with the risk of future adverse advents in HF patients.
- **A BNP level is thus useful when the diagnosis of HF is uncertain and for assessing prognosis.**

Electrocardiography
The 12-lead electrocardiography (ECG) is a critical point of care test to look for evidence of myocardial ischemia or infarction, LVH, arrhythmias, and interventricular conduction delay (e.g., left bundle branch block [LBBB]).

Imaging
Chest Radiography
- The hallmarks of HF on chest radiography (CXR) are cardiomegaly, bilateral pulmonary infiltrates, and pleural effusions (R > L). In addition, the CXR evaluates for other potential causes of dyspnea such as pneumothorax, pneumonia, or chronic lung disease.
- Up to 50% of patients with chronic HF and elevated cardiac filling pressures have clear lung fields on CXR; therefore, this finding should not be used to exclude a diagnosis of HF.

Echocardiography
- The **echocardiogram is a critical component in the evaluation and management of HF.** This imaging test provides information regarding LV and right ventricular (RV) systolic and diastolic function, LVH, valvular disease, pericardial disease, and pulmonary artery pressures.
- Many aspects of disease management and prognosis are determined by the information obtained from the echocardiogram.

Diagnostic Procedures
Myocardial Perfusion Imaging
- Although not a standard test in the evaluation of HF, myocardial perfusion imaging (MPI) with thallium and sestamibi can be used in patients at lower risk for CAD to evaluate for ischemia.
- MPI may be used to direct revascularization in patients with a known ischemic cardiomyopathy by identifying areas of ischemic but viable myocardium (i.e., hibernating myocardium).

Coronary Angiography
- **All patients with unexplained HF and/or who have risk factors for CAD should have an evaluation for ischemia.**
- Coronary angiography is the gold standard for assessing occlusive coronary disease and should be considered unless the patient is a poor candidate (coagulopathy, renal failure, etc.) or the probability of CAD is extremely low.

Cardiac CT and MRI
- These newer imaging modalities may have a role in the initial assessment of HF in the future. Both CT and magnetic resonance angiography could provide a noninvasive approach to evaluate for CAD in new-onset HF.
- Magnetic resonance imaging (MRI) also has potential value in identifying patients with myocarditis or other specific forms of cardiomyopathy (e.g., amyloidosis, sarcoidosis, arrhythmogenic right ventricular dysplasia [ARVD]).
- Additional studies are needed to define the role of these imaging techniques in HF.

Endomyocardial Biopsy
- Routine endomyocardial biopsy for the evaluation of new-onset HF is not recommended. In most cases, the results are nondiagnostic and/or fail to impact management decisions.
- The use of endomyocardial biopsy can be considered in select patients in whom there is clinical suspicion for sarcoidosis, giant cell myocarditis, or amyloidosis.

Treatment of Chronic Heart Failure

- Numerous clinical trials have investigated pharmacologic therapy in chronic HF over the past 30 years. The results of these trials have led to the construction of detailed practice guidelines issued by the American College of Cardiology (ACC), the American Heart Association (AHA), the Heart Failure Society of America (HFSA), and the European Society of Cardiology (ESC) to help optimize outcomes in HF patients.
- The **goals of treatment** are as follows:
  - To improve symptoms, maximize functional status, and improve quality of life.
  - To reduce mortality.
  - To minimize HF hospitalizations.
  - To slow down the progression of disease.
- Patients with ischemic or valvular cardiomyopathy should be evaluated for revascularization (via percutaneous intervention or surgery) and valve repair/replacement, respectively.
- The classification of HF patients into Stages A to D can be used to direct the behavioral, pharmacologic, and device therapy that should be employed to reduce disease progression, hospitalizations, and mortality (Fig. 2).

Medications

Angiotensin-Converting Enzyme Inhibitors
- Angiotensin II is a potent vasoconstrictor that also promotes cardiac fibrosis, myocyte injury, and fluid retention.
- Angiotensin-converting enzyme inhibitors (ACE-I) act by decreasing the conversion of angiotensin I to angiotensin II, thereby attenuating adverse myocardial remodeling and improving renal fluid and electrolyte handling. In addition, ACE-Is increase circulating levels of kinins, which may have beneficial effects in HF.

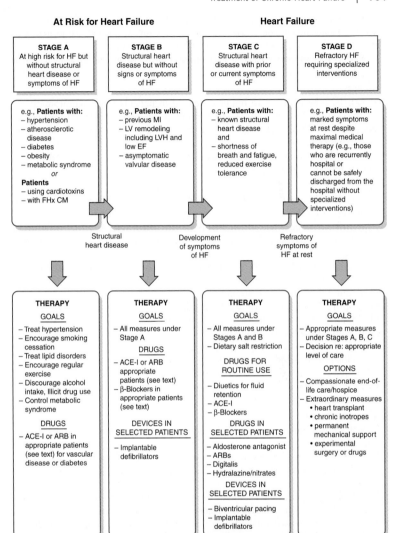

Figure 2. Heart failure (HF) classification by disease stage with appropriate therapeutic goals. ACE-I, angiotensin-converting enzyme inhibitor; ARB, angiotensin receptor blocker; EF, ejection fraction; FMHx CM, family history of cardiomyopathy; LV, left ventricular; LVH, left ventricular hypertrophy; MI, myocardial infarction. (From Hunt S, Abraham WT, Chin MH, et al. ACC/AHA 2005 guideline update for the diagnosis and management of chronic heart failure in the adult: a report of the American College of Cardiology/American Heart Association Task Force on Practice Guidelines. *Circulation* 2005:112:e154–e235, with permission.)

- ACE-Is have become a cornerstone of therapy for patients with systolic dysfunction (EF ≤40%). Clinical trials have demonstrated a survival benefit associated with multiple ACE-Is, suggesting their value in HF is a class effect.
- **All patients with systolic dysfunction should receive ACE-I therapy unless contraindications are present.**

Evidence

- ACE-Is have been shown to improve survival in patients with asymptomatic LV dysfunction (SOLVD prevention trial) and moderate-to-severe HF (SOLVD treatment trial, CONSENSUS-1)[5] and in the setting of post-MI LV dysfunction (SAVE, TRACE, AIRE).[6]
- ACE-Is reduce mortality by ~25% and have favorable effects on hospitalizations, exercise tolerance, and quality of life.

Practical Use

- ACE-Is should be started at a low dose and gradually titrated over several weeks to the dosage levels shown to be effective in the clinical trials (see below).
- Captopril has a short half-life and thus can be useful for the initial titration of ACE-I therapy, particularly in patients with borderline blood pressure or renal function.
- The initial and goal doses of ACE-Is approved for treatment of HF in the United States are as follows:
  - Captopril: 6.25 mg tid → 50 mg tid.
  - Enalapril: 2.5 mg bid → 10 to 20 mg bid.
  - Lisinopril: 2.5 to 5 mg qd → 20 to 40 mg qd.
  - Quinapril: 5 mg bid → 20 mg bid.
  - Ramipril: 1.25 to 2.5 mg qd → 10 mg qd.
  - Trandolapril: 1 mg qd → 4 mg qd.
  - Perindopril: 2 mg qd → 8 to 16 mg qd.
- Serum creatinine and potassium levels should be checked within 2 to 4 weeks of initiating therapy or increasing the dosage.

Adverse Reactions

- ACE-Is are well tolerated, with 85% to 90% of patients able to use these agents long-term.
- The most common adverse reactions associated with ACE-I include cough (10%), hypotension, hyperkalemia, and renal insufficiency. A rare but serious complication is angioedema.
- ACE-Is are teratogenic and should be used with caution in women of childbearing age; they should be **discontinued immediately** if pregnancy is a possibility.
- If possible, nonsteroidal anti-inflammatory drugs (NSAIDs) should be avoided in patients taking ACE-Is because they increase the risk of acute renal failure and hyperkalemia (particularly in the elderly and those with underlying renal insufficiency). NSAIDS also antagonize the beneficial effects of ACE-Is.

Angiotensin Receptor Blockers

- Angiotensin receptor blockers (ARBs) inhibit the RAAS by binding to and inhibiting the type I angiotensin II receptor. In general, comparable hemodynamic and remodeling effects have been seen with these agents when compared with ACE-Is.
- Similar to ACE-Is, ARBs have been shown to provide significant benefits in patients with systolic LV dysfunction.

- **ARBs are an acceptable alternative to ACE-Is in patients intolerant of ACE-I therapy** (because of cough or angioedema). However, the risks of hypotension, hyperkalemia, and renal insufficiency are similar with ACE-Is and ARBs.

Evidence
- ARBs have been shown to benefit patients with chronic HF (CHARM,[7] Val-HeFT[8]) and those with post-MI LV dysfunction (VALIANT).[9] In all of these studies, ACE-I-intolerant patients benefited from ARB therapy, and the magnitude of benefit was similar to that seen with ACE-Is.
- CHARM-Preserved demonstrated a reduction in hospitalizations but no mortality benefit in patients with HF and preserved systolic function (PSF).[10]

Practical Use
- Analogous to ACE-Is, ARBs should be started at a low dose and titrated slowly to goal dosage.
- The initial and goal doses for the ARBs indicated for HF are listed below:
  - Valsartan: 40 mg bid → 160 mg bid.
  - Candesartan: 4 mg qd → 32 mg qd.
- Serum creatinine and potassium levels should be checked within 2 to 4 weeks of initiating therapy or increasing the dose.

Adverse Reactions
- Similar to ACE-Is, hypotension, hyperkalemia, renal insufficiency, and teratogencity can be observed with ARBs. Unlike ACE-Is, ARB therapy is not associated with increased risk of cough.
- The incidence of angioedema is reduced with ARB therapy; however, cases have been reported.

Combination Therapy with ACE-Is and ARBs
- ACE-Is and ARBs attenuate the RAAS through two distinct mechanisms, leading to the hypothesis that combination therapy might provide additional benefit to patients with HF.
- Combination therapy was investigated in subgroups of VALIANT and Val-HeFT and in CHARM-Added.[11] VALIANT showed no benefit of combination therapy, but there was an increased incidence of hyperkalemia and hypotension. CHARM Added demonstrated a 15% reduction in death or hospitalization with combination therapy, whereas Val-HeFT showed benefit only in patients not receiving a β-blocker.
- Accordingly, **the addition of an ARB can be considered in *select* patients already receiving ACE-I and β-blocker therapy who have persistent HF symptoms or recurrent hospitalizations.**
- If combination therapy is employed, vigilant monitoring of potassium and blood pressure is mandatory.
- The combination of an ACE-I, ARB, and aldosterone receptor antagonist should be avoided because of a high risk for hyperkalemia.

β-Adrenergic Receptor Blockers
- Because of their negative inotropic effects, β-blockers were once contraindicated in patients with HF. However, it is now recognized that chronic activation of β-adrenergic receptors can lead to arrhythmias, myocyte apoptosis, and adverse LV remodeling.
- The long-term benefits of β-blocker therapy are now established in patients with chronic HF. **ALL patients with chronic HF and LV systolic dysfunction should receive a β-blocker in the absence of contraindications.**

Evidence

- β-Blockers have been shown to improve survival and HF symptoms in patients with mild, moderate, or severe chronic HF (MERIT-HF,[12] COPERNICUS,[13] US Carvedilol HF trials,[14] and CIBIS I and II[15]) and in the post-MI setting (CAPRICORN[16]).
- Based on data from prospective, randomized trials, **carvedilol**[17] (β_1-, β_2-, α-antagonist), **metoprolol** succinate (β_1-antagonist), or **bisoprolol** (β_1-antagonist) should be used for treatment of chronic HF.

Practical Use

- β-Blockers should be initiated once patients are clinically **euvolemic and already on afterload reducing medications.**
- β-Blocker therapy should be started at a low dose and gradually titrated to the goal dose over a period of several weeks.
- During β-blocker titration, increased fluid retention can occur. This can usually be managed by a temporary increase in diuretic therapy.
- In patients receiving β-blocker therapy who present with decompensated HF, the β-blocker **should be continued at the same or slightly reduced dosage,** as discontinuation has been associated with worse outcomes.
- The initial and goal doses of the recommended β-blockers are listed below:
  - Carvedilol: 3.125 bid → 25 to 50 mg bid.
  - Carvedilol CR: 10 mg qd → 80 mg qd.
  - Metoprolol succinate: 12.5 to 25 mg qd to → 200 mg qd.
  - Bisoprolol: 1.25 mg qd → 5 to 10 mg qd.

Adverse Reactions

- β-Blockers are contraindicated in patients with severe decompensated HF, cardiogenic shock, marked bradycardia (heart rate <40 to 45 bpm), hypotension (systemic blood pressure <90 mm Hg), advanced AV nodal block, or severe bronchospastic lung disease.
- β-Blockers can cause fatigue (usually worse during the first 1 to 2 weeks of therapy), bradycardia/heart block, hypotension, fluid retention, and erectile dysfunction.
- In patients with reactive airway disease, β-blockers can worsen bronchospasm. However, this problem can be minimized by using β_1-selective agents (e.g., metoprolol succinate, bisoprolol).

Aldosterone Antagonists

- The mineralocorticoid aldosterone is now recognized as an important contributor to the pathogenesis of HF. In addition to increasing renal sodium retention, aldosterone has been shown to directly affect the myocardium, promoting fibrosis and adverse remodeling.
- **The use of an aldosterone receptor antagonist is recommended therapy for patients already on ACE-I and β-blockers who have moderate-to-severe HF symptoms and/or frequent HF hospitalizations.**
- An aldosterone antagonist should also be **strongly considered** for patients with an EF of ≤40% after an acute MI.

Evidence

- In the RALES trial, the aldosterone antagonist spironolactone was associated with a 30% reduction in mortality and HF hospitalizations in patients with NYHA Class III to IV HF symptoms and EF of ≤30%.[18]
- The EPHESUS trial studied the selective aldosterone receptor blocker eplerenone in patients with LV dysfunction following an MI.[19] Eplerenone was added to standard

therapy with β-blockers and ACE-I and was found to be associated with an additional 15% reduction in mortality over 1 year.

Practical Use
- Aldosterone receptor antagonists should be started at a low dose in the elderly and in those with impaired renal function.
- **If the baseline potassium level is >5.0 mEq/L or the serum creatinine level is >2.5 mg/dL, then these agents should be avoided because of the risk of life-threatening hyperkalemia.**
- Potassium supplementation should be decreased or stopped when an aldosterone antagonists is initiated.
- After starting therapy, potassium level should be checked within 1 week, and sooner if the patient has a potassium level of >4.5 mEq/L or a serum creatinine level of >1.5 mg/dL prior to initiating therapy.
- The starting and goal doses of the available aldosterone receptor blockers are listed below:
  - Spironolactone: 12.5 to 25 mg qd → 25 mg qd.
  - Eplerenone: 25 mg qd → 25 to 50 mg qd.

Adverse Reactions
- **The most serious adverse event associated with aldosterone blockade is hyperkalemia.** Since the publication of the RALES trial, the number of hospital admissions for hyperkalemia in HF patients has more than doubled. Vigilant monitoring of potassium is mandatory for patients receiving these medications.
- Spironolactone is also associated with gynecomastia in up to 10% of patients; eplerenone is not associated with this side effect.

Digoxin
- Digitalis glycosides were one of the first therapies used in the treatment of HF. Digoxin acts by inhibiting Na-K ATPase, which leads to an increase in intracellular calcium, thereby increasing cardiac contractility.
- **Digoxin should be considered as adjunctive therapy for HF patients already on ACE-I and β-blockers who have persistent HF symptoms, frequent hospitalizations, or chronic atrial fibrillation.**

Evidence
- The largest trial evaluating the effects of digoxin in HF was the DIG trial.[20] This study demonstrated no survival benefit associated with digoxin; however, **HF hospitalizations were reduced.** In post hoc analysis, digoxin levels <1 ng/mL were associated with more favorable outcomes.
- Withdrawal of digoxin from patients taking this medication can result in increased HF symptoms and hospitalizations.[21]

Practical Use
- The standard dose of digoxin for HF is 0.125 to 0.25 mg daily. The use of a loading dose is not necessary for the management of HF. The therapeutic digoxin level is 0.5 to 0.9 ng/mL.
- In patients with renal insufficiency, lower dosing may be necessary to prevent toxicity. The use of 0.125 mg three times per week is often sufficient in these patients.

Adverse Events
- **Digoxin toxicity can be life threatening** and usually manifests with cardiac abnormalities, gastrointestinal disturbances (e.g., nausea, vomiting, diarrhea), or neurologic complaints (e.g., lethargy, altered mental status, visual disturbances). The ECG may

be abnormal (e.g., paroxysmal atrial tachycardia with block, accelerated junction rhythm, bidirectional ventricular tachycardia [VT], atrial fibrillation with regular ventricular response). In severe cases, the patient can present with sustained VT or high-degree AV block.

- The treatment of digoxin toxicity is dependent on the severity of the cardiac manifestations. Electrolyte disorders must be corrected (i.e., potassium and magnesium), and the use of temporary cardiac pacing, phenytoin, and/or digoxin-specific Fab fragments (Digibind) should be considered in select cases. Patients with life-threatening digoxin toxicity require hospitalization and close observation in a monitored setting. A detailed discussion of the treatment of digoxin toxicity is beyond the scope of this book.
- Drug interactions are also common with digoxin. Importantly, amiodarone, verapamil, flecainide, and quinidine may increase digoxin levels by up to 100%.

Hydralazine/Nitrates

- The vasodilator combination of hydralazine and nitrates was the first pharmacologic therapy shown to modify the natural history and reduce mortality in patients with chronic HF (V-HEFT I).[22]
- Although inferior to ACE-I or ARB therapy with respect to mortality, **hydralazine in combination with nitrates can be used as an alternative vasodilator regimen for patients intolerant of ACE-I/ARBs** (usually because of poor renal function or recurrent hyperkalemia).
- **In African American HF patients, hydralazine/nitrates are recommended if persistent HF symptoms are present *despite* use of ACE-I and β-blockers.**

Evidence

- In V-HEFT I, the combination of hydralazine and isosorbide dinitrate was superior to treatment with the α-blocker prazosin despite similar reductions in blood pressure.[22] All patients were also receiving digoxin and diuretics.
- V-HEFT II compared hydralazine/nitrates with enalapril and demonstrated that ACE-I therapy was associated with lower mortality, but other clinical outcomes were similar.[23]
- Subgroup analysis of V-HEFT I and II suggested that African Americans derived particular benefit from hydralazine/nitrate therapy. Recently, the A-HeFT trial confirmed the additive benefit of hydralazine/nitrate therapy in African American patients with Class III to IV HF symptoms who were **already receiving an ACE-I and β-blocker.**[24]

Practical Use

- Hydralazine and nitrates can be administered as a fixed dose combination tablet or as individual components. The dose recommendations are shown below:
  - Combination pill (Bidil): 1 → 2 tablets (20 mg isosorbide dinitrate and 37.5 mg hydralazine) tid.
  - **or**
  - Hydralazine: 12.5 to 25 mg tid → 100 mg tid.
  - **with**
  - Isosorbide mononitrate: 30 → 120 mg qd.
  - **or**
  - Isosorbide dinitrate: 10 → 40 mg tid.

Adverse Reactions

- The most common adverse responses to hydralazine and nitrates are headache, hypotension, and orthostatic symptoms.

- In rare cases, a dose-related drug-induced lupus syndrome can be seen with hydralazine (usually at doses ≥300 mg/day).
- The use of erectile dysfunction agents such as sildenafil and other phosphodiesterase inhibitors must be avoided in patients taking nitrates because of the potential for profound hypotension.
- An additional challenge to the successful use of hydralazine/nitrate therapy is patient compliance because of the large number of pills that must be taken daily.

Diuretics

- Diuretics are the primary medications used for volume control in patients with HF. Despite their ability to relieve congestive HF symptoms, diuretics have not been shown to alter the natural history of HF. In fact, diuretics may be harmful in the long term because of their potential adverse renal and neurohumoral effects.
- Diuretics should always be used in conjunction with dietary sodium and fluid restriction.

Practical Use

- The most commonly used agents in HF include the loop diuretics (furosemide, bumetanide, and torsemide) and the thiazide diuretics (hydrochlorothiazide, chlorthalidone, and metolazone).
- Hydrochlorothiazide and chlorthalidone are mild diuretics that are best suited for patients with mild HF and normal renal function.
- Loop diuretics are more potent and are frequently required in patients with clinical HF. The dose employed is based on volume status, symptom severity, and renal function. The lowest dose necessary to maintain euvolemia should be used. Frequent reassessment of volume status is necessary.
- In patients with significant right-sided volume overload and a poor response to oral furosemide, the use of bumetanide or torsemide should be considered as these drugs have more reliable intestinal absorption.
- The addition of a thiazide diuretic to a loop diuretic can be a useful strategy to facilitate diuresis in patients refractory to loop diuretics. However, significant volume and electrolyte depletion can occur with this combination and thus patients must have close follow-up.
- See Table 2 for conventional and maximal doses of the common diuretics.

Adverse Reactions

- The most common adverse events associated with diuretic therapy are volume contraction (which often manifests as prerenal azotemia and hypotension) and electrolyte disorders (potassium, magnesium, sodium).
- High doses of furosemide have rarely been associated with ototoxicity.
- Diuretic therapy activates the RAAS and the sympathetic nervous system, which can promote further adverse myocardial remodeling.
- Some patients can develop allergic reactions to the sulfa moiety of loop and thiazide diuretics.

Anticoagulation

- Routine anticoagulation is not recommended for patients with LV systolic dysfunction.
- Warfarin should be used in patients with atrial fibrillation or LV thrombus to reduce the risk of thromboembolism.

TABLE 2	Dosing of Diuretics Commonly Used in Heart Failure		
Drug	**Initial Daily Dose**	**Maximal Total Daily Dose**	**Duration of Action**
Loop Diuretics			
Bumetanide	0.5–1 mg IV/PO qd or bid	10 mg	4–6 hours
Furosemide	20–40 mg IV/PO qd or bid	600 mg	6–8 hours
Torsemide	10–20 mg PO qd	200 mg	12–16 hours
Thiazide Diuretics			
Chlorothiazide	250–500 mg PO qd or bid	2,000 mg	6–12 hours
Chlorthalidone	12.5–25 mg PO qd	200 mg	24–72 hours
Hydrochlorothiazide	25 mg qd	200 mg	6–12 hours
Indapamide	2.5 mg qd	5 mg	36 hours
Metolazone	2.5 mg qd	20 mg	12–24 hours
Potassium-Sparing Diuretics			
Amiloride	5 mg qd	20 mg	24 hours
Spironolactone	12.5–25 mg qd	25 mg	2–3 days
Triamterene	50–75 mg bid	200 mg	7–9 hours
Combination Therapy			
Chlorothiazide	200–1,000 mg plus a loop diuretic		
Hydrochlorothiazide	25–100 mg plus a loop diuretic		
Metolazone	2.5–10 mg plus a loop diuretic		

Modified from Hunt S, Abraham WT, Chin MH, et al. ACC/AHA 2005 guideline update for the diagnosis and management of chronic heart failure in the adult: a report of the American College of Cardiology/American Heart Association Task Force on Practice Guidelines. *Circulation* 2005:112:e154–e235.

- Patients with ischemic disease should receive aspirin; however, aspirin should not be given routinely to patients with nonischemic cardiomyopathy (NICM).

Nonpharmacologic Management

- Patient **nonadherence** with medications and diet is a major factor leading to worsened HF symptoms and increased hospitalizations. Therefore, patient education is vital to improve HF outcomes.
- A **low-salt diet** is necessary to avoid excessive fluid accumulation. In patients with mild-to-moderate HF, sodium intake should be restricted to ~2.5 to 3 g/day. Avoidance of foods with high sodium content, such as potato chips, tomato sauce, preserved meats, and fast foods, can help prevent decompensation.
- Patients also need to be educated about **fluid restriction.** For most patients with HF, a 2 to 3 L/day fluid restriction is appropriate; however, in patients with more severe HF or when hyponatremia is present, more aggressive fluid restriction may be required.
- Patients should obtain (or be provided with) a home scale and maintain a record of **daily weights.** Increased weight of >2 or 3 lb from baseline often indicates fluid retention and may warrant adjustment in diuretic dosage.

- **Exercise** in the form of low-impact aerobic activity is recommended for all HF patients in the absence of contraindications. Physical activity can prevent deconditioning and muscle atrophy, both of which worsen HF prognosis. Aggressive weight lifting should be avoided.
- **Smoking cessation** should be emphasized in patients with current tobacco use.
- Patients with HF should have yearly **influenza vaccination** as well as the **pneumococcal pneumonia** vaccination to minimize the risk of pulmonary infections.

Implantable Cardiac Defibrillators

- Arrhythmic sudden cardiac death (SCD) accounts for ~50% of all HF-associated deaths.
- ACE-I, β-blockers, and aldosterone antagonists have all been associated with a reduction in SCD; however, despite these therapies, implantable cardiac defibrillators (ICDs) are associated with improved survival in selected chronic HF patients with reduced systolic function.
- **All patients with an EF of 30% to ≤35%, NYHA Class II or III symptoms, and an estimated survival of >1 year should be considered for placement of an ICD for primary prevention of SCD.**
- Patients with NICM should receive ACE-Is and β-blockers at optimal doses for at least 3 months prior to implanting an ICD, as many of these patients will have significant improvement in LV function with medical therapy.
- Primary prevention ICD implantation should be delayed by 40 days following an acute MI or coronary revascularization.

Evidence

- MADIT-I and MADIT-II established that ICDs reduce mortality by ~1% to 2% per year in selected patients with ischemic cardiomyopathy and an EF of ≤30%.[25]
- Subsequently, the SCD-HeFT study evaluated patients with either ischemic or nonischemic cardiomyopathy and an EF of ≤35% and found that an ICD improved survival in both patient groups.[26]
- The DINAMIT investigated the use of ICD therapy in patients with LV dysfunction within 40 days after acute MI and found no survival benefit with device implantation in this setting.[27]
- Although effective at reducing ventricular ectopy, amiodarone has not been shown to reduce arrhythmic death in patients with HF who have reduced systolic function.
- In general, implantation of a primary prevention ICD is not associated with improved survival during the first 12 to 18 months following insertion.[25,26]

Adverse Events

- Complications associated with ICD implantation include pneumothorax/hemothorax, cardiac rupture, bleeding at the generator site, pericarditis, and device infection.
- Inappropriate shocks occur in 10% to 25% of patients with ICDs, usually related to device sensing of a supraventricular tachycardia (most commonly atrial fibrillation). Device failure is another possible adverse event.
- Some patients report worse quality of life, especially after receiving an ICD shock.

Cardiac Resynchronization Therapy

- LBBB is present in 20% to 30% of patients with HF. Inter- and intraventricular dyssynchrony produced by LBBB can significantly reduce cardiac efficiency and increase mitral regurgitation.

- Implanting an LV pacemaker lead transvenously via the coronary sinus or by a thoracotomy can restore ventricular synchrony.
- Cardiac resynchronization therapy (CRT) should be considered for HF patients with a QRS duration of >120 ms and persistent HF symptoms despite optimal medical therapy. The device can be implanted with or without ICD capabilities.

Evidence
- The two largest clinical trials evaluating the efficacy of CRT were COMPANION[28] and CARE-HF.[29]
- Both studies demonstrated improved HF symptoms and fewer hospitalizations with CRT. CARE-HF also showed a significant 10% absolute risk reduction in mortality in patients receiving CRT (without ICD).

Adverse Events
- CRT devices are associated with the same procedural and infectious complications as described above for ICDs.
- Adverse events unique to CRT include diaphragmatic stimulation from the LV lead and a higher risk of pericardial tamponade from injury to the coronary sinus.
- Technical challenges or inadequate cardiac venous anatomy can preclude percutaneous placement of an LV lead. Such patients often require a surgical approach for placement of the LV lead.

Treatment of Advanced Chronic Heart Failure (Stage D)

General Considerations
- Severe HF symptoms (NYHA Class III or IV) and frequent hospitalizations despite optimal medical therapy.
- Patients with end stage HF represent ~5% of the total HF population; however, they are frequently hospitalized and require close medical attention.
- Potential candidates for heart transplantation and/or mechanical circulatory support (LV assist device [LVAD]) should be identified and referred to a HF specialist.
- Patients should be continued on ACE-I/ARB, β-blockers, aldosterone antagonists, and digoxin as blood pressure and renal function allow.
- Congestive symptoms should be managed with diuretics; however, hypotension, renal dysfunction, and diuretic resistance are frequently encountered in these patients.
- Discussions regarding end-of-life care should occur between patient and provider.

LVADs/Transplantation
- The use of advanced HF therapies such as heart transplantation or LVAD implantation should be considered for patients <65 to 70 years of age with advanced HF refractory to medical therapy who have few comorbidities.
- Cardiopulmonary exercise testing can also be useful. A **VO_2 max of <14 mL O_2/kg/min** has been used to identify patients who might benefit from advanced HF therapy.
- Further discussion of transplantation and LVAD implantation is beyond the scope of this chapter.

Inotropic Therapy
- The use of continuous intravenous inotropic therapy can be considered in select patients with end stage HF and refractory symptoms, particularly those being

considered for transplantation. However, inotropic therapy has been associated with increased mortality and should therefore be initiated with caution.[30]

- The two inotropic agents currently in use are the β-adrenergic agonist dobutamine and the phosphodiesterase inhibitor milrinone. These medications should be initiated only in consultation with a HF specialist.

Hospice

- The 1-year mortality for patients with NYHA Class III to IV HF symptoms ranges from ~50% to 90% depending on patient characteristics. In patients who are not candidates for transplantation or an LVAD, consideration should be given to hospice care for medical and emotional support during the dying process.
- Discussions regarding turning off ICDs at the end of life should be undertaken to avoid unnecessary painful events.

Treatment of Acute Decompensated HF in the Ambulatory Setting

General Considerations

- In contrast to chronic HF, the management of acute decompensated HF (ADHF) is based more on expert opinion than on clinical trial evidence.
- **The primary treatment goals in acute HF syndromes are as follows:**
  - To improve patient symptoms.
  - To identify and treat precipitating factors of decompensation.
  - To minimize cardiac and renal injury.
  - To manage many cases of mild-to-moderate volume overload in the outpatient setting.

Precipitating Factors

- Identifying and treating potential triggers of an HF exacerbation is critical to improving patient outcomes.
- The most common causes of decompensation in patients with established HF include the following:
  - Medication and dietary noncompliance.
  - Arrhythmias (particularly atrial fibrillation or VT).
  - Ischemia.
  - Uncontrolled HTN.
  - Infections (e.g., pneumonia).
  - Substance abuse.
  - Pulmonary embolism.

Hospital Admission

Patients should be considered for hospital admission if they have any of the following:
- Severe symptoms or active myocardial ischemia.
- Uncontrolled or new-onset arrhythmias.
- Hypoxemia.
- Marked tachycardia or bradycardia.
- Worsening renal insufficiency (increased creatinine >0.5 to 1 mg/dL from baseline).
- Suspected severe valve disease.
- Evidence of drug toxicity.

TABLE 3	Outpatient Management of Decompensated Heart Failure (HF)

Mild HF Exacerbation	Moderate HF Exacerbation
• Increase total diuretic dose by 50% and administer bid (e.g., 40 mg qd becomes 40 mg bid) for ~3–5 days • Restrict Na to <2 g/day • Continue ACE-I or ARB and titrate if on low dose • Continue β-blocker • Monitor daily weights at home • Target 1–2 lb weight loss per day • Telephone follow-up in 3–5 days	• Consider ordering BMP • Increase loop diuretic dose by 50% and administer bid for ~7–10 days • If inadequate response after 1–2 days consider addition of metolazone at 2.5–5 mg/day • Restrict Na to <2 g and fluid intake to <2 L • Increase dose of ACE-I/ARB if blood pressure and renal function allow and not on target doses • Consider decreasing β-blocker dose by 50%, but do not discontinue if possible • Monitor daily weights and blood pressure at home • Target 2–3 lb weight loss per day • Telephone follow-up in 3–5 days • Office follow-up with BMP in 1 week

ACE-I, angiotensin-converting enzyme inhibitor; ARB, angiotensin receptor blockers; BMP, basic metabolic panel; Na, sodium.

Evaluation

• For mild HF exacerbations further testing is not usually indicated.
• In moderate HF exacerbations, a BMP should be obtained to assess renal function and electrolyte levels.
• In select patients, a CXR, BNP, and/or CBC should be considered to assess HF severity and to evaluate for anemia or infection.
• If ischemia is suspected, an ECG and troponin level should be obtained.

Management

• The treatment of HF exacerbations involves the use of diuretics and vasodilators.
• Table 3 provides a rational approach to the outpatient management of HF decompensation.

Prognosis

• There are many factors that can help determine prognosis in patients with HF. The following have been associated with worse outcomes in HF:
  • **Patient characteristics:** worse NYHA functional class, older age, inability to tolerate ACE-I or β-blockers, male gender.
  • **HF etiology:** ischemic heart disease.
  • **Lab data:** elevated blood urea nitrogen (BUN) and/or creatinine, hyponatremia, elevated BNP, elevated troponin, low hemoglobin.

- **Echocardiographic data:** lower EF, restrictive diastolic dysfunction, pulmonary HTN.
- **Hemodynamics:** chronically elevated pulmonary capillary wedge pressure, pulmonary HTN.
- **Patient comorbidities:** atrial fibrillation, renal insufficiency, chronic obstructive pulmonary disease (COPD), peripheral arterial disease, cognitive dysfunction.
- **Functional assessment:** decreased VO_2 max, decreased 6-minute walk distance.
- The **Seattle Heart Failure Model** uses several of the above factors to estimate patient survival and can be a useful tool to estimate prognosis in an individual patient. This tool can be accessed online at http://depts.washington.edu/shfm/

HF WITH PRESERVED SYSTOLIC FUNCTION

General Principles

- Up to 50% of patients who present to the hospital with ADHF have normal systolic function on echocardiogram.[3]
- HF with PSF is more common in women, in elderly patients, and in those with HTN.[4]
- Common comorbidities include atrial fibrillation, renal insufficiency, and DM. CAD is less common in this population as compared with those with systolic dysfunction.
- The prognosis for HF with PSF is comparable with HF with systolic dysfunction. The mortality rate at 3 months following index hospitalization is ~10% (Fig. 1) and the 5-year mortality is >50%.

Diagnosis

- Differentiating between diastolic and systolic HF cannot be reliably accomplished without two-dimensional echocardiography.
- Diagnosis is based on echocardiographic criteria and Doppler findings of normal LV systolic function with impaired diastolic relaxation.

Treatment

- The optimal treatment strategy for HF with PSF remains undefined. However, the following approaches are recommended:
  - Control blood pressure.
  - Control heart rate and use warfarin anticoagulation in patients with atrial fibrillation.
  - Use diuretics to treat congestive symptoms, but avoid overdiuresis.
  - Treat underlying ischemia if present.
  - Pending the results of ongoing clinical trials, ACE-Is, ARBs, and β-blockers are considered appropriate therapy for the treatment of HF with PSF.

HYPERTROPHIC CARDIOMYOPATHY

General Principles

Definition
- Hypertrophic cardiomyopathy (HCM) is a genetic cardiomyopathy characterized by asymmetric septal hypertrophy, systolic anterior motion of the mitral valve, and variable degrees of LV outflow tract obstruction.

- Systolic function is usually normal to hyperdynamic, but diastolic function is markedly abnormal.
- The idiopathic form of HCM has an early onset (as early as the first decade of life) without associated HTN.

Pathophysiology

- Many cases of HCM have a genetic component, with mutations in the myosin heavy-chain gene that follow an autosomal-dominant transmission with variable phenotypic expression and penetrance.
- HCM can be classified according to the presence or absence of LV outflow tract obstruction.
- LV outflow obstruction may occur at rest but is enhanced by factors that increase LV contractility or decrease ventricular volume.

Diagnosis

Clinical Presentation

History

- The clinical presentation can be highly variable. In severe cases, patients can become symptomatic early in life, while in other patients the cardiomyopathy can be discovered as an incidental finding later in life.
- Sudden death is most common in children and young adults between the ages of 10 and 35 years and often occurs during periods of strenuous exertion.

Physical Examination

- Physical exam findings include bisferious carotid pulse (in the presence of obstruction).
- Forceful double or triple apical impulse and a coarse systolic outflow murmur localized along the left sterna border that is accentuated by maneuvers that decreased preload (e.g., standing, Valsalva maneuver) may also be found.

Diagnostic Testing

- The ECG may show conduction system disease or low voltage, in contrast to the increased voltage seen with ventricular hypertrophy.
- Two-dimensional echocardiography and Doppler flow studies can establish the presence of significant LV outflow gradient at rest or with provocation.
- Additional risk stratification should be pursued with 24- to 48-hour Holter monitoring and exercise testing.

Treatment

Medications

- Medical therapy can help alleviate symptoms and is directed toward controlling heart rate and reducing contractility. First-line agents are β-blockers and non-dihydropyridine calcium channel blockers. The type 1 antiarrhythmic agent disopyramide can be added in patients with persistent symptoms.
- Diuretics can be helpful, but overdiuresis can worsen outflow tract obstruction, producing hypotension and increased symptoms.

Other Nonpharmacologic Therapies

- Genetic counseling and family screening are recommended for first-degree relatives of patients at high risk for SCD, because the disease is transmitted as an autosomal-dominant trait.

- In patients with refractory symptoms and severe outflow tract obstruction, an alcohol septal ablation or surgical myomectomy can be considered.
- ICD implantation should be strongly considered in patients with syncope, VT, or a family history of SCD.

Surgical Management

- Surgical therapy is useful in the treatment of symptoms but has not been shown to alter the natural history of HCM.
- The most frequently used operative procedure involves septal myotomy-myectomy with or without mitral valve replacement (MVR).
- Alcohol septal ablation, a catheter-based alternative to surgical myotomy-myectomy, seems to be equally effective at reducing obstruction and providing symptomatic relief when compared with the gold standard surgical procedure.
- Cardiac transplantation should be reserved for patients with end stage HCM with symptomatic HF.[31]

RESTRICTIVE CARDIOMYOPATHY

General Principles

Definition

- Restrictive cardiomyopathy results from pathologic infiltration of the myocardium.
- Myocardial infiltration results in abnormal diastolic ventricular filling and varying degrees of systolic dysfunction.

Pathophysiology

- Restrictive cardiomyopathy is most commonly associated with amyloidosis or sarcoidosis.
- Less common causes include glycogen storage diseases, hemochromatosis, endomyocardial fibrosis, and hypereosinophilic syndromes.

Diagnosis

Diagnostic Testing

- Despite increased LV mass by echocardiography, the ECG is often characterized by low voltage.
- In restrictive cardiomyopathy, echocardiography with Doppler analysis may demonstrate thickened myocardium with normal or abnormal systolic function, abnormal diastolic filling patterns, and elevated intracardiac pressure.
- Cardiac catheterization reveals elevated RV and LV filling pressures and a classic dip-and-plateau pattern in the RV and LV pressure tracings.
- RV endomyocardial biopsy may be diagnostic and should be considered in patients in whom a diagnosis is not established.
- It is often difficult to differentiate between restrictive cardiomyopathy and constrictive pericarditis because of similar clinical presentations and hemodynamics, but this distinction is critical as surgical therapy may be effective for constriction.

Treatment

- Therapy targeted at amelioration of the underlying cause should be initiated.
- Cardiac hemochromatosis may respond to reduction of total body iron stores via phlebotomy or chelation therapy with deferoxamine.
- Cardiac sarcoidosis may respond to glucocorticoid therapy, but prolongation of survival with this approach has not been established.
- No therapy is known to be effective in reversing the progression for cardiac amyloidosis.
- Digoxin should be avoided in patients with cardiac amyloidosis because of enhanced susceptibility to digoxin toxicity.

CONSTRICTIVE PERICARDITIS

General Principles

- Constrictive pericarditis may develop as a late complication of pericardial inflammation.
- The noncompliant pericardium causes impairment of ventricular filling and progressive elevation of venous pressure.
- Most cases are idiopathic, but pericarditis after cardiac surgery and mediastinal irradiation are important identifiable causes.
- Tuberculous pericarditis is a leading cause of constrictive pericarditis in some undeveloped countries.
- Constrictive pericarditis is often difficult to distinguish from restrictive cardiomyopathy.

Diagnosis

Clinical Presentation

History

In contrast to cardiac tamponade, the clinical presentation of constrictive pericarditis is insidious, with gradual development of fatigue, exercise intolerance, and venous congestion.

Physical Examination

Physical exam findings include the following:
- JVD with prominent X and Y descents.
- Inspiratory elevation of the jugular venous pressure (Kussmaul's sign).
- Peripheral edema.
- Ascites.
- A pericardial knock during diastole.

Diagnostic Testing

- Echocardiography may reveal pericardial thickening and diminished diastolic filling.
- CT scan or MRI demonstrates pericardial thickening.
- Cardiac catheterization is usually necessary to demonstrate elevated and equalized diastolic pressures in all four cardiac chambers.

Treatment

- Definitive treatment requires complete pericardiectomy, which is accompanied by significant perioperative mortality (5% to 10%) but results in clinical improvement in 90% of patients.
- Patients who are minimally symptomatic can be managed with judicious sodium and fluid restriction and diuretic therapy but must be followed closely to detect hemodynamic deterioration.

CARDIAC TAMPONADE

General Principles

- Cardiac tamponade results from increased intrapericardial pressure secondary to fluid accumulation within the pericardial space.
- Pericarditis of any cause may lead to cardiac tamponade.
- Idiopathic (or viral) and neoplastic forms are the most frequent causes.

Diagnosis

Clinical Presentation

The diagnosis should be suspected in patients with elevated jugular venous pressure, hypotension, pulsus paradoxus, tachycardia, evidence of poor peripheral perfusion, and distant heart sounds.

Diagnostic Testing

- ECG often reveals a tachycardia with low voltage and electrical alternans.
- Echocardiography can confirm the diagnosis of pericardial effusion and demonstrate hemodynamic significance by right atrial and RV diastolic collapse, increased right-sided flows during inspiration, and respiratory variation of the transmitral flow.
- Right heart catheterization is also helpful in determining the hemodynamic significance of a pericardial effusion, especially in patients with a subacute or chronic presentation.
- Hemodynamic findings of elevated, equalized diastolic pressures are present in the patient with cardiac tamponade.

Treatment

- Treatment consists of drainage of the pericardial space via pericardiocentesis or surgical pericardiotomy. Urgent pericardiocentesis should be performed with echocardiographic guidance, if possible.
- **Diuretics, nitrates, and any other preload-reducing agents are absolutely contraindicated for cardiac tamponade.**

REFERENCES

1. American Heart Association. Heart Disease and Stroke Statistics: 2007 Update. Dallas, TX, 2007.
2. Hunt S, Abraham WT, Chin MH, et al. ACC/AHA 2005 guideline update for the diagnosis and management of chronic heart failure in the adult: a report of the American College

of Cardiology/American Heart Association Task Force on Practice Guidelines. *Circulation* 2005;112:e154–e235.

3. Adams KF Jr., Fonarow GC, Emerman CL, et al. Characteristics and outcomes of patients hospitalized for heart failure in the United States: rationale, design, and preliminary observations from the first 100,000 cases in the Acute Decompensated Heart Failure National Registry (ADHERE). *Am Heart J* 2005;149:209–216.

4. Yancy CW, Lopatin M, Stevenson LW, et al. Clinical presentation, management, and in-hospital outcomes of patients admitted with acute decompensated heart failure with preserved systolic function: a report from the Acute Decompensated Heart Failure National Registry (ADHERE) database. *J Am Coll Cardiol* 2006;47:76–84.

5. Garg R, Yusuf S. Overview of randomized trials of angiotensin-converting enzyme inhibitors on mortality and morbidity in patients with heart failure. Collaborative Group on ACE Inhibitor trials. *JAMA* 1995;273:1450–1456.

6. Reynolds G, Hall AS, Ball SG. What have the ACE-inhibitor trials in postmyocardial patients with left ventricular dysfunction taught us? *Eur J Clin Pharmacol* 1996;49 (Suppl 1):S35–S39.

7. Pfeffer MA, Swedberg K, Granger CB, et al. Effects of candesartan on mortality and morbidity in patients with chronic heart failure: the CHARM-Overall programme. *Lancet* 2003;362:759–766.

8. Cohn JN, Tognoni G. A randomized trial of the angiotensin-receptor blocker valsartan in chronic heart failure. *N Engl J Med* 2001;345(23):1667–1675.

9. Pfeffer MA, McMurray JJ, Velazquez EJ, et al. Valsartan, captopril, or both in myocardial infarction complicated by heart failure, left ventricular dysfunction, or both. *N Engl J Med* 2003;349(20):1893–1906.

10. Yusuf S, Pfeffer MA, Swedberg K, et al. Effects of candesartan in patients with chronic heart failure and preserved left-ventricular ejection fraction: the CHARM-Preserved trial. *Lancet* 2003;362:777–781.

11. McMurray JJ, Ostergren J, Swedberg CB, et al. Effects of candesartan in patients with chronic heart failure and reduced left-ventricular systolic function taking angiotensin-converting-enzyme inhibitors: the CHARM-Added trial. *Lancet* 2003;362:767–771.

12. Effect of metoprolol CR/XL in chronic heart failure: metoprolol CR/XL Randomised Intervention Trial in Congestive Heart Failure (MERIT-HF). *Lancet* 1999;353:2001–2007.

13. Packer M, Fowler MB, Roecker EB, et al. Effect of carvedilol on the morbidity of patients with severe chronic heart failure: results of the Carvedilol Prospective Randomized Cumulative Survival (COPERNICUS) study. *Circulation* 2002;106:2194–2199.

14. Packer M, Bristow MR, Cohn, et al. The effect of carvedilol on morbidity and mortality in patients with chronic heart failure. U.S. Carvedilol Heart Failure Study Group. *N Engl J Med* 1996;334:1349–1355.

15. McGavin JK, Keating GM. Bisoprolol: a review of its use in chronic heart failure. *Drugs* 2002;62:2677–2696.

16. Dargie HJ. Effect of carvedilol on outcome after myocardial infarction in patients with left-ventricular dysfunction: the CAPRICORN randomised trial. *Lancet* 2001;357:1385–1390.

17. Torp-Pedersen C, Poole-Wilson PA, Swedberg K, et al. Effects of metoprolol and carvedilol on cause-specific mortality and morbidity in patients with chronic heart failure—COMET. *Am Heart J* 2005;149:370–376.

18. Pitt B, Zannad F, Remme WJ, et al. The effect of spironolactone on morbidity and mortality in patients with severe heart failure. Randomized Aldactone Evaluation Study Investigators. *N Engl J Med* 1999;341(10):709–717.

19. Pitt B, Remme WJ, Zannad F, et al. Eplerenone, a selective aldosterone blocker, in patients with left ventricular dysfunction after myocardial infarction. *N Engl J Med* 2003;348: 1309–1321.

20. The effect of digoxin on mortality and morbidity in patients with heart failure. The Digitalis Investigation Group. *N Engl J Med* 1997;336:525–533.

21. Ahmed A, Gambassi G, Weaver MT, et al. Effects of discontinuation of digoxin versus continuation at low serum digoxin concentrations in chronic heart failure. *Am J Cardiol* 2007;100:280–284.

22. Cohn JN, Archibald DG, Ziesche S, et al. Effect of vasodilator therapy on mortality in chronic congestive heart failure. Results of a Veterans Administration Cooperative Study. *N Engl J Med* 1986;314:1547–1552.

23. Cohn JN, Johnson G, Ziesche S, et al. A comparison of enalapril with hydralazine-isosorbide dinitrate in the treatment of chronic congestive heart failure. *N Engl J Med* 1991;325: 303–310.

24. Taylor AL, Ziesche S, Yancy C, et al. Combination of isosorbide dinitrate and hydralazine in blacks with heart failure. *N Engl J Med* 2004;351:2049–2057.

25. Moss AJ. MADIT-I and MADIT-II. *J Cardiovasc Electrophysiol* 2003;14(Suppl 9):S96–S98.

26. Bardy GH, Lee KL, Mark DB, et al. Amiodarone or an implantable cardioverter-defibrillator for congestive heart failure. *N Engl J Med* 2005;352:225–237.

27. Hohnloser SH, Kuck KH, Dorian P, et al. Prophylactic use of an implantable cardioverter-defibrillator after acute myocardial infarction. *N Engl J Med* 2004;351:2481–2488.

28. Cleland JG, Daubert JC, Erdmann E, et al. The effect of cardiac resynchronization on morbidity and mortality in heart failure. *N Engl J Med* 2005;352:1539–1549.

29. Bristow MR, Saxon LA, Boehmer J, et al. Cardiac-resynchronization therapy with or without an implantable defibrillator in advanced chronic heart failure. *N Engl J Med* 2004;350: 2140–2150.

30. Abraham WT, Adams KF, Fonarow GC, et al. In-hospital mortality in patients with acute decompensated heart failure requiring intravenous vasoactive medications: an analysis from the Acute Decompensated Heart Failure National Registry (ADHERE). *J Am Coll Cardiol* 2005;46:57–64.

31. Firoozi S, Elliot PM, Sharma S, et al. Septal myotomy-myectomy and transcoronary septal alcohol ablation in hypertrophic obstructive cardiomyopathy. A comparison of clinical, haemodynamic and exercise outcomes. *Eur Heart J* 2002;23:1617–1624.

Valvular Heart Disease

Benico Barzilai

Introduction

- As opposed to coronary artery disease, the onset of symptoms in valvular heart disease is often quite insidious with a long period of asymptomatic progression in many patients.
- Symptoms can often be very nonspecific, with fatigue or shortness of breath only with heavy exertion.
- History and physical examination play a prominent role in these patients as they often have physical findings long before the onset of symptoms.
- A generalized approach to the cardiac murmur is presented in Figure 1.[1]
- One recent study suggested significant mitral or aortic valve disease in >10% of patients >80.[2]
- Primary care physicians are frequently the first doctors to recognize the physical findings in these patients. Thus, it is imperative that primary care physicians know when to refer these patients to cardiac specialists.

AORTIC STENOSIS

General Principles

- Aortic stenosis (AS) is usually present for many years before patients become symptomatic.
- There is a long latency with an excellent prognosis until chest pain, syncope, or heart failure develops.
- The operative mortality of isolated aortic valve repair (AVR) is quite good in patients with isolated AS and normal left ventricular (LV) function (1% to 2%), so it is imperative that these patients be followed very closely.

Pathophysiology

- Congenital bicuspid aortic valve disease is the most common cause of severe AS prior to the age of 60.
- After the age of 60, calcific AS of a leaflet valve is the most common cause of AS. Many patients do not develop critical AS until well into their 80s.
- Aortic stenosis produces a pressure gradient between the LV and the aorta, causing pressure overload of the LV. LV compliance is reduced, LV end-diastolic pressure rises, and myocardial oxygen demand is increased.

Diagnosis

Clinical Presentation

History
- As noted, many patients are asymptomatic at first presentation.

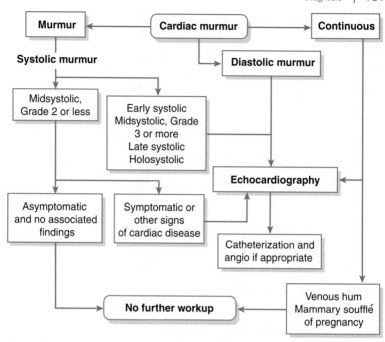

Figure 1. Evaluation of heart murmurs. (Modified from Bonow RO, Carabello BA, Chatterjee K, et al. ACC/AHA 2006 guidelines for the management of patients with valvular heart disease: a report of the American College of Cardiology/American Heart Association Task Force on Practice Guidelines (Writing Committee to Develop Guidelines for the Management of Patients With Valvular Heart Disease): developed in collaboration with the Society of Cardiovascular Anesthesiologists: endorsed by the Society for Cardiovascular Angiography and Interventions and the Society of Thoracic Surgeons. *Circulation* 2006;114:e84–e231.)

- With the development of symptoms (e.g., angina, dizziness/syncope, heart failure), it is imperative that these patients be seen in a timely fashion as the median survival is 1 to 3 years.

Physical Examination
- The physical examination will reveal a harsh mid to late peaking murmur heard over the aortic area but often radiating to carotids and axilla.
- As the severity increases, the murmur peaks later and the aortic second sound (A2) becomes softer.
- The carotid upstroke becomes weaker and is delayed as the significance of AS increases (*pulsus parvus et tardus*).
- An LV heave and a thrill may also be present.

Diagnostic Testing
Electrocardiography
- Electrocardiogram often reveals LV hypertrophy with strain.

TABLE 1	Severity of Aortic Stenosis		
Indicator	Mild	Moderate	Severe
Valve area (cm^2)	>1.5	1.0–1.5	<1.0
Jet velocity (m/s)	<3.0	3.0–4.0	>4.0
Mean gradient (mm Hg)	<25	25–40	>40

Modified from Bonow RO, Carabello BA, Chatterjee K, et al. ACC/AHA 2006 guidelines for the management of patients with valvular heart disease: a report of the American College of Cardiology/American Heart Association Task Force on Practice Guidelines (Writing Committee to Develop Guidelines for the Management of Patients With Valvular Heart Disease): developed in collaboration with the Society of Cardiovascular Anesthesiologists: endorsed by the Society for Cardiovascular Angiography and Interventions and the Society of Thoracic Surgeons. *Circulation* 2006;114:e84–e231.

Imaging
Echocardiography
- The development of quantitative Doppler echocardiography has revolutionized the care of these patients. The aortic valve area and the peak jet across the valve can be determined with accuracy (Table 1).
- Any patient with significant murmur in the aortic region should undergo echocardiography.
- Echocardiography is recommended every 3 years for mild AS, every 1 to 2 years for moderate AS, and at least yearly for severe AS.

Treatment

Medications
- **Statins** have been used to try and retard the progression of AS. One study using atorvastatin in patients with advanced disease showed no benefit.[3] A recent pilot study using rosuvastatin (40 mg) showed mild benefit, but it needs to be reproduced in a multicenter randomized trial.[4]
- **Diuretics** may be useful in treating congestive symptoms but should be used with extreme caution as reduction in LV filling pressure in patients with AS may decrease cardiac output and systemic blood pressure.
- **Nitrates** and other vasodilators should be used carefully in patients with severe AS because these may result in severe hypotension.

Surgical Management
- Aortic valve repair is indicated for symptomatic patients with severe AS.
- Patients who develop an ejection fraction of <50% but who are relatively asymptomatic should be referred for AVR.
- Patients who develop ST depression or hypotension on exercise testing should also be considered for surgery. The exercise test must be performed cautiously with physician supervision.
- Patients with low-gradient AS may benefit from dobutamine echocardiography to differentiate true AS from pseudo AS secondary to low flow.

- All patients require coronary angiography as 50% of patients will have significant coronary artery disease.

Monitoring/Follow-Up

- Aortic stenosis has been shown to progress by an average of 0.1 cm²/year, so patients with valve areas under 1.5 cm² must be followed closely. Some patients progress even faster, particularly those with heavily calcified valves.

AORTIC INSUFFICIENCY

General Principles

Pathophysiology

- Mild aortic insufficiency (AI) is frequently documented by Doppler echocardiography but severe AI requiring operative therapy is relatively uncommon.
- Aortic insufficiency can result from intrinsic valve disease (bicuspid aortic valve, rheumatic heart disease, endocarditis, trauma, lupus, and other connective tissue disease).
- Primary dilatation of the aortic root can also cause severe AI (e.g., Marfan syndrome, aortic dissection, long-standing hypertension, ankylosing spondylitis, and syphilitic aortitis).
- **Chronic severe AI** results in massive (*cor bovinum*) LV dilatation and hypertrophy. Since the ventricle dilates slowly, the regurgitant volume is absorbed by the relatively compliant LV. Chronic severe AI is generally well tolerated. The patient, however, may develop LV dysfunction slowly over time (ejection fraction <50%). It is imperative that patients undergo AVR before irreversible LV dysfunction develops.
- **Severe acute AI** leads to marked increase in LV pressure since the LV is not compliant enough to absorb the regurgitant volume.

Diagnosis

Clinical Presentation

History

Fatigue, dyspnea on exertion, palpitations, and heart failure are the most common symptoms, though many patients may be asymptomatic.

Physical Examination

Physical examination reveals bounding pulses, a wide pulse pressure, and a decrescendo murmur often heard with the patient sitting up or bending forward.

Diagnostic Testing

Electrocardiography

Electrocardiogram reveals LV hypertrophy.

Imaging

Echocardiography

- Any patient with a diastolic murmur should undergo echocardiography.

TABLE 2	Severity of Aortic Insufficiency		
Indicator	Mild	Moderate	Severe
Qualitative			
Angiography	1+	2+	3+ or 4+
Color Doppler jet width (cm)	<0.3	0.3–0.6	>0.6
Quantitative			
Regurgitant volume (mL)	<30	30–59	>0.6
Regurgitant fraction (%)	<30	30–49	>50

Modified from Bonow RO, Carabello BA, Chatterjee K, et al. ACC/AHA 2006 guidelines for the management of patients with valvular heart disease: a report of the American College of Cardiology/American Heart Association Task Force on Practice Guidelines (Writing Committee to Develop Guidelines for the Management of Patients With Valvular Heart Disease): developed in collaboration with the Society of Cardiovascular Anesthesiologists: endorsed by the Society for Cardiovascular Angiography and Interventions and the Society of Thoracic Surgeons. *Circulation* 2006;114:e84–e231.

- The echocardiogram should document the severity of AI, the size of the LV in systole and diastole, and the size of the aortic root (Table 2).

Treatment

Medications
- Initial studies suggested that afterload reduction with nifedipine delayed surgery.[5] However, more recent studies do not support the use of afterload reduction to delay surgery.[6]
- Diuretics and digoxin can be used in symptomatic patients while they are being prepared for surgery.

Other Nonoperative Therapies
Strenuous physical activity should be restricted in patients with AI and associated LV dysfunction. Activities that involve increases in isometric work (lifting heavy objects) are more detrimental than are activities such as walking or swimming.

Surgical Management
- Aortic valve repair is indicated for symptomatic patients with severe AI.
- Patients with the following characteristics should also be referred for surgery:
  - Asymptomatic patients with ejection fraction of <50%.
  - Asymptomatic patients with severe LV dilatation (end-diastolic dimension of ≥75 mm or end-systolic dimension >55 mm).
  - Patients with mild LV dilatation (LV diastolic dimension >60 mm or systolic dimension >40 mm should be followed yearly for progressive LV dilatation).
- Surgery to repair the aortic root is indicated in patients with aortic root >5.0 cm with bicuspid aortic valve. It is imperative that echocardiography be performed yearly in patients with aortic root >4.0 cm. Operative therapy is indicated for an increase of 0.5 cm/year in diameter.

MITRAL STENOSIS

General Principles

Etiology

- Rheumatic heart disease is the most common cause of mitral stenosis (MS), particularly in young women.
- With the decrease in rheumatic heart disease, the prevalence of MS has dropped dramatically.
- Other causes of MS are rare (e.g., congenital, mitral annular calcification).

Pathophysiology

- Low or fixed cardiac output often results in fatigue and dyspnea.
- Significant MS results in elevation of left atrial, pulmonary venous, and pulmonary capillary pressures, with consequent pulmonary congestion.
- The degree of pressure elevation depends on the severity of the obstruction, flow across the valve, diastolic filling time, and presence of effective atrial contraction.

Diagnosis

Clinical Presentation

History
- The onset of symptoms may be quite insidious.
- In addition to dyspnea and fatigue, patients often present with cough and sometimes hemoptysis.
- Symptoms of right heart failure may also occur.
- Symptoms often accompany the development of atrial fibrillation.
- Patients often become symptomatic during pregnancy because of the increased cardiac output.

Physical Examination
- Physical examination reveals a loud S1 and an opening snap in diastole followed by a diastolic rumble (left lateral decubitus).
- A right ventricular heave or loud P2 may also be present.

Diagnostic Testing

Electrocardiography
Electrocardiogram often shows left atrial enlargement and right ventricular hypertrophy.

Imaging
Echocardiography
- Echocardiography can frequently quantify the severity of MS (mean gradient, valve area).
- In some cases, stress echocardiography is performed to assess the gradient during exercise and worsening pulmonary hypertension (Table 3).

Treatment

Medications

- Patients with atrial fibrillation and MS become quite symptomatic, so efforts should be undertaken to maintain normal sinus rhythm.

TABLE 3	Severity of Mitral Stenosis		
Indicator	Mild	Moderate	Severe
Mean gradient (mm Hg)	<5	5–10	>10
Pulmonary pressure (mm Hg)	<30	30–50	>50
Valve area (cm^2)	>1.5	1.0–1.5	<1.0

Modified from Bonow RO, Carabello BA, Chatterjee K, et al. ACC/AHA 2006 guidelines for the management of patients with valvular heart disease: a report of the American College of Cardiology/American Heart Association Task Force on Practice Guidelines (Writing Committee to Develop Guidelines for the Management of Patients With Valvular Heart Disease): developed in collaboration with the Society of Cardiovascular Anesthesiologists: endorsed by the Society for Cardiovascular Angiography and Interventions and the Society of Thoracic Surgeons. *Circulation* 2006;114:e84–e231.

- **Amiodarone** can be used to maintain sinus rhythm.
- **Warfarin** should be given to all patients with atrial fibrillation and MS as the embolic rate is high.
- **Rate control** in patients with chronic atrial fibrillation is essential since tachycardia with shortened diastolic filling time is poorly tolerated (digoxin, β-blockers, and calcium channel blockers).

Surgical Management

- Transesophageal echocardiography may be helpful to assess valve morphology (e.g., mobility of leaflets, calcification) and assist in the determination of the correct procedure.
- Patients with pliable leaflets and little calcium can undergo percutaneous **mitral valvuloplasty.**
- Patients with moderate or severe MS with favorable anatomy and symptoms should undergo valvuloplasty.
- If the patient does not have favorable anatomy, **mitral valve repair or replacement** should be entertained, particularly if the pulmonary artery (PA) pressure is >50 mm Hg at rest.
- If the patient is stress echocardiography can be used to document response to exercise.
- If the PA pressure is >60 mm Hg with exercise or the mean gradient is >25 mm Hg, mitral valve repair or valvuloplasty should be considered.

MITRAL REGURGITATION

General Principles

Epidemiology

- Mitral regurgitation (MR) is a very common with a striking increase in prevalence in patients >65.
- >6% of the patients >65 have moderate MR.

Etiology

- Etiologies frequently requiring operative management include myxomatous degeneration with or without flail leaflet, rheumatic heart disease, connective tissue disorders, and endocarditis.

- Left ventricular dilatation in patients with ischemic and nonischemic cardiomyopathies is also a common cause of MR, but many of these patients are treated medically because of the high operative mortality.

Pathophysiology

- Many patients with normal LV function tolerate chronic severe MR reasonably well.
- These patients will develop progressive left atrial enlargement, which can lead to atrial fibrillation.
- Pulmonary hypertension may develop slowly.
- In patients with acute severe MR, the left atrium may not be compliant enough to absorb the energy from the regurgitant wave. Pulmonary hypertension may develop suddenly in these patients.

Diagnosis

Clinical Presentation

History

- Many patients with chronic severe MR are asymptomatic.
- Patients may present with subtle dyspnea on exertion and fatigue.
- Patients may symptomatically decompensate with the development of atrial fibrillation.

Physical Examination

- Physical examination reveals a holosystolic murmur radiating to the axilla (particularly in patients with degenerative disease and normal LV function).
- Patients with LV dysfunction may have a soft systolic murmur despite the presence of MR.

Diagnostic Testing

Electrocardiography

Electrocardiogram may reveal left atrial enlargement, LV hypertrophy, and possibly right ventricular hypertrophy.

Imaging

Chest Radiography

Chest radiography reveals cardiomegaly, left atrial enlargement, and pulmonary vascular redistribution.

Echocardiography

- The development of color flow Doppler echocardiography has simplified the detection of MR.
- Recent advances in Doppler echocardiography have led to more quantitative indexes of MR, including regurgitant volume, regurgitant fraction, and regurgitant orifice area, as shown in Table 4.

Treatment

Medications

- Afterload reduction with **angiotensin-converting enzyme inhibitors** may improve symptoms, but there is no conclusive evidence that it delays surgery.

TABLE 4	Severity of Mitral Regurgitation		
Indicator	Mild	Moderate	Severe
Qualitative			
Angiographic grade	1+	2+	3+ or 4+
Color Doppler jet area	Small central jet <20% of left atrial area	Central jet 20%–40% of left atrial area	>40% of left atrial area
Quantitative			
Regurgitant volume (mL/beat)	<30	30–59	≥60
Regurgitant fraction (%)	<30	30–49	≥50
Regurgitant orifice area (cm^2)	<0.2	0.2–0.39	>0.40

Modified from Bonow RO, Carabello BA, Chatterjee K, et al. ACC/AHA 2006 guidelines for the management of patients with valvular heart disease: a report of the American College of Cardiology/American Heart Association Task Force on Practice Guidelines (Writing Committee to Develop Guidelines for the Management of Patients With Valvular Heart Disease): developed in collaboration with the Society of Cardiovascular Anesthesiologists: endorsed by the Society for Cardiovascular Angiography and Interventions and the Society of Thoracic Surgeons. *Circulation* 2006;114:e84–e231.

- **Digoxin, β-blockers, and calcium channel blockers** may be used to control the ventricular response in patients with atrial fibrillation.

Surgical Management
- In general, **mitral valve repair** is preferable to **mitral valve replacement.**
- Surgery is indicated for the following:
  - Symptomatic patients with acute severe MR.
  - Patients with severe MR and functional Class II or greater.
  - Asymptomatic patients with severe MR and mild to moderate LV dysfunction (ejection fraction of 30% to 60% or end-systolic dimension ≥40 mm).
  - Surgery can be considered in experienced centers in asymptomatic patients with severe MR and high likelihood of repair (e.g., flail leaflet) (operative mortality <1%).

Monitoring/Follow-Up

Patients with severe MR should be monitored very closely for the onset of symptoms or decrease in LV function if a conservative approach (watchful waiting) is considered. Echocardiography should be done at least yearly.

MITRAL VALVE PROLAPSE

General Principles

- Mitral valve prolapse (MVP) is characterized by prolapse of one or both MV leaflets into the left atrium >2 mm in midsystole.

- With the refinement in the echocardiographic criteria for MVP, the prevalence of MVP is closer to 1% to 5% rather than the 10% originally thought in early studies.
- Many patients with MVP are asymptomatic but many patients have chest pain and palpitations. Some patients have autonomic dysfunction with lightheadedness.
- Patients with thickened leaflets (>5 mm) more frequently have complications of MVP (severe MR, endocarditis, and possible strokes).[7]
- Mitral valve prolapse associated with myxomatous degeneration can lead to ruptured chordae (more often affects men).

Diagnosis

Clinical Presentation

- There seems to be little correlation of the echocardiographic findings and the symptoms of chest pain and palpitations.
- Echocardiography demonstrates systolic prolapse of the mitral leaflets into the left atrium.
- Holter monitoring may reveal atrial and ventricular arrhythmias.

Treatment

- Patients with MVP often respond to low-dose β-blockers (e.g., metoprolol XL 25 mg).
- Calcium channel blockers may be helpful in some patients.
- Endocarditis prophylaxis is no longer recommended for patients with MVP (see below).

ENDOCARDITIS PROPHYLAXIS

In 2007, the American Heart Association (AHA) released its most recent guideline regarding infective endocarditis (IE) prophylaxis; it contains major changes compared with prior guidelines.[8] There is a notable lack of data supporting the use of antibiotic prophylaxis in the setting of dental, gastrointestinal, and genitourinary procedures and evidence of causation is circumstantial. In fact, there has been no prospective, placebo-controlled, multicenter, randomized, double-blind study of the efficacy of IE antibiotic prophylaxis. Based on a synthesis of available data, it is likely that **most cases of IE are not directly caused by dental or other procedures** and that even if antibiotic prophylaxis were completely effective, a very large number of prophylactic doses would be needed to prevent a very small number of cases or IE. **The cumulative risk for IE is much greater with ordinary daily activities** (e.g., chewing, brushing, and flossing). On the other hand, the risks of single-dose antibiotic prophylaxis are quite low but they do exist (e.g., increased antibiotic resistance and rare cases of anaphylaxis). The AHA suggests that there be greater emphasis on oral health in individuals with high-risk cardiac conditions.

The guidelines conclude that **antibiotic prophylaxis is reasonable in very few clinical situations.** Prophylaxis is now recommended (despite the lack of conclusive evidence) **only** for patients undergoing certain dental procedures with cardiac conditions associated with the highest risk of adverse outcome (Table 5). This does **not** include patients with MVP.

- **Only dental procedures that involve manipulation of the gingival tissue or the periapical region** (i.e., near the roots) of teeth or perforation of the oral mucosa warrant prophylaxis. Tooth extractions and cleanings are included. In these instances, prophylactic antibiotics

TABLE 5	Cardiac Conditions with the Highest Risk of Adverse Outcome from Infective Endocarditis

Prosthetic valve or prosthetic material used for valve repair
Previous infective endocarditis
Congenital heart disease (CHD)
Unrepaired cyanotic CHD, including palliative shunts and conduits
Completely repaired CHD with prosthetic material or device, whether placed by
 surgery or by catheter intervention, during the first 6 months after the procedure
Repaired CHD with residual defects at the site or adjacent to the site of a
 prosthetic patch or prosthetic device (which inhibit endothelialization)
Recipients of cardiac transplants who develop cardiac valvulopathy

Modified from Wilson W, Taubert KA, Gewitz M, et al. Prevention of infective endocarditis: guidelines from the American Heart Association. *Circulation* 2007;116:1736–1754.

should be directed against viridans streptococci. Despite known resistance patterns, the recommended regimens for **dental procedures** are as follows:

- **Amoxicillin 2 g PO 30 to 60 minutes before the procedure.**
- **If unable to take PO,** ampicillin 2 g IM/IV **OR** cefazolin 1 g IM/IV **OR** ceftriaxone 1 g IM/IV 30 to 60 minutes before the procedure.
- **If allergic to penicillins,** cephalexin 2 g PO (do not use if there is a history of ana-phylactoid reactions) **OR** clindamycin 600 mg PO **OR** azithromycin/clarithromycin 500 mg PO 30 to 60 minutes before the procedure. Another first- or second-gen-eration cephalosporin may be used in doses equivalent to cephalexin.
- For patients who are **penicillin allergic AND cannot take PO,** cefazolin/ceftriaxone 1 g IM/IV (do not use if there is a history of anaphylactoid reactions) **OR** clindamycin 600 mg IM/IV 30 to 60 minutes before the procedure.
- **Infective endocarditis** prophylaxis may also be reasonable for high-risk patients hav-ing **procedures on the respiratory tract involving incision or biopsy of the respiratory mucosa.** The same regimens recommended above for dental procedures should be used.
- **For procedures on infected skin, skin structures, or musculoskeletal tissue,** it is reasonable that treatment of the infection itself should be active against staphylococci and β-hemolytic streptococci, for example, an antistaphylococcal penicillin or cephalosporin. For patients unable to tolerate penicillins or who are suspected or known to have an oxacillin-resistant *Staphylococcus aureus* (ORSA) infection, van-comycin or clindamycin may be used.
- **Antibiotics solely for the purpose of IE prophylaxis are no longer recommended for gastroin-testinal (including endoscopy) or genitourinary procedures on any patient** (Table 5).

ANTICOAGULATION

- Patients with mechanical prosthetic valves require long-term anticoagulation (target international normalized ratio [INR], 2.5 to 3.5).
- Patients with a higher risk of embolic (mitral valve replacement, atrial fibrillation) should be treated with aspirin (80 to 100 mg/day) though the risk of bleeding is increased, particularly in the elderly.
- Patients undergoing minor surgery or dental procedures do not require discontinu-ation of warfarin.

- However, patients with mechanical valves and atrial fibrillation or prior emboli should receive heparin as a bridge when warfarin is stopped for major surgery.
- In general, warfarin is stopped for 72 hours prior to surgery and heparin is initiated when INR is <2.0.
- Heparin is stopped for 6 hours prior to surgery and reinitiated as soon as feasible postoperatively and continued until the INR is >2.0.
- Low-molecular-weight heparin has been used in small studies. No large randomized studies have been performed, so no official recommendation has been made.

REFERENCES

1. Bonow RO, Carabello BA, Chatterjee K, et al. ACC/AHA 2006 guidelines for the management of patients with valvular heart disease: a report of the American College of Cardiology/ American Heart Association Task Force on Practice Guidelines (Writing Committee to Develop Guidelines for the Management of Patients With Valvular Heart Disease): developed in collaboration with the Society of Cardiovascular Anesthesiologists: endorsed by the Society for Cardiovascular Angiography and Interventions and the Society of Thoracic Surgeons. *Circulation* 2006;114:e84–e231.
2. Nkomo VT, Gardin JM, Skelton TN, Gottdiener JS, Scott CG, Enriquez-Sarano M. Burden of valvular heart diseases: a population-based study. *Lancet* 2006;368:1005–1011.
3. Cowell SJ, Newby De, Prescott RJ, et al. A randomized trial of intensive lipid-lowering therapy in calcific aortic stenosis. *N Engl J Med* 2005;352:2389–2397.
4. Moura LM, Ramos SF, Zamorano JL, et al. Rosuvastatin affecting aortic valve endothelium to slow the progression of aortic stenosis. *J Am Coll Cardiol* 2007;49:554–561.
5. Scognamiglio R, Rahimtoola RH, Fasoli G, Nistri S, Dalla VS. Nifedepine in asymptomatic patients with severe aortic regurgitation and normal left ventricular function. *N Engl J Med* 1994;331:689–694.
6. Evangelista A, Tornos P, Sambola A, Permanyer-Miralda G, Soler-Soler J. Long-term vasodilator therapy in patients with severe aortic regurgitation. *N Engl J Med* 2005;353: 1342–1349.
7. Freed LA, Levy D, Levine RA, et al. Prevalence and clinical outcome of mitral-valve prolapse. *N Engl J Med* 1999;341:1–7.
8. Wilson W, Taubert K, Gewitz M, et al. Prevention of infective endocarditis: Guidelines from the American Heart Association: A guideline from the American Heart Association Rheumatic Fever, Endocarditis, and Kawasaki Disease Committee, Council on Cardiovascular Disease in the Young, and the Council on Clinical Cardiology, Council on Cardiovascular Surgery and Anesthesia, and the Quality of Care and Outcomes Research Interdisciplinary Working Group. *Circulation* 2007;116:1736–1754.

7 Arrhythmia and Syncope

Scott B. Marrus and Timothy W. Smith

GENERAL APPROACH TO ARRHYTHMIAS

Introduction

- The primary care physician will frequently be the first to encounter or suspect an arrhythmia and similarly will continue to care for the patient once the arrhythmia is diagnosed. This chapter focuses on arrhythmia diagnosis and management with an emphasis on issues which arise in the primary care setting.
- The initial approach to any ongoing arrhythmia includes obtaining vital signs and a 12-lead electrocardiogram (ECG). If the patient is unstable (i.e., hypotensive, hypoxic, experiencing chest pain, or dyspnea), immediate treatment according to ACLS (advance cardiac life support) algorithms is necessary.
- Frequently, the clinician is faced with a patient whose symptoms are fleeting and not ongoing. If no ECG tracing from a previous event is available, an arrhythmia can be suspected but not definitively diagnosed. Efforts to confirm or detect the arrhythmia are a large part of the clinical approach to the syndrome.
- If an arrhythmia is suspected, a thorough history and physical exam should be performed.
- The symptoms of arrhythmias are frequently nonspecific and include palpitations, lightheadedness, chest pain, presyncope/syncope, dyspnea, and a sense of anxiety. At the same time, many serious arrhythmias are frequently asymptomatic.
- Frequently, the utility of the history and physical exam is to detect other signs of underlying cardiovascular disease. Fortunately, once an ECG or rhythm monitor recording of the arrhythmia is obtained, a diagnosis can frequently be made.
- In a few cases, such as pre-excitation, the nature of the arrhythmia is evident on a baseline ECG. However, this is the exception, and other tools must be used to obtain a recording of the arrhythmia.

Diagnostic Tools

- Several options are available for the diagnosis of arrhythmias and the correlation of the arrhythmia with the patient's symptoms.
  - **Holter monitor:** an ambulatory ECG monitor that records continuously for 24 or 48 hours. The entire time period is then reviewed for arrhythmias. This approach is useful only in patients with **daily symptoms.**
  - **Event monitor or loop recorder:** an ambulatory ECG monitor which records continuously but saves data only when triggered, either by the patients when they experience symptoms or by predefined criteria such as heart rate. Events are then transmitted via a transtelephonic system for interpretation. This is often the most cost-effective method of identifying arrhythmias and correlating them with symptoms.
  - **Implantable event monitor:** for relatively rare events, an implantable device can be placed.

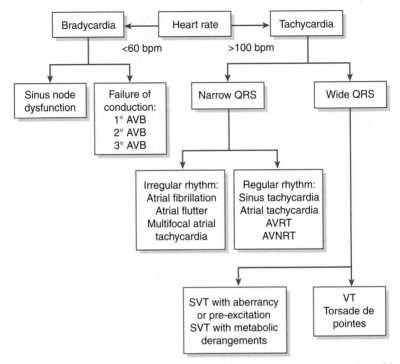

Figure 1. Arrhythmia classification. AVB, atrioventricular block; AVNRT, atrioventricular nodal reentrant tachycardia; AVRT, atrioventricular reentrant tachycardia; bpm, beats per minute; SVT, supraventricular tachycardia; VT, ventricular tachycardia.

Classification

- The categorization of arrhythmias is complex and can include categories based on the underlying electrophysiological mechanisms (reentry, triggered activity, enhanced automaticity), rate, site of origin, and ECG features.
- Although treatment depends primarily on the underlying mechanism, historical terminology and conventions dictate most arrhythmia nomenclature.
- Although there are some inconsistencies, a practical taxonomy for arrhythmias is based on rate and prominent ECG features.
- The first division of this taxonomy is by rate: Tachyarrhythmias are those with a rate >100 beats per minute (bpm), whereas bradyarrhythmias have a rate typically <60 bpm. The terms tachycardia/tachyarrhythmia and bradycardia/bradyarrhythmia are essentially synonymous and will be used interchangeably in this chapter.
- Figure 1 provides an overview of the traditional classification of arrhythmias.

TACHYARRHYTHMIAS

- Tachyarrhythmias exhibit a heart rate >100 bpm and can arise from either supraventricular or ventricular origins.

- Although the appropriate management is dictated by the origin and the mechanism (increased automaticity, reentry, or triggered activity), these details are often not immediately evident.
- For practical purposes, therefore, a distinction is often made between narrow-complex and wide-complex tachycardias (WCT) on the basis of a QRS complex < or >120 ms.

NARROW-COMPLEX TACHYCARDIA

- Narrow-complex tachyarrhythmias invariably originate above or at the atrioventricular (AV) node with a resultant narrow QRS complex that reflects normal activation along the His-Purkinje system.
- Narrow-complex tachycardias are further divided based on the regularity of the rhythm, although this can be difficult to discern at rapid heart rates.
- These arrhythmias include sinus tachycardia, atrial fibrillation (AF), atrial flutter, atrial tachycardias, and various reentrant arrhythmias (e.g., atrioventricular reentrant tachycardia [AVRT], atrioventricular nodal reentrant tachycardia [AVNRT]).

Initial Approach to Narrow-Complex Tachycardia

- The first priority is to check the patient's vital signs and initiate the appropriate ACLS protocol if the patient is unstable.
- In the stable patient, obtain a 12-lead ECG. However, correct identification of the arrhythmia is often difficult with rapid heart rates.
- A helpful approach to tachyarrhythmias is to promote vagal (parasympathetic) activity with either carotid massage or administration of adenosine. This serves to slow down AV nodal conduction, decreasing the rate of the rhythm and frequently allowing identification of the rhythm. In addition, reentrant rhythms which require the AV node for their maintenance will be terminated by these maneuvers.
- **Practical tip to administer a carotid sinus massage:**
  - In the absence of carotid bruits, apply circular pressure to one carotid sinus for 5 seconds.
  - Use caution in patients at risk for myocardial ischemia.
- **Practical tip to administer adenosine:**
  - Give 6 mg **rapid** IV push. Adenosine has a half-life of approximately 9 seconds, so the full dose must be pushed and flushed rapidly. A second dose of 12 mg can be used if the first dose has no effect.
  - Adenosine will cause complete heart block; although typically brief, appropriate resuscitation equipment and personnel should be available.
  - The patient should be warned that adenosine will cause a transient feeling of pre-syncope.
  - Rarely, adenosine can cause severe bronchospasm and severe respiratory distress.

Sinus Tachycardia

General Principles

- Although not an arrhythmia per se, it is important to consider sinus tachycardia when confronted with a rapid, narrow-complex tachycardia.

- Sinus tachycardia is almost invariably a response to an underlying condition such as fever, hypovolemia, pain, anemia, thyrotoxicosis, pulmonary disease, congestive heart failure (CHF), caffeine, illicit drug use/withdrawal, or anxiety.[1]
- In rare cases, however, the sinus tachycardia is genuinely inappropriate and may be due to a reentrant arrhythmia within the sinoatrial (SA) node.[2]

Diagnosis
- Heart rate is typically 150 to 200 bpm.
- ECG will demonstrate P wave with a normal axis and morphology.
- Laboratory evaluation should include underlying causes such as anemia, thyrotoxicosis, and drug intoxication (either medical or illicit).

Treatment
- Treatment is focused on the underlying cause.[1]
- Treatment aimed solely at slowing the heart rate (i.e., β-blockers or calcium channel blockers) is **rarely appropriate** and should be pursued only if the underlying cardiac disease (e.g., valvular disease, coronary artery disease [CAD], CHF) results in intolerance of the elevated heart rate. The increased heart rate frequently represents a compensatory response **which is necessary to maintain cardiac output.**
- It should be emphasized that an inappropriate sinus tachycardia is a rare condition and should be considered only after a rigorous exclusion of secondary causes of tachycardia.

Atrial Fibrillation

General Principles
- AF is the most common sustained arrhythmia with an incidence of ~1% in the general population and ~10% in those >80.[1]
- It is most commonly associated with valvular disease, advanced age, hypertension, CHF, CAD, and mechanical dilatation of the atria.[1,3]
- Hyperthyroidism is the most common noncardiac, treatable cause of AF.
- Frequently described as "lone" (i.e., occurring in the absence of other cardiac disease), "first episode," "recurrent," "paroxysmal" (i.e., recurrent episodes which typically self-terminate), "persistent" (i.e., requiring electrical or chemical cardioversion), and "chronic" (i.e., cannot be converted to normal sinus rhythm).
- AF results in three distinct consequences:
  - The loss of AV synchrony with a resultant decrease in cardiac output due to the lack of the atrial contraction.
  - Increased thromboembolic risk due to blood stasis in the noncontractile atrium.
  - Decreased cardiac output and increased myocardial oxygen demand due to the increased ventricular rate.
- The underlying electrical substrate for AF remains under investigation, although the role of the pulmonary veins as a site of initiation has led to new treatment options (see below).

Diagnosis
- ECG demonstrates chaotic atrial activity without evidence of P waves, although some coarse fibrillation waves may be evident in coarse AF (Fig. 2).

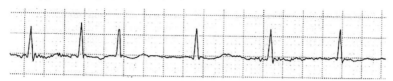

Figure 2. Atrial fibrillation. Note the irregular rhythm and lack of P waves.

- Ventricular rate is typically 140 to 180 bpm but varies substantially depending on rapidity of AV nodal conduction.
- Laboratory evaluation should include tests of thyroid function.

Treatment

- Despite the intuitive appeal of treatment which maintains sinus rhythm, several studies have shown that this strategy is unsuccessful at reducing the morbidity and mortality associated with AF, most likely reflecting the poor success rate of current therapies at maintaining sinus rhythm.[4–6]
- Therefore, current therapy focuses on addressing individually the adverse consequences of AF.
- The two general treatment strategies are often referred to as "rate control," in which the AF rhythm is accepted but the rate is controlled, and "rhythm control," in which efforts are made to maintain sinus rhythm. As discussed below, **both strategies frequently require anticoagulation.**[6]

Control of Ventricular Rate

- Ventricular rate is controlled with medications that slow down AV nodal conduction.
- **β-Blockers and calcium channel blockers** are first-line agents for control of ventricular rate. Choice of specific agents is often determined by other indications or contraindications in a given patient.
- **Digoxin** can also provide control of resting ventricular rate, although it is less effective as reducing ventricular rate during exertion. In addition, digoxin is associated with more side effects than are other agents. Its ideal use is in a patient with LV dysfunction whose ventricular function also benefits from digoxin.
- In some cases, pharmacologic control of ventricular rate proves impossible. In these patients, invasive radio frequency AV node ablation (resulting in complete heart block) with implantation of a permanent pacemaker is an option.

Maintenance of Sinus Rhythm

- Restoration and maintenance of sinus rhythm is a tempting goal but not always readily achievable.
- The aggressiveness with which sinus rhythm is pursued is dictated by patients' overall cardiac function and the degree to which they can tolerate the AF.
- Initial termination of AF is accomplished by synchronized direct current cardioversion (DCCV) with a success rate of ≥80%. DCCV requires sedation and hemodynamic monitoring and should be carried out in facility with emergency resuscitation and airway support available.
- Several medications may result in pharmacologic cardioversion, increase the success rate of DCCV, and improve maintenance of sinus rhythm once cardioversion is accomplished.[1]

- For patients with structural heart disease, preferred agents include amiodarone, sotalol, and dofetilide.
- For patients without structural heart disease, preferred agents include amiodarone, flecainide, and propafenone.
- Amiodarone is typically well tolerated but has several significant long-term side effects. It is therefore less favored for use in young patients who may require decades of therapy.[7]
- Initiation or adjustment of these medications frequently requires inpatient cardiac monitoring and should be performed in consultation with a cardiac electrophysiologist.

AF Ablation/Surgical Treatment Options

- New techniques of catheter-based AF ablation are becoming increasingly successful.
- Should noninvasive attempts to maintain sinus rhythm fail and the patient does not tolerate AF well, invasive ablation techniques can be considered to restore the sinus rhythm.[6]
- Historically, the surgical Cox maze procedure was designed to eliminate AF by creating a pattern of scar lines in the atrium that interrupts the fibrillation. However, this technique is more commonly performed in conjunction with other cardiac operations.
- Minimally invasive catheter-based techniques (such as electrical isolation of the pulmonary veins) may be a more suitable option for patients not requiring cardiac surgery with a success rate of 60% to 80% at experienced centers.
- The details of these techniques continue to undergo rapid development and are beyond the scope of this chapter.
- **Consultation with a cardiac electrophysiologist is warranted for any patient with poorly tolerated AF.**

Thromboembolic Risk

- Although, in theory, restoration of sinus rhythm obviates the need for anticoagulation, several studies have shown that the risk of stroke from atrial thrombi is essentially unchanged by pharmacologic attempts to maintain sinus rhythm.[4,5]
- However, given the risks of anticoagulation, attempts have been made to identify which patients are at high enough risk to justify warfarin therapy.
- Several different indices of thromboembolic risk have been developed. In general, patients with advanced age, CHF, a history of stroke, diabetes, or hypertension are at greater risk of stroke in the context of AF.[4]
- It is essential to ensure the absence of left atrial thrombus **prior to** cardioversion in any patient with AF lasting longer than 48 hours. This can be accomplished with transesophageal echocardiography with visualization of the left atrial appendage; transthoracic echocardiography is not adequate. Alternatively, the patient can be anticoagulated for a period of at least 3 to 4 weeks prior to cardioversion.[4]
- Importantly, the risk of embolic events is highest in the several weeks following cardioversion. Even if the cardioversion is successful with resultant normal electrical activity, restoration of mechanical synchrony requires several weeks. It is therefore essential to continue warfarin anticoagulation for at least 4 weeks following cardioversion.
- It should be emphasized that AF is typically a chronic/recurrent condition. The presumption is therefore that the patient requires permanent anticoagulation unless (a) a contraindication to anticoagulation exists or (b) the patient is clearly at low risk for embolic events.

AF and Pre-excitation (Wolff-Parkinson-White syndrome)

- AF in a patient with an AV bypass tract poses a special risk. In the normal heart, the maximal ventricular rate in AF is limited by the slow conduction of the AV node. When conduction occurs through a bypass tract, the ventricular rate can match the AF rate (400 to 700 bpm) resulting in degeneration into ventricular fibrillation (VF) and cardiovascular collapse.
- The ECG in pre-excited AF is **characterized by an irregularly irregular rate with varying morphologies of a wide-complex QRS.**
- Treatment options include procainamide, amiodarone, or DCCV. AV nodal blocking agents including adenosine, calcium channel blockers, β-blockers, and digoxin should be avoided as they can cause acceleration of the bypass tract conduction. Expert consultation is required for definitive treatment and ablation of the bypass tract.

Perioperative AF

- AF is common in the postoperative patient, especially after cardiac surgery and most specifically valvular surgery. Most episodes are ultimately self-limiting but in the interim pose **the same risks as any other episode of AF.** Because of the potential complications of anticoagulation, prompt DCCV within the first 48 hours of AF is recommended.
- Perioperative treatment with β-blockers has been shown to reduce the incidence of AF.[8]
- In addition, amiodarone is frequently used as either prophylactic treatment or once the AF has occurred.[8]
- Unlike chronic AF, the need for continued therapy should be reevaluated by a cardiologist several months after the operation.

Atrial Flutter

General Principles

- Atrial flutter is sustained reentry within the atria, causing rapid fluttering of the atria.
- Although it is more electrically organized than AF, the atrial transport of blood is still less efficient than normal; flutter thus also has a risk of thromboembolism.
- Many of the same factors that predispose to AF are also related to atrial flutter. It is not uncommon for patients to have both rhythms and transition from one to the other.

Diagnosis

- ECG demonstrates "sawtooth" flutter waves. In typical flutter, these sawtooth waves are most evident in the inferior leads (Fig. 3). In other forms of flutter, various appearances of the flutter waves are possible.
- Flutter waves are typically at a rate of 240 to 340 bpm; 300 bpm is the classic rate.
- Ventricular rate is usually at a 2:1, 3:1, or 4:1 ratio with the atrial rate. Although the ventricular rate may be irregular due to variable conduction block, it is more typically regular with a fixed ratio to the atrial activity.

Treatment

- Medical treatment of atrial flutter is essentially identical to management of AF: control of ventricular rate, management of stroke risk with anticoagulation, and, when possible, maintenance of sinus rhythm.

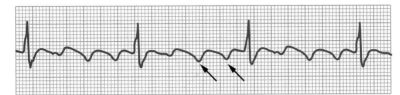

Figure 3. Atrial flutter. This is an example of 3:1 atrial flutter. Note sawtooth-shaped flutter waves (arrows).

- The stereotypical circuit in typical atrial flutter is readily amenable to catheter ablation techniques with a success rate of approximately 90%. However, a significant number of patients subsequently develop AF.[6]

Reentrant Supraventricular Tachycardia (SVT)

General Principles

- Although the term supraventricular tachycardia (SVT) would technically include all rhythms arising above the AV node, it is conventionally applied by cardiologists to a specific group of reentrant rhythms.[9,10]
- SVTs are divided into two main groups based on the anatomy of the reentrant circuit:
  - **AVNRT (AV nodal reentrant tachycardia):** the entire reentrant circuit is contained in the AV node and the immediate surrounding tissue.
  - **AVRT (AV reentrant tachycardia):** the reentrant circuit includes atrial tissue, the AV node, ventricular tissue, and an accessory bypass tract.
- Common features of reentrant rhythms include one branch of the circuit with rapid conduction (and a long refractory period) and another branch with slow conduction (and a short refractory period). With this anatomy, an appropriately timed premature impulse can trigger the reentry and result in continuous cycling of electrical activity in this circuit.
- Different forms of AVRT and AVNRT are characterized by whether the antegrade impulse (forward, i.e., atrial to ventricular) occurs over the "fast" or "slow" pathway. The retrograde impulse (backward, i.e., ventricular to atrial) occurs over the other pathway.
- SVTs result in retrograde P waves as the retrograde signal stimulates the atrium. These rhythms can therefore be further divided into "long RP" in which the (retrograde) P wave occurs significantly after the QRS complex, reflecting retrograde conduction over a slow pathway, or "short RP" in which the (retrograde) P wave occurs rapidly after the QRS.
- AVRT and AVNRT typically occur in patients without other underlying cardiac disease.

Diagnosis

- Clinical presentations include palpitations, dyspnea, syncope, and angina/CHF in patients with underlying cardiac disease.
- Accurate diagnosis of reentrant arrhythmias is frequently, but not invariably, possible from the ECG.

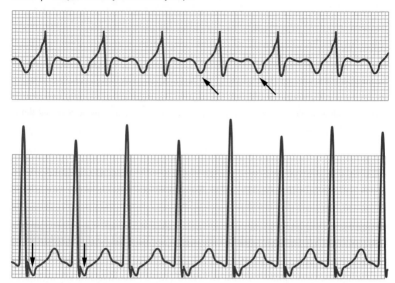

Figure 4. Supraventricular tachycardia. Above, SVT with a long RP interval; note inverted retrograde P waves in lead II (arrows). Below, SVT with a short RP interval; note inverted retrograde P waves in lead II (arrows).

- Reentrant rhythms typically have abrupt onset and termination, in contrast to sinus tachycardia and AF, and exhibit heart rates in the range of 150 to 250 bpm.
- All reentrant SVTs exhibit retrograde P waves which are negative in leads II, III, and aVF, reflecting activation of the atrium in a reverse, caudal-to-cranial direction.
- AVNRT represents approximately 70% of SVTs with AVRT constituting the remainder.[1]
- ECG features of common SVTs are summarized in Figure 4.

Typical AVNRT (50% to 90% of AVNRT):
- Antegrade conduction occurs over the slow pathway and retrograde conduction over the fast pathway.
- As a result, the retrograde P wave occurs within 100 ms of the QRS, making this a "short RP" rhythm. In fact, the RP interval is so brief that typically the P waves are obscured by the QRS or visible only as a pseudo-R in lead V1 or pseudo-S in lead II or III.

Atypical AVNRT:
- Antegrade conduction occurs over the fast pathway and retrograde conduction over the slow pathway.
- As a result, the retrograde P wave is visible between the QRS complexes with a long RP interval.

Orthodromic AVRT (95% of AVRTs):
- Antegrade conduction occurs via the AV node and retrograde conduction over the accessory pathway.
- Most commonly, the RP interval is short due to a fairly rapidly conducting accessory tract. However, a slowly conducting accessory tract is also possible and gives rise to a long RP tachycardia.

Antidromic AVRT:

- This is a WCT but mentioned here for contrast with orthodromic AVRT.
- Antegrade conduction occurs over the accessory pathway with a resultant wide QRS complex.
- AVNRT may be visualized as reentry within the AV node. As a result the tachycardia can continue regardless of events in the atria or ventricles, such as premature ventricular contractions (PVCs), premature atrial contractions (PACs), or bundle branch block. In AVRT, the atrium and ventricle are part of the circuit. Atrial and ventricular events will therefore affect the tachycardia.
- AVRT requires the existence of an accessory tract. Accessory pathways may be "manifest," that is, visible as pre-excited delta waves on the baseline ECG (Wolff-Parkinson-White pattern) or "concealed," that is, lacking evidence of antegrade conduction but capable of retrograde conduction and therefore support of AVRT. A manifest pathway can result in either orthodromic or antidromic AVRT, whereas a concealed pathway is capable only of orthodromic AVRT.

Treatment

- The initial approach to a stable patient with a narrow-complex tachycardia is the use of vagal maneuvers such as the Valsalva maneuver or carotid sinus massage or the administration of adenosine, as discussed above. This will usually result in the termination of the arrhythmia in the case of AVRT and AVNRT.
- Medical treatment consists of AV node blockade with β-blockers, calcium channel blockers, and digoxin.
- DCCV usually terminates the arrhythmia and is required in unstable patients.
- The high success rate (>95%) of catheter ablation makes definitive invasive treatment of these rhythms equally first line with medical management.[9]

Atrial Tachycardia

General Principles

- Atrial tachycardias encompass various intra-atrial arrhythmias, including intra-atrial reentry, automatic tachycardias, and triggered tachycardias.
- These rhythms are almost invariably associated with underlying cardiac disease, chronic obstructive pulmonary disease (COPD), electrolyte imbalances, or digoxin toxicity.[1]

Diagnosis

- ECG features of atrial tachycardia include the following:
  - P wave axis and morphology are **different** from sinus rhythm.
  - Rhythm is typically regular.
  - QRS is usually identical to normal sinus rhythm.
  - An electrophysiology (EP) study is usually required to fully characterize the atrial arrhythmia.

Treatment

- Medical treatment options are focused on treatment of the underlying abnormalities.
- For clinically significant atrial tachycardias, radio frequency catheter ablation is frequently the treatment of choice.

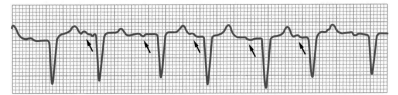

Figure 5. **Multifocal atrial tachycardia.** Note irregular rhythm and P wave with varying morphology and PR interval (arrows).

Multifocal Atrial Tachycardia

General Principles
- Multifocal atrial tachycardia (MAT) is almost invariably associated with COPD or CHF.[11]
- The underlying electrophysiologic mechanism likely involves increased automaticity or triggered activity.

Diagnosis
ECG features of MAT include the following:
- Three or more different P wave morphologies associated with different PR intervals (Fig. 5).
- Atrial rate typically 100 to 130 bpm.

Treatment
- Treatment is focused on the underlying disease with little role for antiarrhythmic medications.
- In cases where treatment is necessary, calcium channel blockers and amiodarone have been shown to have some success.

WIDE-COMPLEX TACHYCARDIAS

- A WCT reflects activation which proceeds through the myocardium *without* use of the His-Purkinje system or does so in a slow and disorganized manner.
- As a result, the QRS is wide due to the slow propagation of the electrical signal. Only a few rhythms generate a wide QRS tachycardia:
  - A ventricular rhythm, that is, ventricular tachycardia (VT).
  - A supraventricular rhythm with aberrancy, that is, an intraventricular conduction delay such as left bundle branch block (LBBB) or right bundle branch block (RBBB).
  - A supraventricular rhythm with excitation through an accessory tract.
  - Metabolic derangements (hyperkalemia or drug toxicity) resulting in a wide QRS.

Initial Approach to a Wide-Complex Tachycardia

- As with narrow-complex tachycardias, the first priority is evaluation of the patient's stability and application of ACLS protocols to the unstable patient.
- The immediate question which must be addressed when confronted with a WCT is whether the rhythm is ventricular in origin or supraventricular with aberrancy or pre-excitation.

- Although the remainder of this discussion will focus on the discrimination between VT and SVT, attention must also be paid to possible metabolic causes of a wide QRS complex, most importantly drug toxicity and hyperkalemia.
- The distinction between VT and SVT with aberrancy is challenging and is not always readily possible. However, several algorithms have been developed to distinguish these possibilities.[12]

Suggestive Features of Ventricular Tachycardia

- Several suggestive features of VT include the following:
  - An extreme rightward axis (−90° to 180°) suggests VT.
  - Slight irregularity or irregularity at the onset of the rhythm suggests VT.
  - A QRS >140 ms in an RBBB-like tachycardia or a QRS >160 ms in a LBBB-like tachycardia suggests VT.
  - The presence of precordial concordance, that is, monomorphic QRS complexes across the precordial leads which are either all entirely positive or all entirely negative suggests VT.
  - The presence of fusion beats (combination of a normal QRS and the ectopic beat) and capture beats (intermittent normal QRS complexes within the tachycardia) indicates AV dissociation and thus indicates VT (Fig. 6).
- In addition, several stepwise algorithms have been developed to distinguish VT from SVT in a WCT.
- The most commonly used criteria are those published by Brugada et al.[13] and are summarized in Table 1. At each step, either the rhythm is identified as VT or one proceeds to the next criterion.
- Although accurate, these criteria are frequently too cumbersome to be applied by those not readily familiar with them. Although the original Brugada criteria demonstrated a sensitivity of 99% and a specificity of 96.5%, further "real-world" studies in which physicians applied these criteria demonstrated a sensitivity of 79% to 92% and a specificity of 44% to 56%.[14]
- A useful rule of thumb is that **any WCT is presumed to be VT until proven otherwise.** This assumption is justified by the fact that up to 80% of WCT in the setting of heart disease is VT.
- This approach is further reinforced by the fact that many of the pharmacological treatments for SVT (adenosine and calcium channel blockers) have the potential to cause degeneration of VT to VF, whereas the treatments for VT (amiodarone and procainamide) are frequently effective and safe for SVT. Therefore, use of VT treatments is preferred if the rhythm is unclear.

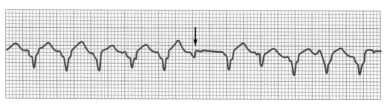

Figure 6. **Ventricular tachycardia.** Note fusion beat (arrow).

TABLE 1	Brugada Criteria for Wide-Complex Tachycardia

- Is there an RS in *any* precordial lead?
  - If no, the rhythm is VT.
- If there is an RS in a precordial lead, measure the time from QRS onset to the nadir of the S wave.
  - If >100 ms, the rhythm is VT.
- Is there evidence of AV dissociation? (i.e., P waves, fusion beats, capture beats)
  - If so, the rhythm is VT.
- Examine the QRS morphology in V1, V2, and V6 for typical VT morphology:
  - RBBB-like pattern (positive QRS polarity in V1 and V2):
    - V1, V2: R or qR indicates VT
  - Other sources also include an RSR′ with R > R′ as indicative of VT
    - V6: rS (i.e., R wave smaller than S wave) indicates VT
  - LBBB-like pattern (negative QRS polarity in V1 and V2):
    - V1, V2: broad initial R wave >40 ms indicates VT

AV, atrioventricular; VT, ventricular tachycardia; LBBB, left bundle branch block; RBBB, right bundle branch block.
Modified from Brugada P, Brugada, J, Mont L, et al. A new approach to the differential diagnosis of a regular tachycardia with a wide QRS complex. *Circulation* 1991;83: 1649–1659.

- **In summary, any WCT should be managed as VT.** Once the patient is stabilized, expert consultation is warranted to clarify the rhythm and future management.

VENTRICULAR ARRHYTHMIAS

- Ventricular arrhythmias encompass a spectrum from single PVCs, couplets and triplets (two to three consecutive PVCs), to VT and VF.
- VT can be described as sustained (definitions vary but are typically defined as >30 seconds in duration or causing hemodynamic collapse requiring immediate cardioversion) or nonsustained (NSVT) (>3 beats but <30 seconds). The abbreviations SVT and NSVT refer to entirely different rhythms despite their similarity. Sustained VT is **not** abbreviated "SVT."
- VT is described as **monomorphic** (in which all of the QRS complexes exhibit the same morphology) or **polymorphic.** Polymorphic VT is closer, both in mechanism and treatment, to VF than to monomorphic VT.
- Management of VT depends on the presence or absence of underlying cardiac disease.
- Reversible causes of VT should be evaluated including cocaine and digitalis intoxication, hypokalemia, hypomagnesemia, and acute ischemia.

Ventricular Arrhythmias in Association with Structural Heart Disease

- VT can be associated with various underlying cardiac diseases, including ischemic cardiomyopathy; nonischemic cardiomyopathy; and infiltrative conditions including amyloidosis, sarcoidosis, either repaired or unrepaired congenital heart disease, and muscular dystrophies.

- Most studies have focused on ischemic and, more recently, nonischemic dilated cardiomyopathies. However, the general approach is applied to cardiomyopathies of other etiologies.

Premature Ventricular Contractions

- PVCs in the context of structural heart disease are associated with an increased risk of sudden cardiac death (SCD).
- However, pharmacological suppression, although effective at reducing the incidence of PVCs, has failed to show a mortality benefit. In fact, use of Class I antiarrhythmics results in an *increased* mortality in the setting of ischemic heart disease.[15,16]
- In light of this, treatment of asymptomatic PVCs themselves is not warranted. Symptomatic PVCs may be treated with β-blockers and other antiarrhythmic agents.

Nonsustained VT

- NSVT in the context of structural heart disease is similarly associated with SCD. As with PVCs, pharmacologic therapy alone does not reduce the incidence of SCD.
- For patients with at least moderately reduced ejection fraction (EF) (typically defined as ≤35%), an implantable cardiac defibrillator (ICD) is warranted for primary prevention, as discussed below, and the presence or absence of NSVT is largely immaterial.

Sustained VT

- Sustained VT requires immediate medical attention. In the unstable patient, termination of the rhythm requires immediate cardioversion.
- In the stable patient, consideration can be given to pharmacologic termination with either amiodarone or lidocaine.
- Unless the rhythm is unequivocally the result of a transient and reversible cause, such as an electrolyte abnormality, ICD therapy is usually indicated.
- Expert consultation is warranted for any sustained VT.

Polymorphic VT

- In the context of ischemic heart disease, polymorphic VT has a worse prognosis than monomorphic VT. Management focuses on treatment of the underlying ischemic disease whenever possible.
- In contrast, other forms of polymorphic VT discussed below require different treatment.

Treatment Options for Ventricular Tachycardia

- After acute termination of the VT, several long-term treatment options are available.
- The first-line treatment is placement of an ICD, which has been shown to reduce mortality when compared with pharmacologic therapy in multiple studies.[17–19]
- Although successful at reducing VT burden, pharmacologic therapy has not been shown to reduce mortality from SCD. As such, its role in treatment is limited to (a) patients with contraindications to ICD placement or (b) patients with an ICD with the intention of reducing the frequency of ICD shocks. First-line medications include amiodarone and sotalol.
- In patients with persistent VT, catheter or surgical ablation procedures can be performed. These procedures are most successful in patients with a well-localized scar rather than a diffuse myocardial process.
- In extreme cases of refractory ventricular arrhythmias, cardiac transplantation can be considered.

VT in Association with Acute Myocardial Ischemia

- The significance of VT in the context of acute myocardial ischemia or infarction depends on the timing of the VT.
- Although VT shortly after acute myocardial infarction (AMI) is a poor prognostic sign with regard to in-hospital mortality, the long-term significance remains unclear. In contrast, late VT portends future malignant arrhythmias.
- One specific form of ischemic arrhythmia, which warrants special mention, is **accelerated idioventricular rhythm** (AIVR). This ventricular rhythm exhibits a wide QRS, a rate between 50 and 120 bpm, and is frequently associated with reperfusion, either spontaneous or medically accomplished. This is a benign rhythm which requires no treatment; there is no long-term prognostic significance of AIVR.

Primary Prevention of Sudden Cardiac Death

- With the increased use of ICDs for termination of potentially fatal ventricular arrhythmias, much attention has been devoted to identifying patients at the greatest risk for SCD.[20]
- The placement of an ICD in patients at high risk for SCD is termed "primary prevention," in contrast to "secondary prevention" in patients who have already experienced either SCD or sustained VT/VF.
- The current ability to identify patients at highest risk for SCD remains limited, as only 30% of patients currently regarded as high risk (i.e., those who receive ICDs) ever experience an aborted arrest and conversely, 50% of SCD occurs in patients not identified as high risk.[21]
- At this point in time, no screening of the general populace is recommended for SCD risk factors beyond standard screening for cardiovascular health.
- Criteria for the placement of an ICD are summarized below in Table 2. Briefly, placement of an ICD for primary prevention is warranted in patients with
  - Ischemic or nonischemic cardiomyopathy and EF <35% with clinical NYHA Class II to III symptoms.
  - EF >35% with NSVT and inducible VT on EP study.

Idiopathic VT Not Associated with Structural Heart Disease

- A minority of ventricular arrhythmias are not associated with obvious structural heart disease, although as our understanding of these diseases progresses, it is frequently discovered that these patients have more subtle molecular or cellular derangements.
- Idiopathic VT is divided into monomorphic and polymorphic VT.
- Monomorphic VT, as found in conditions including repetitive monomorphic VT (RMVT), right ventricular outflow tract VT (RVOT VT), and idiopathic left ventricular VT, has a fairly benign prognosis. In contrast, polymorphic VT, as found in familial catecholaminergic VT, has a more malignant course. The details of these conditions are beyond the scope of this chapter and any VT warrants referral to a cardiac electrophysiologist.

Torsade De Pointes

General Principles

- Torsade de pointes (TdP) (twisting of the points) is a form of polymorphic VT which occurs in association with a baseline prolonged QT interval.

TABLE 2	Selected Indications for Automatic Implantable Cardiac Defibrillator (AICD) Placement

Class I

Cardiac arrest due to VF or VT not due to a reversible cause.

Spontaneous sustained VT in association with structural heart disease.

Syncope of undetermined origin with hemodynamically significant sustained VT induced in EP study not amenable to drug therapy.

Nonsustained VT with CAD, prior MI, LV dysfunction, and inducible VT/VF in EP study.

Class IIa

LV ejection fraction <30%, at least 1 month post-MI and 3 months post-CABG.

Class IIb

Familial and congenital conditions with a high risk of life-threatening ventricular arrhythmias, including hypertrophic cardiomyopathy, long-QT syndrome, Brugada syndrome, and arrhythmogenic right ventricular dysplasia.

Class III

Syncope of undetermined origin without inducible tachyarrhythmias and without structural heart disease.

VF or VT resulting from arrhythmias amenable to surgical or catheter ablation.

VT due to reversible causes, including AMI, electrolyte imbalance, drugs, or trauma.

Significant psychiatric illness precluding reliable follow-up.

Terminal illness with <6 months life expectancy.

Class IV drug-refractory CHF patients who are not candidates for cardiac transplantation.

CABG, coronary artery bypass graft; CAD, coronary artery disease; CHF, congestive heart failure; EP, electrophysiology; LV, left ventricular; MI, myocardial infarction; VF, ventricular fibrillation; VT, ventricular tachycardia.

Class I: Evidence or general agreement that the treatment is useful and effective.

Class IIa: Conflicting evidence or divergence of opinion, with a weight of evidence favoring a benefit.

Class IIb: Conflicting evidence or divergence of opinion, with benefit less well established.

Class III: Evidence or general agreement that the treatment is not effective or is harmful.

Modified from Epstein AE, DiMarco JP, Ellenbogen KA, et al. ACC/AHA/HRS 2008 guidelines for device-based therapy of cardiac rhythm abnormalities. *Circulation* 2008; 117:e350–e408.

- Congenital forms occur in the context of genetic long-QT syndromes (discussed below).
- Most cases occur as the result of acquired QT prolongation due to medications, electrolyte abnormalities (hypokalemia, hypomagnesemia, and hypocalcemia), hypothyroidism, cerebrovascular events, ischemia, or severe CHF.[22]
- In addition, bradycardia (which results in a relatively lengthened QT interval) can exacerbate TdP, although usually this occurs in the context of another precipitating factor.
- Various medications have been associated with a prolonged QT interval. A substantial list of medications (summarized in Table 3) has been associated with QT prolongation, although not invariably with TdP.

TABLE 3	Selected Medications Associated with QT Prolongation

Antiarrhythmic drugs
Quinidine
Procainamide
Disopyramide
Amiodarone
Sotalol
Dofetilide/ibutilide

Psychotropic drugs
Thioridazine
Phenothiazines
Tricyclic antidepressants
Haloperidol
Risperidone
Methadone

Antihistamines
Terfenadine
Astemizole

Antimicrobial drugs
Erythromycin
Clarithromycin
Telithromycin
Azithromycin

Other drugs
Cisapride
Domperidone
Droperidol
Ranolazine
HIV protease inhibitors
Organophosphate insecticides
Cocaine
Arsenic trioxide
Cesium chloride
Some Chinese herbs

- A list of medications associated with QT prolongation and TdP is available at www.qtdrugs.org

Diagnosis
- The ECG appearance of TdP consists of a WCT with a continuously changing axis, giving rise to an undulating appearance (Fig. 7).
- Further laboratory evaluation is focused on electrolyte levels, thyroid function, and myocardial ischemia.

Treatment
- Immediate DCCV is the treatment of choice for an unstable patient with TdP.
- Intravenous magnesium is frequently helpful in terminating stable TdP.
- Avoidance of QT-prolonging medications is crucial in these patients.

Ventricular Fibrillation

VF is a pulseless and **rapidly fatal rhythm without prompt defibrillation** and ACLS management.

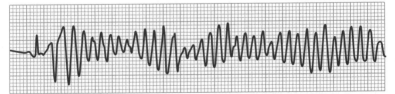

Figure 7. **Torsade de pointes.**

Wolff-Parkinson-White Syndrome and Pre-Excitation

General Principles

- A wide variety of abnormal connections have been described which bypass the normal atria → AV node → bundle of His → Purkinje fiber pattern of excitation.
- The most common and clinically significant of such pathways are Kent bundles, which directly connect atrial and ventricular tissue and are responsible for the Wolff-Parkinson-White syndrome.
- Although other connections exist, their role in arrhythmias is more complex and the Kent bundles serve to illustrate this class of arrhythmias.[1]
- The clinical importance of these pathways is twofold. First, it provides the substrate for reentrant AVRT rhythms (see above). Second, by bypassing the slowed conduction of the AV node, it provides the potential for an atrial arrhythmia such as AF to be conducted at dangerously rapid rates to the ventricle.
- In general, pre-excitation is not associated with other underlying cardiac disease. In the absence of symptoms or a family history of SCD, the occurrence of malignant arrhythmias is rare.

Diagnosis

- The Wolff-Parkinson-White pattern on ECG consists of the following:
  - A short PR interval of <120 ms.
  - A wide QRS interval of >110 to 120 ms, frequently with a slurred upstroke (a delta wave) in some leads.
  - ST-T segment deviation opposite the QRS vector.
- The Wolff-Parkinson-White syndrome consists of the above criteria on the baseline ECG in addition to an SVT (i.e., AVRT).

Treatment

Acute Management

- Acute management is typically required when the patient has developed a reentrant tachycardia or AF with a rapid ventricular response.
- Immediate DCCV is the treatment of choice in the unstable patient.
- Use of AV nodal blocking agents (adenosine, calcium channel blockers, and β-blockers) should be avoided in the case of pre-excited AF since this can result in acceleration of the tachycardia via the accessory pathway.
- IV procainamide or amiodarone can be used safely.

Long-term Management

- In patients without symptoms and at low risk for SCD, treatment may not be necessary.
- Medical treatment options include amiodarone, sotalol, flecainide, or propafenone.
- Radio frequency ablation is 85% to 98% effective at eliminating the bypass tract.

BRADYARRHYTHMIAS

- A heart rate <60 bpm (or according to some, 50 bpm) constitutes bradycardia.
- A considerable variation in normal heart rate has been recorded among healthy patients. Of particular note, trained athletes frequently exhibit heart rates as low as

40 while at rest and can even include sinus pauses and AV nodal blocks. Similarly, heart rates decrease by approximately 24 bpm during sleep.[23]

- As a result of these considerations, it is difficult to define a heart rate alone which warrants treatment. Rather, associated symptoms and the underlying mechanism of the bradycardia must be considered.
- Bradyarrhythmias may result in syncope, lightheadedness, weakness, fatigue, dizziness, or heart failure symptoms.
- Broadly, pathologic bradyarrhythmias result from either a failure of impulse generation by the SA node or by a failure of impulses propagation (i.e., a conduction block).

Sinus Node Dysfunction

General Principles

- **Sick sinus syndrome** is a broad term which encompasses various sinus node dysfunctions.
- One specific form of sick sinus syndrome is known as **tachycardia-bradycardia (or "tachy-brady") syndrome.** This can take the form of almost any combination of tachyarrhythmia and bradyarrhythmia but frequently includes a prolonged sinus pause accompanying the termination of a tachyarrhythmia.
- Sick sinus syndrome can result from either intrinsic fibrosis of the sinus node or extrinsic causes including medications, hypothyroidism, hypothermia, increased intracranial pressure, electrolyte abnormalities, increased vagal tone, ischemia, and surgical trauma.

Diagnosis

- Sick sinus syndrome can have a variety of ECG appearances, including inappropriate sinus bradycardia, sinus pauses, atrial tachyarrhythmias, and inappropriate heart rate responses to exercise.
- Laboratory testing should include thyroid function and electrolyte levels.

Treatment

- Reversible causes and offending medications should be addressed before considering pacemaker implantation. However, if a responsible medication (such as a β-blocker in a patient with CAD) is required, one can consider pacemaker implantation to permit continuation of the medication.
- Indications for pacemaker placement are summarized below in Table 4. They generally include bradycardias that are either of the following:
  - Likely to persist/recur and cause symptoms or
  - Likely to progress to profound bradycardia or asystole.

Conduction Abnormalities

General Principles

- Normal cardiac conduction is initiated at the sinus node and spreads through the atrium to the AV node where it experiences a brief pause before continuing through the His-Purkinje system to activate the ventricular myocardium.

TABLE 4   Selected Indications for Permanent Pacemaker Placement

Class I
  Bradycardia or AVB associated with symptoms
  Third-degree AVB associated with:
    Documented asystole >3 seconds or escape rate <40 bpm
    Neuromuscular disease associated with AVB
  Chronic bifascicular or trifascicular block associated with:
    Intermittent third-degree AVB
    Type-II second-degree AVB
  Congenital third-degree AVB

Class II
  Asymptomatic third-degree AVB with escape rate >40 bpm
  Asymptomatic second-degree Type-II AVB
  Incidental finding of infra-His block on EP study

Class III
  Sinus bradycardia or pauses not associated with symptoms
  Asymptomatic first-degree AVB
  Asymptomatic second-degree Type-I AVB
  AV block expected to resolve

AVB, atrioventricular block; bpm, beats per minute; EP, electrophysiological.
Class I: Evidence or general agreement that the treatment is useful and effective.
Class II: Conflicting evidence or divergence of opinion.
Class III: Evidence or general agreement that the treatment is not effective or is harmful.
Modified from Epstein AE, DiMarco JP, Ellenbogen KA, et al. ACC/AHA/HRS 2008
Guidelines for Device-Based Therapy of Cardiac Rhythm Abnormalities. *Circulation*
2008;117:e350–e408.

- Defects in electrical conduction are described as "atrioventricular block" (AVB) and are categorized based on the behavior of conduction, which typically corresponds to the site/mechanism of the block.
- Causes of AV conduction block are similar to sinus node dysfunction and include fibrosis of the conduction system with age, medications, thyroid disease, infiltrative disease, increased vagal tone, ischemia, and surgical trauma.

Diagnosis

- As with tachyarrhythmias, correlation of symptoms with bradycardia is important and may require the use of ambulatory monitoring. However, the bradyarrhythmia is frequently persistent and readily identified on the 12-lead ECG even at a time that the patient is asymptomatic or minimally symptomatic.
- Laboratory evaluation should include tests of thyroid function and electrolyte levels.
- The ECG features of AV blocks are summarized in Table 5.
- In addition, two special cases of AVB are as follows:
  - 2:1 AVB: Because of the absence of sequential conducted P waves, it is impossible to categorize 2:1 AV block as Type 1 or Type 2. The anatomic level of the block must be inferred.

TABLE 5	Features of Conduction Abnormalities		
Abnormality	**ECG Characteristics**	**Typical Anatomic Location of Block**	**Example**
First-degree AVB	PR interval >120 ms, but without failure of AV conduction (1:1 conduction)	Slowed conduction within the atrium and/or AV node	
Second-degree AVB, Type I (Wenckebach block)	Intermittent failure of AV conduction (A:V > 1:1) Progressively increasing PR interval and (typically) shortening RR interval until a P wave fails to conduct PR interval after the blocked beat is shorter than previous PR interval	High AV node	Note that the nonconducted P wave (arrow) is superimposed on the T wave
Second-degree AVB, Type II	Intermittent failure of conduction; PR interval associated with conducted beats is constant (A:V > 1:1)	His-Purkinje system (infranodal)	
Third-degree AVB	AV dissociation	AV node	

AV, atrioventricular; AVB, atrioventricular block.

- High-grade block: This term describes an AVB with multiple sequential nonconducted P waves. If the block is not associated with intense vagal activity, the anatomic level of the block is usually infranodal.

Treatment

- Reversible causes and offending medications should be addressed before considering pacemaker implantation. However, if a responsible medication (such as a β-blocker in a patient with CAD) is required, one can consider pacemaker implantation to permit continuation of the medication.
- Indications for pacemaker placement are summarized in Table 4.[24]

CONGENITAL ARRHYTHMIAS

Management of congenital arrhythmias is a complex and rapidly evolving field. Any patient suspected of having a congenital arrhythmia syndrome requires evaluation by an experienced specialist.

Brugada Syndrome

- Brugada syndrome is due to mutations in the sodium channel, although the genetics of the disease are complex and incompletely understood.[25]
- Diagnostic criteria continue to evolve but include a typical ECG appearance of ST elevation in leads V1 to V3, an association with spontaneous VT/VF, and a familial pattern.
- Incidence is higher in men than in women and particularly prevalent among Asian males.
- Although pharmacological therapy (usually amiodarone or quinidine) can be considered, affected individuals usually require placement of an ICD for prevention of SCD.

Long QT Syndrome

- To date, mutations in seven genes which generate a congenital QT prolongation have been identified. Subtle differences in clinical features and ECG findings exist among some of these mutations.
- Patients can present with palpitations, syncope, SCD, and TdP.
- Management is complex and depends in part on the genotype of the affected individual. Referral to a cardiac electrophysiologist is warranted in these conditions.[26]

Short QT Syndrome

- Short QT syndrome is a recently described genetic syndrome. To date, mutations in three different potassium channel genes have been associated with short QT syndrome.[27]
- Clinical features include a short QT interval (typically <330 ms when corrected for heart rate), a propensity for AF, and a risk of SCD.
- Optimal medical management for this condition remains undefined. Placement of an ICD is warranted in patients with a personal history or family history of SCD.

Arrhythmogenic Right Ventricular Dysplasia/ Cardiomyopathy (ARVD/ARVC)

- Arrhythmogenic right ventricular dysplasia (ARVD) is characterized by a fibrofatty infiltrate of the right ventricle (although the left ventricle is sometimes involved) with a resultant thinning of the ventricular wall.[28]
- A subset of patients exhibit a familial pattern with mutations in the desmoplakin, plakoglobin, desmoglein, plakophilin-2, or desmocollin (all of which are involved in cell adhesion). Mutations in several other genes as well as mutations at various loci for which the gene is yet to be identified have also been associated with ARVD.
- Naxos disease is an autosomal recessive form of ARVD associated with palmoplantar keratosis and woolly hair.
- Clinical features of ARVD include arrhythmias (most commonly a RVOT VT), syncope, palpitations, and SCD. Despite the involvement of the RV, evidence of RV failure is relatively uncommon.
- Although sotalol and amiodarone may have role in suppressing the ventricular arrhythmias, only ICD placement is likely to reduce the risk of SCD.

Familial Polymorphic Ventricular Tachycardia (Catecholaminergic VT)

- In contrast to TdP, familial polymorphic VT occurs in the absence of QT prolongation. Unlike the other forms of idiopathic VT, this condition is associated with a substantial risk of SCD.
- This syndrome occurs in the absence of apparent cardiac disease and typically manifests as syncope and sudden death; polymorphic VT and VF are most prominent during stress and physical exertion.
- Two genes have been implicated in this condition: the ryanodine receptor (with autosomal dominant transmission) and the calsequestrin 2 gene (with autosomal recessive transmission). Both proteins are involved in calcium handling by the sarcoplasmic reticulum.[29]
- Treatment includes β-blockers, given the catecholamine-induced nature of the arrhythmias. However, even with medical treatment, the incidence of SCD is substantial and ICD placement is typically warranted.

SYNCOPE

General Principles

- Syncope and presyncope can result from a wide variety of mechanisms, including cardiac, neurologic, and metabolic. This section will focus only on the cardiac, and particularly, arrhythmic causes of syncope.
- Studies have estimated that approximately 15% of syncope cases result from arrhythmias. Further, it should be kept in mind that 30% to 50% of cases of syncope have no identifiable cause. Therefore, the diagnostic approach should focus on the identification of high-risk predictors of future events rather than definitive diagnosis of the episode in question.

- Cardiovascular causes of syncope include neurocardiogenic (also known as vasovagal syncope), valvular heart disease, hypertrophic cardiomyopathy, bradyarrhythmias, and tachyarrhythmias.
- Neurocardiogenic syncope is believed to result from a paradoxical bradycardic and/or hypotensive response to a catecholamine surge with resultant syncope.
- Although no findings in the history or physical exam are particularly sensitive or specific, syncope resulting from cardiac arrhythmias tends to occur abruptly and with minimum prodromal symptoms, whereas neurocardiogenic syncope is frequently preceded by a feeling of flushing and lightheadedness.

Diagnosis

- The cardiac evaluation of syncope should include echocardiography and a baseline ECG. Depending on the frequency of events, a Holter or event monitor can be considered to identify a causative arrhythmia.
- The role of tilt-table testing is controversial. This diagnostic test is designed to elicit bradycardia and hypotension in response to gradually increasing the vertical angle of the supine patient and thereby diagnose neurocardiogenic syncope. Sensitivity has been reported as high at 70%; however, 45% to 65% of normal individuals also exhibit a positive response to tilt-table testing, markedly reducing the specificity of this test.[30] In addition, there is a small but distinct risk of cardiac arrest and death.
- The diagnosis of neurocardiogenic syncope can usually be made based on the history and exclusion of other causes without recourse to tilt-table testing.

Treatment

- The management of symptomatic tachyarrhythmias and bradyarrhythmias is covered in the appropriate sections of this chapter.
- Management of neurocardiogenic syncope can be difficult. Although placement of a pacemaker is tempting, the hypotensive response is due to a vasodilatory effect and is *not* a result of the bradycardia. Therefore, patients often continue to have syncope despite control of the bradycardia. Only a subset of patients with an exclusively bradycardic cause of their syncope are likely to benefit from a pacemaker.
- Behavioral modification plays an essential role in the control of neurocardiogenic syncope; patients are educated to avoid environmental triggers and volume depletion. Medications should be reviewed and vasodilatory medications eliminated.
- In selected patients, increased intake of salt and fluids can reduce both orthostatic and neurocardiogenic syncope.
- In general, pharmacologic therapy has been found to be ineffective for neurocardiogenic syncope.[31]
  - β-Blockers (some with intrinsic sympathomimetic activity) have been used, though clinical trial data are conflicting.
  - Midodrine, an α-sympathomimetic drug, may inhibit vasodilation, but there is a risk of hypertension.
  - Some data support a role for selective serotonin reuptake inhibitors (SSRIs), such as paroxetine, and serotonin/norepinephrine reuptake inhibitors (SNRIs), such as venlafaxine.

IMPLANTABLE DEVICES FOR RHYTHM MANAGEMENT

With the increasing prevalence of both pacemakers and implanted defibrillators, it is important for the internist to be familiar with these devices.[32]

Pacemakers

- A pacemaker system consists of one or more electrical leads and a generator containing the battery and processor.
- Pacemaker systems may be either endocardial or epicardial. The more common endocardial system is placed by a percutaneous approach with the electrode leads in a subclavian vein and the generator placed in the subcutaneous pocket near the clavicle. The epicardial system is placed by a surgical approach with the electrodes on the epicardial surface and the generator located either in the upper abdomen or near the clavicle.
- The general principle of all pacemakers is to deliver stimuli which trigger a heartbeat in a pattern which most closely reproduces the normal cardiac activity.
- The full array of algorithms used by modern pacemakers is beyond the scope of this review. However, some general principles of pacemaker function include (for pacemakers programmed in the DDD mode, the most common mode for patients not in AF) the following:
  - If atrial activity is intact, the pacemaker will sense the atrial activity and deliver a ventricular stimulus (if necessary) in response to an atrial P wave.
  - If atrial activity is absent but the intrinsic conduction system is intact, the pacemaker will stimulate the atrium to generate a P wave which is followed by conduction to the ventricle, generating a QRS complex. If the QRS does not occur within a programmed period of time, the pacemaker delivers a ventricular stimulus.
  - If atrial activity is absent and the conduction system is not intact, the pacemaker will deliver stimuli to both the atrium and ventricle with a time delay that simulates the typical P wave and QRS timing.
- Pacemakers can be categorized by the number of leads:
  - **Dual chamber:** the most common configuration. Leads are placed in both the right atrium and the right ventricle. This provides the greatest flexibility of pacemaker modes.
  - **Single chamber:** one lead in the right ventricle. This design is used for patients in whom atrial pacing is not possible, such as chronic AF. Placement of a single atrial lead is an option in patients with an intact conduction system; the frequent progression of disease and subsequent requirement for a ventricular lead may make this an unappealing option.
  - **Biventricular:** In addition to the right atrial and right ventricular leads, a third lead is placed in the coronary sinus to permit independent activation of the left ventricle. This design is used in patients with severe CHF and mechanical dyssynchrony. The selection of patients who will benefit from this device remains under investigation and is beyond the scope of this chapter.
- In addition to the lead configuration, pacemakers and defibrillators are described based on their mode. A five-letter code (although frequently only the first three or four letters are used) describes the sensing and pacing behavior of the device, as summarized in Table 6.

TABLE 6	Implanted Device Modes				
Category	First Letter Chamber paced	Second Letter Chamber sensed	Third Letter Response to sensing	Fourth Letter Programmability	Fifth Letter Antitachycardia function
Letters	O = none; A = atrium; V = ventricle; D = dual (A + V)	O = none; A = atrium; V = ventricle; D = dual (A + V)	O = none; T = triggered; I = inhibited; D = dual (I + T)	O = none; P = simple programming; M = multiprogramming; C = communicating; R = rate-adaptive sensor	O = none; P = pacing; S = shock; D = dual (P and S)

157

- Some common modes of pacemakers include the following:
  - AAI or VVI: simple modes in which the pacemaker will sense and pace the atrium or ventricle at a given rate unless inhibited by endogenous activity.
  - DDDR: a complex mode in which the pacemaker will sense and pace both the atrium and the ventricle in a pattern that attempts to recapitulate normal electrical activity. In addition, a sensor will increase the heart rate if physical activity is detected.
  - VOO: the pacemaker will deliver ventricular pacing a set rate without regard for endogenous activity. This mode has a theoretical risk of R-on-T-induced arrhythmia but is necessary during surgery or other procedures in which electrical interference could cause the pacemaker to fail to pace appropriately.

Pacemaker Management

- Patients with a pacemaker require regular follow-up with an electrophysiologist or cardiologist skilled in pacemaker management. However, the increased use of transtelephonic monitoring has reduced the need for office visits. More sophisticated home-monitoring systems are also being introduced, some utilizing the Internet. Pacemaker batteries require replacement after approximately 3 to 7 years of use, depending on device details and the degree of pacemaker activity.
- Application of a strong magnet will convert any pacemaker to an asynchronous (VOO) mode as long as the magnet is in place over the device. In this mode, the pacemaker will deliver stimuli at a preset rate regardless of sensed cardiac (or extraneous) signals.

Pacemaker Complications and Malfunction
Device Infection

- Device infection is a serious complication and may occur either shortly after implantation or because of seeding of the device at a later time.
- The possibility of endocarditis and device infection must be considered in any patient with bacteremia or signs of local infection at the device site. Explantation of the device is frequently required for definitive treatment.
- In the case of local infection, incision and drainage should be avoided because of the possibility of introducing infection to the device pocket. In general, patients with a possible device infection should be admitted to a facility with experience in this area.

Pacemaker Syndrome

- In the setting of ventricular pacing, some patients experience a syndrome of neck/abdominal pulsations, palpitations, fatigue, dyspnea, and presyncope because of the lack of optimal AV synchrony and resulting decreased cardiac output and increased AV valvular regurgitation.
- Avoiding ventricular-only pacing is the best approach to ameliorating symptoms.

Pacemaker Mediated Tachycardia (PMT)

- Various reentrant arrhythmias may occur which include the pacemaker as part of the circuit despite the use of programming features which minimize this complication. In this situation, application of a magnet to the pacemaker (see above) will interrupt the circuit and terminate the tachycardia.
- Reprogramming may be necessary to prevent recurrences.

Failure to Capture
- Obviously, failure of the pacemaker to stimulate cardiac contraction is a serious malfunction, especially in the pacemaker-dependent patient. In this situation, the first priority is to stabilize the patient with transcutaneous or temporary transvenous pacing if necessary.
- Further evaluation includes consideration of electrolyte disturbances or AMI, both of which can increase the threshold for pacemaker capture. Interrogation of the device will then provide further information regarding device and lead function.

Failure to Sense and Oversensing
- Failure to sense intrinsic cardiac activity results in pacemaker-stimulated beats despite an adequate endogenous rhythm. This rarely presents an acute problem and can be evaluated with device interrogation and expert consultation.
- More seriously, oversensing results when noncardiac signals (diaphragmatic or muscle potentials or environmental signals) are misinterpreted by the device as cardiac activity with a resulting suppression of pacemaker activity. In this case, application of a magnet to the device will result in asynchronous pacing until the problem can be further evaluated.

Automatic Implantable Cardiac Defibrillator (ICD)

- The role of the ICD (also sometimes referred to as automatic implantable cardiac defibrillator) is to continuously monitor the cardiac rhythm and to terminate potentially lethal ventricular arrhythmias.[20]
- Two groups of patients are considered candidates for ICD placement. Patients who have experienced VT/VF and survived warrant ICD placement for secondary prevention of future events. In addition, prophylactic placement of ICDs for prevention of SCD in high-risk patients (primary prevention) has become the standard of care. However, accurate identification of high-risk patients continues to evolve.[24] The current guidelines are summarized in Table 2.
- As with pacemakers, both the more common endocardial and surgical epicardial systems can be placed.
- All ICDs have a basic backup pacing ability. For patients with indications for both a pacemaker and an ICD, a more comprehensive combination device which combines a full array of pacemaker and ICD functions is used.
- To terminate ventricular arrhythmias, ICDs use two techniques:
  - Antitachycardia pacing: a burst of pacing stimuli is delivered at a rate slightly faster than the tachycardia. Frequently, this will interrupt and terminate a reentrant rhythm.
  - Shock delivery: the device is capable of delivering a defibrillatory shock identical in function to external unsynchronized cardioversion.
- Complex and currently imperfect algorithms are used by the device to differentiate VT and VF from atrial arrhythmias. Heart rate remains the most important criterion for detection of ventricular arrhythmias. Inappropriate shocks due to atrial tachyarrhythmias are a risk of ICD therapy.

ICD Management

- Patients should be followed on a regular basis by the electrophysiologist who implanted or who monitors the device.
- Remote follow-up is becoming more common, reducing the frequency of routine office visits.
- Discharge of the ICD is an uncomfortable and alarming experience for the patient. However, it should be remembered that this is the role of the device.
- A single shock does not necessarily require immediate evaluation; however, the patient should contact his or her cardiologist or electrophysiologist at the first opportunity. Multiple shocks or shocks associated with symptoms such as syncope, chest pain, or shortness of breath warrant an immediate emergency department evaluation.

Magnet Application

- Application of a strong magnet to the ICD activates a switch which **disables the anti-tachycardia functions** of the device; it has **no effect on the backup pacing function** (in contrast to the effect of a magnet on the pacemaker as discussed above).
- This is used when the device is delivering shocks inappropriately. With the increased prevalence of devices and, consequently, device malfunction, any facility with ACLS equipment should consider having a magnet available for management of this situation.
- Appropriate magnets can be obtained from the manufacturers of ICDs.

ICD Complications and Malfunction

Device Infection

As with pacemakers, ICD infection is a serious problem and should be managed as discussed above.

Inappropriate Defibrillator Firing/Shock

- The current algorithms used by the ICD to distinguish SVT from VT/VF are imperfect, sometimes resulting in inappropriate shocks for supraventricular rhythms.
- Acute management of this situation includes ECG monitoring to determine the rhythm and application of a magnet if the shocks are inappropriate. Immediate availability of resuscitation personnel and equipment is necessary while the device is inactivated.
- Expert consultation is required to address the reason for the inappropriate therapy.

Failure to Treat VF/VT

Episodes of VF/VT which are not treated by the device require expert consultation for possible reprogramming of the ICD. In the interim, the patient requires monitoring in a facility able to manage these rhythms.

Other Device Concerns

Perioperative Management

- Several concerns arise with pacemaker or ICD function during an operation. Vibrations, pressure, and electrical signals from electrocautery can interfere with normal pacemaker function.
- In general, reprogramming the pacemaker to a DOO/VOO mode and inactivation of the rate-responsive element will prevent these complications. After the procedure, the device should be interrogated to ensure that no damage occurred.

- For thoracic operations, a chest radiography should be performed to confirm that the lead position was not affected.

MRI Imaging
- MRI imaging is contraindicated in patients with a pacemaker or ICD because of the possibility of heating and torque forces on the device itself from the magnetic field as well as potential reprogramming of the device.
- Although investigation into both MRI-compatible devices as well as modification of MRI protocols is underway, a patient with an implanted device should not undergo MRI imaging at this time without consultation with cardiology and radiology.

Radiation Therapy
- Radiation therapy has minimal immediate effect on the device if the beam is not directed directly at or near the pulse generator; however, cumulative radiation doses can result in device damage and warrant regular device interrogation.
- In addition, the shielding effect of the device may reduce the efficacy of the radiation treatment. Consultation with the patient's cardiologist and/or device manufacturer is desirable.

Cardioversion/Defibrillation
- Application of external defibrillation or cardioversion may damage the device. The pads should be applied at a distance from the implanted device and proper device function confirmed once the patient is stabilized.
- **This concern should not prevent the application of appropriate ACLS treatments to the unstable patient.**

Exposure to Environmental EMI
- Electromagnetic interference (EMI) is ubiquitous in the modern world. Common sources include cell phones, antitheft devices, metal detectors, microwave ovens, and high-voltage power lines. However, few cases of significant interference have been reported.
- Patients can limit the potential for interference by not carrying the cell phone in a pocket over the device and using the more distant ear during conversations and by not lingering in the field of antitheft or metal detectors.
- Modern microwave ovens are no longer considered a significant concern (in contrast to early generation ovens).
- Patients exposed to significant electrical signals from industrial equipment should consult their cardiologist.

Driving and Physical Activity
- Few clear guidelines have been published on the issue of physical activity; however, avoidance of contact sports which risk device damage and competitive exertion in patients at risk for arrhythmias is reasonable.
- With regard to driving, physicians should be familiar with local statutes.
- However, it is recommended that patients avoid driving until they are free of VT/VF and ICD shocks for a period of 6 months.

ANTIARRHYTHMIC MEDICATIONS

The generic names, trade names, common indications, and side effects of frequently used antiarrhythmic medications are summarized in Table 7.

TABLE 7	Antiarrhythmic Medications			
Class	Mechanism	Indications	Side Effects	Other Comments
Class Ia	Decreases phase 0 repolarization and inhibits Na and K channels			Prolongs QRS, QT, PR
Quinidine		Atrial fibrillation, flutter, ventricular arrhythmias	Diarrhea, nausea, vomiting, rash, hypotension, fever, tinnitus, blurred vision, headache, thrombocytopenia, lupus-like syndrome	May enhance AV nodal conduction; increases digoxin level and warfarin effects; amiodarone increases quinidine levels; therapeutic range 2–6 mg/L
Procainamide (Pronestyl, Procan)		Ventricular arrhythmias (labeled); atrial arrhythmias (unlabeled)	Drug-induced SLE, GI symptoms, hypotension, rash, insomnia, hepatitis, myopathy, agranulocytosis, heart block/asystole	50%–85% develop ANA; 30%–50% develop SLE; adjust dose for renal dysfunction; therapeutic range 4–10 mg/L (NAPA <20 mg/L)
Disopyramide (Norpace)		Ventricular arrhythmias (labeled); atrial arrhythmias (unlabeled)	Anticholinergic effects, nausea, vomiting, hypotension, hypoglycemia, nervousness	Significant negative inotropic activity; adjust dosage in patients with renal insufficiency, hepatic disease, CHF, and elderly; may enhance AV nodal conduction; therapeutic range 2–6 mg/L

	Mechanism	Indication	Adverse effects	Comments
Class Ib	Decreases phase 0 depolarization and slows down intracardiac conduction			No ECG changes
Lidocaine (Xylocaine)		Acute treatment of ventricular arrhythmias	CNS effects, seizures, coma, psychosis, tremor	Monitor levels for infusions for >24 hours Dependent on hepatic blood flow Therapeutic level 1.5–5 mg/L
Mexiletine (Mexitil)		Ventricular arrhythmias	Cardiac depression, bradycardia/asystole	Should be taken with food; reduce dosage in hepatic dysfunction, CHF, and CrCl >10; therapeutic level 0.5–2 mg/L
Class Ic	Decreases phase 0 depolarization and markedly slows intracardiac conduction		Nausea, vomiting, thrombocytopenia, AV block	Avoid in patients with structural heart disease; prolongs PR and QRS
Fleicainide (Tambocor)		Paroxysmal AF and flutter; paroxysmal SVT (AVNRT); ventricular arrhythmia	Bradycardia, heart block, proarrhythmia	Avoid in patients with CHF; may increase defibrillation threshold; reduce dose in hepatic dysfunction, renal insufficiency, and CHF; therapeutic level 0.2–1 mg/L
Propafenone (Rythmol)		Ventricular arrhythmias (labeled); SVT (unlabeled)	Significant negative inotropy, blurry vision, headache, GI symptoms, neutropenia	May worsen obstructive lung disease; reduce dose in hepatic dysfunction
			Metallic/bitter taste, headache, GI upset, cholestatic jaundice	

(continued)

TABLE 7   Antiarrhythmic Medications (Continued)

Class	Mechanism	Indications	Side Effects	Other Comments
Class II Metoprolol (Lopressor); carvedilol (Coreg); atenolol (Tenormin); esmolol (Brevibloc); and others	β-Adrenergic blockade	HTN; rate control in SVT; ventricular ectopy; angina/CAD	Bradycardia, bronchospasm in predisposed patients, fatigue, CHF exacerbation, hypotension, sexual dysfunction, dizziness	Contraindications: bradycardia, heart block, cardiogenic shock, acute CHF, severe bronchospastic lung disease; may blunt hypoglycemic symptoms
Class III Amiodarone (Cordarone)	K channel inhibition Complex activity at multiple ion channels	Ventricular arrhythmias (labeled); atrial arrhythmias (unlabeled)	Proarrhythmia, torsade de pointes Hyper/hypothyroidism, chemical hepatitis, pulmonary fibrosis, bradycardia, heart block/bradycardia, skin photosensitivity	ECG effects: sinus bradycardia, PR, QRS, and QT prolongation
Dofetilide (Tikosyn)		Maintenance of sinus arrhythmia after cardioversion for AF	Can cause life-threatening ventricular arrhythmia	ECG effect: QTc prolongation; initiation of treatment requires 72 hours inpatient monitoring with QTc measurement after each dose; Only certified cardiologists can prescribe dofetilide

Drug	Mechanism	Indication	Adverse effects	Notes
Sotalol (Betapace)	Combined β-blocker and K-channel blocker	Ventricular arrhythmia (labeled); atrial fibrillation (unlabeled)	Proarrhythmia, including torsade de pointes	ECG effects: sinus bradycardia, QT and PR prolongation; reduce dose in renal dysfunction
Class IV				
Diltiazem (Cardizem)	Calcium channel blockade	Rate control of atrial arrhythmias	Negative inotropy, headache, dizziness, edema, bradycardia, AV block, hypotension	
Verapamil (various)		Rate control of atrial arrhythmia	Negative inotropy, constipation, hypotension, bradycardia, AV block	
Others				
Adenosine (Adenocard)	Depression of AV conduction due to α_1-agonism	Conversion of reentrant SVT	Flushing, dyspnea, chest pressure, nausea, bronchospasm, heart block	May produce transient asystole
Digoxin (Lanoxin)	Increased AV node refractory period due to increased vagal tone	Rate control of AF, atrial flutter, or SVT	Bradycardia, AV block, anorexia, nausea, diarrhea, yellow-green halo around light, blurry vision, confusion, proarrhythmia	ECG effects: PR prolongation, ST depression; toxicity characterized by atrial arrhythmia in conjunction with heart block; toxicity possible at therapeutic levels; toxicity treated with electrolyte correction and use of Digibind; therapeutic levels 1–2 ng/mL

ANA, antinuclear antibody; AV, atrioventricular; AVB, atrioventricular block; AVNRT, atrioventricular nodal reentrant tachycardia; CAD, coronary artery disease; CHF, congestive heart failure; CNS, central nervous system; ECG, electrocardiogram; GI, gastrointestinal; HTN, hypertension; NAPA, n-acetyl procainamide; SLE, systemic lupus erythematosus; SVT, supraventricular tachycardia.

REFERENCES

1. Ellis K, Dresing T. Tachyarrhythmias. In: Griffin BP, Topol EJ, eds. Manual of Cardiovascular Medicine. Philadelphia, PA: Lippincott Williams and Wilkins, 2004:283–313.
2. Yusuf S, Camm, AJ. The sinus tachycardias. *Nat Clin Pract Cardiovasc Med* 2005;2:44–52.
3. Falk RH. Atrial fibrillation. *N Engl J Med* 2001;344:1067–1078.
4. Lip GY, Tse HF. Management of atrial fibrillation. *Lancet* 2007;370:604–618.
5. Wyse DG, Waldo AL, DiMarco JP, et al. A comparison of rate control and rhythm control in patients with atrial fibrillation. *N Engl J Med* 2002;347:1825–1833.
6. Hall MC, Todd DM. Modern management of arrhythmias. *Postgrad Med J* 2006;82: 117–125.
7. Zimetbaum P. Amiodarone for atrial fibrillation. *N Engl J Med* 2007;356:935–941.
8. Mayson SE, Greenspon AJ, Adams S, et al. The changing face of postoperative atrial fibrillation prevention: a review of current medical therapy. *Cardiol Rev* 2007;15:231–241.
9. Ganz LI, Friedman PL. Supraventricular tachycardia. *N Engl J Med* 1995;332:162–173.
10. Delacretaz E. Clinical practice. Supraventricular tachycardia. *N Engl J Med* 2006;354: 1039–1051.
11. McCord J, Borzak, S. Multifocal atrial tachycardia. *Chest* 1998;113:203–209.
12. Eckardt L, Breithardt G, Kirchhof P. Approach to wide complex tachycardias in patients without structural heart disease. *Heart* 2006;92:704–711.
13. Brugada P, Brugada J, Mont L, et al. A new approach to the differential diagnosis of a regular tachycardia with a wide QRS complex. *Circulation* 1991;83:1649–1659.
14. Isenhour JL, Craig S, Gibbs M, et al. Wide-complex tachycardia: continued evaluation of diagnostic criteria. *Acad Emerg Med* 2000;7:769–773.
15. Echt DS, Liebson PR, Mitchell LB, et al. Mortality and morbidity in patients receiving encainide, flecainide, or placebo. The Cardiac Arrhythmia Suppression trial. *N Engl J Med* 1991;324:781–788.
16. Waldo AL, Camm AJ, deRuyter H, et al. Effect of d-sotalol on mortality in patients with left ventricular dysfunction after recent and remote myocardial infarction. The SWORD Investigators. Survival With Oral d-Sotalol. *Lancet* 1996;348:7–12.
17. Bardy GH, Lee KL, Mark DB, et al. Amiodarone or an implantable cardioverter-defibrillator for congestive heart failure. *N Engl J Med* 2005;352:225–237.
18. Moss AJ, Zareba W, Hall WJ, et al. Prophylactic implantation of a defibrillator in patients with myocardial infarction and reduced ejection fraction. *N Engl J Med* 2002;346:877–883.
19. Moss AJ, Hall WJ, Cannom DS, et al. Improved survival with an implanted defibrillator in patients with coronary disease at high risk for ventricular arrhythmia. Multicenter Automatic Defibrillator Implantation Trial Investigators. *N Engl J Med* 1996;335:1933–1940.
20. DiMarco JP. Implantable cardioverter-defibrillators. *N Engl J Med* 2003;349:1836–1847.
21. Zipes DP, Camm AJ, Borggrefe M, et al. ACC/AHA/ESC 2006 guidelines for management of patients with ventricular arrhythmias and the prevention of sudden cardiac death: a report of the American College of Cardiology/American Heart Association Task Force and the European Society of Cardiology Committee for Practice Guidelines (Writing Committee to Develop Guidelines for Management of Patients With Ventricular Arrhythmias and the Prevention of Sudden Cardiac Death): developed in collaboration with the European Heart Rhythm Association and the Heart Rhythm Society. *Circulation* 2006;114:e385–e484.
22. Yap YG, Camm AJ. Drug induced QT prolongation and torsades de pointes. *Heart* 2003;89:1363–1372.
23. Mangrum JM, DiMarco JP. The evaluation and management of bradycardia. *N Engl J Med* 2000;342:703–709.
24. Epstein AE, DiMarco JP, Ellenbogen KA, et al. ACC/AHA/HRS 2008 guidelines for device-based therapy of cardiac rhythm abnormalities: a report of the American College of Cardiology/American Heart Association Task Force on Practice Guidelines (Writing Committee to Revise the ACC/AHA/NASPE 2002 Guideline Update for Implantation of Cardiac Pacemakers and Antiarrhythmia Devices): developed in collaboration with the American Association for Thoracic Surgery and Society of Thoracic Surgeons. *Circulation* 2008;117:e350–e408.

25. Rossenbacker T, Priori SG. The Brugada syndrome. *Curr Opin Cardiol* 2007;22:163–170.

26. Schwartz PJ. Management of long QT syndrome. *Nat Clin Pract Cardiovasc Med* 2005;2: 346–351.

27. Brugada R, Hong K, Cordeiro JM, Dumaine R. Short QT syndrome. *CMAJ* 2005;173: 1349–1354.

28. Kies P, Bootsma M, Bax J, et al. Arrhythmogenic right ventricular dysplasia/cardiomyopathy: screening, diagnosis, and treatment. *Heart Rhythm* 2006;3:225–234.

29. Francis J, Sankar V, Nair VK, Priori SG. Catecholaminergic polymorphic ventricular tachycardia. *Heart Rhythm* 2005;2:550–554.

30. Kapoor WN, Brant N. Evaluation of syncope by upright tilt testing with isoproterenol. A nonspecific test. *Ann Intern Med* 1992;116:358–363.

31. Chen LY, Shen WK. Neurocardiogenic syncope: latest pharmacological therapies. *Expert Opin Pharmacother* 2006;7:1151–1162.

32. Schoenfeld MH. Contemporary pacemaker and defibrillator device therapy: challenges confronting the general cardiologist. *Circulation* 2007;115:638–653.

8

Dyslipidemia

Anne C. Goldberg and Katherine E. Henderson

General Principles

- Lipids are sparingly soluble molecules that include cholesterol, fatty acids, and their derivatives.
- Plasma lipids are transported by lipoprotein particles composed of proteins called **apolipoproteins,** and **phospholipids, cholesterol esters,** and **triglycerides.**
- Human plasma lipoproteins are separated into **five major classes** based on density:
  - Chylomicrons (least dense).
  - Very low-density lipoproteins (VLDLs).
  - Intermediate-density lipoproteins (IDLs).[1]
  - Low-density lipoproteins (LDLs).
  - High-density lipoproteins (HDLs).
  - A sixth class, lipoprotein(a), Lp(a), resembles LDL in lipid composition and has a density that overlaps that of LDLs and HDLs.
- Physical properties of plasma lipoproteins are summarized in Table 1.

Atherosclerosis and Lipoproteins

Nearly 90% of patients with coronary heart disease (CHD) have some form of dyslipidemia. Increased levels of LDL, remnant lipoproteins, and Lp(a) as well as decreased levels of HDL have all been associated with an increased risk of premature vascular disease.[2,3]

Clinical Dyslipoproteinemias

- Most dyslipidemias are multifactorial in etiology and reflect the effects of uncharacterized genetic influences coupled with diet, activity, smoking, alcohol use, and comorbid conditions such as obesity and diabetes mellitus (DM).
- Differential diagnosis of the major lipid abnormalities is summarized in Table 2.
- The major genetic dyslipoproteinemias are reviewed in Table 3.[4–6]

Standards of Care for Hyperlipidemia

- LDL cholesterol–lowering therapy, particularly with hydroxymethylglutaryl-coenzyme A (HMG-CoA) reductase inhibitors, lowers the risk of CHD-related death, morbidity, and revascularization procedures in hypercholesterolemic patients with (secondary prevention)[7–10] or without (primary prevention) known CHD.[10–14]
- Identification and management of high LDL cholesterol is the primary goal of the National Cholesterol Education Program's (NCEP's) third expert report on cholesterol management in adults, or Adult Treatment Program III (ATP III).[15]
- The ATP III executive summary and full report can be viewed online at www.nhlbi.nih.gov/guidelines/cholesterol/.

TABLE 1	Physical Properties of Plasma Lipoproteins[a]		
Lipoprotein	Lipid Composition	Origin	Apolipoproteins
Chylomicrons	TG, 90%; chol, 3%	Intestine	B-48; C-I, C-II, C-III; E
VLDL	TG, 55%; chol, 20%	Liver	B-100; C-I, C-II, C-III; E
IDL	TG, 30%; chol, 35%	Metabolic product of VLDL	B-100; C-I, C-II, C-III; E
LDL	TG, 10%; chol, 50%	Metabolic product of IDL	B-100
HDL	TG, 5%; chol, 20%	Liver, intestine	A-I, A-II, A-IV; C-I, C-II, C-III; E
Lp(a)	TG, 10%; chol, 50%	Liver	B-100; Apo (a)

Chol, cholesterol; HDL, high-density lipoprotein; IDL, intermediate-density lipoprotein; LDL, low-density lipoprotein; Lp(a), lipoprotein(a); TG, triglyceride; VLDL, very low-density lipoprotein.
[a]Balance of particle composition: protein and phospholipid.

Diagnosis

Screening

- Screening for hypercholesterolemia should begin **in all adults age ≥20 years.**
- Screening is best performed with a lipid profile (total cholesterol, LDL cholesterol, HDL cholesterol, and triglycerides) obtained after a 12-hour fast.

TABLE 2	Differential Diagnosis of Major Lipid Abnormalities	
Lipid Abnormality	Primary Disorders	Secondary Disorders
Hypercholesterolemia	Polygenic, familial hyper-cholesterolemia, familial defective apo B-100	Hypothyroidism, nephrotic syndrome
Hypertriglyceridemia	Lipoprotein lipase deficiency, apo C-II deficiency, familial hypertriglyceridemia	Diabetes mellitus, obesity, metabolic syndrome, alcohol use, ora estrogen
Combined hyperlipidemia	Familial combined hyper-lipidemia, Type-III hyperlipoproteinemia	Diabetes mellitus, obesity, metabolic syndrome, hypothyroidism, nephrotic syndrome
Low HDL	Familial alpha lipoproteinemia, Tangier disease, familial HDL deficiency, lecithin: cholesterol acyltrans-ferase deficiency	Diabetes mellitus, metabolic syndrome, hypertriglyceridemia, smoking

HDL, high-density lipoprotein.

TABLE 3 Review of Major Genetic Dyslipoproteinemias

Type of Genetic Dyslipidemia	Typical Lipid Profile	Type of Inheritance Pattern	Phenotypic Features	Other Information
Familial hyper-cholesterolemia (FH)[4]	• Increased total (>300 mg/dL) and LDL (>250 mg/dL) cholesterol • Homozygous form (rare) can have total cholesterol >600 mg/dL and LDL >550 mg/dL	Autosomal dominant	• Premature CAD • Tendon xanthomas • Xanthelasmata • Premature arcus corneae	Because of mutations of the LDL receptor that lead to defective uptake and degradation of LDL
Familial combined hyperlipidemia (FCH)	• High levels of VLDL, LDL, or both • LDL apo B-100 level >130 mg/dL • Similar to FH	Autosomal dominant	• Premature CAD • Patients do *not* develop tendon xanthomas	Genetic and metabolic defects are not established
Familial defective apolipoprotein B-100[5]	• Similar to FH		• Similar to FH	Most of the cases are due to a glutamine for arginine mutation at amino acid 3500 of apo B-100
Type-III hyper-lipoproteinemia (familial dysbeta-lipoproteinemia)[6]	• Symmetric elevations of cholesterol and triglycerides (300–500 mg/dL) • Elevated VLDL to triglyceride ratio (>0.3)	Autosomal recessive	• Premature CAD • Tuberous or tuberoeruptive xanthomas • Planar xanthomas of the palmar creases are essentially pathognomonic	Many homozygotes are normolipidemic and emergence of hyperlipidemia often requires a secondary metabolic factor such as diabetes mellitus, hypothyroidism, or obesity

| Chylomicronemia syndrome | • Most patients have triglyceride levels in the range of 150–500 mg/dL

• Clinical manifestations occur when triglyceride levels exceed 1,500 mg/dL | • Onset before puberty indicates deficiency of lipoprotein lipase or apo C-II, both autosomal recessive

• Familial hypertriglyceridemia is an autosomal-dominant disorder caused by overproduction of VLDL triglycerides and manifests in adults | • Eruptive xanthomas
• Lipemia retinalis
• Pancreatitis
• Hepatosplenomegaly | Familial hypertriglyceridemia and FCH patients may develop chylomicronemia syndrome in the presence of secondary factors such as obesity, alcohol use, or diabetes |

CAD, coronary artery disease; LDL, low-density lipoprotein; VLDL, very-density lipoprotein.

TABLE 4	Major Risk Factors that Modify LDL Goals

Cigarette smoking

Hypertension (blood pressure ≥140/90 mm Hg or on antihypertensive medication)

Low HDL cholesterol (<40 mg/dL)[a]

Family history of premature CHD (CHD in male first-degree relative <age 55 years; CHD in female first-degree relative <age 65 years)

Age (men ≥45 years; women ≥55 years)

CHD, coronary heart disease; HDL, high-density lipoprotein; LDL, low-density lipoprotein.
[a]HDL cholesterol level of ≥60 mg/dL counts as a "negative" risk factor; its presence removes one risk factor from the total count.
Modified from Expert Panel on Detection, Evaluation, and Treatment of High Blood Cholesterol in Adults. Executive summary of the third report of the National Cholesterol Education Program (NCEP) Expert Panel on Detection, Evaluation, and Treatment of High Blood Cholesterol in Adults (Adult Treatment Panel III). *JAMA* 2001;285:2486–2497.

- If a fasting lipid panel cannot be obtained, total and HDL cholesterol should be measured.
- Measurement of fasting lipids is indicated if the total cholesterol level is ≥200 mg/dL or HDL cholesterol level is ≤40 mg/dL.
- If lipids are unremarkable and the patient has no major risk factors for CHD (Table 4), screening can be performed every 5 years.[15]
- Patients hospitalized for an acute coronary syndrome or coronary revascularization should have a lipid panel obtained within 24 hours of admission if lipid levels are unknown.
- Individuals with hyperlipidemia should be evaluated for potential **secondary causes,** including hypothyroidism, DM, obstructive liver disease, chronic renal disease, or nephrotic syndrome, or medications such as estrogens, progestins, anabolic steroids, and corticosteroids.

Risk Assessment

- A major innovation of ATP III is a formal method of CHD risk assessment. ATP III now recognizes **five categories of CHD risk:** very high, high, moderately high, moderate, and lower risk. These CHD risk categories are defined in Table 5.
- DM, noncoronary atherosclerosis (symptomatic cerebrovascular disease, peripheral artery disease, abdominal aortic aneurysm), or multiple risk factors conferring a 10-year CHD risk of >20% are considered **CHD risk equivalents in ATP III.**[16]
- Risk assessment for patients without known CHD or CHD risk equivalents begins with consideration of five risk factors summarized in Table 4.[15]
- A Framingham point score should be determined for any individual with two or more non-LDL cholesterol risk factors. **Framingham point score** algorithms for men and women are summarized in Table 6.[15–17]
- Patients with multiple non-LDL cholesterol CHD risk factors are then divided into those with a **10-year CHD risk of >20%, 10% to 20%, or <10%.**
- Presently, emerging risk factors (e.g., obesity, sedentary lifestyle, prothrombotic and proinflammatory factors, and impaired fasting glucose) do not impact risk assessment, although they may influence clinical judgment when determining therapeutic options.

TABLE 5	ATP III Categories of CHD Risk
Category	**Definition**
Very high risk	CHD and • Multiple risk factors (especially diabetes) • Severe and poorly controlled risk factors (especially continued cigarette smoking) • Multiple risk factors of the metabolic syndrome • Acute coronary syndromes
High risk	CHD or CHD risk equivalent
Moderately high risk	2+ risk factors and 10-year CHD risk of 10%–20%
Moderate risk	2+ risk factors and 10-year CHD risk of <10%
Lower risk	0–1 risk factors

ATP III, Adult Treatment Panel III; CHD, coronary heart disease.
Modified from Grundy SM, Cleeman C, Merz NB, et al. Implications of recent clinical trials for the National Cholesterol Education Program Adult Treatment Panel III Guidelines. *Circulation* 2004;110:227–239.

Treatment

Therapeutic Lifestyle Change

- ATP III thresholds for initiating cholesterol-lowering therapy with **therapeutic lifestyle change** (TLC, diet and exercise) and **hypolipidemic drugs** are summarized in Table 7.[16]
  - All patients requiring cholesterol treatment should implement a diet restricted in total and saturated fat intake in accordance with ATP III recommendations (Table 8).[15]
  - Moderate exercise and weight reduction is also recommended.
  - A registered dietitian may be helpful to plan and start a saturated-fat-restricted and weight-loss-promoting diet.

Treatment Targets

High Risk and Very High Risk

- The ATP III LDL cholesterol treatment target for all **high-risk** patients is <100 mg/dL.[15]
- For CHD patients in the **very high-risk** category, an LDL cholesterol level <70 mg/dL is a therapeutic option.[16]
- An LDL cholesterol level of ≥100 mg/dL is now identified as the threshold for simultaneous treatment with TLC and lipid-lowering agents.[16]
- Based on outcomes in the Heart Protection Study, lipid-lowering drug therapy is also an option for patients with CHD and baseline LDL cholesterol level <100 mg/dL.[10]
- If a high-risk patient has hypertriglyceridemia or low HDL cholesterol, a fibrate or nicotinic acid (niacin) may be added to cholesterol-lowering therapy.[16]

Moderately High Risk

- Patients with two or more non-LDL cholesterol risk factors and a Framingham point score predicting a 10-year CHD risk of 10% to 20% are considered at **moderately high risk** of CHD.

TABLE 6	Estimate of 10-Year Risk (Framingham Point Scores) for Men and Women

Estimate of 10-Year Risk for Men

Age (Years)	Points
20–34	−9
35–39	−4
40–44	0
45–49	3
50–54	6
55–59	8
60–64	10
65–69	11
70–74	12
75–79	13

Total Cholesterol	Points				
	Age 20–39	Age 40–49	Age 50–59	Age 60–69	Age 70–79
<160	0	0	0	0	0
160–199	4	3	2	1	0
200–239	7	5	3	1	0
240–279	9	6	4	2	1
≥280	11	8	5	3	1

	Points				
	Age 20–39	Age 40–49	Age 50–59	Age 60–69	Age 70–79
Nonsmoker	0	0	0	0	0
Smoker	8	5	3	1	1

HDL (mg/dL)	Points	Systolic BP (mm Hg)	Points if Untreated	Points if Treated
≥60	−1	<120	0	0
50–59	0	120–129	0	1
40–49	1	130–139	1	2
<40	2	140–159	1	2
		≥160	2	3

Point Total	10-Year Risk (%)	Point Total	10-Year Risk (%)
<0	<1	9	5
0	1	10	6
1	1	11	8
2	1	12	10
3	1	13	12
4	1	14	16
5	2	15	20
6	2	16	25
7	3	≥17	≥30
8	4		

(continued)

TABLE 6	Estimate of 10-Year Risk (Framingham Point Scores) for Men and Women (*Continued*)

Estimate of 10-Year Risk in Women

Age (Years)	Points
20–34	−7
35–39	−3
40–44	0
45–49	3
50–54	6
55–59	8
60–64	10
65–69	12
70–74	14
75–79	16

Total Cholesterol	Points				
	Age 20–39 Years	Age 40–49 Years	Age 50–59 Years	Age 60–69 Years	Age 70–79 Years
<160	0	0	0	0	0
160–199	4	3	2	1	1
200–239	8	6	4	2	1
240–279	11	8	5	3	2
≥280	13	10	7	4	2

	Points				
	Age 20–39 Years	Age 40–49 Years	Age 50–59 Years	Age 60–69 Years	Age 70–79 Years
Nonsmoker	0	0	0	0	0
Smoker	9	7	4	2	1

HDL (mg/dL)	Points	Systolic BP (mm Hg)	Points if Untreated	Points if Treated
≥60	−1	<120	0	0
50–59	0	120–129	1	3
40–49	1	130–139	2	4
<40	2	140–159	3	5
		≥160	4	6

Point Total	10-Year Risk (%)	Point Total	10-Year Risk (%)
<9	<1	17	5
9	1	18	6
10	1	19	8
11	1	20	11
12	1	21	14
13	2	22	17
14	2	23	22
15	3	24	27
16	4	≥25	≥30

BP, blood pressure; HDL, high-density lipoprotein.
From Expert Panel on Detection, Evaluation, and Treatment of High Blood Cholesterol in Adults. Executive summary of the third report of the National Cholesterol Education Program (NCEP) Expert Panel on Detection, Evaluation, and Treatment of High Blood Cholesterol in Adults (Adult Treatment Panel III). *JAMA* 2001;285:2486–2497, with permission.

TABLE 7	ATP III LDL-C Goals and Thresholds for Therapeutic Lifestyle Changes (TLC) and Drug Therapy		
Category	LDL-C Goal	Start TLC	Start Drug Therapy
Very high risk	<70 mg/dL	Any LDL-C	LDL-C ≥70 mg/dL
High risk	<100 mg/dL	≥100 mg/dL	≥100 mg/dL (consider if baseline LDL-C <100 mg/dL)
Moderately high risk	<130 mg/dL (<100 mg/dL optional)	≥130 mg/dL	≥130 mg/dL (optional if baseline LDL-C 100–129 mg/dL)
Moderate risk	<130 mg/dL	≥130 mg/dL	≥160 mg/dL
Lower risk	<160 mg/dL	≥160 mg/dL	≥190 mg/dL (optional if baseline LDL-C 160–189 mg/dL)

ATP III, Adult Treatment Panel III; LDL-C, low-density lipoprotein cholesterol.
Modified from Grundy SM, Cleeman C, Merz NB, et al. Implications of recent clinical trials for the National Cholesterol Education Program Adult Treatment Panel III Guidelines. *Circulation* 2004;110:227–239.

TABLE 8	Nutrient Composition of the Therapeutic Lifestyle Change (TLC) Diet
Nutrient	Recommended Intake
Saturated fat[a]	<7% of total calories
Polyunsaturated fat	Up to 10% of total calories
Monounsaturated fat	Up to 20% of total calories
Total fat	25–35% of total calories
Carbohydrate[b]	50–60% of total calories
Fiber	20–30 g/day
Protein	Approximately 15% of total calories
Cholesterol	<200 mg/day
Total calories (energy)[c]	Balance energy intake and expenditure to maintain desirable body weight/prevent weight gain

[a]Trans fatty acids are another low-density lipoprotein (LDL)-raising fat that should be kept at a low intake.
[b]Carbohydrate should be derived predominantly from foods rich in complex carbohydrates, including grains (especially whole grains), fruits, and vegetables.
[c]Daily energy expenditure should include at least moderate physical activity (contributing approximately 200 Kcal/day).
From Expert Panel on Detection, Evaluation, and Treatment of High Blood Cholesterol in Adults. Executive summary of the third report of the National Cholesterol Education Program (NCEP) Expert Panel on Detection, Evaluation, and Treatment of High Blood Cholesterol in Adults (Adult Treatment Panel III). *JAMA* 2001;285:2486–, with permission.

- Pharmacotherapy should be initiated if LDL cholesterol level is ≥130 mg/dL.
- ATP III identifies an LDL cholesterol target <100 mg/dL as optional for this group, with drug therapy to be considered for patients with baseline LDL cholesterol 100 to 129 mg/dL.
- Patients with two or more risk factors and a 10-year risk of <10% are candidates for drug therapy when LDL cholesterol remains ≥160 mg/dL despite TLC.[16]

Low Risk

- For **low-risk patients** (0 to 1 risk factors), cholesterol-lowering therapy should be considered if the LDL cholesterol level is ≥190 mg/dL, especially for patients who have undergone a 3-month trial of TLC.
- Patients with very high LDL concentrations (≥190 mg/dL) often have a hereditary dyslipidemia and require treatment with multiple lipid-lowering agents. These patients should be referred to a lipid specialist, and family members should be screened with a fasting lipid battery.
- When LDL cholesterol is 160 to 189 mg/dL, drug therapy should be considered if the patient has a significant risk factor for cardiovascular disease, such as heavy tobacco use, poorly controlled hypertension, strong family history of early CHD, or low HDL cholesterol.[16]

Assessing Response to Therapy

- **Response to therapy should be assessed after 6 weeks** and the dose of medication titrated if the LDL cholesterol treatment target is not achieved.
- The initial dose of a cholesterol-lowering drug should be sufficient to achieve a 30% to 40% reduction in LDL cholesterol.
- If target LDL cholesterol has not been reached after 12 weeks, current therapy should be intensified by further dose titration, adding another lipid-lowering agent, or referral to a lipid specialist.
- Patients at goal should be monitored every 4 to 6 months.

Metabolic Syndrome

- The constellation of abdominal obesity, hypertension, glucose intolerance, and an atherogenic lipid profile (hypertriglyceridemia; low HDL cholesterol; and small, dense LDL cholesterol) characterizes a condition called the **metabolic syndrome.** ATP III diagnostic criteria for the metabolic syndrome are summarized in Table 9.[15,18]
- Approximately 22% of Americans qualify for a diagnosis of the metabolic syndrome by ATP III criteria. Prevalence is increased in older individuals, women, Hispanic Americans, and African Americans.[19]
- Multiple studies have demonstrated the association between cardiovascular events and death and all-cause mortality with the metabolic syndrome.[20]
- ATP III recognizes the metabolic syndrome as a **secondary treatment target** after LDL cholesterol level is controlled.[15]
- The report recommends treating the underlying causes of metabolic syndrome (overweight/obesity, physical inactivity) by implementing weight loss and aerobic exercise and managing cardiovascular risks, such as hypertension, that may persist despite lifestyle changes.[15]

Hypertriglyceridemia

- Recent analyses suggest that hypertriglyceridemia is an **independent cardiovascular risk factor.**[21,22]

TABLE 9	ATP III Diagnostic Criteria for the Metabolic Syndrome

Risk Factor	ATP III[a] Definition
Carbohydrate metabolism	Fasting glucose ≥110 mg/dL (alternatively >100 mg/dL)
Abdominal obesity[b]	Men, waist >40 in Women, waist >35 in
Dyslipidemia	Triglycerides ≥150 mg/dL Men, HDL cholesterol <40 mg/dL Women, HDL cholesterol <50 mg/dL
Hypertension	BP ≥130/85 mm Hg

BMI, body mass index; BP, blood pressure; HDL, high-density lipoprotein.
[a]To qualify for the diagnosis of metabolic syndrome by ATP III criteria, a patient must meet at least three of the five criteria (hyperglycemia, abdominal obesity, high triglycerides, low HDL cholesterol, high BP).
[b]Waist circumferences in Asian and south Asian patients may require different cutpoints.
Modified from Expert Panel on Detection, Evaluation, and Treatment of High Blood Cholesterol in Adults. Executive summary of the third report of the National Cholesterol Education Program (NCEP) Expert Panel on Detection, Evaluation, and Treatment of High Blood Cholesterol in Adults (Adult Treatment Panel III). *JAMA* 2001;285:2486–2497.

- Hypertriglyceridemia is often observed in the metabolic syndrome, and there are many potential etiologies for hypertriglyceridemia, including obesity, DM, renal insufficiency, genetic dyslipidemias, and therapy with oral estrogen, glucocorticoids, or β-blockers.
- The ATP III classification of serum triglyceride levels is as follows[15]:
  - Normal: <150 mg/dL.
  - Borderline-high: 150 to 199 mg/dL.
  - High: 200 to 499 mg/dL.
  - Very high: ≥500 mg/dL
- Treatment of hypertriglyceridemia depends on the degree of severity.
  - For patients with very high triglyceride levels, triglyceride reduction through a very low fat diet (≤15% of calories), exercise, weight loss, and drugs (fibrates, niacin) is the primary goal of therapy to prevent acute pancreatitis.
  - **When patients have a lesser degree of hypertriglyceridemia, controlling the LDL cholesterol level is the primary aim of initial therapy.** TLC is emphasized as the initial intervention to lower triglyceride levels.[15]

Non-HDL Cholesterol

- Non-HDL cholesterol is a secondary treatment target.
- A patient's non-HDL cholesterol level is calculated by subtracting HDL cholesterol from total cholesterol.
- Target non-HDL cholesterol is 30 mg/dL higher than the LDL cholesterol target.
- LDL and non-HDL cholesterol treatment targets for various degrees of cardiovascular risk are summarized in Table 10.[15,16]

Low HDL Cholesterol

- One of the modifications from ATP II includes redefining low HDL cholesterol as <40 mg/dL.

TABLE 10	Comparison of LDL-C and Non-HDL-C Goals by CHD Risk Category	
Category	LDL-C Target (mg/dL)	Non-HDL-C Target (mg/dL)
Very high risk	<70	<100
High risk	<100	<130
Moderately high risk	<130	<160
Moderate risk	<130	<160
Low risk	<160	<190

CHD, coronary heart disease; HDL-C, high-density lipoprotein cholesterol; LDL-C, low-density lipoprotein cholesterol.
Modified from Grundy SM, Cleeman C, Merz NB, et al. Implications of recent clinical trials for the National Cholesterol Education Program Adult Treatment Panel III Guidelines. *Circulation* 2004;110:227–239.

- Low HDL cholesterol is an **independent CHD risk factor** that is identified as a non-LDL cholesterol risk and included as a component of the Framingham scoring algorithm.[23]
- Etiologies for low HDL cholesterol include physical inactivity, obesity, insulin resistance, DM, hypertriglyceridemia, cigarette smoking, high (>60% calories) carbohydrate diets, and certain medications (β-blockers, anabolic steroids, progestins).
- Because therapeutic interventions for low HDL cholesterol are of limited efficacy, ATP III identifies **LDL cholesterol as the primary target of therapy for patients with low HDL cholesterol.**
- Low HDL cholesterol often occurs in the setting of hypertriglyceridemia and metabolic syndrome. Management of these conditions may result in improvement of HDL cholesterol.
- Aerobic exercise, weight loss, smoking cessation, menopausal estrogen replacement, and treatment with niacin or fibrates may elevate low HDL cholesterol.[15]

Lipid-Lowering Therapy and Age
- The risk of a fatal or nonfatal cardiovascular event increases with age, and most cardiovascular events occur in patients 65 years of age and older.
- Secondary prevention trials with the HMG CoA reductase inhibitors have demonstrated significant clinical benefit for patients 65 to 75 years of age.
- The Heart Protection Study failed to show an age threshold for primary or secondary prevention with simvastatin. Patients aged 75 to 80 years at study entry experienced a nearly 30% reduction in major vascular events.[10]
- The PROspective Study of Pravastatin in the Elderly at Risk (PROSPER) trial found a significant reduction in major coronary events among patients aged 70 to 82 years with vascular disease or CHD risks treated with pravastatin.[24]
- **ATP III does not place age restrictions** on treatment of hypercholesterolemia in elderly adults.
- ATP III recommends TLC for young adults (men age 20 to 35 years; women age 20 to 45 years) with an LDL level of ≥130 mg/dL. Drug therapy should be considered in the following high-risk groups:
  - Men who both smoke and have elevated LDL levels (160 to 189 mg/dL).
  - All young adults with an LDL level of ≥190 mg/dL.
  - Those with an inherited dyslipidemia.[15]

Treatment of Elevated Low-Density Lipoprotein Cholesterol

Hydroxymethylglutaryl-Coenzyme A Reductase Inhibitors (Statins)

- Statins (Table 11) are the treatment of choice for elevated LDL cholesterol.[15,25–28]
- The lipid-lowering effect of statins appears within the first week of use and becomes stable after approximately 4 weeks of use.
- Common side effects (5% to 10% of patients) include gastrointestinal (GI) upset (e.g., abdominal pain, diarrhea, bloating, constipation) and muscle pain or weakness, which can occur without creatinine kinase elevations. Other potential side effects include malaise, fatigue, headache, and rash.[25,28]
- Elevations of liver transaminases two to three times the upper limit of normal are dose dependent and reversible with discontinuation of the drug.
  - Liver enzymes should be measured before initiating therapy, at 8 to 12 weeks after dose initiation or titration, then every 6 months.
  - The medication should be discontinued if liver transaminases elevate to more than three times the upper limit of normal.[27]
- Because some of the statins undergo metabolism by the cytochrome P450 enzyme system, taking them in combination with other drugs metabolized by this enzyme system increases the risk of **rhabdomyolysis**.[25,27]
  - Among these drugs are fibrates (greater risk with gemfibrozil), itraconazole, ketoconazole, erythromycin, clarithromycin, cyclosporin, nefazodone, and protease inhibitors.[27]
  - Statins may also interact with large quantities of grapefruit juice to increase the risk of myopathy, although the precise mechanism of this interaction is unclear.
  - Simvastatin can increase the levels of warfarin and digoxin. Rosuvastatin may also increase warfarin levels.

Bile Acid Sequestrant Resins

- Currently available bile acid sequestrant resins include the following:
  - **Cholestyramine:** 4 to 24 g PO/day in divided doses before meals.
  - **Colestipol:** tablets, 2 to 16 g PO/day; granules, 5 to 30 g PO/day in divided doses before meals.
  - **Colesevelam:** 625-mg tablets; three tablets PO bid or six tablets PO daily with food (maximum, seven tablets PO/day).
- Bile acid sequestrants typically lower LDL levels by 15% to 30% and thereby lower the incidence of CHD.[25,28] These agents should not be used as monotherapy in patients with triglyceride levels >250 mg/dL because they can raise triglyceride levels. They may be combined with nicotinic acid or statins.
- Common side effects of resins include constipation, abdominal pain, bloating, nausea, and flatulence.
- Bile acid sequestrants may decrease oral absorption of many other drugs, including warfarin, digoxin, thyroid hormone, thiazide diuretics, amiodarone, glipizide, and statins.
  - Colesevelam interacts with fewer drugs than do the older resins.
  - Other medications should be given 1 hour before or 4 hours after resins.

Nicotinic Acid (Niacin)

- Niacin can lower LDL cholesterol levels by ≥15%, lower triglyceride levels by 20% to 50%, and raise HDL cholesterol levels by up to 35%.[21,29]
- Crystalline niacin is given 1 to 3 g PO/day in two to three divided doses with meals. Extended-release niacin is dosed at night. The starting dose is 500 mg PO, and the

TABLE 11	Currently Available Statins					
Name	Atorvastatin	Fluvastatin	Lovastatin	Pravastatin	Rosuvastatin	Simvastatin
Dose range (mg PO/day)	10–80	20–80	10–80	10–80	5–40	10–80
Triglyceride effect (%)	↓ 13–32	↓ 5–35	↓ 2–13	↓ 3–15	↓ 10–35	↓ 12–36
LDL effect (%)	↓ 38–54	↓ 17–36	↓ 29–48	↓ 19–34	↓ 41–65	↓ 28–46
HDL effect (%)	↑ 4.8–5.5	↑ 0.9–12	↑ 4.6–8	↑ 3–9.9	↑ 10–14	↑ 5.2–10

HDL, high-density lipoprotein; LDL, low-density lipoprotein; ↑, increased; ↓, decreased.

dose may be titrated monthly in 500-mg increments to a maximum of 2,000 mg PO (administer dose with milk or crackers).
- Common side effects of niacin include flushing, pruritus, headache, nausea, and bloating. Other potential side effects include elevation of liver transaminases, hyperuricemia, and hyperglycemia.
  - Flushing may be decreased with the use of aspirin 30 minutes before the first few doses.
  - Hepatoxicity associated with niacin is partially dose dependent and appears to be more prevalent with over-the-counter time-release preparations.
- Avoid use of niacin in patients with gout, liver disease, active peptic ulcer disease, and uncontrolled DM.
  - Niacin can be used with care in patients with well-controlled DM (hemoglobin A_{1c} level ≤7%).
  - Serum transaminases, glucose, and uric acid levels should be monitored every 6 to 8 weeks during dose titration, then every 4 months.

Ezetimibe
- Ezetimibe is currently the only available cholesterol-absorption inhibitor.
- It appears to act at the brush border of the small intestine and inhibits cholesterol absorption.
- The recommended dosing is 10 mg PO once daily. No dosage adjustment is required for renal insufficiency and mild hepatic impairment or in elderly patients.
- Ezetimibe may provide an additional 25% mean reduction in LDL when combined with a statin and provides an approximately 18% decrease in LDL when used as monotherapy.[30–33]
- It is not recommended for use in patients with moderate-to-severe hepatic impairment.
- There appear to be few side effects associated with ezetimibe.
  - In clinical trials, there was no excess of rhabdomyolysis or myopathy when compared with statin or placebo alone.
  - There is a low incidence of diarrhea and abdominal pain compared with placebo. Liver function monitoring is not required with monotherapy because there appears to be no significant impact on liver enzymes when this drug is used alone.
  - Liver enzymes should be monitored when used in conjunction with a statin, as there appears to be a slight increased incidence of enzyme elevations with combination therapy.
- Long-term clinical outcome trials of ezetimibe are ongoing. There have been two short-term surrogate outcome trials suggesting a lack of additive effectiveness with regard to carotid intima-media thickness.[34,35] The clinical utility of these results have been questioned and the matter is currently unresolved.

Treatment of Hypertriglyceridemia
Nonpharmacologic Treatment
- Nonpharmacologic treatments are important in the therapy of hypertriglyceridemia.
- Approaches include the following:
  - Changing oral estrogen replacement to transdermal estrogen.
  - Decreasing alcohol intake.
  - Encouraging weight loss and exercise.

- Controlling hyperglycemia in patients with DM.
- Avoiding simple sugars and very high carbohydrate diets.

Pharmacologic Treatment
- Pharmacologic treatment of isolated hypertriglyceridemia consists of a fibric acid derivative or niacin.
- Statins may be effective for patients with mild-to-moderate hypertriglyceridemia and concomitant LDL cholesterol elevation.[36]

Fibric Acid Derivatives
- Currently available fibric acid derivatives include the following:
  - **Gemfibrozil:** 600 mg PO bid before meals.
  - **Fenofibrate:** typically 48 to 145 mg PO/day.
- Fibrates generally lower triglyceride levels by 30% to 50% and increase HDL levels by 10% to 35%. They can lower LDL levels by 5% to 25% in patients with normal triglyceride levels but may actually increase LDL levels in patients with elevated triglyceride levels.
- Common side effects include dyspepsia, abdominal pain, cholelithiasis, rash, and pruritus. Fibrates may potentiate the effects of warfarin.[25]
- Gemfibrozil given in conjunction with statins may increase the risk of rhabdomyolysis.[27,37–40]

Omega-3 Fatty Acids
- High doses of omega-3 fatty acids from fish oil can lower triglyceride levels.[41,42]
- The active ingredients are eicosapentaenoic acid (EPA) and docosahexaenoic acid (DHA).
- To lower triglyceride levels, 1 to 6 g of EPA plus DHA are needed daily.
- Main side effects are burping, bloating, and diarrhea.
- A prescription form of omega-3 fatty acids is available and is indicated for triglyceride levels >500 mg/dL; four tablets contain about 3.6 g of omega-3 acid ethyl esters and can lower triglyceride levels by 30%.
- In practice, omega-3 fatty acids are being used as an adjunct to statin or other drugs in patients with moderately elevated triglyceride levels.
- The combination of omega-3 fatty acids plus statin has the advantage of avoiding the risk of myopathy seen in the statin-fibrate combination.[43,44]

Treatment of Low High-Density Lipoprotein Cholesterol

- Low HDL cholesterol often occurs in the setting of hypertriglyceridemia and metabolic syndrome. Management of accompanying high LDL cholesterol, hypertriglyceridemia, and the metabolic syndrome may result in improvement of HDL cholesterol.[45]
- **Treatment specifically targeted at raising low HDL cholesterol levels may reduce the risk of cardiovascular events.**[46]
- Nonpharmacologic therapies are the mainstay of treatment including the following:
  - Smoking cessation.
  - Exercise.
  - Weight loss.
- In addition, medications known to lower HDL levels, such as β-blockers, progestins, and androgenic compounds, should be avoided.
- **Niacin is the most effective pharmacologic agent for increasing HDL levels.**[42]

REFERENCES

1. Krauss RM, Lingren RT, Williams PT, et al. Intermediate-density lipoproteins and progression of coronary artery disease in hypercholesterolemic men. *Lancet* 1987;2:62–66.
2. Genest JJ, Martin-Munley SS, McNamara JR, et al. Familial lipoprotein disorders in patients with premature coronary artery disease. *J Am Coll Cardiol* 1992;19:792–802.
3. Kugiyama K, Doi H, Motoyama T, et al. Association of remnant lipoprotein levels with impairment of endothelium-dependent vasomotor function in human coronary arteries. *Circulation* 1998;97:2519–2526.
4. Stone NJ, Levy RI, Fredrickson DS, et al. Coronary artery disease in 116 kindred with familial type II hyperlipoproteinemia. *Circulation* 1974;49:476–488.
5. Innerarity TL, Mahley RW, Weisgraber KH, et al. Familial defective apolipoprotein B-100: a mutation of apolipoprotein B that causes hypercholesterolemia. *J Lipid Res* 1990;31: 1337–1349.
6. Feussner G, Wagner A, Kohl B, et al. Clinical features of type III hyperlipoproteinemia: analysis of 64 patients. *Clin Invest* 1993;71:362–366.
7. Randomised trial of cholesterol lowering in 4444 patients with coronary heart disease: the Scandinavian Simvastatin Survival Study (4S). *Lancet* 1994;344:1383–1389.
8. Sachs FM, Pfeffer MA, Moye LA, et al. The effect of pravastatin on coronary events after myocardial infarction in patients with average cholesterol levels. Cholesterol and Recurrent Events Trial investigators. *N Engl J Med* 1996;335:1001–1009.
9. Prevention of cardiovascular events and death with pravastatin in patients with coronary heart disease and a broad range of initial cholesterol levels. The Long-Term Intervention with Pravastatin in Ischemic Disease (LIPID) Study Group. *N Engl J Med* 1998;339: 1349–1357.
10. Heart Protection Study Collaborative Group. MRC/BHF Heart Protection Study of cholesterol lowering with simvastatin in 20,536 high-risk individuals: a randomised placebo-controlled trial. *Lancet* 2002;360:7–22.
11. Shepherd J, Cobbe SM, Ford I, et al. Prevention of coronary heart disease with pravastatin in men with hypercholesterolemia. West of Scotland Coronary Prevention Study Group. *N Engl J Med* 1995;333:1301–1307.
12. Downs JR, Clearfield M, Weis S, et al. Primary prevention of acute coronary events with lovastatin in men and women with average cholesterol levels: results of AFCAPS/TexCAPS. Air Force/Texas Coronary Atherosclerosis Prevention Study. *JAMA* 1998;279:1615–1622.
13. Sever PS, Dahlöf B, Poulter NR, et al. ASCOT investigators. Prevention of coronary and stroke events with atorvastatin in hypertensive patients who have average or lower-than-average cholesterol concentrations, in the Anglo-Scandinavian Cardiac Outcomes Trial—Lipid Lowering Arm (ASCOT-LLA): a multicentre randomised controlled trial. *Lancet* 2003;361:1149–1158.
14. Colhoun HM, Betteridge DJ, Durrington PN, et al. CARDS investigators. Primary prevention of cardiovascular disease with atorvastatin in type 2 diabetes in the Collaborative Atorvastatin Diabetes Study (CARDS): multicentre randomised placebo-controlled trial. *Lancet* 2004;364:685–696.
15. Expert Panel on Detection, Evaluation, and Treatment of High Blood Cholesterol in Adults. Executive summary of the third report of the National Cholesterol Education Program (NCEP) Expert Panel on Detection, Evaluation, and Treatment of High Blood Cholesterol in Adults (Adult Treatment Panel III). *JAMA* 2001;285:2486–2497.
16. Grundy SM, Cleeman C, Merz NB, et al. Implications of recent clinical trials for the National Cholesterol Education Program Adult Treatment Panel III Guidelines. *Circulation* 2004;110:227–239.
17. Wilson PW, D'Agostino RB, Levy D, et al. Prediction of coronary heart disease using risk factor categories. *Circulation* 1998;97:1837–1847.
18. IDF Worldwide Definition of the Metabolic Syndrome. Available at: http://www.idf.org/home/index.cfm?node=1429. Last accessed August 18, 2009.

19. Ford ES, Giles WH, Dietz WH. Prevalence of metabolic syndrome among US adults: findings from the Third National Health and Nutrition Examination Survey. *JAMA* 2002; 287:356–359.

20. Galassi A, Reynolds K, He J. Metabolic syndrome and risk of cardiovascular disease: a meta-analysis. *Am J Med* 2006;119:812–819.

21. Sarwar N, Danesh J, Eiriksdottir G, et al. Triglycerides and the risk of coronary heart disease: 10,158 incident cases among 262,525 participants in 29 Western prospective studies. *Circulation* 2007;115:450–458.

22. Tirosh A, Rudich A, Shochat T, et al. Changes in triglyceride levels and risk for coronary heart disease in young men. *Ann Intern Med* 2007;147:377–385.

23. Castelli WP, Garrison RJ, Wilson PW, et al. Incidence of coronary heart disease and lipoprotein cholesterol levels: the Framingham Study. *JAMA* 1986;256:2835–2838.

24. Shepherd J, Blauw GJ, Murphy MB, et al. PROSPER study group. PROspective Study of Pravastatin in the Elderly at Risk. Pravastatin in elderly individuals at risk of vascular disease (PROSPER): a randomised controlled trial. *Lancet* 2002;360:1623–1630.

25. Knopp RH. Drug treatment of lipid disorders. *N Engl J Med* 1999;341:498–511.

26. Chong PH. Lack of therapeutic interchangeability of HMG-CoA reductase inhibitors. *Ann Pharmacother* 2002;36:1907–1917.

27. Pasternak RC, Smith SC Jr, Bairey-Merz CN, et al. American College of Cardiology; American Heart Association; National Heart, Lung and Blood Institute. ACC/AHA/NHLBI Clinical Advisory on the Use and Safety of Statins. *Circulation* 2002;106:1024–1028.

28. The Lipid Research Clinics Coronary Primary Prevention Trial results. I. Reduction in incidence of coronary heart disease. *JAMA* 1984;251:351–364.

29. Illingworth DR, Stein EA, Mitchel YB, et al. Comparative effects of lovastatin and niacin in primary hypercholesterolemia. A prospective trial. *Arch Intern Med* 1994;154:1586–1595.

30. Dujovne CA, Ettinger MP, McNeer JF, et al. Efficacy and safety of a potent new selective cholesterol absorption inhibitor, ezetimibe, in patients with primary hypercholesterolemia. *Am J Cardiol* 2002;90:1092–1097.

31. Knopp RH, Gitter H, Truitt T, et al. Effects of ezetimibe, a new cholesterol absorption inhibitor, on plasma lipids in patients with primary hypercholesterolemia. *Eur Heart J* 2003;24:729–741.

32. Gagne C, Bays HE, Weiss SR, et al. Efficacy and safety of ezetimibe added to ongoing statin therapy for treatment of patients with primary hypercholesterolemia. *Am J Cardiol* 2002; 90:1084–1091.

33. Goldberg AC, Sapre A, Liu J, et al. Efficacy and safety of ezetimibe coadministered with simvastatin in patients with primary hypercholesterolemia: a randomized, double-blind, placebo-controlled trial. *Mayo Clin Proc* 2004;79:620–629.

34. Kastelein JJ, Akdim F, Stroes ES, et al. Simvastatin with or without ezetimibe in familial hypercholesterolemia. *N Engl J Med* 2008;358:1431–1443.

35. Taylor AJ, Villines TC, Stanek EJ, et al. Extended-release niacin or ezetimibe and carotid intima-media thickness. *N Engl J Med* 2009 Nov 15. [Epub ahead of print]

36. Brunzell JD. Clinical practice. Hypertriglyceridemia. *N Engl J Med* 2007;357:1009–1017.

37. Rosenson RS. Current overview of statin-induced myopathy. *Am J Med* 2004;116: 408–416.

38. Alsheikh-Ali AA, Kuvin JT, Karas RH. Risk of adverse events with fibrates. *Am J Cardiol* 2004;94:935–938.

39. Jones PH, Davidson MH. Reporting rate of rhabdomyolysis with fenofibrate + statin versus gemfibrozil + any statin. *Am J Cardiol* 2005;95:120–122.

40. Keech A, Simes RJ, Barter P, et al. FIELD study investigators. Effects of long-term fenofibrate therapy on cardiovascular events in 9795 people with type 2 diabetes mellitus (the FIELD study): randomised controlled trial. *Lancet* 2005;366:1849–1861.

41. Nestel PJ, Connor WE, Reardon MF, et al. Suppression by diets rich in fish oil of very low density lipoprotein production in man. *J Clin Invest* 1984;74:82–89.

42. Harris WS, Connor WE, Illingworth DR, et al. Effects of fish oil on VLDL triglyceride kinetics in humans. *J Lipid Res* 1990;31:1549–1558.
43. Maki KC, McKenney JM, Reeves MS, et al. Effects of adding prescription omega-3 acid ethyl esters to simvastatin (20 mg/day) on lipids and lipoprotein particles in men and women with mixed dyslipidemia. *Am J Cardiol* 2008;102:429–433.
44. Barter P, Ginsberg HN. Effectiveness of combined statin plus omega-3 fatty acid therapy for mixed dyslipidemia. *Am J Cardiol* 2008;102:1040–1045.
45. Ballantyne CM, Olsson AG, Cook TJ, et al. Influence of low high-density lipoprotein cholesterol and elevated triglyceride on coronary heart disease events and response to simvastatin therapy in 4S. *Circulation* 2001;104:3046–3051.
46. Singh IM, Shishehbor MD, Ansell BJ. Ligh-density lipoprotein as a therapeutic target: a systematic review. *JAMA* 2007;298:786–798.

Disorders of Hemostasis
Charles S. Eby

General Principles

- Normal hemostasis involves a complex sequence of interrelated reactions that lead to platelet aggregation (primary hemostasis) and activation of coagulation factors (secondary hemostasis) to produce a durable vascular seal.
- **Primary hemostasis** is an immediate but temporary response to vessel injury. Platelets and von Willebrand factor (vWF) interact to form a primary plug.
- **Secondary hemostasis** (coagulation) results in the formation of a fibrin clot (Fig. 1). Injury initiates coagulation by exposing extravascular tissue factor to blood, which initiates activation of factors VII, X, and prothrombin. The subsequent activation of other factors leads to the generation of thrombin, conversion of fibrinogen to fibrin, and formation of a durable clot.[1]

Diagnosis

Clinical Presentation
History
- A detailed history can assess bleeding severity, congenital or acquired status, and primary or secondary hemostatic defects.
- Prolonged bleeding after dental extractions, circumcision, menstruation, labor and delivery, trauma, or surgery may suggest an underlying bleeding disorder.
- Family history may suggest an inherited bleeding disorder.

Physical Examination
- Primary hemostasis defects are suggested by mucosal bleeding and excessive bruising.
  - **Petechiae:** <2 mm subcutaneous bleeding, do not blanch with pressure, typically present in areas subject to increased hydrostatic force: the lower legs and periorbital area (especially after coughing or vomiting).
  - **Ecchymoses:** >3 mm black-and-blue (or violaceous) patches due to rupture of small vessels from trauma.
- Secondary hemostasis defects can produce hematomas (localized masses of clotted/unclotted blood), hemarthroses, or delayed bleeding after trauma or surgery.

Diagnostic Testing
Laboratories
The history and physical exam guide test selection: Initial studies should include platelet count, prothrombin time (PT), activated partial thromboplastin time (aPTT), and peripheral blood smear.

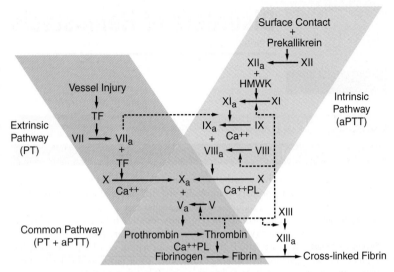

Figure 1. Coagulation cascade. Solid arrows indicate activation and dashed lines indicate additional substrates activated by factor VIIa or thrombin. aPTT, activated partial thromboplastin time; HMWK, high-molecular-weight kininogen; PL phospholipid; PT, prothrombin time; TF, tissue factor.

Primary Hemostasis Tests

- A **low platelet count** requires review of blood smear to rule out platelet clumping artifact (due to the EDTA additive, platelet glycoprotein IIb/IIIa receptor inhibitor drugs), giant platelets, and misclassification of other cells as platelets.
- The **bleeding time** (BT) measures time until bleeding cessation from a standardize skin incision, but it does not quantify the perioperative risk of bleeding.[2] Many factors can prolong the BT: thrombocytopenia, von Willebrand disease (vWD), abnormal capillary or skin integrity, antiplatelet therapy, uremia, liver failure, anemia, and poor technique.
- The **PFA-100** (Dade Behring, Deerfield, Illinois) instrument assesses vWF-dependent platelet activation in flowing citrated whole blood. Most patients with vWD and qualitative platelet disorders have prolonged closure times. Anemia (hematocrit <30%) and thrombocytopenia (platelet count of <100 × 10⁹/L) can cause prolonged closure times.
- **In vitro platelet aggregation** studies measure platelet secretion and aggregation in response to platelet agonists (e.g., adenosine diphosphate [ADP], collagen, arachidonic acid, and epinephrine), and they assist with the diagnosis of qualitative platelet disorders.
- Laboratory evaluation of suspected vWD begins with measurement of **von Willebrand factor antigen** (vWF:Ag) and performance of at least one **vWF activity assay:**
  - **Ristocetin cofactor (vWF:RCo):** Measures vWF-mediated agglutination of control platelets in the presence of ristocetin.
  - **Collagen-binding assay:** Measures vWF affinity for collagen.
  - **"Functional" immunoassay:** Monoclonal antibody to vWF domain that binds to platelets.
  - **vWF multimer analysis** by agarose gel electrophoresis separates vWF multimers by size to classify vWD type 2 subtypes.

TABLE 1	Factor Deficiencies Cause Prolonged Prothrombin Time (PT) and/or Activated Partial Thromboplastin Time (aPTT) That Correct with 50:50 Mix

Abnormal Assay	Suspected Factor Deficiencies
aPTT	XII, XI, IX, or VIII
PT	VII
PT and aPTT	II, V, X, or fibrinogen

Secondary Hemostasis

- **PT:** Measures time to form a fibrin clot after adding thromboplastin (tissue factor and phospholipid) and calcium to citrated plasma.
  - Sensitive to deficiencies of **extrinsic pathway** (factor VII), **common pathway** (factors X and V and prothrombin), and **fibrinogen.**
  - Reporting a PT ratio as an international normalized ratio (INR) reduces interlaboratory variation.[3]
  - Point-of-care instruments accurately measure PT/INR from a drop of whole blood.
- **aPTT:** Measures the time to form a fibrin clot after activation of citrated plasma by calcium, phospholipid, and negatively charged particles.
  - Besides heparin, deficiencies and inhibitors of coagulation factors of the intrinsic pathway (e.g., high-molecular-weight kininogen [HMWK], prekallikrein, factor XII, factor XI, factor IX, and factor VIII), common pathway (e.g., factor V, factor X, and prothrombin), and fibrinogen prolong the aPTT.
- **Thrombin time:** Measures time to form a fibrin clot after addition of thrombin to citrated plasma. Quantitative and qualitative deficiencies of fibrinogen, fibrin degradation products, heparin, and direct thrombin inhibitor (DTI) drugs prolong the thrombin time.
- **Fibrinogen:** The addition of thrombin to dilute plasma and the measurement of a clotting time determine the level of fibrinogen. Conditions causing hypofibrinogen and potential for bleeding include decreased hepatic synthesis, massive hemorrhage, and disseminated intravascular coagulation (DIC).
- **D-dimers** result from plasmin digestion of fibrin. Elevated D-dimer concentrations occur in many disease states that include acute venous thromboembolism, DIC, trauma, and malignancy.
- **Mixing studies** determine whether a factor deficiency or an inhibitor has prolonged the PT or the aPTT. Mixing patient plasma 1:1 with normal pooled plasma (all factor activities = 100%) restores deficient factors sufficiently to normalize or nearly normalize the PT or the aPTT (Table 1). If mixing does not correct the prolonged PT or aPTT, a specific factor inhibitor, a nonspecific inhibitor (e.g., lupus anticoagulant), heparin, or a DTI anticoagulant may have caused the prolongation.

PLATELET DISORDERS

Thrombocytopenia

- Thrombocytopenia is defined as a platelet count of $<140 \times 10^9$/L at Barnes-Jewish Hospital. **In the absence of qualitative platelet defects or vascular damage, spontaneous bleeding often does not occur with platelet counts of $>30 \times 10^9$/L.**
- Thrombocytopenia occurs from decreased production, increased destruction, or sequestration of platelets (Table 2). Many infectious diseases have an

TABLE 2	Classification of Thrombocytopenia

Decreased platelet production	**Increased platelet clearance**
Marrow failure syndromes	Immune-mediated mechanisms
Congenital	Immune thrombocytopenia purpura
Acquired: aplastic anemia, paroxysmal	Thrombotic thrombocytopenia
nocturnal hemoglobinuria	purpura
Hematologic malignancies	Posttransfusion purpura
Marrow infiltration	Heparin-induced thrombocytopenia
Cancer	**Nonimmune mediated**
Granuloma	DIC
Fibrosis	Local consumption (aortic
Primary	aneurysm)
Secondary	Acute hemorrhage
Nutritional	
Vitamin B_{12} deficiency	
Folate deficiency	
Physical damage	
Radiation	
Ethanol	
Chemotherapy	
Increased splenic sequestration	**Infections associated with**
Portal hypertension	**thrombocytopenia**
Felty's syndrome	HIV
Lysosomal storage disorders	HHV-6
Infiltrative hematologic malignancies	Ehrlichiosis
Extramedullary hematopoiesis	*Rickettsia spp.*
	Malaria
	Hepatitis C
	Cytomegalovirus
	Epstein-Barr virus
	Helicobacter pylori
	Escherichia coli O157:H7

association with thrombocytopenia through complex or poorly understood mechanisms.[4]

Immune Thrombocytopenic Purpura

General Principles

- Immune thrombocytopenic purpura (ITP), an acquired autoimmune disorder in which antiplatelet antibodies cause shortened platelet survival and suppress megakaryopoiesis, leads to thrombocytopenia and increased bleeding risk. ITP classification consists of idiopathic (primary) and associated with coexisting conditions (secondary).
- Adult primary ITP has a prevalence of 32 cases per million persons.[5] Secondary ITP occurs less often.
- In ITP, autoantibodies bind to platelet surface antigens and cause premature clearance by the reticuloendothelial system and immune-mediated suppression of

TABLE 3	Drugs Implicated in Immune Thrombocytopenia

Antibiotics
Cephalosporins
  Cefotetan
  Cephalothin
Gentamicin
Linezolid
Penicillins
  Penicillin
  Ampicillin
  Methicillin
Rifampin
Sulfonamides
Trimethoprim
Vancomycin
Anti-inflammatory drugs
Aspirin
Diclofenac
Ibuprofen
Indomethacin
Naproxen
Piroxicam
Sulindac
Tolmetin
Antihistamines
Chlorpheniramine
Cimetidine
Ranitidine
Antiarrhythmics
Amiodarone
Digoxin
Lidocaine
Procainamide
Quinidine

Anticoagulants
Heparin
Low-molecular-weight heparin
Platelet inhibitors
Abciximab
Eptifibatide
Tirofiban
Ticlopidine
Antihypertensives
α-Methyldopa
Acetazolamide
Captopril
Chlorothiazide
Furosemide
Hydrochlorothiazide
Spironolactone
Anticonvulsants
Carbamazepine
Phenytoin
Valproic acid
Other
Acetaminophen
Alemtuzumab
Cocaine
Fludarabine
Gold
Heroin
Iodinated contrast
Quinine
Sulfonylureas
Tricyclic antidepressants

platelet production. Secondary ITP occurs with systemic lupus erythematosus, antiphospholipid antibody syndrome, HIV, hepatitis C virus, *Helicobacter pylori*, and lymphoproliferative disorders.[4]

- **Drug-dependent immune thrombocytopenia** results from drug-platelet interactions prompting antibody binding.[6] Medications linked to thrombocytopenia are listed in Table 3.[7]

Diagnosis

- ITP typically presents as mild mucocutaneous bleeding and petechiae or thrombocytopenia discovered incidentally.
- Primary ITP often has the scenario of isolated thrombocytopenia in the absence of a likely underlying causative disease or medication. **Laboratory tests do not confirm the presence of primary ITP, though they help to exclude some secondary causes.**

- Serologic tests for antiplatelet antibodies generally do not help diagnose ITP because of poor sensitivity and low negative predictive value.[8]
- Diagnosis of ITP **does not typically require bone marrow biopsy and aspirate** studies though these tests help to exclude other causes in select patients such as those with age >60 years and those who do not respond to immune suppression therapy.[9]
- Normalization of platelet counts with discontinuation of suspected drug, and confirmation if thrombocytopenia recurs when rechallenged, supports the diagnosis of drug-induced thrombocytopenia.

Treatment
- The decision to treat primary ITP depends upon the severity of thrombocytopenia and concerns about bleeding.
- Management of secondary ITP may include treatment of the underlying disease and the primary ITP therapy.
- **Initial therapy, when indicated, consists of glucocorticoids** (typically prednisone 1 mg/ kg/day).
- Nonresponders or patients with active bleeding typically also receive intravenous immunoglobulin (IVIG) (1 g/kg × 2 days) or anti-D immunoglobulin (WinRho) if Rh-positive (ineffective postsplenectomy).
- **Most patients respond to therapy with resolution of thrombocytopenia within 1 to 3 weeks.**
- Nonresponders and the 30% to 40% of patients who relapse during a steroid taper have chronic ITP. The therapeutic goals in refractory and relapsed ITP patients consist of a safe platelet count (30–50 × 10^9/L) and minimization of treatment-related toxicities.
- **Two-thirds of patients with refractory ITP will obtain a durable complete response following splenectomy.** Administer pneumococcal, meningococcal, and *Haemophilus influenzae* type B vaccines at least 2 weeks before splenectomy.
- Options for patients unwilling or unable to undergo splenectomy or those who fail splenectomy include prednisone alone or combined with IVIG, and androgen therapy with danazol, other immunosuppressive agents, or anti-CD20 monoclonal antibodies (rituximab).[9,10]
- In 2008, the FDA approved two small-molecule thrombopoietin receptor agonists for treatment of refractory ITP patients with increased bleeding risk. **Romiplostim** (Nplate), dosed SQ weekly, and **eltrombopag** (Promacta), taken orally once a day, produce durable platelet count improvements in a majority of refractory ITP patients beginning 5 to 7 days after initiation. Potential complications include thromboembolic events and bone marrow fibrosis.[11]
- For drug-induced thrombocytopenia, platelet transfusion for severe thrombocytopenia may decrease the risk of bleeding, and IVIG, steroids, and plasmapheresis have uncertain benefit.

Thrombotic Thrombocytopenic Purpura and Hemolytic Uremic Syndrome
General Principles
- Thrombotic thrombocytopenic purpura (TTP) and hemolytic uremic syndrome (HUS) are **thrombotic microangiopathies** (TMA) caused by platelet-vWF aggregates and platelet-fibrin aggregates, respectively, and result in thrombocytopenia, **microangiopathic**

hemolytic anemia (MAHA), and organ ischemia. Typically, clinical and laboratory features permit differentiation of TTP from HUS.

- TMA has an association with DIC, HIV infection, malignant hypertension, vasculitis, organ and stem cell transplant–related toxicity, adverse drug reactions, and, during pregnancy, preeclampsia/eclampsia and HELLP (**H**emolytic anemia, **E**levated **L**iver enzymes, **L**ow **P**latelet count) syndrome.
- Sporadic **TTP** has an incidence of approximately 11.3 cases per 10^6 persons and occurs more frequently in women and African-Americans.[12] HUS usually occurs in outbreaks affecting children. However, adults may present with both typical and atypical variants of HUS.
- Autoantibody-mediated removal of plasma vWF-cleaving protease (ADAMTS13), leading to **elevated levels of abnormally large vWF multimers,** typically causes **sporadic TTP.**[13] The abnormal vWF multimers spontaneously adhere to platelets and may produce occlusive vWF-platelet aggregates in the microcirculation and subsequent microangiopathy. Second-hit events may involve endothelial dysfunction or injury.
- Severe ADAMTS13 deficiency does not cause HUS and other types of TMA, with the exception of some cases associated with HIV and pregnancy.
- **Typical HUS** has an association with *Escherichia coli* (O157:H7) production of Shiga-like toxins.
- **Atypical HUS** has an association with transplantation, endothelial-damaging drugs, and pregnancy.[14] Inherited defects in regulation of the alternative pathway of complement activation cause familial HUS.[15]

Diagnosis

Clinical Presentation

- The complete clinical **pentad** of TTP, present in <30% of cases, includes **consumptive thrombocytopenia, MAHA, fever, renal dysfunction, and fluctuating neurologic deficits.**
- The findings of thrombocytopenia and MAHA should raise suspicion for TTP in the absence of other identifiable causes.
- TTP may occur during pregnancy and postpartum, and in association with HIV infection.
- Patients with autosomal-recessive inherited ADAMTS13 deficiencies have relapsing TTP (Upshaw-Schulman syndrome).
- Diarrhea, often bloody, and abdominal pain often precede typical HUS, and more pronounced renal dysfunction occurs.

Diagnostic Testing

- TMA produce **schistocytes** and thrombocytopenia on blood smears. The findings of anemia, elevated reticulocyte count, low or undetectable haptoglobin, and elevated lactate dehydrogenase support the presence of hemolysis.
- Sporadic TTP has TMA findings, normal PT and aPTT, mild-to-moderate azotemia, very low or undetectable ADAMTS13 enzyme activity, and sometimes an ADAMTS13 inhibitory antibody.
- HUS has TMA and acute renal failure. In typical HUS *E. coli* O157, stool culture has a higher sensitivity than Shiga toxin assays. However, stool samples obtained after diarrhea has resolved reduce the sensitivity of both tests.[16]
- Testing for sporadic or familial HUS should include molecular analysis of complement regulator factor H and I genes through reference laboratories.

Treatment

Thrombotic Thrombocytopenic Purpura

- The mainstay of therapy consists of rapid treatment with **plasma exchange** (PEX) of 1.0 to 1.5 plasma volumes daily. PEX is usually continued for at least 5 days or 2 days after normalization of platelet count and lactate dehydrogenase.
- If PEX is not available or will be delayed, infuse **fresh frozen plasma** (FFP) immediately to replace ADAMTS13.
- Common practice includes the administration of **glucocorticoids:** prednisone, 1 mg/kg PO or methylprednisolone, 1 g IV daily.
- Transfuse red cells based on signs and symptoms of anemia.
- **Platelet transfusion in the absence of severe bleeding is relatively contraindicated because of the potential risk of additional microvascular occlusions.**
- Approximately 90% of treated patients have a remission. Relapses may occur within days to years later after remission.
- Therapy with **rituximab,** an anti-CD20 monoclonal antibody, achieves durable remissions following TTP relapses.[17,18]
- Immunosuppression with cyclophosphamide, azathioprine, or vincristine, and splenectomy may have success in the treatment of refractory or relapsing TTP.[19,20]

Hemolytic Uremic Syndrome

- Treatment of typical HUS remains supportive.
- Familial HUS often leads to chronic renal failure.
- **HUS does not usually improve with PEX.**
- Antibiotic therapy does not hasten recovery or minimize toxicity for HUS associated with infection.
- Atypical HUS associated with calcineurin inhibitors (cyclosporine, tacrolimus) usually responds to drug dose reduction or discontinuation.

Heparin-Induced Thrombocytopenia

General Principles

- Heparin-induced thrombocytopenia (HIT) is an acquired hypercoagulable disorder caused by antibodies targeting heparin and platelet factor 4 (PF4) complexes, which can activate platelets, cause thrombocytopenia, and lead to clot formation through increased thrombin generation.[21]
- HIT typically presents with a decreased platelet count by at least 50% from preexposure baseline, though HIT-associated thrombosis can occur prior to the platelet count drop.
- Exposure to unfractionated heparin (UFH), and less likely with low-molecular-weight heparin (LMWH), and fondaparinux causes HIT.
- HIT complications include venous and arterial thromboses, skin necrosis at injection sites, and acute systemic reactions after IV bolus administration.
- The incidence of HIT varies with clinical setting, anticoagulant formulation, dose, duration of exposure, and previous exposure and it ranges from 0.1% to 1% in medical and obstetric patients receiving prophylactic and therapeutic UFH to >1% to 5% in patients receiving prophylactic UFH after total hip or knee replacements or cardiothoracic surgery.[22]

- Patients exposed only to LMWH have a low incidence of HIT.[23] HIT rarely occurs in association with the synthetic pentasaccharide fondaparinux.[24]

Diagnosis

HIPA antibodies

Clinical Presentation

- Suspect HIT when thrombocytopenia occurs during heparin exposure by any route in the absence of other causes of thrombocytopenia, and when platelet counts recover after cessation of heparin.
- HIT **usually develops between 5 and 14 days of heparin exposure** (typical-onset HIT). Exceptions include **delayed-onset HIT,** which occurs after stopping heparin, and **early-onset HIT,** which starts within the first 24 hours of heparin administration in patients with recent exposure to heparin.[22]
- **HIT rarely causes severe thrombocytopenia and bleeding.**
- **Venous thromboembolic complications occur more often than arterial thromboembolic complications in 30% to 75% of HIT patients.** Thrombosis can precede, be concurrent with, or follow recognition of thrombocytopenia.
- HIT causing venous thrombi at heparin injection sites produces full-thickness skin infarctions sometimes in the absence of thrombocytopenia.
- HIT can cause systemic allergic responses following an IV bolus of heparin characterized by fever, hypertension, dyspnea, and cardiac arrest.

Diagnostic Testing

- For suspected HIT, laboratory tests for **PF4 antibodies** improve diagnostic accuracy. Laboratories use two types of HIT assays: **functional assays** (platelet aggregometry or serotonin release assay to detect activation of control platelets in the presence of patient serum and heparin) and **serologic enzyme immunoassays** (PF4 EIA) to detect PF4 antibodies.
- In comparison, functional assays have higher specificity, whereas serologic tests have higher sensitivity.
- For a low pretest probability of HIT, a functional test should confirm a positive PF4 EIA result.
- For a high clinical suspicion for HIT, despite an initial negative PF4 EIA, the patient should undergo repeat testing.[25]

Treatment

- Since PF4 antibody test results rarely become immediately available, clinical assessment determines initial management.
- A scoring system based on "4Ts" improves diagnostic accuracy: thrombocytopenia, timing, thrombosis, and other explanation for thrombocytopenia.[26]
- When HIT is strongly suspected, begin treatment by **eliminating all heparin exposure.** Patients with thrombosis and those at high risk for thrombosis require alternative anticoagulation with a parenteral DTI, either hirudin (lepirudin) or argatroban (see Chapter 10).
- **Do not substitute LMWH for UFH** because of high rates of cross reactivity with HIT antibodies.
- Perform lower extremity venous compression ultrasound since it often detects deep vein thrombosis in asymptomatic "isolated" HIT patients and the presence of thrombosis mandates longer-duration anticoagulation.[21]

- Start warfarin only after the platelet count normalizes, at an initial low dose, overlapping with a DTI for 5 days, to reduce the risk of limb gangrene due to ongoing hypercoagulable conditions and depletion of protein C and S.
- DTIs prolong the INR and require careful monitoring when transitioning from DTI to warfarin (see Chapter 10).
- The recommended duration of anticoagulation therapy for HIT depends on the clinical scenario: Typically until the platelet count recovers for isolated HIT (without thrombosis) and typical thromboembolism duration for HIT-associated thrombosis (see Chapter 10).

Gestational Thrombocytopenia

- Gestational thrombocytopenia (platelet counts **no lower than 70 × 10⁹/L**) is a benign, mild thrombocytopenia associated with 5% to 7% of otherwise uncomplicated pregnancies.
- Gestational thrombocytopenia occurs in the third trimester of pregnancy. The mother has no symptoms and the fetus remains unaffected.
- Other causes of thrombocytopenia during pregnancy include ITP, preeclampsia, eclampsia, HELLP syndrome, TTP, and DIC.
- Diagnostic testing for gestational thrombocytopenia includes a thorough evaluation for evidence of hemolysis, infection, hypertension, and liver dysfunction to distinguish between these syndromes.

Platelet Transfusion

Platelet Products

- Platelets can be separated from units of donated whole blood (random-donor platelets) or collected by apheresis (single-donor platelets).
- In patients with thrombocytopenia resulting from a platelet production defect, transfusion of either one single-donor apheresis unit or six random-donor units typically produce an **immediate increment of approximately 30 × 10⁹/L.**

Reaction to Platelets

- Removing WBCs from random-donor units by filtration and by apheresis for single-donor units can reduce the risk of febrile reactions, alloimmunization, and refractoriness to platelet transfusion in patients who will require chronic platelet support.
- Platelets are stored at room temperature, which facilitates bacterial replication. Mandated screening for bacterial contamination before the release of stored platelets has reduced severe and fatal platelet transfusion reactions.
- Not using multiparous platelet donors or screening out those with human leukocyte antigen (HLA) antibodies reduces the risk of **transfusion-related acute lung injury** due to donor HLA antibodies that target the recipient leukocytes.

Transfusion Threshold

- Prophylactic platelet transfusion seems appropriate for asymptomatic outpatients with platelet counts of <20 × 10⁹/L and asymptomatic inpatients with platelet counts of <10 × 10⁹/L.

- Patients undergoing a major invasive procedure typically have a platelet transfusion threshold of $<50 \times 10^9$/L. High-risk surgery may warrant prophylactic transfusion to maintain the platelet count at $>100 \times 10^9$/L.
- Bleeding leads to the use of higher platelet transfusion thresholds.
- Shortened platelet survival occurs with sepsis, fever, active bleeding, splenic sequestration, certain drugs, or alloantibody (HLA antigen more likely than platelet specific) development in multiply transfused patients.
- To assess antibody-mediated refractoriness to platelet transfusions, **measure the platelet count before and after 60 minutes of transfusion.** An increment of $<5 \times 10^9$/L suggests that antibody-mediated refractoriness rather than shortened survival due to another mechanism has occurred.
- ABO-compatible platelets, HLA-matched single-donor platelets, or platelets from donors lacking alloantibodies produced by the patients may improve platelet increments.[27]

Thrombocytosis

General Principles

- **Reactive thrombocytosis** may occur in response to recovery from thrombocytopenia, postsplenectomy, iron deficiency, chronic infectious or inflammatory states, and malignancies. Patients with reactive thrombocytosis **do not have an increased risk of bleeding or thrombosis.** Platelet normalization occurs after improvement of the underlying disorder.
- **Essential thrombocythemia** (ET) is a chronic myeloproliferative disorder.
  - Eventual progression to myelofibrosis, acute myeloid leukemia, or myelodysplastic syndrome occurs in a small minority of ET patients.[28]
  - The risk of thrombosis increases with age, prior thrombosis, duration of disease, and other comorbidities.[29]

Diagnosis

Clinical Presentation

- ET may present as an incidental discovery or present with thrombotic or hemorrhagic symptoms.
- Erythromelalgia, due to microvascular occlusive platelet thrombi, presents as intense burning or throbbing of the extremities, typically involving the feet. Cold exposure usually relieves symptoms. Typical signs of erythromelalgia include erythema and warmth of affected digits.
- **Hemorrhage typically occurs with platelet counts of $>1,000 \times 10^9$/L,** and acquired deficiencies of large vWF multimers often accompany hemorrhage patients with ET.[30]
- Approximately 50% of ET patients develop **mild splenomegaly.**

Diagnostic Testing

- 2008 World Health Organization revised criteria for ET require the following:
  - Sustained platelet count of $>450 \times 10^9$/L.
  - Bone marrow biopsy showing increased mature megakaryocytes and no increase in erythropoiesis or granulopoiesis.
  - Chronic myelogenous leukemia, polycythemia vera, and primary myelofibrosis not present according to WHO criteria.

- Presence of JAK2V617F mutation or other clonal marker.[31]
- No evidence for reactive thrombocytosis if clonal marker not present.[32]

Treatment

- Patients requiring platelet reduction therapy include those >60 years, a prior thrombosis or hemorrhage, hypertension, diabetes, smoking, or hyperlipidemia.
- The majority of thrombotic complications occur at modest platelet count elevations. **Treatment typically aims for a platelet count of <400 × 10⁹/L.**
- Platelet-lowering drugs include **hydroxyurea and anagrelide,** or interferon-α in pregnant patients or women in their childbearing years.[33]
  - Limited evidence suggests that long-term hydroxyurea therapy has a very low leukemogenic potential.
  - Anagrelide side effects include palpitations, atrial fibrillation, fluid retention, and headache.
  - Hydroxyurea and anagrelide provide equivalent platelet count control, but anagrelide causes more complications.[34]
- **Platelet pheresis** rapidly lowers platelet counts to manage acute arterial thrombosis.

Qualitative Platelet Disorders

General Principles

- Qualitative platelet disorders present with **mucocutaneous bleeding and excessive bruising** in the setting of an adequate platelet count, normal PT and aPTT, and negative screening tests for vWD.
- Most platelet defects produce prolonged BTs and/or PFA-100 closure times. However, a high clinical suspicion of a disorder in a patient with normal test results should lead to in vitro platelet aggregation studies.
- **Inherited disorders of platelet function** include receptor defects, aberrant signal transduction, cyclo-oxygenase defects, secretory (e.g., storage pool disease) defects, and adhesion or aggregation defects. In vitro platelet aggregation studies can identify patterns of agonist responses consistent with a particular defect such as the rare autosomal-recessive disorders of Bernard-Soulier syndrome (lack of platelet glycoprotein IbIX [vWF receptor]) and Glanzmann thrombasthenia (lack of glycoprotein IIb/IIIa [fibrinogen receptor]).
- **Acquired platelet defects** occur more commonly than do hereditary platelet qualitative disorders.
  - **Conditions associated with acquired qualitative defects** include myeloproliferative diseases, myelodysplasia, acute leukemia, monoclonal gammopathy, metabolic disorders (uremia, liver failure), and cardiopulmonary bypass platelet trauma.
  - **Drug-induced platelet dysfunction** occurs as a side effect of many drugs that include high-dose penicillin, aspirin, and other nonsteroidal anti-inflammatory drugs (NSAIDs), and ethanol. Other drug classes, such as β-lactam antibiotics, β-blockers, calcium channel blockers, nitrates, antihistamines, psychotropic drugs, tricyclic antidepressants, and selective serotonin reuptake inhibitors, cause platelet dysfunction in vitro but rarely cause bleeding.
    - **Aspirin** irreversibly inhibits cyclo-oxygenase-1 and -2. Its effects gradually diminish over 7 to 10 days because of new platelets production.
    - Since **other NSAIDs** reversibly inhibit cyclooxygenase-1 and -2, their effect last only several days. Cyclooxygenase-2 inhibitors have antiplatelet activity

in large doses, but they have a minimal effect on platelets at therapeutic doses.

- **Thienopyridines** (clopidogrel and prasugrel) inhibit platelet aggregation by irreversibly blocking platelet ADP receptor P2Y12.
- **Dipyridamole,** alone or in combination with aspirin, inhibits platelet function by increasing intracellular cyclic adenosine monophosphate.
- **Abciximab, eptifibatide, and tirofiban** block platelet IIb/IIIa-dependent aggregation during management of acute coronary syndrome.
- Certain **foods and herbal products** may affect platelet function including omega-3 fatty acids, garlic and onion extracts, ginger, gingko, ginseng, and black tree fungus.[35] Patients should stop using herbal medications and dietary supplements at least 2 weeks before major surgery.[36]

Treatment

- Conservative management of patients with inherited platelet defects reserves transfusions for major bleeding episodes.
- Anecdotal reports have described successful control of bleeding with recombinant factor VIIa.
- **Treatment of uremic platelet dysfunction** includes the following:
  - Dialysis, to improve uremia.
  - Increase of hematocrit to ≥30%, by transfusion or erythropoietin.
  - **Desmopressin** (diamino-8-D-arginine vasopressin [DDAVP], 0.3 mcg/kg IV), to stimulate release of vWF from endothelial cells.
  - Conjugated estrogens (0.6 mg/kg IV daily for 5 days), which may improve platelet function for up to 2 weeks.
  - Platelets transfusions in actively bleeding patients, though transfused platelets rapidly acquire the uremic defect.
- **Platelet transfusion** compensates for drug-induced platelet dysfunction, except immediately following tirofiban and eptifibatide therapy.
- **Withhold antiplatelet agents for 7 to 10 days before elective invasive procedures.**

INHERITED BLEEDING DISORDERS

Hemophilia A

General Principles

- Hemophilia A is an X-linked recessive coagulation disorder due to mutations in the gene-encoding factor VIII that affects approximately 1 in 5,000 live male births.
- Approximately 40% of cases occur in families with no prior history of hemophilia, reflecting the high rate of spontaneous germ line mutations in the factor VIII gene.[37]
- Factor VIII activity determines bleeding risk: severe (<1%), moderate (1% to 5%), and mild (>5 to 40%).

Diagnosis
Clinical Presentation

- A positive family history (male patients with bleeding disorders on the maternal side of the family tree) can be elicited in up to 75% of male patients who present with abnormal PTT and hemorrhage.

- When due to a spontaneous mutation in the mother, there will be no family history of bleeding.
- Patients with mild or moderate hemophilia may present with hemorrhage only when challenged by trauma or invasive procedures (dental extractions, surgery).
- Severe hemophiliacs present with spontaneous joint, muscle, and GI bleeding. Spontaneous hemarthroses are particularly characteristic. Recurrent hemarthroses can lead to hemophilic arthropathy. Intracranial hemorrhage occurs in a few very severely affected patients in the perinatal period.
- Petechiae and mucosal bleeding is more typical of platelet dysfunction and is, therefore, not characteristic of hemophilia.

Diagnostic Testing
- The PTT is prolonged but insensitive. The PTT may occasionally be normal in those with mild hemophilia.
- PT, BT, and platelet count are normal.
- Factor VIII levels are low.
- Patients who are known to have factor VIII deficiency should always be evaluated for a possible factor VIII inhibitor (using a mixing assay) before an elective surgery or invasive procedure is performed.

Treatment
- The severity of factor VIII deficiency and the type of hemorrhage determine the type of therapy.
- In patients with mild-to-moderate hemophilia A and a minor bleeding episode, **DDAVP** (0.3 mcg/kg IV in 50 to 100 mL normal saline infused over 30 minutes, or 300 mcg intranasally [Stimate, 1.5 mg/mL] dosed every 12 hours) typically increases Factor VIII activity three- to fivefold and has a half-life of 8 to 12 hours. Tachyphylaxis may occur after several doses.[38]
- Patients with mild-to-moderate hemophilia A and major bleeding episodes or those with severe hemophilia A with any hemorrhage require **factor VIII replacement.**
  - Many hemophiliacs infuse **lyophilized factor VIII concentrates** at home. To safeguard from transmission of infectious agents in plasma-derived factor VIII concentrates, donors undergo screening, plasma undergoes nucleic acid testing for pathogens, and the final product undergoes viral inactivation. **Recombinant factor VIII concentrates** have increasingly become available.
  - One to three doses of factor VIII concentrates targeting peak plasma activities of 30% to 50% typically stop mild hemorrhages. Major traumas and surgery require maintenance of factor VIII levels at >80% for extended periods.
  - Plasma factor VIII activity increases approximately 2% for every 1 IU/kg factor VIII concentrate infused. A 50 IU/kg IV bolus would be expected to raise factor VIII activity to approximately 100% over baseline and extended treatment then consists of a 25 IU/kg IV bolus q12 hour.
  - Continuous infusion of factor VIII provides a feasible and efficient alternative to intermittent infusion.[39]
  - Dose adjustments based on peak and trough factor VIII levels ensure adequate hemostasis.
  - Second-line replacement therapies include cryoprecipitate and FFP.

Hemophilia B

- Hemophilia B is an X-linked recessive coagulation disorder secondary to mutations in the gene-encoding factor IX. Hemophilia B affects approximately 1 in 30,000 male births.
- Hemophilia B remains **clinically indistinguishable from hemophilia A,** but the distinction is important, as the therapy consists of **factor IX replacement** with either plasma-derived factor IX or recombinant factor IX.
- **DDAVP does not increase factor IX levels.**
- Postinfusion peak targets, duration of replacement, and laboratory monitoring for treatment of hemophilia B-related bleeding episodes have guidelines similar to those provided for hemophilia A.
- One IU of factor IX replacement per kilogram of body weight typically raises plasma factor IX activity 1%, and factor IX has a half-life of 18 to 24 hours.

Complications of Therapy for Hemophilia

- **Alloantibodies to factor VIII and factor IX (i.e., inhibitors)** in response to replacement therapy develop in approximately 20% and 12% of severe hemophilia A and B patients, respectively. These alloantibodies **neutralize infused factor VIII or factor IX** and prevent correction of the coagulopathy.
- Determining the titer of a factor VIII or factor IX inhibitor, using a laboratory assay that reports inhibitor strength in Bethesda units (BUs), predicts inhibitor behavior and guides therapy.
- **Treatment options** for hemophiliacs with factor VIII or factor IX inhibitors:
  - **Recombinant factor VIIa** dosed at 90 mcg/kg every 2 hours until achievement of hemostasis.[40]
  - **Activated prothrombin complex** concentrate contains partially activated vitamin K-dependent coagulation factors XI, X, and VII and thrombin. The increased risk of thrombotic complications should limit its use.
  - **Large doses of factor VIII or factor IX** concentrates sometimes decrease bleeding in hemophiliacs with weak inhibitors (BU < 5).

Von Willebrand Disease

General Principles
- vWD, **the most common inherited bleeding disorder,** affects an estimated 0.1% of the population.
- vWD results from an inherited **quantitative or qualitative defect of vWF.** Most forms of vWD have an autosomal-dominant inheritance with variable penetrance, although autosomal-recessive forms (types 2N and 3) exist (Table 4).
- vWF circulates as multimers of variable size, and these facilitate adherence of platelets to injured vessel walls and stabilize factor VIII in plasma.
- Classification recognizes three main types of vWD (Table 3)[41]:
  - **Type 1 vWD,** a partial quantitative deficiency of vWF:Ag and activity, accounts for 70% to 80% of cases.
  - **Type 2 vWD includes four subtypes:** 2A, selective loss of large multimers and decreased platelet adhesion; 2B, loss of large and medium multimers due to increased affinity for platelet GPIb; 2M, decreased platelet adhesion without loss of large multimers; and 2N, decreased binding affinity for factor VIII.
  - **Type 3 vWD** has a virtual complete deficiency of vWF.[42]

TABLE 4	Hemostasis Test Patterns in von Willebrand Disease					
	Type I	Type 2a	Type 2b	Type 2m	Type 2n	Type 3
PFA-100 closure time	↑/nl	↑	↑	↑	nl	↑
aPTT	↑/nl	↑/nl	nl/↑	nl/↑	↑/nl	↑
vWF antigen	↓	↓/nl	↓/nl	↓/nl	Normal	Absent
vWF activity	↓	↓↓	↓↓	↓↓	Normal	Absent
Factor VIII:C	↓/nl	↓/nl	↓/nl	↓/nl	↓	↓↓
RIPA	Reduced	Reduced	Enhanced	Reduced	Normal	Absent
Multimetric pattern	Normal	Missing large multimers	Missing large multimers	Normal	Normal	None detected
Inheritance	Dominant	Dominant	Dominant	Dominant	Recessive	Recessive

nl, normal; RIPA, ristocetin-induced platelet aggregation.

Diagnosis

Clinical Presentation

- The characteristic clinical findings consist of mucocutaneous bleeding (epistaxis, menorrhagia, and GI bleeding) and easy bruising.
- Trauma, surgery, or dental extractions may result in life-threatening bleeding in severely affected individuals.
- Patients with mild vWD phenotype may remain undiagnosed into adulthood.[42]

Diagnostic Testing

- If personal and family bleeding histories support a reasonable pretest likelihood of an inherited primary hemostasis or bleeding disorder, **screening for vWD should begin with measurements of vWF antigen and activity and factor VIII activity** (Table 4).
- **vWF:Ag** tests measure circulating vWF protein by immunoassay. A deficiency of vWF:Ag detects types 1 and 3 vWD and low or normal levels may occur with type 2 forms.
- **vWF:RCo** measures vWF-mediated agglutination of control platelets in the presence of ristocetin. A deficiency of vWF (types 1 and 3), vWF mutations that cause a selective loss of large multimers (types 2A and 2B), or defective platelet binding despite a normal multimer pattern (type 2M) causes decreased platelet agglutination.
- Suspect a quantitative vWF defect (type 1) with low vWF and Ag/RCo activity and a vWF:Ag/RCo ratio of >0.7.
- A quantitative deficiency of vWF (types 1 and 3) or vWF mutations that reduce factor VIII binding to vWF (type 2N) may reduce Factor VIII activity.
- Enzyme immunoassays measuring vWF-binding affinity for factor VIII can confirm type 2N diagnosis.
- Suspect type 2 vWD when vWF:Ag/RCo activity has a ratio of <0.7. vWF multimer analysis by gel electrophoresis assesses for the presence (type 2M) or absence (types 2A and 2B) of large vWF multimers, and a ristocetin-induced platelet aggregation test (patient's plasma and platelets plus ristocetin) distinguishes types 2A and 2M (attenuated) from type 2B (exaggerated) platelet aggregation responses.

Treatment

- Management of vWD consists of raising vWF:RCo and factor VIII activities to ensure adequate hemostasis.
- **Minor bleeding in type 1 vWD usually responds to DDAVP.**
  - Test dose administration should confirm clinically acceptable vWF:RCo and factor VIII increments.
  - **vWF:RCo activities of >50% control most hemorrhages.**
  - Recommendations for minor invasive procedures include a DDAVP infusion 1 hour before surgery, followed by infusions every 12 to 24 hours for 2 to 3 days postoperatively, with or without the oral antifibrinolytic drug **aminocaproic acid.**
- DDAVP does not effectively treat some type 2A, 2M, and 2N vWD and all type 3vWD patients. Because of the risk of postinfusion thrombocytopenia, patients with type 2B vWD should not receive DDAVP.
- Severe bleeding and major surgery in vWD patients require **infusion of vWF multimers, available in two brands of factor VIII concentrates** (Alphanate or Humate-P), or cryoprecipitate every 12 to 24 hours to raise vWF:RCo activity to approximately 100% and maintain it between 50% and 100% until sufficient wound repair occurs (typically 5 to 10 days).

ACQUIRED COAGULATION DISORDERS

Vitamin K Deficiency

- Hepatocytes require vitamin K to complete the synthesis (γ-carboxylation) of clotting factors (X, IX, VII, and prothrombin) and the natural anticoagulant proteins C and S.
- **Vitamin K deficiency is usually caused by malabsorption states or poor dietary intake combined with antibiotic-associated loss of intestinal bacterial colonization.** Vitamin K deficiency is suspected when an at-risk patient has a prolonged PT that corrects after a 1:1 mix with normal pooled plasma.
- Vitamin K replacement should be given orally or intravenously.
  - Vitamin K has variable absorption when administered subcutaneously, especially in edematous patients, and intravenous vitamin K carries the risk of anaphylaxis.[43]
  - With adequate replacement therapy, the PT should begin to normalize within 12 hours and should normalize completely in 24 to 48 hours.
- FFP rapidly but temporarily (4 to 6 hours) corrects acquired coagulopathies secondary to vitamin K deficiency. **Patients with coagulopathy who have actively bleeding or who require immediate invasive procedures should receive FFP.**
  - The usual starting dose is 2 to 3 units (400 to 600 mL), with measurement of the PT and aPTT after the infusion to determine the need for additional therapy. Up to 10 to 15 mL/kg may be needed for severe bleeding with significant PT prolongation.
  - Because factor VII has a half-life of only 6 hours, the PT may again become prolonged and require additional FFP, until adequate production of coagulation factors occurs.
  - Vitamin K replacement should be initiated concomitantly with FFP.
- Recommendations for varying degrees of excess INR prolongation due to warfarin are presented in Table 5 of Chapter 10.

Liver Disease

- Liver disease can seriously impair hemostasis because the liver produces coagulation factors, with the exception of vWF.
- Hemostatic abnormalities associated with liver disease typically remain stable unless liver synthetic function rapidly worsens or the patient is not eating normally.
- Other hemostatic complications of liver disease are hyperfibrinolysis, thrombocytopenia due to splenic sequestration, DIC, spontaneous bacterial peritonitis, gastrointestinal hemorrhage, and cholestasis (which impairs vitamin K absorption).
- **Vitamin K replacement** may help shorten the PT in liver dysfunction.
- **FFP is indicated for patients who are bleeding or require an invasive procedure and have abnormal coagulation parameters** (PT or aPTT >1.5 times control).
- **Cryoprecipitate,** a concentrated source of fibrinogen, given at a dose of 1.5 units/10 kg body weight, corrects severe hypofibrinogenemia (<100 mg/dL) in the setting of bleeding or invasive procedures. Periodic measurement of the fibrinogen level determines the need for dosing.
- Reserve platelet transfusions for active bleeding or prior to invasive procedures such as liver biopsies in patients with thrombocytopenia.

Disseminated Intravascular Coagulation

- DIC occurs in a variety of systemic illnesses, including sepsis, trauma, burns, shock, obstetric complications, and malignancies (notably, acute promyelocytic leukemia).
- Exposure of tissue factor to the circulation generates excess thrombin and its consequences: consumption of coagulation factors (including fibrinogen) and regulators (protein C, protein S, and antithrombin), platelet activation, fibrin generation, generalized microthrombi, and reactive fibrinolysis.
- Consequences of DIC include bleeding, organ dysfunction secondary to microvascular thrombi and ischemia, and, less often, large arterial and venous thrombosis.[44]
- Although no one test confirms a diagnosis of DIC, affected patients commonly have **prolonged PT and aPTT, thrombocytopenia, low fibrinogen levels, elevated fibrin degradation products, and a positive D-dimer.**
- DIC treatment consists of supportive care; correction of the underlying disorder if possible; and administration of FFP, cryoprecipitate, and platelets as needed for hypofibrinogenemia and thrombocytopenia.
- Although controversy exists regarding the use of heparin to prevent thrombosis in DIC, large-vessel thrombosis in DIC should be treated with adjusted-dose heparin.
- Recombinant-activated protein C (drotrecogin alpha) can reduce mortality in patients with severe sepsis and DIC but can also cause major hemorrhage.[45]

Acquired Inhibitors of Coagulation Factors

- Acquired inhibitors of coagulation factors may arise *de novo* (**autoantibodies**) or may develop in hemophiliacs (**alloantibodies**) following factor VIII or IX infusions.
- The most common acquired specific inhibitor is directed against factor VIII.
- Patients with coagulation factor inhibitors present with an abrupt onset of bleeding, prolonged aPTT that does not correct after 1:1 mixing, markedly decreased factor VIII activity, and a normal PT.
- Bleeding complications in patients with factor VIII inhibitors (autoantibodies) are managed in the same manner as for hemophiliacs with alloantibodies to factor VIII (see "Inherited Bleeding Disorders" section).

- **Long-term therapy** consists of immunosuppression with cyclophosphamide, prednisone, rituximab, or vincristine to reduce production of the autoantibody.[46]

REFERENCES

1. Lippi G, Favaloro EJ, Franchini M, Guidi GC. Milestones and perspectives in coagulation and hemostasis. *Semin Thromb Hemost* 2009;35:9–22.
2. Gewirtz AS, Miller ML, Keys TF. The clinical usefulness of the preoperative bleeding time. *Arch Pathol Lab Med* 1996;120:353–356.
3. Kirkwood TB. Calibration of reference thromboplastins and standardisation of the prothrombin time ratio. *Thromb Haemost* 1983;49:238–244.
4. Cines DB, Bussel JB, Liebman HA, Luning Prak ET. The ITP syndrome: pathogenic and clinical diversity. *Blood* 2009;113:6511–6521.
5. Frederiksen H, Schmidt K. The incidence of idiopathic thrombocytopenic purpura in adults increases with age. *Blood* 1999;94:909–913.
6. Aster RH, Bougie DW. Drug-induced immune thrombocytopenia. *N Engl J Med* 2007; 357:580–587.
7. Li X, Hunt L, Vesely SK. Drug-induced thrombocytopenia: an updated systematic review. *Ann Intern Med* 2005;142:474–475.
8. Davoren A, Bussel J, Curtis BR, et al. Prospective evaluation of a new platelet glycoprotein (GP)-specific assay (PakAuto) in the diagnosis of autoimmune thrombocytopenia (AITP). *Am J Hematol* 2005;78:193–197.
9. George JN, Woolf SH, Raskob GE, et al. Idiopathic thrombocytopenic purpura: a practice guideline developed by explicit methods for the American Society of Hematology. *Blood* 1996; 88:3–40.
10. Stasi R, Pagano A, Stipa E, Amadori S. Rituximab chimeric anti-CD20 monoclonal antibody treatment for adults with chronic idiopathic thrombocytopenic purpura. *Blood* 2001;98:952–957.
11. Nurden AT, Viallard JF, Nurden P. New-generation drugs that stimulate platelet production in chronic immune thrombocytopenic purpura. *Lancet* 2009;373:1562–1569.
12. Terrell DR, Williams LA, Vesely SK, et al. The incidence of thrombotic thrombocytopenic purpura-hemolytic uremic syndrome: all patients, idiopathic patients, and patients with severe ADAMTS-13 deficiency. *J Thromb Haemost* 2005;3:1432–1436.
13. Furlan M, Robles R, Galbusera M, et al. von Willebrand factor-cleaving protease in thrombotic thrombocytopenic purpura and the hemolytic-uremic syndrome. *N Engl J Med* 1998;339:1578–1584.
14. George JN. The thrombotic thrombocytopenic purpura and hemolytic uremic syndromes: overview of pathogenesis (Experience of The Oklahoma TTP-HUS Registry, 1989–2007). *Kidney Int Suppl* 2009;(112):S8–S10.
15. Atkinson JP, Goodship TH. Complement factor H and the hemolytic uremic syndrome. *J Exp Med* 2007;204:1245–1248.
16. Tarr PI. Shiga toxin-associated hemolytic uremic syndrome and thrombotic thrombocytopenic purpura: distinct mechanisms of pathogenesis. *Kidney Int Suppl* 2009;(112): S29–S32.
17. Zheng X, Pallera AM, Goodnough LT, et al. Remission of chronic thrombotic thrombocytopenic purpura after treatment with cyclophosphamide and rituximab. *Ann Intern Med* 2003;138:105–108.
18. Bresin E, Gastoldi S, Daina E, et al. Rituximab as pre-emptive treatment in patients with thrombotic thrombocytopenic purpura and evidence of anti-ADAMTS13 autoantibodies. *Thromb Haemost* 2009;101:233–238.
19. Ferrara F, Annunziata M, Pollio F, et al. Vincristine as treatment for recurrent episodes of thrombotic thrombocytopenic purpura. *Ann Hematol* 2002;81:7–10.
20. George JN. How I treat patients with thrombotic thrombocytopenic purpura-hemolytic uremic syndrome. *Blood* 2000;96:1223–1229.
21. Alving BM. How I treat heparin-induced thrombocytopenia and thrombosis. *Blood* 2003; 101:31–37.

22. Warkentin TE, Greinacher A, Koster A, et al. American College of Chest Physicians. Treatment and prevention of heparin-induced thrombocytopenia: American College of Chest Physicians Evidence-Based Clinical Practice Guidelines (8th Edition). *Chest* 2008;133:340S–380S.

23. Ban-Hoefen M, Francis C. Heparin induced thrombocytopenia and thrombosis in a tertiary care hospital. *Thromb Res* 2009;124:189–192.

24. Warkentin TE, Maurer BT, Aster RH. Heparin-induced thrombocytopenia associated with fondaparinux. *N Engl J Med* 2007;356:2653–2655.

25. Chan M, Malynn E, Shaz B, Uhl L. Utility of consecutive repeat HIT ELISA testing for heparin-induced thrombocytopenia. *Am J Hematol* 2008;83:212–217.

26. Lo GK, Juhl D, Warkentin TE, et al. Evaluation of pretest clinical score (4 T's) for the diagnosis of heparin-induced thrombocytopenia in two clinical settings. *J Thromb Haemost* 2006;4:759–765.

27. Hod E, Schwartz J. Platelet transfusion refractoriness. *Br J Haematol* 2008;142:348–360.

28. Harrison CN. Essential thrombocythaemia: challenges and evidence-based management. *Br J Haematol* 2005;130:153–165.

29. Harrison CN, Gale RE, Machin SJ, Linch DC. A large proportion of patients with a diagnosis of essential thrombocythemia do not have a clonal disorder and may be at lower risk of thrombotic complications. *Blood* 1999;93:417–424.

30. Budde U, Scharf RE, Franke P, et al. Elevated platelet count as a cause of abnormal von Willebrand factor multimer distribution in plasma. *Blood* 1993;82:1749–1757.

31. Baxter EJ, Scott LM, Campbell PJ, et al. Cancer Genome Project. Acquired mutation of the tyrosine kinase JAK2 in human myeloproliferative disorders. *Lancet* 2005;365:1054–1061.

32. Tefferi A, Vardiman JW. Classification and diagnosis of myeloproliferative neoplasms: the 2008 World Health Organization criteria and point-of-care diagnostic algorithms. *Leukemia* 2008;22:14–22.

33. Storen EC, Tefferi A. Long-term use of anagrelide in young patients with essential thrombocythemia. *Blood* 2001;97:863–866.

34. Harrison CN, Campbell PJ, Buck G, et al. United Kingdom Medical Research Council Primary Thrombocythemia 1 Study. Hydroxyurea compared with anagrelide in high-risk essential thrombocythemia. *N Engl J Med* 2005;353:33–45.

35. Basila D, Yuan CS. Effects of dietary supplements on coagulation and platelet function. *Thromb Res* 2005;117:49–53.

36. Hodges PJ, Kam PC. The peri-operative implications of herbal medicines. *Anaesthesia* 2002;57:889–899.

37. Mannucci PM, Tuddenham EG. The hemophilias—from royal genes to gene therapy. *N Engl J Med* 2001;344:1773–1779.

38. Mannucci PM. Desmopressin (DDAVP) in the treatment of bleeding disorders: the first 20 years. *Blood* 1997;90:2515–2521.

39. DiMichele D, Neufeld EJ. Hemophilia. A new approach to an old disease. *Hematol Oncol Clin North Am* 1998;12:1315–1344.

40. Hedner U. Recombinant factor VIIa (Novoseven) as a hemostatic agent. *Semin Hematol* 2001;38:43–47.

41. Sadler JE, Budde U, Eikenboom JC, et al. Working Party on von Willebrand Disease Classification. Update on the pathophysiology and classification of von Willebrand disease: a report of the Subcommittee on von Willebrand Factor. *J Thromb Haemost* 2006;4:2103–1214.

42. Mannucci PM. How I treat patients with von Willebrand disease. *Blood* 2001;97:1915–1919.

43. Crowther MA, Douketis JD, Schnurr T, et al. Oral vitamin K lowers the international normalized ratio more rapidly than subcutaneous vitamin K in the treatment of warfarin-associated coagulopathy. A randomized, controlled trial. *Ann Intern Med* 2002;137:251–254.

44. Levi M, Ten Cate H. Disseminated intravascular coagulation. *N Engl J Med* 1999;341:586–592.

45. Dhainaut JF, Yan SB, Joyce DE, et al. Treatment effects of drotrecogin alfa (activated) in patients with severe sepsis with or without overt disseminated intravascular coagulation. *J Thromb Haemost* 2004;2:1924–1933.

46. Wiestner A, Cho HJ, Asch AS, et al. Rituximab in the treatment of acquired factor VIII inhibitors. *Blood* 2002;100:3426–3428.

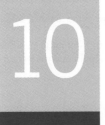

10 Venous Thromboembolism and Anticoagulation Therapy

Roger D. Yusen and Brian F. Gage

General Principles

Definitions

- **Venous thromboembolism (VTE)** refers to the presence of **deep vein thrombosis (DVT)** or pulmonary embolism (PE).
- **Superficial thrombophlebitis** may occur in any superficial vein.
- **Antiphospholipid antibody (APA) syndrome** diagnosis requires the presence of at least one clinical and one laboratory criterion[1]:
  - **Clinical criteria** consist of (a) the occurrence of arterial or venous thrombosis in any tissue or organ and (b) pregnancy morbidities (unexplained late fetal death; premature birth complicated by eclampsia, preeclampsia, or placental insufficiency; and at least three unexplained consecutive spontaneous abortions).
  - **Laboratory criteria** consist of persistent (at least 12 weeks apart) detection of autoantibodies (lupus anticoagulant [LA], anticardiolipin antibody, and β_2-glycoprotein-1 antibodies) that react with negatively charged phospholipids.
  - The APA syndrome may include other features, such as thrombocytopenia, valvular heart disease, livedo reticularis, neurologic manifestations, and nephropathy.

Anatomy

- The anatomic location of DVT and PE may affect prognosis and treatment recommendations.
- Thromboses can be classified as **deep** or **superficial** and as **proximal** or **distal**.
  - To emphasize its deep vein location, the term **femoral vein** has replaced the term **superficial femoral vein**.
  - **Proximal** lower extremity DVTs occur in or superior to the popliteal vein (or the confluence of tibial and peroneal veins), whereas **distal** DVTs occur inferior to the popliteal vein (or the confluence of tibial and peroneal veins).
- Location in the pulmonary arterial system characterizes **PEs** as **central** (main pulmonary artery, lobar, or segmental) or **distal**.

Etiology/Pathophysiology

- Symptomatic DVTs most commonly develop in the lower limbs.
- Untreated calf vein DVTs may propagate proximally.
- **Without treatment, approximately 50% of patients with proximal lower extremity DVT develop PE.**
- DVTs in the proximal lower extremities and pelvis produce most PEs.
- DVTs that occur in upper extremities, often secondary to an indwelling catheter, may also cause PE.
- DVT may occur concomitantly with superficial thrombophlebitis.

- **Superficial thrombophlebitis** occurs in association with varicose veins, trauma, infection, and hypercoagulable disorders.
- Other causes of pulmonary arterial occlusion include in situ thrombi (e.g., sickle cell disease), marrow fat embolism, amniotic fluid embolism, pulmonary artery sarcoma, and fibrosing mediastinitis.

Risk Factors

- Venous thromboemboli have an increased incidence under conditions of **stasis, hypercoagulability, and/or venous endothelial injury.**
  - Acute illnesses that lead to prolonged **immobilization** (trauma, surgery, and other major medical illnesses) predispose to development of VTE.
  - Hypercoagulable states may have an inherited or acquired etiology.
    - **Acquired hypercoagulable states** may arise secondary to malignancy, nephrotic syndrome, estrogen use, and pregnancy.
    - Both **heparin-induced thrombocytopenia** (see "Heparin-Induced Thrombocytopenia" section in Chapter 9) and the **APA syndrome** (see Chapter 28) can cause arterial or venous thrombi. At least 10% of patients with systemic lupus have LAs; however, most patients with LAs do not have SLE.
- **Inherited thrombophilic disorders** are suggested by a history of spontaneous VTE at a young age (<50 years), recurrent VTE, VTE in first-degree relatives, thrombosis in unusual anatomic locations, and recurrent fetal loss.
  - The most common inherited risk factors for VTE include two gene polymorphisms (**factor V Leiden** and **prothrombin gene G20210A**); deficiencies of the natural anticoagulants **protein C, protein S,** and **antithrombin; dysfibrinogenemia;** and **hyperhomocysteinemia.**
  - **Homocystinuria,** caused from deficiency of cystathionine-β-synthase, leads to extremely high plasma homocysteine levels and arterial and venous thromboembolic events that begin in childhood. More commonly, milder homocysteine elevations arise from an interaction between genetic mutations that affect enzymes involved in homocysteine metabolism and acquired factors such as inadequate folate consumption.[2]
- Unusual spontaneous venous thromboses, such as cavernous sinus thrombosis, mesenteric vein thrombosis, or portal vein thrombosis, may be the initial presentation of paroxysmal nocturnal hemoglobinuria or myeloproliferative disorders.
- **Spontaneous (idiopathic) thrombosis,** despite the absence of an inherited thrombophilia and detectable autoantibodies, predisposes patients to future thromboses.[2]

Prevention

Prevention, by identifying patients at high risk of thromboembolism and instituting prophylactic measures, remains the ideal strategy for reducing the morbidity and mortality of VTE. After an initial VTE, short- and long-term secondary prevention strategies remain paramount.

Diagnosis

Clinical Presentation

- **DVT** has neither sensitive nor specific symptoms and signs. However, pretest assessment of the probability of a DVT provides useful information when combined with the results of compression ultrasound or a D-dimer test, or both, in determining whether to exclude or accept the diagnosis of DVT or perform additional imaging studies.[3]
  - DVT may produce pain and edema in the affected extremity.

- **Superficial thrombophlebitis** presents as a tender, warm, erythematous, and often palpable thrombosed vein. Accompanying DVT may produce additional symptoms and signs.
- **PE** has neither sensitive nor specific symptoms and signs.
  - PE may produce shortness of breath, chest pain (pleuritic), hypoxemia, hemoptysis, pleural rub, new right-sided heart failure, and tachycardia.[4]
  - Validated **clinical risk factors** for a PE in outpatients who present to an emergency department include signs and symptoms of DVT, high suspicion of PE by the clinician, tachycardia, immobility in the past 4 weeks, history of VTE, active cancer, and hemoptysis.[5]
  - **Clinical suspicion of DVT or PE should lead to objective testing.**

Differential Diagnosis

- The differential diagnosis for **unilateral lower extremity** symptoms and signs of **DVT,** such as swelling and pain, includes Baker cyst, hematoma, venous insufficiency, postphlebitic syndrome, lymphedema, sarcoma, arterial aneurysm, myositis, cellulitis, rupture of the medial head of the gastrocnemius, and abscess.
- **Bilateral lower extremity edema** often suggests the presence of heart, renal, or liver failure.
- Additional diseases to consider in association with **lower extremity pain** include musculoskeletal and arteriovascular disorders.
- The **differential diagnosis of symptoms and signs of PE** includes dissecting aortic aneurysm, myocardial ischemia, heart failure, pneumonia, acute bronchitis, bronchocarcinoma, pericardial or pleural disease, and costochondritis.

Diagnostic Testing

Laboratory Studies
D-Dimer

- **D-dimers,** cross-linked fibrin degradation products, may increase during acute illness or VTE.
- Assays used to measure D-dimers differ in accuracy.
- D-dimer testing for DVT or PE has a low positive predictive value and specificity; **patients with an elevated D-dimer require further evaluation.**
- A sensitive quantitative D-dimer assay has a negative predictive value high enough to exclude a **DVT** in conjunction with a low (objectively defined) clinical probability and/or a negative noninvasive test.[6,7]
- A negative D-dimer in combination with low pretest probability can exclude almost all **PEs.**[8]
- In the setting of a moderate-to-high clinical pretest probability (e.g., patients with cancer), a negative D-dimer does not have sufficient negative predictive value for excluding the presence of **DVT or PE.**[9,10]

Hypercoagulability Testing

- Signs and symptoms of the APA syndrome should lead to laboratory evaluation (Table 1).
  - Serologic tests (immunoglobulin G and immunoglobulin M β_2-glycoprotein-1 antibodies and immunoglobulin G and immunoglobulin M cardiolipin antibodies) or clotting assays (LA) detect APAs.
  - Performing both serologic and clotting assays improves sensitivity.
  - Although it does not predispose to bleeding, an LA may prolong the activated partial thromboplastin time (aPTT) or prothrombin time/international normalized ratio (PT/INR).

TABLE 1	Laboratory Evaluation of Thrombophilic States
Inherited Thrombophilia	**Laboratory Assessment**
Prothrombin gene mutation G20210A	G20210A mutation
Partial protein C deficiency	Protein C activity
Partial protein S deficiency	Free protein S antigen, protein S activity
Partial antithrombin deficiency	Antithrombin heparin cofactor activity
Factor V Leiden	Activated protein C resistance, if positive confirm with factor V Leiden PCR
Hyperhomocysteinemia	Fasting plasma homocysteine level
Acquired Thrombophilias	**Laboratory Assessment**
Antiphospholipid antibody syndrome	Anticardiolipin antibody, β_2-glycoprotein-1, lupus anticoagulant
Paroxysmal nocturnal hemoglobinuria	RBC or WBC flow cytometry for loss of CD55, CD59
Myeloproliferative disorder	JAK-2 mutation

PCR, polymerase chain reaction; RBC, red blood cell; WBC, white blood cell.

- To assess for **paroxysmal nocturnal hemoglobinuria** in the setting of unusual spontaneous venous thromboses, perform flow cytometry to detect missing antigens on red cells or leukocytes.

Imaging
DVT-Specific Testing
- Initial diagnostic testing for symptomatic acute DVT should consist of a **noninvasive test,** typically **compression ultrasound** (called **duplex examination** when performed with Doppler testing).[11]
  - Compression ultrasound has low sensitivity for detecting **calf DVT** and may fail to visualize parts of the deep femoral vein, parts of the upper extremity venous system, and the pelvic veins.
  - The presence of an **old DVT** on compression ultrasound may make new DVT harder to detect.
  - Noninvasive testing has a low sensitivity in **asymptomatic** patients.
  - **Simplified compression ultrasound** limited to only the common femoral vein in the groin and the popliteal vein (down to the trifurcation of the calf veins) has lower sensitivity than does a complete proximal lower extremity venous examination.
    - Repeating simplified noninvasive tests within 10 days improves sensitivity.
    - Concerns about unreliable noninvasive test results or patient follow-up should lead to complete noninvasive testing or venography.
  - **Serial testing** can improve the diagnostic yield. If a patient with a clinically suspected lower extremity DVT has a negative initial noninvasive test result, one can withhold anticoagulant therapy and repeat testing 3 to 14 days later.
  - Lower extremity venous compression ultrasonography provides useful information in a patient with a suspected PE who has a nondiagnostic ventilation/perfusion (V/Q) or chest computed tomography (CT) scan, or when the clinician has a high suspicion of PE in the setting of a negative diagnostic test. Detection of

a proximal DVT serves as a surrogate marker for PE, and this scenario may not require further pulmonary imaging. (see "Pulmonary Embolism-Specific Testing" section).

- In addition to assessing for DVT, compression ultrasound, magnetic resonance (MR) venography, and CT venography may detect other pathology (see "Differential Diagnosis" section).
- **Venography,** the gold-standard technique for diagnosing DVT, requires placement of an IV catheter, administration of iodinated contrast, and exposure to radiation.
  - Patients with suspected DVT should first undergo noninvasive testing.
  - Contraindications to venography include renal dysfunction and dye allergy.
- **Magnetic resonance imaging** (MRI) has shown good sensitivity for acute, symptomatic proximal DVT in small studies.
- **CT venography** testing for DVT commonly occurs in conjunction with a contrast-enhanced spiral CT testing for PE.[12,13]
  - CT venography allows for visualization of the veins in the abdomen, pelvis, and proximal lower extremities.
- **PE-protocol CT** for evaluation of patients with suspected DVT has lower accuracy than the CT used for suspected PE.[12,13]

Pulmonary Embolism-Specific Testing

- **Nondefinitive tests** such as electrocardiography (e.g., right-sided strain pattern, with characteristic S wave in lead I and Q wave in lead III, and T wave inversion in lead III), troponin and brain natriuretic peptide levels, blood gases, and chest radiography may help determine the pretest probability, focus the differential diagnosis, and assess the cardiopulmonary reserve, but they do not rule in or rule out PE with acceptable certainty.
- **Unless an objectively low clinical probability of PE combined with a negative test (e.g., D-dimer) occur, the suspicion of PE requires further evaluation.**
- **Contrast-enhanced spiral (helical) chest CT:**
  - PE-protocol chest CT requires IV administration of iodinated contrast and exposure to radiation.
  - Contraindications to PE-protocol CT include renal dysfunction and dye allergy.
  - **Multidetector CT** has better sensitivity than single-detector CT for evaluating patients with suspected PE.
  - Used according to standardized protocols in conjunction with expert interpretation, spiral CT has good accuracy for detection of large (proximal) PEs, but it has lower sensitivity for detecting small (distal) emboli.[12]
  - Lower extremity compression ultrasonography may provide additional useful information, though negative D-dimer and multidetector chest CT tests exclude most PE.[14]
  - **Clinical suspicion discordant with the objective test finding** (e.g., high suspicion with a negative CT scan, or low suspicion with a positive CT scan) **should lead to further testing.**
  - Advantages of CT scan over V/Q scan include more diagnostic results (positive or negative), with fewer indeterminate or inadequate studies, and the detection of alternative diagnoses, such as dissecting aortic aneurysm, pneumonia, and malignancy.
- **V/Q scanning:**
  - V/Q scanning requires administration of radioactive material (via both inhaled and IV routes).
  - V/Q scans may be classified as normal, nondiagnostic (i.e., very low probability, low probability, intermediate probability), or high probability for PE.

- V/Q scanning remains most useful in a patient with a normal chest radiograph, because nondiagnostic V/Q scans frequently occur in the setting of an abnormal chest radiograph.
- Use of clinical suspicion improves the accuracy of V/Q scanning; in patients with normal- or high-probability V/Q scans and matching pretest clinical suspicion, V/Q testing has a positive predictive value of 96%.[15]
- **MR angiography:**
  - MRI requires IV administration of a nonionic contrast agent (e.g., gadolinium).
  - MRI appears to be sensitive for diagnosing acute PE, though large studies have not been performed, and the PIOPED III study aims to better define the accuracy of MRI.
- **Pulmonary angiography:**
  - Angiography requires placement of a pulmonary artery catheter, infusion of IV contrast, and exposure to radiation.
  - Similar to venography and PE-protocol CT scanning, contraindications to angiography include renal dysfunction and dye allergy.
  - Less invasive tests have mostly replaced pulmonary angiography over the past decade.
- **Echocardiography** to assess cardiopulmonary reserve and evidence of end-organ damage (right ventricular dysfunction) in patients with PE has a role in decision making regarding the use of thrombolytic therapy.
- **Additional laboratory tests** such as B-type natriuretic peptide (BNP) and troponin have prognostic value, though they do not rule in or rule out PE.[16]

Treatment

- **VTE therapy** should aim to prevent recurrent VTE, consequences of VTE (i.e., postphlebitic syndrome [pain, edema, and ulceration], pulmonary arterial hypertension, and death), and complications of therapy (e.g., bleeding and heparin-induced thrombocytopenia).
- Clinicians should perform standard baseline laboratory tests (i.e., complete blood cell count, PT, and aPTT) before starting anticoagulants.
- Unless contraindications exist, **initial treatment of VTE should consist of parenteral anticoagulation,** either with IV or SC unfractionated heparin (UFH), SC low-molecular-weight heparin (LMWH), or SC pentasaccharide (fondaparinux).

Anticoagulant Therapy

Warfarin

- Warfarin is an oral anticoagulant that **inhibits reduction of vitamin K to its active form** and leads to depletion of the vitamin K-dependent clotting factors II, VII, IX, and X and proteins C and S (see Fig. 1 of Chapter 9).
- Although warfarin has good oral absorption, it requires 4 to 5 days to achieve the full anticoagulant effect.
- The initial INR rise primarily reflects warfarin-related depletion of factor VII; the depletion of factor II takes several days because of its relatively long half-life.
- Because of the rapid depletion of the anticoagulant protein C and slower onset of anticoagulant effect, patients might develop increased hypercoagulability during the first few days of warfarin therapy if warfarin is not combined with a parenteral anticoagulant.[17]
- The typical recommended **starting dose** of warfarin is 5 mg PO daily but depends upon age and habitus (e.g., approximately 3 mg in older, petite patients; approximately 7 mg

TABLE 2	Warfarin Nomogram	
Day	International Normalized Ratio (INR)	Dosage (mg)
2	<1.5	5
	1.5–1.9	2.5
	2.0–2.5	1.0–2.5
	>2.5	0
3	<1.5	5–10
	1.5–1.9	2.5–5.0
	2–3	0–2.5
	>3	0
4	<1.5	10
	1.5–1.9	5
	2–3	0–3
	>3	0
5	<1.5	10
	1.5–1.9	7.5–10.0
	2–3	0–5
	>3	0

Starting dose 5 mg PO daily on day 1.
Modified from Crowther MA, Harrison L, Hirsh J. Reply: warfarin: less may be better. *Ann Intern Med* 1997;127:333.

in younger, robust patients). Patients with polymorphisms in genes for cytochrome P-450 2C9 or vitamin K epoxide reductase likely benefit from cautious warfarin initiation (see www.WarfarinDosing.org). The INR is used to adjust dosing (Table 2).[18]

- **Treatment of DVT/PE with warfarin requires overlap therapy with a parenteral anticoagulant;** in combination with warfarin, patients should receive a parenteral anticoagulant (UFH, LMWH, or pentasaccharide) **for at least 4.5 days and until they achieve INRs of at least 2.0 for 2 consecutive days.**[19]
- For most indications, warfarin has a **target INR** of 2.5 and a **therapeutic range** of 2 to 3.
- Patients with **mechanical heart valves** often require a higher level of anticoagulation (e.g., INR target range, 2.5 to 3.5) (Table 3).
- **Warfarin nomogram dosing** has more success than does nonstandardized dosing (Table 2).

TABLE 3	Anticoagulation with Artificial Heart Valves	
Material	Type/Location	INR Target
Tissue	Any	2.5 for 3 months, then ASA 325 mg lifelong
Mechanical[a]	St. Jude aortic	2.5
	St. Jude mitral	3
	Caged ball/caged disc	3

ASA, acetylsalicylic acid; INR, international normalized ratio.
[a]Add ASA for any caged valve, known or suspected coronary artery disease, h/o prior stroke, or mitral valve repair.

- **INR monitoring** should occur frequently during the first month of therapy (e.g., twice weekly for 1 to 2 weeks, then weekly for 2 weeks, and then less frequently).
  - Patients receiving a stable warfarin dose should have INR monitoring performed monthly, though patients with labile INRs should have more frequent monitoring (e.g., weekly).
  - The addition or discontinuation of medications, especially antifungal agents or antibiotics, should trigger more frequent INR monitoring.
- **Long-term anticoagulation with SC LMWH or fondaparinux** provides a treatment option for compliant patients who have unacceptable INR lability, or those with LA and difficulty monitoring because of an elevated baseline INR.

Unfractionated Heparin
- **UFH** comes from porcine intestinal mucosa.
- UFH catalyzes the inactivation of thrombin and factor Xa by antithrombin.
- At usual doses, UFH prolongs the thrombin time and aPTT, and it has a minimal effect on the PT/INR.
- Because the anticoagulant effects of UFH normalize within hours of discontinuation and **protamine sulfate** reverses it even faster, UFH is the anticoagulant of choice for patients with increased risk of bleeding.
- Abnormal renal function does not typically affect UFH dosing.
- For **DVT prophylaxis,** the typical dosage is 5,000 units SC every 8 to 12 hours. Prophylactic UFH therapy does not require aPTT monitoring, since it has a low bleeding risk and it typically does not significantly prolong the aPTT.
- For **therapeutic anticoagulation,** UFH is usually administered IV with a bolus followed by continuous infusion.
  - **Nomogram-driven weight-based dosing** provides a more rapid and reliable prolongation of the aPTT into the therapeutic range than does nonnomogram dosing.[20]
  - Bleeding risks lead to the use of different-intensity nomograms for different types of patients; patients with VTE often receive larger boluses and higher initial drip rates than do patients with unstable angina who use aspirin and other medications that increase bleeding.
  - **Treatment doses of UFH may be administered subcutaneously:** initial dose of 333 U/kg SC, followed by a fixed dose of 250 U/kg every 12 hours.[21]

Low-Molecular-Weight Heparin
- **LMWHs** are produced by chemical or enzymatic cleavage of UFH.
- Since LMWH inactivates factor Xa to a greater extent than it does thrombin (IIa), LWMH minimally prolongs the aPTT.
- Extensive clinical trials have confirmed the efficacy and safety of weight-based SC LMWH for the treatment of VTE.
- Given a linear dose response, LMWH does not typically require factor Xa monitoring.
  - In patients experiencing renal dysfunction, obesity, or pregnancy, factor Xa level monitoring may be prudent.
  - For therapeutic anticoagulation, peak factor Xa levels, measured 4 hours after an SC dose, should be 0.6 to 1.0 IU/mL for every12-hour dosing and 1.0 to 2.0 IU/mL for every24-hour dosing.[22]
- Different LMWH preparations have different dosing recommendations (Table 4).
- **Given the renal clearance of LMWHs, they are generally contraindicated in patients with CrCl of <10 mL/min, and patients with a CrCl of <30 mL/min require dose adjustments**

TABLE 4	Low-Molecular-Weight Heparin (LMWH) and Pentasaccharide Dosages for Treatment of Venous Thromboembolism

Drug	Dosage
Enoxaparin	Outpatient: 1 mg/kg SC q12 hours Inpatient: 1 mg/kg SC q12 hours *or* 1.5 mg/kg SC q24 hours
Tinzaparin	175 IU/kg SC daily[a]
Dalteparin	200 IU/kg SC daily[b]
Fondaparinux	5 mg SC daily for weight <50 kg, 7.5 mg SC daily for weight 50–100 kg, and 10 mg SC daily for weight >100 kg

IU, anti-Xa units; for enoxaparin, 1 mg = 100 anti-Xa units.
[a]U.S. Food and Drug Administration (FDA)-approved for treatment of PE without DVT.
[b]Not an FDA-approved indication. Two hundred IU/kg SC daily for month 1, followed by 150 IU/kg SC daily during months 2–6 for patients with cancer undergoing prolonged LMWH therapy.
Caution with use of fondaparinux, tinzaparin, dalteparin, or enoxaparin for pregnancy, morbid obesity, or end stage renal disease (CrCl <30 mL/min); anti-Xa level monitoring is recommended in these settings.

(e.g., enoxaparin 1 mg/kg once daily instead of twice daily). Dose adjustments may also be required in patients with cachexia or morbid obesity, or in women who are pregnant.

- Although initial LMWH overlap therapy with warfarin is typically converted to sole PO warfarin long-term therapy, patients with cancer may have reduced recurrent VTE when treated long-term with LMWH rather than warfarin at a slightly reduced dose.[23]
- **Protamine only partially reverses LMWH.**
- Because of the SC dosing route, LMWH facilitates outpatient VTE therapy.
- Patients selected for outpatient DVT therapy should have: no other indications for hospitalization (i.e., complications of VTE), low risk for VTE recurrence and bleeding, adequate cardiopulmonary reserve, adequate instruction and understanding of the warning signs of bleeding and VTE recurrence, access to a telephone and transportation, ability to inject the drug or a responsible caretaker, and adequate outpatient follow-up with a health care provider who can manage frequent lab testing, complications, etc.[24]
- **Pregnant** women with VTE (and without artificial heart valves) may undergo **long-term anticoagulation with SC LMWH.** Pregnant patients should undergo Factor Xa level monitoring.
- LMWH provides a long-term alternative to vitamin K antagonist treatment in patients who have clearly **failed oral anticoagulation** (objectively confirmed new VTE despite consistently therapeutic INRs).
- In patients with cancer, LMWH (e.g., dalteparin 200 IU/kg once daily for 1 month, followed by 150 IU/kg for 5 months) lowers the VTE recurrence rates compared with standard coumarin therapy (INR of 2 to 3).[23]

Fondaparinux
- Fondaparinux, a **synthetic pentasaccharide that is structurally similar to the region of the heparin molecule, binds antithrombin** and functions as a selective inhibitor of factor Xa.

- Because fondaparinux inhibits factor Xa and does not inhibit thrombin, it does not significantly prolong the aPTT.
- Large clinical trials have confirmed the efficacy and safety of weight-based subcutaneously dosed fondaparinux for the treatment of VTE.
- Similar to the LMWHs, fondaparinux does not require **factor Xa monitoring,** except for patients with significant renal dysfunction.
- Fondaparinux may be used for outpatient VTE therapy.
- The recommended dose for VTE therapy ranges from 5 to 10 mg SC daily, depending on weight (Table 4).[25,26]

Other Treatments

- **Leg elevation** reduces edema associated with DVT.
- **Ambulation** is encouraged for patients with DVT, especially after improvement of pain and edema, though strenuous lower extremity activity should initially be avoided.
- **Fitted graduated compression stockings** help to reduce the high incidence of postphlebitic syndrome in patients with lower extremity DVT.
- **Superficial thrombophlebitis** associated with IV infusion therapy does not require systemic anticoagulation, and treatment of discomfort may consist of oral NSAIDs.
  - For patients with spontaneous superficial thrombophlebitis, nonextensive disease does not clearly require systemic anticoagulation. Treatment with low-dose LMWH (e.g., enoxaparin 40 mg SQ qd) for 8 to 12 days may lower the short-term incidence of deep and superficial VTE.[27]
  - Extensive superficial thrombophlebitis should undergo systemic anticoagulation for at least 4 weeks.[28]
  - Recurrent superficial thrombophlebitis may be treated with anticoagulation or vein stripping.[29]

Duration of Anticoagulation

- **Duration of anticoagulation** decisions require individualization based on patient preferences and assessment of the patient's added risk of recurrent VTE off anticoagulant therapy versus the added risk of bleeding complications from continued anticoagulation.[30]
- Patients with a **first episode of VTE due to reversible risk factors** (e.g., surgery, major trauma) have a low risk of recurrence (<6%/year) and guidelines recommend 3 months of anticoagulation.[28]
- Guidelines recommend a minimum of 3 months of anticoagulant therapy for patients with a **first episode of idiopathic VTE** associated with less compelling and transient risk factors, such as prolonged travel, oral contraceptive pills/hormone replacement therapy, or minor injury.[28]
- For patients with unprovoked proximal lower extremity DVT or PE, guidelines recommend consideration of long-term anticoagulation, especially in willing patients with no major risk factors for bleeding and achievable good anticoagulant monitoring.
- For patients with a strong preference for less frequent INR monitoring, guidelines recommend low-intensity therapy (INR range 1.5 to 2.0) with less frequent monitoring over discontinuation of therapy.[28]
- For patients with **cancer and VTE,** they should undergo anticoagulation until cancer resolution or development of a contraindication. For patients with **a first VTE and one inherited hypercoagulable risk factor,** guidelines recommend a longer-duration anticoagulation that depends on the type **of thrombophilia.**

- **Heterozygous factor V Leiden** or heterozygous prothrombin 20210A do not necessitate because the increased odds of recurrence is 1.6 and 1.4 with these factors, respectively.
- Deficiency of protein S, protein C, or AT III carries a greater risk of recurrence than of heterozygous factor V Leiden or heterozygous prothrombin 20210A so the former necessitate longer treatment.[31]
- Patients with a **first VTE and antiphospholipid antibodies or two inherited risk factors** should receive a longer course of anticoagulation (e.g., 12 months) and indefinite therapy should be considered.
- Guidelines recommend that patients with **isolated calf vein DVT** or **upper extremity DVT** often undergo short-duration (e.g., 3 months) anticoagulation.
- Patients with **recurrent idiopathic VTE** should receive anticoagulation indefinitely, unless a contraindication develops, or patient preferences dictate otherwise.
- Patients with a history of VTE, especially those with ongoing risk factors, should possibly receive temporary prophylactic anticoagulation (e.g., low-dose LMWH SQ) during **periods of increased VTE risk,** including surgery, trauma, immobilization, prolonged air travel, hospitalization for medical illnesses, and postpartum.

Special Therapy

- **Inferior vena cava (IVC) filters** are mainly indicated for acute DVT when there are **absolute contraindications to anticoagulation** (e.g., active bleeding, severe thrombocytopenia, and urgent surgery) **or recurrent thromboemboli despite therapeutic anticoagulation.**
  - Although prophylactic IVC filters in patients with acute DVT/PE reduce the risk of recurrent PE, **a reduction in overall mortality has not been demonstrated,** and they do increase DVT recurrence.[32]
  - Relative indications for IVC filters include primary or metastatic CNS cancer or limited cardiopulmonary reserve after a DVT/PE.
  - **In patients who had IVC filters placed because of temporary contraindications to anticoagulation, anticoagulation therapy should be added when safe, to reduce the risk of filter-related thromboses.**
  - Several types of removable IVC filters exist and can provide a temporary physical barrier against emboli from the lower extremities, but they increase the risk of DVT recurrence. Filter removal requires a second procedure.
- **Catheter embolectomy,** often combined with local thrombolytic therapy, can treat large, acute PE and DVT.

Risk Management and Complications

- **Bleeding is the major complication of anticoagulation.**
  - Up to 2% of patients who receive short-term UFH, LMWH, or pentasaccharide for VTE therapy experience major bleeding.
  - For patients receiving chronic oral coumarin therapy (INR 2 to 3), the annual incidence of major bleeding is approximately 1% to 3%.
  - Concomitant use of antiplatelet agents increases the risk of bleeding.
- **Major bleeding in a patient with an acute VTE should lead to the discontinuation of anticoagulation and consideration of IVC filter placement. Reinitiation of standard-duration anticoagulation should occur after the bleeding concerns have resolved.**
- **Asymptomatic INR elevation on warfarin:**
  - Asymptomatic minor INR elevations of <5 should be managed by holding or reducing warfarin dose until the INR returns to the appropriate range and then resuming warfarin at a lower dose (Table 5).

TABLE 5	Treatment of Elevated INR >5 (Besides Stopping All Antithrombotic Therapy)	
Bleeding	**INR**	**Action**
None	5–9	Evaluate for food and drug interactions and for dosing or laboratory errors Repeat INR in 1–4 days If INR rising or at high risk for bleeding, give vitamin K 1–2.5 mg PO
	>9	Evaluate for food and drug interactions and for dosing or laboratory errors Repeat INR in 12–24 hours and in 48 hours Vitamin K 2–10 mg PO; repeat vitamin K as needed
Minor	Any	Vitamin K 1–5 mg PO or IVPB INR q8–24 hours; repeat vitamin K as needed If bleeding not controlled in 24 hours, treat as major bleeding
Major	Any	Vitamin K 10 mg IV over 10–20 minutes FFP (2–3 units) or factor VII concentrate Repeat INR in 6–12 hours and continue vitamin K and FFP until INR remains normal AND bleeding has stopped Surgical intervention for hemostasis

FFP, fresh frozen plasma; INR, international normalized ratio.

- Moderate (INR ≥5 but <9) elevation of the INR in asymptomatic patients should be treated by holding one or more warfarin doses. Treatment with oral vitamin K1 1 to 5 mg probably does not reduce the risk of hemorrhage in this setting (as compared with warfarin cessation alone) but lowers the INT.[33]
- Severe (INR >9) elevation of the INR should be treated with vitamin K (e.g., oral vitamin K1 2 to 10 mg) unless the INR is likely to be spurious.[34]
- **Bleeding with warfarin** (Table 6)[35]:
- Serious hemorrhages should be treated with vitamin K (10 mg) by slow IV infusion and fresh frozen plasma (FFP). Because of the long half-life of warfarin (approximately 36 hours, depending on genotype), vitamin K should be repeated every 8 or 12 hours to prevent INR rebound.
- Although expensive and potentially thrombogenic, recombinant factor VIIa may stop life-threatening bleeding.[36]
- **For patients receiving parenteral anticoagulants:**
- **Discontinuation usually restores normal hemostasis.**
- With moderate-to-severe bleeding, give **FFP.**
- For patients receiving UFH who develop major bleeding, heparin can be completely reversed by infusion of **protamine sulfate** in situations where the potential benefits outweigh the risks (e.g., intracranial bleed, epidural hematoma, and retinal bleed).
- After IV administration, UFH serum concentrations decline rapidly because of a short half-life. Likewise, the amount of protamine required decreases over time.
- **Approximately 1 mg protamine sulfate IV neutralizes 100 units of UFH,** up to a maximum dose of 250 mg. **For major bleeding associated with LWMH,** protamine sulfate has

| TABLE 6 | HEMORR₂HAGES Score |

Risk Factor[a]	Definition
Hepatic or renal disease	Albumin <3.6, CrCl <30 mL/min
ETOH (alcohol) abuse	
Malignancy	
Older age	>75 years
Reduced platelets/ platelet function	Plt <75 K, on ASA or clopidogrel
Rebleeding	2 points for prior major bleed, 1 point for prior minor bleed
Hypertension	SBP >160 mm Hg
Anemia	HCT <30%
Genetic factors	Presence of VKORC1 or CYP2C9 SNPs
Excessive fall risk	
Stroke	Prior ischemic stroke

HEMORR₂HAGES Score	Bleeding Rate per 100 Patient Years Warfarin (95% CI)
0	1.9 (0.6–4.4)
1	2.5 (1.3–4.3)
2	5.3 (3.4–8.1)
3	8.4 (4.9–13.6)
4	10.4 (5.1–18.9)
>5	12.3 (5.8–23.1)

ASA, acetylsalicylic acid; CI, confidence interval; CrCl, creatinine clearance; HCT, hematocrit; Plt, platelet; SBP, systolic blood pressure; SNP, single nucleotide polymorphism.
[a]One point for each bleeding risk factor, except a prior major bleed (2 points).
Modified from Gage BF, Yan Y, Milligan PE, et al. Clinical classification schemes for predicting hemorrhage: results from the National Registry of Atrial Fibrillation (NRAF). *Am Heart J* 2006;151:713–719.

less efficacy compared with its effect on UFH since it neutralizes only approximately 60% of LMWH.[37] Protamine does not reverse pentasaccharide (e.g., fondaparinux).
- **For patients with very serious bleeding receiving fondaparinux,** concentrated factor VIIa may be used with caution.
- If possible, **anticoagulants should be avoided in patients about to undergo neuraxial procedures** (lumbar puncture and epidural/spinal anesthesia, and epidural catheter removal) because of the risk of development of **epidural hematomas and subsequent spinal cord compression** and paralysis.[37]
- **Occult gastrointestinal or genitourinary bleeding** is a relative and not absolute contraindication to anticoagulation, though its presence prior to or during anticoagulation warrants an investigation for underlying disease.
- **Warfarin-induced skin necrosis,** associated with rapid depletion of protein C may occur during initiation of warfarin therapy.
  - Necrosis occurs most often in areas with a high percentage of adipose tissue, such as breast tissue, and it can be life threatening.

- Therapeutic anticoagulation with an immediate-acting anticoagulant (UFH, LMWH, etc.) and/or avoidance of "loading doses" of warfarin prevents warfarin-induced skin necrosis.
- **Warfarin is absolutely contraindicated in early (i.e., first trimester) pregnancy** because of the risk of **teratogenicity,** and it is often avoided during the entire pregnancy because of the **risk of fetal bleeding,** though it is safe for infants of nursing mothers.
- **Osteoporosis** may occur with long-term heparin or warfarin use.[38]

Special Considerations

- Perioperative management of anticoagulation requires close coordination with the surgical service (see Chapter 2) to address timing of interventions and therapeutic changes with the aim of thromboembolism prevention and avoidance of bleeding.
- **Invasive procedures** require discontinuation of warfarin.
  - **To achieve a preoperative INR of <1.5, stop warfarin therapy 4 to 5 days before an invasive procedure.**
  - In situations where a clinician aims to minimize the patient's time off therapeutic anticoagulation, parenteral anticoagulation should be initiated when the INR becomes subtherapeutic, approximately 3 days after the last warfarin dose but it should be stopped 6 to 24 hours prior to the procedure, depending on the half-life of the parenteral drug.
  - In some instances, intravenous UFH is the preferred choice of bridging therapy (e.g., pregnant woman with a mechanical heart valve undergoing a procedure).
  - If an INR of around 1.7 is acceptable for the procedure, the warfarin dose can be halved for 4 days preoperatively.[39]
  - After the procedure, resume warfarin (at the previous dose) and/or parenteral anticoagulation as soon as hemostasis and bleeding risk reach an acceptable level, typically within 24 hours.

Follow-Up

For a suspicious clinical presentation, **testing for intrinsic hypercoagulable risk factors ideally should wait until the patient is in stable health and off anticoagulation therapy** for at least 2 weeks to avoid false-positive results for nongenetic testing.

- If reasons exist to screen for hypercoagulable risk factors, collect blood for activated protein C resistance/factor V Leiden and LA. Blood collection for protein C, protein S, and antithrombin testing should occur before initiating anticoagulation. Although normal protein C, protein S, and antithrombin tests rule out congenital deficiencies, abnormally low results require confirmation through repeat testing (off therapy) or screening first-degree relatives to rule out a temporary deficiency related to the acute thrombosis.
- For patients with suspected lower extremity DVT, an initial negative compression ultrasound, and no satisfactory alternative explanation, **serial compression ultrasonography** in 3 to 14 days can improve the diagnostic yield.
- If patient preferences or contraindications lead to the withholding of anticoagulant therapy for **calf DVT,** we recommend further evaluation with **a repeat compression ultrasonography** to assess for proximal extension, which would mandate therapy.
- Testing for PE in patients with DVT and testing for DVT in patients with PE will produce many positive findings; such testing rarely affects therapy. However, baseline

results may provide useful comparison data for patients who return with symptoms of VTE, though studies have not determined the cost-effectiveness of this practice.

• Prolongation of anticoagulation duration in patients with residual thrombosis on **compression ultrasonography at the end of standard duration anticoagulation** for proximal DVT reduces VTE recurrence but can cause hemorrhage.[40]

REFERENCES

1. Miyakis S, Lockshin MD, Atsumi T, et al. International consensus statement on an update of the classification criteria for definite antiphospholipid syndrome (APS). *J Thromb Haemost* 2006;4:295–306.

2. Seligsohn U, Lubetsky A. Genetic susceptibility to venous thrombosis. *N Engl J Med* 2001;344:1222–1231.

3. Wells PS, Anderson DR, Bormanis J, et al. Value of assessment of pretest probability of deep-vein thrombosis in clinical management. *Lancet* 1997;350:1795–1798.

4. Wells PS, Ginsberg JS, Anderson DR, et al. Use of a clinical model for safe management of patients with suspected pulmonary embolism. *Ann Intern Med* 1998;129:997–1005.

5. Wells PS, Anderson DR, Rodger M, et al. Excluding pulmonary embolism at the bedside without diagnostic imaging: management of patients with suspected pulmonary embolism presenting to the emergency department by using a simple clinical model and D-dimer. *Ann Intern Med* 2001;135:98–107.

6. Stein PD, Hull RD, Patel KC, et al. D-dimer for the exclusion of acute venous thrombosis and pulmonary embolism: a systematic review. *Ann Intern Med* 2004;140:589–602.

7. Wells PS, Owen C, Doucette S, et al. Does this patient have deep vein thrombosis? *JAMA* 2006;295:199–207.

8. Ginsberg JS, Wells PS, Kearon C, et al. Sensitivity and specificity of a rapid whole-blood assay for D-dimer in the diagnosis of pulmonary embolism. *Ann Intern Med* 1998; 129:1006–1011.

9. Lee AY, Julian JA, Levine MN, et al. Clinical utility of a rapid whole-blood D-dimer assay in patients with cancer who present with suspected acute deep venous thrombosis. *Ann Intern Med* 1999;131:417–423.

10. Goldstein NM, Kollef MH, Ward S, Gage BF. The impact of the introduction of a rapid D-dimer assay on the diagnostic evaluation of suspected pulmonary embolism. *Arch Intern Med* 2001;161:567–571.

11. Tapson VF, Carroll BA, Davidson BL, et al. The diagnostic approach to acute venous thromboembolism. Clinical practice guideline. American Thoracic Society. *Am J Respir Crit Care Med* 1999;160:1043–1066.

12. Stein PD, Fowler SE, Goodman LR, et al; PIOPED II Investigators. Multidetector computed tomography for acute pulmonary embolism. *N Engl J Med* 2006;354:2317–2327.

13. Rathbun SW, Raskob GE, Whitsett TL. Sensitivity and specificity of helical computed tomography in the diagnosis of pulmonary embolism: a systematic review. *Ann Intern Med* 2000;132:227–232.

14. Righini M, Le Gal G, Aujesky D, et al. Diagnosis of pulmonary embolism by multidetector CT alone or combined with venous ultrasonography of the leg: a randomised non-inferiority trial. *Lancet* 2008;371:1343–1352.

15. Value of the ventilation/perfusion scan in acute pulmonary embolism. Results of the prospective investigation of pulmonary embolism diagnosis (PIOPED). The PIOPED Investigators. *JAMA* 1990;263:2753–2759.

16. Lega JC, Lacasse Y, Lakhal L, Provencher S. Natriuretic peptides and troponins in pulmonary embolism: a meta-analysis. *Thorax* 2009;64(10):869–875. Jun 11. [Epub ahead of print]

17. Sallah S, Thomas DP, Roberts HR. Warfarin and heparin-induced skin necrosis and the purple toe syndrome: infrequent complications of anticoagulant treatment. *Thromb Haemost* 1997;78:785–790.

18. Crowther MA, Harrison L, Hirsh J. Reply: warfarin: less may be better. *Ann Intern Med* 1997;127:333.
19. Warkentin TE, Greinacher A, Koster A, Lincoff AM; American College of Chest Physicians. Treatment and prevention of heparin-induced thrombocytopenia: American College of Chest Physicians Evidence-Based Clinical Practice Guidelines (8th Edition). *Chest* 2008;133:340S–380S.
20. Raschke RA, Reilly BM, Guidry JR, et al. The weight-based heparin dosing nomogram compared with a "standard care" nomogram. A randomized controlled trial. *Ann Intern Med* 1993;119:874–881.
21. Kearon C, Ginsberg JS, Julian JA, et al; Fixed-Dose Heparin (FIDO) Investigators. Comparison of fixed-dose weight-adjusted unfractionated heparin and low-molecular-weight heparin for acute treatment of venous thromboembolism. *JAMA* 2006;296:935–942.
22. Hirsh J, Lee AY. How we diagnose and treat deep vein thrombosis. *Blood* 2002;99: 3102–3110.
23. Lee AY, Levine MN, Baker RI, et al; Randomized Comparison of Low-Molecular-Weight Heparin versus Oral Anticoagulant Therapy for the Prevention of Recurrent Venous Thromboembolism in Patients with Cancer (CLOT) Investigators. Low-molecular-weight heparin versus a coumarin for the prevention of recurrent venous thromboembolism in patients with cancer. *N Engl J Med* 2003;349:146–153.
24. Yusen RD, Haraden BM, Gage BF, et al. Criteria for outpatient management of proximal lower extremity deep venous thrombosis. *Chest* 1999;115:972–979.
25. Büller HR, Davidson BL, Decousus H, et al; Matisse Investigators. Fondaparinux or enoxaparin for the initial treatment of symptomatic deep venous thrombosis: a randomized trial. *Ann Intern Med* 2004;140:867–873.
26. Büller HR, Davidson BL, Decousus H, et al; Matisse Investigators. Subcutaneous fondaparinux versus intravenous unfractionated heparin in the initial treatment of pulmonary embolism. *N Engl J Med* 2003;349:1695–1702.
27. Superficial Thrombophlebitis Treated By Enoxaparin Study Group. A pilot randomized double-blind comparison of a low-molecular-weight heparin, a nonsteroidal anti-inflammatory agent, and placebo in the treatment of superficial vein thrombosis. *Arch Intern Med* 2003;163:1657–1663.
28. Kearon C, Kahn SR, Agnelli G, et al. American College of Chest Physicians. Antithrombotic therapy for venous thromboembolic disease: American College of Chest Physicians Evidence-Based Clinical Practice Guidelines (8th Edition). *Chest* 2008;133:454S–545S.
29. Mannucci PM, Boyer C, Wolf M, et al. Treatment of congenital antithrombin III deficiency with concentrates. *Br J Haematol* 1982;50:531–535.
30. Kearon C, Ginsberg JS, Kovacs MJ, et al; Extended Low-Intensity Anticoagulation for Thrombo-Embolism Investigators. Comparison of low-intensity warfarin therapy with conventional-intensity warfarin therapy for long-term prevention of recurrent venous thromboembolism. *N Engl J Med* 2003;349:631–639.
31. Segal JB, Brotman DJ, Necochea AJ, et al. Predictive value of factor V Leiden and prothrombin G20210A in adults with venous thromboembolism and in family members of those with a mutation: a systematic review. *JAMA* 2009;301:2472–2485.
32. PREPIC Study Group. Eight-year follow-up of patients with permanent vena cava filters in the prevention of pulmonary embolism: the PREPIC (Prevention du Risque d'Embolie Pulmonaire par Interruption Cave) randomized study. *Circulation* 2005;112:416–422.
33. Crowther MA, Ageno W, Garcia D, et al. Oral vitamin K versus placebo to correct excessive anticoagulation in patients receiving warfarin: a randomized trial. *Ann Intern Med* 2009;150:293–300.
34. Gunther KE, Conway G, Leibach L, Crowther MA. Low-dose oral vitamin K is safe and effective for outpatient management of patients with an INR >10. *Thromb Res* 2004;113: 205–209.
35. Gage BF, Yan Y, Milligan PE, et al. Clinical classification schemes for predicting hemorrhage: results from the National Registry of Atrial Fibrillation (NRAF). *Am Heart J* 2006;151:713–719.

36. Crowther MA, Berry LR, Monagle PT, Chan AK. Mechanisms responsible for the failure of protamine to inactivate low-molecular-weight heparin. *Br J Haematol* 2002;116:178–186.

37. Horlocker TT, Wedel DJ, Benzon H, et al. Regional anesthesia in the anticoagulated patient: defining the risks (the second ASRA Consensus Conference on Neuraxial Anesthesia and Anticoagulation). *Reg Anesth Pain Med* 2003;28:72–197.

38. Gage BF, Birman-Deych E, Radford MJ, et al. Risk of osteoporotic fracture in elderly patients taking warfarin: results from the National Registry of Atrial Fibrillation 2. *Arch Intern Med* 2006;166:241–246.

39. Marietta M, Bertesi M, Simoni L, et al. A simple and safe nomogram for the management of oral anticoagulation prior to minor surgery. *Clin Lab Haematol* 2003;25:127–130.

40. Prandoni P, Prins MH, Lensing AW, et al; AESOPUS Investigators. Residual thrombosis on ultrasonography to guide the duration of anticoagulation in patients with deep venous thrombosis: a randomized trial. *Ann Intern Med* 2009;150:577–585.

Common Pulmonary Complaints

Peter G. Tuteur

Introduction

The lungs have both respiratory and nonrespiratory functions.
- Respiratory functions:
  - Ventilation: the movement of gas in and out of the lung structure.
    - Minute ventilation (VE): volume of gas exhaled per minute.
    - Alveolar ventilation (VA): the movement of gas in and out of perfused alveolae per minute.
  - Respiration: the exchange of gases at the alveolar level (O_2 and CO_2).
- Nonrespiratory functions:
  - Acid-base balance; change in VA is inversely related to $PaCO_2$. Change in $PaCO_2$ is inversely related to the effect on the pH.
  - Synthesis, activation and inactivation of biologically active molecules.
  - Hemostatic function.
  - Lung defense mechanisms.
- The anatomy of the lungs serves their functions well. The simple cartoon depicts the ventilatory apparatus (airways) and the respiratory apparatus (alveoli and adjacent vascular structures). Typically, when these structures are altered by disease, function is impaired, and symptoms develop. Most pulmonary symptoms are included in the following categories:
- Shortness of breath (exercise intolerance, breathlessness).
- Cough.
- Expectoration (sputum, blood).
- Wheezing (also consider stridor).
- Chest pain (discomfort, ache, tenderness).

The Focused Pulmonary Physical Examination

- Initially one evaluates extrathoracic sites looking for sinus tenderness, potentially obstructing posterior pharyngeal tissue, tracheostomy site (open or healed), and conjunctivitis as seen in sarcoid or Sjögren's syndrome.
- Directing one's attention to the thorax, one observes breathing depth, regularity, and symmetry.
- Palpation of the chest wall might identify a focal or diffuse area of tenderness directing the examiner to consider diagnoses such as costochondritis, unexpected rib fracture, or even pulmonary embolism.
- Auscultation should be performed listening to both phases of ventilation, inspiration and expiration. Furthermore, this should take place during both tidal volume breathing and forceful expiration preceded by a deep inspiration.

• If cough develops regularly following deep inspiration, an interstitial pulmonary process becomes an important item in the differential diagnosis.

Auscultated Pulmonary Sounds

• Adventitious (added) sounds are crackles, gurgles, or wheezes.
• When **wheezing** is heard during a prolonged expiratory phase of a force expiratory volume maneuver, airway narrowing is present and so focuses the subsequent workup.
• **Crackles** (rales) are intermittent sounds typically occurring during inspiration and are most meaningfully evaluated following a deep forceful expiration. These sounds might be considered "pulmonary opening snaps" produced when previously collapsed lung structures (airways or alveoli) open during the inspiratory phase. Awareness of the timing is critical for determining an appropriate differential diagnosis.
  • Crackles heard early in inspiration represent openings of previously collapsed larger airways as occurs in cystic fibrosis, bronchiectasis, and chronic bronchitis.
  • Late inspiratory crackles represent openings of previously collapsed distal structures such as alveoli or terminal bronchioles often abnormal in interstitial pulmonary processes or bronchiolitis obliterans.
• Gurgles are produced when fluid (mucus, blood) is present in the airways and gas moves through them. Modification of the gurgles location or character following forceful cough confirms this notion.

DYSPNEA

General Principles

Shortness of breath or dyspnea (the subjective sensation of breathlessness) is a highly nonspecific symptom occurring in most primary pulmonary, cardiac, and some musculoskeletal disorders.

Etiology

• Cardiac causes:
  • Acute cardiac dyspnea is often related to either **pulmonary edema** secondary to CHF or as a result of myocardial infarction.
  • **Valvular disease,** specifically left-sided diseases including critical aortic stenosis and mitral stenosis, can lead to dyspnea.
  • **Constrictive pericarditis** may result in exertional dyspnea and peripheral edema.
• Pulmonary diseases:
  • **Vocal cord dysfunction** may result in symptoms that can be difficult to distinguish from those of asthma. Clues include central wheezing, which occurs on inspiration and on expiration.
  • **Tracheal stenosis** may occur as a result of tracheal injury from prior intubation or result from inflammation due to Wegener's granulomatosis or relapsing polychondritis.
  • **Asthma** causes episodic or waxing or waning dyspnea.
  • **Chronic obstructive pulmonary disease** (COPD) is a common cause of dyspnea.
  • **Interstitial lung disease** may result in dyspnea and progressive pulmonary disability.
  • **Chest wall deformities,** such as kyphoscoliosis, may result in dyspnea because of mechanical reduction of lung volumes, diminished respiratory compliance, and mechanical muscle disadvantage.

- **Neuromuscular diseases** often lead to dyspnea due to muscular weakness. Later in life, respiratory difficulties may develop in polio survivors, particularly those who had respiratory paralysis during acute illness.
- **Pleural effusion** frequently has dyspnea as a primary symptom.
- **Pulmonary hypertension** causes dyspnea on exertion.
- Extrapulmonary causes:
  - Massive ascites.
  - Severe anemia may cause marked dyspnea likely from reduced oxygen-carrying capacity or high-output cardiac state.
  - Anxiety disorders.
  - Obesity.

Diagnosis

Clinical Presentation

History

- Assess the degree of disability; inquire whether dyspnea is present at rest or only with activity.
- Determine whether dyspnea is constant or episodic.
- Ask about edema, orthopnea, or paroxysmal nocturnal dyspnea.
- Inquire about a history of angina and cardiovascular risk factors.
- Elicit a smoking history as well as a thorough occupational exposure history.
- To aid in the differential diagnosis detailing associated characteristics is important. Table 1 will serve as a guideline.

TABLE 1	Characteristics of Shortness of Breath

Character	Meaning
Increases when supine	• Phrenic nerve (diaphragmatic) dysfunction • Left ventricular failure and congestive heart failure
Increases with exercise	• Ventilatory limitation: chronic obstructive pulmonary disease, asthma, bronchiectasis, cystic fibrosis • Respiratory limitation: pulmonary embolism, pulmonary hypertension, left to right shunt • Cardiac dysfunction • Neuromuscular weakness • Interstitial pulmonary process
Sudden versus slow onset	• Acute disease versus chronic disease
Episodic	• Asthma, gastroesophageal reflux disease, sinusitis, aspiration, bronchiectasis, exacerbation of chronic bronchitis
At altitude	• Impairment of oxygen gas exchange • Anemia • Altitude-associated pulmonary edema • Cardiac dysfunction
Breathlessness associated with emersion—hot tub, swimming pool, bath tub	• Diaphragmatic dysfunction

Physical Examination
- Elevated pulse and respiratory rate are nonspecific but suggest organic disease.
- Posture (leaning forward with the arms tripoding), accessory muscle use, and pursed lip breathing suggest COPD.
- Look for nasal polyps and purulent nasal discharge.
- Signs of current or past ear or nasal cartilage inflammation may suggest tracheal involvement from relapsing polychondritis or Wegener's granulomatosis.

Diagnostic Testing
Plain Chest Radiography
- A chest radiography (CXR) should be one of the initial diagnostic evaluations.
- Attention should be paid to the presence of effusion, edema, and lung volume size (reduced vs. enlarged).
- Location of lung involvement is also helpful for diagnosis:
  - Lower-lobe involvement is characteristic of idiopathic pulmonary fibrosis, rheumatologic disease, and asbestosis.
  - Mid- and upper-lung zone development is associated with granulomatous diseases and silicosis.

Computed Tomography
- Detects approximately 10% of cases of idiopathic fibrosis not visible on CXR.
- When performed with contrast it may reveal chronic thromboembolic disease.

Echocardiography
When pulmonary disease is not present, echocardiography can reveal evidence of left ventricular dysfunction and valvular disease.

Pulmonary Function Test
Refer to the detailed section later in this chapter.

COUGH

General Principles

- Cough is the sudden exhalation of lung gas mixture.
- The first response to the initiation of a cough reflex is deep inhalation followed by glottic closure and then maximum forceful expiratory maneuver. This may or may not be associated with the expectoration of phlegm, sputum (mucoid or purulent), or blood.
- Cough may be initiated by afferent stimulation of the upper airways structures such as the posterior pharynx, response to an inhaled irritant by larger airways, activation of stretch receptors of alveolar wall, and stimulation of the diaphragm either from above or below.

Etiology
- Identifying the etiology of cough is often a significant challenge.
- When the etiology is not immediately obvious, causes to consider include cough equivalent asthma, sinusitis, gastroesophageal reflux disease (GERD), nonbacterial (fungal) endobronchial infection, and interstitial pulmonary processes.
- A differential diagnosis is present in Table 2.

TABLE 2	Causes of Cough

Site of Cough Initiation	Potential Associated Conditions
Upper extrathoracic airways	
Posterior pharynx	• Sinusitis, tumor
Epiglottis	• Epiglottis (with sore throat)
Vocal cords	• Polyps, voice abuse
Trachea	• Aspiration, GERD
	• Status posttracheostomy, dynamic
	• Compression of trachea
Large airways	
Intrathoracic trachea	• Stricture
Large named bronchi	• Bronchitis, bronchiectasis, cystic fibrosis, asthma
Alveolar walls	Interstitial pulmonary processes:
	• Uremia
	• Iveolar proteinosis
	• Radiation
	• Oxygen toxicity
	• Viral
	• Sarcoidosis
	• Hemosiderosis
	• Malignancy or myeloma
	• Idiopathic
	• Tuberculosis
	• Fungal
	• Allergic or amyloid
	• Collagen vascular disease
	• Eosinophilic granuloma
	• Drugs or dust
Diaphragm	• Pleural effusion
	• Subpleural pulmonary infection/infarction
	• Subdiaphragmatic process (abscess, peritonitis)

Diagnosis

Clinical Presentation

History

- Recognition of the type and amount of expectoration often leads to a specific diagnosis.
- Nonproductive cough implies either a chronic irritating factor or an interstitial process potentially as simple as a viral pneumonitis or as complex as inflammation and/or scarring of the alveolar walls.
- When mucus production is reported (and even if present it is not always reported because of the social stigmata related to spitting), an inflammatory process (acute vs. chronic) likely is present that may be associated with infection (purulent sputum).

Physical Examination
- Examine the ears for otitis, which is a rare cause of cough.
- Examine the nose for evidence of mucopurulent secretions, sinus tenderness, boggy turbinates, or polyps, all of which suggest postnasal drip and perhaps a predisposition to asthma.
- Postnasal drip may also cause a cobblestone appearance of the tonsillar pillars.
- The throat should also be examined for signs of bulbar neurologic dysfunction.

Diagnostic Testing
- Obtain a **CXR.** If it is abnormal, focus on directed evaluation of the abnormality. If it is normal, obtaining sputum cytology, microbiological stains, and cultures is neither warranted nor cost-effective.
- **Sinus computed tomography (CT) scan** provides superior imaging and is no more expensive than plain radiography, but there is no validation of its predictive value. Sensitivity is probably very good but specificity is uncertain.
- **Pulmonary function tests** (PFTs) should be obtained if the prior workup is otherwise negative and symptoms do not resolve.

Treatment

When possible, therapy should be directed by diagnosis.

Postnasal Drip (Upper Airway Cough Syndrome)
- In the absence of infectious symptoms, begin therapy with a first-generation oral antihistamine such as azatadine maleate (1 mg bid) and a sustained-release decongestant.
- Nonsedating antihistamines do not appear to be effective.[1]
- Response usually occurs within 1 week and is confirmatory of the diagnosis.
- If therapy is unsuccessful in relieving symptoms in 2 weeks, consider obtaining a sinus CT scan.[2]

Postviral Bronchial Hyperreactivity
- This tends to be resistant to therapy but fortunately is self-limited.
- Ipratropium bromide (two puffs q4 to 6 hour) is significantly more effective than placebo in reducing cough in this entity.[3]
- Evidence for efficacy of inhaled steroids and oral steroids is weaker, but they can be given if cough persists despite ipratropium use.
- Resistant cough should be treated with antitussives and reassurance.

Angiotensin-Converting Enzyme Inhibitors
- Discontinuing angiotensin-converting enzyme (ACE) inhibitors often results in relief of symptoms in less than a week, and virtually all patients are better in 4 weeks.[4]
- Changing ACE inhibitors is unlikely to be effective as this is a class effect.
- Alternatives such as angiotensin receptor blockers (ARBs) can be used.

HEMOPTYSIS

General Principles

- Coughing up blood from a pulmonary source is called hemoptysis. On occasion, hemoptysis is confused with hematemesis or the expectoration of blood from a nasopharyngeal source. Blood originates from the bronchial circulation in most cases but has a pulmonary arterial source in pulmonary arteriovenous malformations, Rasmussen's aneurysms in tuberculous cavities, and the diffuse alveolar hemorrhage syndromes of autoimmune origin.

Significance
- Hemoptysis is an infrequent complaint for those who seek primary care but is of great concern to the patient. When present in small amounts, the greatest concern is about **lung cancer.** When there is a large amount, the event itself is frightening to the patient and the physician.

Etiology
- Conditions typically associated with hemoptysis include the following:
  - Carcinoma of the lung.
  - Necrotizing pneumonitis.
  - Tuberculosis.
  - Bronchiectasis.
  - Hereditary hemorrhagic telangiectasia (Osler-Weber-Rendu syndrome).
  - Bronchiectasis.
  - Cystic fibrosis.
- Of note, hemoptysis associated with anticoagulation therapy or hypocoagulable disease states usually develops only when there is an underlying pulmonary pathology.

Diagnosis

Clinical Presentation

History
- Obtain an estimate of the volume of hemoptysis. If the history suggests acute hemoptysis of ≥2 oz, refer the patient immediately to a hospital emergency department.
- Ask about the appearance of the sputum:
  - Frothy pink sputum suggests congestive heart failure or mitral stenosis.
  - Purulent sputum with fevers and chills suggests pneumonia.
  - Chronic sputum with streaks of blood suggests bronchitis.
  - Chronic large-volume purulent sputum punctuated by episodes of frank blood suggests bronchiectasis.
- The presence of chest pain may accompany pulmonary embolism, lung cancer involving the parietal pleura, and pneumonia.
- Determine the smoking history and obtain an occupational history, specifically addressing asbestos exposure.

Physical Examination
- Fever suggests an infectious cause.
- Examine the nasopharynx carefully to rule out an upper-airway source of bleeding.
- Halitosis may accompany lung abscess.
- Auscultate the chest for signs of consolidation (pneumonia), a pleural rub (pulmonary infarction, pneumonia), or a localized wheeze (bronchial obstruction by a neoplasm).
- Synovitis and rash may suggest vasculitis.
- Telangiectasia on face, lips, tongue, and fingers may indicate hereditary hemorrhagic telangiectasia and coexistent pulmonary.

Diagnostic Testing

Laboratory Evaluation
- Obtain a complete blood cell count (including platelets), prothrombin time, and partial thromboplastin time.
- Examine the urine for microscopic hematuria and red-cell casts that may suggest a vasculitic pulmonary-renal syndrome and obtain a serum creatinine.
- Send sputum for Gram stain, acid-fast stain, culture, and cytologic examination.
- In cases in which pulmonary vasculitis is a consideration, obtain antinuclear antibodies and antineutrophil cytoplasmic antibodies.

Imaging
- The chest radiograph can localize infiltrate or mass. Volume loss or atelectasis suggests bronchial obstruction. Pulmonary cavitation may occur with lung abscess, tuberculosis, or cavitary cancer.
- High-resolution CT with contrast is the best method for diagnosis of bronchiectasis. It is also excellent for the diagnosis of aspergilloma and may detect a broncholith or arteriovenous malformation.

Bronchoscopy
- Fiberoptic bronchoscopy should be performed in all patients with an abnormal CXR and less than massive hemoptysis. The diagnostic sensitivity varies from study to study depending on the population evaluated but at best is localizing or diagnostic in approximately half.[5,6]
- Identification of the bleeding site is three times as likely if bronchoscopy is done within 48 hours.[7]

Treatment

- The treatment of small-volume hemoptysis is directed at the underlying disease process.
- Hemoptysis that is associated with chronic bronchitis and bronchiectasis should be treated with antibiotics and antitussives.
- Massive hemoptysis can be lethal and generally demands aggressive evaluation and treatment.[8]
- The treatment of other diagnoses producing hemoptysis is beyond the scope of this chapter.

NONCARDIAC CHEST PAIN

General Principles

- Noncardiac chest pain is that due to causes other than heart disease. Often referred to as atypical chest pain, it is generally used to include all chest pain that is not caused by coronary disease. Noncardiac chest discomfort is quite common in ambulatory practice. Its greatest importance lies in the concern it causes to patient and physician alike that significant heart disease underlies the symptom.

Etiology

- This discussion assumes that the presence of coronary disease has been evaluated and ruled out. The remaining common causes involve the chest wall, pleura, and esophagus. Diseases of the gallbladder, pancreas, and large and small bowel and psychiatric disorders account for a majority of the remainder. Esophageal pain can easily be confused with coronary ischemia and is most often due to reflux or spasm. Gallbladder pain may radiate to the chest.

Chest Wall Disorders
- Musculoskeletal pain is more common than neurogenic pain.
- Costochondral and chondrosternal pain is frequently the result of exercise, injury, or inflammation of obscure cause.
- Rib fracture may occur from direct trauma.
- Intercostal or pectoral muscle strain may occur from exercise.
- Nerve pain may be a result of pre-eruption herpes zoster or postviral or idiopathic neuritis.

Pleural Disorders
- Viral pleuritis may follow coxsackie B infection.
- Pneumonia is often accompanied by pleural inflammation and sometimes pain.
- Systemic lupus erythematosus is often complicated by pleural involvement producing pain.
- Pulmonary infarction occurs in a minority of cases of pulmonary embolism and is often accompanied by pain.

Diagnosis

Clinical Presentation

History
- If one is notified of acute severe pain by phone, refer the patient to an emergency department for initial evaluation of coronary artery disease, aortic dissection, and pulmonary embolism, any of which may be rapidly fatal; office evaluation is not appropriate.
- **Musculoskeletal** pain is of widely varying duration, from a few seconds to days. The patient may notice that it hurts to touch.
- **Neurologic** pain is less likely to be increased by thoracic movement, but neck, arm, and shoulder movement may worsen nerve root irritation or thoracic outlet compression.
- **Pleuritic** pain is typically sharp and aggravated by inspiration and cough, but less so by movement. An exception is the pleural pain component that may accompany pericarditis.
- **Esophageal** pain is classically improved or relieved with antacids or H_2 blockers, and the duration is typically longer than that caused by angina. However, it may be dull or heavy rather than burning and may radiate to the neck or arm.
- **Gallbladder pain** is usually of acute onset, associated with nausea and vomiting, and felt in the right upper quadrant or epigastrium. It may improve with nitroglycerin.
- **Pancreatitis** usually presents with severe epigastric pain with radiation to the back, nausea, and vomiting.

Physical Examination
- Most patients who present to the office with noncardiac chest pain look well.
- Tachycardia may accompany any of the acute illnesses and is characteristic of pulmonary embolism and infarction.
- Palpate the chest wall for tenderness; although characteristic of musculoskeletal pain, it may also be present in empyema, pleurodynia, and rarely pulmonary infarction.

- Percuss and auscultate for dullness or hyperresonance; the former may herald pleural effusion or consolidation, the latter pneumothorax.
- Palpate the abdomen for right upper quadrant tenderness and a Murphy's sign.
- Inspect the skin for the eruption of herpes zoster.
- Examine the cervical and thoracic spine for any signs of tenderness and determine if pain is worsened by cervical spine motion or vertical compression.

Diagnostic Testing

- Although patients may need no further evaluation given their presentation, obtaining a normal electrocardiogram (ECG) may be worth its cost in providing the patient with reassurance.
- If chest wall tenderness follows trauma or is accompanied by systemic symptoms, rib films may show evidence of fracture or malignancy.
- Pain that is radicular and unremitting may warrant magnetic resonance imaging (MRI) of the cervical or thoracic spine.
- If the symptoms suggest pleuropulmonary infection, obtain a CXR.
- Nonpleuritic pain without an obvious origin should prompt evaluation for a gastrointestinal source.

Treatment

- Treatment is directed at the specific diagnosis that is responsible for the chest pain.
- Treat musculoskeletal pain with nonsteroidal anti-inflammatory medication, which may also be helpful for nonspecific neuritis.

PULMONARY FUNCTION TESTS

General Principles

- Further evaluation of the above symptoms and signs is aided by objective assessment of pulmonary function.
- Pulmonary function tests (PFTs) neither provide a specific diagnosis nor determine "disability." They simply quantitatively measure a degree of impairment of both ventilation and respiration.
- In general, these measurements are performed at rest but can also be performed under the stress of exercise often uncovering more subtle impairment.
- Also, in the pulmonary function laboratory, one can assess ventilatory muscle function and determine the potential therapeutic effect of aerosolized bronchodilator medication and supplemental oxygen.
- The various PFTs available may be categorized as follows (Table 3):
  - Spirometry—forced vital capacity (FVC), forced expiratory volume in 1 second (FEV_1), the ratio of FEV_1 to FVC, and peak expiratory flow (PEF).
  - Lung volumes—total lung capacity (TLC), residual volume (RV), functional residual capacity (FRC), and expiratory reserve volume (ERV).
  - Diffusing capacity of the lung for carbon monoxide (DLCO).
  - Arterial blood gas analysis (ABG).
  - Six-minute walk/oxygen assessment.
  - Cardiopulmonary exercise study.
  - Airway challenge testing (methacholine challenge).

TABLE 3	Pulmonary Function Tests			
Test	**Graphic Representation**	**Numerical Data**	**Indication**
Spirometry	• Flow/volume loop • Volume versus time plot	• FEV_1 • FEV • FEV_1/FVC	• Screen for impairment • Establish baseline prior to nonpulmonary intervention that may change pulmonary function (chemotherapy, amiodarone, inhaled insulin) • Follow the course of pulmonary disease with or without therapeutic intervention • Preoperative assessment
Lung volumes	• Pressure/volume • Flow/pressure	• TLC • RV • FRC • ERV	• Confirm restrictive abnormality • Determine air trapping and/or hypoventilation • Measure early effect of obesity
Diffusing capacity		• DLCO • DLCO corrected • DLCO/V_A	• Noninvasive assessment of gas exchange
Arterial blood gas analysis		• PaO_2 • $PaCO_2$ • pH • $\Delta PA\text{-}aO_2$	• Assessment of adequacy of arterial oxygenation • Assessment of alveolar ventilation • Assessment of acid-base status • Assessment of O_2 gas exchange efficiency
Co-oximetry		• COHb • SaO_2	• Assessment of exposure to products of combustion (cigarette smoking) • Direct measurement of oxygen saturation that considers the level of COHb and methemoglobin

Test	Measurements	Purpose/Indications
O_2 assessment/6-minute walk	• SpO_2 during exercise • Blood pressure during exercise • FEV_1 before and after exercise • Effect of supplemental oxygen and determination of quantity required to maintain adequate oxygenation • Distance walked in 6 minutes	• Quantified need for supplemental oxygen • Determine change of FEV_1 associated with exercise • Quantify distance walked in 6 minutes
CPXT	• ECG • Heart rate • Oxygen consumption (VO_2 max) • Carbon dioxide production (VCO_2) • VE	• Determination of what physiologic impairment(s) is associated with exercise intolerance • Aid in differentiation of the role of cardiac, ventilatory, and respiratory factors causing work limitation
Methacholine challenge test	• Serial FEV_1 after increasing methacholine concentrations	• PC_{20} = identifying the concentration of methacholine required to reduce FEV_1 by 20% • Need to objectify the presence or absence of bronchial reactivity

COHb, carboxyhemoglobin; CPXT, cardiopulmonary exercise test; DLCO, diffusing capacity of the lung for carbon monoxide; ERV, expiratory reserve volume; FEV_1, forced expiratory volume in 1 second; FRC, functional residual capacity; FVC, forced vital capacity; $PaCO_2$, arterial partial pressure of carbon dioxide; PaO_2, arterial partial pressure of oxygen; $\Delta PA\text{-}aO_2$, alveolar-arterial oxygen gradient; RV, residual volume; SaO_2, arterial oxygen saturation; SpO_2, oximetric arterial oxygen saturation; TLC, total lung capacity; V_A, alveolar volume; VCO_2, carbon dioxide production; VE, minute ventilation; VO_2, oxygen consumption.

Interpretation

Many pulmonary function studies are effort dependent; therefore, the first step of PFT interpretation is to assess the validity of the measured values. Specifically, one asks, did the technician/patient interaction result in maximum patient effort? The general definition of validity is that the two best attempts are within 5% of each other. When this is not the case, all may not be lost because the best test still represents a minimum level of the patient's function, albeit probably less than the true maximum value. Table 4 discusses the interpretation of basic PFTs.

Predicted Values

Predicted values are based on age, gender, height, and race. Normal range is generally considered to be 80% to 120% of the mean predicted value. Measured values are compared with the predicted range aiding the interpretive process.

Ordering Appropriate Tests

It is neither medically appropriate nor legally acceptable to just order "pulmonary function tests." Specific test designation is required. To do so most successfully, one must clearly keep in mind the clinical question stimulating an order for pulmonary function studies. Spirometry alone may be appropriate to screen for impairment of function but insufficient for a patient with advance disease whose care may require information regarding the severity of the obstructive abnormality, the acute affect of bronchodilator administration, the presence or absence of air trapping, and the need for supplemental oxygen. When determining whether cardiac dysfunction is contributing to exercise intolerance, a cardiopulmonary exercise test (CPXT) may help. In contrast, if one is monitoring for a potential drug side effect causing impairment of gas exchange, rest and exercise ABG analysis alone may provide all the needed information.

DLCO
- DLCO, on the other hand, may be less helpful, for example, in the person administered amiodarone.
- If a baseline value is determined when the dysrhythmia is still present and/or congestive heart failure is incompletely resolved, the DLCO may be elevated because of mild pulmonary hypertension resulting in the perfusion of previously unperfused lung apices.
- Similarly, when the dysrhythmia is controlled and the heart failure resolved, the DL will fall. Interpretation of whether the fall of DLCO is secondary to improvement of the disease by the treatment drug or is a side effect of that agent may be impossible.
- The DLCO is influenced by many factors as outlined in Table 5.

Contingency Ordering

The collection of meaningful information may become more efficient if one anticipates potential abnormalities to be determined on PFTs and request additional tests should such abnormalities be identified. For example:
- If FEV_1 >80% predicted, perform additional spirometry after the administration of aerosolized bronchodilator.

TABLE 4 Pulmonary Function Test Interpretation

Type of Physiologic Abnormality	Criteria	Qualitative Interpretation
Obstructive ventilatory defect	Decreased FEV_1/FEV	Decreased FEV_1/FEV **with** normal FEV_1 = **minimal** obstructive ventilatory defect
	Decreased FEV_1	FEV_1 70%–79% = **mild** obstructive ventilatory defect FEV_1 60%–69% = **moderate** obstructive ventilatory defect FEV_1 50%–59% = **moderately severe** ventilatory defect FEV_1 35%–49% = **severe** ventilatory defect ≤34% = **very severe** ventilatory defect
	Increased airways resistance (Raw)	
	Decreased conductance (Gaw)	
Bronchial reactivity	Increased FEV_1 after administration of aerosolized bronchodilator	>12% and 200 mL increase from baseline
	Methacholine challenge test	>20% FEV_1 fall at a concentration of methacholine ≤8 mg/mL
Restrictive ventilatory defect	Decreased total TLC (plethysmography)	TLC 65%–79% = **mild** restrictive ventilatory defect TLC 50%–64% = **moderate** restrictive ventilatory defect TLC ≤ 49% = **severe** restrictive ventilatory defect FVC ≤ 79% suggests a restrictive abnormality; valid decreased TLC is required for confirmation
	Decreased TLC (dilution)	Dilution technique for measurement of TLC is less specific than plethysmography because of underestimation in the face of obstruction
Combined obstructive venti-latory defect and restrictive ventilatory defect	Decreased FEV_1 and FEV_1/FEV and TLC	Discount severity of obstructive ventilatory defect in face of restrictive ventilatory defect Restrictive ventilatory defect same criteria as above

(continued)

237

TABLE 4 Pulmonary Function Test Interpretation *(Continued)*

Type of Physiologic Abnormality	Criteria	Qualitative Interpretation
Impairment of gas exchange at rest	Increased $\Delta PA\text{-}aO_2$	Identify upper limits of normal of $\Delta PA\text{-}aO_2$ as standardized for age $\Delta PA\text{-}aO_2 \leq 10$ mm Hg above the age-adjusted upper limit = **mild** impairment of gas exchange $\Delta PA\text{-}aO_2$ 11–20 mm Hg above the age-adjusted upper limit = **moderate** $\Delta PA\text{-}aO_2 > 20$ mm Hg above the age-adjusted upper limit = **severe** impairment of gas exchange
Impairment of gas exchange during exercise	Increased $\Delta PA\text{-}aO_2$	Normal response of $\Delta PA\text{-}aO_2$ to exercise is a lowering of $\Delta PA\text{-}aO_2$ from resting baseline to during (not after) exercise If $\Delta PA\text{-}aO_2$ increases during exercise, functional obliteration of pulmonary capillary bed is strongly suspected
O_2 assessment	SpO_2	Possible impairment of gas exchange exists when SpO_2 falls $\geq 3\%$ during exercise When SpO_2 is $\leq 88\%$, supplemental oxygen is usually required
Assessment for physiologic consequence of right-to-left shunt	Measurement of PaO_2 after breathing 100% O_2 in a closed system for 20 minutes or longer	A right-to-left shunt is likely if PaO_2 does not reach ≥ 600 mm Hg following 100% O_2 breathing
Ventilatory muscle function	Supine spirometry	Diaphragmatic dysfunction is suggested by >20% fall of FEV_1 and FVC assuming the supine position as compared to similar measurements in the sitting or standing position
	MIP MEP MVV	Global muscle dysfunction is suggested by proportionately low MVV (MVV = $FEV_1 \times 40$) and decreased MIP and MEP

FEV_1, forced expiratory volume in 1 second; FVC, forced vital capacity; MEP, maximum expiratory pressure; MIP, maximum inspiratory pressure; MVV, maximum voluntary ventilation; PaO_2, arterial partial pressure of oxygen; $\Delta PA\text{-}aO_2$, alveolar-arterial oxygen gradient; SpO_2, oximetric arterial oxygen saturation; TLC, total lung capacity.

TABLE 5	Factors Influencing DLCO

Increases DLCO	Decreases DLCO
Polycythemia (increased hemoglobin)	Anemia
CHF (increased blood flow to apices)	Interstitial pulmonary process
Obesity	Decreased gas exchanging surface (emphysema)
Quiescent asthma	Increased volume of lungs with areas of low V/Q
Pulmonary hypertension	Increased carboxyhemoglobin
	Decreased lung volume

CHF, congestive heart failure; DLCO, diffusing capacity of the lung for carbon monoxide; V/Q, ventilation/perfusion ratio.

- If SpO_2 <94%, perform an ABG while patient is breathing room air at rest.
- If FEV_1 <80%, perform TLC measurement.
- If SpO_2 <90% at rest, perform oxygen assessment/6-minute walk test.

Radiographic Studies

A detailed discussion of radiographic studies is not within the scope of this work. Table 6 should serve as a guideline for the usefulness of available studies.

TABLE 6	Radiographic Studies for Pulmonary Complaints	

Study	Radiation Dose	Use/Indication
Standard PA and lateral CXR	Trivial	Screening, following longitudinal changes
CT of chest without contrast	Minimum but significant	Excellent for detailing parenchymal processes
CT of chest with contrast	Minimum but significant	Excellent for detailing parenchymal process and its relation to vascular structures
CT of chest with pulmonary embolism protocol	Small but significant	Most sensitive test for identifying pulmonary embolism
High-resolution CT of chest	Small but significant	Best for defining interstitial process
MRI chest	None	Assessment of foci of activity: inflammation and malignancy
Ventilation/ perfusion scan	Small but significant	Less specific and sensitive alternative to PE protocol CT to identify pulmonary embolism

CT, computed tomography; CXR, chest radiography; PE, pulmonary embolism.

REFERENCES

1. Spencer CM, Faulds D, Peters DH. Cetirizine. A reappraisal of its pharmacological properties and therapeutic use in selected allergic disorders. *Drugs* 1993;46:1055–1080.
2. Irwin RS, Baumann MH, Bolser DC, et al. Diagnosis and management of cough executive summary: ACCP evidence-based clinical practice guidelines. *Chest* 2006;129:1S–23S.
3. Braman SS. Postinfectious cough: ACCP evidence-based clinical practice guideline. *Chest* 2006;129:138S–146S.
4. Dicpinigaitis PV. Angiotensin-converting enzyme inhibitor-induced cough: ACCP evidence-based clinical practice guidelines. *Chest* 2006;129:169S–173S.
5. O'Neil KM, Lazarus AA. Hemoptysis. Indications for bronchoscopy. *Arch Intern Med* 1991;151:171–174.
6. McGuinness G, Beacher JR, Harkin TJ, et al. Hemoptysis: prospective high-resolution CT/bronchoscopic correlation. *Chest* 1994;105:1155–1162.
7. McCalley SW. Clinical efficacy of early and delayed fiberoptic bronchoscopy in patients with hemoptysis. *Am Rev Respir Dis* 1982;125:269–270.
8. Jean-Baptiste E. Clinical assessment and management of massive hemoptysis. *Crit Care Med* 2001;28:1642–1647.

12 Chronic Obstructive Pulmonary Disease and Asthma

Warren Isakow

CHRONIC OBSTRUCTIVE PULMONARY DISEASE

General Principles

Definition

Chronic obstructive pulmonary disease (COPD) is defined by the American Thoracic Society (ATS) as "a preventable and treatable disease state characterized by airflow limitation that is not fully reversible. The airflow limitation is usually progressive and is associated with an abnormal inflammatory response of the lungs to noxious particles or gases, primarily caused by cigarette smoking. Although COPD affects the lungs, it also produces significant systemic consequences."[1]

Classification

COPD is a complex disease in which patients may have components of chronic bronchitis, emphysema, and even asthma:

- **Chronic bronchitis** is defined clinically as chronic cough, productive of at least two tablespoons of sputum, for 3 months in each of 2 successive years, in a patient in whom other causes of chronic productive cough have been excluded.
- **Emphysema** is a pathological definition referring to permanent enlargement of the airspaces distal to the terminal bronchioles, accompanied by destruction of their walls and without obvious fibrosis.
- **Asthma** differs from COPD in that the airflow limitation is reversible, although some patients with asthma do develop poorly reversible airflow limitation. However, asthma is a different disease entity with regard to pathogenesis and therapeutic response and will be addressed separately.

Epidemiology and Risk Factors

- COPD is currently the fourth leading cause of morbidity and mortality in the United States and is projected to be the third leading cause by 2020.[2]
- Approximately 4% to 6% of adult white males and 1% to 3% of adult white females have COPD, and it is estimated that 20 million adults in the United States have COPD, the majority of whom have chronic bronchitis.
- Risk factors for COPD are presented in Table 1.

TABLE 1	Risk Factors for Chronic Obstructive Pulmonary Disease (COPD)
Major COPD Risk Factors	**Comments**
Cigarette smoking: active and passive	15%–20% of smokers develop airflow obstruction
	Smoking results in accelerated age-related lung decline of 80–100 mL/year compared to 20–30 mL/year in nonsmokers
α_1-Antitrypsin deficiency	Significant lung disease usually develops only in smokers
	Panacinar emphysema
	Bronchiectasis
	Liver manifestations: cirrhosis
	Skin manifestations: panniculitis
Air pollution	Could be responsible for differences in urban and rural death rates
	Particulates more important than photochemical pollutants
Occupational exposures	Dust exposure causes mucus hypersecretion
	Gold miners, farmers, grain handlers, cement workers, cotton workers

Diagnosis

Clinical Presentation

- COPD is an insidious disease, and dyspnea usually does not develop until the FEV_1 (forced expiratory volume in 1 second) is ≤60% of predicted. The etiology of the dyspnea is multifactorial and includes the following:
  - Expiratory airflow obstruction with air trapping.[3]
  - Hyperinflation that produces abnormalities in chest wall and respiratory muscle function.[4]
  - Mucus hypersecretion.
  - Bronchoconstriction.
  - Maldistribution of ventilation causes frequency dependence and abnormalities in gas exchange.
  - Deconditioning.
  - Nutritional abnormalities and weight loss.

History

- Important symptoms of COPD include the following:
  - Dyspnea.
  - Chronic cough.
  - Sputum production.
  - Chest tightness.
  - Wheezing (occasionally).
  - History of "exacerbations" of the patient's symptoms, requiring antibiotic therapy or even hospitalization.

TABLE 2	Grading the Severity of COPD	
Severity of COPD	Postbronchodilator FEV_1/FVC Ratio	FEV_1 (% Predicted)
Mild	<0.7	>80
Moderate	<0.7	50–80
Severe	<0.7	30–50
Very severe	<0.7	<30

COPD, chronic obstructive pulmonary disease; FEV_1, forced expiratory volume in 1 second; FVC, forced vital capacity.
Modified from Rabe KF, Hurd S, Anzueto A, et al. Global strategy for the diagnosis, management, and prevention of chronic obstructive pulmonary disease: GOLD executive summary. *Am J Respir Crit Care Med* 2007;176:532–555.

- Attention should also be paid to ominous symptoms of weight loss, recurrent hemoptysis, or hoarseness. These symptoms should precipitate a thorough search for concurrent malignancy.

Physical Examination
- Signs on physical examination are often present only with more advanced disease and include the following:
  - Wheezing.
  - Barrel-shaped chest (hyperinflation).
  - Pursed lip breathing.
  - Accessory muscle use.
  - Hoover's sign (inward movement of the lower costal margin with inspiration).
  - Peripheral edema from cor pulmonale.
- Clubbing is not a physical exam finding that occurs in COPD and, if present, a search for another cause is indicated.

Pulmonary Function Tests
- The crucial step in the diagnosis of obstructive lung disease is pulmonary function testing (PFT), including spirometry.
- Spirometry is the only reliable means for diagnosing COPD and importantly also classifies the severity of the disease.[1]
- The sine qua non for making the diagnosis of obstructive lung disease is a reduced ratio of the FEV_1 to the forced vital capacity (FVC).
- The grading of COPD severity by PFTs is presented in Table 2.
- A comprehensive pulmonary assessment often includes other testing of pulmonary function (Table 3). These become particularly important as disease severity increases, especially the oxygen evaluation.

The BODE Index
- The BODE index[5] is a relatively new multidimensional grading system to provide a better composite picture of disease severity and includes the following parameters:
  - Body mass index (BMI).
  - FEV_1.
  - Dyspnea, graded by the Medical Research Council dyspnea scale (Table 4).
  - Exercise tolerance (6-minute walk distance).

TABLE 3	Pulmonary Function Testing in COPD
Test	**Comments**
Spirometry both pre- and postbronchodilator	Useful to make the diagnosis Able to grade disease severity Useful to follow patients serially A significant response to bronchodilator (FEV_1 increase by >12% and 200 mL) is more suggestive of reactive airway disease
Lung volumes by body plethysmography, helium dilution, or nitrogen washout	Useful to detect air trapping (elevated residual volume) and hyperinflation (elevated total lung capacity)
DLCO	Tends to be very low in emphysema, less severely decreased with chronic bronchitis
Arterial blood gases	Should be performed with moderate or severe impairment to assess for resting hypoxemia and detect hypercapnia
Oxygen evaluation (6-minute walk test)	Useful to detect oxyhemoglobin desaturation with exercise Provides an assessment of resting and exertional oxygen needs Quantifies the distance the patient can walk

COPD, chronic obstructive pulmonary disease; FEV_1, forced expiratory volume in 1 second; DLCO, diffusing capacity of the lung for carbon monoxide.

- The Medical Research Council index is better at predicting the risk of death, from any cause, compared with the FEV_1 alone (Table 4).
- The highest possible score is 10 points, with lower scores indicating a lower risk of death (Table 5).

Laboratory Studies

- α_1-Antitrypsin levels should be checked in patients with the following problems[6]:
  - Premature onset of COPD or severe impairment before the age of 50.

TABLE 4	The Medical Research Council (MRC) Dyspnea Scale
Grade	**Degree of Breathlessness Related to Activity**
1	Not troubled by breathlessness except on strenuous exercise
2	Short of breath when hurrying or walking up a slight hill
3	Walks slower than contemporaries on level ground because of breathlessness, or has to stop for breath when walking at own pace
4	Stops for breath after walking about 100 m or after a few minutes on level ground
5	Too breathless to leave the house, or breathless when dressing or undressing

Adapted from Fletcher CM, Elmes PC, Fairbairn MB, et al. The significance of respiratory symptoms and the diagnosis of chronic bronchitis in a working population. *BMJ* 1959;2:257–266.

TABLE 5	The BODE Index			
	Point on BODE Index			
Variable	**0**	**1**	**2**	**3**
FEV$_1$ (% predicted)	≥65	50–64	36–49	≤35
6-minute walk distance (m)	≥350	250–349	150–249	≤149
MRC dyspnea scale	0–1	2	3	4
BMI	>21	≤21		

BMI, body mass index; FEV$_1$, forced expiratory volume in 1 second; MRC, Medical Research Council.
Adapted from Celli BR, Cote CG, Marin JM, et al. The body-mass index, airflow obstruction, dyspnea, and exercise capacity index in chronic obstructive pulmonary disease. *N Engl J Med* 2004;350:1005–1012.

- Predominance of basilar emphysema.
- A family history of α$_1$-antitrypsin deficiency or early onset emphysema.
- Chronic bronchitis with airflow obstruction in a patient who never smoked.
- Unexplained bronchiectasis or cirrhosis.
- Genetic phenotyping should be performed if the α$_1$-antitrypsin level is low.
- Imaging studies, such as chest radiographs (CXR), are also helpful in evaluating hyperinflation and in excluding concomitant disease (e.g., lung cancer). Routine chest computed tomography (CT) scanning is not indicated in the care of patients with COPD.

Treatment

General Management
- An overview of the general management of COPD is given in Figure 1.[7,8]
- Each component of this management plan will be discussed in detail below.

Smoking Cessation
- The beneficial effect of smoking cessation is well demonstrated by the Lung Health Study.[9] Subjects who continued to smoke experienced higher yearly declines in lung function than did sustained quitters.
- Therefore, smoking cessation has the potential to preserve lung function, reduce symptoms, and decrease mortality. Nicotine addiction causes a state of dependence; effective smoking cessation measures require a multidisciplinary approach.[10]

Patient Education
- It is important that patients understand the nature, chronicity, treatment options, and prognosis of COPD. Educational materials are available from the American Lung Association (http://www.ALA.org).

Health Maintenance
- Yearly influenza vaccination is recommended for all patients, as well as a pneumococcal vaccine every 5 years. Yearly CXR should be performed.

Medications
Short-Acting Bronchodilators
- Metered-dose inhalers (MDIs) that contain a β$_2$-agonist, an anticholinergic agent, or both, can result in improvement of airflow obstruction and hyperinflation, less dyspnea,

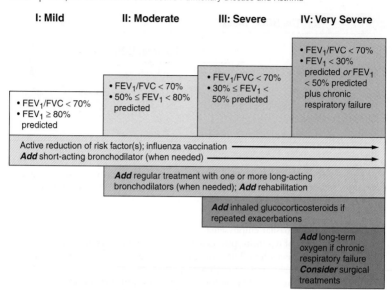

| I: Mild | II: Moderate | III: Severe | IV: Very Severe |

• FEV₁/FVC < 70%
• FEV₁ ≥ 80% predicted

• FEV₁/FVC < 70%
• 50% ≤ FEV₁ < 80% predicted

• FEV₁/FVC < 70%
• 30% ≤ FEV₁ < 50% predicted

• FEV₁/FVC < 70%
• FEV₁ < 30% predicted *or* FEV₁ < 50% predicted plus chronic respiratory failure

Active reduction of risk factor(s); influenza vaccination
Add short-acting bronchodilator (when needed)

Add regular treatment with one or more long-acting bronchodilators (when needed); *Add* rehabilitation

Add inhaled glucocorticosteroids if repeated exacerbations

Add long-term oxygen if chronic respiratory failure
Consider surgical treatments

Figure 1. **Therapy at each stage of COPD, the GOLD guidelines.** COPD, chronic obstructive pulmonary disease; FEV₁, forced expiratory volume in 1 second; FVC, forced vital capacity. (Modified from Rabe KF, Hurd S, Anzueto A, et al. Global strategy for the diagnosis, management, and prevention of chronic obstructive pulmonary disease: GOLD executive summary. *Am J Respir Crit Care Med* 2007;176:532–555, with permission.)

and potentially fewer exacerbations in patients, regardless of reversibility on bronchodilator testing. Commonly used inhalers for COPD are detailed in Table 6.

- These agents are the mainstay of therapy in COPD, and patients should use two to four puffs every 4 to 6 hours.[11]
- Combination therapy with both agents is appropriate in patients with more severe disease.[12]
- Proper MDI technique should be verified at outpatient visits and if patients have difficulty, a spacer device may prove beneficial. Nebulized agents may also be used in patients with poor technique.

Long-Acting Bronchodilators
- Current societal guidelines endorse the regular use of long-acting agents to improve symptoms and quality of life and reduce exacerbations in COPD.[1] Numerous formulations are available (Table 6).
- The long-acting β₂-agonists salmeterol, formoterol, and arformoterol produce bronchodilation for up to 12 hours, potentially reducing nocturnal symptoms. There is good randomized controlled trial data that salmeterol is effective in reducing the frequency of exacerbations.[13]
- Tiotropium is a long-acting anticholinergic agent which can improve airflow over a 24-hour period. Clinical studies show that this agent also relieves dyspnea, reduces exacerbation frequency, and improves quality of life.[14]
  - There is preliminary data that this agent may attenuate the decline of lung function with time.

TABLE 6 Commonly Used Inhalers in COPD

Drug Name	Trade Names	Formulation	Adult Dose	Comments
Albuterol	Proventil Ventolin Proventil-HFA Ventolin-HFA Accuneb ProAir HFA	MDI: 90 mcg/spray NEB: 2.5 mg/3 mL	2 puffs INH q4–6 hour prn 2.5 mg NEB q4–6 hour prn	Short-acting β_2-agonist
Levalbuterol	Xopenex Xopenex-HFA	HFA: 45 mcg/puff NEB: 0.31, 0.63, or 1.25 mg/3 mL	1–2 puffs INH q4–6 hour prn 0.63 mg NEB q6–8 hour prn	Short-acting β_2-agonist
Ipratropium bromide	Atrovent Atrovent HFA	MDI: 17 mcg/spray	2 puffs INH q4–6 hour prn	Short-acting anticholinergic
Albuterol/ipratropium bromide	Combivent	MDI: 120/21 mcg/spray	1–2 puffs INH q6 hour	Combination short-acting β_2-agonist and short- acting anticholinergic
Salmeterol	Serevent	DPI: 50 mcg/blister	1 INH q12 hour	Long-acting β_2-agonist
Formoterol	Foradil	DPI: 12 mcg/INH	1 INH q12 hour	Long-acting β_2-agonist
Arformoterol tartrate	Brovana	NEB: 15 mcg/2 mL	1 NEB q12 hour	Long-acting β_2-agonist
Tiotropium	Spiriva	DPI: 18 mcg	1 INH q24 hour	Long-acting anticholinergic
Fluticasone propionate/ salmeterol	Advair	DPI: 100 mcg/50 mcg 250 mcg/50 mcg 500 mcg/50 mcg	1 INH q12 hour	Combination of an inhaled corticosteroid and a long-acting β_2-agonist

COPD, chronic obstructive pulmonary disease; DPI, dry powder inhaler; HFA, hydrofluoroalkane; INH, inhalation; MDI, metered-dose inhaler;
NEB, nebulizer solution or nebulized.

- Short-acting anticholinergic agents should not be used in conjunction with this agent.
- Many patients with severe COPD are managed with combinations of short-acting bronchodilators (SABDs) and long-acting bronchodilators (LABDs) to relieve dyspnea.

Methylxanthines
- Theophylline use has declined recently in view of its potential toxicity; however, this long-acting oral bronchodilator can be used as add-on therapy in patients who are still dyspneic despite maximal inhaled bronchodilator use.[15]
- Theophylline has multiple drug interactions, and drug levels need to be monitored routinely and whenever potentially interacting medications are added to a patient's regimen. Therapeutic range is between 6 and 12 mg/L.
- Side effects include anxiety, tremor, nausea, and vomiting.
- Toxicity can be manifest by tachyarrhythmias and seizures.

Corticosteroids
- Inhaled corticosteroids are used in COPD to attenuate the inflammatory component of the disease (Table 6). The largest randomized controlled trial recently published did not confirm a mortality benefit over 3 years with these agents.[13]
- However, there is clinical data that inhaled corticosteroids are effective at reducing exacerbation frequency and improving quality of life.
- The Global Initiative for Chronic Obstructive Lung Disease (GOLD) guidelines support using inhaled corticosteroids in patients with severe disease and frequent exacerbations.[7,8] The ATS/European Respiratory Society (ERS) guidelines support their use in patients with persistent symptoms despite maximal bronchodilation.[1]
- Higher pneumonia rates were described in the "TORCH trial" and this needs further investigation.[13] Patients should be educated to wash their mouths out after using inhaled steroids to reduce thrush and hoarseness.
- A brief trial of oral steroids may benefit as many as 30% of patients with COPD with wheezing, frequent exacerbations, or severe impairment. An objective improvement in FEV_1 should be evident to justify maintenance therapy with an oral steroid. Doses in the range of 40 mg/day for 1 to 2 weeks are used and then tapered off as soon as possible.
- Response to an oral steroid increases the likelihood of response to an inhaled corticosteroid.
- Chronic use of oral steroids is discouraged because of the systemic side effects including osteoporosis, hyperglycemia, risk of peptic ulcer disease, immunosuppression, and cataracts.

Pulmonary Rehabilitation
- Dyspnea significantly impairs quality of life in COPD; pulmonary rehabilitation comprises a multidimensional continuum of services aimed at improving functional status both physically and psychologically. Rehabilitation programs can reduce exacerbation frequencies and significantly improve quality of life and ability to perform activities of daily living (ADLs).[16]
- Any patient with moderate COPD should be considered for referral to a comprehensive pulmonary rehabilitation program, particularly those with persistent dyspnea on maximal pharmacologic therapy, frequent exacerbations and hospital admissions, and impaired functional status and quality of life.
- These programs consist of the following:
  - Graded exercise programs to enhance functionality.

- These typically occur three times a week with a goal of 30 minutes of continuous aerobic activity. Patients are exercised on tracks, treadmills, and bicycles and also perform arm ergometry and light weight lifting to promote upper body strength.
  - Attention is also paid to increasing flexibility. Patients are monitored with pulse oximetry and oxygen is titrated during the exercise program. The workload is gradually increased until patients reach 80% of their maximum heart rate or breathlessness.
- Nutrition and psychosocial support and counseling.
- Oxygen assessments and potentially noninvasive cardiac stress testing should be performed prior to initiation of a rehabilitation program in patients at risk for significant coronary artery disease.

Oxygen Therapy

- Oxygen therapy has been shown to reduce mortality in hypoxemic patients with COPD and also improve physical and mental function.[17,18]
- Arterial blood gases (ABGs) should be obtained to document whether hypoxemia is present when breathing room air. Pulse oximetry is then useful to perform routine checks after a baseline oxyhemoglobin saturation is obtained.
- The indications for oxygen therapy as derived from the Nocturnal Oxygen Therapy Trial Group (NOTT) are as follows:
  - PaO_2 <55 mm Hg or SpO_2 <88% at rest.
  - PaO_2 <56 to 59 mm Hg or SpO_2 <89% if there is p pulmonale, cor pulmonale, or HCT >55%.
  - With exercise if accompanied by desaturation to levels above.
  - With sleep if accompanied by desaturation to levels above.
- Desaturation is common during sleep in patients with COPD, so formal overnight oximetry with oxygen titration may be helpful. If this is not available, patients are generally told to increase their resting oxygen setting by 1 L during sleep.
- Many patients develop worsening hypoxemia during acute exacerbations of COPD. These supplemental requirements may decrease after treatment of the exacerbation, so a follow-up oxygen evaluation should be performed 1 to 3 months later.
- Prescriptions for oxygen should specify the oxygen dose (L/min) for rest, exercise, and sleep as well as the delivery system.
- There are three main forms of oxygen delivery for patients:
  - **Oxygen concentrators:** These are large devices which are normally placed in the patient's home for home use. Patients need an additional portable mode of delivery which is discussed below.
  - **Compressed gas:** It is a portable form of therapy but can occasionally be difficult to carry or push around because of the size and weight of the gas canisters.
  - **Liquid oxygen:** This is the most expensive but most mobile form of therapy for patients.
- The oxygen is normally delivered to the patient via a continuous-flow, dual-prong nasal cannula.
- Patients with COPD rarely require very high concentrations of oxygen, which necessitate the use of a reservoir system with an oxymizer device.
- Demand pulse systems that deliver oxygen only during inspiration are also available.

Surgical Options

- **Bullectomy** can be performed in patients with dyspnea in whom a bulla or bullae occupy at least 50% of a hemithorax and compress the normal lung.

- **Lung volume reduction surgery** can have excellent spirometric and functional outcomes in highly selected patients with severe emphysema (FEV$_1$ <35%) and apical target areas which consist of poorly functioning and volume-occupying lung which can be surgically resected.[19]
- **Lung transplantation** can be performed in patients who have severe obstruction (FEV$_1$ <25%), hypercapnia, pulmonary hypertension, and marked limitation of ADLs, but who are young without significant comorbidities.[20]

Replacement Therapy

- Augmentation therapy with α_1-antitrypsin is available and is indicated in patients with α_1-antitrypsin deficiency, obstructive lung disease, and who have quit smoking.[21]
- Hepatitis vaccination should be performed prior to starting therapy.
- The efficacy of this therapy has been supported by observational studies. The therapy is expensive and is given intravenously, weekly, biweekly, or monthly.

MANAGEMENT OF ACUTE EXACERBATIONS OF COPD

General Principles

- Acute exacerbations are a common occurrence in patients with COPD and tend to occur more frequently in those patients who continue to smoke.
- These episodes are characterized by a change in the patient's baseline dyspnea, cough and/or sputum production beyond day-to-day variability, and sufficient to warrant a change in management.
- Exacerbations are often precipitated by viral or bacterial respiratory infections as well as air pollution, and account for a significant portion of the costs of managing COPD due to frequent physician visits, hospitalization, and time away from work.[22]

Diagnosis

- Patients who are experiencing exacerbations often have worsening of their hypoxemia and hypercapnia during these episodes; evaluation is indicated to identify patients who may require hospitalization.
- Evaluation should focus on the severity of the dyspnea; the patients' ability to sleep, eat, and care for themselves; and underlying comorbidities.
- Physical exam findings of altered mental status, hemodynamic abnormalities, increased accessory muscle use, and significant comorbidities should prompt hospitalization.
- A CXR should also be performed in these patients.

Treatment

- Management, whether pursued as an outpatient or as an inpatient, consists of maximization of bronchodilator therapy, corticosteroids[23] (oral prednisone at a dose of 40 mg/day for 7 to 10 days), and antibiotics if there is evidence for purulent sputum.
- The antibiotic chosen can be narrow spectrum to cover *Haemophilus influenzae*, *Moraxella* spp., or *Streptococcus pneumoniae* in patients who do not have recent nosocomial risk factors.
- Gram-negative organisms are not unusual in patients with severe COPD, comorbid illnesses, and recurrent exacerbations, so coverage should be broadened in patients with these risk factors.

ASTHMA

General Principles

- Asthma is a chronic inflammatory disorder of the airways in which many cell types play a role, in particular mast cells, eosinophils, and T lymphocytes.
- In susceptible individuals, this inflammation causes recurrent episodes of wheezing, breathlessness, chest tightness, and cough particularly at night and/or in the early morning. These symptoms are usually associated with widespread but variable airflow limitation that is at least partly reversible either spontaneously or with treatment.[24,25]
- The inflammation also causes an associated increase in airway responsiveness to a variety of stimuli.

Diagnosis

Clinical Presentation

History

- The patient's medical history is of critical importance in establishing the probable diagnosis of asthma and also identifying characteristic triggers for exacerbations of the patient's symptoms. Asthma may have its onset in infancy through adulthood, and the symptoms may be intermittent or persistent.[26]
- The history at the initial visit and all subsequent visits should focus on the following features:
  - Presence of cough, which can occasionally be productive of yellow sputum and classically is worse at night or in the early morning.[27]
    - Wheezing.
    - Shortness of breath.
    - A feeling of "chest tightness."
    - Nocturnal awakenings.
    - A history of episodic symptoms.
    - History of allergic/atopic disease.
    - Prior therapeutic response to asthma medications.
    - Triggers of asthma:
      - Exercise.
      - Allergen or environmental exposure (cold air, strong odors, mold, dust, pollen).
      - Gastroesophageal reflux disease.
    - History of missed work/school days.
    - Prior history of hospitalization and intubation.
    - Tobacco abuse.
    - History of aspirin sensitivity.
    - History of sinusitis.

Physical Examination

- Important features to note include the length of the expiratory phase, the presence of wheezing, allergic rhinitis (pale, boggy nasal mucus membranes), and nasal polyps.
- Patients with more severe airflow obstruction may exhibit tachypnea, accessory muscle use, have no wheezing due to poor air movement, and can ultimately develop a pulsus paradoxus.

TABLE 7	Common Mimics of Asthma

Diffuse airway obstruction
- COPD
- α_1-Antitrypsin deficiency
- Bronchiectasis
- Cystic fibrosis
- Bronchiolitis obliterans
- Tracheobronchomalacia

Localized airway obstruction
- Endobronchial tumor
- Carcinoid tumor
- Endobronchial foreign body
- Extrinsic airway compression

Laryngeal obstruction
- Vocal cord dysfunction

Other
- CHF
- Churg-Strauss syndrome
- Pulmonary embolism
- Sarcoidosis
- Allergic bronchopulmonary aspergillosis

CHF, congestive heart failure; COPD, chronic obstructive pulmonary disease.

Differential Diagnosis

- Many of the conditions in Table 7 can be differentiated from asthma by the absence of reversibility with bronchodilators, review of the flow volume loop, and consideration of the temporal course and onset of the symptoms.
- Occasionally, laboratory testing can help identify some of the other mimics of asthma.

Diagnostic Testing

- The diagnosis of asthma is based on history and clinical course, objective PFT, and serial monitoring of lung function and occasionally needs to be confirmed by bronchoprovocation testing.
- An objective measurement of airflow obstruction is therefore essential in the diagnosis and management of asthma.

Spirometry

- Patients with asthma can occasionally have normal pulmonary function and typically will develop episodes of variable airflow obstruction.
- Patients with persistent asthma normally have features of airway obstruction on spirometry, manifested by one or more of the following:
  - A reduced FEV_1:FVC ratio below 70%.
  - Reductions in the FEV_1, the degree depending on asthma severity.
  - Reversibility with bronchodilator testing, defined as an **FEV_1 or FVC increase of >12% and 200 mL from baseline.**

- If spirometry is normal, bronchoprovocation testing with methacholine may identify patients with airway hyperresponsiveness.[28] This test is not specific for asthma; however, a negative test result makes the diagnosis less likely.

Peak Expiratory Flow Rate Monitoring

- Peak expiratory flow rate (PEFR) monitoring is helpful in making the diagnosis of asthma and in outpatient management of the disease.[29]
- The clinician should be aware that this test is very effort and technique dependant. Patients can identify their personal bests and be educated on the appropriate management when their PEFR starts decreasing.
- Significant variability in PEFR occurs in asthmatic individuals, and the absence of this feature may make the diagnosis less likely.

Laboratory Studies

- A **CXR** should be performed in patients with late-onset asthma and difficult to control asthma and at the initial evaluation. This helps differentiate asthma from some of the common conditions which can mimic the disease.
- A **complete blood cell count** (CBC) should be performed at the initial evaluation to detect eosinophilia.
- **Allergy testing** (skin testing and in vitro testing) can occasionally be useful in patients with immunoglobulin E (IgE)-mediated asthma. An absolute **IgE level** should also be checked at the initial evaluation and in patients with difficult to control asthma.
- A limited **sinus CT** is useful in patients with prominent sinus symptoms.

Treatment

Severity Classification and Management of Asthma

- The current NIH/NHLBI guidelines, updated in 2007, are an extremely useful resource for clinicians to guide asthma management[24,25] (refer to Tables 8 and 9).
- **The major goals of asthma therapy are as follows:**
  - Freedom from symptoms (including nocturnal symptoms).
  - No limitation of daily activities including exercise.

TABLE 8	Classification of Asthma Severity				
Asthma Severity	Days with Symptoms	Nights with Symptoms	PEF or FEV$_1$	PEF Variability	Step for Initiating Treatment[a]
Severe	Continual	Frequent	≤60%	>30%	Step 4 or 5
Moderate	Daily	≥5/month	>60% to <80%	>30%	Step 3
Mild	3–6/week	3–4/month	≥80%	20%–30%	Step 2
Intermittent	≤2/week	≤2/month	≥80%	<20%	Step 1

[a]See Table 9.
Modified from National Asthma Education and Prevention Program Expert Panel Report 3 (EPR3): Guidelines for the Diagnosis and Management of Asthma. Full Report 2007. National Heart, Lung, and Blood Institute, 2007. National Institutes of Health publication 08-4051.

TABLE 9	Stepwise Approach for Managing Asthma in Adults
Step 6	Daily medications: • Inhaled steroid (high dose) **AND** • Long-acting inhaled β_2-agonist **AND** • Oral steroid Consider: Omalizumab for patients who have allergies
Step 5	Daily medications: • Inhaled steroid (high dose) **AND** • Long-acting inhaled β_2-agonist Consider: Omalizumab for patients who have allergies
Step 4	Daily medications: • Inhaled steroid (medium dose) **AND** • Long-acting inhaled β_2-agonist Alternatives: Inhaled steroid (medium dose) plus either leukotriene modifier or theophylline
Step 3	Daily medication: • Inhaled steroid (medium dose) **OR** • Inhaled steroid (low dose) **AND** • Long-acting inhaled β_2-agonist Alternatives: Inhaled steroid (low dose) plus either leukotriene modifier or theophylline
Step 2	Daily medication: • Inhaled steroid (low dose) is preferred Alternatives: Nedocromil, cromolyn, leukotriene modifier, or sustained-release theophylline
Step 1	No daily medication needed
All patients	**Quick relief** with a short-acting bronchodilator: inhaled β_2-agonist (2–4 puffs) as needed for symptoms

Modified from National Asthma Education and Prevention Program Expert Panel Report 3 (EPR3): Guidelines for the Diagnosis and Management of Asthma. Full Report 2007. National Heart, Lung, and Blood Institute, 2007. National Institutes of Health publication 08-4051.

- Minimization of acute exacerbations and emergency visits.
- Optimization of lung function.
- Minimal medication side effects and tailoring of medications to individual patient profiles.
- To attain these goals, periodic patient visits are necessary; patient as well as caregiver education is critical to prevent clinical deterioration.
- Visits should be utilized to review symptoms and medication usage, especially short-acting bronchodilators, and to obtain an objective assessment of lung function and educate.

General Approach

- The stepwise approach only provides general guidelines to assist clinical decision making, and clinicians should tailor medications to the needs of individual patients.
- Control of symptoms should be obtained as rapidly as possible. Either start with aggressive therapy (e.g., add a course of oral steroids or a higher dose of inhaled steroids to the therapy that corresponds to the patients' initial step of severity) or start at the step that corresponds to the patients' initial severity and step up treatment, if necessary.
- A course of oral steroids (maximum of 60 mg/day) may be needed at any time and at any step.
- Treatment should be reviewed every 1 to 6 months and therapies gradually withdrawn if possible to the least medication necessary to maintain control.
- Inadequate control is indicated by increased use of short-acting β_2-agonists.
- Patients with exercise-induced bronchospasm should take two to four puffs of an inhaled β_2-agonist 5 to 30 minutes before exercise.
- LABDs should not be used as monotherapy in persistent asthma.[30]
- Leukotriene-modifying agents (montelukast, zafirlukast, and zileuton) can be used as add-on therapy in patients with persistent asthma to improve asthma control and potentially reduce the dose of inhaled corticosteroid.[31]
- Omalizumab, a recombinant humanized monoclonal anti-IgE antibody, has been shown to reduce asthma exacerbations and improve asthma control symptoms in poorly controlled, moderate-to-severe persistent asthma.[32] Potential candidates for omalizumab must have allergy testing to document sensitization to a perennial allergen. The therapy is expensive, and the drug is dosed based on patient weight and IgE levels.
- Medications commonly used for asthma are detailed in Table 10.

Asthma Education

- Develop a partnership with the patient and family.
- Provide training on self-management skills.
- Provide information about asthma including the following:
  - Details about chronicity of the disease.
  - Need for medications.
  - Role of short-acting β_2-agonists.
  - Importance of communication.
- Teach and discuss inhaler and spacer techniques.
- Discuss environmental control measures.
- Address misconceptions, fears, and patient's financial concerns.
- Develop an action plan for exacerbations.

Initial Outpatient Treatment of Asthma Exacerbations

- Patients experiencing severe asthma exacerbations should receive systemic corticosteroids.
- In addition, an inhaled β_2-agonist by nebulization (1 dose every 20 minutes) may be needed.
- Oxygen should be administered to keep the oxygen saturation at >90%.
- Patients with a history of prior intubation and those who do not respond to initial therapy should be considered for hospital admission.

TABLE 10	Medications Commonly Used for Asthma

Drug Name	Trade Names	Formulation	Adult Dose
Short-acting β₂-agonists			
Albuterol	Proventil	MDI: 90 mcg/spray	2 INH q4–6 hour prn
	Ventolin	NEB: 2.5 mg/3 mL	2.5 mg NEB q4–6 hour
	Proventil-HFA		prn
	Ventolin-HFA		
	Accuneb		
	ProAir HFA		
	Generic		
Levalbuterol	Xopenex	HFA: 45 mcg/puff	1–2 INH q4–6 hour prn
	Xopenex-HFA	NEB: 0.31, 0.63, or	0.63 mg NEB q6–8 hour
		1.25 mg/3 mL	prn
Pirbuterol	Maxair	MDI: 200 mcg/INH	1–2 INH q4–6 hour prn
Long-acting β₂-agonists			
Salmeterol	Serevent	DPI: 50 mcg/blister	1 INH q12 hour
Formoterol	Foradil	DPI: 12 mcg/capsule	1 INH q12 hour
Combination inhaled corticosteroid with a long-acting β₂-agonist			
Fluticasone propionate/ salmeterol	Advair	DPI: 100/50, 250/50, 500/50 mcg/INH	DPI: 1 INH q12 hour
	Advair HFA	HFA: 45/21, 115/21, 230/21 mcg/INH	HFA: 2 INH q12 hour
Budesonide/ formoterol fumarate dihydrate	Symbicort	Inhalation aerosol: 80/4.5 mcg/INH 160/4.5 mcg/INH	2 INH q12 hour

Drug Name	Low Dose	Medium Dose	High Dose
Inhaled corticosteroids (comparative daily dosages)			
Beclomethasone dipropionate 40 mcg/spray 80 mcg/spray	160–480 mcg 40 mcg: 4–12 INH 80 mcg: 2–6 INH	480–800 mcg 40 mcg: 12–20 INH 80 mcg: 6–10 INH	>800 mcg 40 mcg: >20 INH 80 mcg: >10 INH
Budesonide DPI: 180 mcg/ spray	180–360 mcg 1–2 INH	360–540 mcg 2–3 INH	>540 mcg >3 INH
Flunisolide 250 mcg/spray	500–1,000 mcg 2–4 INH	1,000–2,000 mcg 4–8 INH	>2,000 mcg >8 INH
Fluticasone MDI: 44, 110, 220 mcg/spray	88–264 mcg 44 mcg: 2–6 INH 110 mcg: 2 INH	264–660 mcg 110 mcg: 2–6 INH	>660 mcg 110 mcg: >6 INH 220 mcg: >3 INH
Triamcinolone acetonide 100 mcg/spray	400–1,000 mcg 4–10 INH	1,000–2,000 mcg 10–20 INH	>2,000 mcg >20 INH

(*continued*)

TABLE 10	Medications Commonly Used for Asthma (*Continued*)		
Drug	**Formulation**	**Adult Dose**	**Comments**
Leukotriene modifiers			
Montelukast (Singulair)	10-mg tablets	10 mg PO daily	Blocks leukotriene D_4
Zafirlukast (Accolate)	10-mg tablets 20-mg tablets	20 mg PO q12 hour	Food decreases bioavailability Take 1 hour before or 2 hours after meals
Zileuton (Zyflo)	600-mg tablets	600 mg PO q6 hour	Monitor ALT levels Inhibits 5-lipoxygenase
Other agents			
Theophylline Bronkodyl Uniphyl Elixophyllin Slo-bid Slo-Phyllin Theo-24 Theo-Dur Theolair	Multiple including liquid, capsules, sustained-release tablets	300–600 mg/day divided bid to tid	Multiple drug interactions Narrow therapeutic index Follow levels frequently (goal levels of 5–15 mcg/mL) Phosphodiesterase inhibitor
Cromolyn (Intal)	MDI: 800 mcg/ spray	2 INH qid	One dose prior to exercise or allergen exposure provides prophylaxis for 1 hour
Nedocromil (Tilade)	MDI: 1.75 mg/ spray	2 INH qid	One dose prior to exercise or allergen exposure provides prophylaxis for 1 hour

MDI, metered-dose inhaler; HFA, hydrofluoroalkane; NEB, nebulizer solution or nebulized; DPI, dry powder inhaler; INH, inhalation.

- In addition, the presence of a pulsus paradoxus >12 mm Hg, PEFR or FEV_1 <50% predicted, hypoxemia, and normocapnia despite tachypnea or hypercapnia ($PaCO_2$ >42 mm Hg) should trigger hospital admission.
- The management of the hospitalized patient with an asthma exacerbation will not be discussed here, except to highlight the need for patient education prior to discharge, a written patient action plan, PEFR meter use reinforcement, and planning for outpatient follow-up.[33]

CYSTIC FIBROSIS

General Principles

- Cystic fibrosis (CF) is the most common lethal genetic disease in Caucasians, with an incidence of 1 in 3,200 live births in the United States.
- Although it is less common in non-Caucasians, the diagnosis needs to be considered in patients of diverse backgrounds. The diagnosis of CF is typically made during childhood, but 8% of patients are diagnosed during adolescence or adulthood.
- With improved therapy, the median survival has been extended to approximately 36.5 years in 2005.

Pathophysiology

- CF is an autosomal recessive disorder that is caused by mutations of the cystic fibrosis transmembrane conductance regulator (CFTR) protein, located on chromosome 7.[34] CFTR protein normally regulates and participates in the transport of electrolytes across epithelial cell membranes.[35]
- There is considerable phenotypic variation in disease expression that occurs primarily as a result of the specific genetic mutation. >1,500 mutations in the CFTR domain on chromosome 7 have been identified which can result in defective protein production, processing, regulation, and conduction.
- The primary clinical manifestations of the disease are related to abnormal electrolyte transport; however, there are still elements that are poorly understood.
- The abnormal airway secretions in patients with CF predispose the patient to chronic infection and chronic colonization with organisms such as *Staphylococcus aureus* and mucoid strains of gram-negative organisms such as *Pseudomonas aeruginosa*. The chronic infection results in chronic airway inflammation and ultimately bronchiectasis.

Diagnosis

- The diagnosis of CF is based on clinical and family history in combination with persistently elevated concentrations of sweat chloride (the main laboratory confirmation used), or genetic confirmation revealing two known disease-causing CF mutations or nasal transepithelial potential difference measurements that are typical of CF.[36]
- Atypical patients may lack classic symptoms and signs or have normal sweat tests. Although genotyping may assist in the diagnosis, it alone cannot establish or rule out the diagnosis of CF.

Pulmonary Manifestations

- Pulmonary symptoms lead to the consideration of the diagnosis of CF in 50% of cases.
- Symptoms typically include cough and purulent sputum production with dyspnea ensuing as the disease progresses. Almost all patients eventually develop chronic sinopulmonary disease, bronchiectasis, and obstructive lung disease.
- Acute pulmonary exacerbations, characterized by fevers, cough, increased sputum volume and purulence, malaise, and weight loss, may lead to significant deterioration and subsequent hospitalization.
- Airway colonization occurs early in life in patients with CF and the colonizing flora tends to change with time.

- *S. aureus* tends to colonize younger patients, and in older individuals, it is replaced by mucoid strains of *P. aeruginosa.*
- Additional respiratory problems include episodes of hemoptysis, pneumothorax, and allergic bronchopulmonary aspergillosis.

Extrapulmonary Manifestations

- Extrapulmonary manifestations of CF include exocrine pancreatic insufficiency, seen in 90% of patients, resulting in fat malabsorption; deficiency of fat-soluble vitamins A, D, E, and K; and malnutrition.
- CF involvement of the gastrointestinal (GI) tract causes considerable problems including steatorrhea, constipation, impaction, distal ileal obstruction syndrome, volvulus, intussusception, and rectal prolapse.
- CF also affects the endocrine pancreas manifested as diabetes mellitus and pancreatitis. Significant hepatobiliary complications include the development of cirrhosis with portal hypertension, cholelithiasis, and cholecystitis.
- Male patients with CF tend to be infertile due to an absence of the vas deferens, whereas female patients may have fertility problems due to amenorrhea and abnormally thick cervical mucus production.[37]
- Many individuals with CF suffer from growth retardation, osteopenia, and osteoporosis and can develop a CF-associated arthropathy as well as hypertrophic osteoarthropathy.[38] Digital clubbing appears in childhood in virtually all symptomatic patients.

Differential Diagnosis

- All adult patients with unexplained **bronchiectasis** should be considered as possible cases of undiagnosed CF and should have sweat testing performed.
- **Primary ciliary dyskinesia** or immunoglobulin deficiency may lead to bronchiectasis, sinusitis, and infertility, but few GI symptoms and no sweat electrolyte abnormalities are present.
- Men with **Young's syndrome** have bronchiectasis, sinusitis, and azoospermia but the respiratory disease is usually mild, and GI symptoms or sweat manifestations are not present.
- **Shwachman syndrome,** consisting of pancreatic insufficiency and cyclic neutropenia, may also lead to lung disease, but sweat chloride concentrations are normal and the neutropenia is distinguishing.

Diagnostic Testing

Skin Sweat Testing

- Using a standardized quantitative pilocarpine iontophoresis, this method remains the gold standard for the diagnosis of CF.
- A sweat chloride concentration of >60 mmol/L is consistent with the diagnosis of CF.[39]
- The diagnosis should be made only if there is an elevated sweat chloride concentration on two separate occasions in a patient with a typical phenotype or with a history of CF in a sibling.
- Borderline sweat test results (40 to 60 mmol/L sweat chloride) or nondiagnostic test results in the setting of high clinical suspicion should also lead to repeat sweat testing, nasal potential difference testing, or genetic testing.
- Abnormal sweat chloride concentrations are rarely detected in non-CF patients (e.g., Addison's disease and untreated hypothyroidism). Sweat testing should only be performed in centers with experience of this test and who perform the test regularly.

Genetic Testing
- Genetic tests have detected >1,200 CF mutations on chromosome 7. The most common CFTR mutation in patients is ΔF508.
- Most commercially available probes are quite sensitive but test for only a minority of the known CF mutations, although they are able to identify >90% of the abnormal CF genes in Ashkenazi Jews.
- For patients to have clinical disease, two of the recessive genes must be abnormal.

Nasal Potential Difference
Nasal potential difference measurements can be performed at experienced centers and are able to detect the abnormal epithelial chloride secretion that is typical of CF.[40]

Other Tests
Other tests may be supportive of the diagnosis of CF and clinically useful, although they are not absolutely diagnostic.
- **CXR** may show hyperinflation and upper lobe predominant bronchiectasis.
- **PFTs** typically show expiratory airflow obstruction with air trapping and hyperinflation. Impairments of gas exchange also occur and can progress to hypoxemia and hypercapnia.
- **Sputum cultures** typically identify *P. aeruginosa* and *S. aureus*, or both, and sputum sensitivity testing is useful for directing therapy.
- Testing for **malabsorption** is often not formally performed, because clinical evidence, steatorrhea, low fat-soluble vitamin levels (A, D and E), and a prolonged prothrombin time (vitamin K) as well as a clear response to pancreatic enzyme treatment are usually considered sufficient for diagnosing exocrine insufficiency.
- Testing for sinusitis or infertility, especially obstructive azoospermia in males, would also be supportive of the diagnosis of CF.

Treatment

- The goals of CF therapy include improving quality of life and functionality, decreasing the number of exacerbations and hospitalizations, avoiding complications associated with therapy, and decreasing mortality.[41] A major focus of therapy is on airway clearance and controlling infections.
- Care at comprehensive CF core centers is recommended. These centers are designed to address the multiple organ system involvement typical of the disease and are typically staffed by pulmonary specialists who lead teams of nurses, nutritionists, and social workers to help the patients live with a chronic illness.
- Specialty consultation with gastroenterologists, endocrinologists, and occasionally interventional radiologists may be required during the course of care of each individual patient.

Nonpharmacologic Treatment
- **Mucus mobilization/airway clearance** can be accomplished using various airway clearance techniques, including postural drainage with chest percussion and vibration, with or without mechanical devices (flutter valves, high-frequency chest oscillation vests, low and high positive expiratory pressure devices, etc.), and breathing and coughing exercises.[42]
- **Pulmonary rehabilitation** and exercise is recommended as it improves secretion mobilization and functional status.

- **Oxygen therapy** is indicated in patients with CF, based on the same criteria as in patients with COPD. Rest and exercise oxygen assessments should be performed as clinically indicated.

Pharmacologic Treatment

- **Bronchodilators** such as β_2-agonists (Table 6) are used to treat the reversible components of airflow obstruction and help facilitate mucus clearance. Many patients with CF have acute improvements in FEV_1 as well as symptomatic improvement with bronchodilators.[43] These agents are contraindicated in the rare patient with associated paradoxical deterioration of airflow after their use.
- **Recombinant human deoxyribonuclease** ("DNase," dornase alfa, Pulmozyme) digests extracellular DNA, decreasing the viscoelasticity of the sputum.
  - Dornase alpha improves pulmonary function and decreases the incidence of respiratory tract infections that require parenteral antibiotics.[44]
  - The recommended dose of dornase alfa (Pulmozyme) is 2.5 mg/day inhaled using a jet nebulizer.
  - Adverse effects may include pharyngitis, laryngitis, rash, chest pain, and conjunctivitis.
- **Hypertonic saline,** inhaled bid to qid, can be used as an additional regimen in patients already using bronchodilators and dornase alpha. Clinical trials have shown improved mucus clearance, small improvements in lung function, and fewer exacerbations requiring antibiotic therapy.[45] A 7% saline solution is used and should be preceded by an inhaled bronchodilator to offset the bronchospasm that can occur from this therapy. This is a relatively new modality in CF care, and patient selection for this time-consuming therapy is still evolving.
- **Antibiotic therapy** forms an integral component of the care of patients with CF. The airways become colonized in most patients with CF and the typical pathogens in adulthood include *P. aeruginosa* and *S. aureus.*
  - **Sputum cultures** are critically important to provide the clinician with an idea which antibiotics are effective against the colonizers/pathogens during acute exacerbations.
  - In addition, routine sputum cultures are useful in identifying other colonizers which can impact outcomes in patients with CF, including the following:
    - *Burkholderia cepacia.*
    - *Achromobacter xylosoxidans.*
    - *Stenotrophomonas maltophilia.*
    - *Aspergillus* spp.
    - Methicillin-resistant *S. aureus* (MRSA).
    - Nontuberculous mycobacteria (*Mycobacterium avium complex* and *Mycobacterium abscessus*).
  - **Aerosolized antibiotics** are frequently used in patients with CF. Inhaling aerosolized tobramycin (300 mg nebulized bid for 28 days on, alternating with 28 days off) using an appropriate nebulizer and compressor improves pulmonary function, decreases the density of *P. aeruginosa*, and decreases the risk of hospitalization.[46] Patients with pan-resistant *P. aeruginosa* species may sometimes benefit from inhaled colistin therapy.
  - **Macrolide antibiotic therapy** with azithromycin, used chronically three times per week in patients rigorously screened for concurrent nontuberculous mycobacterial disease, has been shown to improve lung function and reduce exacerbations, most likely on the basis of an anti-inflammatory effect.[47]

- **Systemic glucocorticoids** are indicated only for refractory lung disease that has demonstrated subjective (less dyspnea) and objective (decreased airflow obstruction or improved exercise tolerance, or both) benefit during a trial period. Short courses of glucocorticoid therapy may be helpful to some patients, but long-term therapy should be avoided to minimize the side effects, which include glucose intolerance, osteopenia, and growth retardation. There is very little data to support the use of inhaled corticosteroids in patients with CF, unless they have concomitant asthma.
- **Vaccinations** including a yearly influenza vaccine and a pneumococcal vaccine every 5 years are recommended.

Lung Transplantation

- Most patients with CF die from pulmonary disease.
- An FEV_1 <30% of the predicted normal value, marked alveolar gas exchange abnormalities (resting hypoxemia or hypercapnia), evidence of pulmonary hypertension, or increased frequency or severity of pulmonary exacerbations should lead to consideration of lung transplantation as a treatment option.[48]
- The suppurative nature of the lung disease in CF mandates that bilateral transplantation be performed.
- Survival rates of 40% to 60% at 5 years are standard.

Treatment of Extrapulmonary Disease

- **Pancreatic enzyme supplementation** should be instituted after pancreatic insufficiency and malabsorption have been demonstrated. Enzyme dose is titrated to achieve one to two semisolid stools per day. Enzymes are taken immediately before meals and snacks.
  - Dosing of pancreatic enzymes should be initiated at 500 units lipase/kg/meal and should not exceed 2,500 units lipase/kg/meal.
  - High doses (6,000 units lipase/kg/meal) have been associated with chronic intestinal strictures.
- **Vitamin supplementation** is recommended, especially the fat-soluble vitamins that are not well absorbed in the setting of pancreatic insufficiency. Vitamins A, D, E, and K can all be taken orally on a regular basis. Iron deficiency anemia requires iron supplementation. Osteopenia should be aggressively treated.
- Sinusitis regimens are used in the typical fashion.
- Pancreatic endocrine dysfunction, specifically diabetes mellitus, is treated with insulin in the standard fashion, but typical diabetic dietary restrictions are liberalized (high-calorie diet with unrestricted fat) to encourage appropriate growth and weight maintenance.

Acute CF Exacerbations

- Acute exacerbations of CF pulmonary disease are marked by dyspnea, increasing cough, increased mucus production, and worsening of spirometry.
- Very mild exacerbations can be treated with oral antibiotics if the colonizer remains susceptible to an orally available agent. Typical drugs for susceptible staphylococcal species include dicloxacillin, trimethoprim-sulfamethoxazole, or doxycycline.
- However, most patients with exacerbations will require initiation of IV antibiotics. Choice of these agents is dictated by the sputum sensitivities, if available. Combination therapy with a semisynthetic penicillin, a third- or fourth-generation cephalosporin, a carbapenem or a quinolone, and an aminoglycoside is the typical therapy recommended during acute exacerbations.

- Synergy testing of resistant isolates at specialized centers may allow for more effective antibiotic selection; however, the benefits of this approach remain unproven. The presence of MRSA on sputum culture testing often necessitates addition of vancomycin or linezolid.
- The duration of antibiotic therapy is dictated by the clinical response. Typically, antibiotics are given for 10 to 14 days.
- Dosing of many antibiotics needs to be altered in patients with CF because of altered pharmacokinetics and volumes of distribution in these patients. For example, cefepime is often dosed at 2 g IV q8 hour.
- Once daily IV tobramycin dosing is as effective as and simpler than multiple daily-dose regimens but requires monitoring of peak and trough levels closely.[49] Patients need to be monitored for side effects, including ototoxicity and renal dysfunction.
- Home IV antibiotic therapy is common, administered through a peripherally inserted central catheter (PICC) line, subclavian Hohn catheter, or an established Port-A-Cath.
- Initial hospitalization is recommended to allow access to comprehensive therapy and diagnostic testing as well as establishment of appropriate dosing and monitoring of the aminoglycoside.

Special Problems

- ***B. cepacia complex:*** Acquisition of this organism is associated with accelerated decline of lung function and shortened survival in patients with CF. In addition, colonization with this organism is a contraindication to lung transplantation at some centers because of the resistance patterns of this pathogen.[50] Patients colonized by *Burkholderia* spp. should be kept separated from other patients with CF (different clinic days, different floors in the hospital).
- **Allergic bronchopulmonary aspergillosis** can occur in patients with CF.[51]
- **Nontuberculous mycobacteria,** normally *Mycobacterium avium-intracellulare* (MAI) and rarely *M. abscessus,* can infect patients with CF. Treatment decisions depend on symptoms, radiographic appearances, and pulmonary function. In general, the same therapies are required as in patients with non-CF bronchiectasis.
- **Hemoptysis** in CF is common, especially small amounts of blood during pulmonary exacerbations. Massive hemoptysis is usually treated with IV antibiotics, airway control and ventilatory support if needed, and radiographic embolization of the bronchial arteries feeding the site of hemoptysis. Embolization may need to be repeated because of the extensive bronchial collaterals that patients with CF develop. Limited pulmonary resection is a last resort.
- **Pneumothorax** in patients with CF tends to occur as lung function worsens. Treatment consists of chest tube drainage. For persistent air leaks, pleurodesis may be required.
- Women with CF who become pregnant normally tolerate the pregnant state well as long as their lung function is not severely impaired with associated pulmonary hypertension.[52] Close monitoring of lung function and glycemic control is needed.

Monitoring

- Spirometry is the best objective measurement of lung function in CF, and routine spirometric monitoring is recommended. A significant decline in spirometry, even in the absence of increased symptoms, mandates intensification of therapy.
- Sputum cultures and sensitivity testing should also be sent from outpatient visits.

- HbA$_{1c}$ monitoring of diabetic patients is advised.
- Yearly vitamin levels (vitamin A, E) as well as bone densitometry is recommended.

REFERENCES

1. Celli BR, Macnee W, Agusti A, et al. Standards for the diagnosis and treatment of patients with COPD: a summary of the ATS/ERS position paper. *Eur Respir J* 2004;23:932–946.
2. Barnes PJ. Chronic obstructive pulmonary disease. *N Engl J Med* 2000;343:269–280.
3. Hogg JC, Chu F, Utokaparch S, et al. The nature of small-airway obstruction in chronic obstructive pulmonary disease. *N Engl J Med* 2004;350:2645–2653.
4. O'Donnell DE. Ventilatory limitations in chronic obstructive pulmonary disease. *Med Sci Sports Exerc* 2001;33:S647–S655.
5. Celli BR, Cote CG, Marin JM, et al. The body-mass index, airflow obstruction, dyspnea, and exercise capacity index in chronic obstructive pulmonary disease. *N Engl J Med* 2004;350:1005–1012.
6. Stoller JK, Aboussouan LS. Alpha1-antitrypsin deficiency. *Lancet* 2005;365:2225–2236.
7. Fabbri L, Pauwels RA, Hurd S. Global strategy for the diagnosis, management and prevention of chronic obstructive pulmonary disease: GOLD executive summary updated 2003. *COPD* 2004;1:105–141.
8. Rabe KF, Hurd S, Anzueto A, et al. Global strategy for the diagnosis, management, and prevention of chronic obstructive pulmonary disease: GOLD executive summary. *Am J Respir Crit Care Med* 2007;176:532–555.
9. Anthonisen NR, Connett JE, Kiley JP, et al. Effect of smoking intervention and the use of inhaled anticholinergic bronchodilator on the rate of decline of the FEV$_1$. The Lung Health Study. *JAMA* 1994;272:1497–1505.
10. The Tobacco Use and Dependence Clinical Practice Guideline Panel, Staff and Consortium Representatives: a clinical practice guideline for treating tobacco use and dependence. A US Public Health Service report. *JAMA* 2000;283:3244–3254.
11. Ram FS, Sestini P. Regular inhaled short acting beta2 agonists for the management of stable chronic obstructive pulmonary disease: Cochrane systematic review and meta-analysis. *Thorax* 2003;58:580–584.
12. Combivent Inhalation Aerosol Study Group. In chronic obstructive pulmonary disease, a combination of ipratropium and albuterol is more effective than either agent alone: an 85-day multicenter trial. *Chest* 1994;105:1411–1419.
13. Calverley P, Anderson JA, Celli B, et al. Salmeterol and fluticasone propionate and survival in chronic obstructive pulmonary disease. *N Engl J Med* 2007;356:775–789
14. Brusasco V, Hodder R, Miravitlles M, et al. Health outcomes following treatment for six months with once daily tiotropium compared with twice daily salmeterol in patients with COPD. *Thorax* 2003;58:399-404. Erratum in *Thorax* 2005;60:105.
15. Ram FS, Jardin JR, Atallah A, et al. Efficacy of theophylline in people with stable chronic obstructive pulmonary disease: a systematic review and meta-analysis. *Respir Med* 2005;99: 135–144.
16. American Thoracic Society. Pulmonary rehabilitation—1999. *Am J Respir Crit Care Med* 1999;159:1666–1682.
17. NOTT Group. Continuous or nocturnal oxygen therapy in hypoxemic COPD. *Ann Intern Med* 1980;93:391–398.
18. Crockett AJ, Cranston JM, Moss JR, et al. Domiciliary oxygen for chronic obstructive pulmonary disease. *Cochrane Database Syst Rev* 2000;CD001744.
19. Fishman A, Martinez F, Naunheim K, et al. A randomized trial comparing lung volume reduction surgery with medical therapy for severe emphysema. *N Engl J Med* 2003;348: 2059–2073.
20. Nathan SD. Lung transplantation: disease-specific considerations for referral. *Chest* 2005; 127;1006–1016.
21. Stoller JK, Aboussouan LS. Alpha1-antitrypsin deficiency. 5: Intravenous augmentation therapy: current understanding. *Thorax* 2004;59:708–712.

22. Connors AF Jr, Dawson NV, Thomas C, et al. Outcomes following acute exacerbations of severe chronic obstructive lung disease. The SUPPORT investigators. *Am J Respir Crit Care Med* 1996;154:959–967.

23. Niewoehner DE, Erbland ML, Deupree RH, et al. Effect of systemic glucocorticoids on exacerbations of chronic obstructive pulmonary disease. Department of Veterans Affairs Cooperative Study Group. *N Engl J Med* 1999;340:1941–1947.

24. National Asthma Education and Prevention Program Expert Panel Report 3 (EPR-3): Guidelines for the Diagnosis and Management of Asthma. Summary Report 2007. Bethesda, MD: National Heart, Lung, and Blood Institute, 2007. National Institutes of Health publication 08-5846. Available at: http://www. nhlbi.nih.gov/guidelines/asthma/index.htm. Last accessed: November 24, 2009.

25. National Asthma Education and Prevention Program Expert Panel Report 3 (EPR-3): Guidelines for the Diagnosis and Management of Asthma. Full Report 2007. Bethesda, MD: National Heart, Lung, and Blood Institute, 2007. Publication 08-4051. Available at: http://www.nhlbi.nih.gov/guidelines/asthma/ index.htm. Last accessed: November 24, 2009.

26. Yunginger JW, Reed CE, O'Connell EJ, et al. A community-based study of the epidemiology of asthma. Incidence rates, 1964–1983. *Am Rev Respir Dis* 1992;146:888–894.

27. Irwin RS, Curley FJ, French CL. Chronic cough: the spectrum and frequency of causes, key components of the diagnostic evaluation, and outcome of specific therapy. *Am Rev Respir Dis* 1990;141:640–647.

28. Crapo RO, Casaburi R, Coates AL, et al. Guidelines for methacholine and exercise challenge testing—1999. *Am J Respir Crit Care Med* 2000;161:309–329.

29. Cowie RL, Revitt SG, Underwood MF, Field SK. The effect of a peak flow-based action plan in the prevention of exacerbations of asthma. *Chest* 1997;112:1534–1538.

30. Nelson HS, Weiss ST, Bleecker ER, et al. The Salmeterol Multicenter Asthma Research Trial: a comparison of usual pharmacotherapy for asthma or usual pharmacotherapy plus salmeterol. *Chest* 2006;129:15–26.

31. Phipatanakul W, Greene C, Downes SJ, et al. Montelukast improves asthma control in asthmatic children maintained on inhaled corticosteroids. *Ann Allergy Asthma Immunol* 2003;91:49–54.

32. Soler M, Matz J, Townley R, et al. The anti-IgE antibody omalizumab reduces exacerbations and steroid requirement in allergic asthmatics. *Eur Respir J* 2001;18:254–261.

33. Rodrigo GJ, Rodrigo C, Hall JB. Acute asthma in adults: a review. *Chest* 2004;125: 1081–1102.

34. Rommens JM, Iannuzzi MC, Kerem B, et al. Identification of the cystic fibrosis gene: chromosome walking and jumping. *Science* 1989;245:1059–1065.

35. Denning GM, Estedgaard LS, Cheng SH, et al. Localization of cystic fibrosis transmembrane conductance regulator in chloride secretory epithelia. *J Clin Invest* 1992;89:339–349.

36. Stern RC. The diagnosis of cystic fibrosis. *N Engl J Med* 1997;336:487–491.

37. Dodge JA. Male fertility in cystic fibrosis. *Lancet* 1995;346:587–588.

38. Haworth CS, Selby PL, Webb AK, et al. Low bone mineral density in adults with cystic fibrosis. *Thorax* 1999;54:961–967.

39. Davis PB, DelRio S, Munts JA, et al. Sweat chloride concentration in adults with pulmonary disease. *Am Rev Respir Dis* 1983;138:34–37.

40. Alton EW, Currie D, Logan-Sincleair R, et al. Nasal potential difference: a clinical diagnostic test for cystic fibrosis. *Eur Respir J* 1990;3:922–926.

41. Yankaskas JR, Marshall BC, Sufian B, et al. Cystic fibrosis adult care: consensus conference report. *Chest* 2004;125:1S–39S.

42. Hardy KA, Anderson BD. Noninvasive clearance of airway secretions. *Respir Care Clin N Am* 1996;2:323–345.

43. Cropp GJ. Effectiveness of bronchodilators in cystic fibrosis. *Am J Med* 1996;100:19S–29S.

44. Fuchs HJ, Borowitz DS, Christiansen DH, et al. Effect of aerosolized recombinant human DNase on exacerbations of respiratory symptoms and on pulmonary function in patients with cystic fibrosis. The Pulmozyme Study Group. *N Engl J Med* 1994;331:637–642.

45. Elkins MR, Robinson M, Rose BR, et al. A controlled trial of long-term inhaled hypertonic saline in patients with cystic fibrosis. *N Engl J Med* 2006;354:229–240.
46. Ramsey BW, Pepe MS, Quan JM, et al. Intermittent administration of inhaled tobramycin in patients with cystic fibrosis. *N Engl J Med* 1999;340:23–30.
47. Saiman L, Marshall BC, Mayer-Hamblett N, et al. Azithromycin in patients with cystic fibrosis chronically infected with *Pseudomonas aeruginosa*: a randomized controlled trial. *JAMA* 2003;290:1749–1756.
48. Yankaskas JR, Mallory BG Jr. Lung transplantation in cystic fibrosis: consensus conference statement. *Chest* 1998;113:217–226.
49. Smyth A, Tan KH, Hyman-Taylor P, et al. Once versus three times daily regimes of tobramycin treatment for pulmonary exacerbations of cystic fibrosis—the TOPIC study: a randomized controlled trial. *Lancet* 2005;365:573–578.
50. Chaparro C, Maurer J, Gutierrez C, et al. Infection with *Burkholderia cepacia* in cystic fibrosis: outcome following lung transplantation. *Am J Respir Crit Care Med* 2001;163: 43–48.
51. Stevens DA, Moss RB, Kurup VP, et al. Allergic bronchopulmonary aspergillosis in cystic fibrosis-state of the art: Cystic Fibrosis Foundation Consensus Conference. *Clin Infect Dis* 2003;37:S225–S664.
52. Goss CH, Rubenfeld GD, Otto K, Aitjen ML. The effect of pregnancy on survival in women with cystic fibrosis. *Chest* 2003;124:1460–1468.

13

Interstitial Lung Diseases and Pulmonary Hypertension

Raksha Jain and Murali M. Chakinala

INTERSTITIAL LUNG DISEASE

General Principles

- The interstitial lung diseases (ILDs), also known as the diffuse parenchymal lung diseases, are a heterogeneous group of disorders characterized by infiltration of cellular and noncellular material into the lung parenchyma.
- The role of the primary care physician is to recognize the presentation of an ILD, start the initial workup, know when to involve the pulmonary specialist, and be aware of disease course and treatment options.
- The terminology for the ILDs is somewhat of a misnomer. ILDs not only affect the interstitial compartment of the lungs but also involve the alveoli, microvasculature, and small airways.
- There are >100 distinct types of ILDs, yet no universal classification system exists.[1]
- Treatment of many of the ILDs is difficult and relies on immunosuppressive agents that are not always beneficial.
- Referral for lung transplantation should be considered when appropriate.

Epidemiology

- The prevalence of ILDs is estimated to be 80.9 per 100,000 in males and 67.2 per 100,000 in females.[2]
- Idiopathic pulmonary fibrosis (IPF) is the most common form, accounting for 25% to 35% of cases.[1]
- Sarcoidosis and connective tissue disease (CTD)–related ILDs are the next most prevalent.

Pathophysiology

- Mechanisms of these diseases are not well understood.
- Theories include injury to the alveolar epithelium which results in inflammation and an abnormal host response that may ultimately lead to fibrosis.
- The collagen deposition leads to stiff lungs with poor distensibility, resulting in a restrictive ventilatory pattern and worsening gas exchange.
- Pulmonary hypertension may be a late complication in the disease course.

Diagnosis

Classification

- There is no universal classification scheme for the ILDs; however, they can be categorized on the basis of etiology and presentation.

- Histopathology is shared across different diseases and must be considered in context with clinical information before making a final diagnosis.
- Diagnosis is based on a combination of clinical presentation, radiographic findings, and histopathologic specimens (Table 1).
- A general approach to the diagnosis of ILD is presented in Figure 1.[3]

Clinical Presentation

History

- History is an extremely important component of the evaluation of ILDs.
- Demographics can be helpful (e.g., lymphangioleiomyomatosis [LAM] is most common in young women).
- Temporal course of symptoms should be noted. For example, acute interstitial pneumonia (AIP), cryptogenic organizing pneumonia (COP), acute eosinophilic pneumonia (AEP), and alveolar hemorrhage syndromes develop quite rapidly (days to weeks), whereas IPF, nonspecific interstitial pneumonitis (NSIP), hypersensitivity pneumonitis (HP), and sarcoidosis have a more insidious onset (months to years).
- The most common presenting symptom is dyspnea on exertion. Cough is also common. Nonpulmonary symptoms, such as dysphagia, Raynaud's phenomenon, myalgias, and arthralgias, point toward an underlying connective tissue disorder.
- The age of onset of disease is highly variable.
- Active smoking is associated with respiratory bronchiolitis-ILD (RB-ILD), desquamative interstitial pneumonia (DIP), and pulmonary Langerhans cell histiocytosis (PLCH).
- Occupational and environmental exposures can reveal disorders such as HP and pneumoconiosis.
- History of drug use such as amiodarone or treatment with chemotherapy agents and radiation may reveal an underlying cause.
- Family history may also be important (i.e., familial form of IPF).

Physical Examination

- The hallmark feature of ILD, specifically IPF, is dry "Velcro" crackles upon auscultation of the lungs and clubbing of the nails.
- Systemic findings of fever, joint pains, and rashes are more indicative of an associated CTD or sarcoidosis.
- Findings of a CTD, including cutaneous telangectasias, sclerodactyly, arthritis, myositis, and joint deformities, may be present on examination.

Diagnostic Testing

Laboratory Tests

- Laboratory tests should be interpreted in the appropriate clinical setting (Table 2).
- Angiotensin-converting enzyme level for sarcoidosis is generally not useful due to its low sensitivity and specificity.

Pulmonary Function Tests

- Pulmonary function tests (PFTs) should include spirometry, lung volumes, diffusion capacity, and exercise oximetry as well as an arterial blood gas in certain circumstances.
- PFTs classically show a restrictive ventilatory defect: low total lung capacity, low vital capacity, low forced expiratory volume in 1 second (FEV_1), and low forced vital capacity (FVC) but normal or high FEV_1/FVC.[4]
- Abnormal gas exchange is often evident with a low diffusion capacity of the lung for carbon monoxide (DLCO) and **hypoxemia, particularly with exercise.**
- Elevated DLCO is consistent with alveolar hemorrhage.

TABLE 1	Classification Scheme for the Interstitial Lung Diseases (ILDs)

Category	Disease
Idiopathic interstitial pneumonias	Acute interstitial pneumonitis (AIP)/diffuse alveolar damage (DAD), previously known as Hamman-Rich syndrome
	Idiopathic pulmonary fibrosis (PF)/usual interstitial pneumonia (UIP)
	Nonspecific interstitial pneumonitis (NSIP)
	Cryptogenic organizing pneumonitis (COP)/bronchiolitis obliterans organizing pneumonia (BOOP)
	Respiratory bronchiolitis-interstitial lung disease (RB-ILD)
	Desquamative interstitial pneumonia (DIP)
	Lymphocytic interstitial pneumonia (LIP)
Occupational/ environmental	Hypersensitivity pneumonitis (HP)
	Pneumoconiosis
	Heavy metal disease (e.g., cobalt)
	Berylliosis
	Asbestosis
	Silicosis
	Noxious gas/fumes/vapors
Immune-related	Connective tissue disease–related—systemic lupus erythematosus, rheumatoid arthritis, scleroderma/ systemic sclerosis, polymyositis, and dermatomyositis
	Vasculitis—Wegener's granulomatosis, Churg-Strauss, microscopic polyangiitis
	Goodpasture syndrome
Eosinophilic interstitial lung disease	Acute eosinophilic pneumonia (AEP)
	Chronic eosinophilic pneumonia (CEP)
Treatment-related	Drugs (see www.pneumotox.com)—amiodarone, nitrofurantoin
	Chemotherapy—bleomycin
	Radiation-induced
Malignancy	Lymphangitic carcinomatosis
	Bronchoalveolar cell carcinoma
	Amyloidosis
Others	Sarcoidosis
	Lymphangioleiomyomatosis (LAM)
	Pulmonary alveolar proteinosis (PAP)
	Pulmonary Langerhans cell histiocytosis (PLCH) (formerly known as eosinophilic granulomatosis)
	Neurofibromatosis

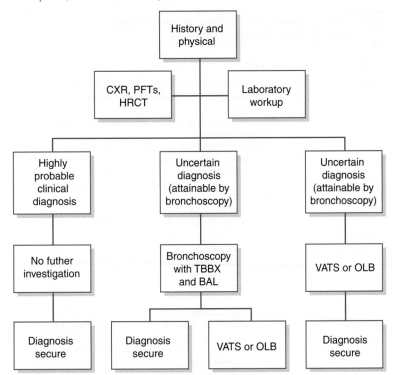

Figure 1. Approach to diagnosing interstitial lung diseases. BAL, bronchoalveolar lavage; CXR, plain chest radiography; HRCT, high-resolution computed tomography; OLB, open lung biopsy; PFTs, pulmonary function tests; TBBX, transbronchial biopsy; VATS, video-assisted thoracoscopic surgery. (Modified from British Thoracic Society. The diagnosis and treatment of diffuse parenchymal lung disease in adults. *Thorax* 1999;54:S1–S28.)

- Diseases such as sarcoidosis, HP, PLCH, and LAM are associated with an obstructive ventilator pattern because of airway involvement.

Radiographic Studies
Plain Chest Radiography
- A chest radiography (CXR) can be helpful in revealing an ILD but is not typically a diagnostic study.
- It can be normal in up to 10% of patients with clinically significant ILDs.[5]
- Radiographic patterns that may be associated with ILDs include the following[1,4]:
  - Small lung volumes: IPF- and CTD-related.
  - Preserved or large lung volumes: HP, LAM, PLCH, chronic obstructive pulmonary disease with ILD, neurofibromatosis-associated ILD.
  - Upper lobe predominance: sarcoidosis, silicosis.
  - Lower lobe predominance: IPF.
  - Peripheral zone predominance: COP, chronic eosinophilic pneumonia (CEP).
  - Migratory infiltrates: COP, HP, eosinophilic pneumonia.

TABLE 2	Helpful Blood and Urine Tests to Evaluate ILDs

Laboratory Test	Interpretation
Complete blood count	Eosinophilia may support eosinophilic pneumonia or a drug-related ILD. Acute anemia may support alveolar hemorrhage.
Creatine kinase, aldolase, anti-Jo1 antibody	Elevated levels support polymyositis or dermatomyositis in patients with muscle pain.
Urinary sediment	RBC casts or dysmorphic RBCs may suggest a systemic vasculitis.
Antinuclear antibody, rheumatoid factor, antiribonucleic protein antibody, anticentromere antibody, antitopoisomerase antibody	Elevated results *may* support a CTD-related ILD.
C-ANCA, P-ANCA	Positive C-ANCA followed by the detection of antiproteinase 3 antibody supports Wegener's granulomatosis. Positive P-ANCA followed by the detection of antimyeloperoxidase antibody supports microscopic polyangiitis or Churg-Strauss syndrome.
Antiglomerular basement membrane antibody	A positive result in a patient with alveolar hemorrhage is diagnostic for Goodpasture syndrome.
Hypersensitivity pneumonitis serum precipitins	Results should be interpreted on the basis of clinical context. Sensitivity and specificity are variable.

C-ANCA, cytoplasmic antineutrophilic cytoplasmic antibody; CTD, connective tissue disease; ILD, interstitial lung disease; P-ANCA, perinuclear antineutrophilic cytoplasmic antibody; RBC, red blood cell.
Modified from Raghu G, Brown KK. Interstitial lung disease: clinical evaluation and keys to an accurate diagnosis. *Clin Chest Med* 2004;25:409–419.

Chest Computed Tomography
- High-resolution computed tomography (CT) (HRCT) is the most helpful radiographic test to evaluate ILDs and will also help guide location for lung biopsy and possible mediastinal lymph node sampling.
- Patterns on HRCT that may be associated with ILDs include the following[1,4]:
  - Reticular lines with honeycombing and traction bronchiectasis: IPF, CTD-related, asbestosis, sarcoidosis.
  - Nodules: pneumoconiosis, malignancy, rheumatoid arthritis (RA), Wegener's granulomatosis (WG), HP, sarcoidosis (nodular pattern particularly along bronchovascular bundles is common in sarcoidosis).
  - Cystic disease: LAM and PLCH.
  - Honeycombing: IPF, asbestosis, CTD-related, chronic HP.

- Ground-glass opacities: alveolar hemorrhage, HP, AIP, drug-induced diseases, pulmonary alveolar proteinosis (PAP), NSIP.
- Multi-focal consolidation: COP or secondary bronchiolitis obliterans organizing pneumonia (BOOP).
- Hilar/mediastinal lymphadenopathy: sarcoidosis, berylliosis, silicosis.
- "Crazy paving": PAP.

Lung Biopsy
- Biopsy is indicated to provide a definitive diagnosis before initiating therapy, to predict prognosis, to assess disease activity, and to exclude neoplastic or infectious processes that may mimic an ILD.
- There are three routes for lung biopsies: transbronchial lung biopsy via **bronchoscopy,** wedge biopsy via **open thoracotomy** or open lung biopsy, and biopsy via **video-assisted thoracoscopic surgery (VATS).**
- Bronchoscopy may be a useful minimally invasive way of gaining information about the ILDs.
  - **Bronchoalveolar lavage** (BAL) may help diagnose eosinophilic lung disease, PAP, and alveolar hemorrhage.
  - **Transbronchial biopsies** (TBBX) provide small tissue samples of lung parenchyma but may be useful in diagnosing certain diseases, especially ones that have a bronchovascular predilection, such sarcoidosis and lymphangitic carcinomatosis.
  - Other diseases that can diagnosed by TBBX include eosinophilic lung diseases, COP, AIP, and PLCH.
- Surgical lung biopsies, both open and VATS, have a high sensitivity for diagnosing ILDs because of larger tissue sampling that provides better evaluation of small airways and distal alveolar architecture. The diagnostic yield is estimated to be 92% and morbidity and mortality are relatively low at 2.5% and 0.3%, respectively. The choice between open thoracotomy and VATS is typically based on the expertise of the surgeon. Surgical lung biopsy can be deferred if a clinical diagnosis can be made with great certainty.[2]
- ILD pathology is frequently inhomogeneous. Thus, large specimens typically >2 cm in diameter from more than one lobe of the lung are ideal. It is best to sample from areas of active disease yet relatively preserved lung, as opposed to areas of dense fibrosis or honeycombing.
- Relative **contraindications** to a surgical lung biopsy include radiologic evidence of end-stage lung disease with honeycombing, serious cardiovascular disease, advanced age, mechanical ventilatory support with high O_2 requirements, or **when management will not be altered by pathologic information.**

Treatment

Idiopathic Interstitial Pneumonias
- There are six idiopathic interstitial pneumonias classified on the basis of histopathology (Tables 3 and 4).[2,6]
- A surgical lung biopsy is often needed to determine specific disease.
- **Known etiologies should be excluded,** for example, CTD, drugs, or pneumoconiosis.

Idiopathic Pulmonary Fibrosis
- This is the most common ILD.
- It typically affects patients >50 years of age and men much more commonly than women.

TABLE 3	American Thoracic Society/European Respiratory Society Criteria for Diagnosis of IPF without a Surgical Lung Biopsy
Major criteria (must have all four)	• Exclusion of known causes of ILDs (drugs, exposures, CTDs) • Abnormal PFTs: restrictive ventilatory defect (low vital capacity) and abnormal gas exchange (low DLCO or increased $P(A-a)O_2$ gradient or decreased PaO_2) • Bibasilar reticular abnormalities with minimal ground-glass opacities on HRCT • Transbronchial lung biopsy or BAL showing no features to support an alternative diagnosis
Minor criteria (must have three of four)	• Age >50 years • Insidious onset of otherwise unexplained dyspnea • Duration of illness ≥3 months • Bibasilar inspiratory crackles ("dry" or "Velcro")

BAL, bronchoalveolar lavage; CTD, connective tissue disease; DLCO, diffusing capacity of the lung for carbon monoxide; HRCT, high-resolution computed tomography; ILD, interstitial lung disease; IPF, idiopathic pulmonary fibrosis; PFTs, pulmonary function tests. Modified from American Thoracic Society. Idiopathic pulmonary fibrosis: diagnosis and treatment. International consensus statement. American Thoracic Society (ATS) and the European Respiratory Society (ERS). *Am J Respir Crit Care Med* 2000;161:646–664.

- Diagnosis of IPF can be made without a surgical lung biopsy (see Table 3).
- Distinguishing IPF from fibrotic NSIP may be very difficult.
- Corticosteroids are typically first-line therapy but show improvement only in 10% to 30% of patients.[5] The role of other immunosuppressants is disappointing and unclear.
- Early referral for lung transplantation is advised, if no contraindications exist.

Nonspecific Interstitial Pneumonia
- NSIP is a pattern of lung response to a variety of injuries.
- Diseases associated with NSIP include CTD such as scleroderma, rheumatoid arthritis, and polymyositis-dermatomyositis.
- Presentation is similar to IPF although NSIP may be a more subacute presentation, and patients may have signs and symptoms of a CTD.
- CXR is similar to other idiopathic interstitial pneumonias and HRCT characteristically shows ground-glass opacities with varying degrees of fibrosis.
- There are **three histologic subtypes:** cellular (type I), fibrosing (type II), and mixed (type III). Cellular NSIP shows diffuse inflammatory cell infiltration without significant collagen deposition whereas fibrosing NSIP shows alveolar septal thickening with fibroblastic proliferation and collagen deposition.
- NSIP, especially cellular and mixed types, responds to immunosuppressive therapy and has significantly better prognosis than IPF.[7]

TABLE 4 Summary of Features of the Idiopathic Interstitial Pneumonias

	IPF	NSIP	DIP and RB-ILD	COP/BOOP	AIP	LIP
Duration	Chronic (>12 months)	Subacute to chronic (months to years)	Subacute (weeks to months)	Subacute (<3 months)	Abrupt (1–2 weeks)	Chronic (>12 months)
HRCT findings	Peripheral, subpleural, basal predominance; Reticular opacities; Architectural distortion; Traction bronchiectasis; Honeycombing; Minimal "ground-glass"; Temporally heterogeneous with areas of end-stage honeycombing and adjacent unaffected areas	Peripheral subpleural, basal, symmetric; Ground-glass attenuation/consolidation; Lower lobe volume loss; Occasional subpleural sparing	DIP: diffuse ground-glass opacities in the middle and lower lungs; RB-ILD: bronchial wall thickening; centrilobular nodules; patchy ground-glass opacities	Subpleural or peribronchial; Patchy consolidation; Nodules	Diffuse and bilateral; Ground-glass opacities often with lobular sparing	Diffuse; Centrilobular nodules; Ground-glass attenuation; Septal and bronchovascular thickening; Thin-walled cysts
Treatment	Poor response to corticosteroids or cytotoxic agents	Corticosteroids and steroid-sparing agents	**Smoking cessation;** effectiveness of corticosteroids unknown	Corticosteroids	Effectiveness of corticosteroids unknown	Corticosteroids
Prognosis	5-year mortality = 80%; median survival 2–3 years after diagnosis	Cellular NSIP: 5-year mortality <10% (median survival >10 years) Fibrotic NSIP: 5-year mortality = 10% (median survival 6–8 years)	DIP: 5-year mortality <5% RB-ILD: no deaths reported	5-year mortality <5% (deaths are rare)	60% mortality in <6 months	Limited data

AIP, acute interstitial pneumonia; BOOP, bronchiolitis organizing pneumonia; COP, cryptogenic organizing pneumonia; DIP, desquamative interstitial pneumonia; HRCT, high-resolution computed tomography; IPF, idiopathic pulmonary fibrosis; LIP, lymphocytic interstitial pneumonia; NSIP, nonspecific interstitial pneumonitis; RB-ILD, respiratory bronchiolitis-interstitial lung disease.
Modified from King TE. Clinical advances in the diagnosis and therapy of the interstitial lung diseases. *Am J Respir Crit Care Med* 2005;172:268–279.

Cryptogenic Organizing Pneumonia
- COP is defined histologically by BOOP, which encompasses collagenous granulation tissue in the lumens of small airways and alveolar ducts with surrounding alveolar chronic inflammation.
- It classically presents like pneumonia, but the patient fails to respond to antibiotics.
- BOOP may be caused by drugs, inhalational exposures, or infection. COP can be diagnosed only if known causes of BOOP are excluded.
- The diagnosis can usually be made by transbronchial biopsy.
- CXR and HRCT show patchy peripheral infiltrates that may be migratory.
- This disease tends to be steroid responsive but has a high rate of relapse (up to 50%).[5]

Sarcoidosis

- This is the second most common ILD.
- It is a multisystem disorder most commonly affecting the lungs and is characterized by the presence of **noncaseating epitheliod granulomas.**
- Infectious granulomatous disease should be ruled out before initiating therapy.
- HRCT typically reveals nodular infiltrates in a lymphatic distribution with an **upper and midlung predominance.**
- Mediastinal and bilateral hilar lymphadenopathy is common.
- First-line treatment is steroids, but when and in whom to initiate therapy is still controversial. Generally, steroids for chronic ILD are not initiated unless disease fails to remit after an extended period of time (e.g., 12 to 18 months).
- Guidelines for use of steroid sparing agents are also unclear.

Hypersensitivity Pneumonitis

- HP has been referred to as an **"extrinsic allergic alveolitis."**
- It is a disease of inflammation caused by repeated inhalation of an inciting agent in a sensitized host.
- Presentation can be acute, subacute, or chronic depending on the type and level of exposure to the offending agent.
- Common forms of HP include bird fancier's disease, farmer's lung disease, and "hot tub lung," but dozens of others have been reported.
- HRCT is variable and includes centrilobular nodules, ground-glass opacities, or extensive honeycombing.
- Treatment includes removal of the offending exposure. Steroids can be used if very symptomatic.

Wegener's Granulomatosis

- WG is a **necrotizing granulomatous vasculitis** of the upper and lower respiratory tract and can cause a rapidly progressive glomerulonephritis.
- Presentations include sinusitis, epistaxis, ulcers, hemoptysis, and dyspnea.
- Specificity of cytoplasmic antineutrophilic cytoplasmic antibody (C-ANCA) testing is 99% but requires confirmation as an antibody to proteinase 3. Sensitivity ranges from 30% to 60%. There is a strong correlation between C-ANCA and disease activity.[5]
- Radiographic features are variable but include heterogeneous pulmonary infiltrates and pulmonary nodules.
- Pathologic specimens include the presence of inflammatory masses with necrotic areas and granulomatous vasculitis.

- The mainstay of treatment is oral cyclophosphamide plus corticosteroids. Remission is achieved in 75% of patients. If untreated, WG follows a rapidly fatal course.[5]

Eosinophilic Syndromes

- There are a variety of eosinophilic lung diseases including acute and chronic eosinophilic pneumonia (AEP and CEP, respectively), allergic bronchopulmonary aspergillosis, Churg-Strauss syndrome, and idiopathic hypereosinophilic syndrome.
- AEP typically has an acute, severe presentation characterized by diffuse infiltrates which often responds to corticosteroids.
- CEP is a slow, progressive disease that may have severe pulmonary and systemic symptoms. Radiographic findings commonly show peripheral pulmonary infiltrates. BAL eosinophils are often >50%, and peripheral eosinophilia is typical. The disease is responsive to corticosteroids but may relapse in approximately 50% of patients.

Pulmonary Alveolar Proteinosis

- The disease is characterized by the accumulation of periodic acid Schiff positive, lipid-rich proteinaceous material in the alveolar spaces.
- Granulocyte macrophage colony-stimulating factor (GM-CSF) mutations or acquired inactivating antibodies play a critical role in the pathogenesis.
- Disease onset is typically gradual.
- CXR shows a diffuse alveolar filling process.
- HRCT shows diffuse ground-glass opacities in a pattern referred to as "crazy paving."
- BAL demonstrates a thick milky effluent secondary to the large amount of proteinaceous material.
- Spontaneous recovery occurs in >25% of patients. Corticosteroids have no clear benefit.[5] Subcutaneous GM-CSF has shown some benefit. In patients with severe respiratory failure, whole-lung lavage with saline is necessary.

Lymphangioleiomyomatosis

- It is a rare cystic disease which causes progressive airflow obstruction in young women.
- Pneumothoraces are common.
- HRCT shows numerous uniform thin-walled cysts.
- Treatment options include antiestrogen agents or oophorectomy.

Pulmonary Langerhans Cell Histiocytosis

- PLCH is a disease that features activation and proliferation of Langerhans cells.
- >90% of cases occur in smokers.[5]
- Symptoms of cough and dyspnea typically occur insidiously.
- CXR shows diffuse micronodular infiltrates.
- HRCT shows numerous irregular cysts and centrilobular nodules.
- Smoking cessation is beneficial. Corticosteroid therapy early in the disease may be helpful.

Follow-Up and Monitoring

- Monitoring of the clinical course with clinical, radiographic, and physiologic parameters may be useful, especially if the patient is being treated. A battery of information including PFTs, arterial blood gas, and HRCT should be obtained at baseline and at regular intervals to assess progression or remission.

- Bone density assessment should be considered on an annual or twice-yearly basis for patients receiving chronic steroid therapy, especially patients with additional risk factors, and aggressive prevention and treatment of osteoporosis.
- Patients with a positive tuberculosis skin test (PPD) should be considered for isoniazid (INH) prophylaxis prior to the initiation of steroid and immunosuppressive therapy.
- Because untreated uveitis can lead to blindness, all patients with sarcoid should regularly receive a detailed ophthalmologic evaluation.
- Patients with ILD should be considered for intermittent echocardiographic monitoring for the development of pulmonary hypertension.

PULMONARY HYPERTENSION

General Principles

- Pulmonary hypertension (PH) is frequently encountered during the evaluation of respiratory or cardiac conditions.
- While PH can occur in the setting of **acute** conditions (e.g., pulmonary embolism, pulmonary edema, acute respiratory distress syndrome), **chronic** PH should prompt an evaluation to determine its origins and guide therapy.
- Internists and primary care physicians should be aware of basic pulmonary physiology, the differential diagnosis of PH, and how to evaluate the condition in order to identify which patients need therapeutic intervention.

Physiology of Pulmonary Circulation

- The pulmonary circulation's main role is to deliver deoxygenated blood from the right side of the heart into close proximity of the alveolar sacs to facilitate oxygen uptake into the bloodstream.
- Diffusion of oxygen from the alveolar sacs onto circulating blood cells occurs through a redundant parallel capillary network.
  - The vascular bed has tremendous surface area and capacitance.
  - Pulmonary circulatory system is a low-pressure circuit capable of handling the entire cardiac output as well as significant increases in blood flow during exertion.
- Autoregulation of arterioles through vasoconstriction and vasodilation matches ventilation and perfusion, which minimize shunting (i.e., low ventilation and high perfusion) and dead space (i.e., high ventilation and low perfusion).
- Vascular resistance is the ratio between the pressure decline across a circuit and the amount of blood flow through the circuit. Pulmonary vascular resistance (PVR) is calculated as:

$$PVR = \frac{\text{Mean PAP} - \text{mean PAOP}}{CO}$$

PAP = pulmonary artery pressure
PAOP = pulmonary artery occlusion (wedge) pressure
CO = cardiac output

- A low pulmonary vascular resistance allows the right ventricle to normally be a thin-walled chamber that is incapable of acutely generating high pressures (i.e., >50 mm Hg).
- **Normal mean PAP is <25 mm Hg and normal PVR is <2 "Wood units"** (or 150 to 250 dyn·sec·cm^{-5} or <15 to 25 MPa·sec·m^{-3}). One Wood unit (80 dyn·sec·cm^{-5} or 8 MPa·sec·m^{-3}) equals the PVR of an average healthy person presuming mean

PAP = 13 mm Hg, PCOP = 8, and CO = 5 L/min ([13 − 8]/5 = 1 mm Hg·min/L = 1 Wood unit). PVR measurements can be converted to an index by dividing by the body surface area in m^2.

Nomenclature and Pathophysiology

- PH is generically defined as **_mean_ PAP ≥25 mm Hg at rest or ≥30 mm Hg during exercise.**
- There are five categories of PH delineated in the 2003 Venice classification scheme (Table 5).[8]
- Mechanisms leading to PH differ among categories:
  - **Group I** encompasses conditions distinguished by **severe vascular remodeling** (see below).
  - **Group II** patients largely develop passive PH from elevated "downstream" pressures in the left side of the heart.
  - **Group III** patients encounter lung destruction as a result of underlying lung disease and/or vascular remodeling due to chronic hypoxemia.
  - **Group IV** diseases result from progressive obliteration of vasculature due to embolization of "foreign" material.
  - **Group V** conditions have variable mechanisms for developing PH, including vasculature compression, lung destruction, or vascular remodeling.
- **Pulmonary arterial hypertension (PAH)** is a category of diseases that share pathobiology resulting from **vasoconstriction, endothelial and smooth cell proliferation,** and **in situ thrombosis.**
  - Defined as elevated pulmonary artery pressures in the setting of normal LV filling pressures (i.e., PAOP ≤15 mm Hg).
  - Notable for severely elevated pulmonary artery pressures that can ultimately result in right ventricular failure.
  - Most common type is associated with collagen vascular diseases, particularly progressive systemic sclerosis or scleroderma.
- **Pulmonary venous hypertension** is the most frequently encountered type of PH in western countries, whereas PH associated with lung disease and/or hypoxemia is second most common.

Diagnosis

Clinical Presentation

- The core problem in PH is the deranged relationship between the flow of blood (i.e., the cardiac output) through the pulmonary vasculature and the pressures generated. This relationship is represented by the calculated PVR (see above).
- Initially, pulmonary pressures rise as the PVR is climbing, but most patients will be asymptomatic and the RV compensates through hypertrophy. Patients eventually become symptomatic due to limitations of cardiac output during periods of exertion.
  - Most common complaints are **dyspnea** and **diminished exercise tolerance.**
  - Patients also report **palpitations** during activity, which is the self-perception of tachycardia required to meet cardiac output demands during activity.
  - **Hoarseness** can also be encountered because of left recurrent laryngeal nerve compression by the enlarging pulmonary artery (i.e., Ortner's syndrome).
- As the condition progresses with additional increase in the PVR and RV afterload, peak cardiac output declines further until even resting cardiac output is depressed.

TABLE 5	2003 Venice Revised Classification of Pulmonary Hypertension

Group I: Pulmonary artery hypertension
Idiopathic pulmonary arterial hypertension (IPAH)
Familial pulmonary arterial hypertension (FPAH)
Associated with other diseases
   Collagen vascular diseases
   Congenital systemic to pulmonary shunts
   Portal hypertension
   Drugs and toxins
   HIV infection
   Other (glycogen storage diseases, Gaucher disease, hereditary hemorrhagic telangiectasia, hemoglobinopathies, myeloproliferative disorders, and splenectomy)
Associated with significant venous or capillary involvement
   Pulmonary veno-occlusive disease
   Pulmonary capillary hemangiomatosis

Group II: Pulmonary venous hypertension
Left-ventricular disease
Left-atrial disease
Left-sided valvular heart disease

Group III: Pulmonary hypertension associated with lung disease and/or hypoxia
Chronic obstructive lung disease
Interstitial lung disease
Alveolar-hypoventilation disorders
Sleep-disordered breathing
Chronic exposure to high altitude

Group IV: Pulmonary hypertension due to chronic thrombotic and/or embolic disease
Thromboembolic obstruction of proximal and/or distal arteries
Other types of pulmonary embolism: tumor, foreign material, parasites

Group V: Miscellaneous
Sarcoidosis
Pulmonary Langerhans' cell histiocytosis
Mediastinal compression of pulmonary arteries: tumor, adenopathy, fibrosing mediastinitis

Modified from Rubin LJ. Diagnosis and management of pulmonary arterial hypertension: ACCP evidence-based clinical guidelines. *Chest* 2004;126:7S–10S.

- **Fatigue** and **syncope** herald overt right heart failure exhibited by **lower extremity edema,** ascites, and early satiety/right upper quadrant pain from hepatic congestion.
- Ultimately, dilation of the RV and displacement of interventricular septum encroach upon the LV leading to impaired LV filling and precipitous decline in cardiac output.
- **The leading cause of death in patients with PAH is right heart failure.**

Diagnostic Testing

- Objectives for evaluation of chronic PH are to delineate the type of PH, identify contributory factors, and gauge its severity.
- PH should be considered in the following situations:
  - Unexplained dyspnea or diminished exercise tolerance
  - Isolated right heart failure
  - Risk factors for PAH (i.e., kindred with familial PAH, systemic sclerosis)
  - Incidentally discovered on echocardiogram
  - Suggestive ECG findings:
    - Right axis deviation
    - Right atrial enlargement (P wave taller than 2.5 mm in inferior leads)
    - Right ventricular hypertrophy (prominent R wave in V_1/V_2 or prominent S wave in V_5/V_6)
    - Right ventricular strain (ST-T segment depression and T-wave inversions in right precordial leads or pattern of S wave in I with Q-wave and T-wave inversion in III)
- Prominent central pulmonary arteries on CXR.
- An algorithm for evaluating PH is outlined in Figure 2. The evaluation can be done concurrently if echocardiography confirms the suspicion of PH.
- Patients with severe PH, which is considered discordant to degree of underlying cardiac or pulmonary conditions, require evaluation to exclude additional causes of PH as outlined in Figure 2.

Right Heart Catheterization

Before beginning therapy for PAH, right heart catheterization should be done to:
- Confirm elevated pulmonary artery and right heart pressures.
- Exclude left heart disease (i.e., normal LV filling pressures).
- Screen for missed left-to-right shunts.
- Infer prognosis by magnitude of right atrial pressure elevation and cardiac index depression.[9]

Vasodilator Challenge

- Perform an acute vasodilator challenge in PAH patients that are not in extreme right heart failure.
- Avoid if mean right atrial pressures are >20 mm Hg or cardiac indexes are <1.5 L/min/m.[2]
- Vasodilators of choice include inhaled nitric oxide, IV epoprostenol, and IV adenosine.
- Significant response is a **decline in mean pulmonary artery pressure ≥10 mm Hg to a concluding mean pulmonary artery pressure ≤40 mm Hg with stable or improved cardiac output.**[10]

Functional Assessment

- **Before beginning therapy for PAH, patients should have baseline functional assessments** performed to assist with longitudinal monitoring.
- The World Health Organization functional classification is detailed in Table 6. Prognosis is considerably worse for patients in functional Class III or IV than for patients in functional Class I or II.
- Unencouraged **6-minute walk test:** distance covered during a 6-minute walk has correlated with functional class in idiopathic pulmonary arterial hypertension patients.[11]

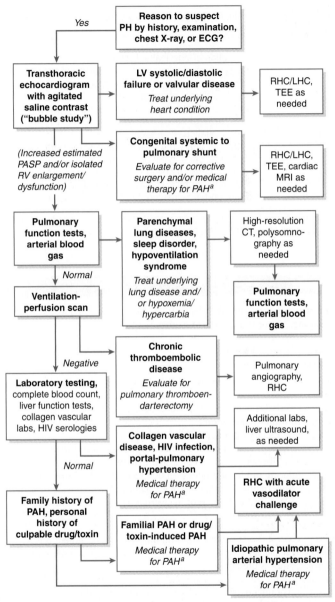

Figure 2. Diagnostic algorithm for the evaluation of pulmonary hypertension. [a]Prior to medical therapy, patients should complete right heart catheterization and baseline functional assessments. CT, computed tomography; ECG, electrocardiogram; LHC, left heart catheterization; LV, left ventricle; PAH, pulmonary artery hypertension; PASP, pulmonary artery systolic pressure; PH, pulmonary hypertension; RHC, right heart catheterization; RV, right ventricle; TEE, transesophageal echocardiogram.

TABLE 6	World Health Organization Functional Classification Scheme
Class I:	No limitation of physical activity Ordinary physical activity does not cause undue dyspnea or fatigue, chest pain, or near syncope.
Class II:	Slight limitation of physical activity Ordinary physical activity causes undue dyspnea or fatigue, chest pain, or near syncope.
Class III:	Marked limitation of physical activity Less than ordinary physical activity causes undue dyspnea or fatigue, chest pain, or near syncope.
Class IV:	Inability to perform any physical activity without symptoms Dyspnea and/or fatigue may be present at rest and discomfort is increased by any physical activity.

Modified from Rubin LJ. Diagnosis and management of pulmonary arterial hypertension: ACCP evidence-based clinical guidelines. *Chest* 2004;126:7S–10S.

Treatment

The treatment approach in PAH depends on the specific diagnosis, as mechanisms for developing PAH vary widely across categories (Table 5).

Treatment of Group I PAH

General Therapies
- Avoid vasoconstrictive substances: over-the-counter decongestants, nicotine, and cocaine.
- Avoid strong Valsalva maneuvers that can induce syncope: heavy lifting or straining during micturition or defecation.
- Avoid excessive dietary salt intake (2 to 3 g/day).
- Routine vaccinations against influenza and *Streptococcus pneumoniae*.
- Avoid pregnancy because of historically high maternal mortality.
- Minimize exposure to high altitudes (>5,000 feet), including airline travel.
- In patients with right-to-left shunts (e.g., patent foramen ovale or atrial septal defects), use filters on IVs to prevent inadvertent systemic air embolization.

Conventional Therapies
- **Diuretics** to control excess volume and minimize RV encroachment on LV.
- **Long-term oxygen therapy** to maintain SaO_2 >90% at all times, unless a right-to-left intracardiac shunt is present.
- **Warfarin** is recommended for patients without contraindications to chronic anticoagulation. Recommendation is stronger for idiopathic pulmonary arterial hypertension patients.[10] Caution must be exercised in patients with systemic sclerosis, cirrhosis/portal hypertension, and certain patients with congenital systemic to pulmonary shunts because of unique bleeding tendencies.
- **Digoxin** has weak inotropic effects on the RV but can also assist with management of tachyarrhythmias.

Pulmonary Vasomodulators
- Calcium-channel blockers:
  - Beneficial for only a very small minority of patients with PAH and **should _not_ be used without confirming vasoresponsiveness with an acute vasodilator challenge** (see above).[10]
  - Titrated to maximum tolerated dose over several weeks with close monitoring for side effects, such as fatigue, hypotension, and edema.
- Three classes of specific pulmonary vasomodulators: **endothelin-receptor antagonists, phosphodiesterase 5 inhibitors, and prostacyclin analogues** (i.e., prostanoids) are detailed in Table 7.
  - Choice of initial therapy is based on severity of condition, individual's psychosocial makeup, and comorbidities.
  - See Figure 3 for suggested treatment algorithm.[12]
    o The more advanced someone's condition, the more likely to need continuous prostanoid infusion.
    o Combining agents from different classes can be considered if treatment response to single agent is suboptimal.[12]

Interventional Therapies
Atrial Septostomy
- Percutaneously created right-to-left shunt in the inter-atrial septum.
- Indicated for severe, medically refractory right heart failure.[6]
- Net increase in oxygen delivery (DO$_2$) through augmentation of cardiac output (CO), in spite of lower oxygen saturations:

$$DO_2 = [(1.34 \times \text{hemoglobin} \times SaO_2) + PaO_2 \times .0031] \times CO \times 10$$

SaO$_2$ = systemic oxygen saturation
PaO$_2$ = partial pressure of oxygen dissolved in blood

Closure of Systemic to Pulmonary Shunt
- Percutaneous and surgical options, depending on type and size of defect.
- Determination requires calculation of net direction of shunting.
- Generally, shunts can be closed if ratio of pulmonary blood flow to systemic blood flow (Q_p/Q_s) is >1.5.
- The role of preclosure medical therapy is still evolving.

Lung Transplantation
- Indicated for PAH patients in advanced functional class despite maximal medical therapy.[13]
- Single or bilateral lung transplants can be done if there are no significant cardiac defects.
- Heart-lung transplantation required for patients with complex defects, including ventricular septal defects.
- RV recovers systolic function within the first few months of surgery.
- Thirty-day and 1-year survival is lower for the PAH group, but long-term results (median 4.5 years) are comparable to other transplanted groups.[14]

Treatment of Groups II to V PH
Group II
- Group II patients should receive appropriate therapy to lower left-sided filling pressures and optimize LV function in order to minimize "passive" PH.

TABLE 7 Vasomodulator Therapy for Pulmonary Arterial Hypertension

Drug Class	Drug	Route	Indication	Dose	Toxicity/Adverse Effects
Endothelin-receptor antagonists	Bosentan	PO	Classes III–IV	125 mg bid	Hepatotoxicity, teratogenicity, edema
Phosphodiesterase-5 inhibitors	Ambrisentan	PO	Classes II–IV	5–10 mg qd	Hepatotoxicity, teratogenicity, edema
	Sildenafil	PO	Classes I–IV	20 mg tid	Headache, hypotension, dyspepsia, epistaxis
Prostanoids	Iloprost	INH	Classes II–IV	2.5–5 mcg 6–9×/day	Headache, cough, syncope
	Treprostinil	SC, IV	Classes II–IV	Continuous infusion with variable dose	Extremity pain, headache, diarrhea, site pain (SC), skin abscess (SC), catheter complications (IV)
	Epoprostenol	IV	Classes III–IV	Continuous infusion with variable dose	Catheter complications, jaw pain, diarrhea, headache, extremity pain, skin flushing, rash

INH, inhalation; IV, intravenously; PO, by mouth; SC, subcutaneously.

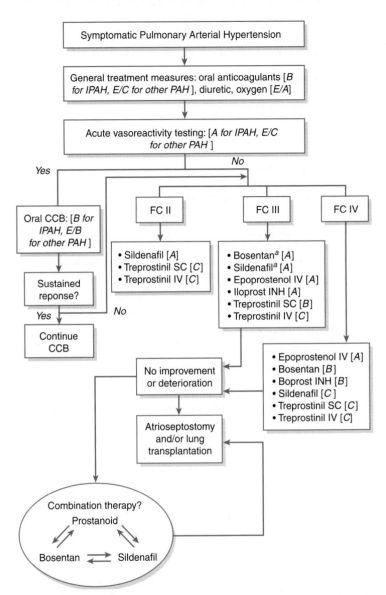

Figure 3. PAH treatment algorithm. [a]Not in order of preference. *A,* strong recommendation based on level of evidence and net benefit; *B,* moderate recommendation based on level of evidence and net benefit; *C,* weak recommendation based on level of evidence and net benefit; *E/A,* strong recommendation based on expert opinion only; *E/B,* moderate recommendation based on expert opinion only; *E/C,* weak recommendation based on expert opinion only. CCB, calcium channel blocker; FC, functional class (see Table 6); IPAH, idiopathic pulmonary artery hypertension; IV, intravenously; PAH, pulmonary artery hypertension; SC, subcutaneously. (From Badesch DB, Abman SH, Simonneau G, et al. Medical therapy for pulmonary arterial hypertension: updated ACCP evidence-based clinical practice guidelines. *Chest* 2007;131:1917–1928, with permission.)

- Therapeutic choices vary on the basis of underlying LV problem and are beyond the scope of this chapter.
- Diuretics to remove excess fluid.
- Antihypertensive agents to lower LV afterload.
- Rate-control agents to extend diastolic filling time.
- Inotropes to augment LV contractility.
- Interventional treatments:
  - Coronary revascularization
  - Valve repair
  - Restoration of sinus rhythm
  - LV augmentation therapy
- **There is no proven role for pulmonary vasomodulators.**

Group III

- Group III patients need therapy to minimize deleterious effects of lung disease on PH.
- Bronchodilators for management of airways disease.
- Appropriate immunomodulatory therapy for specific interstitial disease.
- Long-term oxygen therapy is essential if SaO_2 is $\leq 89\%$ or PaO_2 is ≤ 59.
  - Patients should be tested at rest and during exercise.
  - Patients not meeting criteria during daytime should be evaluated while sleeping; supplemental oxygen if SaO_2 is $\leq 88\%$ or PaO_2 is ≤ 55, especially when polycythemia is present.
- Patients with sleep-disordered breathing (i.e., obstructive sleep apnea) can develop mild PH and should receive appropriate treatment, most commonly noninvasive positive pressure ventilation (NIPPV). If hypoventilation coexists, hypercarbia can cause significant PH and should also be treated with NIPPV.
- Patients with alveolar hypoventilation syndromes, notable for severe hypercarbia and hypoxemia (e.g., central hypoventilation, chest wall diseases), can develop severe chronic PH and should be treated with NIPPV.
- **No proven role for pulmonary vasomodulators.**

Groups IV and V

- Group IV patients need careful evaluation to determine extent and location of vascular occlusions, which are most commonly venothromboemboli. Patients who have significant proximal vessel involvement (i.e., at least at the segmental vessel level) should be offered pulmonary thromboendarterectomy.[13]
- Management of Group V patients depends on the specific condition.

REFERENCES

1. Ryu JH, Daniels CE, Hartman TE, et al. Diagnosis of interstitial lung diseases. *Mayo Clin Proc* 2007;82:976–986.
2. King TE. Clinical advances in the diagnosis and therapy of the interstitial lung diseases. *Am J Respir Crit Care Med* 2005;172:268–279.
3. British Thoracic Society. The diagnosis, assessment and treatment of diffuse parenchymal lung disease in adults. *Thorax* 1999;54:S1–S30.
4. Raghu G, Brown KK. Interstitial lung disease: clinical evaluation and keys to an accurate diagnosis. *Clin Chest Med* 2004;25:409–419.
5. George RB, Light RW, Matthay MA, Matthay RA, eds. Diffuse interstitial and alveolar lung diseases. Chest Medicine: Essentials of Pulmonary and Critical Care Medicine. 6th Ed. Philadelphia, PA: Lippincott Williams & Wilkins, 2006:262–313.

6. American Thoracic Society. Idiopathic pulmonary fibrosis: diagnosis and treatment. International consensus statement. American Thoracic Society (ATS) and the European Respiratory Society (ERS). *Am J Respir Crit Care Med* 2000;161:646–664.
7. Kim DS, Collard HR, King TE. Classification and natural history of the idiopathic interstitial pneumonias. *Proc Am Thorac Soc* 2006;3:285–292.
8. Rubin LJ. Diagnosis and management of pulmonary arterial hypertension: ACCP evidence-based clinical guidelines. *Chest* 2004;126:7S–10S.
9. D'Alonzo GE, Barst RJ, Ayres SM, et al. Survival in patients with pulmonary arterial hypertension: results from a national prospective registry. *Ann Intern Med* 1991;115:343–349.
10. Badesch DB, Abman SH, Ahearn GS, et al. Medical therapy for pulmonary arterial hypertension: ACCP evidence-based clinical guidelines. *Chest* 2004;126:35S–62S.
11. Miyamoto S, Nagaya N, Satoh T, et al. Clinical correlates and prognostic significance of six-minute walk test in patients with primary pulmonary hypertension: comparison with cardiopulmonary exercise testing. *Am J Respir Crit Care Med* 2000;161:487–492.
12. Badesch DB, Abman SH, Simonneau G, et al. Medical therapy for pulmonary arterial hypertension: updated ACCP evidence-based clinical practice guidelines. *Chest* 2007;131:1917–1928.
13. Doyle RL, McCrory D, Channick RN, et al. Surgical treatments/interventions for pulmonary arterial hypertension: ACCP evidence-based clinical practice guidelines. *Chest* 2004;126:63S–71S.
14. Trulock EP, Christie JD, Edwards LB, et al. Registry of the International Society for Heart and Lung Transplantation: twenty-fourth official adult lung and heart-lung transplantation report—2007. *J Heart Lung Transplant* 2007;26:782–795.

14

Sleep Disorders
Tonya D. Russell

Introduction

Sleep disorders are a common problem among the primary care population. One survey of a primary care population estimated that 60% of patients exhibited symptoms consistent with at least one sleep disorder. Within this population, 23.6% of patients reported symptoms consistent with obstructive sleep apnea (OSA) syndrome, 32.3% of patients reported symptoms consistent with insomnia, and 29.3% of patients reported symptoms consistent with restless legs syndrome (RLS).[1]

OBSTRUCTIVE SLEEP APNEA

General Principles

Epidemiology
- The prevalence of OSA, as defined by an apnea-hypopnea index (AHI) >5 events per hour, is estimated to be 24% of men and 9% of women.
- The prevalence of obstructive sleep apnea-hypopnea syndrome (OSAHS), as defined by an AHI >5 in association with daytime sleepiness, is 4% of men and 2% of women.[2]

Pathophysiology
- Obstructive apneas and hypopneas result from excessive soft tissue or structural abnormalities of the upper airway resulting in cessation of breathing (apneas) or decreased airflow (hypopneas) during sleep.
- Obstructive events can be associated with snores, arousals from sleep, and oxygen desaturations.

Medical Complications
- Patients with OSA are more likely to be hypersomnolent.
- Patients with OSAHS have an increased risk of motor vehicle collisions.[3,4]
- OSAHS increases the risk for hypertension, with the risk increasing with the severity of the OSA.[5,6] Treatment of OSA can improve the control of hypertension, but it may take several weeks before the effects are seen.[7–10]
- Patients with severe untreated OSAHS (AHI >30) have a higher risk of fatal and nonfatal cardiovascular events when compared with healthy controls and patients with severe OSAHS treated with continuous positive airway pressure (CPAP).[11] There was no difference in other cardiovascular risk factors between the untreated and the CPAP treated severe OSAHS groups.
- There is increased risk of congestive heart failure in patients with OSA.[12]

- OSA is associated with an adjusted hazard ratio of 1.97 for risk of stroke or death from any cause.[13]
- Studies have demonstrated impaired glucose tolerance and increased insulin resistance in patients with OSA even when controlled for obesity.[14,15] Treatment of OSA with CPAP has been demonstrated to improve glycemic control.[16]

Diagnosis

Clinical Presentation
- Common signs and symptoms of OSA are outlined in Table 1.[17]
- Other conditions that result in muscle hypotonia, increased weight, or craniofacial abnormalities may be associated with OSA, such as hypothyroidism, acromegaly, or Down syndrome.
- Alcohol and medications with sedative properties can worsen OSA because of decreased muscle tone and increased arousal threshold.

Diagnostic Testing
- The gold standard for diagnosing OSA is with an overnight polysomnogram.
  - Typically, the monitoring includes electroencephalogram, electrooculogram, and electromyogram leads for sleep staging.
  - In addition, respiratory effort is monitored by thoracic and abdominal belts, as well as airflow via thermistor or pressure transducer.
  - Electrocardiogram and oxygen saturations are recorded, and in situations in which hypoventilation is a concern, transcutaneous carbon dioxide levels may be monitored.
- Currently, portable polysomnographic monitoring devices are not recommended for unattended studies (i.e., a technician is not available by the bedside).
- Polysomnogram studies are often performed as split studies. Per the American Academy of Sleep Medicine recommendations, if a patient has an AHI >40 events per hour during the first 2 hours of sleep, a CPAP titration can be started during the same study.[18]
- The severity of OSA can be defined as outlined in Table 2.[19]

TABLE 1	Signs and Symptoms of OSAHS

Obesity
Snoring
Awakening snorting or gasping
Witnessed apneas
Excessive daytime somnolence
Morning headaches
Large neck circumference (>40 cm^3)
Unrefreshing sleep
Poorly controlled hypertension
Craniofacial abnormalities (micrognathia, retrognathia, macroglossia)
Nocturnal oxygen desaturations
Hypercapnia not explained by other etiology

OSAHS, obstructive sleep apnea-hypopnea syndrome.

TABLE 2	Severity of OSA Based on Sleepiness and Apnea-Hypopnea Index	
	Sleepiness	Apnea-Hypopnea Index
Mild	Sedentary activities only	5–15 events/hour
Moderate	Meetings, concerts, presentations	15–30 events/hour
Severe	Driving, conversation, eating	>30 events/hour

Modified from American Academy of Sleep Medicine Task Force. Sleep-related breathing disorders in adults: recommendations for syndrome definition and measurement techniques in clinical research. *Sleep* 1999;22:667–689.

Treatment

Continuous Positive Airway Pressure

- CPAP is the standard therapy for OSAHS. It is typically initiated for home use after a CPAP titration has been performed in a sleep center. During titrations, CPAP is usually increased to relieve snoring, as well as continued obstructive apneas and hypopneas.
- Autotitrating positive airway pressure (APAP) devices are available. These machines titrate through a range of pressures on the basis of algorithms within the device to determine snoring and changes in airflow.
- Several studies have shown that APAP is as effective as CPAP in treating OSAHS.
  - In patients who require a wide range of pressures to resolve their OSAHS and have trouble tolerating higher pressures during the entire night (i.e., a patient who requires lower pressures in the lateral position or during nonrapid eye movement sleep and higher pressures in the supine position or during rapid eye movement sleep), APAP may be a more tolerable option.
  - However, APAP is probably not a good option for patients with significant comorbid conditions.[20]
- Patients who have difficulty in tolerating CPAP may prefer bi-level positive airway pressure devices.
- Potential side effects and barriers to use of CPAP, as well as potential remedies, are outlined in Table 3.

Surgery

- Patients who want to consider surgery for OSAHS should be evaluated by an otolaryngologist to determine whether the area of upper airway obstruction is amenable to surgery.
- **Tracheotomy** can be curative for OSA, as the area of upper airway obstruction is bypassed.
- **Uvulopalatopharyngoplasty** is a common surgery performed for OSA. Response to surgery varies from 40% to 60% depending upon how surgical success is defined.
- Patients with higher AHIs are less likely to respond.
- Complications can include voice changes, foreign body sensation, and nasal reflux.[21]
- **Laser-assisted uvulopalatoplasty** differs from uvulopalatopharyngoplasty in that the tonsils and pharyngeal pillars are not excised. Currently, the recommendations for use of laser-assisted uvulopalatoplasty **are only in primary snoring, not OSA.**[22]
- Patients being considered for surgical treatment for snoring or OSA should undergo evaluation with overnight polysomnogram prior to surgery. If OSA is present on the

TABLE 3	Complications Related to CPAP and Potential Remedies
Complication	**Remedy**
Excessive nasal dryness/ epistaxis	Use humidifier
Excessive nasal congestion	Decrease humidity; nasal steroids
Mouth dryness	Use humidifier; full face mask
Eye dryness	Ensure good mask fit to limit air leaks
Claustrophobia	Use lower profile masks such as nasal pillows
Aerophagia	Lowest possible therapeutic pressure; APAP
Frequent mask leaks	Refit with new mask; shave facial hair
Skin breakdown	Proper mask fit to prevent excessive tightening of head gear

APAP, autotitrating positive airway pressure; CPAP, continuous positive airway pressure.

baseline study, a postsurgical polysomnogram should be performed to document resolution of the OSAHS.[23]

Dental Devices

- Oral appliances can be used to treat OSA. Overall, the success rate is approximately 50%, although patients with more severe OSA seem to be less likely to respond.
- Complications from oral appliances include temperomandibular joint pain, tooth and gum irritation, and occlusal changes, although most complications are temporary.
- Dental devices should be fitted by practitioners specializing in dental sleep medicine.
- Patients being considered for dental appliances for snoring or OSA should undergo evaluation with overnight polysomnogram before starting therapy. If OSA is present on the baseline study, a repeat polysomnogram should be performed with the appliance in place to document resolution of the OSAHS.[24]

Medical Therapy

- Weight reduction should be encouraged in obese patients.
- Treatment of underlying endocrine disorders, such as hypothyroidism and acromegaly, should be pursued.
- Patients should limit alcohol, sedatives, and narcotics, which could worsen OSA.
- In patients with continued sleepiness despite adequate therapy other potential causes for the daytime somnolence, as outlined in Table 4, should be considered.

TABLE 4	Differential Diagnosis for Excessive Daytime Somnolence

Sleep disordered breathing—obstructive or central sleep apnea
Restless legs syndrome/periodic limb movement disorder
Insufficient sleep time
Environmental sleep disturbance
Narcolepsy
Idiopathic hypersomnia

- Modafinil is a stimulant medication approved for use in patients with continued daytime sleepiness despite adequate therapy of OSAHS with CPAP and no other obvious cause for sleepiness.[25]

INSOMNIA

General Principles

- Insomnia typically encompasses the complaint of inability to fall asleep or maintain sleep.
- While approximately one third of the general population has experienced insomnia at some point, of those patients with severe insomnia, approximately 80% have reported symptoms for more than a year.[26]
- Table 5 lists causes of insomnia and their associated characteristics.

Diagnosis

Clinical Presentation

- A thorough history to determine sleep schedule, sleep hygiene, confounding factors, such as underlying medical conditions or mental disorders, and medication use should be performed.
- In addition, a description of the sleep environment should be obtained to assess for environmental disturbances.
- Symptoms suggestive of other sleep disorders, which could cause fragmentation of sleep (RLS, periodic limb movement disorder, or sleep disordered breathing), should be elicited.

TABLE 5	Causes of Insomnia and Associated Characteristics
Cause	Characteristic
Restless legs syndrome	Uncomfortable sensation in legs interfering with ability to fall asleep
Pain	Any underlying condition associated with chronic pain
Mental disorder	Underlying depression or anxiety
Adjustment insomnia	Associated with acute stressor
Inadequate sleep hygiene	Poor sleep habits, i.e., irregular sleep times; excessive caffeine, nicotine, or alcohol use; using the bedroom for nonsleep-related activities
Psychophysiologic insomnia	Increased arousal, frequent inability to "turn off thoughts"
Idiopathic insomnia	Occurring since childhood
Drug or substance abuse	Chronic use of pain medicines, stimulants, alcohol, or sedative hypnotics
Circadian rhythm disturbance	Advanced or delayed sleep phase

Diagnostic Testing

- Polysomnogram should be performed if another underlying sleep disorder is suspected.
- Sleep logs and interviews of bed partners may give additional data regarding the underlying sleep disturbance.[27]
- An actigraph is a wristwatch-type device that measures movement and therefore can act as a surrogate for assessing sleep. Actigraphy may be useful in monitoring treatment effect in patients with insomnia, although it may underestimate the total sleep time as compared with polysomnography.[28]

Treatment

Medication

- Over-the-counter medications are frequently used by patients to treat insomnia. Table 6 lists common over-the-counter medications and their potential side effects. There are no strong data to support the efficacy of these agents.[29]
- The prescription medications that are approved for treatment of insomnia are the **benzodiazepine receptor agonists** and the **melatonin receptor agonists.** Of these, eszopiclone (nonbenzodiazepine hypnotic) and ramelteon (melatonin agonist) are the only ones FDA approved for long-term use. The benzodiazepine receptor agonists are considered controlled substances, whereas the melatonin receptor agonists are not.[29]
- Frequently, sedating antidepressants are also prescribed for insomnia in off-label use, although data supporting their use are lacking. Table 7 outlines the prescription medications for insomnia as well as some of the potential side effects.[29]
- Treatment of underlying medical or mental conditions which could be contributing to insomnia should be instituted.

TABLE 6	Over-the-Counter Medications for Insomnia and Their Side Effects	
Medication	**Dosage**	**Side Effects**
Antihistamine (diphenhydramine)	25–75 mg	Hangover effect, dizziness, anticholinergic effects (dry mouth, urinary retention, delirium)
Melatonin	0.3–5 mg	Fatigue, headache, drowsiness, possible vasoconstriction
Valerian root	1.5–3 g of herb or root 400–900 mg of aqueous extract	Dizziness, headache, excitability, hepatic toxicity (in combination products)
Alcohol	Self-dosing	Impaired cognition and motor skills, anterograde amnesia; although initially sedating, as alcohol is metabolized it can cause fragmentation of sleep

TABLE 7 — Prescription Medications Used for Insomnia

Medication	Class	Dosage	Half-Life	Side Effects
Temazepam	Benzodiazepine	7.5–30 mg	11 hours	Hangover effect, anterograde amnesia, rebound insomnia, withdrawal symptoms
Eszopiclone	Nonbenzodiazepene	1–3 mg	6 hours	Hangover effect, headache, dizziness, possible impaired memory at peak concentrations
Zolpidem		5–10 mg	4 hours	
Zolpidem extended release		6.25–12.5 mg	4 hours	
Zaleplon		5–10 mg	1 hour	
Ramelteon	Melatonin receptor agonist	8 mg	1–3 hours	Dizziness, headache, fatigue, somnolence
Trazodone	Antidepressant	50–100 mg	6–12 hours	Headache, somnolence, rebound insomnia, priapism
Amitriptyline	Tricyclic antidepressant	25–100 mg	10–26 hours	Somnolence, dizziness, dry mouth, arrhythmias
Mirtazapine	Antidepressant	7.5–45 mg	20–40 hours	Somnolence, dry mouth, increased weight

TABLE 8	Components of Cognitive Behavioral Therapy for Insomnia
Component	**Description**
Sleep hygiene education	Avoiding excessive caffeine, alcohol, nicotine; optimizing sleeping environment
Stimulus control	Consistent wake-up time, out of bed during prolonged awakenings, reserving the bedroom for sleeping, avoiding napping
Sleep restriction	Minimize the amount of time spent in bed not sleeping
Imagery	Form a relaxing image which helps prevent intrusive thoughts from interfering with sleep
Muscle relaxation	Progressive relaxation of muscle groups to relieve muscle tension

Nonpharmacologic Therapy

- Cognitive behavioral therapy (CBT) encompasses a wide variety of techniques aimed at breaking the cycle of insomnia.[30] Table 8 describes various components of CBT for insomnia.
- CBT has been shown to be beneficial in improving the nighttime and daytime symptoms associated with insomnia.[31–33]

RESTLESS LEGS SYNDROME

General Principles

Epidemiology

- Prevalence of RLS is estimated to be between 2.5% and 15% of the population.
- The severity of symptoms can be highly variable.
- In some patients with RLS, there is a hereditary link.[34]

Pathophysiology

- The role of dopamine in RLS has been most strongly supported by the improvement of symptoms with dopamine agonists.[35]
- Iron is necessary for the rate-limiting step in dopamine synthesis. Therefore, low iron levels may decrease dopamine synthesis.[36] Ferritin levels <50 mcg/L have been associated with increased severity of RLS. Iron supplementation is recommended in the setting of RLS when ferritin is <50 mcg/L.[37]

Diagnosis

- RLS is a clinical diagnosis in which the four essential criteria, as outlined in Table 9, are met.[38]
- Periodic limb movements are frequently seen on the polysomnograms of patients with RLS, although a polysomnogram is not required to make the diagnosis of RLS.
- RLS can be associated with other underlying conditions such as pregnancy, uremia, and anemia.

TABLE 9	Clinical Criteria for Restless Legs Syndrome

Urge to move legs associated with an uncomfortable sensation in legs
The urge to move legs or the uncomfortable sensation is worsened during periods of inactivity
Movement temporarily improves or relieves the urge to move or uncomfortable sensation in the legs
Symptoms are worse in the evening

Modified from Allen RP, Picchietti D, Hening WA, et al. Restless legs syndrome: diagnostic criteria, special considerations, and epidemiology. A report from the restless legs syndrome diagnosis and epidemiology workshop at the National Institutes of Health. *Sleep Medicine* 2003;4:101–119.

- Pharmacologic agents such as caffeine, nicotine, alcohol, dopamine antagonists, diphenhydramine, serotonin reuptake inhibitors, and tricyclic antidepressants may worsen RLS.[39]

Treatment

- Lifestyle modification to avoid the above mentioned precipitants should be attempted.
- Dopaminergic agents are the mainstay of therapy.[39]
- Gabapentin at a starting dose of 600 mg and titrated up to 2,400 mg as needed resulted in improvement in RLS symptoms without significant side effects.[40]
- Benzodiazepines and opioids can also be effective in treating RLS symptoms.
- Supplementation of iron in iron-deficient patients.

REFERENCES

1. Kushida CA, Nichols DA, Simon RD, et al. Symptom-based prevalence of sleep disorders in an adult primary care population. *Sleep Breath* 2000;4:11–15.
2. Young T, Palta M, Dempsey J, et al. The occurrence of sleep-disordered breathing among middle-aged adults. *N Engl J Med* 1993;328:1230–1235.
3. Young T, Blustein J, Finn L, Palta M. Sleep-disordered breathing and motor vehicle accidents in a population-based sample of employed adults. *Sleep* 1997;20:608–613.
4. Terán-Santos J, Jiménez-Gómez A, Cordero-Guevara J, et al. The association between sleep apnea and the risk of traffic accidents. *N Engl J Med* 1999;340:847–851.
5. Nieto FJ, Young T, Lind BK, et al. Association of sleep-disordered breathing, sleep apnea, and hypertension in a large community-based study. *JAMA* 2000;282:1829–1836.
6. Peppard PE, Young T, Palta M, Skatrud J. Prospective study of the association between sleep-disordered breathing and hypertension. *N Engl J Med* 2000;342:1378–1384.
7. Becker HF, Jerrentrup A, Ploch T, et al. Effect of nasal continuous positive airway pressure treatment on blood pressure in patients with obstructive sleep apnea. *Circulation* 2003; 107:68–73.
8. Logan AG, Tkacova R, Perlikowski SM, et al. Refractory hypertension and sleep apnoea: effect of CPAP on blood pressure and baroreflex. *Eur Respir J* 2003;21:241–247.
9. Robinson GV, Smith DM, Langford BA, et al. Continuous positive airway pressure does not reduce blood pressure in nonsleepy hypertensive OSA patients. *Eur Respir J* 2006; 27:1229–1235.
10. Campos-Rodriguez F, Grilo-Reina A, Perez-Ronchel J, et al. Effect of continuous positive airway pressure on ambulatory BP in patients with sleep apnea and hypertension: a placebo-controlled trial. *Chest* 2006;129:1459–1467.

11. Marin JM, Carrizo SJ, Vicente E, Agusti AGN. Long-term cardiovascular outcomes in men with obstructive sleep apnoea-hypopnoea with or without treatment with continuous positive airway pressure: an observational study. *Lancet* 2005;365:1046–1053.

12. Shahar E, Whitney C, Redline S, et al. Sleep-disordered breathing and cardiovascular disease: cross-sectional results of the Sleep Heart Health Study. *Am J Respir Crit Care Med* 2001;163:19–25.

13. Yaggi HK, Concato J, Kernan WN, et al. Obstructive sleep apnea as a risk factor for stroke and death. *N Engl J Med* 2005;353:2034–2041.

14. Ip MSM, Ng MTM. Obstructive sleep apnea is independently associated with insulin resistance. *Am J Respir Crit Care Med* 2002;165:670–676.

15. Punjabi NM, Shahar E, Redline S, et al. Sleep-disordered breathing, glucose intolerance, and insulin resistance: the Sleep Heart Health Study. *Am J Epidemiol* 2004;160:521–530.

16. Babu AR, Herdegen J, Fogelfeld L, et al. Type 2 diabetes, glycemic control, and continuous positive airway pressure in obstructive sleep apnea. *Arch Intern Med* 2005;165:447–452.

17. Kushida CA, Efron B, Guilleminault C. A predictive morphometric model for the obstructive sleep apnea syndrome. *Ann Intern Med* 1997;127:581–587.

18. Kushida CA, Littner MR, Morgenthaler T, et al. Practice parameters for the indications for polysomnography and related procedures: an update for 2005. *Sleep* 2005;28:499–521.

19. American Academy of Sleep Medicine Task Force. Sleep-related breathing disorders in adults: recommendations for syndrome definition and measurement techniques in clinical research. *Sleep* 1999;22:667–689.

20. Berry RB, Parish JM, Hartse KM. The use of auto-titrating continuous positive airway pressure for treatment of adult obstructive sleep apnea. *Sleep* 2002;25:148–173.

21. Sher AE, Schechtman KB, Piccirillo JF. The efficacy of surgical modifications of the upper airway in adults with obstructive sleep apnea syndrome. *Sleep* 1996;19:156–177.

22. Littner M, Kushida CA, Hartse K, et al. Practice parameters for the use of laser-assisted uvulopalatoplasty: an update for 2000. *Sleep* 2001;24:603–619.

23. Thorpy M, Chesson A, Derderian S, et al. Practice parameters for the treatment of obstructive sleep apnea in adults: the efficacy of surgical modifications of the upper airway. *Sleep* 1996;19:152–155.

24. Ferguson KA, Cartwright R, Rogers R, Schmidt-Nowara W. Oral appliances for snoring and obstructive sleep apnea: a review. *Sleep* 2006;29:244–262.

25. Morgenthaler TI, Kapen S, Lee-Chiong T, et al. Practice parameters for the medical therapy of obstructive sleep apnea. *Sleep* 2006;29:1031–1035.

26. Sateia MJ, Doghramji K, Hauri PJ, Morin CM. Evaluation of chronic insomnia. *Sleep* 2000;23:243–308.

27. Chesson A, Hartse K, McDowell Anderson W, et al. Practice parameters for the evaluation of chronic insomnia. *Sleep* 2000;23:237–241.

28. Valliéres A, Morin CM. Actigraphy in the assessment of insomnia. *Sleep* 2003;26:902–906.

29. Morin AK, Jarvis CI, Lynch AM. Therapeutic options for sleep-maintenance and sleep-onset insomnia. *Pharmacotherapy* 2007;27:89–110.

30. Morgenthaler TI, Kramer M, Alessi C, et al. Practice parameters for the psychological and behavioral treatment of insomnia: an update. An American Academy of Sleep Medicine report. *Sleep* 2006;29:1415–1419.

31. Harvey AG, Sharpley AL, Ree MJ, et al. An open trial of cognitive therapy for chronic insomnia. *Behav Res Ther* 2007;45:2491–2501.

32. Edinger JD, Wohlgemuth WK, Radtke RA, et al. Cognitive behavioral therapy for treatment of chronic primary insomnia—a randomized controlled trial. *JAMA* 2001;285:1856–1864.

33. Morin CM, Bootzin RR, Buysse DJ, et al. Psychological and behavioral treatment of insomnia: update of recent evidence (1998–2004). *Sleep* 2006;29:1398–1414.

34. Masood A, Phillips B. Epidemiology of restless legs syndrome. In: Chokroverty S, Hening W, Walters A, eds. Sleep and Movement Disorders. Philadelphia, PA: Elsevier Science, 2003:316–321.

35. Henning WA, Allen RP, Earley CJ, et al. An update on the dopaminergic treatment of restless legs syndrome and periodic limb movement disorder. *Sleep* 2004;27:560–583.
36. Allen RP, Earley CJ. Dopamine and iron in the restless legs syndrome. In: Chokroverty S, Hening W, Walters A, eds. Sleep and Movement Disorders. Philadelphia, PA: Elsevier Science, 2003:333–340.
37. Sun ER, Chen CA, Ho G, et al. Iron and the restless legs syndrome. *Sleep* 1998;21:381–387.
38. Allen RP, Picchietti D, Hening WA, et al. Restless legs syndrome: diagnostic criteria, special considerations, and epidemiology. A report from the restless legs syndrome diagnosis and epidemiology workshop at the National Institutes of Health. *Sleep Med* 2003;4:101–119.
39. Hening WA. Current guidelines and standards of practice for restless legs syndrome. *Am J Med* 2007;120:S22–S27.
40. Garcia-Borreguero D, Larrosa O, de la Llave Y, et al. Treatment of restless legs syndrome with gabapentin: a double-blind, crossover study. *Neurology* 2002;59:1573–1579.

15 Pleural Effusion and Solitary Pulmonary Nodule

Devin P. Sherman, Martin L. Mayse, and
Thomas M. De Fer

PLEURAL EFFUSION

General Principles

Definition

- A pleural effusion is the abnormal accumulation of fluid in the pleural space.
- The pleural space normally contains only a small amount of fluid that is not radiographically apparent.
- Effusions are categorized into two types: transudates and exudates. This differentiation is defined with laboratory testing (see later) and identifies effusions secondary to diseases that do not directly damage the pleural surfaces (transudates) versus diseases that do directly damage the pleural surfaces. This designation is important since the management of the two types of effusions is distinctly different.
  - **Transudative pleural effusions** result from the alteration of hydrostatic and oncotic factors that increase the formation or decrease the absorption of pleural fluid (e.g., increased mean capillary pressure [heart failure] or decreased oncotic pressure [cirrhosis or nephrotic syndrome]).
  - **Exudative pleural effusions** occur when damage or disruption of the normal pleural membranes or vasculature (e.g., tumor involvement of the pleural space, infection, inflammatory conditions, or trauma) leads to increased capillary permeability or decreased lymphatic drainage.
- When transudative effusions are identified, the underlying systemic disease should also be identified (congestive heart failure [CHF], liver disease, kidney disease) and treatment should be directed toward the primary disorder.
- Exudative effusions frequently indicate a process (malignancy, infection, etc.) that directly injures the pleura and deserves further investigation and therapy, typically focused on the pleural space.

Etiology

Pleural effusions occur in a wide variety of disease states; however, **90% of pleural effusions are the result of only five diseases**[1]:
- CHF (36%).
- Pneumonia (22%).
- Malignancy (14%).
- Pulmonary embolism (PE) (11%).
- Viral disease (7%).

Diagnosis

Clinical Presentation

The underlying cause of the effusion typically dictates the symptoms, although patients may be asymptomatic. Pleural inflammation, abnormal pulmonary mechanics, and worsened alveolar gas exchange produce symptoms and signs of disease.

- Inflammation of the parietal pleura leads to pain in locally (intercostal) involved areas or referred (phrenic) distributions (shoulder).
- Dyspnea is frequent and may be present out of proportion to the size of the effusion.
- Cough can occur.

History and Physical Examination

- Unfortunately, a definitive diagnosis based upon pleural fluid analysis is possible in less than half of all effusions. Therefore, it is important to define the clinical setting of a pleural effusion with a thorough history and physical examination to aid in diagnosis.
- Obtain a detailed **history with review of systems** to identify symptoms of CHF, underlying malignancy, PE, myocardial infarction, surgery or trauma, connective tissue diseases, or other underlying or recent infections.
- **Social history** focused on smoking history and possible TB exposures.
- **Family history** focused on malignancy, heart disease, and connective tissue diseases.
- **Signs of a pleural effusion on physical exam** include dullness to chest percussion, decreased or absent tactile fremitus, and decreased breath sounds. A shifted trachea or a pleural rub may be present. The physical exam should also focus on signs of potential underlying diseases, such as CHF or pneumonia that could cause an effusion.

Diagnostic Testing

Prior to any invasive diagnostic or therapeutic procedure, the patient should undergo imaging to confirm the presence, character, and size of the effusion.

Chest Radiography

- Pleural effusions are often initially detected by chest radiography (CXR).
- Effusions are seen as blunting of the costophrenic angle or opacification of the base of the hemithorax without the loss of volume of the hemithorax (which would suggest atelectasis) or the presence of air bronchograms (which would suggest pneumonia).
- CXR can also detect masses or infiltrates that may give clues to an etiology.
- Decubitus chest films are frequently obtained to demonstrate that at least a portion of the fluid is not loculated and amenable to thoracentesis (Table 1 and Fig. 1).

Chest Computed Tomography

- Computed tomography (CT) with contrast given by PE protocol is recommended if PE is suspected.
- It can be used to further define masses, lymphadenopathy, or other abnormal findings on CXR.
- CT with contrast given by standard protocol (in which the images are timed such that the contrast bolus is in the systemic vasculature) helps differentiate pleural fluid from lung masses and atelectatic lung; it also serves to identify and define the extent of pleural fluid thickening and pleural nodularity.

TABLE 1	Indications for Thoracentesis

- Pleural effusion of unknown etiology
- Fever in setting of long-standing pleural effusion
- Air-fluid level in the pleural space
- Rapid change in size of effusion
- Concern that empyema is developing

Thoracic Ultrasonography
- Ultrasound is one of the best modalities to assess for pleural fluid loculations.
- It provides real-time guidance for pleural procedures and can reduce both the complications and failure rate of thoracentesis.

Thoracentesis
Once a pleural effusion has been identified, the clinician must decide whether to sample the pleural fluid for either diagnostic or therapeutic benefit, or both. Table 1

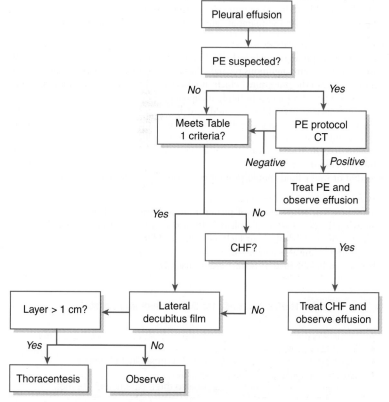

Figure 1. Evaluation of the unknown pleural effusion. CHF, congestive heart failure; CT, computed tomography; PE, pulmonary embolism.

TABLE 2	Light's Criteria for Definition of an Exudate[1]

An exudate is defined by meeting any one or more of the following criteria:
- Serum to effusion protein ratio of >0.5
- Serum to effusion LDH ratio of >0.6
- Effusion LDH level of >200 or >2/3 of the upper value of normal for serum LDH

A transudate is defined when none of these three parameters are met

LDH, serum lactate dehydrogenase.

shows indications for thoracentesis while Figure 1 is a schematic for the evaluation of an unknown effusion.
- If a patient has significant symptoms of dyspnea, cough, pain, or a supplemental oxygen requirement, a therapeutic thoracentesis is warranted.
- Thoracentesis can be performed safely, in the absence of disorders of hemostasis, on effusions that demonstrate a thickness >10 mm on a lateral decubitus film.
- Loculated effusions can be localized with ultrasonography or CT scan.
- The most common serious complications of thoracentesis are pneumothorax, bleeding, and introduction of infection into the pleural space.
- Proper technique and sonographic guidance minimize the risk of complications.

Pleural Fluid Appearance
- Pleural fluid appearance may be helpful in diagnostic and therapeutic considerations.
- Red-tinged or serosanguinous pleural effusions indicate the presence of blood. This is either due to the procedure (which should clear with continued aspiration) or due to the primary disorder (commonly malignancy, PE, or trauma).
- The presence of gross blood should lead to the measurement of a pleural fluid hematocrit. Hemothorax is defined as a pleural fluid blood hematocrit ratio of >0.5, and chest tube drainage should be implemented.
- Malodorous fluid or frank pus is consistent with an empyema, and tube thoracostomy should occur immediately.
- Turbid or milky fluid should prompt evaluation for chylothorax (see later).

Initial Pleural Fluid Laboratories
- The most important aspect of pleural fluid analysis is the laboratory evaluation, allowing the designation of a pleural effusion as either transudate or exudate using Light's criteria[1,2] (Table 2) or Heffner's criteria[3] (Table 3).
- Based upon clinical suspicion, other laboratory tests on the pleural fluid, as outlined below, can be obtained to further aid in diagnosis.

TABLE 3	Heffner's Criteria for Definition of an Exudate[2]

An exudate is defined by meeting any one or more of the following criteria:
- Pleural fluid protein is >2.9 g/dL
- Pleural fluid LDH level is >0.45 times the upper limit of normal
- Pleural fluid cholesterol level is >45 g/dL

A transudate is defined when none of these three parameters are met

LDH, serum lactate dehydrogenase.

- Of note, in patients who have an exudative effusion by chemical criteria, but clinical suspicion for heart, liver, or kidney disease is high, then a serum to pleural fluid albumin gradient should be checked. A gradient of >1.2 g/dL suggests that the pleural fluid is likely due to CHF, liver, or kidney disease.[4]

Light's Criteria

- The most frequently used criteria for defining pleural fluid as either exudate or transudate is Light's criteria.[1]
- These criteria have a 97.9% sensitivity for detecting an exudative effusion.[5]
- At the time of thoracentesis, a simultaneous measurement of serum lactate dehydrogenase (LDH) and protein must be sampled to properly use the following criteria.

Heffner's Criteria

- Heffner's criteria have a similar sensitivity to Light's criteria (98.4%).[3]
- They have the benefit of not requiring simultaneous blood work for interpretation.

Other Laboratory Testing
Differential Cell Count

- High cell counts are more typically seen in exudative effusions (however, this is not a component of Light's criteria).
- A high **neutrophil count** is suggestive of an infectious process, especially bacterial, and should prompt consideration of an empyema.[6]
- **Eosinophilia** (>10% of total nucleated cell count) is suggestive of air or blood in the pleural space.[7] If neither of these is present, consideration should be given to fungal or parasitic infection, drug-induced disease, PE, asbestos-related disease, and Churg-Strauss syndrome.[8]
- **Lymphocytosis** (>50% of the total nucleated cell count) is suggestive of malignancy or tuberculosis.[6]
- **Mesothelial cells,** when present, argue against the diagnosis of tuberculosis.
- **Plasma cells** in abundance suggest multiple myeloma.

Routine Gram Stain with Culture and AFB Culture

- Routine stains should be obtained to quickly determine if an effusion is infected and to direct antibiotic therapy if indicated (Table 4).
- Staining for acid-fast bacilli and culture for tuberculosis are performed when clinically indicated.

TABLE 4	Indication for Tube Thoracostomy in Parapneumonic Effusions

Radiographic
- Pleural fluid loculation
- Effusion filling more than half of hemithorax
- Air-fluid level present

Microbiologic
- Pus in pleural space
- Positive gram stain for microorganisms
- Positive pleural fluid cultures

Chemical
- Pleural fluid pH level of <7.2
- Pleural fluid glucose level of <60 mg/dL

Glucose
- A concentration <60 mg/dL is probably due to tuberculosis, malignancy,[9] rheumatoid arthritis,[10] or a parapneumonic effusion.[11]
- For parapneumonic effusions, with a glucose level <60 mg/dL, tube thoracostomy should be considered (Table 4).

pH
- Pleural fluid with a low pH usually corresponds to a low glucose and a high LDH; otherwise, the low pH may be due to poor sample collection technique (proper pH testing on pleural fluid involves anaerobic collection in a heparinized syringe and stored on ice).
- A pH level of <7.3 is seen with empyema, tuberculosis, malignancy, collagen vascular disease, or esophageal rupture.
- For parapneumonic effusions with a pH level of <7.2, tube thoracostomy should be considered (Table 4).[8,12]

Cytology
- Cytology is positive in approximately 60% of malignant effusions.[13]
- Priming the fluid collection bag with unfractionated heparin may increase the yield.
- Of note, the volume of pleural fluid analyzed does not impact the yield of cytologic diagnosis.[14]

Amylase
- An elevation in amylase suggests pancreatic disease, malignancy, or esophageal rupture but should not be routinely measured unless there is a clinical suspicion.[15]
- Malignancy and esophageal rupture have salivary amylase elevations and not pancreatic amylase elevations.

Triglycerides
- Turbid or milky fluid should prompt an investigation for chylothorax.
- The fluid should be centrifuged. If the cloudiness clears, then the appearance was merely secondary to cells and debris.
- If the supernatant does not clear and instead remains turbid, then pleural lipids should be checked.
- Elevation in triglyceride levels (>110 mg/dL) suggests that a chylothorax is present,[2,8] usually due to a disruption of the thoracic duct from trauma, surgery, or malignancy (i.e., lymphoma). Chylomicrons in the pleural fluid will confirm this.

Other Diagnostic Procedures
- When there is increased clinical suspicion for a certain diagnosis, other invasive procedures may be useful.
- **Closed pleural biopsy** typically adds little to the diagnostic yield of thoracentesis, except in the diagnosis of tuberculosis. For tuberculous effusions, pleural fluid cultures alone are positive in only 20% to 25% of cases. However, the combination of pleural fluid studies and pleural biopsy (demonstrating granulomata or organisms) is 90% sensitive in establishing TB as the etiology of the effusion.
- **Diagnostic thoracoscopy** has largely replaced closed pleural biopsy. Thoracoscopy allows visually directed biopsies, thus increasing the diagnostic yield for malignancy, while maintaining the high diagnostic yield for TB possible with closed pleural biopsy.

Effusion Classification
Transudative Effusions
- Transudative pleural effusions usually have low protein and LDH. The glucose level is usually similar to the serum level, and the pH level is generally higher than blood pH.

- Most transudates are clear, straw colored, nonviscous, and odorless.
- White blood cell count is usually <100 cells/high-power field, and the red blood cell count is usually <10,000 cells/high-power field.
- Transudates should lead to further evaluation of the heart, liver, and kidney with therapy directed accordingly.

Exudative Effusions
- Exudative pleural effusions usually have high protein or LDH values and meet one of Light's criteria as described above.
- Diagnosis of the etiology of the pleural fluid should proceed with a careful history and physical examination followed by pleural fluid analysis.
- There is a broad differential for exudative pleural effusions, and once a diagnosis is determined, therapy should be directed toward the cause.

Parapneumonic Effusions and Empyema
- Parapneumonic effusions are exudates that develop secondary to pulmonary infections.
- Patients with pneumonia should undergo rapid diagnostic testing because an infected pleural space (empyema) needs to be treated without delay.
- Parapneumonic effusions and empyema should be managed with tube drainage when indicated based on the size, presence of loculations, gross appearance of the fluid, or biochemical analysis of the pleural fluid (Table 4).[12]
- Antibiotics should be administered broadly and then narrowed as directed by culture data.
- Multiple chest tubes are sometimes required to adequately drain the pleural space.
- Failure to adequately and quickly drain the pleural space can lead to organization of the pleural fluid and formation of a thick pleural "rind" which may necessitate surgical removal known as **decortication.**

Malignant Pleural Effusions
- Malignant pleural effusions arise from tumor involvement of the pleura or mediastinum.
- In addition, patients with cancer are at increased risk of pleural effusions from other secondary causes such as PE, postobstructive pneumonia, chylothorax, and drug and radiation reactions.
- It may be appropriate for some patients with stable effusions without significant symptoms to avoid further invasive procedures and observe only.

TREATMENT

Therapeutic Thoracentesis
- This intervention may improve patient's comfort and relieve dyspnea.
- Repeated thoracenteses are reasonable if they achieve symptomatic relief and if fluid reaccumulation is slow.
- The rapid removal of >1 L of pleural fluid may result in re-expansion pulmonary edema and is discouraged.
- Unfortunately, 95% of malignant effusions recur, and the median time to recurrence is <1 week.

Chemical Pleurodesis
- Pleurodesis is an effective procedure indicated for a recurrent pleural effusion in a patient whose symptoms were relieved with initial drainage but has rapid reaccumulation.

- Chemical sclerosant is instilled into the pleural space to promote fusion of the visceral and parietal pleura (pleurodesis).
- Chemicals used for pleurodesis are talc, doxycycline or minocycline, and bleomycin (considered less effective and more expensive).
- Systemic analgesics and lidocaine added to the sclerosing agent should be used to reduce the significant discomfort associated with this procedure.[16]
- If chest tube drainage remains high (>100 mL/day), >2 days after the initial pleurodesis, a second dose of sclerosing agent can be administered.

Chronic Indwelling Pleural Catheter

- This technique can provide good symptomatic control of an effusion via intermittent patient-controlled drainage.
- The Pleurex catheter is better at controlling symptoms than doxycycline pleurodesis.[17]
- Furthermore, repeated drainage leads to pleurodesis in roughly 50% of patients, allowing the catheter to be removed.

Pleurectomy or Pleural Abrasion

- Removal of the pleural lining or mechanical trauma to the pleural lining to promote pleurodesis.
- Requires thoracotomy and should be reserved for patients with a good prognosis who have had ineffective pleurodesis by other means.

Chemotherapy and Mediastinal Radiotherapy

May control effusions in responsive tumors, such as lymphoma or small-cell bronchogenic carcinoma.

SOLITARY PULMONARY NODULE

General Principles

- The **solitary pulmonary nodule** (SPN) is defined as a ≤3 cm isolated, spherical, well-circumscribed lesion completely surrounded by aerated lung without associated atelectasis, hilar enlargement, or pleural effusion.[18,19]
- A lesion of >3 cm is referred to as **pulmonary mass** and the probability of malignancy is much higher.[18,19] Some authorities also distinguish **subcentimeter nodules** as <8 to 10 mm, which are much less likely to be malignant.[18]
- The large majority of SPNs are discovered incidentally on plain CXR or chest CT obtained for other reasons.[18]
- The prevalence of SPNs is highly dependent on the characteristics of the population studied (e.g., age, smoking status) and the technique used (i.e., CXR or CT). It has been reported to range from 0.2% to 7% for CXRs and 8% to 51% for CT.[18,20–22] Some SPNs detected on CXR will be false positives.
- Importantly, **long-term survival is dramatically better after resection of a malignant SPN compared with that of advanced lung cancer.**

Etiology

The rate of malignancy in patients with SPNs varies greatly depending on study populations and methods of detection used. There are certain characteristics that increase the risk of malignancy and these will be discussed below. Table 5 outlines a differential diagnosis for the SPN.

TABLE 5	Partial Differential Diagnosis of the Solitary Pulmonary Nodule

Neoplastic
Malignant
  Primary lung cancer
    Adenocarcinoma (including the
      bronchoalveolar variant)
    Squamous cell
    Small cell
    Large cell
    Carcinoid
  Metastatic (e.g., breast, colorectal,
    germ cell, head & neck,
    melanoma, prostate, renal cell)
  Lymphoma
Benign
  Hamartoma

Vascular
AV malformation
Hemangioma
Focal hemorrhage
Pulmonary infarct

Inflammatory
Sarcoidosis
Wegener granulomatosis
Rheumatoid arthritis

Infectious
Granulomatous
  Tuberculosis
  Nontuberculous mycobacteria
  Histoplasmosis
  Coccidioidomycosis
  Cryptococcosis
  Aspergillosis
  Blastomycosis
Round pneumonia
Lung abscess/septic embolus
Parasitic (e.g., ascariasis,
  dirofilariasis, echinococcosis,
  and paragonimiasis)

Other
Healed or nonspecific granulomas
Nonspecific inflammation or fibrosis
Round atelectasis
Bronchogenic cyst
Intrapulmonary lymph node
Lipoid pneumonia
Pulmonary sequestration
Amyloid

Diagnosis

Clinical Presentation

- Most patients with an SPN will be asymptomatic with regard to the nodule itself. Age, smoking status, history of extrathoracic cancer, and history of prior lung cancer are perhaps the most important historical features that increase the likelihood that an SPN is malignant.[18,19,23–26]
- Patients should also be asked about constitutional symptoms that may be due to malignancy or infection such as fever, chills, sweats, weight loss, anorexia, weakness, fatigue, and malaise.
- The physical examination is usually normal with regard to the SPN. Nonetheless, a careful pulmonary examination is indicated.

Diagnostic Testing

Chest Radiography
CXR factors suggestive of malignancy are as follows[18,20,23,24,27]:
- **Likelihood of malignancy increases rapidly with size.** Those <1 cm are not usually malignant, but SPNs of >2 cm often are malignant.
- **Upper lobe lesions,** particularly on the right, are more likely to be malignant.

- **Irregular or spiculated margins** increase the likelihood of malignancy. Smooth margins are more likely to be benign and scalloped margins have intermediate likelihood.
- **Stippled and/or eccentric calcifications** are associated with malignancy. Laminated, central, and dense calcifications suggest a granuloma, whereas the "popcorn" pattern suggests hamartoma. Patients with obviously benign calcifications need not be evaluated further.
- The **doubling time** for malignant SPNs is usually between 20 and 300 days, often <100 days. One doubling time equates to an approximate 30% increase in diameter. On the basis of these assumptions, most authorities agree that **SPNs that are stable in size for 2 years are very unlikely to be malignant. Because of the importance of growth rate, it is critical to compare with previous CXRs or CTs.** Slowly growing bronchoalveolar cancers are known to exist and they may subsequently become more aggressive. This seems to be particularly true of lesions with a "ground-glass" appearance, and lengthier follow-up may be indicated in these cases.[28]

The American College of Chest Physicians (ACCP) recommends that clinicians **estimate the pretest probability of malignancy before ordering further imaging studies or biopsy.**[18] This may be done qualitatively using all of the factors discussed above as appropriate. Several prediction models have been developed.[23,29,30] The prediction model developed by Swensen et al. has been validated but is no more accurate than expert clinician assessment.[31] In this model, the independent predictors are age (OR 1.04 for each year); smoking, current or past (OR 2.2); history of cancer diagnosed ≥5 years ago (OR 3.8), patients with cancer diagnosed <5 years ago were excluded; nodule diameter (OR 1.14 for each mm); spiculation (OR 2.8); and upper lobe (OR 2.2).[23]

Chest Computed Tomography

High-resolution chest CT is clearly more sensitive and specific for detection and characterization of SPNs. **The ACCP recommends that all patients with an indeterminate SPN on CXR have high-resolution CT of the chest preformed.**[18] If there are any prior chest CTs, these should obviously be reviewed. In addition to the radiographic features discussed above, CT characteristics suggestive of malignancy include the following[18-20,27,32,33]:

- Vascular convergence.
- Dilated bronchus leading into the nodule.
- Pseudocavitation.
- Thick (>15 mm), irregular walled cavitation.
- Dynamic contrast enhancement >15 Hounsfield units (HU).
- Fat attenuation (−40 to −120 HU) is strongly suggestive of hamartoma or lipoma. Some metastatic malignancies (e.g., liposarcoma or renal cell carcinoma) may occasionally contain fat.

Positron Emission Tomography

Fluorodeoxyglucose positron emission tomography (**^{18}F-FDG PET**) may also be used to further characterize SPNs.[34] Reviews have estimated the sensitivity to be 87% to 96.8% and specificity to be 77.8% to 83%.[35] Sensitivity is less for subcentimeter (<8 to 10 mm) SPNs. It is important to recognize that false negatives can occur and if clinical suspicion still exists, a biopsy should be strongly considered. **The ACCP recommends ^{18}F-FDG PET for patients with low-to-moderate pretest probability and an SPN of >8 to 10 mm with indeterminate (i.e., not clearly benign) CT characteristics.**[18] In some centers, PET and CT can be combined in a single scan.

Further Evaluation

Once the clinical and imaging characteristics are known, the choice of subsequent management can be a close call between risk and benefit. Alternatives include observation with serial radiographs, biopsy, and surgery. Each of these has advantages and disadvantages that depend greatly on the likelihood of malignancy.

- **Observation** is appropriate for those with a very low likelihood of malignancy (<5%). Reasonable follow-up consists of serial high-resolution CT scans at 3, 6, 12, and 24 months. Any evidence of growth is presumptive evidence of malignancy. If the lesion is stable after 2 years then the risk of malignancy is very low.[18]
- Observation with serial CT scans may also be appropriate for SPNs of >8 to 10 mm: (1) with low likelihood (<30 to 40%) of malignancy and a negative ^{18}F-FDG PET scan or dynamic contrast enhancement of <15 HU; (2) a nondiagnostic biopsy and a negative ^{18}F-FDG PET scan; (3) the patient declines aggressive evaluation.[18]
- **Biopsy** is recommended for SPNs of >8 to 10 mm in patients who would be appropriate candidates for surgical cure when (1) the clinical likelihood of malignancy and results of imaging studies are not in agreement (e.g., high clinical suspicion but a negative ^{18}F-FDG PET scan); (2) a specific treatment is available for a benign diagnosis (e.g., fungal infection); (3) the patient wants biopsy confirmation prior to committing to surgery (this may be most useful when the risks of surgery are high).[18]
  - Usually the preferred biopsy technique is **CT-guided transthoracic needle aspiration,** especially for more peripheral lesions. Sensitivity and specificity is variable and depends on multiple factors including lesion size, expertise of the radiologist, availability of a onsite cytopathologic examination, needle size, and number of needle passes.[18,19,27,32,36–38] The reported rate of pneumothorax is variable, ranging from approximately 12% to 44%. Most do not require chest tube placement. Factors associated with pneumothorax include increased lesion depth, smaller SPN size, emphysema, smaller needle-pleural angle, lateral biopsy site, and lesion site near a fissure.[18,39–44]
  - **Bronchoscopic biopsy** may be a viable alternative in specific situations (e.g., central lesions, lesions adjacent to a bronchus, an air bronchogram in the lesion) and there is available expertise.[18] Electromagnetic navigation bronchoscopic biopsy is an emerging technique for peripheral lesions.[45]
- **Surgical management** is recommended for indeterminate SPNs of >8 to 10 mm in appropriate surgical candidates when (1) the clinical likelihood is moderate to high; (2) ^{18}F-FDG PET is positive; and (3) the patient prefers to undergo a definitive procedure.[18] There are typically two surgical options:
  - **Thoracotomy** is the most definitive approach particularly for more centrally located SPNs that are not accessible by other techniques.
  - **Video-assisted thorascopic surgery (VATS)** is a minimally invasive technique with a lower mortality rate. It is usually the preferred method for SPNs in the peripheral third of the lung.

REFERENCES

1. Light RW, Macgregor MI, Luchsinger PC, et al. Pleural effusions: the diagnostic separation of transudates and exudates. *Ann Intern Med* 1972;77:507–513.
2. Light RW. Pleural Diseases. 5th Ed. Philadelphia, PA: Lippincott Williams & Wilkins, 2007.
3. Heffner JE, Brown LK, Barbieri CA. Diagnostic value of tests that discriminate between exudative and transudative pleural effusions. Primary Study Investigators. *Chest* 1997;111:970–980.

4. Roth BJ, O'Meara TF, Cragun WH. The serum-effusion albumin gradient in the evaluation of pleural effusions. *Chest* 1990;98:546–549.

5. Romero S, Candela A, Martin D, et al. Evaluation of different criteria for the separation of pleural transudates from exudates. *Chest* 1993;104:399–404.

6. Light RW, Erozan YS, Ball WC Jr. Cells in pleural fluid. Their values in differential diagnosis. *Arch Intern Med* 1973;132:854–860.

7. Spriggs AI, Boddington MM. The Cytology of Effusions: Pleural, Pericardial, and Peritoneal and of Cerebrospinal Fluid. 2nd Ed. New York: Grune & Stratton, 1968.

8. Light RW. Clinical practice. Pleural effusions. *N Engl J Med* 2002;346:1971–1977.

9. Balbir-Gurman A, Yigla M, Nahir AM, et al. Rheumatoid pleural effusion. *Semin Arthritis Rheum* 2006;35:368–373.

10. Rodriguez-Panadero F, Lopez Mejias J. Low glucose and pH levels in malignant pleural effusions. Diagnostic significance and prognostic value in respect to pleurodesis. *Am Rev Respir Dis* 1989;139:663–667.

11. Heffner JE, Brown LK, Barbieri C, et al. Pleural fluid chemical analysis in parapneumonic effusions. A meta-analysis. *Am J Respir Crit Care Med* 1995;151:1700–1708.

12. Colice GL, Curtis A, Deslauriers J, et al. Medical and surgical treatment of parapneumonic effusions: an evidence-based guideline. *Chest* 2000;118:1158–1171.

13. Prakash UB, Reiman HM. Comparison of needle biopsy with cytologic analysis for the evaluation of pleural effusion: analysis of 414 cases. *Mayo Clin Proc* 1985;60:158–164.

14. Sallich SM, Sallach JA, Vazquez E, et al. Volume of pleural fluid required for diagnosis of pleural malignancy. *Chest* 2002;122:1913–1917.

15. Branca P, Rodriguez RM, Rogers JT, et al. Routine measurement of pleural fluid amylase is not indicated. *Arch Intern Med* 2001;161:228–232.

16. Walker-Renard PB, Vaughn LM, Sahn SA. Chemical pleurodesis for malignant pleural effusions. *Ann Intern Med* 1994;120:56–64.

17. Putman JB, Light RW, Rodriguez RM, et al. A randomized comparison of indwelling pleural catheter and doxycycline pleurodesis in the management of malignant pleural effusion. *Cancer* 1999;86:1992–1999.

18. Gould MK, Fletcher J, Iannettoni MD, et al. Evaluation of patients with pulmonary nodules: when is it lung cancer? ACCP evidence-based clinical practice guidelines (2nd edition). *Chest* 2007;132:108S–130S.

19. Ost D, Fein AM, Feinsilver SH. Clinical practice. The solitary pulmonary nodule. *N Engl J Med* 2003;348:2535–2542.

20. Wahidi MM, Govert JA, Goudar RK, et al. Evidence for the treatment of patients with pulmonary nodules: when is it lung cancer?: ACCP evidence-based clinical practice guidelines (2nd edition). *Chest* 2007;132:94S–107S.

21. Henschke CI, McCauley DI, Yankelevitz DF, et al. Early Lung Cancer Action Project: overall design and findings from baseline screening. *Lancet* 1999;354:99–105.

22. Holin SN, Dwork RE, Glaser S, et al. Solitary pulmonary nodules found in a community-wide chest roentgenographic survey. *Am Tuberc Pulm Dis* 1959;79:427–439.

23. Swensen SJ, Silverstein MD, Ilstrup DM, et al. The probability of malignancy in solitary pulmonary nodules. Application to small radiologically indeterminate nodules. *Arch Intern Med* 1997;157:849–855.

24. Gould MK, Ananth L, Barnett PG. A clinical model to estimate the pretest probability of lung cancer in patient with solitary pulmonary nodules. *Chest* 2007;131:383–388.

25. Schultz EM, Sanders GD, Trotter PR, et al. Validation of two models to estimate the probability of malignancy in patients with solitary pulmonary nodules. *Thorax* 2008;63:335–341.

26. Mery CM, Pappas AN, Bueno R, et al. Relationship between a history of antecedent cancer and the probability of malignancy for a solitary pulmonary nodule. *Chest* 2004;125: 2175–2181.

27. Winer-Muram HT. The solitary pulmonary nodule. *Radiology* 2006;239:34–49.

28. Aoki T, Nakata H, Watanabe H, et al. Evolution of peripheral lung adenocarcinomas: CT findings correlated with histology and tumor doubling time. *AJR Am J Roentgenol* 2000; 174:763–768.

29. Gurney JW. Determining the likelihood of malignancy in solitary pulmonary nodules with Bayesian analysis. Part I. Theory. *Radiology* 1993;186:405–413.

30. Gurney JW, Lyddon DM, McKay JA. Determining the likelihood of malignancy in solitary pulmonary nodules with Bayesian analysis. Part II. Application. *Radiology* 1993;186:415–422.

31. Swensen SJ, Silverstein MD, Edell ES, et al. Solitary pulmonary nodules: clinical prediction model versus physicians. *Mayo Clin Proc* 1999;74:319–329.

32. Jeong YJ, Yi CA, Lee KS. Solitary pulmonary nodules: detection, characterization, and guidance for further diagnostic workup and treatment. *AJR Am J Roentgenol* 2007;188:57–68.

33. Swensen SJ, Viggiano RW, Midthun DE, et al. Lung nodule enhancement at CT: multicenter study. *Radiology* 2000;214:73–80.

34. Herder GJ, van Tinteren H, Golding RP, et al. Clinical prediction model to characterize pulmonary nodules: validation and added value of 18F-fluorodeoxyglucose positron emission tomography. *Chest* 2005;128:2490–2496.

35. Gould MK, Maclean CC, Kuschner WG, et al. Accuracy of positron emission tomography for diagnosis of pulmonary nodules and mass lesions: a meta-analysis. *JAMA* 2001;285:914–924.

36. Lacasse Y, Wong E, Guyatt GH, et al. Transthoracic needle aspiration biopsy for the diagnosis of localized pulmonary lesions: a meta-analysis. *Thorax* 1999;54:884–893.

37. Wallace MJ, Krishnamurthy S, Broemeling LD, et al. CT-guided percutaneous fine-needle aspiration biopsy of small (≤1 cm) pulmonary lesions. *Radiology* 2002;225:823–828.

38. Ohno Y, Hatabu H, Takenaka D, et al. CT-guided transthoracic needle aspiration biopsy of small (<20 mm) solitary pulmonary nodules. *AJR Am J Roentgenol* 2003;180:1665–1669.

39. Kazerooni EA, Lim FT, Mikhail A, et al. Risk of pneumothorax in CT-guided transthoracic needle aspiration biopsy of the lung. *Radiology* 1996;198:317–375.

40. Cox JE, Chiles C, McManus CM, et al. Transthoracic needle aspiration biopsy: variable that affect risk of pneumothorax. *Radiology* 1999;212:165–168.

41. Yeow KM, See LC, Lui KW, et al. Risk factors for pneumothorax and bleeding after CT-guided percutaneous coaxial cutting needle biopsy of lung lesions. *J Vasc Interv Radiol* 2001;12:1305–1312.

42. KO JP, Shepard JO, Drucker EA, et al. Factors influencing pneumothorax rate at lung biopsy: are dwell time and angle of pleural puncture contributing factors? *Radiology* 2001;218:491–496.

43. Saji H, Nakamura H, Tsuchida T, et al. The incidence and the risk of pneumothorax and chest tube placement after percutaneous CT-guided lung biopsy: the angle of the needle trajectory is a novel predictor. *Chest* 2002;121:1521–1526.

44. Yeow KM, Su IH, Pan KT, et al. Risk factors of pneumothorax and bleeding: multivariate analysis of 660 CT-guided coaxial cutting needle lung biopsies. *Chest* 2004;126:748–754.

45. Eberhardt R, Anantham D, Herth F, et al. Electromagnetic navigation diagnostic bronchoscopy in peripheral lung lesions. *Chest* 2007;131:1800–1805.

16 Diabetes Mellitus
Rashmi S. Mullur and Ernesto Bernal-Mizrachi

General Principles

- Diabetes mellitus (DM) is characterized by hyperglycemia resulting from defects in insulin secretion, insulin action, or both.
- Chronic hyperglycemia is associated with long-term damage of various organs, especially the eyes, kidneys, nerves, heart, and blood vessels.
- DM is a chronic illness that requires precise medical care focused on glycemic control, regulation of blood pressure, lipid lowering therapy, preventative care, and patient self-education.
- Management of diabetic emergencies such as ketoacidosis and hyperosmolar syndrome will not be covered in this manual.

Classification

Type 1 DM
- Type 1 DM is identified by β-cell destruction leading to absolute insulin deficiency.[1]
- Type 1 DM accounts for only 5% to 10% of those with diabetes.
- It results from a **cellular-mediated autoimmune destruction of the β-cells** of the pancreas.
- Immune markers now identified in these patients include islet cell autoantibodies, autoantibodies to insulin, autoantibodies to glutamic acid decarboxylase, and autoantibodies to the tyrosine phosphatases IA-2 and IA-2β.
- One or more of these autoantibodies are present in 85% to 90% of individuals and it has strong human leukocyte antigen associations.
- Immune-mediated diabetes commonly occurs in childhood and adolescence, but it can occur at any age. In adults, this disorder is commonly referred to late-onset autoimmune diabetes.
  - The rate of β-cell destruction is variable; in some adults, full destruction of β-cells can take years.
- Eventually, these individuals become **dependent on insulin for survival and are at risk for ketoacidosis.**
- Patients are rarely obese at the time of diagnosis, but the presence of obesity does not exclude the diagnosis.
- Physicians should be mindful of immune-mediated type 1 DM in patients with a history of other autoimmune disorders such as Graves disease, Hashimoto thyroiditis, Addison disease, vitiligo, celiac sprue, autoimmune hepatitis, myasthenia gravis, and pernicious anemia.

Type 2 DM
- Type 2 DM is the **most common form of diabetes,** accounting for up to 90% of all cases of DM.
- This form of diabetes includes all individuals who have insulin resistance and have relative insulin deficiency.

- **Most patients will not need insulin therapy to survive** and can be managed with oral hypoglycemic agents; however, there is growing evidence that long-standing type 2 DM is associated with impaired β-cell function and the need for treatment with insulin.[2]
- **Most patients are obese or have an increased percentage of abdominal body fat,** which can worsen insulin resistance.
- **Ketoacidosis rarely occurs** in these patients but can arise in the setting of another illness or infection.
- These patients frequently go undiagnosed for years, and patients are at increased risk of developing macrovascular and microvascular complications due to chronic hyperglycemia.
- The risk of developing type 2 DM increases with age, obesity, and lack of physical activity or women with a prior diagnosis of gestational diabetes mellitus (GDM).
- The frequency varies in different racial and ethnic subgroups and it has a **strong genetic predisposition;** however, the genetics are complex and not clearly defined.

Other Types of DM
Monogenetic Defects of the β-Cell
These forms of diabetes are characterized by the onset of hyperglycemia at an early age and are referred to as maturity-onset diabetes of the young.[3]
- They are characterized by impaired insulin secretion with no minimal or no defects in insulin action.
- They are inherited in an autosomal dominant pattern.

Diseases of the Exocrine Pancreas
- Any condition that results in injury to the pancreas can cause diabetes.
- Trauma, pancreatectomy, and acquired illnesses such as pancreatitis, infection, and pancreatic carcinoma can result in insulin deficiency.
- Inherited conditions such as cystic fibrosis and hemochromatosis will also damage β-cells and impair insulin secretion.

Drug- or Chemical-Induced Diabetes
- Toxins and intravenous pentamidine can permanently destroy pancreatic β-cells.[4]
- Patients receiving α-interferon have been reported to develop diabetes associated with islet cell antibodies.[5]

Endocrinopathies
Endocrine disorders such as Cushing disease and acromegaly results in the secretion of hormones that antagonize insulin action and result in impaired glucose tolerance and insulin resistance.

Gestational Diabetes Mellitus
- GDM complicates up to 4% of all pregnancies.
- Women with GDM are at higher risk for developing type 2 DM later in life; women with a history of GDM should be evaluated yearly for the onset of diabetes.

Diagnosis

- For diabetes, there is **no distinction between tests used for screening and diagnosis.**
- Testing in asymptomatic individuals should follow these guidelines:
  - **All adults who are overweight (body mass index [BMI] >25 kg/m²) and have additional risk factors** (Table 1).

TABLE 1	Risk Factors for Diabetes Mellitus

Physical inactivity
First-degree relative with diabetes
Members of a high-risk ethnic population (e.g., African-American, Latino, Native American, Asian American, Pacific Islander)
Women who delivered a baby weighing >9 lb or were diagnosed with GDM
Hypertension (>140/90 mm Hg or on therapy for hypertension)
HDL cholesterol level >35 mg/dL (0.90 mmol/L) and/or a triglyceride level >250 mg/dL (2.82 mmol/L)
Women with polycystic ovarian syndrome
Impaired glucose tolerance or impaired fasting glucose on previous testing
Other clinical conditions associated with insulin resistance (e.g., severe obesity, acanthosis nigricans)
History of cerebrovascular disease

GDM, gestational diabetes mellitus; HDL, high-density lipoprotein.

- In the absence of the above criteria, testing of diabetes should begin at age 45 years.
- If results are normal, testing should be repeated at least at 3-year intervals, with more frequent testing, if clinically indicated.
- Upon diagnosis, the initial evaluation should include a complete medical history that addresses the following:
  - Classifying the type of diabetes.
  - Identifying the presence of diabetic complications.
  - Reviewing previous treatments.
  - Forming a comprehensive management plan targeting glycemic, lipid, cardiovascular, and nutritional goals.

Emerging Diagnostic Criteria for Diabetes

- For a number of years, the hemoglobin A_{1c} has been recognized as an accurate, precise measure of chronic glycemic levels and correlates well with the risk of diabetes complications.
- **Hemoglobin A_{1c} test is now the diagnostic test of choice for diabetes.**[6]
- Diabetes should be diagnosed when hemoglobin A_{1c} level is >6.5%.
  - Diagnosis should be confirmed with a repeated hemoglobin A_{1c} test.
  - Confirmation is not required in symptomatic subjects with plasma glucose levels at >200 mg/dL.
  - If hemoglobin A_{1c} testing is not possible, previously recommended diagnostic methods are acceptable including fasting plasma glucose (FPG) or oral glucose tolerance test (OGTT).
- The previously described clinical states "prediabetes, impaired fasting glucose, and impaired glucose tolerance" are no longer clinically relevant because they do not clearly identify the chronic risk of hyperglycemia.
- Those with hemoglobin A_{1c} levels that do not meet diagnosis for diabetes but are elevated to >6.0% should receive counseling on preventative measures such as nutrition, lifestyle modification, and an increase in physical activity.

- In addition to lifestyle counseling, metformin may be considered in those who are at very high risk for developing diabetes, such as the following[7]:
  - A history of combined impaired fasting glucose and impaired glucose tolerance.
  - Hemoglobin A_{1c} level of >6%.
  - Hypertension (HTN).
  - Low high-density lipoprotein (HDL) cholesterol or elevated triglycerides.
  - Family history of diabetes in a first-degree relative.
  - Obese and age <60 years.

Traditional Diagnostic Criteria for Diabetes

- Patients must meet ONE of the following current criteria to meet the diagnosis of diabetes:
  - **FPG of >126 mg/dL** (7.0 mmol/L).
    - Fasting is defined as no caloric intake for at least 8 hours.
  - **Symptoms of hyperglycemia and a random plasma glucose of >200 mg/dL** (11.1 mmol/L).
    - Classic symptoms of hyperglycemia include polyuria, polydipsia, and unexplained weight loss.
  - **OGTT 2-hour plasma glucose of >200 mg/dL** (11.1 mmol/L).
    - The patient should receive a glucose load containing the equivalent of 75 g anhydrous glucose dissolved in water.

Type 1 Diabetes

- People with type 1 diabetes typically present with acute symptoms of diabetes and markedly elevated blood glucose levels, and are diagnosed soon after the onset of hyperglycemia.
- Measurement of islet autoantibodies can identify patients at risk for developing type 1 diabetes.
  - Widespread testing of asymptomatic individuals is not currently recommended.
  - In the setting of clinical research, testing may be appropriate in high-risk populations, such as the following:
    - Patients with prior transient hyperglycemia.
    - Relatives with type 1 diabetes.

Gestational Diabetes

- Women should be evaluated for their individual GDM risk at the first prenatal visit[8] (Table 2).

TABLE 2	Assessing Risk for Gestational Diabetes
Very High Risk	**Low Risk**
Severe obesity	Age <25 years
Prior history of GDM or delivery of large-for-gestational-age infant	Weight normal before pregnancy
Presence of glycosuria	Member of an ethnic group with a low prevalence of diabetes
Diagnosis of PCOS	No known diabetes in first-degree relatives
Strong family history of type 2 diabetes	No history of abnormal glucose tolerance
	No history of poor obstetrical outcome

GDM, gestational diabetes mellitus; PCOS, polycystic ovarian syndrome.

- Women at very high risk for GDM should be screened for diabetes as soon as possible after the confirmation of pregnancy.
- Women at low risk do not need to be screened.
- All women who have a greater than low risk of GDM should undergo GDM testing at 24 to 28 weeks of gestation.
- Because women with a history of GDM have a higher risk of developing type 2 diabetes, they should be screened for diabetes at 6 to 12 weeks postpartum, using nonpregnant OGTT criteria.
- Two approaches may be followed for GDM screening at 24 to 28 weeks.

Two-Step Approach
- Perform initial screening by measuring plasma or serum glucose 1 hour after a 50-g oral glucose load.
- After 50-g load, a glucose threshold of >140 mg/dL identifies approximately 80% of women with GDM; the sensitivity is further increased to approximately 90% by a threshold of >130 mg/dL.
- Perform a diagnostic 100-g OGTT on a separate day in women who exceed the chosen threshold on 50-g screening.

One-Step Approach
- Perform a diagnostic 100-g OGTT in all women to be tested at 24 to 28 weeks.
- Should be performed in the morning after an overnight fast of at least 8 hours.
- To make a diagnosis of GDM, at least two of the following plasma glucose values must be found:
  - Fasting: >95 mg/dL.
  - 1 hour: >180 mg/dL.
  - 2 hour: >155 mg/dL.
  - 3 hour: >140 mg/dL.

Treatment

- Patients should receive care from a physician-coordinated team including, but not limited to, physicians, certified diabetic nurse educators, dietitians, pharmacists, and mental health professionals with expertise and a special interest in diabetes.
- All treatment plans should emphasize the role of the patient as the primary component of care with emphasis on self-management education.
  - In developing a management plan, consideration should be given to the patient's age, school/work schedule, physical activity, eating patterns, social situation and personality, cultural factors, and other medical conditions.

Glycemic Goals
- Glycemic control should be assessed by both capillary blood glucose (CBG) and A_{1c} values.
- Data have shown that targeting the following goals for glycemic control is associated with the lowest risk of long-term complications for both type 1 and type 2 DM.[9,10]
  - **Preprandial CBG values between 90 and 130 mg/dL.**
  - **Postprandial CBG values 180 mg/dL.**
  - **Hemoglobin A_{1c} values <7% or as close to normal while avoiding hypoglycemia.**
- For GDM, recent consensus guidelines target the following values[11]:
  - Preprandial CBG: <95 mg/dL, and

EITHER
- 1-hour postprandial CBG: <140 mg/dL

OR
- 2-hour postprandial CBG: <120 mg/dL.
- Goals should be individualized and may vary based on the following:
  - Duration of diabetes.
  - Age/life expectancy.
  - Comorbid conditions.
  - Known cardiovascular disease (CVD) or advanced microvascular complications.
  - Hypoglycemia unawareness.
  - Individual patient considerations.

Self-Monitoring of Capillary Blood Glucose

- For patients using noninsulin therapy, medical nutrition therapy (MNT), or less-frequent insulin therapy, self-monitoring of capillary blood glucose (SMBG) should occur at least once daily.
- For patients using multiple-daily insulin injections or insulin pump therapy, SMBG should occur at least three times daily.
- Physicians should review records of SMBG at every visit to titrate and adjust medical therapy.
- Continuous glucose monitoring, used along with intensive insulin regimens, has been shown to be useful in the management of adults with type 1 DM, especially those with hypoglycemia unawareness and/or frequent hypoglycemic episodes.[12]

Hemoglobin A_{1c}

- **The hemoglobin A_{1c} level should be measured at least two times a year in patients who are meeting treatment goals without hypoglycemia and have stable glycemic control.**
- **It should be measured quarterly in patients whose therapy has changed or who are not meeting glycemic goals.**
- Point-of-care testing for hemoglobin A_{1c} allows for timely decisions on therapy changes, when needed.[13]
- For any individual patient, the frequency of hemoglobin A_{1c} testing is dependent on the clinical situation and the judgment of the clinician.
- Limitations of hemoglobin A_{1c} testing:
  - Inaccurate hemoglobin A_{1c} values may result from the following factors:
    - Conditions that affect erythrocyte turnover.
    - Hemoglobin variants.
    - Recent blood transfusions.
  - Does not provide a measure of glycemic variability or hypoglycemia.
- Other measures of chronic glycemia such as fructosamine are available, but linkage to average glucose control and prognostic significance are not clear at this time.

Medical Nutrition Therapy

- **All patients with diabetes and prediabetes should undergo medical nutrition counseling** under the guidance of a registered clinical dietician.[14]
- In overweight and obese insulin-resistant individuals, **modest weight loss** has been shown to reduce insulin resistance.[15]
  - Both low-carbohydrate or low-fat calorie-restricted diets may be effective up to 1 year.[16]

- For patients on low-carbohydrate diets, monitor lipid profiles, renal function, and protein intake and adjust hypoglycemic therapy as needed.
- **Saturated fat intake should be <7% of total calories** and trans-fat intake should be limited.
- Carbohydrate intake:
  - Monitoring carbohydrate intake through carbohydrate counting, exchanges, or estimation is a key strategy in achieving glycemic control.
  - **The recommended dietary allowance for digestible carbohydrate is 130 g/day.** This is based on the amount of glucose required for central nervous system function without additional reliance on glucose production from protein and fat stores.
- Sweeteners and sugar alcohols:
  - FDA-recommended nonnutritive sweeteners are acesulfame potassium, aspartame, neotame, saccharin, and sucralose.
  - All have been shown to be safe for people with diabetes and women during pregnancy. Reduced calorie sweeteners.
  - FDA-approved sugar alcohols are erythritol, isomalt, lactitol, maltitol, mannitol, sorbitol, xylitol, tagatose, and hydrogenated starch hydrolysates.
  - The use of sugar alcohols may cause diarrhea, especially in children.
- Alcohol intake:
  - Adults with diabetes should **limit alcohol intake to less than one drink per day** for women and <2 drinks per day for men.
- Vitamins and supplements:
  - Routine supplementation with antioxidants (such as vitamins E and C and carotene) is not advised.
  - Data on routine chromium supplementation is not conclusive and is not currently recommended.

Bariatric Surgery

- Bariatric surgery should be considered for adults with BMI of >35 kg/m^2 and type 2 diabetes, especially if the diabetes is difficult to control with lifestyle and pharmacologic therapy.[17]
  - Currently, there is insufficient evidence to recommend surgery in patients with a BMI of <35 kg/m^2 outside of a research protocol.
  - There may be glycemic effects of intestinal bypass procedures that are independent of effects on weight.
- Longer-term concerns of bariatric surgery include vitamin and mineral deficiencies, osteoporosis, and hypoglycemia from insulin hypersecretion, although the latter effect is rare.

Physical Exercise

- Regular exercise can improve blood glucose, reduce cardiovascular risk, and further weight loss.
- Structured exercise regimens in patients with type 2 diabetes have been shown to decrease the hemoglobin A_{1c} level independent of changes in BMI.[18]
- **People with diabetes should exercise for >150 min/week.**
- Prior to recommending a program of physical activity, physicians should assess risk factors for coronary artery disease (CAD). Currently, screening asymptomatic diabetic patients remains unclear, and providers should use their clinical judgment for each individual case.
- Carbohydrate intake and medication adjustments will need to be addressed to avoid hypoglycemia, especially in individuals taking insulin and/or insulin secretagogues.

- For patients with proliferative diabetic retinopathy or severe nonproliferative diabetic retinopathy, vigorous aerobic or resistance exercise is contraindicated due to the risk of triggering vitreous hemorrhage or retinal detachment.[19]
- For patients with severe peripheral neuropathy, non–weight-bearing activities such as swimming, bicycling, or arm exercises are typically better tolerated.

Immunizations

- Influenza and pneumonia are associated with higher mortality and morbidity in people with diabetes.
- Diabetic patients are at increased risk of the bacteremic form of pneumococcal infection and nosocomial bacteremia.[20]
- The Centers for Disease Control and Prevention's Advisory Committee on Immunization Practices recommends **influenza and pneumococcal vaccines for all individuals with diabetes.**[21]
  - Influenza vaccine should be administered yearly.
  - Pneumococcal polysaccharide vaccine should be administered to all diabetic patients of >2 years of age.
  - A one-time revaccination is recommended for individuals >65 years of age previously immunized when they were <65 years of age if the vaccine was administered >5 years ago.
  - Other indications for repeat vaccination include nephrotic syndrome, chronic kidney disease, and immunocompromised states.

Hypoglycemia

- **The preferred treatment of hypoglycemia is 15 to 20 g of glucose,** although any form of carbohydrate that contains glucose can be used.
- Fats should be avoided acutely because they can prolong the acute glycemic response.[22]
- Patients should be instructed to recheck their CBG level 15 minutes after treatment.
  - If this shows continued hypoglycemia, the treatment should be repeated.
  - Once CBG level returns to normal, the individual should consume a meal or snack to prevent recurrence of hypoglycemia.
- Severe hypoglycemia is defined as hypoglycemia that requires the assistance of another person and cannot be treated with oral carbohydrate due to patient confusion or unconsciousness.
- **Patients with a history of severe hypoglycemia should be prescribed glucagon,** and caregivers or family members of these individuals should be instructed on proper administration.
- **Hypoglycemia unawareness** is characterized by repetitive hypoglycemia that results in a deficiency of the protective counter-regulatory hormone and autonomic responses.
- Individuals with hypoglycemia unawareness should have higher glycemic goals temporarily to partially reverse hypoglycemia unawareness and reduce risk of future episodes.[23]

Psychosocial Assessment

- Individual psychological and social issues can impair a patient's ability to adhere to a diabetes treatment regimen.[24]
- Self-management is often limited by attitudes toward the illness, personal expectations, patient's mood and affect, quality of life, psychiatric history, and financial, social and emotional resources.

- Indications for referral to a mental health specialist familiar with diabetes management are as follows:
  - Noncompliance with medical regimen.
  - Depression with the possibility of self-harm.
  - Debilitating anxiety (alone or with depression).
  - Indications of an eating disorder.
  - Cognitive functioning that significantly impairs judgment.
- Adjusting treatment regimens to assess barriers to adherence may improve overall quality of care.

Management of Hyperglycemia

- In type 2 diabetes, there are a number of modifiable environmental factors that play a role in disease development.
- Interventions that target obesity, a sedentary lifestyle, and nutrition have been shown to have a beneficial effect on hyperglycemia.
- In addition to these factors, a number of oral antidiabetic agents are very useful in early disease.

Oral Agents

- The primary target and effectiveness of each class of oral antidiabetic agent will be summarized here.
- As disease progresses in a type 2 diabetic, there are numerous combinations of therapies that can be individualized to meet a glycemic target.

Metformin

- It is the only biguanide in clinical use.
- The primary effect is to decrease hepatic glucose output and lower fasting glycemia.
- **Therapy with metformin as a single agent will lower hemoglobin A$_{1c}$ levels by approximately 1.5%.**[25]
- It is generally well tolerated, but some patients do note gastrointestinal symptoms as a common side effect. This can be avoided by slow-dose titration.
  - Metformin is contraindicated in patients with renal dysfunction because it can increase the risk of lactic acidosis.
  - Other risk factors for lactic acidosis in which metformin should be discontinued include hypovolemia, serious infection, tissue hypoxia, alcoholism, and severe cardiopulmonary disease.
  - Recent studies suggest that metformin is safe unless the GFR falls below 30 mL/min.[26]

Sulfonylureas

- Sulfonylureas (SUs) enhance endogenous insulin secretion.
- They are similar to metformin in efficacy and lower hemoglobin A$_{1c}$ levels by approximately 1.5%.
- The **primary adverse effect is hypoglycemia;** it can be severe and prolonged, especially in elderly patients or those with liver or renal disease. Patients who are known to skip meals should not take SU because of an increased risk of hypoglycemia.
- Glyburide, a first-generation SU, is associated with a higher-risk hypoglycemia than other SU and is no longer recommended as a first-line antidiabetic agent.
- Second-generation SUs (gliclazide, glimepiride, glipizide, and their extended formulations) are the preferred agents of this class of antidiabetic drugs.
- Weight gain is common after initiation of therapy.

- Although the hypoglycemic effect is quite rapid, studies have shown that an SU alone is inferior to the use of a thiazolidinedione (TZD) or metformin alone.[27]

Glinides

- These drugs also stimulate endogenous insulin secretion but bind to a different site within the SU receptor.
- They have a shorter circulating half-life than SU and are administered more frequently.
  - Because of their short half-life, they are **less likely to cause prolonged hypoglycemia.**
  - They are a good choice for patients who would otherwise tolerate a SU but have had hypoglycemia because of variable meal times and/or skipped meals.
- There are two currently available glinides on the market: repaglinide and nateglinide.
- Repaglinide is almost as effective as metformin or SU at decreasing hemoglobin A_{1c} level by 1.5%, but nateglinide is somewhat less potent.[28]
- The risk of weight gain is similar to that with most SUs.

α-Glucosidase Inhibitors

- α-Glucosidase inhibitors decrease the digestion and absorption of polysaccharides in the small intestine.
- These agents are effective at lowering postprandial glucose levels without causing hypoglycemia, but they are not as effective as metformin or SU at decreasing the hemoglobin A_{1c} level.
- The most common side effects are malabsorption and weight loss.
- Many patients report increased gas production and gastrointestinal symptoms, which result in the patients discontinuing this agent.

Thiazolidinediones

- TZDs are peroxisome proliferator–activated receptor γ-agonists.
- There are two TZDs currently available in the United States, **rosiglitazone** and **pioglitazone.**
- The primary mechanism of action of TZD is to increase the sensitivity of muscle, liver, and fat to insulin.
- **When used alone, they have been shown to lower the hemoglobin A_{1c} level by 0.5% to 1.4%.**
- The most common side effects are weight gain and fluid retention. Given this, there is also a twofold greater risk of congestive heart failure.[29]
- Several **meta-analyses suggest an increase in risk for myocardial infarction** with rosiglitazone.[30] When looking at the risk of using pioglitazone, studies have found no significant effects on primary CVD outcome.[31] While the meta-analyses conducted are not conclusive in assessing potential cardiovascular risk, physicians are advised to be cautious in patients with known CVD.
- Other concerning effects of TZDs include an increase in fracture risk and lower bone mineral density, especially in postmenopausal women.[32]
- Currently, TZDs can be used as monotherapy or in combination with metformin, SU, glinides, and/or insulin.

Dipeptidyl Peptidase-4 Inhibitors

- The gut insulinotropic hormones, **incretins,** include glucagon-like peptide-1 (GLP-1) and glucose-dependent insulinotropic peptide (GIP).[33]
- Both hormones are rapidly degraded by the enzyme dipeptidyl peptidase-4 (DPP-4).
- DPP-4 inhibitors have been shown to enhance the effects of GLP-1 and GIP, increasing glucose-mediated insulin secretion and suppressing glucagon secretion.
- Currently, **sitagliptin** is the only oral DPP-4 inhibitor available in the United States; there is another compound, **vildagliptin,** available in Europe, with many others now in development.

- **They have been shown to lower hemoglobin A$_{1c}$ level by 0.6% to 0.9%.**
- They are very well tolerated and have few side effects.
- It is currently approved for use as monotherapy or in combination with metformin or TZDs.

Other Noninsulin Therapies

Amylin Agonists

- Pramlintide, a synthetic analogue of the β-cell hormone amylin, has been shown to slow down gastric emptying, inhibit glucagon production, and decrease postprandial hyperglycemia.[34]
- It is administered **subcutaneously** before meals.
- **On average, it can decrease the hemoglobin A$_{1c}$ levels by 0.5% to 0.7%.**
- Like exenatide, the major side effects are gastrointestinal, predominantly nausea which tends to improve over time. **Weight loss** is associated with treatment and may be secondary to gastrointestinal side effects.
- **Pramlintide is approved for use only as adjunctive therapy with insulin,** regular or rapid-acting analogues.

Glucagon-Like Peptide-1 Agonists

- GLP-1 is a peptide produced by the small intestine that has been shown to potentiate glucose-stimulated insulin secretion.[35]
- **Exenatide,** a synthetic GLP-1 agonist, binds to the GLP-1 receptor on the pancreatic β-cell and is currently the only approved GLP-1 agonist available.
- It is administered as a twice-daily **subcutaneous injection.**
- **It has been shown to lower hemoglobin A$_{1c}$ levels by 0.5% to 1%.**
- Additional actions of exenatide include suppressing glucagon secretion and slowing down gastric motility.
- There is a high incidence of gastrointestinal side effects including nausea, vomiting, or diarrhea, but the majority of these symptoms resolve over time. Exenatide is **associated with weight loss,** which may be a result of its gastrointestinal side effects.
- Recent studies suggest an increased risk of pancreatitis associated with use of GLP agonists, but there are only a small number of cases reported at this time. It is not clear if this is a direct result of exenatide use and will need to be investigated over time.
- Exenatide is approved for use with SU, metformin, and/or a TZD.

Insulin

- **Insulin remains the most effective medication in the treatment of hyperglycemia.**
- Standard insulin preparations can be divided into two basic categories: intermediate acting and short acting.
  - **Intermediate-acting insulin** (i.e., NPH) is administered once or twice daily to provide basal insulin levels that suppress hepatic glucose production. Because NPH has a peak onset of activity of 6 to 8 hours, there can be some associated hypoglycemia when using this for basal insulin coverage.
  - **Short-acting insulin** (i.e., regular) has a peak onset of activity of 3 to 4 hours and is often used in combination with NPH to provide mealtime coverage.
- Conventional insulin therapy describes the use of simpler insulin regimens such as single daily injections, two injections per day of regular and NPH insulin, and mixed together and given in fixed amounts.
- **Intensive insulin therapy describes more complex regimens that combine basal insulin with rapid-acting insulin three or more times daily to cover meals.**

Type 1 Diabetes

- Insulin is the mainstay of treatment of type 1 diabetes and all patients should be managed cooperatively with an endocrinologist.
- **The majority of patients with type 1 diabetes will be maintained on intensive insulin therapy with multiple daily injections.**
- Since the arrival of both rapid- and long-acting insulin analogs, intensive glucose control in patients with type 1 diabetes is less associated with prolonged hypoglycemia.[36]
- Both **insulin glargine and detemir** are long-acting insulin analogs that have very modest peaks of activity, making them **ideal to provide a continuous basal insulin** level in a type 1 diabetic patient.
  - Dosing for insulin glargine is typically once daily, but in certain cases, patients may require twice-daily dosing.
  - Dosing for insulin detemir is twice daily.
- The resulting rapid-acting insulins available are **insulin lispro, aspart, and glulisine.**[37]
  - All have an onset of action within 5 to 15 minutes, peak action at 30 to 90 minutes, and a duration of action of 2 to 4 hours.
  - **These agents decrease postprandial hyperglycemia.**
  - They have been shown to reduce the frequency of hypoglycemia.
  - Rapid-acting insulin should be injected **immediately before meals** and the doses can be rapidly adjusted to match the hyperglycemia and carbohydrate intake in most type 1 diabetic patients.
- Most newly diagnosed patients with type 1 diabetes can be **started on a total daily dose of 0.2 to 0.4 units of insulin per kilogram per day, although most will ultimately require 0.6 to 0.7 units per kilogram per day.**
- Designing a **multiple daily injection** regimen should occur in collaboration with an endocrinologist, diabetes educator, and nutritionist to clearly assess the needs of the individual.
- **As a general rule of thumb, approximately half of the total daily dose should be given as a basal insulin, and the remainder is given as short- or rapid-acting insulin, divided before meals.**

Type 2 Diabetes

- Patients with persistent hyperglycemia despite oral hypoglycemic therapy may require the addition of insulin to their regimen or the transition to an insulin-based regimen alone.
- By using a combination of insulin and oral medications, studies have shown that insulin is effective in suppressing hepatic glucose production, improving the effectiveness of the oral agents, and decreasing the patients overall hyperinsulinemia.[38]
- Basal insulin, given once bedtime, is used commonly at bedtime to supplement oral hypoglycemic drug therapy.
  - This can be done with NPH or, the **long-acting insulin analog, glargine.** Because of the need for twice-daily dosing, detemir is infrequently used for this purpose.
  - **A safe starting dose is typically 10 units or 0.2 units/kg.**
  - This dose should be titrated up to achieve an FPG level of 90 to 130 mg/dL.
  - If nocturnal hypoglycemia or symptomatic hypoglycemia occurs in patients taking bedtime NPH, the dose should be decreased or the patient should be switched to insulin glargine.
- For most type 2 diabetic patients, supplementation of their oral hypoglycemic regimen with basal insulin is usually adequate to achieve glycemic goals.
- For some patients no longer responding to oral agents, preprandial boluses are necessary. These patients should be transitioned to an insulin-based regimen with the guidance of an endocrinologist.

Prevention and Management of Diabetes Complications

Cardiovascular Disease

- CVD remains the biggest cause of morbidity and mortality in patients with diabetes.
- Diabetes is an independent risk factor for CVD, and patients with type 2 diabetes typically have concomitant risk factors such as HTN and hyperlipidemia.

Hypertension

- HTN in diabetic patients is both a risk factor for CVD and microvascular complications.
- Typically, in type 1 diabetes, HTN is often the result of underlying nephropathy, whereas in type 2 diabetes, it is usually a result of weight, lifestyle, and other metabolic risk factors.
- The diagnostic cutoff for HTN is lower in diabetic patients because of the synergistic effect of high blood pressure and hyperglycemia on CVD. **HTN in a diabetic patient is defined as a blood pressure of >130/80 mm Hg.**
- Previous trials have shown that there is a clear reduction in the prevalence of CAD events, stroke, and development of nephropathy when patients are treated to a blood pressure of <130/80 mm Hg.[39,40]
- There are no well-controlled trials of nonpharmacologic therapies for the treatment of HTN in patients with diabetes, but given their benefit in nondiabetic patients, the following can be use in conjunction with medical therapy:
  - Reducing sodium intake.
  - Reducing excess body weight.
  - Increasing consumption of fruits, vegetables, and low-fat dairy products.
  - Avoiding excessive alcohol consumption.
  - Increasing activity levels.
- Pharmacologic therapies for lowering blood pressure should include regimens based on medications that are effective in both controlling HTN and reducing cardiovascular events.
- **Inhibitors of the renin-angiotensin system are especially useful in the treatment of diabetic patients with HTN and should be considered a first-line agents.**[41]
  - Angiotensin-converting enzyme (ACE) inhibitors and angiotensin receptor blockers (ARBs) have been shown to reduce CVD outcomes.
  - For patient with type 2 diabetes and significant nephropathy, ARBs were superior to calcium channel blockers in reducing heart failure.
- Most patients with HTN and diabetes will require multidrug therapy to reach treatment goals.
- During pregnancy, patients with diabetes should have a target blood pressure goal of systolic blood pressure 110 to 129 mm Hg and diastolic blood pressure 65 to 79 mm Hg.[42]
  - Treatment with ACE inhibitors and/or ARBs is contraindicated.
  - Antihypertensive drugs known to be safe in pregnancy include methyldopa, labetalol, diltiazem, clonidine, and prazosin.

Dyslipidemia

- Many clinical trials have shown the benefit of pharmacologic therapy in diabetic patients both for primary prevention and on outcomes in patients with concomitant CAD.
- The most common lipid abnormalities seen in diabetes include low levels of HDL cholesterol and elevated triglyceride levels.

- Lifestyle intervention, including medical nutrition therapy, increased physical activity, weight loss, and smoking cessation, may allow some patients to reach lipid goals.
  - Nutrition counseling should focus on reducing saturated fat, cholesterol, and transunsaturated fat intake in the diet.
  - Improved glycemic control can improve dyslipidemia in patients with very high triglycerides.
- **For most patients with diabetes, the primary goal of therapy is to lower LDL cholesterol level to a target goal of <100 mg/dL** (2.60 mmol/L).
  - Multiple studies have shown that statins are the drugs of choice for LDL cholesterol lowering.[43]
- **In high-risk patients with a history of acute coronary syndromes or cardiovascular events, studies have shown that therapy with high doses of statins to achieve LDL cholesterol level of <70 mg/dL led to a significant reduction in further events.**[44]
- If the HDL cholesterol level is <40 mg/dL, niacin can be used to raise the HDL cholesterol level, but it can significantly increase the blood glucose level at high doses.
- The ADA and American College of Cardiology discussed the use of apolipoprotein B (apo B) in patients with diabetes in a 2008 consensus panel.[45]
  - For patients who are high risk for CAD and diabetes, in whom the LDL cholesterol goal would be <70 mg/dL, apo B should be measured. A target level is <80 mg/dL.
  - For patients on statins with an LDL goal of <100 mg/dL, apo B should be targeted to <90 mg/dL.

Antiplatelet Therapy
- **In diabetic patients, aspirin is recommended for primary and secondary prevention of cardiovascular events.**
- In previous clinical trials, many varied dosages have been used (from 75 to 325 mg/day).
- The United States Preventive Services Task Force (USPSTF) recommends aspirin use when 5-year CVD risk is ≥3% (i.e., Framingham score). It should be considered in men >40 years of age, postmenopausal women, and younger patients with CVD risk factors, such as diabetes.[46]
- The use of clopidogrel in diabetic patients, who are aspirin intolerant or as adjunctive therapy with aspirin, demonstrated a decrease in secondary CVD events.[47]

Smoking Cessation
- Studies of patients with diabetes have shown a much higher risk of CVD and premature death in smokers.
- Smoking results in earlier development of microvascular complications.
- Physicians should routinely assess tobacco use and encourage cessation.

Screening and Treatment
- Diabetic patients often have atypical presentations of CAD, and screening the diabetic population for CAD is quite controversial.
- Some studies have shown that using a risk factor-based approach to the initial diagnostic evaluation may fail to identify patients with silent ischemia.[48]
- Newer studies reveal that intensive medical therapy is equivalent to revascularization in diabetic patients. There is significant controversy over screening asymptomatic diabetic patients.[49]
- The most recent data demonstrated no clinical benefit of routine screening in asymptomatic type 2 diabetic patients with normal ECGs.

- Currently, the recommendation is to assess cardiovascular risk factors annually in all diabetic patients and to treat accordingly. The pertinent risk factors are as follows:
  - Dyslipidemia.
  - HTN.
  - Smoking.
  - Positive family history of premature coronary disease.
  - Presence of micro- or macroalbuminuria.

Nephropathy
- Diabetic nephropathy remains one of the leading causes of end stage renal disease (ESRD).
- Microalbuminuria, defined as albuminuria in the range of 30 to 299 mg/24 hours, is the earliest stage of diabetic nephropathy in both type 1 and type 2 diabetes.
  - It is a known CVD risk factor.
  - Patients who progress to gross proteinuria are more likely to develop end stage renal disease.
- Studies have shown that intensive glycemic control can delay the onset of microalbuminuria as well as the progression from microalbuminuria to macroalbuminuria.[50]
- In addition, studies have shown that lower systolic blood pressure after treatment with an ACE-inhibitor or ARBs can reduce the development of nephropathy.[51,52]
  - Using a combination of drugs that block the rennin-angiotensin-aldosterone system can provide additional decreases in albuminuria, but the long-term combined effects of these drugs have not yet been investigated.
- Patients with progressive nephropathy despite optimal glycemic and blood pressure control and therapy with ACE-I and/or ARBs should be referred for further evaluation by a nephrologist and should consider dietary protein restriction.
- **The preferred method for screening for microalbuminuria is a random spot collection of urine with a calculation of the albumin:creatinine ratio.**
  - Two out of three measurements within 3 to 6 months should be elevated prior to diagnosis of albuminuria.
  - Exercise, infection, fever, heart failure, hyperglycemia, and HTN may elevate urinary albumin excretion over baseline values.
- **Serum creatinine should be measured at least yearly in patients with diabetes,** regardless of the degree of urine albumin excretion. Creatinine should be used to estimate GFR and to stage the level of CKD, if present.

Retinopathy
- The prevalence of diabetic retinopathy correlates with the duration of diabetes.
- It is a frequent cause of blindness in diabetic patients; other eye disorders, such as glaucoma and cataracts, also occur at an earlier age and more frequently in diabetic patients.
- Intensive glycemic control has been shown to prevent and delay the progression of diabetic retinopathy.
- The primary reason for aggressive retinal screening in diabetic patients is the treatment benefit from laser photocoagulation surgery. Numerous studies have shown that it is very effective in preventing vision loss but cannot reverse any existing visual defect.
- Retinopathy is estimated to take at least 5 years to develop after the onset of hyperglycemia.[53]
  - Patients with type 1 diabetes should have an initial comprehensive, dilated eye examination within 5 years after the onset of diabetes.

TABLE 3	Risk Factors for Ulcers and Amputations

Previous amputation
Past foot ulcer history
Peripheral neuropathy
Foot deformity
Peripheral vascular disease
Vision impairment
Diabetic nephropathy (especially patients on dialysis)
Poor glycemic control
Cigarette smoking

- Patients with type 2 diabetes should have an initial comprehensive, dilated eye examination soon after diagnosis.
- Subsequent examinations for both type 1 and type 2 diabetic patients are repeated annually if there is no documented retinopathy. Examinations should occur more frequently if retinopathy is progressing.

Neuropathy
There are numerous neurologic manifestations of diabetes, but the most prevalent are chronic sensorimotor diabetic polyneuropathy (DPN) and autonomic neuropathy.

Foot Care
- Major causes of morbidity and mortality in diabetic patients with neuropathy include amputation and foot ulceration.
- Risk factors for ulcers or amputations are shown in Table 3.
- **All diabetic patients should have a comprehensive foot examination yearly.**
  - Physicians should document any history of previous foot ulceration or amputation, neuropathic or peripheral vascular symptoms, impaired vision, tobacco use, and foot care practices.
  - The assessment should include the following:
    - General inspection of skin integrity and musculoskeletal deformities.
    - Documentation of pedal pulses and history of claudication.
    - Neurologic examination to identify loss of protective sensation using a 10-g monofilament.
- **A diagnostic ankle-brachial index (ABI) should be performed in any patient with symptoms of peripheral arterial disease.**[54]
  - Screening ABI be performed in patients >50 years of age.
  - Screening ABI should be considered in patients <50 years of age who have other peripheral arterial disease risk factors (e.g., smoking, HTN, hyperlipidemia, or duration of diabetes >10 years).
- **Patients should be counseled on the importance of foot care, appropriate footwear, and the risk associated with impaired sensation.**
  - Patients with loss of protective sensation should be instructed to visually inspect their feet daily.
- Nail care and debridement of calluses should be performed by a foot care specialist or health professional.
- Foot ulcers and wound care may require care by a podiatrist, orthopedic or vascular surgeon, or rehabilitation specialist experienced in the management of individuals with diabetes.

TABLE 4	Clinical Manifestations of Diabetic Autonomic Neuropathy

Resting tachycardia (>100)
Exercise intolerance
Orthostatic hypotension (a fall in systolic blood pressure >20 mm Hg
  upon standing)
Constipation and/or gastroparesis
Erectile dysfunction
Hypoglycemic autonomic failure

Peripheral Neuropathy
- As mentioned above, diabetic patients should be screened annually for DPN by measuring ankle reflexes, pinprick sensation, vibration perception (using a 128-Hz tuning fork), and 10-g monofilament pressure sensation at the distal plantar aspect of both great toes and metatarsal joints.
- **Loss of monofilament perception and reduced vibration perception can predict the development of foot ulcers.**[55]
- The primary treatment of diabetic neuropathy is optimal glycemic control.
- Patients with painful DPN may benefit from pharmacological treatment of their symptoms with tricyclic drugs and anticonvulsants.

Autonomic Neuropathy
- A careful history and physical examination is the most helpful tool in the diagnosis of autonomic neuropathy.
- Common clinical manifestations of autonomic neuropathy are presented in Table 4.
- Gastroparesis should be suspected in individuals with erratic glucose control or with upper gastrointestinal symptoms without other identified cause. The treatment of gastroparesis symptoms may improve with dietary changes and prokinetic agents.
- Treatments for erectile dysfunction often involves phosphodiesterase type 5 inhibitors. More invasive therapies, such as intracorporeal or intraurethral prostaglandins, vacuum devices, or penile prostheses, are often required and should be co-managed with a professional specializing in erectile dysfunction.

REFERENCES

1. American Diabetes Association. Diagnosis and classification of diabetes mellitus. *Diabetes Care* 2009;32:S62–S67.
2. Butler AE, Janson J, Bonner-Weir S, et al. Beta-cell deficit and increased beta-cell apoptosis in humans with type 2 diabetes. *Diabetes* 2003;52:102–110.
3. Fajans SS, Bell GI, Bowden DW, et al. Maturity onset diabetes of the young (MODY). *Diabet Med* 1996;13:S90–S95.
4. Bouchard P, Sai P, Reach G, et al. Diabetes mellitus following pentamidine-induced hypoglycemia in humans. *Diabetes* 1982;31:40–45.
5. Fabris P, Betterle C, Floreani A, et al. Development of type 1 diabetes mellitus during interferon alfa therapy for chronic HCV hepatitis. *Lancet* 1992;340:548.
6. ADA position statement: International Expert Committee report on the role of the A_{1c} assay in the diagnosis of diabetes. *Diabetes Care* 2009;32:1327–1334.
7. Knowler WC, Barrett-Connor E, Fowler SE, et al. Reduction in the incidence of type 2 diabetes with lifestyle intervention or metformin. *N Engl J Med* 2002:346:393–403.

8. American Diabetes Association: Gestational diabetes mellitus (Position Statement). *Diabetes Care* 2004;27:S88–S90.

9. The effect of intensive treatment of diabetes on the development and progression of long-term complications in insulin-dependent diabetes mellitus. The Diabetes Control and Complications Trial Research Group. *N Engl J Med* 1993;329:977–986.

10. Effect of intensive blood-glucose control with metformin on complications in overweight patients with type 2 diabetes (UKPDS 34). UK Prospective Diabetes Study (UKPDS) Group. *Lancet* 1998;352:854–865.

11. Metzger BE, Buchanan TA, Coustan DR, et al. Summary and recommendations of the Fifth International Workshop-Conference on Gestational Diabetes Mellitus. *Diabetes Care* 2007;30:S251–S260.

12. The Juvenile Diabetes Research Foundation Continuous Glucose Monitoring Study Group. Continuous glucose monitoring and intensive treatment of type 1 diabetes. *N Engl J Med* 2008;359:1464–1476.

13. Miller CD, Barnes CS, Phillips LS, et al. Rapid A_{1c} availability improves clinical decision-making in an urban primary care clinic. *Diabetes Care* 2003;26:1158–1163.

14. Franz MJ, Bantle JP, Beebe CA, et al. Evidence-based nutrition principles and recommendations for the treatment and prevention of diabetes and related complications. *Diabetes Care* 2002;25:148–198.

15. Klein S, Sheard NF, Pi-Sunyer X, et al. Weight management through lifestyle modification for the prevention and management of type 2 diabetes: rationale and strategies: a statement of the American Diabetes Association, the North American Association for the Study of Obesity, and the American Society for Clinical Nutrition. *Diabetes Care* 2004;27: 2067–2073.

16. Stern L, Iqbal N, Seshadri P, et al. The effects of low-carbohydrate versus conventional weight loss diets in severely obese adults: one-year follow-up of a randomized trial. *Ann Intern Med* 2004;140:778–785.

17. Buchwald H, Estok R, Fahrbach K, et al. Weight and type 2 diabetes after bariatric surgery: systematic review and meta-analysis. *Am J Med* 2009;122:248–256.

18. Boulé NG, Kenny GP, Haddad E, et al. Meta-analysis of the effect of structured exercise training on cardiorespiratory fitness in Type 2 diabetes mellitus. *Diabetologia* 2003;46: 1071–1081.

19. Aiello LP, Wong J, Cavallerano J, et al. Retinopathy. In: Ruderman N, Devlin JT, Kriska A, eds. Handbook of Exercise in Diabetes. 2nd Ed. Alexandria, VA: American Diabetes Association, 2002:401–413.

20. Smith SA, Poland GA. Use of influenza and pneumococcal vaccines in people with diabetes. *Diabetes Care* 2000;23:95–108.

21. Available at: http://www.cdc.gov/vaccines/recs/. Last accessed: July 21, 2009.

22. Gannon MC, Nuttall FQ. Protein and diabetes. In: Franz MJ, Bantle JP, eds. American Diabetes Association Guide to Medical Nutrition Therapy for Diabetes. Alexandria, VA: American Diabetes Association, 1999:107–125.

23. Cryer PE, Davis SN, Shamoon H. Hypoglycemia in diabetes. *Diabetes Care* 2003;26: 1902–1912.

24. Young-Hyman D. Psychosocial factors affecting adherence, quality of life, and well-being: helping patients cope. In: Bode B, ed. Medical Management of Type 1 Diabetes. 4th Ed. Alexandria, VA: American Diabetes Association, 2004:162–182.

25. DeFronzo R, Goodman A. The Multicenter Metformin Study Group: Efficacy of metformin in patients with non-insulin-dependent diabetes mellitus. *N Engl J Med* 1995;333: 541–549.

26. Shaw JS, Wilmot RL, Kilpatrick ES. Establishing pragmatic estimated GFR thresholds to guide metformin prescribing. *Diabet Med* 2007;24:1160–1163.

27. Kahn SE, Haffner SM, Heise MA, et al. Glycemic durability of rosiglitazone, metformin, or glyburide monotherapy. *N Engl J Med* 2006;355:2427–2443.

28. Rosenstock J, Hassman DR, Madder RD, et al. Repaglinide versus nateglinide monotherapy: a randomized, multicenter study. *Diabetes Care* 2004;27:1265–1270.

29. Singh S, Loke YK, Furberg CD. Thiazolidinediones and heart failure: a teleoanalysis. *Diabetes Care* 2007;30:2248–2254.

30. Nissen SE, Wolski K. Effect of rosiglitazone on the risk of myocardial infarction and death from cardiovascular causes. *N Engl J Med* 2007;356:2457–2471.

31. Dormandy JA, Charbonnel B, Eckland DJA, et al. Secondary prevention of macrovascular events in patients with type 2 diabetes in the PROactive Study (PROspective pioglitAzone Clinical Trial in macroVascular Events): a randomized controlled trial. *Lancet* 2005;366: 1279–1289.

32. Meier C, Kraenzlin ME, Bodmer M, et al. Use of thiazolidinediones and fracture risk. *Arch Intern Med* 2008;168:820–825.

33. Raz I, Hanefeld M, Xu L, et al. Efficacy and safety of the dipeptidyl peptidase-4 inhibitor sitagliptin as monotherapy in patients with type 2 diabetes mellitus. *Diabetologia* 2006;49: 2564–2571.

34. Riddle M, Frias J, Zhang B, et al. Pramlintide improved glycemic control and reduced weight in patients with type 2 diabetes using basal insulin. *Diabetes Care* 2007;30:2794–2799.

35. Kendall DM, Riddle MC, Rosenstock J, et al. Effects of exenatide (exendin-4) on glycemic control and weight over 30 weeks in patients with type 2 diabetes treated with metformin and a sulfonylurea. *Diabetes Care* 2005;28:1083–1091.

36. Ratner RE, Hirsch IB, Neifing JL, et al. Less hypoglycemia with insulin glargine in intensive insulin therapy for type 1 diabetes. U.S. Study Group of Insulin Glargine in Type 1 Diabetes. *Diabetes Care* 2000;23:639–643.

37. Hirsch IB. Insulin analogues. *N Engl J Med* 2005;352:174–183.

38. Riddle MC, Rosenstock J, Gerich J. The treat-to-target trial: randomized addition of glargine or human NPH insulin to oral therapy of type 2 diabetic patients. *Diabetes Care* 2003;26:3080–3086.

39. Tight blood pressure control and risk of macrovascular and microvascular complications in type 2 diabetes: UKPDS 38: UK Prospective Diabetes Study Group. *BMJ* 1998;317:703–713.

40. Adler AI, Stratton IM, Neil HA, et al. Association of systolic blood pressure with macrovascular and microvascular complications of type 2 diabetes (UKPDS 36): prospective observational study. *BMJ* 2000;321:412–419.

41. Major outcomes in high-risk hypertensive patients randomized to angiotensin converting enzyme inhibitor or calcium channel blocker vs diuretic: the Antihypertensive and Lipid-Lowering Treatment to Prevent Heart Attack Trial (ALLHAT). *JAMA* 2002;288:2981–2997.

42. Sibai BM. Treatment of hypertension in pregnant women. *N Engl J Med* 1996;335: 257–265.

43. Heart Protection Study Collaborative Group: MRC/BHF Heart Protection Study of cholesterol-lowering with simvastatin in 5963 people with diabetes: a randomised placebo-controlled trial. *Lancet* 2003;361:2005–2016.

44. Nissen SE, Tuzcu EM, Schoenhagen P, et al. Effect of intensive compared with moderate lipid-lowering therapy on progression of coronary atherosclerosis: a randomized controlled trial. *JAMA* 2004;291:1071–1080.

45. Brunzell JD, Davidson M, Furberg CD, et al. Consensus statement from the American Diabetes Association and the American College of Cardiology Foundation. *Diabetes Care* 2008;31:811–822.

46. US Preventive Services Task Force. Aspirin for the primary prevention of cardiovascular events: recommendation and rationale. *Ann Intern Med* 2002;136:157–160.

47. Bhatt DL, Marso SP, Hirsch AT, et al. Amplified benefit of clopidogrel versus aspirin in patients with diabetes mellitus. *Am J Cardiol* 2002;90:625–628.

48. Scognamiglio R, Negut C, Ramondo A, et al. Detection of coronary artery disease in asymptomatic patients with type 2 diabetes mellitus. *J Am Coll Cardiol* 2006;47:65–71.

49. Boden WE, O'Rourke RA, Teo KK, et al. Optimal medical therapy with or without PCI for stable coronary disease. *N Engl J Med* 2007;356:1503–1516.

50. Effect of intensive therapy on the development and progression of diabetic nephropathy in the Diabetes Control and Complications Trial: the Diabetes Control and Complications (DCCT) Research Group. *Kidney Int* 1995;47:1703–1720.

51. Remuzzi G, Macia M, Ruggenenti P. Prevention and treatment of diabetic renal disease in type 2 diabetes: the BENEDICT study. *J Am Soc Nephrol* 2006;17:S90–S97.
52. Brenner BM, Cooper ME, de Zeeuw D, et al. Effects of losartan on renal and cardiovascular outcomes in patients with type 2 diabetes and nephropathy. *N Engl J Med* 2001;345: 861–869.
53. Klein R, Klein BE, Moss SE, et al. The Wisconsin epidemiologic study of diabetic retinopathy. II. Prevalence and risk of diabetic retinopathy when age at diagnosis is <30 years. *Arch Ophthalmol* 1984;102:520–526.
54. American Diabetes Association: Peripheral arterial disease in people with diabetes (Consensus Statement). *Diabetes Care* 2003;26:3333–3341.
55. Boulton AJ, Vinik AI, Arezzo JC, et al. Diabetic neuropathies: a statement by the American Diabetes Association. *Diabetes Care* 2005;28:956–962.

17

Endocrine Diseases
William E. Clutter

Evaluation of Thyroid Function

Thyroid-Stimulating Hormone

- **Plasma thyroid-stimulating hormone (TSH) assay is the initial test of choice in most patients with suspected thyroid disease.**
- TSH levels are elevated in even mild primary hypothyroidism and are suppressed to <0.1 μU/mL in even subclinical hyperthyroidism (i.e., thyroid hormone excess too mild to cause symptoms). **A normal TSH level excludes hyperthyroidism and primary hypothyroidism.**
- TSH levels usually are within the reference range in secondary hypothyroidism and are not useful for detection of this rare form of hypothyroidism.
- Abnormal TSH levels are not specific for clinically important thyroid disease, which should usually be **confirmed by plasma thyroid hormone measurement.**
- TSH is mildly elevated (up to 20 μU/mL) in some euthyroid patients with non-thyroidal illnesses and in subclinical hypothyroidism.
- TSH levels may be suppressed to <0.1 μU/mL in nonthyroidal illness, in subclinical hyperthyroidism, in some euthyroid elderly patients, and during treatment with dopamine or high doses of glucocorticoids.
- TSH levels remain <0.1 μU/mL for some time after hyperthyroidism is corrected.

Free Thyroxine

- Measurement of free T4 confirms the diagnosis of clinical hypothyroidism in patients with elevated plasma TSH and confirms the diagnosis and assesses the severity of hyperthyroidism when plasma TSH is <0.1 μU/mL.
- It is also used to diagnose secondary hypothyroidism and adjust thyroxine therapy in patients with pituitary disease.
- Most laboratories measure free T4 by one of several types of immunoassay.
- **Measurement of total plasma T4 alone is not adequate,** because thyroxine-binding globulin (TBG) levels are altered in many circumstances.

Effect of Nonthyroidal Illness

- Many illnesses alter thyroid tests without causing true thyroid dysfunction. These changes must be recognized to avoid mistaken diagnosis and therapy.[1]
- **The low T3 syndrome occurs in many illnesses,** during starvation, and after trauma or surgery.
  - Conversion of T4 to T3 is decreased and plasma T3 levels are low.
  - It may be an adaptive response to illness, and thyroid hormone therapy is not beneficial.
- The low T4 syndrome occurs in severe illness.
  - It may be due to decreased TBG levels, inhibition of T4 binding to TBG, or suppressed TSH secretion.

TABLE 1	Effects of Drugs on Thyroid Function Tests

Effect	Drug
Decreased free and total T4	
True hypothyroidism (TSH elevated)	Iodine (amiodarone, radiographic contrast)
	Lithium
Inhibition of TSH secretion	Glucocorticoids
	Dopamine
Multiple mechanisms (TSH normal)	Phenytoin
Decreased total T4 only	
Decreased TBG (TSH normal)	Androgens
Inhibition of T4 binding to TBG (TSH normal)	Furosemide (high doses)
	Salicylates
Increased free and total T4	
True hyperthyroidism (TSH <0.1 μU/mL)	Iodine (amiodarone, radiographic contrast)
Inhibited T4–T3 conversion (TSH normal)	Amiodarone
Increased free T4 only	
Displacement of T4 from TBG in vitro (TSH normal)	Unfractionated heparin, low–molecular-weight heparin
Increased total T4 only	
Increased TBG (TSH normal)	Estrogens, tamoxifen

T3, triiodothyronine; T4, thyroxine; TBG, thyroxine-binding globulin; TSH, thyroid-stimulating hormone.

- TSH levels decrease early in severe illness, sometimes to <0.1 μU/mL.
- During recovery they rise, sometimes to levels higher than the normal range (but rarely higher than 20 μU/mL).

Effects of Drugs
- Iodine-containing drugs (e.g., amiodarone, radiographic contrast media) may cause hyperthyroidism or hypothyroidism in susceptible patients.
- Many drugs alter thyroid function tests, especially plasma T4, without causing true thyroid dysfunction (Table 1).
- In general, plasma TSH levels are a reliable guide to determining whether true hyperthyroidism or hypothyroidism is present.

HYPOTHYROIDISM

General Principles

- Primary hypothyroidism (due to disease of the thyroid itself) accounts for >90% of cases.[2]

- Hypothyroidism is readily treatable and should be suspected in any patient with compatible symptoms, especially in the presence of a goiter or a history of radioactive iodine (RAI) therapy or thyroid surgery.
- **Chronic lymphocytic thyroiditis (Hashimoto disease) is the most common cause** and may be associated with Addison disease and other endocrine deficits.[3]
- Its prevalence is greatest in women and increases with age.
- **Iatrogenic hypothyroidism** due to thyroidectomy and RAI therapy is also a common cause.
- Transient hypothyroidism occurs in **postpartum thyroiditis and subacute thyroiditis,** usually after a period of hyperthyroidism.
- **Drugs** that may cause hypothyroidism include iodine, lithium, α-interferon, interleukin-2, and thalidomide.
- **Secondary hypothyroidism** due to TSH deficiency is uncommon but may occur in any disorder of the pituitary or hypothalamus. It rarely occurs without other evidence of pituitary disease.

Diagnosis

Clinical Presentation

- Most symptoms of hypothyroidism are nonspecific and develop gradually.
- They include cold intolerance, fatigue, somnolence, poor memory, constipation, menorrhagia, myalgias, and hoarseness.
- Signs include slow tendon-reflex relaxation, bradycardia, facial and periorbital edema, dry skin, and nonpitting edema (myxedema).
- Mild weight gain may occur, but hypothyroidism does not cause obesity.
- Rare manifestations include hypoventilation, pericardial or pleural effusions, deafness, and carpal tunnel syndrome.

Diagnostic Testing

- Laboratory findings may include hyponatremia and elevated plasma levels of cholesterol, triglycerides, and creatine kinase.
- The ECG may show low-voltage and T-wave abnormalities.
- Thyroid imaging with ultrasound or radionuclide scan is not useful in diagnosis of hypothyroidism.
- **In suspected primary hypothyroidism, TSH is the best initial diagnostic test.**
  - A normal value excludes primary hypothyroidism, and a markedly elevated value (>20 μU/mL) confirms the diagnosis.
  - If plasma TSH is elevated moderately (5 to 20 μU/mL), plasma free T4 should be measured.
  - A low free T4 confirms clinical hypothyroidism.
  - **A clearly normal free T4 with an elevated plasma TSH indicates subclinical hypothyroidism,** in which thyroid function is impaired but increased secretion of TSH maintains plasma T4 levels within the reference range.
    - These patients may have nonspecific symptoms that are compatible with hypothyroidism and a mild increase in serum cholesterol and low-density lipoprotein cholesterol levels.
    - They develop clinical hypothyroidism at a rate of 2.5%/year.
- **If secondary hypothyroidism is suspected because of evidence of pituitary disease, plasma free T4 should be measured.**

- Plasma TSH levels are usually within the reference range in secondary hypothyroidism and cannot be used alone to make this diagnosis.
- **Patients with secondary hypothyroidism should be evaluated for other pituitary hormone deficits and for a mass lesion of the pituitary or hypothalamus.**
- In severe nonthyroidal illness, the diagnosis of hypothyroidism may be difficult.
  - Plasma total T4 and free T4 measured by routine assays may be low.
  - Plasma TSH is still the best initial diagnostic test.
  - Marked elevation of plasma TSH (>20 μU/mL) establishes the diagnosis of primary hypothyroidism.
  - A normal TSH value is strong evidence that the patient is euthyroid, except when there is evidence of pituitary or hypothalamic disease, in which case free T4 should be measured.
  - Moderate elevations of plasma TSH (<20 μU/mL) may occur in euthyroid patients with nonthyroidal illness and are not specific for hypothyroidism.

Treatment

Thyroid Hormone Replacement

- Thyroxine is the drug of choice.
- The average replacement dose is 1.6 μg/kg PO qd and most patients require doses between 75 and 150 μg qd.
  - Young and middle-aged patients should be started on 100 μg daily.
  - In otherwise healthy elderly patients, the initial dose should be 50 μg daily.
  - Patients with heart disease should be started on 25 μg daily and monitored carefully for exacerbation of cardiac symptoms.
- The need for lifelong treatment should be emphasized.
- Thyroxine should be taken 30 minutes before a meal, since dietary fiber interferes with its absorption, and should not be taken with medications such as calcium or iron supplements that affect its absorption.

Follow-Up and Dose Adjustment

- In primary hypothyroidism, the goal of therapy is to maintain plasma TSH within the normal range.
  - After 6 to 8 weeks, plasma TSH should be measured. The dose of T4 then should be adjusted in 12- to 25-μg increments at intervals of 6 to 8 weeks until plasma TSH is normal.
  - Thereafter, annual TSH measurement is adequate to monitor therapy.
  - **Overtreatment,** indicated by a plasma TSH below the normal range, should be avoided, as it **increases the risk of osteoporosis and atrial fibrillation.**
- **In secondary hypothyroidism, plasma TSH cannot be used to adjust therapy.**
  - The goal of therapy is to maintain the plasma free T4 near the middle of the reference range.
  - The dose of T4 should be adjusted at 6- to 8-week intervals until this goal is achieved.
  - Thereafter, annual measurement of plasma free T4 is adequate to monitor therapy.
- Coronary artery disease may be exacerbated by treatment of hypothyroidism. The dose should be increased slowly, with careful attention to worsening angina, heart failure, or arrhythmias.

Difficult to Control Hypothyroidism

- Difficulty in controlling hypothyroidism is most often due to poor compliance with therapy. Observed therapy may be necessary in some cases.
- Other causes of increasing T4 requirements include the following:
  - Malabsorption due to intestinal disease.
  - Drugs that interfere with T4 absorption (e.g., calcium carbonate, ferrous sulfate, cholestyramine, sucralfate, aluminum hydroxide).
  - Other drug interactions that increase T4 clearance (e.g., rifampin, carbamazepine, phenytoin) or block conversion of T4 to T3 (amiodarone).
  - Pregnancy, in which T4 requirement increases in the first trimester.
  - Gradual failure of remaining endogenous thyroid function after treatment of hyperthyroidism.

Subclinical Hypothyroidism

- Subclinical hypothyroidism should be treated with T4 if any of the following is present[4]:
  - Symptoms compatible with hypothyroidism
  - Goiter
  - Hypercholesterolemia that warrants treatment
  - Plasma TSH >10 μU/mL.
- Untreated patients should be monitored annually, and T4 should be started if symptoms develop or serum TSH increases to >10 μU/mL.

Pregnancy

- Thyroxine dose increases by an average of 50% in the first half of pregnancy.[5]
- In women with primary hypothyroidism, plasma TSH should be measured as soon as pregnancy is confirmed and monthly thereafter through the second trimester.
- The thyroxine dose should be increased as needed to maintain plasma TSH within the normal range.

Urgent Therapy

- Urgent therapy is rarely necessary for hypothyroidism.
- Most patients with hypothyroidism and concomitant illness can be treated in the usual manner; however, **hypothyroidism may impair survival in critical illness** by contributing to hypoventilation, hypotension, hypothermia, bradycardia, or hyponatremia. Such patients should be admitted to the hospital for therapy of hypothyroidism and the concomitant illness.
- Confirmatory tests should be obtained before thyroid hormone therapy is started in a severely ill patient, including serum TSH and free T4.
- T4, 50 to 100 μg IV, can be given every 6 to 8 hours for 24 hours, followed by 75 to 100 μg IV daily until oral intake is possible.
- **Such rapid correction is warranted only in extremely ill patients.**
- Vital signs and cardiac rhythm should be monitored carefully to detect early signs of exacerbation of heart disease.
- Hydrocortisone, 50 mg IV every 8 hours, usually is recommended during rapid treatment with thyroid hormone on the grounds that replacement of thyroid hormone may precipitate adrenal failure.

HYPERTHYROIDISM

General Principles

- Hyperthyroidism should be suspected in any patient with compatible symptoms, as it is a readily treatable disorder that may become highly debilitating.
- **Graves disease** causes most cases of hyperthyroidism, especially in young patients.[6] This autoimmune disorder may also cause two signs that are not found in other causes of hyperthyroidism: proptosis (exophthalmos) and pretibial myxedema.
- **Toxic multinodular goiter** (MNG) is a common cause in older patients.
- Unusual causes include iodine-induced hyperthyroidism, usually precipitated by drugs (e.g., amiodarone or radiographic contrast media), thyroid adenomas (which present as a single nodule), subacute thyroiditis (painful tender goiter with transient hyperthyroidism), postpartum thyroiditis (nontender goiter with transient hyperthyroidism), and surreptitious ingestion of thyroid hormone.
- TSH-induced hyperthyroidism is extremely rare.

Diagnosis

Clinical Presentation

- Symptoms include heat intolerance, weight loss, weakness, palpitations, oligomenorrhea, and anxiety.
- Signs include brisk tendon reflexes, fine tremor, proximal weakness, stare, and eyelid lag.
- Cardiac abnormalities may be prominent, including sinus tachycardia, atrial fibrillation, and exacerbation of coronary artery disease or heart failure.
- In the elderly, hyperthyroidism may present with only atrial fibrillation, heart failure, weakness, or weight loss, and a high index of suspicion is needed to make the diagnosis.
- Presence of proptosis or pretibial myxedema indicates Graves disease (although many patients with Graves disease lack these signs).
- Palpation of the thyroid can determine whether a diffuse or nodular goiter is present; most hyperthyroid patients with a diffuse nontender goiter have Graves disease.
- History of recent pregnancy, neck pain, or iodine administration suggests causes other than Graves disease.
- The differential diagnosis is presented in Table 2.

TABLE 2	Differential Diagnosis of Hyperthyroidism
Signs	**Diagnosis**
Diffuse, nontender goiter	Graves disease (rarely postpartum silent thyroiditis)
Multiple thyroid nodules	Toxic multinodular goiter
Single thyroid nodule	Thyroid adenoma
Tender painful goiter	Subacute thyroiditis
Normal thyroid gland	Graves disease (rarely postpartum thyroiditis or factitious hyperthyroidism)

Diagnostic Testing

- **Plasma TSH is the best initial diagnostic test.**
  - If plasma TSH is <0.1 μU/mL, plasma free T4 should be measured to determine the severity of hyperthyroidism and as a baseline for therapy.
  - If plasma free T4 is elevated, the diagnosis of clinical hyperthyroidism is established.
  - If plasma TSH is <0.1 μU/mL but free T4 is normal, the patient may have clinical hyperthyroidism due to elevation of plasma T3 alone; in this case plasma T3 should be measured.
  - This combination of test results may also be due to suppression of TSH by nonthyroidal illness.
    - A third-generation TSH assay with a detection limit of 0.01 μU/mL may be helpful in patients with suppressed TSH and nonthyroidal illness.
    - Most patients with clinical hyperthyroidism have plasma TSH levels that are <0.01 μU/mL in such assays, whereas nonthyroidal illness rarely suppresses TSH to this degree.
  - **Subclinical hyperthyroidism** may lower TSH to <0.1 μU/mL, and therefore suppression of TSH alone does not confirm that symptoms are due to hyperthyroidism.
    - Subclinical hyperthyroidism is present when the plasma TSH is suppressed to <0.1 μU/mL but the patient has no symptoms that are definitely caused by hyperthyroidism and plasma levels of T4 and T3 are normal.[7]
- In rare cases, 24-hour **RAI uptake** (RAIU) is needed to distinguish Graves disease or toxic MNG (in which RAIU is elevated) from postpartum thyroiditis, iodine-induced hyperthyroidism, or factitious hyperthyroidism (in which RAIU is very low).

Treatment

- Some forms of hyperthyroidism (subacute or postpartum thyroiditis) are transient and require only symptomatic therapy.
- Three methods are available for definitive therapy: RAI, thionamides, and subtotal thyroidectomy, none of which controls hyperthyroidism rapidly.
- During treatment, patients are followed by clinical evaluation and measurement of plasma free T4. **Plasma TSH is useless in assessing the initial response to therapy,** as it remains suppressed until after the patient becomes euthyroid.
- Regardless of the therapy used, all patients with Graves disease require lifelong follow-up for recurrent hyperthyroidism or development of hypothyroidism.

Symptomatic Therapy

- β-adrenergic antagonists are used to relieve such symptoms as palpitations, tremor, and anxiety until hyperthyroidism is controlled by definitive therapy or until transient forms of hyperthyroidism subside.
- The initial dose of atenolol, 25 to 50 mg daily, is adjusted to alleviate symptoms and tachycardia.
- β-adrenergic antagonist therapy should be reduced gradually, then stopped as hyperthyroidism is controlled.
- Verapamil at an initial dose of 40 to 80 mg tid can be used to control tachycardia in patients with contraindications to β-adrenergic antagonists.

Thionamides

- Methimazole and propylthiouracil (PTU) inhibit thyroid hormone synthesis.[8]
- PTU also inhibits extrathyroidal conversion of T4 to T3.
- Once thyroid hormone stores are depleted (after several weeks to months), T4 levels decrease.
- These drugs have no permanent effect on thyroid function.
- In the majority of patients with Graves disease, hyperthyroidism recurs within 6 months after therapy is stopped.
  - Spontaneous remission of Graves disease occurs in approximately one third of patients during thionamide therapy, and, in this minority, no other treatment may be needed. Remission is more likely to occur in mild, recent-onset hyperthyroidism.
- Initiation of therapy:
  - Before starting therapy, patients must be warned of side effects and precautions.
  - Usual starting doses are PTU, 100 to 200 mg PO tid, or methimazole, 10 to 40 mg PO daily; higher initial doses can be used in severe hyperthyroidism.
- Follow-up:
  - Restoration of euthyroidism takes up to several months.
  - Patients are evaluated at 4-week intervals with assessment of clinical findings and plasma free T4.
  - If plasma free T4 levels do not fall after 4 to 8 weeks, the dose should be increased.
  - Doses as high as PTU, 300 mg PO qid, or methimazole, 60 mg PO daily, may be required.
  - Once the plasma free T4 level falls to normal, the dose is adjusted to maintain plasma free T4 within the normal range.
  - No consensus exists on the optimal duration of therapy, but periods of 6 months to 2 years are used most commonly. Regardless of the duration of therapy, patients must be monitored carefully for recurrence of hyperthyroidism after the drug is stopped.
- Side effects are most likely to occur within the first few months of therapy.
  - Minor side effects include rash, urticaria, fever, arthralgias, and transient leukopenia.
  - **Agranulocytosis** occurs in 0.3% of patients who are treated with thionamides.
  - Other life-threatening side effects include **hepatitis, vasculitis, and drug-induced lupus erythematosus.**
  - These complications usually resolve if the drug is stopped promptly.
  - Patients must be warned to stop the drug immediately if jaundice or symptoms suggestive of agranulocytosis (e.g., fever, chills, sore throat) develop and to contact their physician promptly for evaluation.
  - Routine monitoring of the white blood cell count is not useful for detecting agranulocytosis, which develops suddenly.

Radioactive Iodine Therapy

- A single dose permanently controls hyperthyroidism in about 90% of patients, and further doses can be given if necessary.
- A pregnancy test is done immediately before therapy in potentially fertile women.
- Usually, 24-hour RAIU is measured and used to calculate the dose.
- Thionamides interfere with RAI therapy and should be stopped at least 3 days before treatment.
- If iodine treatment has been given, it should be stopped at least 2 weeks before RAI therapy.

- Most patients with Graves disease are treated with 8 to 10 mCi, although treatment of toxic MNG requires higher doses.
- Follow-up:
  - Usually, several months are needed to restore euthyroidism.
  - Patients are evaluated at 4- to 6-week intervals, with assessment of clinical findings and plasma free T4.
  - If thyroid function stabilizes within the normal range, the interval between follow-up visits is increased gradually to annual intervals.
  - If symptomatic hypothyroidism develops, T4 therapy is started.
  - Mild hypothyroidism after RAI therapy may be transient, and asymptomatic patients can be observed for further 4 to 6 weeks to determine whether hypothyroidism will resolve spontaneously.
  - If symptomatic hyperthyroidism persists after 6 months, RAI treatment is repeated.
- Side effects:
  - **Hypothyroidism occurs in more than half of patients within the first year** and continues to develop at a rate of approximately 3%/year thereafter.
  - A slight rise in plasma T4 may occur in the first 2 weeks after therapy, owing to release of stored hormone. This development is important only in patients with severe cardiac disease, which may worsen as a result. Such patients should be treated with thionamides to restore euthyroidism and to deplete stored hormone before treatment with RAI.
  - No convincing evidence has been found that RAI has a clinically important effect on the course of Graves' eye disease.
  - It does not increase the risk of malignancy.
  - No increase in congenital abnormalities has been found in the offspring of women who conceive after RAI therapy and the radiation exposure to the ovaries is low, comparable to that from common diagnostic radiographs. Concern for potential teratogenic effects should not influence physicians' advice to patients.

Subtotal Thyroidectomy

- This procedure provides long-term control of hyperthyroidism in most patients.
- **Surgery may trigger a perioperative exacerbation of hyperthyroidism** and patients should be prepared for surgery by one of two of the following methods.
  - A thionamide is given until the patient is nearly euthyroid. Supersaturated potassium iodide (SSKI), 40 to 80 mg (1 to 2 drops) PO bid, is then added, and surgery is scheduled 1 to 2 weeks later. Both drugs are stopped postoperatively.
  - Atenolol, 50 to 100 mg daily, and SSKI, 1 to 2 drops PO bid, are started 1 to 2 weeks before surgery is scheduled. The dose of atenolol is increased, if necessary, to reduce the resting heart rate below 90 beats/minute. Atenolol, but not SSKI, is continued for 5 to 7 days after surgery.
- Follow-up:
  - Patients should be evaluated 4 to 6 weeks after surgery, with assessment of clinical findings and plasma free T4 and TSH.
  - If thyroid function is normal, the patient is seen at 3 and 6 months, then annually.
  - If symptomatic hypothyroidism develops, T4 therapy is started.
  - Mild hypothyroidism after subtotal thyroidectomy may be transient, and asymptomatic patients can be observed for a further 4 to 6 weeks to determine whether hypothyroidism will resolve spontaneously.
  - Hyperthyroidism persists or recurs in 3% to 7% of patients.

- **Complications of thyroidectomy include hypothyroidism in 30–50% of patients and hypoparathyroidism in perhaps 3%.**
  - Rare complications include permanent vocal cord paralysis due to recurrent laryngeal nerve injury and perioperative death.
  - The complication rate appears to depend on the experience of the surgeon.

Choice of Definitive Therapy

- **In Graves disease, RAI therapy is the treatment of choice for almost all patients.** It is simple, highly effective, and causes no life-threatening complications.
- It cannot be used in pregnancy. **PTU should be used to treat hyperthyroidism in pregnancy** but it provides long-term control of hyperthyroidism in fewer than one half of patients and carries a small risk of life-threatening side effects.
- Thyroidectomy should be used only in patients who refuse RAI therapy and who relapse or develop side effects with thionamide therapy.

Other Causes of Hyperthyroidism

- Toxic MNG and toxic adenoma should be treated with RAI (except in pregnancy).
- Transient forms of hyperthyroidism due to thyroiditis should be treated symptomatically with atenolol.
- Iodine-induced hyperthyroidism is treated with thionamides and atenolol until the patient is euthyroid.
- Although treatment of some patients with amiodarone-induced hyperthyroidism with glucocorticoids has been advocated, nearly all patients with amiodarone-induced hyperthyroidism respond well to thionamide therapy.[9]
- **Subclinical hyperthyroidism increases the risk of atrial fibrillation in the elderly and predisposes to osteoporosis in postmenopausal women and should be treated in these groups of patients.** Whether other patients should be treated is unclear.

Urgent Therapy

- Urgent therapy is warranted when hyperthyroidism exacerbates heart failure or coronary artery disease and in rare patients with severe hyperthyroidism complicated by fever and delirium.[10] Such patients should be admitted to the hospital for therapy.
- PTU, 300 mg PO every 6 hours, should be started immediately.
- Iodide (SSKI, 1 to 2 drops PO every 12 hours) should be started 2 hours after the first dose of PTU to inhibit thyroid hormone secretion rapidly.
- Propranolol, 40 mg PO every 6 hours (or an equivalent dose of a parenteral β-adrenergic antagonist), should be given to patients with angina or myocardial infarction, and the dose should be adjusted to prevent tachycardia.
- Propranolol may benefit some patients with heart failure and marked tachycardia but can further impair left ventricular function. In patients with clinical heart failure, it should be given only with careful monitoring of left ventricular function.
- Plasma free T4 is measured every 3 to 4 days, and treatment with iodine is discontinued when free T4 approaches the normal range.
- RAI therapy should be scheduled 2 weeks after iodine is stopped.

Hyperthyroidism in Pregnancy

- **RAI is contraindicated in pregnancy,** and therefore patients should be treated with PTU.
- The dose should be adjusted to maintain the plasma free T4 near the upper limit of the normal range to avoid fetal hypothyroidism.

- The dose required often decreases in the later stages of pregnancy.
- Atenolol, 25 to 50 mg PO daily, can be used to relieve symptoms while awaiting the effects of PTU.
- The fetus and neonate should be monitored carefully for hyperthyroidism.

EUTHYROID GOITER

- The diagnosis of euthyroid goiter is based on palpation of the thyroid and on evaluation of thyroid function.
- If the thyroid is enlarged, the examiner should determine whether the enlargement is diffuse or multinodular or whether a single nodule is present. **All three forms of euthyroid goiter are common, especially in women.**
- Imaging studies, such as thyroid scans or ultrasonography, provide no useful additional information about goiters that are diffuse or multinodular, and should not be performed in these patients.
  - Furthermore, **20% to 60% of people have nonpalpable thyroid nodules that are detectable by ultrasound.**
  - **These nodules rarely have any clinical importance** but their incidental discovery may lead to unnecessary diagnostic testing and treatment.[11]

Diffuse Goiter

- Almost all euthyroid diffuse goiters in the United States are due to chronic lymphocytic thyroiditis (Hashimoto's thyroiditis).[4]
- As Hashimoto disease may also cause hypothyroidism, plasma **TSH should be measured even in patients who are clinically euthyroid.**
- Small diffuse goiters usually are asymptomatic, and therapy is seldom required. The patient should be monitored regularly for the development of hypothyroidism.

Multinodular Goiter

- MNG is common in older patients, especially women.
- Most patients are asymptomatic and require no treatment.
- In a few patients, hyperthyroidism (toxic MNG) develops.
- In rare patients, the gland compresses the trachea or esophagus, causing dyspnea or dysphagia, and treatment is required.
  - Thyroxine treatment has less, if any, effect on the size of MNGs and is rarely indicated.
  - RAI therapy reduces gland size and relieves symptoms in most patients.[12]
  - Subtotal thyroidectomy can also be used to relieve compressive symptoms.
- The risk of malignancy in MNG is low, comparable to the frequency of incidental thyroid carcinoma in clinically normal glands.
- Evaluation for thyroid carcinoma with needle biopsy is warranted only if one nodule is disproportionately enlarged.

Single Thyroid Nodules

- **Single thyroid nodules are usually benign but a small number are thyroid carcinomas.**[13]
- Clinical findings that increase the likelihood of carcinoma include the presence of cervical lymphadenopathy, a history of radiation to the head or neck in childhood,

and a family history of medullary thyroid carcinoma or multiple endocrine neoplasia syndromes type 2A or 2B. A hard fixed nodule, recent nodule growth, or hoarseness due to vocal cord paralysis also suggests malignancy. However, **most patients with thyroid carcinomas have none of these risk factors,** and nearly all single thyroid nodules should be evaluated with needle aspiration biopsy.

- Patients with thyroid carcinoma should be managed in consultation with an endocrinologist.
- Nodules with benign cytology should be reevaluated periodically by palpation and biopsied again if they enlarge.
- T4 therapy has little or no effect on the size of single thyroid nodules and is not indicated.
- **Imaging studies cannot distinguish benign from malignant nodules and are not necessary for the evaluation of a palpable thyroid nodule.**
- The management of nonpalpable thyroid nodules discovered incidentally by ultrasound is controversial.[14]

ADRENAL FAILURE

General Principles

- Adrenal failure may be due to disease of the adrenal glands (primary adrenal failure, Addison disease), with deficiency of cortisol and aldosterone and elevated plasma adrenocorticotropic hormone (ACTH) or due to ACTH deficiency caused by disorders of the pituitary or hypothalamus (secondary adrenal failure) with deficiency of cortisol alone.[15]
- Findings in adrenal failure are nonspecific and, without a high index of suspicion, the diagnosis of this potentially lethal but readily treatable disease is easily missed.
- Adrenal failure should be suspected in patients with hypotension (including orthostatic hypotension), persistent nausea, weight loss, hyponatremia, or hyperkalemia.[16]

Primary Adrenal Failure

- Primary adrenal failure is often due to autoimmune adrenalitis, which may be associated with other endocrine deficits (e.g., hypothyroidism).[17]
- Infections of the adrenal gland such as tuberculosis and histoplasmosis may cause adrenal failure.
- Hemorrhagic adrenal infarction may occur in the postoperative period, in coagulation disorders and hypercoagulable states, and in sepsis (i.e., Waterhouse-Friderichsen syndrome).
  - Adrenal hemorrhage often causes abdominal or flank pain and fever; CT scan of the abdomen reveals high-density bilateral adrenal masses.
- Adrenoleukodystrophy causes adrenal failure in young males.
- In patients with AIDS, adrenal failure may develop because of disseminated cytomegalovirus, mycobacterial or fungal infection, adrenal lymphoma, or treatment with ketoconazole, which inhibits steroid hormone synthesis.

Secondary Adrenal Failure

- **Secondary adrenal failure is most often due to glucocorticoid therapy;** ACTH suppression may persist for a year after therapy is stopped.
- Any disorder of the pituitary or hypothalamus can cause ACTH deficiency but usually other evidence of these disorders can be seen.

Diagnosis

Clinical Presentation

- Symptoms include anorexia, nausea, vomiting, weight loss, weakness, and fatigue.
- Orthostatic hypotension and hyponatremia are common.
- Usually symptoms are chronic, but shock that is fatal unless treated promptly may develop suddenly. Often, this adrenal crisis is triggered by illness, injury, or surgery.
- Hyperpigmentation (due to marked ACTH excess) and hyperkalemia and volume depletion (due to aldosterone deficiency) occur only in primary adrenal failure.

Diagnostic Testing

- **The short cosyntropin stimulation test is used for diagnosis.**
  - Cosyntropin, 250 µg, is given IV or IM and plasma cortisol is measured 30 minutes later.
  - The normal response is a stimulated plasma cortisol >20 µg/dL.
  - This test detects primary and secondary adrenal failure, except within a few weeks of onset of pituitary dysfunction (e.g., shortly after pituitary surgery).
- The distinction between primary and secondary adrenal failure usually is clear.
  - Hyperkalemia, hyperpigmentation, or other autoimmune endocrine deficits indicate primary adrenal failure, whereas deficits of other pituitary hormones, symptoms of a pituitary mass (e.g., headache, visual field loss), or known pituitary or hypothalamic disease indicate secondary adrenal failure.
  - If the cause is unclear, the plasma ACTH level distinguishes primary adrenal failure (in which it is markedly elevated) from secondary adrenal failure.
  - Evidence of adrenal enlargement or calcification on abdominal CT indicates that the cause is infection or hemorrhage.
  - Patients with secondary adrenal failure should be tested for other pituitary hormone deficiencies and should be evaluated for a pituitary or hypothalamic tumor.

Treatment

Adrenal Crisis

- **Adrenal crisis with hypotension must be treated immediately.**
- These patients should be admitted to the hospital for therapy and be evaluated for an underlying illness that precipitated the crisis.
- If the diagnosis of adrenal failure is known, hydrocortisone, 100 mg IV every 8 hours, should be given, and 0.9% saline with 5% dextrose should be infused rapidly until hypotension is corrected.
  - The dose of hydrocortisone is decreased gradually over several days as symptoms and any precipitating illness resolve, and then is changed to oral maintenance therapy.
  - Mineralocorticoid replacement is not needed until the dose of hydrocortisone is <100 mg/day.
- If the diagnosis of adrenal failure has not been established, a single dose of dexamethasone, 10 mg IV, should be given, and a rapid infusion of 0.9% saline with 5% dextrose should be started.
  - A cosyntropin stimulation test should be performed.
  - Dexamethasone is used because it does not interfere with subsequent measurements of cortisol.

- After the 30-minute plasma cortisol measurement, hydrocortisone, 100 mg IV every 8 hours, should be given until the test result is known.

Outpatient Maintenance Therapy

- **All patients with adrenal failure require cortisol replacement with prednisone.**
- Most patients with primary adrenal failure also require replacement of aldosterone with fludrocortisone.
- Prednisone, 5 mg PO every morning, should be started.
  - Patients should initially be evaluated every 1 to 2 months.
  - The dose of prednisone is adjusted to eliminate symptoms and signs of cortisol deficiency or excess, with most patients requiring between 4 mg every morning to as much as 5 mg every morning and 2.5 mg every evening.
  - Eventually, annual follow-up is adequate **unless an acute illness develops.**
  - Concomitant therapy with rifampin, phenytoin, or phenobarbital accelerates glucocorticoid metabolism and increases the dose requirement.
- During illness, injury, or the perioperative period, the dose of prednisone must be increased.
  - **For minor illnesses,** the patient should double the dose for 3 days. If the illness resolves, the maintenance dose is resumed. **Vomiting requires immediate medical attention,** with IV glucocorticoid therapy and IV fluid. Patients can be given a prefilled syringe of dexamethasone, 4 mg, to be self-administered IM for vomiting or severe illness if medical care is not immediately available.
  - **For severe illness** or injury, hydrocortisone, 50 mg IV every 8 hours, should be given, with the dose tapered as severity of illness wanes. The same regimen is used in patients who are undergoing surgery, with the first dose of hydrocortisone given preoperatively. Usually, the dose can be reduced to maintenance therapy 3 to 4 days after uncomplicated surgery.
- In primary adrenal failure, fludrocortisone, 0.1 mg PO qd, should be given, along with liberal salt intake.
  - During follow-up visits, supine and standing blood pressure and serum potassium should be monitored.
  - The dose of fludrocortisone is adjusted to maintain blood pressure and serum potassium within the normal range; the usual dose is 0.05 to 0.2 mg PO qd.
- Patients should be educated in management of their disease, including adjustment of prednisone dose during illness. They should wear a medical identification tag or bracelet.

CUSHING SYNDROME

General Principles

- Cushing syndrome (the clinical effects of increased glucocorticoid hormone) is most often iatrogenic due to therapy with glucocorticoid drugs.
- ACTH-secreting pituitary microadenomas (Cushing disease) account for approximately 80% of cases of endogenous Cushing syndrome.
- Adrenal tumors and ectopic ACTH secretion account for the remainder.
- Clinical features include truncal obesity, rounded face, fat deposits in the supraclavicular fossae and over the posterior neck, hypertension, hirsutism, amenorrhea, and depression.
- More specific findings include thin skin, easy bruising, reddish striae, proximal muscle weakness, and osteoporosis.

- Diabetes mellitus may develop in some patients.
- Hyperpigmentation or hypokalemic alkalosis suggests Cushing syndrome because of ectopic ACTH secretion.

Diagnosis

- The diagnosis is based on increased cortisol excretion and lack of normal feedback inhibition of ACTH and cortisol secretion.[18]
- **Overnight dexamethasone suppression test can be done as a screening test.**
  - 1 mg dexamethasone given PO at 11:00 PM; plasma cortisol measured at 8:00 AM the next day; normal plasma cortisol level <2 μg/dL.
- If the overnight dexamethasone suppression test is abnormal, 24-hour urine cortisol should be measured. **24-hour urine cortisol** measurement can also be done as a screening test.
- Both tests are very sensitive, and **a normal value virtually excludes the diagnosis.**
- If the 24-hour urine cortisol is more than four times the upper limit of the reference range in a patient with compatible symptoms, the diagnosis of Cushing syndrome is established.
- In patients with milder elevations of urine cortisol, a **low-dose dexamethasone suppression test** should be performed.
  - Dexamethasone, 0.5 mg PO every 6 hours, is given for 48 hours, starting at 8:00 AM.
  - Urine cortisol is measured during the last 24 hours and plasma cortisol is measured 6 hours after the last dose of dexamethasone.
  - Failure to suppress plasma cortisol to <2 μg/dL and urine cortisol to less than the normal reference range is diagnostic of Cushing syndrome.
- Testing should not be done during severe illness or depression, which may cause false-positive results.
- Phenytoin therapy also causes false-positive dexamethasone suppression test results by accelerating metabolism of dexamethasone.
- **Random plasma cortisol levels are not useful for diagnosis,** because the wide range of normal values overlaps that of Cushing syndrome.
- After the diagnosis of Cushing syndrome is made, tests to determine the cause should be done in consultation with an endocrinologist.

Treatment

- The treatment of hypercortisolism is dependent on its cause and a complete discussion of management is beyond the scope of this chapter.
- Stopping exogenous glucocorticoids when possible is clearly indicated.
- Other treatments usually require the assistance of an endocrinologist or neurosurgeon.

INCIDENTAL ADRENAL NODULES

General Principles

- Adrenal nodules are a common incidental finding on abdominal imaging studies.
- **Most incidentally discovered nodules are benign adrenocortical tumors** that do not secrete excess hormone, but the differential diagnosis includes adrenal adenomas that cause

Cushing syndrome or primary hyperaldosteronism, pheochromocytoma, adreno-cortical carcinoma, and metastatic cancer.[19]

Diagnosis

Clinical Presentation
- The patient should be evaluated for symptoms and signs of Cushing syndrome.
- Hypertension suggests the possibility of primary hyperaldosteronism or pheochromocytoma.
- Episodes of headache, palpitations, and sweating suggest pheochromocytoma.
- Hirsutism suggests the possibility of an adrenocortical carcinoma.

Diagnostic Testing
- The imaging characteristics of the nodule may suggest a diagnosis (e.g., benign adrenocortical nodule) but are not specific enough to obviate further evaluation.[20]
- Patients who have potentially resectable cancer elsewhere and in whom an adrenal metastasis must be excluded may require positron emission tomography scanning.
- In other patients, the diagnostic issue is whether a syndrome of hormone excess or an adrenocortical carcinoma is present.
- Plasma potassium, fractionated metanephrines, and dehydroepiandrosterone sulfate should be measured, and an overnight dexamethasone suppression test should be performed.

Treatment

- Patients with hypertension and hypokalemia should be evaluated for primary hyperaldosteronism by measuring the ratio of plasma aldosterone (in ng/dL) to plasma renin activity (in ng/mL/hr) in a single blood sample.
  - This sample can be obtained from an ambulatory patient without special preparation.
  - If the ratio is <20, the diagnosis of primary hyperaldosteronism is excluded, whereas a ratio of >50 makes the diagnosis very likely.
  - Patients with an intermediate ratio should be further evaluated in consultation with an endocrinologist.
- Abnormalities of cortisol secretion should be evaluated further.
- If there is clinical or biochemical evidence of a pheochromocytoma, the nodule should be resected after appropriate α-adrenergic blockade with phenoxybenzamine.
- Elevation of plasma dehydroepiandrosterone sulfate or a large nodule suggests adrenocortical carcinoma.
- A policy of resecting all nodules >4 cm in diameter appropriately treats the great majority of adrenal carcinomas while minimizing the number of benign nodules removed unnecessarily.[21]
- Most incidental nodules are <4 cm in diameter, do not produce excess hormone, and do not require therapy.
- At least one repeat imaging procedure 3 to 6 months later is recommended to ensure that the nodule is not enlarging rapidly (which would suggest an adrenal carcinoma).

HYPERCALCEMIA

General Principles

- Approximately 50% of serum calcium is ionized (free) and the remainder is complexed, primarily to albumin.
- Changes in serum albumin alter total calcium concentration without affecting the clinically relevant ionized calcium level and if serum albumin is abnormal, clinical decisions should be based on **albumin-corrected or ionized calcium levels.**
- Calcium metabolism is regulated by parathyroid hormone (PTH) and metabolites of vitamin D.
- PTH increases serum calcium by stimulating bone resorption, increasing renal calcium reabsorption, and promoting renal conversion of vitamin D to its active metabolite calcitriol (1,25-dihydroxyvitamin D [1,25(OH)$_2$D]).
  - Serum calcium regulates PTH secretion by a negative feedback mechanism; hypercalcemia suppresses PTH release.
- Vitamin D is converted by the liver to 25-hydroxyvitamin D [25(OH)D], which in turn is converted by the kidney to 1,25(OH)$_2$D.
  - The latter metabolite increases serum calcium by promoting intestinal calcium absorption and plays a role in bone formation and resorption.
- Other factors that raise serum calcium include PTH-related peptide, which acts on PTH receptors, and some cytokines produced by plasma cells and lymphocytes.[22]

Etiology

- The major causes of hypercalcemia are listed in Table 3.
- >95% of cases are due to primary hyperparathyroidism or malignancy.
- **Primary hyperparathyroidism:**
  - Causes most cases of mild hypercalcemia in ambulatory patients.
  - It is a common disorder, especially in elderly women. **Approximately 85% of cases are due to an adenoma of a single gland,** 15% to enlargement of all four glands, and 1% to parathyroid carcinoma.
  - Familial syndromes that include primary hyperparathyroidism (e.g., the multiple endocrine neoplasia syndromes) cause enlargement of all four glands.
- **Malignancy** causes most severe, symptomatic hypercalcemia. Common causes of malignant hypercalcemia include the following:
  - Breast carcinoma (which is usually metastatic to bone when hypercalcemia occurs)

TABLE 3	Major Causes of Hypercalcemia

Common
  Primary hyperparathyroidism
  Malignancy
Uncommon
  Sarcoidosis, other granulomatous diseases
  Drugs
  Vitamin D toxicity
  Lithium
  Calcium carbonate (milk-alkali syndrome)
  Hyperthyroidism

- Squamous carcinoma of the lung, head and neck, or esophagus (which may produce humoral hypercalcemia without extensive bone metastases)
- Multiple myeloma
- Renal, bladder, and ovarian carcinoma may also cause hypercalcemia
- **Most malignant hypercalcemia is due to secretion of PTH-related peptide by the tumor,** except for myeloma, in which hypercalcemia is mediated by cytokines.
- Other causes of hypercalcemia are uncommon and are almost always suggested by the history or physical examination.[23]
  - Thiazide diuretics cause persistent hypercalcemia only in patients with increased bone turnover, for example, due to mild primary hyperparathyroidism.
  - Sarcoidosis and other granulomatous disorders may cause hypercalcemia by excessive synthesis of $1,25(OH)_2D$.
  - Familial benign hypercalciuric hypercalcemia is a rare autosomal dominant disorder that causes asymptomatic hypercalcemia from birth. It is due to a genetic defect in the calcium-sensing receptor on parathyroid cells and should be suspected if there is a family history of asymptomatic hypercalcemia.

Diagnosis

Clinical Presentation

- **Most symptoms of hypercalcemia are present only if serum calcium is above 12 mg/dL.**
- In the majority of patients, mild, asymptomatic hypercalcemia is found incidentally.
- The history and physical examination should focus on duration of hypercalcemia (if >6 months without obvious cause, primary hyperparathyroidism is almost certain), history of renal stones, symptoms and signs of malignancy, evidence for any of the unusual causes of hypercalcemia (e.g., calcium supplements, vitamin D, or lithium), and family history of hypercalcemia or other components of multiple endocrine neoplasia syndromes.
- Mild hypercalcemia causes polyuria. Polyuria combined with nausea and vomiting may cause marked dehydration, which impairs calcium excretion and may cause rapidly worsening hypercalcemia.
- Severe hypercalcemia may cause renal failure and chronic hypercalcemia may cause nephrolithiasis (not seen in hypercalcemia of malignancy).
- GI symptoms include anorexia, nausea, vomiting, and constipation.

Diagnostic Testing

- Decreased bone density (and rarely a specific bone disorder, osteitis fibrosa) can result from chronic hyperparathyroidism.
- Neurologic findings include weakness, fatigue, confusion, stupor, and coma.
- ECG manifestations include a shortened QT interval.
- Mildly elevated serum calcium levels should be repeated and the serum albumin-corrected and ionized calcium should be measured to determine whether hypercalcemia is actually present.
- The serum intact PTH level should be measured.
  - If serum PTH is elevated in a patient with hypercalcemia, the diagnosis of primary hyperparathyroidism is confirmed.
  - Intact PTH is suppressed to below the reference range or to the lower part of the reference range in all other causes of hypercalcemia except familial benign hypercalcemia.

- If the PTH level is suppressed, evaluation for other causes of hypercalcemia should be directed by clinical findings and may include a chest radiography, bone scan, and serum and urine protein electrophoresis.
- Severe symptomatic hypercalcemia is usually due to malignancy and the cancer is almost always clinically apparent.
- Vitamin D intoxication can be confirmed by measurement of elevated serum levels of 25(OH)D and the diagnosis of sarcoidosis as the cause of hypercalcemia is supported by elevated serum levels of 1,25(OH)$_2$D.
- In rare cases in which the diagnosis remains unclear, measurement of serum levels of PTH-related peptide may help confirm or exclude malignancy.

Treatment

- Patients with symptoms of hypercalcemia or serum calcium levels >13 mg/dL should be admitted to the hospital for evaluation and therapy.
- Treatment of severe hypercalcemia includes measures that increase calcium excretion and decrease resorption of calcium from bone. The purpose is to relieve symptoms while the cause of hypercalcemia is found and treated.

Extracellular Fluid Volume Restoration

- Severely hypercalcemic patients are almost always dehydrated and the first step in therapy is extracellular fluid (ECF) volume repletion with 0.9% saline to restore the glomerular filtration rate and promote calcium excretion.
- At least 3 to 4 L should be given in the first 24 hours and a positive fluid balance of at least 2 L should be achieved.

Saline Diuresis

- After ECF volume is restored, infusion of 0.9% saline (100 to 200 mL/hr) promotes calcium excretion.
- Serum electrolytes, calcium, and magnesium should be measured every 6 to 12 hours.
- **Furosemide adds little** to the effect of saline diuresis and may prevent adequate restoration of ECF volume. It should not be given unless clinical evidence of heart failure develops.

Zoledronic Acid

- Zoledronic acid is a bisphosphonate that inhibits bone resorption and should be used if symptoms persist or the serum calcium continues to be >12 mg/dL after initial volume repletion.
- A dose of 4 mg in 100 mL 0.9% saline is infused over 15 minutes.
- Serum calcium should be measured daily.
- Hypercalcemia abates gradually over several days and remains suppressed for 1 to 2 weeks.
- Treatment can be repeated when hypercalcemia recurs.
- Side effects include asymptomatic hypocalcemia, hypomagnesemia, hypophosphatemia, and transient low-grade fever.

Glucocorticoids

- **Steroids are effective in hypercalcemia due to myeloma, sarcoidosis, and vitamin D intoxication.**
- The initial dose is prednisone, 20 to 50 mg PO bid or its equivalent.

- It may take 5 to 10 days for serum calcium to fall.
- After serum calcium stabilizes, the dose should be gradually reduced to the minimum needed to control symptoms of hypercalcemia.

Management of Primary Hyperparathyroidism

- The most effective therapy for primary hyperparathyroidism is parathyroidectomy.
- However, in the asymptomatic majority of patients, surgery may not be indicated.
- The natural history of asymptomatic hyperparathyroidism is not fully known but in many patients the disorder has a benign course, with little change in clinical findings or serum calcium for years.
- The major concern in these patients is the possibility of progressive loss of bone mass and increased risk of fracture.
- Deterioration of renal function is also possible but unlikely in the absence of nephrolithiasis. Currently, it is impossible to predict the patients in whom problems will develop.
- **Indications for parathyroidectomy** include the following:
  - Symptoms due to hypercalcemia
  - Nephrolithiasis
  - Hip or spine bone mass by dual-energy radiography >2.5 standard deviations below the gender-specific mean peak bone mass (a T score < −2.5)
  - Serum calcium >1 mg/dL above the upper end of the reference range
  - Age <50 years
  - Infeasibility of long-term follow-up[24]
- Surgery is a reasonable choice in otherwise healthy patients even if they do not meet these criteria, because experienced surgeons have a success rate of 90% to 95% with low perioperative morbidity and correction of hyperparathyroidism is followed by an increase in bone mass and a decrease in the risk of fracture.
- Preoperative localization of an adenoma by sestamibi scan may permit a limited neck dissection, which further decreases the risk of complications.
- Asymptomatic patients who do not meet criteria for parathyroidectomy or who refuse surgery can be followed by assessing clinical status, serum calcium and creatinine levels, and bone mass at 1- to 2-year intervals.[25]
- Surgery should be recommended if any of the above criteria develop or if there is progressive decline in bone mass or renal function.

HYPERPROLACTINEMIA

General Principles

- The major causes of hyperprolactinemia are presented in Table 4.
- In women, the most common causes of pathologic hyperprolactinemia are prolactin-secreting pituitary microadenoma (i.e., an adenoma with a diameter of <1 cm) and idiopathic hyperprolactinemia.
- In men, the most common cause is prolactin-secreting macroadenoma.
- Hypothalamic or pituitary lesions that cause deficiency of other pituitary hormones often cause hyperprolactinemia by compressing the pituitary stalk.
- In women, hyperprolactinemia causes amenorrhea or irregular menses and infertility.
  - Approximately only one half of these women have **galactorrhea.**
  - Prolonged estrogen deficiency increases the risk of osteoporosis.

TABLE 4	Major Causes of Hyperprolactinemia

Pregnancy and lactation
Prolactin-secreting pituitary adenoma (prolactinoma)
Idiopathic hyperprolactinemia
Drugs
Dopamine antagonists (phenothiazines, metoclopramide, methyldopa)
Others (verapamil, cimetidine, some antidepressants)
Interference with synthesis or transport of hypothalamic dopamine
Hypothalamic lesions
Pituitary macroadenomas
Primary hypothyroidism
Chronic renal failure

- In men, hyperprolactinemia causes androgen deficiency and infertility but not gynecomastia.
  - Mass effects of a large pituitary tumor (e.g., headaches, visual field loss) and hypopituitarism are common in men with hyperprolactinemia.

Diagnosis

Clinical Presentation
- The history and physical should include symptoms and signs of prolactin excess, pituitary mass effect, and hypothyroidism.
- A careful medication history should be obtained.

Diagnostic Testing
- Hyperprolactinemia is common in young women and plasma prolactin should be measured in women with amenorrhea, whether or not galactorrhea is present.
- Mild elevations should be confirmed by repeat measurements.
- Laboratory evaluation should include plasma TSH and a pregnancy test.
- **Prolactin levels >200 ng/mL occur only in prolactinomas,** and levels between 100 and 200 ng/mL strongly suggest this diagnosis.
- **Levels <100 ng/mL may be due to any cause except prolactin-secreting macroadenoma** and such levels in a patient with a large pituitary mass indicate that it is not a prolactinoma.
- Testing for hypopituitarism is needed only in patients with a macroadenoma or hypothalamic lesion and should include measurement of plasma free T4, a cosyntropin stimulation test (see Adrenal Failure section, above), and measurement of plasma testosterone in men.
- MRI of the pituitary should be performed in most cases, as nonfunctional pituitary or hypothalamic tumors may present with mild hyperprolactinemia.

Treatment

Microadenomas and Idiopathic Hyperprolactinemia
- Most patients are treated because of infertility or to prevent estrogen deficiency and osteoporosis.

- Some women may be observed without therapy by periodic follow-up of prolactin levels and symptoms.
- In most patients, hyperprolactinemia does not worsen and prolactin levels sometimes return to normal.
- **Enlargement of microadenomas is rare.**
- Dopamine agonists suppress plasma prolactin and restore normal menses and fertility in most women.
  - Initial doses are **bromocriptine,** 1.25 to 2.5 mg PO every hour with a snack, or **cabergoline,** 0.25 mg twice per week.
  - Doses are adjusted by measurement of plasma prolactin at 2- to 4-week intervals to the lowest dose that suppresses prolactin to the normal range. Maximally effective doses are 2.5 mg bromocriptine tid and 1.5 mg cabergoline twice per week.
  - Initially, patients should use barrier contraception, as fertility may be restored quickly.
  - Side effects include nausea and orthostatic hypotension, which can be minimized by increasing the dose gradually and usually resolve with continued therapy. Side effects are less severe with cabergoline.
- Women who want to become pregnant should be managed in consultation with an endocrinologist.
- Women who do not want to become pregnant should be followed with clinical evaluation and plasma prolactin every 6 to 12 months.
  - Every 2 years, plasma prolactin should be measured after bromocriptine has been withdrawn for several weeks to determine whether the drug still is needed.
  - Follow-up imaging studies are not warranted unless prolactin levels increase substantially.
  - Transsphenoidal resection of prolactin-secreting microadenomas is used only in the rare patients who do not respond to or cannot tolerate bromocriptine. Prolactin levels usually return to normal but up to one-half of patients relapse.

Prolactin-Secreting Macroadenomas

- **Such lesions should be treated with a dopamine agonist,** which usually suppresses prolactin levels to normal, reduces tumor size, and improves or corrects abnormal visual fields in some 90% of cases.
- The dose is adjusted as described as above, except that if mass effects are present, the dose should be increased to maximally effective levels over a period of several weeks.
- Visual field tests, if initially abnormal, should be repeated 4 to 6 weeks after therapy is started.
- Pituitary imaging should be repeated 3 to 4 months after initiation of therapy.
- If tumor shrinkage and correction of visual abnormalities are satisfactory, therapy can be continued indefinitely, with periodic monitoring of plasma prolactin.
- The full effect on tumor size may take >6 months.
- Further imaging probably is not warranted unless prolactin levels rise despite therapy.
- **Transsphenoidal surgery is indicated to relieve mass effects and to prevent further tumor growth** if the tumor does not shrink or if visual field abnormalities persist during dopamine agonist therapy. However, the likelihood of surgical cure of hyperprolactinemia due to a macroadenoma is low, and most patients require further therapy with a dopamine agonist.

- Women with prolactin-secreting macroadenomas should not become pregnant unless the tumor has been resected surgically, as the risk of symptomatic enlargement during pregnancy is 15% to 35%. Barrier contraception is essential during dopamine agonist treatment.

MALE HYPOGONADISM

General Principles

- The testes have two distinct but related roles:
  - Secretion of testosterone (the major androgen) by the Leydig cells, which produce and maintain sexual characteristics.
  - Production of spermatozoa by the seminiferous tubules, a process that requires high local concentrations of testosterone.
- The testes are regulated by the pituitary gland, which secretes the gonadotropins, luteinizing hormone (LH), and follicle-stimulating hormone.
- Gonadotropin secretion is regulated by the hypothalamus via secretion of LH-releasing hormone and by negative feedback by gonadal hormones.
- Hypogonadism due to disease of the testes results in diminished feedback on the pituitary and increased secretion of gonadotropins.
- If hypogonadism is due to disorders of the pituitary or hypothalamus, serum gonadotropin levels are within or below the reference range.
- Male hypogonadism may present with androgen deficiency or infertility because of oligospermia (low sperm count).
- Androgen deficiency is always associated with infertility, but oligospermia often occurs in men with normal testosterone levels.

Etiology

- Male hypogonadism may be due to disorders of the testes or due to dysfunction of the pituitary or hypothalamus (Table 5).

TABLE 5	Major Causes of Androgen Deficiency
Testicular disorders	
Klinefelter syndrome	
Orchitis (mumps, other viruses)	
Trauma	
Drug (including alcohol)	
Autoimmune testicular failure	
Hypothalamic pituitary dysfunction	
Congenital luteinizing hormone–releasing hormone deficiency (Kallmann syndrome)	
Hyperprolactinemia	
Cushing syndrome	
Other pituitary or hypothalamic disorders	
Chronic illness	
Combined defects	
Hepatic cirrhosis	
Chronic renal failure	

- Cirrhosis and chronic renal failure also impair gonadotropin secretion and testicular function.

Testicular Disorders

- **Klinefelter syndrome** (47, XXY karyotype) occurs in approximately 1 in 500 male births.
  - Seminiferous tubules fail to develop normally, and because of this, the testes are small and firm with no spermatogenesis.
  - The degree of androgen deficiency ranges from mild to severe.
  - Klinefelter syndrome usually presents as delayed puberty or persistent gynecomastia after puberty.
- **Viral orchitis** in adults, most often due to mumps, can cause testicular atrophy. It usually causes infertility alone, but androgen deficiency occurs in severe cases.
- **Alcohol** causes testicular dysfunction directly and by causing hepatic cirrhosis.
- **Drugs** that impair androgen synthesis or action include ketoconazole, cimetidine, and spironolactone.
- Infertility without androgen deficiency is usually **idiopathic** but may be due to milder forms of the disorders that cause androgen deficiency or due to cryptorchidism that was not corrected early in childhood.
- Azoospermia (complete absence of sperm in the ejaculate) with normal testosterone levels may be due to obstruction or absence of the vas deferens.

Hypothalamic Pituitary Dysfunction

- Any disorder of the hypothalamus or pituitary may cause androgen deficiency alone or combined with other pituitary hormone deficiencies.
- **Hyperprolactinemia** in men is usually due to a prolactin-secreting pituitary macroadenoma.
- **Kallmann syndrome** (congenital deficiency of LH-releasing hormone) presents as failure of puberty. Other pituitary hormones are usually intact. Most patients have anosmia (lack of sense of smell).

Diagnosis

Clinical Presentation

- The history should include the age at onset of puberty, libido, potency and frequency of intercourse, frequency of shaving, testicular injury or infection, past fertility, medications, and chronic illnesses.
- Physical signs may include testicular atrophy (testes <15 mL in volume or <4 cm in greatest diameter), decreased facial and body hair, gynecomastia, and lack of sense of smell.
- Impotence (erectile dysfunction) with a normal libido is usually due to neurologic or vascular disorders or drugs rather than due to androgen deficiency.

Diagnostic Testing

- Androgen deficiency is confirmed by measurement of serum **testosterone.**
- If testosterone is low, serum **LH** should be measured.
- An elevated serum LH indicates a testicular cause of androgen deficiency.
- If LH is not elevated, hypothalamic or pituitary dysfunction is responsible, and serum **prolactin** should be measured, secretion of other pituitary hormones should be assessed, and the pituitary and the hypothalamus should be imaged.

• Men with infertility but normal serum testosterone levels should be evaluated by semen analysis.
  • The most important characteristic is sperm concentration, with the normal range considered to be >20 million/mL.
  • Interpretation is complicated by variability of the sperm count in normal men.
  • Oligospermia should be confirmed by at least two semen analyses.

Treatment

• Androgen deficiency can be treated by injected or topical testosterone.
  • **Testosterone ester** (testosterone enanthate or cypionate) can be given at a dose of 150 to 250 mg IM every 2 weeks. In most men, a dose of 200 mg is satisfactory.
  • **1% testosterone gel** can be applied topically. The starting dose is 5 g once daily.
  • Side effects of androgens include acne and gynecomastia.
  • Men older than age 50 years should undergo regular screening for prostate cancer.
  • Patients should be followed at 6- to 12-month intervals, with assessment of their clinical response.
  • Measurement of serum testosterone is necessary only if there is an inadequate clinical response to therapy.
• Infertility due to testicular disorders such as idiopathic oligospermia is correctable only by assisted reproduction techniques.
  • Patients with azoospermia and normal levels of testosterone and gonadotropins should be evaluated for obstruction of the vas deferens in consultation with a urologist.
  • Patients with hypogonadism due to pituitary or hypothalamic disorders who desire fertility should be referred to an endocrinologist for treatment.

HIRSUTISM

General Principles

• Hirsutism is the growth of dark terminal hair in a woman in a male pattern.
• It is a common complaint and may indicate **androgen excess.** However, there is a broad range of hair growth in normal women, and many patients with hirsutism have no evidence of androgen excess.
• Even slight increases in androgen production can cause noticeable hair growth in women.
• More severe androgen excess causes **virilization.**
• The major issue in evaluating hirsutism is to exclude the possibility that a woman is one of the small minority with a serious cause (such as Cushing syndrome or an ovarian or adrenal tumor).

Etiology

• Androgen excess can originate from the ovaries or adrenals. Exogenous androgens can also cause hirsutism.
• **By far the most common cause is the polycystic ovary syndrome,** which includes hirsutism, infertility, and amenorrhea or irregular menses that are not due to another identifiable disorder.
  • These patients do not ovulate regularly.
  • Hirsutism and menstrual irregularity usually begin at puberty.

- A wide range of abnormality is found in this syndrome, from mild hirsutism alone (sometimes called idiopathic hirsutism) to amenorrhea with enlarged ovaries.
- These women are **resistant to insulin** and the resulting high insulin levels play a role in stimulating ovarian androgen production.
- Rare ovarian tumors may produce hirsutism.
- Adrenal causes of hirsutism include Cushing disease, congenital adrenal hyperplasia, and, rarely, adrenal carcinoma.

Diagnosis

Clinical Presentation

- The history should include the age at onset of hirsutism, symptoms of virilization, any abnormality of menses, and fertility.
- The physical examination should include the extent of hair growth, signs of Cushing syndrome or virilization, and palpation for ovarian enlargement.
  - Signs of virilization like frontal and temporal balding, laryngeal enlargement and deepening of the voice, increased muscle mass, and clitoral enlargement are common features of virilization and suggest a serious underlying cause.

Diagnostic Testing

- **Serum total and free testosterone should be measured.**
- Testing for Cushing syndrome should be performed if there are any symptoms or signs to suggest this disorder.
- Multiple ovarian cysts are a common finding in women with normal menses and no hirsutism; ultrasound of the ovaries should not be performed unless an ovarian tumor is suspected.
- Almost all patients with no evidence of virilization and mild elevation of free testosterone have a disorder that falls within the spectrum of polycystic ovary syndrome. They can be treated for this without further evaluation.
- Patients with evidence of virilization or with serum total testosterone levels >200 ng/dL may have an ovarian or adrenal tumor and should be further evaluated in consultation with an endocrinologist.

Treatment

- Patients with mild hirsutism may not require medical therapy if cosmetic measures such as plucking or shaving produce a satisfactory result.
- The response of hair growth to drug therapy is slow and often incomplete.
- **Oral contraceptives** suppress ovarian androgen production and may improve hirsutism.
- In women with the polycystic ovary syndrome, drugs that improve insulin resistance may reduce androgen production and improve menstrual abnormalities and fertility.
  - **Metformin,** 500 to 1,000 mg bid, can be used in patients with normal renal function.[26]
  - It should be started at a dose of 500 mg daily and the dose gradually increased over a several-week period.
  - Side effects include diarrhea, nausea, and abdominal cramps.
  - Lactic acidosis is very rare in patients with serum creatinine of <1.5 mg/dL.
  - Patients should be followed at 3- to 6-month intervals, with assessment of hair growth, menstrual regularity, and serum-free testosterone.

- **Spironolactone,** 25 to 100 mg bid, is an androgen and aldosterone antagonist that can reduce excess hair growth.[27]
  - Side effects include irregular menses, nausea, and breast tenderness.
  - It should not be used in patients with renal dysfunction because it may cause hyperkalemia.
  - It should not be used by women desiring fertility.
  - Combination therapy with an oral contraceptive may be more effective and allows regular menses.
  - Patients should be followed at 3- to 6-month intervals, with assessment of hair growth, menstrual regularity, and serum potassium.

REFERENCES

1. Adler SM, Wartofsky L. The nonthyroidal illness syndrome. *Endocrinol Metab Clin North Am* 2007;36:657–672.
2. Roberts CG, Ladenson PW. Hypothyroidism. *Lancet* 2004;363:793–803.
3. Pearce EN, Farwell AP, Braverman LE. Thyroiditis. *N Engl J Med* 2003;348:2646–2655.
4. Surks MI, Ortiz E, Daniels GH, et al. Subclinical thyroid disease: scientific review and guidelines for diagnosis and management. *JAMA* 2004;291:228–238.
5. Abalovich M, Amino N, Barbour LA. Management of thyroid dysfunction during pregnancy and postpartum: an Endocrine Society Clinical Practice Guideline. *J Clin Endocrinol Metab* 2007;92:S1–S47.
6. Cooper DS. Hyperthyroidism. *Lancet* 2003;362:459–468.
7. Cooper DS. Approach to the patient with subclinical hyperthyroidism. *J Clin Endocrinol Metab* 2007;92:3–9.
8. Cooper DS. Antithyroid drugs. *N Engl J Med* 2005;352:905–917.
9. Osman F, Franklyn JA, Sheppard MC, Gammage MD. Successful treatment of amiodarone-induced thyrotoxicosis. *Circulation* 2002;105:1275–1277.
10. Nayak B, Burman K. Thyrotoxicosis and thyroid storm. *Endocrinol Metab Clin North Am* 2006;35:663–686.
11. Topliss D. Thyroid incidentaloma: the ignorant in pursuit of the impalpable. *Clin Endocrinol (Oxf)* 2004;60:18–20.
12. Weetman AP. Radioiodine treatment for benign thyroid diseases. *Clin Endocrinol (Oxf)* 2007;66:757–764.
13. Wang SH, Arscott P, Wu P, Baker JR Jr. No apparent damage in the thyroid of transgenic mice expressing antiapoptotic FLIP. *Thyroid* 2006;16:1–33.
14. Ross DS. Nonpalpable thyroid nodules—managing an epidemic. *J Clin Endocrinol Metab* 2002;87:1938–1940.
15. Arlt W, Allolio B. Adrenal insufficiency. *Lancet* 2003;361:1881–1893.
16. Dorin RI, Qualls CR, Crapo LM. Diagnosis of adrenal insufficiency. *Ann Intern Med* 2003;139:194–204.
17. Ten S, New M, Maclaren N. Clinical review 130: Addison's disease 2001. *J Clin Endocrinol Metab* 2001;86:2909–2922.
18. Newell-Price J, Bertagna X, Grossman AB, Nieman LK. Cushing's syndrome. *Lancet* 2006;367:1605–1617.
19. Young WF Jr. Clinical practice. The incidentally discovered adrenal mass. *N Engl J Med* 2007;356:601–610.
20. Udelsman R, Fishman EK. Radiology of the adrenal. *Endocrinol Metab Clin North Am* 2000;29:27–42.
21. Young WF Jr. Management approaches to adrenal incidentalomas. A view from Rochester, Minnesota. *Endocrinol Metab Clin North Am* 2000;29:159–185.
22. Strewler GJ. The physiology of parathyroid hormone-related protein. *N Engl J Med* 2000; 342:177–185.

23. Jacobs TP, Bilezikian JP. Clinical review: rare causes of hypercalcemia. *J Clin Endocrinol Metab* 2005;90:6316–6322.
24. Bilezikian JP, Potts JT Jr, Fuleihan Gel-H, et al. Summary statement from a workshop on asymptomatic primary hyperparathyroidism: a perspective for the 21st century. *J Clin Endocrinol Metab* 2002;87:5353–5361.
25. Bilezikian JP, Silverberg SJ. Clinical practice. Asymptomatic primary hyperparathyroidism. *N Engl J Med* 2004;350:1746–1751.
26. Moghetti P, Castello R, Negri C, et al. Metformin effects on clinical features, endocrine and metabolic profiles, and insulin sensitivity in polycystic ovary syndrome: a randomized, double-blind, placebo-controlled 6-month trial, followed by open, long-term clinical evaluation. *J Clin Endocrinol Metab* 2000;85:139–146.
27. Moghetti P, Tosi F, Tosti A, et al. Comparison of spironolactone, flutamide, and finasteride efficacy in the treatment of hirsutism: a randomized, double blind, placebo-controlled trial. *J Clin Endocrinol Metab* 2000;85:89–94.

18

Nutrition and Obesity
Mariko K. Johnson and Shelby A. Sullivan

General Definitions

Macronutrients
- Provide energy.
- Consist of protein, carbohydrate, and fat.

Micronutrients
- Do not provide energy.
- Consist of vitamins and minerals.

Essential Nutrients
Nutrients not synthesized by the body and therefore completely supplied by the diet.

Malnutrition
- May refer to a state of overnutrition or undernutrition.
- For the purposes of this chapter, will refer to a state of undernutrition.

Obesity
Results from macronutrient overnutrition though obese patients may have micronutrient deficiencies.

General Principles

Undernutrition
- Deficiency of one or more nutrients.
- Occurs when nutrient availability fails to meet metabolic requirements.
- May result from inadequate nutrient intake, malabsorption, increased metabolic demands, ineffective substrate use, or any combination of these.
- Overall incidence of undernutrition in the United States is not well-defined but in hospitalized patients may be as high as 69%.[1]
- Results in loss of skeletal and cardiac muscle function, impairment of immune function, apathy, depression, and prolonged hospital stays.
- Death can occur when weight falls to two thirds of ideal body weight.[2]
- Risk factors for undernutrition include advanced age, chronic medical illnesses, drug-nutrient interactions, low socioeconomic status, and social isolation.

Overnutrition
- Excess of one or more nutrients.
- Occurs when nutrient intake exceeds nutrient expenditure.
- Generally results from excessive nutrient intake.
- Although macronutrients may be consumed in excess, micronutrient intake may be inadequate.

Office Assessment

- Includes a general medical history including a careful diet history, physical examination, and screening for undernutrition and overnutrition.
- Further history may be elicited and ancillary tests may be ordered as needed.

Medical History

- Complete diet history.
  - Ask open-ended questions and be nonjudgmental.
  - Have the patient fill out an eating pattern questionnaire (e.g., "Eating Pattern Questionnaire" from the American Medical Association[3]).
  - Have the patient fill out a food diary for 3 to 7 days (e.g., "Food and Activity Diary" from the American Medical Association, a Web-based diary developed by the United States Department of Agriculture [USDA] is also available[4]).
- Evaluation of medical and psychiatric illnesses as well as surgical procedures that may affect energy or nutrient intake, absorption, or expenditure.
- Medications that may interact with nutrient absorption or cause weight gain.
- Family history of conditions such as obesity, diabetes, and hyperlipidemia.
- Evaluation of psychosocial environment and substance abuse (alcoholism) that may predispose to micronutrient deficiencies.
- Review of systems with attention to appetite and changes in weight.

Physical Examination

- Vital signs: Blood pressure, heart rate, temperature, height, weight, and a calculation of body mass index.
- **Body mass index (BMI)** = weight $(kg)/height^2$ (m^2).
  - Underweight: BMI <18.5 kg/m^2.
  - Normal weight: BMI 18.5 to 25.0 kg/m^2.
  - Overweight: BMI >25 kg/m^2.
  - Obesity: BMI >30 kg/m^2.
  - Morbid obesity: BMI >40 kg/m^2.
- A BMI outside of the normal range is associated with increased morbidity.
- A subjective assessment of fat and muscle mass can be made visually by the examiner.
- The skin, hair, and oral cavity may hold additional clues to micronutrient deficiencies.

Screening for Undernutrition

- Unintentional weight loss of 10% of body weight in the past 3 months.
- BMI <18.5 kg/m^2.

Screening for Overnutrition

- BMI >25 kg/m^2.

Further Evaluation in Undernutrition

- If undernutrition is present, the evaluating physician should consider factors that affect nutrient intake, absorption, and metabolism (Table 1).
- Physical examination in the malnourished patient should focus on general appearance, skin, hair, nails, mucus membranes, and the neurologic system.
- Laboratory assessment in the malnourished patient may include individual micronutrient levels and evaluation of systemic disease if suspected (e.g., thyroid function, HIV status).

TABLE 1	Causes of Malnutrition	
Inadequate Nutrient Intake	**Malabsorption**	**Altered Metabolism**
Limited finances	Pancreatic insufficiency	Fever
Ill-fitting dentures	Regional enteritis	Sepsis
Oral ulcers	Celiac disease	Cancer cachexia
Dysphagia	Whipple disease	AIDS wasting syndrome
Gastric ulcer	Gastrectomy	
Pulmonary disease with poor mechanics	Small-bowel resection	
Depression	Bariatric surgery	
Anorexia nervosa	Protein-losing enteropathy	

- Serum albumin level is not generally recommended, as a depressed level is not specific for malnutrition. It is often depressed in overhydration, acute illness, or chronic liver, renal, or cardiopulmonary disease.

Further Evaluation in Overnutrition

- If obesity is present, the evaluating physician should consider factors that affect intake and ability to perform physical exercise, and remember that obese patients may have micronutrient deficiencies.
  - What quantity and type of foods are being consumed?
  - What type of lifestyle does the patient lead?
  - Is there evidence for secondary causes of obesity including genetic syndromes, hypothyroidism, insulinoma, or Cushing syndrome?
- Physical examination in the obese patient should focus on distribution of body fat and identification of comorbid conditions.
  - Distribution of body fat can be evaluated via waist to hip ratio although this is not routinely done in many offices and has significant operator variability.
  - Comorbid conditions include insulin resistance, male hypogonadism, polycystic ovarian syndrome, cardiovascular disease, obstructive sleep apnea, gallstone disease, osteoarthritis, as well as gastrointestinal and reproductive cancers.
  - Physical examination should be focused accordingly.
- Laboratory assessment in the obese patient should aim to assess comorbidities and rule out secondary causes if suspected.
  - At minimum laboratory assessment should include a fasting lipid panel and fasting blood glucose in addition to blood pressure monitoring.

Dietary Guidelines

Dietary Reference Intakes

- Estimates of daily nutrient intakes that can be used for planning and assessing diets for healthy individuals.
- Consist of four reference intakes:
  - Estimated average requirement (EAR).
  - Recommended dietary allowance (RDA).

- The tolerable upper limit (UL).
- Adequate intake (AI).
- Current DRIs can be found on the USDA website.[4]

Estimated Average Requirement
Estimated daily intake of essential nutrients adequate to meet the nutritional needs of 50% of the individuals in a specific age and gender group.

Recommended Dietary Allowances
- Estimated daily intake of essential nutrients adequate to meet the nutritional needs of practically all (97% to 98%) individuals in a specific age and gender group.
- Is 2 standard deviations above the EAR.
- If the EAR for a given nutrient cannot be established through sufficient scientific data, the RDA for that nutrient cannot be established.
- When the RDA cannot be established, the AI is used instead.

Adequate Index
- When sufficient data are not available to estimate an average requirement, an AI is set.
- The AI is used as a goal for the nutrient intake of individuals and is based on observed or experimental calculations.

Tolerable Upper Limit
- The daily upper limit of intake of essential nutrients safe for most individuals.
- Data are lacking for many nutrients and therefore lack of an UL at this time does not mean that one does not exist.

USDA Dietary Guidelines for Americans

- Developed by the USDA and the Department of Health and Human Services and revised every 5 years, most recently in 2005.
- Generally encourage Americans to eat fewer calories, be more active, and to make wiser food choices.
- Guidelines note populations with special needs in the Executive Summary.
- Guidelines are the basis of the food guide pyramid.

USDA Food Guide Pyramid

- The USDA food guide pyramid was first released in 1992 and was revised in 2005 and emphasizes the following:[5]
  - *Personalization:* a personalized recommendation of the kinds and amounts of food to eat each day can be found at www.mypyramid.gov.
  - *Gradual improvement:* the slogan "Steps to a Healthier You" suggests that individuals can benefit from taking small steps to improve their diet and lifestyle each day.
  - *Physical activity:* the picture of steps and the person climbing them reminds us of the importance of daily physical activity.
  - *Variety:* symbolized by the six color bands representing the five food groups of MyPyramid and oils.
  - *Moderation:* represented by the narrowing of each food group from bottom to top. The wider base stands for foods with little or no solid fats, added sugars, or caloric sweeteners. These should be selected more often to get the most nutrition from calories consumed.

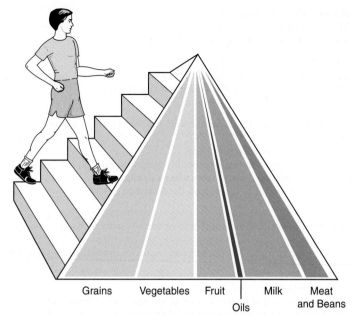

Grains   Vegetables   Fruit   Milk   Meat and Beans
Oils

Figure 1. United States Department of Agriculture Food Guide Pyramid.

- *Proportionality:* shown by the different widths of the food group bands. The widths suggest how much food a person should choose from each group. The widths are just a general guide, not exact proportions.
- The USDA Web site (www.mypyramid.gov) (last accessed December 1, 2009) contains links to "MyPyramid Plan," "MyPyramid Tracker," and "Steps to a Healthier Weight" which provide patients with individualized diet and exercise plans; "Executive Summary" provides guidelines for populations with special needs (Fig. 1).

Other Diets
The Mediterranean diet, Asian diet, and Atkins diet are examples of other existing diets but will not be discussed further here.

Calculating Energy Requirements
Energy
- Total energy expenditure = basal metabolic rate (BMR) + the energy expenditure of activity + the thermic effect of food.
- The thermic effect of food is a small percentage of total energy expenditure and is largely ignored when energy requirements are estimated.
- **Harris-Benedict equations** estimate BMR on the basis of gender, height, age, and weight.
  - Male: BMR (kcal) = 66.5 + (13.8 × weight in kg) + (5 × height in cm) − (6.8 × age in years)
  - Female: BMR (kcal) = 655 + (9.6 × weight in kg) + (1.9 × height in cm) − (4.7 × age in years)

TABLE 2	Energy Requirements Based on BMI

BMI	Energy Requirements (kcal/kg/d)
<15	36–45
15–19	31–35
20–29	26–30
≥30	15–25

BMI, body mass index.

- Energy needs are then calculated by multiplying BMR by an activity factor between 0.8 and 1.8 that adjusts for the stress of various medical conditions and for the level of activity.
- Table 2 can be used for an easy reference to determine energy requirements.

Macronutrients

- Macronutrients provide energy and include fat, carbohydrate, and protein
- Full DRIs for macronutrients are available at the USDA Web site[4]

Protein

- Components of protein.
  - Essential and nonessential amino acids.
    ○ Essential amino acids are histidine, isoleucine, leucine, lysine, methionine/cystine, phenylalanine/tyrosine, threonine, tryptophan, and valine.
- Types of protein.
  - Complete proteins contain all essential amino acids and are derived from animal sources and select plant sources such as soy, quinoa, Spirulina, buckwheat, hemp seed, and amaranth.
  - Incomplete proteins do not contain all essential amino acids.
- Sources of protein.
  - Include meat, dairy products other than cream and butter, and plant products such as grains, legumes, and vegetables.
- Plant proteins can be ingested in combination so that their amino acid patterns become complementary.
  - Vegans can meet requirements when grains, legumes, and leafy greens are combined.
- The RDA for protein intake in young healthy adults of both sexes is 0.8 g/kg body weight/day. The average American's daily protein intake far exceeds the RDA.
- Protein requirements increase during growth, pregnancy, lactation, and rehabilitation.

Carbohydrate

- Components of carbohydrate.
  - Carbohydrates are composed of saccharide units.
- Types of carbohydrate.
  - Complex carbohydrates.
    ○ Polysaccharides.
    ○ Include starch which is digestible.
    ○ Include fiber which is indigestible.

- Sugars
  - Monosaccharides (glucose, fructose), disaccharides (sucrose, lactose, maltose), or oligosaccharides.
  - Sucrose and lactose are the primary dietary sugars.
- Sources of carbohydrate.
  - Carbohydrates are primarily derived from plant sources.
- Carbohydrates typically comprise 45% to 65% total daily calories.

Fiber

- Fiber intake for males is 30 to 38 g/day and for females is 21 to 29 g/day
- Most Americans do not consume the recommended amount of fiber and may benefit from supplementation.

Soluble Fiber

- Soluble in water and fermentable by intestinal bacteria.
- Pectin, gum, mucilages, and some hemicelluloses are considered soluble fibers.
- Benefits of soluble fiber.
  - Delayed gastric emptying, slowed intestinal transit, and decreased glucose absorption with benefits in obese patients.
  - Improvement in glycemic control in diabetic patients.
  - A decrease in luminal wall tension (pain and cramps) and diarrhea in irritable bowel syndrome.
  - Binding of fatty acids, cholesterol, and bile acids leading to lower serum lipid levels and atherosclerosis prevention.
- Sources of soluble fiber.
  - Found in all plant sources (whole grains, legumes, and prunes are very good sources).
  - Found in commercially available sources such as psyllium (Metamucil) and methylcellulose (Citrucel).

Insoluble Fiber

- Insoluble in water and not fermented by intestinal bacteria.
- Cellulose, lignin, and some hemicelluloses are considered insoluble fibers.
- Benefits of insoluble fiber.
  - Insoluble fibers increase intestinal transit and increase fecal bulk, providing a laxative effect.
  - May reduce the rates of diverticulosis and colonic neoplasms.
- Sources of insoluble fiber.
  - Found in certain plant sources (whole grains, flax seed, and certain vegetables such as celery, potato skin, and green beans are good sources).

Fat

- Components of fat.
  - Glycerol backbone with three fatty acid chains.
- Categorization of fat.
  - Fatty acid chain length: short-chain, medium-chain, and long-chain fatty acids.
  - Degree of hydrogen saturation of the fatty acid chains:
    - Polyunsaturated (multiple unsaturated sites).
    - Monounsaturated (a single unsaturated site).
    - Saturated (completely saturated).

- Ability of the body to synthesize the fat: essential or nonessential.
  - Essential fatty acids are omega-3 α-linolenic acid and omega-6 linoleic acid.
  - All other fatty acids are nonessential.
- Increasing saturation is associated with increasing risk of coronary artery disease.
- Unsaturated fatty acids may be hydrogenated to form transfats (see below).
- Polyunsaturated fats are divided into n-6 and n-3 fatty acids according to their molecular structure.
- A high ratio of n-6 fatty acid to n-3 fatty acid intake may be atherogenic.
- Fat should comprise no >35% of total daily calories.
- Saturated fat should comprise no >7% of total daily calories.

Transfats
- Made by hydrogenating vegetable oils.
- Hydrogenation solidifies the oils and increases the shelf life and flavor of the foods that contain them.
- Contribute to increased blood low-density lipoprotein (LDL) cholesterol, decreased blood high-density lipoprotein (HDL) cholesterol, and coronary artery disease.
- Transfat should comprise no >1% of total daily calories.

Cholesterol
- Dietary fats and cholesterol are packaged into lipoproteins for delivery to the tissues.
- Lipoproteins are classified into five groups according to their density.
  - LDL
  - HDL
  - VLDL (very low-density lipoprotein).
  - IDL (intermediate density lipoprotein).
  - Chylomicrons (triacylglycerol-rich lipoproteins).
- LDL, VLDL, IDL, and chylomicrons carry cholesterol to the tissues.
- HDL returns cholesterol from the tissues to the liver.
- LDL cholesterol carries 70% of serum cholesterol.
- HDL cholesterol carries 20% to 30% of serum cholesterol and levels are inversely correlated with the risk of heart disease.
- Lipid-modifying drugs have been developed and can improve serum lipid profiles. These are discussed in detail in chapter 8.
- Reduced saturated fat, transfat and cholesterol intake, weight loss, and dietary adjuncts such as soluble fiber, plant sterols and stanols, and soy protein may decrease LDL cholesterol levels.
- Aerobic exercise, weight loss, smoking cessation, omega-3 fatty acid intake, reduced saturated and transfat intake, increased soluble fiber intake, and drinking one to two servings of red wine daily have been associated with increased HDL levels.
- Cholesterol intake should be <300 mg/day (Table 3).

Health Risks of Fat and Cholesterol
- Saturated fat, transfat, and cholesterol intake have been linked to coronary artery disease and reduced intake of these substances is recommended.
- Monounsaturated fats (when substituted for saturated fat) have beneficial effects on the cholesterol profile decreasing LDL and triglyceride levels while increasing HDL.
- The ratio of n-6 to n-3 fatty acid intake contributes to the pro- or antiatherogenic properties of polyunsaturated fats (when substituted for saturated fat).

TABLE 3	Dietary Sources of Fats	
Type of Fat	Food Source	Atherogenicity
Saturated fats	Dairy and meat products	High
Monounsaturated fats	Olive and canola oils, avocado, nuts	Low
Polyunsaturated fats (n-6)	Margarines, vegetable oils	High
Polyunsaturated fats (n-3)	Seed oils (linseed, rapeseed, soya, and walnut oils)	Low
	Nuts, green leafy vegetables	
	Fatty fish (tuna, salmon, sardines, mackerel, herring) and fish oils	
Transfats	Vegetable shortening, margarine, cookies, and snack foods	High
Cholesterol	Egg yolks, dairy and meat products	High

Other Energy Sources

Alcohol
- Is structurally similar to carbohydrate.
- Each gram of ethanol yields 7 kcal and can be a significant source of empty calories.
- The alcohol contents in one 1.5-oz shot of hard liquor, one 12-oz beer, and one 5-oz glass of wine are roughly equivalent.
- One serving of an alcoholic beverage provides 14 to 20 g ethanol (100 to 140 calories) plus additional calories found in additives such as cream, sodas, or fruit juices.
- Ethanol is known to increase HDL in serum; thus, moderate ethanol use may convey a cardioprotective effect.
- Alcohol interferes with thiamine absorption and formation of its active metabolite.

Macronutrient Substitutes

Artificial Sweeteners and Sugar Substitutes
- Provide sweetness with a reduction in calories.
- Five artificial sweeteners have been approved by the U.S. Food and Drug Administration (FDA): saccharin, aspartame, acesulfame, sucralose, and neotame (Table 4).

Fat replacements
- Olestra is a mixture of hexa-, hepta-, and octaesters of sucrose with long-chain fatty acids.
  - Imparts taste indistinguishable from fat yet is too large to be absorbed.
  - Currently found primarily in snack foods such as chips.
  - Side effects.
    ○ Cramping, flatulence, and diarrhea from fat malabsorption.
    ○ Poor absorption of fat-soluble vitamins because they are excreted with olestra.

TABLE 4	Current Artificial Sweeteners				
Chemical Name	Trade Name	Year of Approval (Limited/Full)	Sweetness[a]	Health Concerns	Heat Stable?
Saccharin	Sweet 'N Low	Available before creation of the FDA	300×	Bladder cancer. FDA required a warning label until 2001 when research showed that the urine precipitate found in laboratory animals was not found in humans. Still banned or restricted in certain countries.	Yes
Aspartame	NutraSweet Equal Canderel	1981/1996	200×	Brain cancer. Must be avoided by patients with phenylketonuria because phenylalanine is a metabolite of aspartame.	No
Acesulfame K	Sunett Sweet One	1988/2003	200×	None to date	Yes
Sucralose	Splenda	1998/1999	600×	None to date	Yes
Neotame	None	2002/2002	7,000–13,000×	None to date	Intermediate

[a]As compared to sucrose.

Micronutrients

Vitamins
- Essential organic compounds that are required to maintain growth, metabolism, and overall health.
- Fat-soluble (vitamins A, D, E, K) or water-soluble (all other vitamins) (Table 5).

Minerals
- Inorganic compounds that do not supply energy (Table 6).
- Important in regulating metabolism, tissue catabolism, and anabolism.
  - Cellular regulation and fluid balance.
  - Coenzymes and cofactors.
  - Bone and tooth formation.

Drug-Nutrient Interactions

- Food can enhance or impede medication effects.
- Medication can influence food and nutrient intake, absorption, metabolism, and excretion.
- It is beyond the scope of this chapter to list all possible interactions; however, some common interactions may be found in Table 7.

Dietary Supplements

- Products (other than tobacco) intended to supplement the diet that bear or contain one or more of the following dietary ingredients: a vitamin, a mineral, an herb or other botanical, an amino acid, a dietary substance for use by man to supplement the diet by increasing the total daily intake, or a concentrate, metabolite, constituent, extract, or combination of these ingredients (Table 8).
- Americans spend billions of dollars annually on supplements.
- Product labels must include ingredient labeling (name, part of plant for herbs, quantity of each ingredient and strength), the words dietary supplement, and nutritional labeling.
- **Supplements do not require FDA approval** and therefore vary greatly in strength, potency, and purity.
  - Some products may contain no active ingredient.
  - Contamination with pesticides, drugs, or heavy metals may occur, and it is the burden of the FDA to show that a product is not safe.
- Supplements may interact with other dietary supplements or prescription medications.
- Nonspecific side effects such as GI distress, headache, allergic reactions, and medication interactions have been described for all supplements.
- Long-term effects of supplementation are not known.

Complementary and Alternative Medicine

- Complementary and alternative medicine is a group of diverse medical and health care systems, practices, and products that are not presently considered to be part of conventional medicine.

TABLE 5	Water- and Fat-Soluble Vitamins			
Vitamin	Function	Source	Deficiency	Toxicity
A	Visual pigments Cell differentiation Gene regulation	Liver, fish Yellow-orange vegetables + fruits Green leafy vegetables	Night blindness Hyperkeratotic skin Xerophthalmia/ blindness	Dermatitis Increased intracranial pressure Bone pain/hypercalcemia Liver fibrosis Birth defects in pregnancy
D	Calcium homeostasis Bone metabolism	Fortified milk Herring, salmon, sardines, liver	Osteomalacia	Hypercalcification of bone Kidney stones Soft tissue calcification Hypercalcemia
E	Membrane antioxidant	Vegetable oils Wheat germ, rice bran Nuts, seeds	Neuropathy Myopathy	Bleeding
K	Clotting Calcium metabolism	Green leafy vegetables Olive and soybean oils	Coagulopathy Bleeding dyscrasia	Interferes with warfarin Hemolytic anemia with IV
C	Biosynthesis of collagen and carnitine Metabolism of drugs and steroids	Citrus fruits Green vegetables	Scurvy (poor wound healing, bleeding diathesis)	Osmotic diarrhea False positive FOBT Oxalate and UA kidney stones (hypothetical) Increased Fe absorption in patients with Fe overload
B₁ (Thiamine)	Coenzyme for oxidative decarboxylations of 2-keto acids and transketolations	Brewer's yeast Meats (especially pork) Sunflower seeds, wheat germ, nuts, legumes Enriched grain products	Beriberi: High-output CHF (wet) Peripheral neuro- pathy (dry) Wernicke's encephalopathy	Excessive IV or IM: Convulsion Cardiac arrhythmias Anaphylactic shock

(continued)

TABLE 5	Water- and Fat-Soluble Vitamins (Continued)			
Vitamin	**Function**	**Source**	**Deficiency**	**Toxicity**
B₂ (Riboflavin)	Coenzyme in redox reactions of fatty acids and the TCA cycle	Liver, meats Brewer's yeast Dairy products and eggs Fortified cereals Broccoli, spinach, mushrooms	Cheilosis Glossitis Angular stomatitis Corneal vascularization Anemia Personality changes	None
B₃ (Niacin)	Precursor of NAD and NADP which are important in redox rxns	Meat, poultry, fish Dairy products and eggs Fortified cereals Fortified flour Corn, potato Noncitrus fruits and juices	Pellagra: Diarrhea Dermatitis Confusion or dementia	Histamine-induced exacerbations of asthma and PUD Liver toxicity Elevated serum uric acid Glucose intolerance
B₆ (Pyridoxine)	Coenzyme in amino acid metabolism Heme and neurotransmitter synthesis	Liver Oatmeal Bananas Chicken Potatoes Wheat germ, rice	Dermatitis Glossitis Peripheral neuropathy Convulsions Anemia Personality changes	Sensory neuropathy
B₁₂ (Cobalamin)	Coenzyme in metabolism of propionate, amino acids, and single carbon fragments	Clams, oysters, crab, tuna Liver, beef	Megaloblastic anemia Depression Neuropathy Psychosis Glossitis	None

Nutrient	Function	Sources	Deficiency	Toxicity
Folic acid	Coenzyme in single carbon metabolism	Fortified cereals Brewer's yeast Legumes Leafy green vegetables Citrus fruit and juices Meat, poultry, fish	Megaloblastic anemia Diarrhea Fatigue Depression Confusion Glossitis	None May correct the bone marrow effects of B_{12} deficiency without correcting its neurologic manifestations
Biotin	Coenzyme for carboxylations Important in gluconeogenesis and fatty acid synthesis	Cereals Egg yolks (whites contain avidin which binds biotin plus reduces bioavailability) Liver, soy Brewer's yeast Nuts, legumes	Anorexia Paresthesias Depression/hallucinations Dermatitis, hair loss	None
Pantothenic acid	Coenzyme for fatty acid metabolism	Meat, liver, fish, poultry Milk products + egg yolks Legumes Whole grain cereals Brewer's yeast	Paresthesias Ataxia Muscle cramps Depression Hypoglycemia	None
Choline	Precursor for acetylcholine and phospholipids	Soybeans Milk products + egg yolks Peanuts Whole grain cereals Potatoes, tomatoes Bananas and oranges	Fatty liver Elevated transaminases	Hypotension Cholinergic diaphoresis Diarrhea Salivation

CHF, congestive heart failure; FOBT, fecal occult blood testing; NAD, nicotinamide adenine dinucleotide; NADP, nicotinamide adenine dinucleotide phosphate; PUD, peptic ulcer disease; TCA, tricarboxylic acid; UA, uric acid.

TABLE 6	Minerals			
Mineral	Function	Source	Deficiency	Toxicity
Calcium	Component of bones and teeth Signal transduction Muscle contraction Clotting	Dairy products Sardines, clams, oysters Turnips, mustard greens Legumes Broccoli	Rickets Osteoporosis Tetany	Milk-alkali syndrome Kidney stones Impaired iron absorption
Phosphorus	Component of bones and teeth, cell membranes, phospholipids, ATP	Meat, poultry, fish Eggs Dairy products Legumes Nuts, grains, chocolate	Rickets Rhabdomyolysis Paresthesia/ataxia Hemolysis Acidosis	Hypocalcemia Tetany
Magnesium	Component of bones Role in nerve conduction Protein synthesis Enzyme activation	Nuts, legumes Grains, corn Peas, carrots Seafood Brown rice	Depression Muscle weakness Tetany Convulsions Growth failure	Osmotic diarrhea Flushing Double vision Slurred speech Weakness, paralysis Cardiopulmonary failure
Potassium	Water and electrolyte balance Cell membrane transfer	Fruits Potato Beans Wheat bran Dairy products Eggs	Weakness Apathy Cardiac arrhythmias Paralysis	Cardiac arrhythmia Cardiac arrest
Iron	Oxygen transport	Organ meats, meat Clams, oysters Molasses Nuts, legumes, seeds Leafy green vegetables Enriched grains and cereals	Microcytic anemia Listlessness and fatigue Impaired cognitive development	GI distress Hemochromatosis

	Function	Sources	Deficiency	Toxicity
Zinc	Cofactor in metabolism Protein synthesis Collagen formation Alcohol detoxification Taste and smell	Oysters Wheat germ Beef, liver, poultry Whole grains	Growth retardation Abnormal taste and smell Changes in skin, hair, and nails	GI distress Anemia from copper deficiency (competitive absorption) Pulmonary fibrosis
Copper	Utilization of iron stores Lipid, collagen, pigment, and neurotransmitter synthesis	Liver, meat, fish Shellfish Whole grains Legumes Eggs	Anemia Growth retardation Skin/hair abnormalities Mental deterioration Osteopenia Myopathy Cardiomyopathy	GI distress Mental deterioration Hemolytic anemia Liver failure Renal dysfunction Nausea and vomiting Neuropathy Dermatitis
Selenium	Protects against free radicals	Grains Meats, poultry, fish Dairy products		Renal failure Dermatitis Pulmonary cancer
Chromium	Regulation of blood glucose	Mushrooms, prunes, asparagus Organ meats Whole grains and cereals	Glucose intolerance Lipid abnormalities	
Iodine	Thyroid hormone synthesis	Iodized table salt Saltwater seafood Sunflower seeds Mushrooms	Goiter Hypothyroidism	Thyroid dysfunction Acneiform rash
Manganese	Brain and bone function Collagen	Liver, eggs Wheat bran Legumes Nuts Lettuce, blueberries, pineapple	Impaired growth Skeletal abnormalities Impaired CNS function	Neurotoxicity Parkinsonian-like symptoms Pneumoconiosis
Molybdenum	Metabolism of purines and pyrimidines	Seafood, poultry, meat Soybeans, lentils Buckwheat Oats, rice bread	Neurologic abnormalities	Fetal abnormalities Chronic toxicity: bone, kidney, nerve, and muscle dysfunction
Fluoride	Maintenance of teeth and bones	Fluorinated drinking water Fish, meat Legumes Grains	Dental caries Bone disorders	Mottled teeth Acute toxicity: acidosis, cardiac arrhythmias, death

ATP, adenosine triphosphate; CNS, central nervous system; GI, gastrointestinal.

TABLE 7	Important Food/Nutrient and Medication Interactions	
Food/Nutrient	**Medication**	**Interaction**
Grapefruit juice	Carbamazepine Calcium channel blockers Cyclosporin Saquinavir Astemizole Statins Cisapride Buspirone Clomipramine Benzodiazepines Tacrolimus	Increases medication concentrations Mediated by suppression of the P-450 enzyme CYP3A4 Effect lasts 24 hours Drugs with high presystemic metabolism are affected the most
Tyramine-containing foods: Aged cheese, overripe fruit, spoiled foods, fermented/dry salami or sausage, soy sauce, marmite-concentrated yeast extract, sauerkraut, fava and broad beans, banana peel, tap beer	Monoamine oxidase inhibitors Furazolidone Isoniazid Procarbazine	Leads to hypertensive crisis Mediated by release of norepinephrine by culprit foods and MAOIs Suggested upper limit of tyramine is 6 mg/day
Potassium supplements	Spironolactone Triamterene Amiloride	Can cause hyperkalemia

Nutrient	Drug	Effect
Vitamin K-rich foods: Dark leafy green vegetables, soybean, canola, cottonseed, olive oils	Warfarin Phenindione	Suppresses warfarin effect Intake permitted but should be consistent
Vitamin B_6	Hydralazine Isoniazid Chloramphenicol Cycloserine	Inhibits absorption of vitamin B_6
Fat-soluble vitamins	Cholestyramine Colestipol Mineral oil	Inhibits absorption of fat-soluble vitamins
Folic acid	Sulfasalazine Phenytoin Primidone Colestipol Cholestyramine Methotrexate Pyrimethamine Nitrofurantoin Trimethoprim	Inhibits absorption of folic acid
Vitamin B_{12}	Histamine-2 receptor antagonists Proton pump inhibitors Chloramphenicol Cycloserine	Inhibits absorption of vitamin B_{12}

TABLE 8	Common Dietary Supplements				
Functional Food	Structure Function	Natural Sources (All May be Found in Dietary Supplements)	Potential Benefits	Grade of Evidence for Benefit[a]	Potential Side Effects
Creatine	Nitrogenous organic acid Involved in the transfer of phosphate to ADP Provides energy for muscle activity	Synthesized by the body Food sources (meat, milk, and fish)	Improved athletic performance Hyperlipidemia Cardiac diseases Muscular and neuromuscular diseases	C C C C	Asthma exacerbation Liver and kidney toxicity Muscle breakdown Electrolyte imbalances Altered glycemic control Stroke Decreased function of vitamins A, D, E, and K
Coenzyme Q10	Benzoquinone Cofactor in electron transport Antioxidant	Food sources (fish, fish oils, nuts, meats)	Hypertension Neurodegenerative and muscular diseases Cardiac diseases Mitochondrial diseases Cancer Migraines HIV Kidney failure Diabetes	B C C C C C C C D	Organ damage during exercise Liver toxicity Thyroid dysfunction Platelet dysfunction Hypoglycemia
Glucosamine	Amino sugar Component of cartilage	Synthesized by the body	Osteoarthritis Venous insufficiency Inflammatory bowel disease Rheumatoid arthritis	D A# C C C	Allergic potential in those with shellfish allergies Hypertension Palpitations Cataracts Bleeding Altered glycemic control

				A#	
Chondroitin	Glycosaminoglycan Component of cartilage	Cartilage	Osteoarthritis Ophthalmologic uses Coronary disease Psoriasis Interstitial cystitis	B C C C	Hair loss Breathing difficulties Hypertension Asthma exacerbation Bleeding Edema Bone marrow suppression
Lipoic acid	Antioxidant Cofactor in glucose metabolism	Synthesized by the body Food sources (organ meats, beef, yeast, broccoli, spinach)	Neuropathy Glucose utilization Neurodegenerative disorders	B ? ?	Malodorous urine Hypoglycemia Biotin deficiency
Omega-3 fatty acids: α-linolenic acid eicosa-pentaenoic acid docosa-hexaenoic acid	Polyunsaturated fatty acid with a carbon-carbon double bond in the ω-3 position Anti-inflammatory	Food sources: Wild-caught oily fish (salmon, herring, mackerel, anchovies, sardines) Flaxseed Mussels and clams Eggs from free-range chickens Kiwifruit Walnuts	Secondary prevention of CV disease Hypertension Hypertrigly-ceridemia Primary prevention of CV disease Protection from cyclosporine toxicity Varicose veins ADHD Developmental and learning problems Arthritis	A A A B B C C C C	Hemorrhagic risk at high doses Impairment of glycemic control in diabetics Immunosuppression Increase in LDL cholesterol in some patients

(continued)

TABLE 8	Common Dietary Supplements (*Continued*)				
Functional Food	Structure Function	Natural Sources (All May be Found in Dietary Supplements)	Potential Benefits	Grade of Evidence for Benefit[a]	Potential Side Effects
Probiotics: *Lactobacillus* spp. *Bifidobacterium* spp.	Beneficial bacteria or yeasts Reconstitute the gut flora after disruption caused by stressors such as antibiotics, toxins, or disease preventing harmful bacteria from taking over	Food sources: Dairy products Probiotic fortified foods	Chronic pouchitis Antibiotic-associated diarrhea	B C	None

[a]National Institutes of Health grade of evidence for benefit
A: Strong scientific evidence for this use
B: Good scientific evidence for this use
C: Unclear scientific evidence for this use
D: Fair scientific evidence against this use
F: Strong scientific evidence against this use
The most recent grade of evidence for glucosamine and chondroitin in osteoarthritis was assigned before publication of the GAIT trial. Clegg DO, Reda DJ, Klein MA, et al. Glucosamine, chondroitin sulfate, and the two in combination for painful knee osteoarthritis. *N Engl J Med* 2006;354:795–808.
? NIH evidence grading unavailable at this time.
ADHD, attention deficit hyperactivity disorder; ADP, adenosine diphosphate; LDL, low-density lipoprotein.

- Overseen by the National Center for Complementary and Alternative Medicine, a branch of the National Institutes of Health.
- Encompasses healing techniques (acupuncture, massage, prayer, meditation) as well as dietary supplements.
- Some common complementary and alternative medicine dietary supplements are listed in Table 9.

Obesity and Approaches to Weight Loss

Obesity

- >60% of Americans are overweight, >30% are obese, and approximately 5% are morbidly obese,[6] and these rates have more than doubled in the past 20 years.
- Obesity is associated with many comorbidities including diabetes mellitus, hypertension, hyperlipidemia, atherosclerosis, gout, cardiovascular disease, and sleep apnea.
- Lifestyle changes (diet and exercise) are the cornerstones of weight loss, though medications and surgery can be considered when diet and exercise fail in certain populations.

Approaches to Weight Loss

- Consist of therapeutic lifestyle modifications, bariatric surgery, and medications.
- Treatment decisions must take into account each patient's readiness for change (motivation, stress levels, time availability) and barriers to change.

Lifestyle Modification

- **Decreasing caloric intake.**
  - Set small goals—start with one or two small changes that the patient agrees to.
  - Recommend substitutions (e.g., baked potato instead of french fries).
  - Encourage more low-calorie foods at meals and for snacks.
  - Recommend eating regular meals.
  - Do not deny patients their favorite foods, but stress the importance of portion control.
  - Discuss triggers to eating.
  - For more information on healthy choices and portion control, consider referral to a nutritionist/dietician.
- **Increasing physical activity.**
  - Helps sustain weight loss.[7]
  - Activity should be recorded in an activity diary.
  - Encourage 30 to 60 minutes of moderate physical activity on most days of the week.
  - Encourage activities that your patient enjoys.
  - Incorporate exercise into daily activities (e.g., walking to do nearby errands, ride your bike to work, walk the dog, take the stairs instead of the elevator).

Bariatric Surgery

- Used as an adjunct to and not as a substitute for therapeutic lifestyle changes.
- Indications.
  - BMI >40 kg/m^2 or BMI 35 to 40 kg/m^2 with life-threatening cardiopulmonary disease, severe diabetes, or lifestyle impairment AND
  - Failure to achieve weight loss with other treatment modalities.

TABLE 9	Popular Herbal and Botanical Dietary Supplements		
Name	**Common Names**	**Reported Indications for Use**	**Adverse Side Effects**
Echinacea purpurea *E. angustifolia* *E. pallida*	American or purple coneflower	Colds, flu, or other infections, wound care	No toxic effects
Valeriana officinalis	Valerian, all-heal, garden heliotrope	Insomnia, anxiety, headaches, depression	Headaches, dizziness, fatigue
Tanacetum parthenium	Feverfew, bachelor's buttons, featherfew	Fevers, headaches, stomachaches, toothaches, insect bites, infertility, menstrual and childbirth problems, migraines, rheumatoid arthritis, psoriasis, allergies, asthma, tinnitus, nausea, dizziness	Aphthous ulcers, mucosal irritation, loss of taste, rebound headaches, anxiety, joint pain, uterine contractions, and miscarriage
Ginkgo biloba	Gingko, fossil tree, maidenhair tree, Japanese silver apricot, kew tree, yinhsing	Asthma, bronchitis, tinnitus, dementia, claudication, sexual dysfunction, multiple sclerosis	Headache, dizziness Increased bleeding risk, seizures or death if uncooked seeds are consumed
Hypericum perforatum	St. John's wort, goat weed, Klamath weed, Hypericum	Depression, anxiety, sleep disorders	Photosensitivity, anxiety, dry mouth, dizziness, headache, sexual dysfunction, many drug interactions
Serenoa repens	Saw palmetto, cabbage palm, American dwarf palm tree	Benign prostatic hypertrophy, hormone imbalances, bladder disorders, decreased sex drive, pelvic pain, hair loss	Decreased sex drive, breast tenderness

Piper methysticum	Kava-kava, awa, kava pepper	Anxiety, insomnia, menopausal symptoms	Liver failure, dystonia, many drug interactions, drowsiness, yellow skin
Panax ginseng	Asian ginseng, ginseng	Recovery from illness, energy enhancement, erectile dysfunction, hepatitis C, menopausal symptoms, hypertension, diabetes	Headaches, insomnia, breast tenderness, menstrual irregularities, hypertension, hypoglycemia
Cimicifuga racemosa	Black cohosh, black snake root, macrotys, bugbane, bugwort, rattle root, rattle weed	Rheumatism, menopausal symptoms, menstrual irregularities, labor induction, premenstrual syndrome	Headaches, weight disturbances, possible link to hepatitis, may be unsafe for pregnant women and women with a history of breast cancer
Ephedra ≥40 species	Chinese ephedra, Ma Huang	Increased energy, weight loss	Stroke, myocardial infarction, sudden death, hypertension, insomnia, anxiety, psychosis, worsening of kidney disease, diabetes
Pausinystalia yohimbe	Yohimbe bark, yohimbine	Aphrodisiac, erectile dysfunction	Hypertension, insomnia, palpitations, anxiety, headache, drug interactions (MAOIs, SSRIs, TCAs), kidney failure

MAOIs, monoamine oxidase inhibitors; SSRIs, serotonin reuptake inhibitors; TCAs, tricyclic antidepressants.

- Contraindications.
  - History of medical noncompliance.
  - Psychiatric illness.
  - High risk of death during the procedure.
- Requires involvement of a team of medical, surgical, psychiatric, and nutrition experts.
- Most common current techniques include laparoscopic adjustable gastric banding and Roux-en-Y gastric bypass; less common techniques include biliopancreatic diversion and biliopancreatic diversion with duodenal switch.
- Patients should be aware of multiple complications and risks associated with the procedure.
- Complication rates are lower at centers with more experience.

Medications

- Indications:
  - BMI >30 kg/m^2 or BMI >27 kg/m^2 with concomitant obesity-related risk factors or diseases.
  - Unable to achieve weight loss goal despite therapeutic lifestyle changes.
  - No contraindications to use.
- Weight loss medications are meant to be used as an adjunct to and not as a substitute for therapeutic lifestyle changes.
- They should be discontinued if the patient has not responded within 1 to 2 months.
- The use of such a medication should be considered long-term (if not life-long) in patients who respond, as patients will regain weight quickly if the drug is stopped.
- Medications approved for short-term use (phentermine, diethylpropion, benzphetamine, phendimetrazine) are not typically used because of their limitations on duration of use and addictive properties and will not be discussed further here.

Sibutramine (Meridia or Reductil)

- Central reuptake inhibitor of norepinephrine and serotonin thought to act centrally by suppressing appetite.
- Studies have shown that patients who take sibutramine and make therapeutic lifestyle changes will lose about 4% more weight than patients making therapeutic lifestyle changes alone.[8]
- Increases heart rate and blood pressure.
- Carries a risk of serotonin syndrome when combined with MAOIs, triptans, and opioids.
- Contraindications include poorly controlled hypertension, coronary artery disease, angina, arrhythmias, congestive heart failure, stroke, transient ischemic attacks, seizure disorder, severe liver or kidney disease, and concomitant use of monoamine oxidase inhibitors (MAOIs).
- Modest efficacy and cardiac effects have limited its use.
- Is a schedule IV controlled substance in the United States.
- Costs approximately $1,600 per year of treatment at recommended doses.

Orlistat (Xenical)

- Works by inhibiting pancreatic lipase and reducing the absorption of fat.
- Inhibits fat absorption by 30% at recommended doses.
- Studies have shown that patients who take orlistat and make therapeutic lifestyle changes will lose about 4% more weight than patients making therapeutic lifestyle changes alone.[8]

- Contraindicated in patients with malabsorption syndromes.
- Side effects include diarrhea, bowel incontinence, flatulence, and oily spotting.
- Interferes with absorption of fat-soluble vitamins and a multivitamin should be taken to prevent deficiency.
- Costs approximately $2,600 per year of treatment at recommended doses.

Orlistat (Alli)
- A half-strength over-the-counter version of Xenical became available under the trade name *Alli* in June 2007.
- Inhibits fat absorption by 25% as compared with 30% for full-strength Xenical.
- Side effects are the same as for Xenical and are still significant despite the reduced dose.
- Costs approximately $500 to $700 per year depending on the dose used.

Internet Nutrition Resources

- USDA food pyramid, http://www.mypyramid.gov
- American Medical Association, http://www.ama-assn.org
- American Dietetic Association, http://www.eatright.org
- National Center for Complementary and Alternative Medicine, http://nccam.nih.gov
- American Botanical Council, http://www.herbalgram.org
- Office of Dietary Supplements, http://dietary-supplements.info.nih.gov
- Food and Nutrition Information Center, http://www.nal.usda.gov/fnic
- U.S. Food and Drug Administration, http://www.fda.gov

REFERENCES

1. Weinsier RL, Hunker EM, Krundieck CL, et al. Hospital malnutrition: a Prospective evaluation of general medical patients during the course of hospitalization. *Am J Clin Nutr* 1979;32:418.
2. Kotler DP, Wang J, Pierson RN. Studies of body composition in patient with the acquired immunodeficiency syndrome. The United Nations University Press: Food and Nutrition Bulletin 1989;11:55–60.
3. Eating Pattern Questionnaire. American Medical Association. 2003. Available at: http://www.ama-assn.org/ama1/pub/upload/mm/433/weight.pdf. Last accessed December 1, 2009.
4. Dietary Guidance. DRI Tables. National Agricultural Library. United States Department of Agriculture. Available at: http://fnic.nal.usda.gov/nal_display/ index.php?info_center=4&tax_level=3&tax_subject=256&topic_id=1342&level3_id=5140. Last accessed December 1, 2009.
5. http://www.mypyramidtracker.gov/. Last accessed 12/1/09.
6. Ogden CL, Carroll MD, Curtin LR, et al. Prevalence of overweight and obesity in the United States, 1999–2004. *JAMA* 2006;295(13):1549–1555.
7. Pavlou KN, Krey S, Steffee WP. Exercise as an adjunct to weight loss and maintenance in moderately obese subjects. *Am J Clin Nutr* 1989;203(2):1115–1123.
8. Padwal R, Li SK, Lau DC. Long-term pharmacotherapy for overweight and obesity: a systematic review and meta-analysis of randomized controlled trials. *Int J Obes Relat Metab Disord* 2003;27:1437–1446.

19

Laboratory Assessment of Kidney and Urinary Tract Disorders

Ying Chen, Vikrant Rachakonda, and Michelle C. L. Cabellon

Urinalysis

Introduction

The initial evaluation of renal and urinary tract disease includes urinalysis. Urinalysis consists of two components:

- **Macroscopic examination:** The macroscopic examination includes dipstick evaluation, which yields information regarding the physical and chemical properties of a urine sample, whereas microscopy provides for evaluation of formed elements in the urine.
- **Microscopic evaluation** of the urinary sediment: A microscopic evaluation of urine sediment should be performed in the presence of abnormal renal function, macroscopic examination with hematuria or proteinuria, or clinical concern for urinary tract infection.

Specimen Collection and Testing Procedure

- Urine samples should be examined within 2 hours of collection, as urea breakdown into ammonia results in alkaline urine. This promotes cell lysis and cast degradation.
- Ideally, samples should be collected from midstream catch of an early morning specimen. Alternatively, bladder catheterization, either transurethral or suprapubic, may be used.
- First perform dipstick testing to interpret colorimetric reaction results. It is important to assess the color and clarity of urine as well.
- For microscopic evaluation, collect 10 to 12 mL of a freshly voided specimen and centrifuge at 1,500 to 3,000 rpm for 3 to 5 minutes. Then remove approximately 0.5 mL of supernatant using a pipette, and resuspend the sediment pellet in the remaining supernatant. Apply one or two drops of this solution onto a clean glass slide and cover with a cover slip. View the sample with phase-contrast microscopy at 100$\times$ and 400$\times$ magnification to examine the formed elements in the urine.

Physical and Chemical Properties of Urine

Color

- Normal urine should appear pale to yellow in color, whereas dilute specimens are lighter in color, and concentrated urine has an amber appearance.
- **Red urine** is seen with hematuria, hemoglobinuria, and myoglobinuria. The presence of blood on dipstick testing without red blood cells (RBCs) on microscopy is suggestive of myoglobinuria. Consumption of foods with red color may also yield red urine; drugs including phenytoin and rifampin may also color the urine red.
- **Brown or black urine** may be seen with copper poisoning and alkaptonuria (where urine turns from yellow to black upon standing).

Clarity
- Normal urine is clear.
- Turbid urine is seen with organisms, cells, and casts in the urine. Urinary tract infections usually produce turbid urine.
- Other causes include hematuria, lipiduria, and metabolic disease (oxaluria, uricosuria).

Odor
- Normal urine does not have a strong odor.
- Foul-smelling urine may be encountered with urinary tract infections.
- Diabetic ketoacidosis is associated with fruity odor, and gastrointestinal-vesical fistulas may result in a fecal odor to urine.

Specific Gravity
- Specific gravity refers to the relative density of urine with respect to water.
- Normal values range from 1.005 to 1.020.
- Specific gravity ≥ 1.020 is consistent with concentrated urine in the setting of dehydration; higher values suggest glycosuria or other osmotically active substances in the urine.
- Values ≤ 1.005 suggest dilute urine, which may be seen in water intoxication and diabetes insipidus.
- Proteinuria (>7 g/dL) may cause falsely elevated specific gravity, and falsely decreased values may be seen with urine pH <6.5.

Urine pH
- The normal urine pH ranges from 4.5 to 8.0.
- Acidic urine is associated with metabolic acidosis (i.e., starvation ketosis, diabetic ketoacidosis), dehydration, and large protein loads.
- Carbon dioxide retention with compensatory metabolic alkalosis can decrease urine pH, and extrarenal bicarbonate losses (i.e., diarrhea) may promote urinary acidification.
- Alkaline urine is typically seen in renal tubular acidosis.
- Urea-splitting organisms (i.e., *Proteus* spp.) can raise urinary pH.
- Similarly, prolonged storage of urine results in conversion of urea to ammonia, and urinary pH increases.

Glucose
- In patients with preserved renal function and normal serum glucose concentrations, urine glucose is typically absent.
- Dipstick analysis can provide qualitative information regarding the presence or absence of glycosuria.
- More specific techniques are required to quantify glycosuria, however.
- Urine glucose may be seen in diabetes mellitus, liver disease, pancreatic disease, Fanconi syndrome, and Cushing syndrome.

Protein
- Urine dipstick is the main screening test for proteinuria, but it is only sensitive to protein concentrations >20 mg/dL (roughly equivalent to 300 mg/day).
- The test is a pH-based assay, and albumin is the primary protein identified.
- False-positive results may be seen with highly concentrated specimens, alkaline urine, or high urinary concentration of penicillin, cephalosporins, or iodinated radiocontrast agents.

- False-negative tests are associated with dilute urine and nonalbumin proteins, including immunoglobulins and amyloid.
- A sulfosalicylic acid test may be used to identify nonalbumin proteins.

Hemoglobin
- The dipstick can detect as few as four RBCs per high-power microscopic field (HPF).
- Free hemoglobin or myoglobin in urine, as can be seen with hemolysis or rhabdomyolysis, catalyzes the same dipstick reaction. These conditions should be suspected when the urine dipstick is positive for occult blood in the absence of RBCs on microscopic examination of the urine sediment.
- False-negative tests result from the presence of substances such as ascorbic acid (ingestion of >200 mg/day vitamin C) that diminish the oxidizing potential of the reagent strip.
- Detection of hematuria by dipstick should always be confirmed by microscopic examination of the urine. The presence of dysmorphic RBCs or RBC casts (an "active" urine sediment) or the coexistence of proteinuria suggests that the hematuria is of glomerular origin.

Leukocyte Esterase
- The detection of leukocyte esterase relies on the release of esterases from granulocytes.
- The sensitivity of a positive leukocyte esterase is variable depending on the population studied.
- False-positive results are seen when significant delay occurs between sampling and testing; false-positive results can also occur with contamination by vaginal cells.
- False-negative results occur with inhibition of granulocyte function, including glycosuria and high urinary concentrations of antibiotics.

Urine Nitrite
- Urine dipstick testing depends on bacterial conversion of urinary nitrates into nitrite.
- While many gram-negative bacteria can reduce nitrates to nitrite, certain organisms, including *Enterococcus* spp., *Neisseria gonorrhoeae*, and mycobacteria, do not; this may result in "false-negative" results.
- False-negative results are also seen with insufficient bladder incubation time, low urinary nitrate excretion, and reduction of nitrates to nitrogen by bacteria.
- Both leukocyte esterase and nitrite testing must be combined with microscopic examination and clinical context to accurately diagnose urinary tract infections.

Microscopic Examination of Urine
Red Blood Cells
- Three RBCs or more/HPF is consistent with at least microscopic hematuria.
- **Dysmorphic RBCs** are suggestive of glomerular disease, whereas normal RBCs suggest bleeding from the lower genitourinary tract.
- Hematuria is discussed in further detail in Chapter 21.

White Blood Cells
- Urinary white blood cells (WBCs) are associated with either infection or inflammation.
- Pyuria is defined as more than five WBCs/HPF.
- Extraurinary inflammation, as seen in appendicitis, can result in pyuria.

- Urine **eosinophils** may be seen in allergic interstitial nephritis, but this finding is neither sensitive nor specific. Urine eosinophils are also present with parasitic infection of the urinary tract (schistosomiasis), cholesterol emboli, chronic pyelonephritis, and prostatitis. Eosinophiluria is identified with Hansel staining of the urine.

Epithelial Cells
- Various types of epithelial cells are commonly encountered on urine microscopy.
- **Squamous epithelial cells** are large, flat cells with central nuclei; they are found in the distal urinary tract and are almost always contaminants.
- **Transitional epithelial cells** are small, pear-shaped cells lining the bladder and ureters. They may be seen after bladder catheterization but are also found in genitourinary malignancy.
- **Renal tubular epithelial cells** are notable for large nuclei; their presence suggests renal tubular injury.
- **Oval fat bodies** are lipid-laden renal epithelial cells. They are identified by the presence of a "Maltese cross" on polarized light microscopy. Their presence is suggestive of nephrotic syndrome.

Casts
Casts form when proteins secreted into the tubular lumen capture other intraluminal debris (lipids, cells, bacteria). They often take the shape of the tubular lumen.
- **Hyaline casts:** Hyaline casts are formed by Tamm-Horsfall protein secreted by tubular epithelium into the tubular lumen. Tamm-Horsfall proteins accumulate into casts under states of dehydration or acidic urine.
- **Granular casts:** These are formed by Tamm-Horsfall proteins and products of cellular breakdown. "Muddy brown" granular casts are seen in acute tubular necrosis and are composed of debris from tubular epithelial cell destruction.
- **RBC casts:** RBC casts are easily identified as tubular, orange-red structures on light microscopy. Their presence indicates glomerular hematuria.
- **WBC casts:** WBC casts consist of WBCs and tubular proteins trapped in the tubular lumen. These are seen with interstitial inflammation, including pyelonephritis, allergic interstitial nephritis, and occasionally with glomerulonephritis.
- **Waxy casts:** These casts are formed from the degradation of other casts. They are smooth, well-defined structures visible without polarized light. Waxy casts are mainly seen in chronic kidney disease (CKD).
- **Fatty casts:** These are characterized by "Maltese crosses" visible under polarized light. Fatty casts are seen with ethylene glycol poisoning and nephrotic syndrome.

Organisms
- Bacteriuria is frequently encountered, as many urine specimens are not collected under sterile conditions. The clinical context of this finding aids in determining the presence of infection.
- Common bacterial causes of urinary tract infection include *E. coli*, *Staphylococcus saprophyticus* (especially in menstruating females), *Enterococcus* spp., Group B Streptococcus, and other gram-negative bacillus infections (e.g., *Klebsiella* spp., *Citrobacter* spp., and *Pseudomonas* spp.).
- Antimicrobial therapy is guided by urine Gram's stain, culture, and sensitivity testing.
- *Candida* spp. are frequently seen as contaminants from genital secretions or indwelling Foley catheter colonization.

Crystals
- A discussion of pathologic urinary crystals and nephrolithiasis may be found in Chapter 21.
- Crystals are often present as artifacts on microscopy, however.
- Acidic urine can result in precipitation of calcium oxalate and various urate stones.
- Alkaline urine can result in precipitation of triple phosphate, calcium carbonate, and calcium oxalate stones.
- Crystals may form from precipitation of drugs and drug metabolites (e.g., anti-retroviral agents, acyclovir, and sulfonamides).

Assessment of Renal Function

Creatinine as a Marker of Renal Function
- Creatinine is a metabolite of skeletal muscle that is freely filtered at the glomerulus and undergoes no significant tubular reabsorption. It is secreted to a small degree by the renal tubules into the urine. Its production is relative to an individual's muscle mass.
- As expected, aging and weight loss contribute to reduced creatinine production rates.
- In patients with normal renal function, >90% of creatinine elimination occurs by glomerular filtration. As renal function declines, up to 50% of creatinine elimination occurs by tubular secretion.
- Subsequently, **all estimates of renal function based on creatinine overestimate actual function,** and the degree of overestimation increases with worsening renal function.
- Serum creatinine (S_{Cr}) varies inversely with glomerular filtration rate (GFR). Any elevation of S_{Cr} above the normal range (0.6 to 1.2 mg/dL) should alert the physician to the presence of reduced GFR and renal insufficiency.
- Changes in plasma creatinine are not linearly related to renal function. For example, an increase in creatinine from 1.0 to 1.5 signifies a greater decline in renal function than an increase from 2.0 to 2.5.

Estimation of GFR
- Because S_{Cr} is a function of muscle mass and is dependent on age, gender, and size, it can often be **difficult to assess the degree of renal impairment from S_{Cr} alone.**
- Renal function, or GFR, can be clinically assessed more accurately by calculating or measuring the creatinine clearance (CrCl). This estimation of GFR is **accurate only if the S_{Cr} is stable and in steady state.**
- As renal disease progresses toward end stage, these methods become less accurate as creatinine is increasingly secreted by the diseased proximal tubules, causing overestimation of true GFR.
- The equations below are very useful in adjustment of drug doses and for quick estimation of kidney function, but they may underestimate true GFR in healthy patients, and they are less accurate in very obese or very elderly patients. In these cases, a 24-hour urine measurement of creatinine may be the test of choice.

The Cockcroft-Gault CrCl Formula[1]
- The Cockcroft-Gault formula was derived from studies on adult inpatient male patients. Problems with this formula include estimation of lean body weight and overestimation of true GFR with worsening renal function.

$$CrCl \text{ (mL/min)} = [(140 - Age) \times \text{lean body weight (kg)} \times (.85 \text{ if female})]/(72 \times S_{Cr})$$

- It takes age, ideal body weight, and gender into account to estimate GFR from a measurement of S_{Cr}.
- This formula estimates CrCl in mL/min (normal: 100 to 125 mL/min for males and 85 to 100 mL/min for females).
- This rapid estimation of GFR is useful in adjustment of drug dosages for decreased renal function based on S_{Cr}.

The Modification of Diet in Renal Disease Equations[2]

- The modification of diet in renal disease equation was developed in an outpatient CKD population, and in patients with GFR <60 mL/min/1.73 m^2 the equation accurately estimates renal function. **In patients with normal renal function, however, the modification of diet in renal disease is not useful.** It has not been validated in patients >70 years of age or in hospitalized patients.[1–4]

$$GFR = 186 \times S_{Cr}^{-1.154} \times age^{-0.203} \times (1.210 \text{ if black}) \times (0.742 \text{ if female})$$

- The abbreviated equation uses age, serum creatinine, gender, and race (black vs. other).

24-Hour Urine Collection for CrCl

- Patients should be instructed to discard their first morning urine and then begin the 24-hour urine collection, ending the collection with inclusion of the following morning's first void.
- The amount of total creatinine in the collection can be used to assess the adequacy of the collection; an adequate 24-hour urine collection contains 15 to 20 mg/kg creatinine for females and 20 to 25 mg/kg for males.
- Accuracy may be altered by incorrect collection of the urinary specimen or hypersecretion of creatinine in advanced kidney disease.

Determination of Chronicity

- The diagnosis of CKD is suggested by a stable elevated S_{Cr} for greater than a few months.
- Acute kidney injury (AKI) should be assessed urgently because it can often be reversed. The diagnosis of AKI is suggested by a history of sudden onset (days to weeks before presentation) of hypertension, edema, hematuria, or proteinuria.
- Further investigation in the determination of AKI versus chronic kidney injury (CKI) includes urinalysis and renal ultrasound. The finding of symmetrically small kidneys (<10 cm) on ultrasound images favors CKD, with the notable exceptions of diabetic nephropathy, polycystic kidney disease, amyloidosis, and HIV nephropathy, in which the kidneys may be enlarged.
- In patients with clearly established AKI, an acute deterioration of renal function must prompt an evaluation for causes of superimposed CKD, which are usually reversible.

Proteinuria

- Patients with normal renal function excrete <150 mg of total protein or <30 mg of albumin in 24 hours.[5]
- **Proteinuria defined as urinary protein excretion >150 mg/day.** It is usually initially detected by reagent dipstick, which indicates the presence of albumin in the urine. The urine dipstick is sensitive to protein concentrations >20 mg/dL, which is roughly equal to 300 mg/day. Hence, **any proteinuria detected on dipstick should be further evaluated.**

- Quantification of proteinuria aids in classification of severity. Nephrotic syndrome refers to the pentad of urine protein excretion >3 g/day, hypoalbuminemia <3.5 g/dL, edema, hypercholesterolemia, and lipiduria. **Nephrotic-range proteinuria refers to urine protein excretion >3 g/day** without the other findings.

24-Hour Urine Collection for Protein

- Accurately quantify the amount of daily protein excretion in the urine.
- Concurrent collection of urine creatinine should also be done to ensure the completeness of the collection. The amount of creatinine excreted stays relatively constant at 15 to 20 mg/kg for females and 20 to 25 mg/kg for males with stable weight and diet.
- Many patients have significant difficulty collecting all urine during the 24-hour period.

Spot Urine Protein-Creatinine Ratio

- Rapidly estimate the amount of protein excretion in 24 hours.[4]
- This test uses a random spot urine sample for protein (mg/dL) and creatinine (mg/dL) concentrations to calculate urine protein-creatinine ratio. **The resulting unitless ratio closely approximates the amount of daily protein excretion in g/1.73 m² body surface area.** A normal ratio is <0.15 (<150 mg/day).
- Although this test is **far less cumbersome** to perform than the 24-hour urine collection, the results **can be unreliable in patients at either extremes of muscle mass.** Also, this test is not as accurate for predicting conditions that cause variable amounts of proteinuria per day (e.g., postural proteinuria or diabetic nephropathy).

Diagnostic Approach

- A positive dipstick test should be repeated at least once at a 1-week interval. Once confirmed on a second dipstick, urine protein excretion should be quantified.
- Conditions that are associated with functional proteinuria, such as fever, emotional stress, heavy physical exercise, or acute medical illness, should be excluded before the test is repeated.
- Functional proteinuria is usually transient and is most likely related to changes in renal hemodynamics. If the proteinuria is transient, no further investigation is required.

History and Physical Examination

- Focus on signs and symptoms of conditions associated with proteinuria, such as hypertension, diabetes mellitus, or connective tissue diseases.
- Medications should be reviewed.
  - **Nonsteroidal anti-inflammatory drugs** are associated with a variety of renal diseases and should be discontinued in the presence of proteinuria pending further evaluation.
- Clinical features of malignancies, especially multiple myeloma and lymphoma, should be sought. Furthermore, solid organ malignancies are associated with glomerulonephritis.
- Findings consistent with infections, such as HIV, viral hepatitis, and bacterial endocarditis, should be evaluated, as all these can cause glomerular disease.

Microscopic Examination of the Urine Sediment

- Should be done once proteinuria is considered persistent (positive dipstick on more than one occasion).
- Urine sediment should be carefully examined for other signs of glomerular disease such as hematuria, RBC casts, and oval fat bodies.

Laboratory Testing

- Includes complete blood count (CBC), basic metabolic profile, albumin, and a 24-hour urine collection for protein. Abnormal values of renal function tests or proteinuria >150 mg/24 hours suggest intrinsic renal disease.
  - Patients >30 years of age should also have a serum and urine protein electrophoresis to exclude paraproteinemia, which may be caused by multiple myeloma or amyloidosis.
- **Orthostatic proteinuria** is defined as proteinuria with <75 mg of urinary protein excretion while recumbent.
  - This condition has a good prognosis, is uncommon in patients >30 years of age, and can be diagnosed with a split urine collection for protein.
  - Total urinary protein does not usually exceed 1.5 g/day.

Nephrology Referral

- Major indications for nephrology referral are as follows:
  - Estimated GFR <60 mL/min/1.73 m^2.
  - Estimated GFR >60 mL/min/1.73 m^2 but with an associated known renal disease (e.g., polycystic kidney disease) or with an otherwise unexplained elevated serum creatinine.
  - Evidence of nephrotic syndrome.
  - Persistent nonnephrotic proteinuria with normal renal function, with or without associated microscopic hematuria.
  - Macroscopic hematuria with negative urologic evaluation.
  - Persistent microscopic hematuria, usually with some associated proteinuria.
  - Malignant hypertension.
  - Hyperkalemia.
- Data suggests that many patients with CKD are referred late in the course of their disease, often after complications from CKD have arisen. This results in metabolic and hematologic mismanagement, as well as loss of early preparation for dialysis, including preemptive fistula or other access placement.
- Early referral allows for a timely renal biopsy, if indicated, which may alter management and outcome.
- Early referral also allows for risk factor modification, including strict hypertension and glycemic control, lipid management, and smoking cessation. Early initiation of possible disease-modifying therapy, such as angiotensin-converting enzyme inhibitors, is more likely to occur under the care of a supervising nephrologist.

REFERENCES

1. Levey AS, Bosch JP, Lewis JB, et al. A more accurate method to estimate glomerular filtration rate from serum creatinine: a new prediction equation. Modification of Diet in Renal Disease Study Group. *Ann Intern Med* 1999;130:461–470.
2. Poggio ED, Wang X, Greene T, et al. Performance of the modification of diet in renal disease and Cockcroft-Gault equations in the estimation of GFR in health and in chronic kidney disease. *J Am Soc Nephrol* 2005;16:459–466.
3. Rule AD, Larson TS, Bergstralh EJ, et al. Using serum creatinine to estimate glomerular filtration rate: accuracy in good health and chronic kidney disease. *Ann Intern Med* 2004;141:929–937.
4. National Kidney Foundation. K/DOQI clinical practice guidelines for chronic kidney disease: evaluation, classification, and stratification. *Am J Kidney Dis* 2002;39(2 suppl 1):S1–S266.
5. Wingo CS, Clapp WL. Proteinuria: potential causes and approach to evaluation. *Am J Med Sci* 2000;320:188–194.

20 Acute Kidney Injury, Glomerulopathy, and Chronic Kidney Disease

Ying Chen, Vikrant Rachakonda, and Michelle C.L. Cabellon

ACUTE KIDNEY INJURY

General Principles

- Acute kidney injury (AKI) is a clinical syndrome denoted by an abrupt decline (over days to a few weeks) in glomerular filtration rate (GFR) sufficient to decrease the elimination of nitrogenous waste products (urea and creatinine) and other uremic toxins.[1]
- Clinically, AKI is often further divided into oliguric (<500 mL/day) or nonoliguric (>500 mL/day) AKI.[2]
- It has been suggested that AKI complicates 5% of all hospital and 30% of all ICU admissions.[3]
- AKI needs to be quickly recognized and the underlying etiology determined.

Etiology and Pathophysiology

The etiologies of AKI can be divided into three major groups on the basis of the anatomic nature of the lesion: prerenal, intrinsic, and postrenal.

Prerenal Azotemia

- Prerenal azotemia refers to conditions that lead to impaired renal perfusion with a resultant fall in glomerular capillary filtration pressure. The renal parenchymal function is generally preserved.
- The most common scenario of diminished renal perfusion is in the setting of **reduced effective extracellular volume,** which results in production of concentrated urine with a low urine sodium (<10 mmol/L) and a concentrated urine (urine osmolality >500 mOsm/kg). It includes:
  - Hypovolemia
  - Decreased cardiac output:
    - The presence of AKI in the setting of severe heart failure has been termed the **cardiorenal syndrome.**
    - It is often exacerbated by the use of angiotensin converting enzyme (ACE) inhibitors and diuretics.
  - Liver cirrhosis
- However, **preferential renal vasoconstriction** may lead to a prerenal state in certain situations, even with normal or elevated systemic blood pressure (BP), including:
  - Nonsteroidal anti-inflammatory drugs (NSAIDs).
  - ACE inhibitors and angiotensin receptor blockers (ARBs).
  - Calcineurin inhibitors (e.g., cyclosporine and tacrolimus).
- **Radiocontrast agents**:
  - This typically occurs in patients with underlying renal impairment.

TABLE 1	Some Causes of Toxic Acute Tubular Necrosis
Exogenous Toxins	**Endogenous Toxins**
Drugs (e.g., gentamicin, amphotericin B, acyclovir)	Hemoglobin and myoglobin
Recreational drugs (e.g., cocaine, phencyclidine [PCP], amphetamine)	Uric acid
Radiocontrast	Immunoglobulin light chains
Toxic chemicals (e.g., ethylene glycol, carbon tetrachloride)	
Biologic poisonous material (e.g., snake venom)	

From Agha IA. Acute Renal Failure. In: Agha IA, Green GB (eds). Washington Manual Nephrology Subspecialty Consult. Philadelphia, PA: Lippincott Williams & Wilkins, 2004: 37–55, with permission.

- Other risk factors include the following[4]:
  - Diabetic nephropathy
  - Advanced age (>75 years)
  - Congestive heart failure
  - Volume depletion
  - High or repetitive doses of radiocontrast agent
  - High osmolar contrast agents
- **Endotoxin** associated with bacterial infection is also associated with prerenal AKI.

Intrinsic Renal Causes of Acute Renal Kidney Injury

- The most common cause of AKI due to intrinsic renal disease is acute tubular necrosis (ATN).
  - Common causes of ATN are listed in Table 1.
  - ATN is usually considered to be due to ischemic or nephrotoxic injury.[5,6]
  - The most important toxic materials that lead to ATN are drugs.[7]
- However, other important disease processes such as glomerular disease, acute interstitial nephritis, and small vessel disease (e.g., vasculitis, renal atheroembolism) may also lead to AKI.

Postrenal Failure

- Ureteral obstruction (e.g., calculus, tumor, clot, sloughed papillae, and external compression).
- Bladder outlet obstruction (e.g., prostatic hypertrophy, neurogenic bladder, carcinoma, and urethral stricture).

Diagnosis

Clinical Presentation

History
- **Urine history:**
  - Establish urine volume and recent trends.
  - Elicit any history of hematuria, proteinuria, dysuria, or pyuria.

- Urgency, frequency, dribbling, and incontinence, especially in elderly men, may direct to benign prostatic hypertrophy.
- **Drug history:**
  - Look for nephrotoxins such as NSAIDs, ACE inhibitors, ARBs, aminoglycosides, or radiocontrasts.
  - It should include over-the-counter formulations and herbal remedies or recreational drugs.
- **Volume status:**
  - History of thirst or orthostatic lightheadedness may point toward intravascular depletion.
  - Weight gain, ankle swelling, orthopnea, or paroxysmal nocturnal dyspnea may signify fluid retention.
  - Look for the possible causes of **fluid loss:**
    - Gastrointestinal losses: diarrhea, vomiting, and prolonged nasogastric drainage.
    - Renal losses: diuretics and osmotic diuresis in hyperglycemia.
    - Dermal losses: burns and extensive sweating.
    - Third spacing: acute pancreatitis, ascites, and muscle trauma.
- Exclude **infections.**
- Other potential causes:
  - Chronic liver disease may cause **hepatorenal syndrome.**
  - Hepatitis C with purpura may suggest cryoglobulinemia.
  - Arthralgias, skin rash, and oral ulcers may suggest a connective tissue disorder.
  - Sinusitis, cough, and hemoptysis may alert the physician to the possibility of Wegener granulomatosis (WG) or Goodpasture syndrome.
  - A history of recent sore throats or significant skin infections may suggest acute poststreptococcal glomerulonephritis.
  - Low back pain and anemia may suggest multiple myeloma.

Physical Examination
- Orthostatic vital signs, mucous membrane and skin turgor, and examination of jugular veins can assess the patient's fluid balance. Looking for sacral edema in a patient in a supine position is important.
- The presence of S3, pulmonary crackles, and pitting edema suggests volume overload.
- The presence of abdominal bruits suggests renovascular disease.
- Pelvic examination in females and rectal examination in both females and males may detect a cause of postrenal obstruction.
- The kidney can be palpable in cases of hydronephrosis or polycystic kidney disease.

Diagnostic Testing
Laboratories
Urinalysis and Urine Sediment
- Routine dipstick and microscopic analysis of urine should always be done and are often helpful in determining the cause of AKI.
  - Prerenal AKI: hyaline casts.
  - ATN: muddy brown granular casts, epithelial cells, and epithelial cell casts.
  - Glomerulonephritis: dysmorphic red blood cells (RBCs) and RBC casts.
  - Acute interstitial nephritis: eosinophils, other white blood cells (WBCs), and WBC casts.
- Usually, the urine is bland in prerenal and uncomplicated postrenal AKI while an abnormal urinalysis and active sediment suggest an intrinsic renal cause.

TABLE 2	Laboratory Tests in the Differentiation of Oliguric Prerenal Azotemia from Oliguric Intrinsic Acute Tubular Necrosis

Diagnosis	U/P_{Cr}	U_{Na}	FE_{Na} (%)	U_{osm}	Plasma BUN/Cr
Prerenal azotemia	>40	<20	<1	>500	>20
Oliguric ATN	<20	>40	>1	<350	<10–15

FE_{Na}, fractional excretion of sodium; Plasma BUN/Cr, plasma blood urea nitrogen to creatinine ratio; U_{Na}, urine sodium concentration; U_{osm}, urine osmolality; U/P_{Cr}, urine to plasma creatinine ratio.

Assessment of Renal Function

- In prerenal states, the kidney avidly retains sodium, usually resulting in low urine sodium and a **fractional excretion of sodium (FE$_{Na}$)** of <1%. FE_{Na} is particularly helpful in oliguric AKI (Table 2).

$$FE_{Na} = [(U_{Na} \times P_{Cr})/(P_{Na} \times U_{Cr})] \times 100$$

where U = urine, P = plasma, Na = sodium, and Cr = creatinine.

- Because loop diuretics force natriuresis, calculation of FE_{Na} is misleading in patients who are taking these agents. The **fractional excretion of urea (FE$_{urea}$)** of <30% is suggestive of prerenal azotemia (Table 2).

$$FE_{urea} = [(U_{urea} \times P_{Cr})/(BUN \times U_{Cr})] \times 100$$

where U_{urea} = urine urea, P = plasma, BUN = blood urea nitrogen (mg/dL), and Cr = creatinine.

Imaging

Ultrasonography

- Ultrasonography exhibits high sensitivity (90% to 98%) but a lower specificity (65% to 84%) for the detection of urinary tract obstruction.[5]
- It can also measure the echotexture (increased echogenicity suggests more chronic damage) and kidney size (a marked difference may suggest renovascular disease).

Computed Tomography

Compared with renal ultrasonography, computed tomography is superior in the evaluation of ureteral obstruction since it can define the level of obstruction and demarcate retroperitoneal fibrosis or a retroperitoneal mass.

Diagnostic Procedures

Renal biopsy is reserved for patients in whom the cause of intrinsic AKI is unclear; therefore, a nephrology referral is indicated.

Treatment

Nondialytic Therapy

- **Volume expansion.** Prompt and effective restoration of effective circulatory volume is the key in prerenal azotemia.
- **Avoidance of nephrotoxins.**
  - Contrast media should be used cautiously.
  - ACE inhibitors, ARBs, and NSAIDs should be held.

- **Electrolyte management**
  - **Hyperkalemia** is a potentially lethal complication of AKI.
    - Rule out pseudohyperkalemia by repeating the serum electrolytes. Consider drawing the sample without the use of a tourniquet or fist clenching.
    - If the patient has thrombocytosis or marked leukocytosis, the sample may be drawn in a heparinized tube.
    - Obtain a stat ECG and arterial blood gases (ABG) (if acidosis is a concern).
    - Review the patient's medication list and stop all exogenous K^+ and potentially offending drugs.
    - **Acute treatment** consists of the following:
      - **Calcium gluconate** 10%, 10 mL IV over 2 to 3 minutes decreases cardiac membrane excitability. The effect occurs in minutes but lasts only 30 to 60 minutes. It can be repeated after 5 to 10 minutes if the ECG does not change. Use with extreme caution in patients receiving digoxin.
      - **Insulin,** 10 to 20 units IV, causes an intracellular shift of K^+ in 10 to 30 minutes. The effect lasts for several hours. Glucose, 50 to 100 g IV (1 to 2 ampules D50), should also be administered to prevent hypoglycemia.
      - **NaHCO₃,** 1 ampule IV can also be used to cause an intracellular shift of K^+, and the effect can last several hours. This treatment should probably be reserved for patients with severe hyperkalemia and metabolic acidosis. Patients with end-stage renal disease (ESRD) seldom respond and may not tolerate the Na^+ load.
      - **β₂-Adrenergic agonists** can be used to cause an intracellular shift of K^+.
      - **Diuretics** (e.g., furosemide 40 to 120 mg IV) enhance K^+ excretion provided renal function is adequate.
      - **Cation exchange resins** (sodium polystyrene sulfonate, Kayexalate) enhance K^+ excretion from the gastrointestinal tract. Kayexalate may be given PO (20 to 50 g in 100 to 200 mL 20% sorbitol) or as a retention enema (50 g in 200 mL 20% sorbitol). The effect may not be evident for several hours and lasts 4 to 6 hours. Doses may be repeated every 4 to 6 hours as needed.
      - **Dialysis** may be necessary for severe hyperkalemia when other measures are ineffective and for patients with renal failure.
  - Hyperphosphatemia and hypocalcemia are also common in AKI.
- **Acid-base disorders.** Metabolic acidosis is a common complication of AKI. If severe, alkali therapy may be required.
  - Severe acidosis (pH <7.20) may require treatment with parenteral NaHCO₃. Rapid infusion should be considered only for very severe acidosis.
  - The bicarbonate deficit may be calculated as follows:

$$[HCO_3^-] \text{ deficit (mEq/L)} = [0.5 \times \text{body weight (kg)}] - (24 - \text{measured } [HCO_3^-])$$

  - Overaggressive correction should be avoided to prevent overshoot alkalosis.
  - Hypernatremia and fluid overload can occur with NaHCO₃ administration.
  - Serum electrolytes should be followed closely.
- **Nutrition support.** This may be the most important facet of conservative care.
- Treatment for specific causes of AKI.
  - Immunosuppressive agents for glomerulonephritis or vasculitis.
  - Systemic anticoagulation for renal artery or vein thrombosis.
  - Plasmapheresis for hemolytic uremic syndrome/thrombotic thrombocytopenic purpura.

Dialytic Therapy for Acute Renal Failure

- Indications for initiation of dialytic support in acute renal failure include the following:
  - Severe hyperkalemia, metabolic acidosis, or volume overload refractory to medical therapy.
  - Uremic syndrome:
    - Uremic pericarditis
    - Encephalopathy
    - Neuropathy
    - Bleeding
    - Need to start total parental nutrition (volume/solute issue)
  - Overdose/intoxications
  - Refractory hypercalcemia
  - Refractory hyperuricemia

GLOMERULOPATHY

General Principles

- Numerous inflammatory and noninflammatory diseases affect the glomerulus and lead to alterations in glomerular permeability and selectivity resulting in proteinuria and, in some cases, hematuria.
- The glomerulus may be primarily affected or may be damaged as part of a multisystem disease, most frequently systemic lupus erythematosus (SLE) or vasculitis.

Diagnosis

Clinical Presentation

Asymptomatic

Isolated Proteinuria

- This refers to the presence of 150 mg to 3 g of urinary protein per day, as measured in a 24-hour urine collection.
- **Microalbuminuria** is defined as the excretion of 30 to 300 mg albumin per day. This measurement is used to identify diabetic subjects at risk of developing nephropathy and to assess cardiovascular risk, for example, in patients with hypertension (HTN).

Isolated Hematuria

- Hematuria is classified as either microscopic, referring to more than two RBCs per high power field (HPF) in spun urine, or macroscopic, referring to visible brown/red urine not associated with pain.
- Glomerular hematuria is confirmed by the presence of dysmorphic RBCs and RBC casts in the urine sediment.

Nephritic Syndrome

- This is a clinical syndrome with **proteinuria <3 g/day, edema, hematuria with RBC casts,** renal failure with or without oliguria, and HTN.
- Common glomerular diseases present as nephritic syndrome include the following:
  - Poststreptococcal glomerulonephritis (GN)
  - Other postinfectious diseases: endocarditis, abscess, shunt.

- IgA nephropathy
- Lupus nephritis
- Focal segmental glomerulosclerosis (FSGS)
- Membranoproliferative GN (type I and type II)

Nephrotic Syndrome
- It is defined as **proteinuria >3 g/day,** hypoalbuminemia <3.5 g/dL, hyperlipidemia, lipiduria, and edema.
- It is pathognomonic of glomerular disease.
- The major causes of nephrotic syndrome include the following:
  - Minimal change disease (MCD)
  - FSGS
  - Membranous nephropathy (MN)
  - Membranoproliferative GN (type I and type II)
  - Cryoglobulinemic membranoproliferative GN
  - Amyloidosis
  - Diabetic nephropathy
- The nephrotic syndrome is also associated with an increased risk of atherosclerosis, thromboembolic events, and infectious complications:
  - Hypercoagulability is due to the excretion of antithrombotic proteins, including proteins C and S, and antithrombin III. Venous thromboembolic disease is more common than arterial thrombosis.
  - Increased risk of infection is due to excretion of immunoglobulins.

Rapidly Progressive Glomerulonephritis
- Rapidly progressive glomerulonephritis (RPGN) is an acute presentation of GN that **advances to ESRD in days to weeks.**
- The key pathologic finding in RPGN is extensive formation of extracapillary crescents in over half of the glomeruli. The term is used interchangeably with **crescentic GN.**
- It is frequently classified into three categories on the basis of pathologic/immunologic features:
  - Antineutrophil cytoplasmic antibody (ANCA)–associated/pauci-immune:
    o Wegener granulomatosis (cytoplasmic ANCA)
    o Microscopic polyangiitis (perinuclear ANCA)
    o Pauci-immune crescentic GN (perinuclear ANCA)
  - Antiglomerular basement membrane–mediated:
    o Goodpasture syndrome
  - Immune-complex mediated:
    o Lupus nephritis
    o Poststreptococcal GN
    o IgA nephropathy/Henoch-Schönlein purpura

Chronic Glomerulonephritis
- Chronic glomerulonephritis is a slowly progressive glomerular disease that **leads to ESRD over a period of months to years.**
- It is suggested by HTN, proteinuria >3 g/day, chronic renal insufficiency, and small, atrophic, smooth kidneys.

History
- Ask about symptoms including pitting edema, periorbital edema, foamy urine, and hematuria.

- Some causes of GN have a familial nature like Alport syndrome (renal failure associated with hearing loss). There are uncommon familial forms of IgA nephropathy, FSGS, and hemolytic uremic syndrome.
- Certain drugs and toxins may cause glomerular disease:
  - NSAIDs are associated with MCD
  - Penicillamine, NSAIDs, and mercury are associated with MN.
  - Heroin is associated with FSGS.
  - Cyclosporine, tacrolimus, and mitomycin C are associated with hemolytic uremic syndrome.
- The review of systems should cover multisystem diseases associated with glomerular disease such as HTN, diabetes mellitus (DM), SLE, amyloid, and vasculitis.
- Recent or persistent infections may also associate with different glomerular diseases (especially poststreptococcal infection, infective endocarditis, etc.).
- Various malignancies are also associated with glomerular diseases.

Physical Examination
- In the patient with nephrosis, a pathognomonic feature is edema distributed in the periorbital region in the mornings. Facial edema is most often absent in heart failure or in patients with liver cirrhosis due to the inability of these patients to lie flat.
- Xanthelasmas may be present due to hyperlipidemia associated with nephrotic syndrome.
- Muehrcke bands (white bands in fingernails parallel to the lunula) may also be present from hypoalbuminemia in patients with nephrotic syndrome.
- Palpable purpura may be seen in cryoglobulinemia, vasculitis, or SLE.

Differential Diagnosis
Minimal Change Disease
- MCD is defined by the presentation of nephrotic syndrome, the absence of histologic glomerular abnormality by light microscopy, and podocyte foot process effacement by electron microscopy.
- The peak incidence is in children 2 to 7 years of age, but the disease may occur at any age.
- Most cases are idiopathic. Secondary causes include the following:
  - Hypersensitivity induced by NSAIDs
  - Lithium treatment
  - Non-Hodgkin lymphoma
- Urine sediment is usually bland. Complement levels are normal. Renal biopsy is required for diagnosis, especially in adults.
- Complications of MCD include infection, peritonitis in ascitic fluid, thromboembolism, and acute renal failure, especially in the setting of hypovolemia.[8]

Focal Segmental Glomerulosclerosis
- Histopathologically, FSGS is defined by segments of sclerosis in only a portion (segmental) of some glomeruli (focal). Foot process effacement and interstitial fibrosis are common, with a degree that correlates with poorer prognosis.[9]
- Primary idiopathic FSGS:
  - The most common cause of idiopathic nephrotic syndrome in adults. The disease is markedly more common in African-Americans, and the mean age of onset is 20 years.
  - FSGS presents most often as the nephrotic syndrome but may also present as persistent nonnephrotic range proteinuria, HTN, microscopic hematuria, and renal insufficiency at the time of presentation in 20% to 30%.

- There is frequent progression to ESRD (up to 50% in 10 years).
- Diagnosis requires renal biopsy.
- Treatment is controversial. Standard therapy begins with high-dose corticosteroids. The use of other immunosuppressive agents in steroid-resistant patients remains controversial.
- Secondary FSGS:
  - HIV-associated nephropathy:
    o Up to 95% of cases occur in African-Americans.
    o Renal ultrasound shows enlarged kidneys with increased echogenicity.
    o The collapsing form of FSGS is most notably associated with HIV.
  - Reduced renal mass (unilateral renal agenesis, renal ablation, renal allograft)
  - Sickle cell anemia
  - Heroin-associated nephropathy
  - Chronic vesicoureteral reflux
  - Morbid obesity
  - Congenital cyanotic heart disease

Membranous Nephropathy
- MN is a glomerular disease characterized by subepithelial immune deposits of IgG and complement along the glomerular basement membrane. It is associated with a marked increase in glomerular permeability to protein, which is manifested clinically as nephrotic syndrome.[10]
- MN represents the most common cause of idiopathic nephrotic syndrome in adults >60 years of age and the second most common cause (after FSGS) of the nephrotic syndrome in all adults.
- Most cases are idiopathic, but MN occurs in association with a variety of conditions:
  - Autoimmune diseases, including SLE and type 1 DM
  - Hepatitis B, hepatitis C, and HIV
  - Malignancies, including lung, stomach, breast, colon, or prostate adenocarcinoma; nonHodgkin lymphoma; and leukemia
  - Associated drugs: NSAIDs, gold, penicillamine
- Eighty percent of patients with MN present with overt nephrotic syndrome; the other 20% present with nonnephrotic proteinuria. Microscopic hematuria may be seen in up to 50% of adults. Serum complement levels are normal in idiopathic MN.
- The incidence of deep vein thrombosis, especially renal vein thrombosis, is more common in MN than in other forms of the nephrotic syndrome.
- Renal biopsy is required to make the diagnosis.

Membranoproliferative Glomerulonephritis
- Membranoproliferative glomerulonephritis (MPGN) is characterized by diffuse mesangial proliferation, thickening of the capillary wall, subendothelial immune deposits, and hypercellularity. Most cases are associated with circulating immune complexes and hypocomplementemia.
- Based on the histomorphologic pattern, there are three types of MPGN.
  - Type 1: discrete immune deposits in the mesangium and subendothelial space.[11]
  - Type 2: continuous, ribbonlike deposits along the basement membranes of the glomeruli, tubules, and Bowman capsule. It is often called dense-deposit disease.[12]
  - Type 3: subepithelial deposits are prominent and there is complex disruption of the glomerular basement membrane. It is also immune mediated, like type 1.[13]

- Most adults who present with MPGN type I have underlying hepatitis C.[11]
- **Hepatitis C-associated MPGN** is characterized by the findings as below:
  - Frequent cryoglobulinemia
  - Associated arthritis
  - Low levels of C3 or C4
  - Low levels of rheumatoid factor
  - Skin leukocytoclastic vasculitis

IgA Nephropathy and Henoch-Schönlein Purpura
- IgA nephropathy is a mesangial proliferative GN characterized by diffuse mesangial deposition of IgA.
- IgA nephropathy is **the most common cause of idiopathic GN in the world.**
- The clinical presentation of IgA nephropathy ranges from asymptomatic microscopic hematuria with variable degrees of proteinuria and episodic macroscopic hematuria, to uncommonly, rapidly progressive crescentic disease. Hematuria concurrent with upper respiratory tract infection is seen within 1 to 2 days, which distinguishes IgA nephropathy from poststreptococcal GN, in which the hematuria is delayed by 2 to 3 weeks.
- Twenty-five percent to thirty percent of patients develop ESRD within 20 years of diagnosis.[14]
- Half of patients have increased serum IgA levels, but levels do not correlate with disease activity.
- Henoch-Schönlein purpura, a systemic small vessel vasculitis with mesangial and extrarenal vascular IgA deposits that presents with arthralgia, purpuric skin rash, abdominal pain, or gastrointestinal bleeding. It predominantly affects children. It may be pathogenetically related to IgA nephropathy.[15]

Glomerulonephritis in Multisystem Disorders
Renal Disease in Systemic Lupus Erythematosus
- Lupus nephritis is an immune complex-mediated complication of SLE that presents in various histologic patterns described in a World Health Organization classification (Table 3).
- Renal biopsy is almost always indicated for initial diagnosis as well as any relapsing disease, as classification can change throughout time and knowledge of this may change management.
- World Health Organization classification of lupus nephritis.
  - Patients in Classes I and II have good prognoses and minimal or no clinical presenting features.

TABLE 3	WHO Classification of Lupus Nephritis
Class	**Definition**
I	Normal or minimal pathology
II	Mesangial nephropathy
III	Focal segmental proliferative GN (<50% glomeruli affected)
IV	Diffuse proliferative GN (≥50% glomeruli affected)
V	Membranous GN

GN, glomerulonephritis; WHO, World Health Organization.

- Patients in Classes III, IV, and V present similarly, usually with nephrotic-range proteinuria and hematuria and sometimes with rapidly declining renal function.
- Lupus nephritis accounts for a large portion of morbidity and mortality among patients with SLE despite advances in early diagnosis and treatment.
- Serum complement levels are usually low because of classic complement pathway activation.

Poststreptococcal GN
- Poststreptococcal GN is an immune complex-mediated GN with renal deposition of complement C3 and IgG in subepithelial "humps"; it is associated with low serum C3, CH50 after infection with nephritogenic strains of group A or sometimes, group C streptococci.[16]
- Poststreptococcal GN is principally a disease of children, occurring 1 to 3 weeks after pharyngitis or impetigo.
- The clinical presentation consists of dark urine and edema, often with HTN, and sometimes with oliguria.
- Classic laboratory tests include antibodies to streptococcal antigens (antistreptolysin O and anti-DNase B) and hypocomplementemia.

Wegener Granulomatosis
- WG is a granulomatous necrotizing small-vessel vasculitis affecting the upper and lower respiratory tracts and kidneys.
- Clinical features include sinusitis, nasopharyngeal mucosal ulceration, hemoptysis, purpura, and renal involvement.
- C-ANCAs are positive in 65% to 90% of patients with active, systemic WG. Serum complement levels are normal.

Goodpasture Disease
- Goodpasture disease is suggested by the clinical presentation of a pulmonary renal syndrome consisting of hemoptysis, pulmonary infiltrates, and/or RPGN.
- It is characterized by focal necrotizing crescentic GN in association with circulating antiglomerular basement membrane antibodies in the blood and linear staining of IgG along the glomerular basement membrane.
- Approximately 30% of patients with Goodpasture disease are P-ANCA positive.

Amyloidosis
- Amyloidosis is characterized by the deposition of extracellular fibrillar materials of various types in tissues and organs. Renal amyloidoses include immunoglobulin light chain (AL) and systemic secondary (AA) amyloidoses.
- The AL form is most commonly seen in patients with systemic idiopathic amyloidosis or multiple myeloma.
- Clinical features include proteinuria with or without microscopic hematuria, renal insufficiency, and monoclonal light chains detected by serum and urine protein electrophoresis.
- Congo red stain will leave an apple-green birefringence if AL amyloid is present on biopsy specimen.

Diagnostic Testing

Laboratories
- The routine laboratories should include assessment of renal function (blood urea nitrogen [BUN], serum Cr), urinalysis (UA) and microscopic examination of the urine sediment.

TABLE 4	Serologic Tests for Glomerulonephritis

Glomerular Disease	Serologic Tests
Lupus nephritis	ANA, anti–double-stranded DNA antibody
Cryoglobulinemia	Cryoglobulins and rheumatoid factor
Goodpasture disease	Anti-GBM antibody
Vasculitis	ANCAs
Poststreptococcal GN	Antistreptolysin-O antibody
Hepatitis-associated MPGN	Hepatitis B and C serologies
HIV-associated nephropathy	HIV antibodies
Amyloidosis and light chain deposition disease	Serum and urine protein electrophoresis

ANA, antinuclear antibody; ANCA, antineutrophil cytoplasmic antibody; GBM, glomerular basement membrane; GN, glomerulonephritis; HIV, human immunodeficiency virus; MPGN, membranoproliferative glomerulonephritis.

- The amount of urine protein should be quantified. For most cases, a spot urine protein to creatinine ratio can give an accurate assessment of grams of protein per 24 hours.
- The presence or absence of RBC casts or dysmorphic RBCs will help diagnosis.
- Certain serologic tests should be considered (Table 4).
- Measurement of C3, C4, and CH50 is particularly helpful in limiting the differential diagnosis (Table 5).

Imaging
Renal ultrasound is invaluable in the workups of glomerulopathy.
- Ensure the presence of two kidneys.
- Rule out obstruction or anatomic abnormalities.
- Assess kidney size. Atrophic small kidneys (<9 cm) suggest chronic kidney disease (CKD) and should limit use of kidney biopsy or aggressive immunosuppressive therapies.

TABLE 5	Complement Measurements in Glomerulonephritis	

Pathway Affected	Complement Changes	Glomerular Disease
Classical pathway activation	C3 ↓, C4 ↓, CH50 ↓	Lupus nephritis Mixed essential cryoglobulinemia MPGN type 1
Alternate pathway activation	C3 ↓, C4 normal, CH50 ↓	Poststreptococcal GN GN associated with other infections Hemolytic uremic syndrome MPGN type II

GN, glomerulonephritis; MPGN, membranoproliferative glomerulonephritis.
Modified from Feehally J, Floege J, Johnson RJ. Comprehensive Clinical Nephrology. 3rd Ed. Philadelphia, PA: Mosby, 2007.

• Large kidneys (>14 cm) can be seen in nephrotic syndrome associated with diabetes, amyloid, or HIV infection.

Diagnostic Procedures

A renal biopsy is usually required to establish diagnosis and treatment of most glomerular diseases. It requires a nephrology referral.

Treatment

• General treatment of glomerular disease addresses control of proteinuria, edema, HTN, and hyperlipidemia.
• Patients with proteinuria should be treated with **ACE inhibitors and/or angiotensin receptor blockers (ARBs)** to a goal proteinuria of <1 g/day. Toxicities with these agents include hyperkalemia and rising serum Cr (elevation ≤30% is acceptable).
• **Aggressive HTN control** is essential for patients with glomerular disease. Blood pressure goals are <130/80 mm Hg and can be achieved with a combination of diuretics and the above agents.
• Edema is controlled with dietary **sodium restriction** and **judicious use of diuretics.**
• Treatment of hyperlipidemia consists of the use of **statins.**
• Specific treatments of the various glomerulopathies are complex and require a nephrology consultation.
  • Corticosteroids are the mainstay of therapy for MCD.
  • Therapy for the underlying disorder is first-line management for FSGS. Secondary FSGS is most often not responsive to therapy.
  • Disease-specific therapy for MN is controversial but classically consists of alternating days of high-dose corticosteroids and daily cytotoxic therapy, such as cyclophosphamide.
  • Corticosteroids play a minimal role in the treatment of MPGN and have not been studied in adults.
  • Treatment of IgA nephropathy is based on severity of hematuria, proteinuria, GFR, and histopathology. Immune-modulating agents can be used in patients who continue to have refractory proteinuria.[8]
  • Management of poststreptococcal GN is generally supportive. Treatment of streptococcal infection with penicillin should be included even if no persistent infection is present in order to decrease antigenic load.
  • The treatment of lupus nephritis is highly dependent on the type and severity. Classes I and II generally do not require specific therapy. Treatment for Classes III to V is uncertain but typically includes corticosteroids and immunosuppressives.
  • Steroids and cytotoxic agents are used for WG and Goodpasture disease. Initial treatment of Goodpasture disease is also aimed at reducing the circulating antiglomerular basement membrane antibodies by daily plasmapheresis.

CHRONIC KIDNEY DISEASE

General Principles

• According to current estimates, approximate 6.2 million American adults have CKD. The most common causes of CKD and ESRD are DM and HTN.
• Risk factors for CKD include age; low income/education; African American, American Indian, Hispanic, Asian, or Pacific Islander; and family history of CKD, DM, HTN,

autoimmune diseases, systemic infections, urinary tract infections/obstruction/nephrolithiasis, cancer, prior AKI, reduction in kidney mass, and exposure to certain drugs and toxins.[17]

- Identifying and treating CKD early is critical, as disease progression is associated with increased mortality, hospitalization, and cardiovascular events.
- Most patients with CKD have a progressive fairly constant decline in GFR over time. However, some patients may experience stabilization or remission.
- The rate of decline for an individual patient can be somewhat difficult to predict but is known to be dependent on the type of kidney disease. Other factors associated with a faster rate of decline include African-American race, lower baseline kidney function, male gender, and older age.[17]
- Acute declines in GFR are not unusual in the course of CKD and may be caused by factors such as volume depletion, radiocontrast, NSAIDs, some antibiotics (e.g., aminoglycosides, amphotericin B), ACE inhibitors and ARBs, cyclosporine and tacrolimus, and urinary tract obstruction.
- There is a strong association between CKD and cardiovascular disease. Modifiable risk factors (e.g., HTN, dyslipidemia, DM, and tobacco use) should be treated aggressively.

Definition

- According to the 2003 National Kidney Foundation guidelines on Chronic Kidney Disease, CKD is defined as either kidney damage or decreased GFR for at least 3 months duration.[17]
- Markers of kidney damage include proteinuria, urinary tract abnormalities on imaging, and abnormal urinary sediment or urinary chemistries.

Classification

- The National Kidney Foundation staging for CKD is presented in Table 6.[17]
- The goals of management of Stages 1 and 2 CKD are prevention of disease progression and treating underlying etiologies of kidney damage.
- Goals of treatment of Stage 3 CKD include treating complications of CKD that present at this level of dysfunction.
- Goals of treatment of Stage 4 CKD are treating complications of CKD and planning for initiation of renal replacement therapy.
- As discussed in Chapter 19, GFR may be estimated by the Modification of Diet in Renal Disease equation:

$$GFR = 186 \times S_{Cr}^{-1.154} \times age^{-0.203} \times (1.210 \text{ if black}) \times (0.742 \text{ if female})$$

Diagnosis

- The basic diagnostic evaluation is discussed in detail in Chapters 19 and in the preceding sections of this chapter.
- Identifying the specific type of kidney disease involved dictates its treatment and prognosis.
- Renal function should be assessed to determine the stage of disease. The rate of decline of renal function can be assessed by ongoing measurements of serum Cr (e.g., plotting the inverse of serum Cr against time). The rate of decline can subsequently be used to estimate the interval to the onset of kidney failure.[17]
- Those things that can accelerate the rate of decline of renal function should be identified and treated or eliminated, if possible (e.g., DM and HTN, see below).

TABLE 6	Staging of Chronic Kidney Disease		
Stage	Description	GFR (mL/min/1.73 m^2)	Action
1	Kidney damage with normal GFR	>90	Diagnosis and treatment; slow progression
2	Kidney damage with mildly decreased GFR	60–89	Estimate progression
3	Moderately decreased GFR	30–59	Evaluate and treat complications
4	Severely decreased GFR	15–29	Prepare for renal replacement therapy
5	Kidney failure	<15 or dialysis	Renal replacement therapy

GFR, glomerular filtration rate.
Modified from National Kidney Foundation. K/DOQI clinical practice guidelines for chronic kidney disease: evaluation, classification, and stratification. *Am J Kidney Dis* 2002;39(2 suppl 1): S1–S266.

- Patients with diabetes should be screened annually for diabetic kidney disease.
- Screening should consist of spot urine albumin/Cr ratio, serum Cr, and estimation of GFR.
- **Microalbuminuria** is defined as an albumin/Cr ratio of 30 to 300 mg/g.[18]
- **Macroalbuminuria** is defined as an albumin/Cr ratio of >300 mg/g.
- Symptoms and signs of the complications of renal dysfunction must be identified.
  - Uncontrolled HTN can accelerate decline in renal function by increasing intraglomerular pressure. Furthermore, inappropriate sodium retention exacerbates HTN in patients with CKD. The Seventh Report of the Joint National Committee on Prevention, Detection, Evaluation, and Treatment of High Blood Pressure (JNC 7) recommends a BP goal of <130/80 mm Hg.[19]
  - **Anemia** of CKD is due to decreased erythropoietin production that usually occurs once GFR is <30 mL/min/1.73 m^2. Anemia is associated with poorer outcomes in CKD.[20]
  - **Secondary hyperparathyroidism** occurs as an adaptation to (1) phosphorus retention due to decreased GFR and (2) hypocalcemia due to reduced 1-alpha hydroxylation to active vitamin D. Elevated parathyroid hormone (PTH) can result in increased bone turnover, placing patients at high risk for bone fractures. Serum levels of calcium, phosphorus, and intact plasma PTH should be measured in all patients with CKD and GFR <60 mL/min/1.73 m^2. Dual energy x-ray absorptiometry should be done in patients with fractures and those with risk factors for osteoporosis.[21]
  - **Metabolic acidosis** may develop because with decreasing GFR the kidney is less effective in excreting acid loads. Acidosis is present in most patients when the estimated GFR is below 30 mL/min/1.73 m^2. Deleterious effects of metabolic acidosis include bone demineralization, insulin resistance, and increased protein catabolism. Serum

bicarbonate is used as a surrogate marker of acidosis and should be measured with increasing frequency as CKD progresses.[21]
- Because of the strong association between CKD and cardiovascular disease, modifiable risk factors (e.g., HTN, dyslipidemia, DM, and tobacco use) should be identified.
  - Dyslipidemia is common in CKD and patients should be **screened for dyslipidemia with a fasting lipid profile annually.**[22]
  - Those with hyperlipidemia should be evaluated for potential causes such as nephrosis, hypothyroidism, excess alcohol consumption, chronic liver disease, and medications.

Treatment

- Treatment of CKD is multifaceted and includes the following:
  - Specific therapy directed at the etiology of the kidney disease (see above).
  - Slowing the loss of kidney function.
  - Treatment of the complications of loss of kidney function.
  - Prevention and treatment of cardiovascular disease and its risk factors (covered in detail in the appropriate chapters).
  - Preparation for renal replacement therapy.
  - Renal replacement therapy (beyond the scope of this chapter).

Hypertension

- Lifestyle modifications are often insufficient to achieve BP goals in CKD and multiple antihypertensives are often required to meet BP goals.
- Control of HTN is particularly important in patients with diabetes.
- **ACE inhibitors and ARBs** are the agents of choice.[23,24] They reduce intraglomerular pressures and hence slow the progression of renal dysfunction.
  - After starting ACE inhibitors or ARBs, serum K^+ and Cr levels should be checked within 1 to 2 weeks. An increase in potassium of up to 30% is acceptable after starting these agents.
  - Repeat measurements after dose increases.
- **Diuretics** are often effective adjuvant agents for BP control.[23,24]
  - Thiazide diuretics are ineffective once GFR is <30 mL/min/1.73 m^2, while higher doses of loop diuretics can reduce BP.
  - Reasonable starting doses include furosemide 40 mg PO bid or bumetanide 1 mg PO bid.

Diabetes Mellitus

- In patients with type 1 and type 2 DM lowering HbA_{1c} levels to approximately 7.0% reduces the development of microalbuminuria.[18]
- Reducing the HbA_{1c} to approximately 7.0% may also reduce the rate of decline of GFR.
- Refer to the Chapter 16 for details regarding the treatment of DM.

Dyslipidemia

- Treatment of the dyslipidemia in CKD should follow the guidelines set by the Adult Treatment Panel III (ATP III) of the National Cholesterol Education Program (NCEP).[22,25]
- Currently, many consider ESRD to be coronary artery disease equivalent.
- Refer to the Chapter 8 for details on the treatment of dyslipidemia.

Anemia

- Treatment with **erythropoiesis-stimulating agents** (ESAs) usually begins once the hemoglobin (Hgb) is <10 g/dL.
  - Initial treatment options include epoetin alfa at 50 to 100 units/kg SC three times per week or darbepoetin alfa 0.45 mcg/kg SC every one to two weeks. Subsequent dosing should be guided by changes in hemoglobin levels.
  - Rates of Hgb increase are dose-dependent usually <1 g Hgb/week.
- Hgb should be measured at least monthly during ESA treatment to prevent fluctuation outside the goal range.
- The goal Hgb range is 11 to 12 g/dL. Recent studies have demonstrated that Hgb >13 g/dL in patients with CKD may result in increased risk of myocardial ischemia, stroke, blood clots, and death.[20,26]
- **Iron stores should be repleted** before initiating ESA therapy and should continue to be monitored during ESA therapy for ongoing depletion (every 3 months).
  - Goals include ferritin >200 ng/mL and transferring saturation >20% in non-dialysis CKD patients.[20]
  - Repletion can be in oral or IV form. Ferrous sulfate 325 mg PO bid-tid can be trialed. Oral formulations are best absorbed in an acid environment on an empty stomach; hence patients on antireflux medications may require increased doses. For absorption reasons as well as side effects, IV iron is often required.
  - If response to oral iron is inadequate, or if patients cannot tolerate oral iron, then iron dextran may be given intravenously. This is usually prescribed in a nephrologist's office, with a 25-mg test dose given first to monitor for adverse events. If tolerated, 500 to 1,000 mg is given IV. Other IV preparations such as iron sucrose or sodium ferric gluconate can also be used, but these require several smaller doses over several days to total 1 g of iron.

Secondary Hyperparathyroidism

- Treatment of secondary hyperparathyroidism is geared, in a stepwise fashion at (1) reducing phosphorus intake, (2) replacing vitamin D levels, and (3) vitamin D analogue treatment. Target levels for PTH are presented in Table 7.
- **Phosphorus intake** can be reduced by either dietary restriction or phosphate binders.[21]
  - Dietary intake should be limited to 800 to 1,000 mg/day.
  - Calcium-based binders may be used if dietary restriction of phosphate is insufficient.
  - The total dose of elemental calcium provided by the calcium-based phosphate binders should not exceed 1,500 mg/day.
- **Vitamin D deficiency should be corrected.**[21]
  - In Stages 3 and 4 CKD patient if the plasma intact PTH is above the target range for the stage of CKD (Table 7), serum 25-hydroxy vitamin D should be measured.
  - If the serum level is <30 ng/mL, supplementation with ergocalciferol should be initiated.
  - Vitamin D insufficiency (16 to 30 ng/mL) is treated with ergocalciferol 50,000 IU PO monthly for 6 months.
  - Mild deficiency (5 to 15 ng/mL) is treated with ergocalciferol 50,000 IU PO weekly for 4 weeks and then 50,000 IU monthly for 5 months.
  - Severe deficiency (<5 ng/mL) is treated with ergocalciferol 50,000 IU PO weekly for 12 weeks and then 50,000 IU monthly for 3 months.
  - Vitamin D levels should be reassessed at the conclusion of treatment.

TABLE 7	Target PTH Goals in CKD	
CKD Stage	Intact PTH Goal	Frequency of PTH Measurement in Untreated Patients
Stage 3	35–70 pg/mL	Yearly
Stage 4	70–110 pg/mL	Every 3 months

CKD, chronic kidney disease; PTH, parathyroid hormone.
Modified from National Kidney Foundation. K/DOQI clinical practice guidelines for bone metabolism and disease in chronic kidney disease. *Am J Kidney Dis* 2003;42(4 suppl 3): S1–S201.

- Once the patient is replete, continue supplementation with a vitamin D-containing multivitamin.
- If the serum levels of corrected total calcium exceed 10.2 mg/dL, discontinue all forms of vitamin D therapy.
- If PTH levels continue to be above goal (Table 7) in Stage 3 or 4 CKD patients who are vitamin D replete, **active vitamin D treatment** can be used to further reduce PTH levels.[21]
  - Therapy with an active oral vitamin D sterol (e.g., calcitriol) is indicated when serum levels of 25-hydroxy vitamin D are >30 ng/mL and plasma levels of intact PTH are above the target range for the CKD stage (Table 7). The typical starting dose of calcitriol is 0.25 μg PO daily.
  - Vitamin D sterol should be given only to patients with serum levels of corrected total calcium <9.5 mg/dL and serum phosphorus <4.6 mg/dL.
  - During treatment serum levels of calcium and phosphorus should be monitored at least every month after initiation of therapy for the first 3 months and then every 3 months thereafter. Plasma PTH levels should be measured at least every 3 months for 6 months and every 3 months thereafter. Active vitamin D therapy should be held if PTH falls below the target range, calcium is >9.5 mg/dL, or phosphorus is >4.6 mg/dL.
  - Vitamin D sterol treatment is also indicated for dialysis patient with PTH >300 ng/mL. Intact PTH, ionized calcium, and phosphorus should be often measured. The intact PTH should not be reduced to absolutely normal levels, as this may result in adynamic bone disease.

Metabolic Acidosis
- In Stages 3 to 5 CKD the goal total CO_2 is ≥22 mEq/L.[21]
- When total CO_2 is <20 mEq/L alkali salts, such as sodium bicarbonate 650 to 1,300 mg PO bid-tid, may be started.

Nutrition
- Patients with Stage 3 and Stage 4 CKD may benefit from nutritional consultation.
- Nutritional goals are summarized in Table 8 but individualized patient therapy is most appropriate.
- While current recommendations suggest reducing dietary protein intake to minimize urea production, patients with CKD are at increased risk of malnutrition. Hypoalbuminemia is a marker of increased mortality in ESRD patients, and low

TABLE 8	Nutrition Goals for Patients with Stages 3 and 4 CKD
Nutritional Item	**Goal**
Sodium	2 g/day
Protein	0.6–0.75 g/kg/day
Total calories	35 kcal/kg/day
Phosphorus	800–1,000 mg/day
Potassium	2–3 g/day

Modified from Clinical practice guidelines for nutrition in chronic renal failure. K/DOQI, National Kidney Foundation. *Am J Kidney Dis* 2000;35(6 suppl 2):S1–S140.

serum albumin is a contraindication to peritoneal dialysis. Current guidelines recommend measuring albumin every 1 to 3 months.[27]

Referral

- Patient referral to a nephrologist should always occur once GFR is less 30 mL/min/1.73 m^2; furthermore, referral may also be appropriate in patients with Stage 3 CKD in whom further decline is anticipated.
- Late nephrology referral is associated with poorer outcomes and increased cost of care.
- Patients with Stage 4 CKD should be referred for early vascular access for hemodialysis.
  - Arteriovenous fistulas are preferred for hemodialysis, as they have lower risks of infection, lower incidence of dysfunction, and higher flow rates than arteriovenous grafts (AVGs). Arteriovenous fistulas require an average of 3 to 4 months to mature after placement.
  - AVGs are preferred to indwelling catheters, as these have lower risks of infection and better flow rates compared with catheters. AVGs require approximately 3 to 6 weeks to mature before use.
- Nephrology consultation may aid in guiding the decision to initiate renal replacement therapy.
  - In diabetic CKD, dialysis may be advised once GFR is <15 mL/min/1.73 m^2.
  - In nondiabetic CKD, dialysis may be advised once GFR is <10 mL/min/1.73 m^2.
  - Signs and symptoms of uremia, HTN, and volume overload may contribute to a decision to initiate dialysis at higher GFR.
  - Malnutrition in the setting of a higher GFR may drive the decision to initiate early dialysis.

REFERENCES

1. Feehally J, Floege J, Johnson RJ. Comprehensive Clinical Nephrology. 3rd Ed. Philadelphia, PA: Mosby, 2007:755.
2. Feehally J, Floege J, Johnson RJ. Comprehensive Clinical Nephrology. 3rd Ed. Philadelphia, PA: Mosby, 2007:771.
3. Hou SH, Bushinsky DA, Wish JB, et al. Hospital-acquired renal insufficiency: a prospective study. *Am J Med* 1983;74:243.
4. Lin J, Bonventre JV. Prevention of radiocontrast nephropathy. *Curr Opin Nephrol Hypertens* 2005;14:105–110.

5. Schrier RW, Wang W, Poole B, Mitra A. Acute renal failure: definitions, diagnosis, pathogenesis, and therapy. *J Clin Invest* 2004;114:5–14.

6. Bonventre JV, Weinberg JM. Recent advances in the pathophysiology of ischemic acute renal failure. *J Am Soc Nephrol* 2003;14:2199–2210.

7. Agha IA. Acute Renal Failure. In: Agha IA, Green GB (eds). Washington Manual Nephrology Subspecialty Consult. Philadelphia, PA: Lippincott Williams & Wilkins, 2004:37–55.

8. Feinstein EI, Chesney RW, Zelikovic I. Peritonitis in childhood renal disease. *Am J Nephrol* 1988;8:247–265.

9. Chun MJ, Korbet SM, Schwatz MM, Lewis EJ. FSGS in nephrotic adults: presentation, prognosis, and response to therapy of the histologic variants. *J Am Soc Nephrol* 2004;15: 2169–2177.

10. Cattran DC. Idiopathic membranous glomerulonephritis. *Kidney Int* 2001;59:1983–1994.

11. Johnson RJ, Gretch DR, Yamabe H, et al. Membranoproliferative glomerulonephritis associated with hepatitis C virus infection. *N Engl J Med* 1993;328:465–470.

12. Smith RJ, Alexander J, Barlow PN, et al. New approaches to the treatment of dense deposit disease. *J Am Soc Nephrol* 2007;18:2447–2456.

13. Strife CF, Lackson EC, McAdams AJ. Type III membranoproliferative glomerulonephritis: long-term clinical and morphologic evaluation. *Clin Nephrol* 1984;21:323–334.

14. Barratt J, Feehally J. Treatment of IgA nephropathy. *Kidney Int* 2006;69:1934–1938.

15. Rai A, Nast C, Adler S. Henoch-Schönlein purpura nephritis. *J Am Soc Nephrol* 1999;10: 2637–2644.

16. Balter S, Benin A, Pinto SW, et al: Epidemic nephritis in Nova Serrana, Brazil. *Lancet* 2000; 355:1776–1780.

17. KDOQI, National Kidney Foundation. KDOQI clinical practice guidelines for chronic kidney disease: evaluation, classification, and stratification. *Am J Kidney Dis* 2002;39(2 suppl 1):S1–S266.

18. KDOQI, National Kidney Foundation. KDOQI clinical practice guidelines and clinical practice recommendations for diabetes and chronic kidney disease. *Am J Kidney Dis* 2007; 49(2 suppl 2):S12–S154.

19. Chobanian AV, Bakris GL, Black HR, et al. The seventh report of the joint national committee on prevention, detection, evaluation, and treatment of high blood pressure: the JNC 7 Report. *JAMA* 2003;289:2560–2572.

20. KDOQI, National Kidney Foundation. KDOQI clinical practice guideline and clinical practice recommendations for anemia in chronic kidney disease: 2007 update of hemoglobin target. *Am J Kidney Dis* 2007;50:471–530.

21. KDOQI, National Kidney Foundation. KDOQI clinical practice guidelines for bone metabolism and disease in chronic kidney disease. *Am J Kidney Dis* 2003;42(4 suppl 3): S1–S201.

22. KDOQI, National Kidney Foundation. KDOQI clinical practice guidelines for management of dyslipidemias in patients with kidney disease. *Am J Kidney Dis* 2003;41(4 suppl 3): S1–S91.

23. KDOQI, National Kidney Foundation. KDOQI clinical practice guidelines on hypertension and antihypertensive agents in chronic kidney disease. *Am J Kidney Dis* 2004;43(5 suppl 1): S1–S290.

24. Toto RD. Treatment of hypertension in chronic kidney disease. *Semin Nephrol* 2005;25: 435–439.

25. Expert Panel on Detection, Evaluation, and Treatment of High Blood Cholesterol in Adults. Executive summary of the third report of the National Cholesterol Education Program (NCEP) expert panel on detection, evaluation, and treatment of high blood cholesterol in adults (Adult Treatment Panel III). *JAMA* 2001;285:2486–2497.

26. Singh AK, Szczech L, Tang KL, et al. Correction of anemia with epoetin alfa in chronic kidney disease. *N Engl J Med* 2006;355:2085–2098.

27. KDOQI, National Kidney Foundation. KDOQI clinical practice guidelines for nutrition in chronic renal failure. *Am J Kidney Dis* 2000;35(6 suppl 2):S1–S140.

21

Hematuria and Nephrolithiasis

Ying Chen, Jawad Munir,
Vikrant Rachakonda, and Steven Cheng

HEMATURIA

General Principles

- Hematuria, or blood in the urine, can occur at any site of the genitourinary tract. Hematuria may be associated with serious underlying disease and thus requires thorough investigation.
- Hematuria is classified as **gross (macroscopic) or microscopic.**
  - Gross (macroscopic) hematuria is visible as red, pink, or cola-colored urine.
  - Microscopic hematuria is defined by the American Urological Association (AUA) as three or more red blood cells (RBCs)/high power field (HPF) from two of three urine specimens in patients at low risk of serious urologic disease and from one of three urine specimens in patients with risk factors for significant urologic pathology (Table 1).[1,2]
  - The prevalence of microscopic hematuria ranges from 0.19% to 21%[1,3] depending on the population studied. Prevalence is highest in older men.[4]
- Etiologies of hematuria classically fall into either glomerular or nonglomerular sources (Table 2). The former can be differentiated from the latter by the detection of dysmorphic RBCs or RBC casts in the urine, or the coexistence of significant proteinuria.
- No cause of microscopic hematuria is found in at least 8% to 10% of patients.[2]
- The U.S. Preventative Services Task Force recommends against screening asymptomatic patients for bladder cancer with tests for microscopic hematuria (i.e., urine dipstick or microscopic analysis) or with urine cytology.

Diagnosis

Clinical Presentation

History

- The differential diagnosis of **nonglomerular** hematuria is broad. Patients may be entirely asymptomatic except for hematuria or they may have associated symptoms, which aid in diagnosis.
  - Colicky pain at the costovertebral angle or flank with radiation to the groin usually indicates a ureteral stone.
  - A history of dysuria or urinary frequency suggests a urinary tract infection (UTI), which is usually accompanied by leukocytes or bacteria in the urine.
  - Urinary hesitancy, dribbling, or weak urinary stream accompanies bladder outlet obstruction from a stone, enlarged prostate, or tumor.
  - A family history of nephrolithiasis and a history of inflammatory bowel disease or bowel resection (hyperoxaluria) should also be sought when stones are a consideration.

TABLE 1	Risk Factors for Significant Urologic Pathology in Patients with Microscopic Hematuria

Age >40 years
History of smoking
History of gross hematuria
History of urologic disorder or disease
Occupation exposure to benzenes or aromatic amines
Recurrent urinary tract infection
Irritative voiding symptoms
History of high-dose cyclophosphamide use
History of pelvic irradiation
Analgesic abuse

Modified from Grossfeld GD, Litwin MS, Wolf JS Jr, et al. Evaluation of asymptomatic microscopic hematuria in adults: the American Urological Association best practice policy—part II: patient evaluation, cytology, voided markers, imaging, cystoscopy, nephrology evaluation, and follow-up. *Urology* 2001;57:604–610.

- A history of heavy physical activity may explain transient (<48 hours) microscopic hematuria.
- Patients with polycystic kidney disease usually also have a family history of this disease.
- A history of sickle cell disease or sickle cell trait should be obtained in African-American patients, as vascular sickling, particularly in the renal medulla, can cause RBC extravasation.
- Assess for risk factors for serious urologic pathology, including gross hematuria, occupational exposures, tobacco use history, and high-dose cyclophosphamide use (Table 1).
- Travel history may elicit an evaluation for schistosomiasis.
- The presence of hematuria along with a history that may suggest **glomerular disease** should prompt referral to a nephrologist.
- A history of hematuria 1 to 2 weeks after pharyngitis or skin infection suggests poststreptococcal glomerulonephritis.
- Bacterial infectious endocarditis, sepsis, abscesses, or infection of an indwelling foreign body such as a ventriculoatrial shunt can be associated with a proliferative glomerulonephritis. Other infectious diseases such as viral hepatitis (hepatitis B and C) and syphilis can also cause a variety of glomerulopathies.
- IgA nephropathy can present with episodic gross hematuria in the setting of upper respiratory infections.
- Immune complex–mediated glomerular diseases such as systemic lupus erythematosus or systemic vasculitis can present with arthritis, arthralgias, fever, or rashes.
- A family history of deafness and renal failure is a feature of hereditary nephritis or Alport syndrome.
- As many of these glomerular diseases are associated with **acute kidney injury** and require specific treatment, a nephrologist should be involved early in the care of patients presenting with glomerular hematuria.
- Patients taking systemic anticoagulant medications present with hematuria only if there is an underlying nonglomerular lesion that necessitates further evaluation, such as a stone, tumor, or infection.[3,5]

TABLE 2	Causes of Microscopic Hematuria	

Origin of Hematuria		Causes
Nonglomerular	Upper urinary tract (renal, vascular, ureteral)	Pyelonephritis Nephrolithiasis Renal cell carcinoma Polycystic kidney disease Hypercalciuria or hyperuricosuria Renal pelvis/ureteral transitional cell carcinoma Renal trauma Interstitial nephritis Renal infarction/renal vein thrombosis/arteriovenous malformation Papillary necrosis Renal tuberculosis Ureteral stricture with hydronephrosis Sickle cell disease
	Lower urinary tract (bladder, prostate, urethra)	Cystitis Prostatitis Urethritis Bladder cancer Prostate cancer Benign bladder and ureteral polyps Urethral or meatal stricture Trauma Schistosomiasis
Glomerular		IgA nephropathy Thin basement disease Primary or secondary glomerulonephritis
Uncertain		Exercise hematuria "Benign" unexplained recurrent microscopic hematuria

Modified from Cohen RA, Brown RS. Clinical practice. Microscopic hematuria. *N Engl J Med* 2003;348:2330–2338.

- Exposure to cyclophosphamide may lead to hemorrhagic cystitis and, less commonly, bladder cancer, even after cessation of the medication.

Physical Examination
- Start with measurement of blood pressure and assessment of volume status. The presence of edema and hypertension strongly favors glomerular causes of hematuria.
- Fever, costovertebral tenderness, or suprapubic tenderness to palpation may suggest infection.

- Abdominal examination may reveal masses consistent with bladder enlargement or polycystic kidneys.
- Rashes, arthritis, or heart murmurs can often be found with systemic vasculitis, autoimmune glomerulonephritis, and infectious endocarditis-related glomerulonephritis.
- Digital rectal examination should be performed to evaluate for gastrointestinal bleeding, prostate masses, or prostatic tenderness.
- Vaginal examination should be performed in women to exclude vaginal bleeding.

Diagnostic Testing

Laboratories

- The **urinalysis** is used to determine whether the hematuria is glomerular or nonglomerular.
- The presence of dysmorphic RBCs or RBC casts ("active" urine sediment) or the coexistence of proteinuria suggests that the blood is coming from the glomerulus of the kidney.
- Include an assessment of renal function with serum creatinine (S_{Cr}). An elevated S_{Cr} in the presence of hematuria requires urgent investigation of renal disease.
- Hemoglobin electrophoresis should be obtained in African American patients with hematuria without prior diagnosis of sickle cell disease or sickle trait.
- If pyuria or bacteriuria is present on urinalysis, urine culture should be obtained to look for infection. If the urine culture is positive, then repeat urinalysis should be performed 6 weeks after appropriate antimicrobial therapy for resolution of hematuria.
- The presence of proteinuria on urine dipstick warrants quantification of protein excretion (see Chapter 19). A urine protein/creatinine ratio >0.3 or a 24-hour urine protein excretion >300 mg suggests a renal source of bleeding. Nephrology consultation should be obtained.
- Urine cytology is less sensitive than cystoscopy for bladder cancer but more specific.[3]
- Laboratory evaluation for glomerular hematuria includes HIV testing, viral hepatitis serologies, rapid plasma reagin (RPR), antinuclear antibody, antineutrophil cytoplasmic antibody, antiglomerular basement membrane antibodies, complement levels, and cryoglobulins.
- In patients at risk for bladder and ureteral malignancies, urine cytology should be obtained. If cytology reveals cells suspicious for malignancy, cystoscopy is warranted.
- In 2001, the AUA proposed the following algorithm for evaluating asymptomatic microscopic hematuria; this is presented in Figures 1 and 2.[2,6]

Imaging

- Imaging should be performed in patients with no evidence of glomerular disease or UTI. Imaging modalities include ultrasound, intravenous urography (IVU), and computed tomography (CT) scanning. Renal and perirenal infections or abscesses may also be evaluated with CT.
- CT scan is the preferred modality for imaging both renal stones (94% to 98% sensitivity) and solid masses. Masses <3 cm, which may be missed by IVU or renal ultrasound, are visualized by CT scan.[2] Disadvantages include exposure to radiation, risk of contrast-induced nephropathy, cost, and risk of fetal morbidity in pregnancy.
- Ultrasonography can be effective in characterizing solid versus cystic renal lesions but size detection is limited to masses >3 cm in size.[3] Sensitivity for stones is poor.[2] Ultrasound is the safest of urinary tract imaging modalities and is preferred in pregnancy.[3]

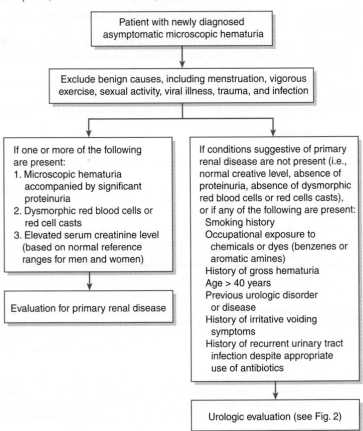

Figure 1. Initial evaluation of asymptomatic microscopic hematuria. (From Grossfeld GD, Wolf JS, Litwin MS, Hricak H, Shuler CL, Agerter DC, Carroll P. Evaluation of asymptomatic microscopic hematuria in adults: the American Urological Association best practice policy recommendations. Part II: patient evaluation, cytology, voided markers, imaging, cystoscopy, nephrology evaluation, and follow-up. Urology 2001;57(4), with permission.)

- IVU is traditionally the initial imaging modality of the upper urinary tract. While more sensitive than ultrasound for detecting renal and ureteral transitional cell carcinoma, it cannot distinguish between solid and cystic lesions.[2] IVU often requires additional imaging by either ultrasound or CT scan. Other disadvantages include radiation exposure and risk of contrast-induced nephropathy.
- In patients with microscopic hematuria, it is recommended that all patients 40 years and older, as well as patients <40 years of age with risk factors for serious urologic disease, undergo cystoscopy.[2] Furthermore, patients with urine cytology suspicious for malignancy should have cystoscopy.
- In cases in which cystoscopy reveals bleeding from only one ureteral orifice, hematuria may be explained by unilateral vascular lesions such as arteriovenous fistula,

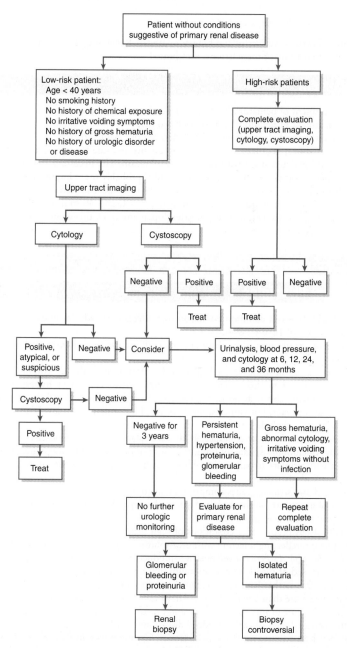

Figure 2. Urologic evaluation of asymptomatic microscopic hematuria. (From Grossfeld GD, Wolf JS, Litwin MS, Hricak H, Shuler CL, Agerter DC, Carroll P. Evaluation of asymptomatic microscopic hematuria in adults: the American Urological Association best practice policy recommendations. Part II: patient evaluation, cytology, voided markers, imaging, cystoscopy, nephrology evaluation, and follow-up. Urology 2001;57(4), with permission.)

hemangioma, or varices of the kidney or ureter. Renal angiography may be performed to document these lesions, if indicated.

Treatment

- The treatment of hematuria is entirely dependent on the cause.
- The treatment of nephrolithiasis is discussed below.
- The treatment of glomerulonephritis is detailed in Chapter 20.
- As noted above, in at least 8% to 10% of patients no cause for microscopic hematuria will be determined with the initial evaluation. The necessary follow-up for these patients is not entirely clear. Follow-up is probably more important in those with risk factors (Table 1). The AUA recommends repeat urinalysis, urine cytology, and blood pressure measurement at 6, 12, 24, and 36 months for those at higher risk.[2] Obviously, if symptoms develop at any time, this would prompt further evaluation.

NEPHROLITHIASIS

General Principles

- Nephrolithiasis is a common condition that affects men twice as often as women (lifetime risk of 12% vs. 6%).[7]
- The peak age of onset is the third decade, with increasing incidence until the age of 60.
- The prevalence of stone disease is increased in both sexes in the last two decades.
- Risk factors for nephrolithiasis include family history, primary hyperparathyroidism, renal tubular acidosis, recurrent UTIs, inflammatory bowel disease, obesity, gout, diabetes, hot climates, high protein, high-sodium diet, low fluid intake, and perhaps a high dietary fructose.[7,8]
- **Calcium stones account for approximately 80% of all stones** and are composed of calcium oxalate, calcium phosphate, or both.[9] Calcium stones are usually idiopathic but can occur with primary hyperparathyroidism, medullary sponge kidney, or distal renal tubular acidosis.
- Uric acid and struvite stones comprise the majority of the remainder.
- **Uric acid stones** form in the setting of uric acid overproduction, low urinary volumes, and persistently acid urine pH.
- **Struvite stones** occur under conditions of high urinary pH and increased ammonia production, reflecting infection with urea-splitting organisms (e.g., *Proteus mirabilis*, *Klebsiella* spp.). *Escherichia coli* does not produce urease.[9,10] Struvite stones are usually composed of magnesium ammonium phosphate (struvite) or carbonate apatite and are often in the shape of a "staghorn," as they grow rapidly and typically extend to involve more than one renal calyx. They often occur in paraplegic or quadriplegic patients because of increased predisposition to UTIs. Staghorn calculi are associated with increased rates of chronic kidney disease and death.
- **Cystine stones** account for <1% of all stones. Cystine stones arise from an inherited disorder of dibasic amino acid renal transport, resulting in an excess cystine in the urine. Cystine is relatively insoluble in urine and often crystallizes to form radiopaque stones.[11]

Diagnosis

Clinical Presentation

- The clinical spectrum of nephrolithiasis ranges from incidental radiologic diagnosis of otherwise asymptomatic disease to severe symptoms, such as flank pain (renal colic), hematuria, UTIs, or even renal failure.
- **Asymptomatic disease:** Patients with nephrolithiasis may remain asymptomatic for years. They usually become symptomatic if a stone causes obstruction in the urinary tract.
- **Renal colic:** Renal colic is typically abrupt in onset, colicky in nature, and localized to the flank area. The pain often radiates into the groin and the testicles or labia. Hematuria, urinary frequency, urgency, nausea, and vomiting are common associated symptoms. Staghorn calculi do not generally present in this fashion.[10]
- **Hematuria:** Trauma to the urinary tract by passage of a stone leads to hematuria. It may be gross or microscopic and can occur even in asymptomatic patients.
- **Renal failure:** Acute renal failure may result if the obstruction is bilateral or if it obstructs a solitary functional kidney.
- Patients with staghorn calculi may be asymptomatic but others can present with recurrent UTIs, gross hematuria, abdominal pain, fever, and urosepsis.[10]
- Even in classic presentations of acute renal colic, it is important to rule out other conditions which may mimic this condition, including acute appendicitis, intestinal obstruction, ectopic pregnancy, and cholecystitis.

Diagnostic Testing

Laboratories

- **Laboratory studies** should include an assessment of renal function with serum creatinine and serum electrolytes, including calcium.
- A urinalysis is mandatory.
- Hexagonal cystine crystals may be detected on microscopic examination of the urine.[11]

Imaging

- **Plain radiography** may visualize radiopaque stones but it is clearly limited by its inability to detect radiolucent stones or provide additional data regarding the urinary tract.
- **IVU** is more sensitive but entails administration of nephrotoxic contrast.
- These studies have largely been replaced by the **spiral CT scan** (without contrast), which is currently the gold standard for the diagnosis of nephrolithiasis.[2]
- In patients who cannot receive radiation, including pregnant women, an ultrasound may be useful to rule out significant hydronephrosis. However, the presence of small stones may go undetected with ultrasound and the exact level of obstruction may not be clearly delineated.

Metabolic Evaluation of Nephrolithiasis

- All patients with kidney stones should have an assessment of their **serum calcium levels, stone composition,** and **dietary intake.**
- Patients with recurrent calcium stones or a single noncalcium stone should undergo more extensive evaluations, including at least **two 24-hour urine studies** for measurement of urine volume, pH, calcium, urate, oxalate, citrate, creatinine, and sodium.
- These urine studies should not be performed within 3 to 4 weeks of an acute stone episode or in the presence of a UTI.

- The urinary findings in patients with **idiopathic calcium stones** may include hypercalciuria, hyperuricosuria, hyperoxaluria, and hypocitraturia.
  - Hypercalciuria is present in approximately 50% of patients with calcium stones.
  - Calcium stones may also precipitate around a uric acid nidus in patients with hyperuricosuria, even in the absence of hypercalciuria.
- A quantitative 24-hour urine for cystine should be collected if the composition of the stone is unknown.

Treatment

Acute Management

- The treatment of acute renal colic consists of analgesia, relief of obstruction, and control of infection if present.
- The urine should be strained to retrieve the stone for analysis.
- The rate of spontaneous stone passage is dependent on stone size (and location). If the stone is <5 mm, conservative management is adequate, as 80% to 90% of these stones pass spontaneously.[12,13]
- Stones 5 to 7 mm pass spontaneously only 50% of the time, and stones >7 mm rarely pass spontaneously.
- Stones <7 mm can be managed conservatively if there is no evidence of obstruction or infection and the pain is controllable with oral analgesic agents.
- Fluid administration should be titrated to achieve a urine output of roughly 2 L/day to assist with the passage of the stone.
- Nifedipine and peripheral α-blockers may improve the rate of stone passage (referred to as "medical expulsive therapy").[14]
- If there is evidence of hydronephrosis or multiple stones, a follow-up imaging study, such as a spiral CT, is warranted.[14]
- Complete obstruction, UTI, urosepsis, or uncontrollable pain is indication for expedited stone removal.
  - A urology consultation should be obtained in these circumstances.
  - Treatment modalities include extracorporeal shockwave lithotripsy, percutaneous nephrolithotomy, ureteroscopic removal, surgery, and chemolysis.[14]

Dietary Modification

- Dietary counseling should be provided to **all** patients with kidney stones to prevent further stone formation.
- **Fluid intake** should be increased to achieve increased urine flow rates and to lower the urine solute concentration. Some suggest a target urine volume of >2 L daily. This often requires a fluid intake of at least 2.5 L/day.
- **Dietary calcium** intake should be kept within the normal range (800 to 1,000 mg/day). Calcium restriction may result in impaired bone mineralization and **may actually increase the risk for nephrolithiasis** by increasing the absorption and urinary excretion of oxalate.[9,15]
- To decrease urinary calcium, a **low-sodium diet** (100 mEq or 2.3 g/day) should be followed.[9]
- A **low-oxalate diet** may decrease urinary oxalate.[9] Oxalate is present in beets, rhubarb, spinach, greens, okra, tea, chocolate, cocoa, and nuts.
- A **low-protein diet** increases urine pH, decreases uric acid excretion, and may also decrease urinary calcium excretion.[9]

Specific Stone Types

Calcium Stones

Urinary abnormality identified with 24-hour urine studies and treated as follows:

- **Hypercalciuria** (>4 mg/kg/day) is most often due to increased gastrointestinal absorption of calcium but may also be caused by impaired renal tubular calcium reabsorption or excessive skeletal resorption as in primary hyperparathyroidism.
  - Patients should maintain a normal calcium intake (800 to 1,000 mg/day).
  - They should ensure adequate fluid intake and restrict sodium intake to 2,300 mg/day.
  - Thiazide diuretics (e.g., hydrochlorothiazide 25 to 50 mg PO daily) increase renal calcium reabsorption and are frequently used in this setting.[9,16]
- **Hyperuricosuria** (>0.75 g/24 hours in men; >0.7 g/24 hours in women) may also result in calcium stone formation as uric acid crystals may serve as a nidus for calcium oxalate or calcium phosphate precipitation.
  - Allopurinol, 300 mg PO daily, has been shown to decrease calcium stone formation in the setting of hyperuricosuria.[9]
- **Hyperoxaluria** (>40 mg/day) often responds to dietary restriction.
  - Patients with small bowel malabsorption due to intrinsic disease (e.g., inflammatory bowel disease) or jejunoileal bypass may absorb excessive oxalate, resulting in enteric hyperoxaluria.
  - Dietary restriction of oxalate and oxalate binders such as oral calcium citrate or cholestyramine may be useful.
  - A 24-hour urine collection should be obtained within 2 to 4 weeks of initiating supplemental dietary calcium therapy to monitor for hypercalciuria.
  - Primary hyperoxaluria is due to a genetic enzymatic defect in amino acid metabolism in which excess oxalate is produced. These patients have nonenteric hyperoxaluria that does not respond to dietary manipulation.
- **Hypocitraturia** (<250 mg/24 hours in men; <300 mg/24 hours in women) is a frequent finding.
  - Citrate is a potent inhibitor of calcium oxalate precipitation.
  - Citrate excretion can be enhanced by therapy with potassium citrate, starting at a dose of 20 mEq PO tid.[9]
  - Lemon juice is an inexpensive and well-tolerated source of dietary citrate and increases urinary citrate excretion. Four ounces of lemon juice in 2 L of water per day may be useful in patients with borderline low urinary citrate. However, more recent evidence suggests that lemonade may be insufficient to increase urinary citrate and decrease pH.[8]

Uric Acid Stones

- Conservative therapy involves maintenance of urine volumes of >2 L/day through oral hydration, dietary protein/purine restriction (i.e., meat, fish, and poultry), and alkalinization of urine to pH 6.5 to 7.0 with an oral alkali preparation, such as potassium citrate.
- Allopurinol, 300 mg PO qd, can be used if these measures fail.[17]
- Probenecid and other uricosuric drugs should be avoided, as they may increase the risk of uric acid or calcium stones.

Cystine Stones

- In general, patients with cystine stones should be followed by a nephrologist.
- These stones are resistant to lithotripsy and often require surgical stone extraction.

- High fluid intake (3 to 4 L/day) and consistent alkalinization (pH >7.5, potassium citrate, sodium citrate, and sodium bicarbonate) are need to substantially affect solubility and are difficult for patients to achieve.
- Cystine and methionine dietary restriction is impractical.
- Cystine-binding drugs (e.g., penicillamine, α-mercapto propionylglycine/tiopronin, and perhaps captopril) may be necessary.[11]

Struvite Stones

- For antimicrobial treatment to be effective, the infected stone must be removed surgically, percutaneously, or by extracorporeal shockwave lithotripsy.
- For poor surgical candidates, chemolysis is possible but it is unlikely to be effective on its own.[10]

REFERENCES

1. Grossfeld GD, Litwin MS, Wolf JS, et al. Evaluation of asymptomatic microscopic hematuria in adults: the American Urological Association best practice policy—part I: definition, detection, prevalence, and etiology. *Urology* 2001;57:599–603.
2. Grossfeld GD, Litwin MS, Wolf JS Jr, et al. Evaluation of asymptomatic microscopic hematuria in adults: the American Urological Association best practice policy–part II: patient evaluation, cytology, voided markers, imaging, cystoscopy, nephrology evaluation, and follow-up. *Urology* 2001;57:604–610.
3. Cohen RA, Brown RS. Clinical practice. Microscopic hematuria. *New Engl J Med* 2003;348: 2330–2338.
4. Mariani AJ, Mariani MC, Macchioni C, et al. The significance of adult hematuria: 1,000 hematuria evaluations including a risk-benefit and cost-effectiveness analysis. *J Urol* 1989; 141:350–355.
5. Culclasure TF, Bray VJ, Hasbargen JA. The significance of hematuria in the anticoagulated patient. *Arch Intern Med* 1994;154:649–652.
6. Grossfeld G, Wolf JS, Litwin M, et al. Asymptomatic microscopic hematuria in adults: summary of the AUA best practice policy recommendations. *Am Fam Physician* 2001;63: 1145–1154.
7. Curhan GC. Epidemiology of stone disease. *Urol Clin North Am* 2007;34:287– 293.
8. Tracy CR, Pearle MS. Update on the medical management of stone disease. *Curr Opin Urol* 2009;19:200–204.
9. Delvecchio FC, Preminger GM. Medical management of stone disease. *Curr Opin Urol* 2003;13:229–233.
10. Healy KA, Ogan K. Pathophysiology and management of infectious staghorn calculi. *Urol Clin North Am* 2007;34:363–374.
11. Mattoo A, Goldfarb DS. Cystinuria. *Semin Nephrol* 2008;28:181–191.
12. Miller OF, Kane CJ. Time to stone passage for observed ureteral calculi: a guide for patient education. *J Urol* 1999;162:688–690.
13. Coll DM, Varanelli MJ, Smith RC. Relationship of spontaneous passage of ureteral calculi to stone size and location as revealed by unenhanced helical CT. *AJR Am J Roentgenol* 2002; 178:101–113.
14. Preminger GM, Tiselius HG, Assimos DG, EAU/AUA Nephrolithiasis Guideline Panel. 2007 guideline for the management of ureteral calculi. *J Urol* 2007;178:2418–2434.
15. Borghi L, Schianchi T, Meschi T, et al. Comparison of two diets for the prevention of recurrent stones in idiopathic hypercalciuria. *N Engl J Med* 2002;346:77–84.
16. Escribano J, Balaguer A, Pagone F. Pharmacological interventions for preventing complications in idiopathic hypercalciuria. *Cochrane Database Syst Rev* 2009;(1):CD004754.
17. Cameron MA, Sakhaee K. Uric acid nephrolithiasis. *Urol Clin North Am* 2007;34:335–346.

22 General Infectious Disease

F. Matthew Kuhlmann and Thomas C. Bailey

GENERAL CONSIDERATIONS

Principles Of Therapy

Various infections are covered in this chapter; however, this section is not a comprehensive overview of all common infections encountered in primary care. It should be noted that some processes, such as hepatitis, are covered elsewhere.

Diagnostic Consideration

- Perhaps the most difficult question to answer in assessing a patient with a potentially infectious complaint is determining **whether the patient truly has an infection,** and if so, with which type of organism.
- Infections can be classified into broad categories such as bacterial, viral, fungal, mycobacterial, or parasitic. The history and physical examination are critical in this regard and should account for travel history, work exposure, and the underlying health of the patient.
- The importance in determining the etiology of the disease process is highlighted by the **ever-increasing burden of drug resistance** in all pathogens.
- Antimicrobial resistance is frequently attributed to overprescribing of antimicrobials.[1]

Antimicrobial Selection

Once the decision has been made to prescribe antimicrobials, the following factors should be addressed:
- Local epidemiology of various pathogens
- Local susceptibility patterns
- Drug-drug interactions
- Tolerability
- Pharmacokinetics and pharmacodynamics
- Cost

Follow-Up Assessment

Some patients do not respond as anticipated to the prescribed therapy; in this situation, one should consider the following:
- Is the suspected agent correct?
- Were the drug and the dosage correct?
- Did the patient take the medication?

- Has a complication, such as an abscess, developed?
- Is a resistant pathogen present?
- Is there a noninfectious complication?

RESPIRATORY TRACT INFECTIONS

The discussion in this section will focus on diagnosing and treating acute and chronic sinusitis, pharyngitis, bronchitis, and community-acquired pneumonia (CAP).

Acute Sinusitis

General Principles

- Excessive secretions or mucosal edema prevents drainage and ventilation of the sinus cavities.
- Predisposing conditions include viral upper respiratory tract infections (URIs), allergic rhinitis, dental disease, pressure changes (e.g., air flights), swimming, and conditions affecting the normal nasal anatomy such as nasal polyps.
- **Acute sinusitis is generally caused by viruses** infecting the upper respiratory tract. Uncommonly (0.5% to 2% of URIs), viral URIs develop into acute bacterial sinusitis requiring antibiotic treatment.[2]
- Bacterial sinusitis is usually caused by pneumococci, *Moraxella catarrhalis,* and non-typeable *Haemophilus influenzae. Staphylococcus aureus* is a less frequent cause.

Diagnosis

- Distinguishing viral from bacterial sinusitis is difficult as there are no historical or examination findings that can clearly differentiate between the two infections (Table 1).
- Patients with viral or bacterial sinusitis may complain of nasal congestion, purulent nasal discharge, anosmia, facial pain, headache, fever, or pressure when bending over.
- Physical examination findings include nasal turbinate edema, sinus tenderness, purulent drainage from the nasal sinus or in the posterior oropharynx, and failure of transillumination of the hard palate.
  - Transillumination is difficult to perform, has poor interobserver variability, and is of relatively low yield.
  - Tenderness over the bridge of the nose suggests ethmoid sinus disease.
- Ultrasound, radiography, and CT scan are of little use in the outpatient setting.[3] Their benefit lies in diagnosing complications or more severe sinusitis.
- Sinus aspirate is not indicated for uncomplicated sinusitis.
- Concerning symptoms warranting more aggressive treatment and monitoring include frontal or sphenoidal disease, erythema, periorbital swelling, and mental status changes.

TABLE 1	Distinguishing Bacterial from Viral Acute Sinusitis
Bacterial	**Viral**
Symptoms lasting >10 days	Symptoms resolve in 7–10 days
Symptoms worse after 5–7 days	
Purulent nasal discharge	Thin, translucent discharge

- Complications of acute sinusitis include osteomyelitis ("Pott's puffy tumor"), orbital extension, cavernous sinus thrombosis, and central nervous system invasion with meningitis or abscess formation.
- These complications are rare and occur on the order of 1 in 10,000 cases.
- In patients with diabetes and acidosis, one would need to consider mucormycosis.

Treatment

- Nonpharmacological means such as humidity and nasal washes have shown little benefit in clinical trials.
- Decongestants are frequently helpful and alone may be the only therapy necessary.
  - Topical nasal sprays should not be used for >5 days as this may lead to rebound symptoms (e.g., phenylephrine, oxymetazoline).
- As viral etiologies are the most common, **antimicrobials are frequently overused and are associated with minimal benefit** and increased risk of side effects in patients with acute sinusitis.
  - The decision to use antimicrobials should be based on the patient's history and on clinical judgment. Narrow spectrum and inexpensive agents are preferred.
- **When antimicrobials are indicated, use of first-line agents for 7 to 10 days is appropriate.** These are as follows:
  - Amoxicillin 500 to 875 mg every 8 hours.
  - Doxycycline 100 mg every 12 hours for 1 day followed by 50 mg every 12 hours.
  - Trimethoprim-sulfamethoxazole (160/800) one tablet orally every 12 hours.
  - Azithromycin 500 mg daily for 3 to 5 days; this is more costly.
- For serious disease:[2]
  - Amoxicillin/clavulanic acid (500/125 mg every 8 hours or 2,000 mg/125 mg every 12 hours).
  - Fourth generation quinolone (e.g., moxifloxacin 400 mg daily).
  - Ceftriaxone 1 g IV daily.
- Surgery is indicated for patients with sinusitis due to zygomyces.

Chronic Sinusitis

General Considerations

- The European Academy of Allergology and Clinical Immunology (EAACI) defines chronic sinusitis as typical signs and symptoms of sinusitis with radiographic findings with symptoms lasting >12 weeks.[4]
- Chronic sinusitis results from refractory obstruction.
- Underlying asthma and allergy are significant risk factors for this disease; this is evidenced by variations in cytokine profiles between noninfectious and infectious chronic sinusitis.
- The microbiologic flora typically includes gram-negative organisms such as *Pseudomonas aeruginosa* and anaerobic bacteria.
- Dematiaceous fungi and *Aspergillus* spp. have been implicated in chronic allergic rhinosinusitis.[5]

Diagnosis

- The diagnosis is largely based on clinical and endoscopic findings.
- Patients frequently have nasal polyposis.
- Complete blood count showing absolute eosinophilia >500 cells/mL may be suggestive.

- Markers of chronic inflammation may be useful such as C-reactive protein and erythrocyte sedimentation rate.
- Culture of the sinuses is rarely indicated.
- Radiographic imaging for uncomplicated chronic sinusitis is rarely indicated.
- Concerning signs requiring referral include unilateral signs (e.g., polyp or mass), bleeding, diplopia, maxillary paresthesia, orbital swelling, or disease in an immunocompromised person.[6]

Treatment

- **Topical steroids** are the mainstay of treatment and their benefit has been shown in randomized trials.
- Allergen avoidance for allergic individuals may be beneficial.
- The EAACI found **insufficient evidence to advocate for the use of antibiotic treatment.**[4]
- Should antibiotics be used, coverage should include anaerobic species and the duration is typically 4 to 6 weeks of treatment. Amoxicillin-clavulanate is typical first-line coverage.

Pharyngitis

General Principles

- Sore throat is a frequent complaint of patients and perhaps the most concerning diagnosis is **Group A streptococcal (GAS) pharyngitis.** This disease is most concerning based on its association with acute rheumatic fever and potential for suppurative complications.[7] This section will focus on infections due to GAS, but consider the following:
  - **Respiratory viruses account for the greatest majority of cases,** including adenovirus, parainfluenza virus, rhinovirus, and respiratory syncytial virus amongst others.
  - In addition to GAS, rare causes of bacterial pharyngitis include *Neisseria gonorrhoeae, Corynebacterium diphtheriae,* anaerobes, and *Arcanobacterium haemolyticum*—the latter of which causes a rash similar to scarlet fever in young adults. Mycoplasma and *Chlamydia* spp. have also been implicated.
- GAS is the etiologic agent associated with scarlet fever and acute rheumatic fever. Although the incidence of these sequelae has decreased dramatically in recent decades in developed nations, the reason for this is a subject of debate.
- Treatment for viral pharyngitis supportive.
- GAS pharyngitis **usually resolves spontaneously** within 3 to 4 days.

Diagnosis

- GAS usually presents in children during the winter and spring, accounting for only 5% to 10% of cases of pharyngitis in adults.
  - Typical symptoms include fever, sore throat, cervical lymphadenopathy, and the absence of cough.
  - Symptoms such as coryza, ulcerative lesions, viral exanthema, and diarrhea suggest an alternative diagnosis.
- There is often a history of exposure to GAS in close contacts.
- Physical examination findings include fever, erythematous tonsils with or without exudate, a petechial rash on the palate, scarlatiniform rash, swollen uvula, and tender anterior cervical lymphadenopathy.
- Appropriately obtained samples are crucial for diagnostic accuracy of rapid antigen tests and throat cultures. Neither test is able to distinguish between acute GAS infection and colonization in the setting of viral pharyngitis.

- Serologic tests are indicative of prior infections and are not useful in acute infections.
- **A negative rapid antigen test is sufficient to exclude streptococcal infection in adults;** however, culture for GAS may be considered as the rapid test's sensitivity approaches, but does not equal, that of culture.

Treatment

- Treatment is indicated in the setting of appropriate historical and examination findings along with positive culture or rapid antigen testing.
  - In most circumstances, urgent therapy is not needed.
  - The benefits of treatment include prevention of the spread of disease, avoidance of complications such as tonsillar abscess or rheumatic fever, and slight decrease in the duration of symptoms.
- Treatment to prevent the major sequelae of GAS infection is effective up to 9 days after the development of symptoms.
- The only therapy proven in clinical trials to reduce the development of rheumatic fever is intramuscular penicillin (PCN) given as 1.2 million units of benzathine PCN for one dose.
- Other oral options include PCN V 500 mg two to three times daily for 10 days (or 250 mg three or four times daily), erythromycin, clindamycin, and lastly, first generation cephalosporins.
- Treatment or screening of asymptomatic close contacts is generally not necessary; one exception would be patients diagnosed with rheumatic fever.
- Patients are generally no longer contagious after 24 hours of treatment with PCN.[8]

Acute Bronchitis

General Principles

- Acute bronchitis is defined as airway inflammation with cough and without evidence of pneumonia.[9]
- **Viruses account for the majority of cases** and include influenza, adenovirus, respiratory syncytial virus, parainfluenza, coronavirus, rhinovirus, and human metapneumovirus.
- The role of bacteria in acute bronchitis is unknown, but implicated species include *Bordetella pertussis, Chlamydia* spp., and *Mycoplasma* spp.
- Rates of pertussis have been slowly increasing due to waning immunity in an aging population.[10]
  - It is now recommended by the Centers for Disease Control and Prevention (CDC) to substitute the tetanus vaccine with the tetanus-diphtheria-acellular pertussis vaccine (tetanus and diphtheria combined with acellular pertussis) for patients with unclear vaccination histories.
- Disease results from inflammation within the bronchi in response to the invading organism.
- Cough is generally the most prominent sign and lasts for at least 5 days and up to 21 days.
  - Productive sputum results from sloughing of the bronchial epithelium and is not necessarily an indication of a bacterial rather than a viral infection.
  - Many patients experience a decrease in their FEV_1 (forced expiratory volume in 1 one second) but the long-term effects are unknown.
  - Deterioration of a patient's respiratory status may occur in patients with underlying lung disease.
  - Overt pneumonia can develop as complication of acute bronchitis.

- Recurrent visits to the primary physician are common.
- The differential diagnosis includes pneumonia, asthma, bronchiectasis, and acute exacerbations of chronic bronchitis.

Diagnosis

- The general presentation is a young person with cough; fever may or may not be present. Patients generally lack tachypnea and tachycardia.
- On examination, young patients typically lack rales and egophony. This does not hold true in elderly patients who can present atypically with pneumonia.
- A rapid test for influenza is indicated when this treatable disease is present at high proportions in the local community.
- In younger patients without evidence of pneumonia by history or examination, radiography is not indicated.
  - In elderly patients, radiography to help rule out pneumonia is warranted.
- Patients with atypical bacterial infections are generally younger and present with subacute disease and symptoms that may last up to 6 weeks.
  - Testing for cold agglutinins with a titer >1:64 or mycoplasma IgM titers after 7 days of illness may assist in the diagnosis.
  - Pertussis (whooping cough) presents with paroxysmal cough with or without posttussive emesis. The characteristic "whoop" is generally not present in previously immunized patients.
  - In these patients, nasopharyngeal culture, polymerase chain reaction (PCR), or direct fluorescent antibodies will assist in the diagnosis.

Treatment

- **Antimicrobials are generally not indicated,** as their use does not have any significant impact on disease course in randomized trials. **Abuse of antimicrobials in the setting of acute bronchitis is unfortunately all too common.**
- Treatment is largely supportive in most patients.
- Treatment can be directed at underlying pathogens, such as neuraminidase inhibitors for influenza (see below) or macrolides for pertussis.
- Although there is no evidence based on clinical trials, the use of inhaled $\beta2$ agonists or inhaled corticosteroids may be of benefit over a 7-day period. This may be especially true in patients with underlying lung disease.
- Acute exacerbations of chronic bronchitis are covered in Chapter 12.

Influenza

General Principles

- Influenza is a common viral illness that has received much press recently due to concerns about avian or pandemic flu (H5N1). Throughout history it has caused epidemic disease from year to year. Of concern is its ability to cause outbreaks in institutional settings such as nursing homes and hospitals.[11]
- Two important concepts in influenza pathogenesis are antigenic shift and antigenic drift.
  - **Antigenic shift** refers to changes in the hemagglutinin or neuraminidase strain (e.g., from H3N2 to H5N2).
  - **Antigenic drift** refers to minor antigenic changes within a strain reflecting seasonal variation. Because of antigenic drift, yearly vaccination is warranted.
  - The vaccine strain is predicted by epidemiological data of circulating virus.

- Influenza outbreaks occur in the late fall and winter in North America. The virus is transmitted by aerosolized droplets and invades the respiratory epithelium.
- Complications, in particular staphylococcal pneumonia or exacerbations of underlying disease, are a frequent cause of morbidity and mortality.

Diagnosis

- During epidemics, the diagnosis is made largely on clinical grounds. Patients present with nonspecific findings of fever, myalgias, malaise, cough, and headache, usually sudden in onset.[12]
- Viral culture is the gold standard for diagnosis of influenza; however, **rapid antigen testing** has proven useful in clinical settings and can decrease the overuse of antibiotics.

Treatment

- Effective therapy should be initiated as soon after symptoms have begun to be effective (within 48 hours of symptom onset).
- Rimantadine and amantadine are active against influenza A only.
  - They work by blocking the M2 ion channel preventing viral entry and replication in the cellular nucleus.
  - Often they cause neuropsychiatric side effects, especially in elderly patients.
  - Resistance has been increasing as well, and for this reason **the CDC no longer recommends their use.**[13]
- Zanamivir and oseltamivir are active against both influenza A and B by inhibiting neuraminidase.
  - Resistance is uncommon but does occur.
  - Zanamivir's use is limited due to its inhalational route of delivery.
  - Oseltamivir can cause nausea, and recently was noted to be associated with severe delirium.
- Effective treatment begins with prevention.
  - All at risk and interested persons in addition to health care professionals should receive influenza vaccination.
  - The CDC offers yearly guidelines as the vaccine becomes available.

Community-Acquired Pneumonia

General Principles

- The discussion in this section is centered on the diagnosis and management of patients with pneumonia in the ambulatory setting. The provider should take note that differences exist in the management of patients with hospital-acquired pneumonia, nursing home pneumonia, and health care–associated pneumonia.[14]
- Guidelines are available through the Infectious Diseases Society of America (www.idsociety.org).
- Despite significant improvements in the management of critically ill patients in recent years, CAP remains the eighth leading cause of mortality in the United States, with rates increasing after the age of 55.
- **Cigarette smoking is the strongest independent risk factor for invasive pneumococcal disease.**
- **The most typical pathogens in outpatient settings are *Streptococcus pneumoniae*, *M. pneumoniae*, *C. pneumoniae*, and *H. influenzae*** (not type B).
- *M. pneumoniae* is the most common pathogen in patients <50 years old.

- Other atypical causes include *Legionella* spp., *S. aureus, Klebsiella pneumoniae,* and *Pseudomonas aeruginosa,* the latter two being more common in alcoholics.
- Other factors to be considered include seasonality (respiratory syncytial virus and influenza), travel history (severe acute respiratory syndrome coronavirus), other exposures, and bioterrorism threats (anthrax, plague, and tularemia).

Diagnosis

History
- The diagnosis of CAP largely rests upon identifying the appropriate signs and symptoms along with an infiltrate on chest radiography.
- Typical historical findings include the acute onset of fever and cough with productive sputum. Malaise, anorexia, chills, and abdominal complaints are also frequent findings.
- Travel and exposure history may increase one's suspicion for unusual pathogens such as tuberculosis (TB), psittacosis, fungal infections, tularemia, or unusual viral infections.
  - In such cases, therapy should include treatment directed toward the suspected pathogen as well as empiric therapy for more common causes of CAP.
  - Once the pathogen is known, therapy should be directed solely at that particular agent.

Physical Examination
- Rales or egophony are usually present.
- Tachypnea and hypotension are ominous findings and warrant more rapid evaluation.
- Elderly patients often lack typical signs and symptoms and may present with more subtle findings such as altered mental status or hypothermia.

Diagnostic Testing
- Blood cultures should be obtained if patients are to be hospitalized in an intensive care unit, have failed prior antimicrobial therapy, have immunodeficient states, functional asplenia, cavitary disease, or pleural effusion on radiography, or have underlying liver, lung, or hematological disease.
  - Routine blood cultures in outpatient settings are rarely positive and add to the cost of treatment; however, their use is important in epidemiological studies of local disease patterns.
- Sputum cultures and Gram stains are useful only when quality specimens can be obtained.
- Other considerations:
  - Urinary testing for pneumococcus or *Legionella* spp. is not routinely indicated.
  - Legionella testing should be done in epidemic settings or when history strongly suggests the diagnosis (e.g., alcoholism, severe disease, or endemic settings).
  - Patients who have stayed in hotels or were on cruises in the prior 2 weeks should undergo sputum culture for *Legionella* spp.
  - Legionella test should also be considered in the elderly, the immunocompromised, alcoholics, and when hyponatremia or liver test abnormalities are present.

Treatment

- **Consideration of local resistance patterns is paramount** to determining appropriate initial empiric antimicrobial therapy.
- The decision on site of care should be based on illness severity scores such as the PORT (Pneumonia Patient Outcomes Research Team) score.[15]

- The majority of cases of pneumonia can be managed in the outpatient setting.
- These risk indicators should not be used alone in determining site of care as the provider's clinical judgment always supersedes.
- The inability to care for oneself, tolerate oral antimicrobials, or have reliable follow-up care may influence one's decision to admit a patient for treatment.

Antimicrobial Therapy
- **Treatment should always be tailored to provide narrow coverage if the etiologic agent is known.**
- In the absence of known comorbidities or high prevalence of local resistance in an otherwise healthy patient, macrolide therapy (azithromycin 500 mg PO for one dose and then 250 mg PO daily for 5 days, clarithromycin 500 mg PO twice daily, and erythromycin 250 mg PO every 6 hours) provides adequate coverage.
  - Doxycycline (100 mg PO every 12 hours) is an appropriate second-line agent.
  - **Fluoroquinolone use is discouraged in this setting.**
- For patients with underlying chronic conditions such as heart disease or diabetes, malignancy, asplenia, or immunosuppression, alternative agents can be used.
  - **Prior use of a first-line agent in the preceding 3 months dictates the need for alternative agents.**
- Respiratory fluoroquinolones (levofloxacin 500 mg PO daily, moxifloxacin 400 mg PO daily) are the simplest drugs to administer.
- β-lactam antibiotics combined with a macrolide are also appropriate.
- The preferred β-lactam is high-dose amoxicillin/clavulanate (2 g/125 mg every 12 hours or amoxicillin 1 g three times daily).
  - The minimum duration of therapy is 5 days. Patients should be afebrile for 48 to 72 hours and clinically improving before stopping treatment.
  - Failure to respond to initial antimicrobial therapy should prompt a systematic approach to uncovering the reason for failure.
- Complications include development of empyema, bronchiolitis obliterans with organizing pneumonia, extrapulmonary disease, resistant pathogens or atypical pathogens not covered by the initial therapy, drug fever, or misdiagnosis of a non-infectious process such as pulmonary embolism, cardiac disease, or vasculitis.
- Follow-up chest radiography is indicated in nonresponding patients with the caveat that radiographic findings typically lag behind clinical improvement. Evidence of worsened disease or new complications is sought on repeat chest radiography.
- All patients aged 13 to 64 years should be offered HIV testing. This is especially true in the absence of other comorbid conditions.
- Vaccination to prevent severe invasive pneumococcal disease is advisable for all patients 65 years of age or older.
- **Smoking cessation should be strongly encouraged.**

LATENT INFECTIONS

- The majority of systemic viral infections are acquired during childhood. These include human herpes virus 6 (HHV-6), cytomegalovirus (CMV), varicella virus, and others. These can cause primary or recurrent infections in adults.
- This section will focus on Epstein-Barr virus (EBV) and varicella-zoster virus (VZV) as they cause common infections and complications into adulthood. Please refer to Chapter 23 for a discussion of herpes simplex virus.

Epstein-Barr Virus (Mononucleosis)

General Principles

- Symptomatic EBV infection typically occurs in older children and adolescents. Young children are generally asymptomatic.
- EBV is spread by close human contact via saliva but is not especially contagious. Sexual transmission may also occur.
- Viral shedding can occur for months after infection.
- By adulthood the vast majority of the population is seropositive.

Diagnosis

- **Mononucleosis** refers to a broader syndrome of fever, malaise/fatigue, pharyngitis, cervical lymphadenopathy, and splenomegaly. Some have relatively mild symptoms and some present with only fever and lymphadenopathy.
  - Primary CMV infection, a closely related virus, has been implicated as an additional causative agent.
  - Primary infection with human immunodeficiency virus (HIV) has caused a similar syndrome.
- Other findings may include splenomegaly, rash (especially following administration of ampicillin or amoxicillin, others have also been described), and rarely neurologic manifestations (e.g., Guillain-Barré syndrome, meningitis, encephalitis, neuritis).
- **Absolute lymphocytosis with atypical lymphocytes** on complete blood count is usually seen.
- Hepatic function tests are often abnormal, typically in a cholestatic pattern, and are self-limited.
- **Heterophile antibodies** (e.g., Monospot) are usually positive early in the disease.

Treatment

- Treatment is typically supportive.
  - Acyclovir has some activity against EBV but has **no clinical benefit and its use is not recommended.**
  - Corticosteroids may be used to abate severe complications including autoimmune manifestations or airway narrowing due to lymphadenopathy.
- Complications include thrombocytopenia, Guillain-Barré syndrome, and splenic rupture.
- Prolonged convalescence is not necessary.
  - Patients should avoid contact sports for a minimum of 3 weeks from the time of diagnosis, and longer if splenomegaly persists.[16]

Varicella-Zoster Virus

General Principles

- VZV is the etiologic agent of chicken pox (primary infection usually in childhood) and shingles (herpes zoster, reactivation usually in adulthood).
- Rarely VZV presents as a disseminated disease in immunosuppressed hosts, which is rapidly fatal, presenting with vague initial complaints usually including abdominal pain.
- Chicken pox in adults is rare and usually follows exposure to an infected child.
  - The classic rash is described as "dew drops on a rose petal."
  - Fever is usually present.

- Latent infection after primary infection occurs in sensory nerve ganglia.
- Over a lifetime, zoster develops in approximately 30% of patients with a history of chicken pox. It is more common in patients <60 years of age.[17]
- Complications of zoster infections include encephalitis, zoster ophthalmicus, myelitis, retinitis, postherpetic neuralgia, and postherpetic itch.

Diagnosis

- Diagnosis of shingles is based largely on clinical grounds.
- A dermatomal vesicular rash with marked pain is the hallmark of zoster.
- Trigeminal zoster raises the concern for **zoster ophthalmicus,** a potential sight threatening lesion.
  - Lesions on the tip of the nose (Hutchinson's sign) or around the eye are highly suggestive for this process and require urgent referral to an ophthalmologist.
- If diagnostic uncertainty exists, culture or PCR of vesicular fluid can yield the diagnosis.
- Rash is not essential in zoster, an entity known as **zoster sine herpete,** and is usually associated with dermatomal muscular weakness.
- The **Ramsay Hunt syndrome** (herpes zoster oticus) is associated with reactivation in the geniculate ganglia and is diagnosed as facial palsy with mucocutaneous lesions (ear, side of tongue).[18]

Treatment

Antivirals

- Primary VZV can be adequately treated with acyclovir, valacyclovir, or famciclovir to prevent more serious complications of primary infection including VZV pneumonia.
- Immunocompromised patients and those with VZV pneumonia should be admitted to receive parenteral therapy.
- In general, zoster ophthalmicus requires initial parenteral therapy.
- **Oral therapy for uncomplicated disease should be initiated within 48 hours but benefit can be seen up to 72 hours after development of symptoms.**
  - Typical regimens include acyclovir 800 mg PO five times daily, valacyclovir 1,000 mg three times daily, or famciclovir 500 mg PO three times daily, all for 7 days.
- Topical therapy is of minimal benefit.
- **Steroid use is controversial.**

Pain Management

- Pain management is the most significant part of treatment and **early aggressive treatment may decrease the risk of developing postherpetic neuralgia.**
  - Tricyclic antidepressants and opioid analgesics are the mainstays of therapy.
  - Gabapentin or pregabalin may also be considered.
- Once postherpetic neuralgia has developed, effective treatments include the following:
  - Tricyclic antidepressants (e.g., amitriptyline, nortriptyline, and desipramine)
  - Anticonvulsants (e.g., gabapentin, pregabalin, and valproic acid)
  - Opioids
- For postherpetic neuralgia, other means such as topical capsaicin (0.025% cream five times daily), neural blockade, and topical lidocaine have been used.
- Referral to a pain specialist may be required.

Vaccination

- The live attenuated varicella vaccine (e.g., Varivax) has been used in children for several years.

- As a result, concern has arisen that adults will experience waning immunity because of lack of recurrent exposure to the virus. This has led to efforts to develop a vaccine for the prevention of zoster infections.
- The currently licensed vaccine (Zostavax) is a higher-dose version of the pediatric vaccine, a live attenuated vaccine.
- The vaccination has been shown to decrease the incidence of herpes zoster and postherpetic neuralgia.[19]
- The Advisory Committee on Immunization Practices recommends its use for all nonimmunocompromised individuals 60 years of age and older.[20]

TRAVEL MEDICINE

- The recent growth in international travel has lead to further study and development of travel medicine practice guidelines. Primary care physicians should be able to provide advice for low-risk travel destinations, but referral to a practitioner competent in travel medicine may be warranted.[21]
- Pretravel assessment focuses on prevention and should include a detailed assessment of risk for exposure to various diseases, an assessment of potential for personal injury, and how these various processes may interact with the patient's underlying health.
- The pretravel counseling session also provides an opportunity for updated recommended adult vaccinations.
- Specific topics to discuss include management of traveler's diarrhea, malaria prophylaxis and insect avoidance, and personal safety amongst other more specific concerns depending on the patient's destination.
- Topics relating to personal safety are beyond the scope of this discussion but include sexual risk, road safety, sun and heat exposure, evacuation insurance, and high-altitude illness.
- Travel counseling depends on the destination; recommendations for specific destinations for U.S. travelers can be obtained at the CDC's Web site (http://wwwn.cdc.gov/travel/default.aspx). Additional advisories related to travel destinations can be obtained through the U.S. Department of State's Web site (www.travel.state.gov).

Malaria

- Malaria is commonly caused by *Plasmodium falciparum* and *P. vivax* with *P. falciparum* causing more severe disease and *P. vivax* causing relapsing disease. Other species include *P. ovale* and *P. malariae.*
- Malaria presents as a nonspecific illness with severe fevers, chills, headache, nausea, vomiting, and myalgia.
  - Infection with *P. falciparum* is a medical emergency. Diagnosis currently rests on finding parasites on a blood smear.
- **The most important aspect of malaria prevention is avoidance of mosquito bites.**
  - This includes use of insect repellants, bed nets, wearing long sleeve shirts and pants, and avoiding outdoor exposure during feeding times of anopheles mosquitoes (from dusk through dawn).
- Malaria is the most common preventable infection in the returned traveler and inappropriate chemoprophylaxis is the most common reason for developing disease.

TABLE 2	Common Agents for Malaria Prophylaxis for Travelers from the United States	
Drug	**Dosing**	**Precautions**
Chloroquine	500 mg (salt) PO weekly Start: 1–2 weeks prior to travel Finish: 4 weeks after travel	Itching, bitter taste, retinal or visual field deficits
Atovaquone/ proguanil	250/100 mg PO daily Start: 1–2 days prior to travel Finish: 1 week after travel	Gastrointestinal upset
Mefloquine	250 mg PO weekly Start: 1 week prior to travel Finish: 4 weeks after travel	Night terrors Caution with seizures, psychosis, depression, or cardiac conduction disturbances
Doxycycline	100 mg PO daily Start: 1–2 days prior to travel Finish: 4 weeks after travel	Photosensitivity Contraindicated in children and pregnancy

- The choice of chemoprophylactic drugs depends on the patient's risk, drug resistance at the destination, and side effect profiles of various regimens.
  - Information on local resistance patterns is available through the CDC Web site or by calling the malaria hotline (770-488-7788).
- **Chloroquine** phosphate 500 mg (salt) by mouth weekly starting 1 week prior to travel and continuing through 4 weeks after returning home is the first-line agent for prophylaxis given its low cost, beneficial side effect profile, and safety in pregnancy. However, due to the frequency of drug resistance, its use is limited.
- Prophylaxis with **primaquine** is rarely indicated except for in long-term travelers to high-risk areas. This should not be administered unless the patient is known not to be G6PD deficient.
- Other drugs to be considered are listed in Table 2.
- Treatment should be initiated promptly along with hospital admission and consultation with a specialist in the setting of severe disease.
  - Information can also be obtained via the CDC's malaria hotline (770-488-7788).
  - Indicators of severe disease are altered mental status, hemodynamic instability, bleeding, jaundice, renal failure, disseminated intravascular coagulation, acidosis, hemoglobinuria, and parasitemia >5%.[22]
- Treatment regimens for active disease are beyond the scope of this discussion, as this usually requires inpatient care.

Traveler's Diarrhea

General Principles
- Traveler's diarrhea is usually a benign, self-limited illness of 3 to 5 days duration, but its sudden onset during travel can be quite disruptive. **It is by far the most common illness of travelers.**

- Prevention is the most important aspect of care.[21]
- **Common pathogens include the following:**
  - Enterotoxigenic *Escherichia coli*
  - *Salmonella* spp.
  - *Campylobacter* spp.
  - *Shigella* spp.
  - Norovirus has been associated with several travel-related outbreaks.
- Other pathogens include parasites, of which *Giardia lamblia* is the most common, *Aeromonas* spp., *Vibrio* spp., and *Plesiomonas* spp.

Diagnosis

- True disease is defined as three loose stools or more in 24 hours along with fever, nausea, vomiting, or abdominal cramping.
- Postinfectious irritable bowel syndrome is also common, often due to disruption of the normal gastrointestinal lining.
- Specific diagnostic testing is generally necessary only in those with severe symptoms (e.g., hypovolemia, bloody diarrhea, fever, severe abdominal pain), the elderly, immunocompromised, and those with recent antibiotic use.
- **Fecal leukocyte testing** of uncertain value.
- **Stool cultures** are very often negative but should probably be done in those with bloody diarrhea, inflammatory bowel disease, and in the immunocompromised and food handlers.
- **Ova and parasite testing** is also not routinely necessary but should be considered in those with more chronic symptoms, who travel to endemic areas, daycare workers, men who have sex with men, and waterborne outbreaks.

Treatment

- Maintaining adequate hydration.
  - The patients should be advised that if they are unable to drink fluids, they should seek prompt local medical attention.
  - Likewise, if fever or blood in the stool is present, local medical care should be sought.
- For patients without fever or blood in their stool, diarrhea can be managed symptomatically with **loperamide. Bismuth subsalicylate** can be used as a second-line agent.
- **Antimicrobial agents** can shorten the duration of disease by up to a day.
  - This may be significant for travelers on brief vacations.
  - First-line therapy has been with **fluoroquinolones** (ciprofloxacin 500 mg PO twice daily for 1 to 3 days).
  - Resistance, particularly to *Campylobacter* spp. in Asia, has been increasing.
  - Azithromycin 1,000 mg for one dose is a second-line agent.
  - Rifaximin, a poorly absorbed antimicrobial, has been undergoing investigation.

Prevention

- Prevention can be attained by avoiding contaminated food and water.
  - Practices such as boiling or filtering water and avoidance of raw foods or foods prepared in unsanitary conditions can be difficult as travelers are often in situations in which declining food is considered offensive.
  - Encouraging common-sense practices as eating thoroughly cooked or peeled foods and drinking only bottled or filtered water will minimize the incidence of disease.

- **Antibiotic prophylaxis is considered to be of no or minimal benefit** in preventing traveler's diarrhea.

Vaccinations for Travelers

- Several vaccines are available for travelers depending on their destination. Information available at www.cdc.gov.
- Familiarity with their indications and contraindications is important in recommending their use. The general risk for acquiring a particular infection is on the order of <1 per 1,000 visits.[21]
- Documentation of any prior and current vaccinations is important; often this information is needed by the traveler to gain access to various locations.
- One should also consider the nature of the vaccine (live attenuated, vaccine components) and its relation to the host prior to administration as well as immune interference between vaccines when administering multiple simultaneous or sequential vaccines.
- **As a general rule, live vaccines are contraindicated in pregnancy.**

Specific Vaccinations

Yellow Fever

- This vaccine is often required to enter countries.
- Proper handling is important and it can only be administered by licensed vaccine centers. It is a live attenuated virus.
- Vaccine-associated adverse event are more common and occur more frequently in previously nonimmune and older individuals.
  - The most serious are yellow fever associated viscerotropic and neurologic disease. These can be life threatening.
- Its use is contraindicated in those with thymus disorders and immunosuppression is a relative contraindication.
- In addition, the safety of yellow fever vaccination during pregnancy has not been established and the vaccine should be administered to a pregnant woman only if travel to an endemic area is unavoidable and if an increased risk for exposure exists.

Cholera

This vaccine is no longer produced in the United States as the risk to an individual traveler is low.

Hepatitis A

- Although hepatitis A is usually a self-limited disease, its acquisition can be disruptive to travel. Fulminant hepatitis A does occur but it is rare.
- It is generally recommended to receive this vaccination and even partial vaccination in those unable to receive the full series due to time constraints has benefit.

Hepatitis B

- Given its widespread use in the United States, many travelers will have already received the full series.
- The risk of acquiring disease in short-term travel is very low.

Meningococcus

- This vaccine is now routinely recommended for many persons living in the United States.

- Its use should be considered in travelers to the meningitis belt of Sub-Saharan Africa and pilgrims to the Hajj.
- Although relatively safe, cases of Guillain-Barré syndrome have been linked to this vaccine.

Rabies
- Use of this vaccine is highly dependent on the particulars of a patient's travel.
- It should be considered for those who will be exposed to potentially infected animals (monkeys and dogs) and when it will be difficult to seek immediate medical care.

Japanese Encephalitis
- This vaccine is indicated in travelers with prolonged exposure to endemic areas.
- It is associated with hypersensitivity reactions upon receipt.

Typhoid
- This vaccine is indicated in travelers to endemic areas who will be exposed to poor sanitary conditions.
- Their protection is incomplete and travelers must continue to practice avoidance behaviors.

Other Vaccines
- Some patients may require **polio** vaccination or booster vaccination.
- Nonpregnant individuals who have not received a measles booster should also receive an additional **measles-mumps-rubella** vaccination.
- Tetanus-diphtheria-acellular pertussis booster should also be administered.
- In addition, one may consider placing a tuberculin skin test (Mantoux PPD) prior to travel for certain high-risk travelers who may be exposed to TB.

DIARRHEAL ILLNESS

General Principles
- Acute infectious diarrhea remains a substantial public health concern as noted by several recalls of contaminated foods.
- The CDC notes that the incidence of infections due to *Campylobacter* spp., *Listeria monocytogenes, Shigella* spp., and *Yersinia enterocolitica* has been declining but those due to *Vibrio* spp. and *Salmonella* spp. have, respectively, increased or remain unchanged.[23]
- In the United States, the annual incidence of diarrheal illness approaches 1.4 episodes per person.
- Recently, infections due to *Clostridium difficile* have become more virulent and their significance in nosocomial infections and as adverse events related to antibiotic overuse is becoming better understood.[24]
- Perhaps the most commonly used definition states that diarrhea is an increase in stool liquidity along with an increase in frequency to three or more stools daily.[25]
- Acute diarrhea lasts <14 days, whereas chronic diarrhea lasts >30 days. The intervening period is defined as persistent diarrhea.
- In the United States, elderly patients account for the majority of the mortality associated with diarrheal illness, approximately 50% to 75% of the total deaths.[26]

Etiology
Viral
- **Rotavirus** diarrhea is a self-limited disease of 3 to 5 days duration. Diagnostic assays are available. Newer vaccines have been approved that do not carry a risk of intussusception.

- **Norovirus** (formerly known as the Norwalk virus) is associated with disease outbreaks, particularly on cruise ships. This relatively common cause has agent a predilection for the winter and spring.

Bacterial

- Several different strains of **_Escherichia coli_** cause diarrheal illness.
  - Enterotoxigenic forms are the most common cause of traveler's diarrhea.
  - Shiga-toxin producing strains such as 0157:H7 are important in causing hemolytic uremic syndrome (HUS).
  - Outbreaks have been associated with undercooked meats and packaged produce.
- **Salmonella** infection is often associated with poultry and eggs, but outbreaks have occurred with varied food sources.
  - Reptiles often carry the bacteria and such strains have been associated with severe disease in children.
  - _S. typhi_ and _S. paratyphi_ are the agents associated with typhoid fever.
  - _S. enteritidis_ and _S. typhimurium_ commonly cause diarrheal disease in the United States.
- **Shigella** transmission is from person to person and outbreaks have been associated with reptiles, day care centers, and various food sources. Initial watery diarrhea becomes mucoid and bloody.
- **_C. jejuni_** is perhaps the most common form of infectious diarrhea in the United States. It usually comes from contaminated chickens. _C. coli_ and other less common species can also cause diarrheal illness. This infection has been associated with Guillain-Barré syndrome and reactive arthritis.
- **_Y. enterocolitica_** infection has been associated with outbreaks in puppies. Often, patients have evidence of mesenteric adenitis.
- **_L. monocytogenes_** is a particularly virulent infection associated with consumption of unpasteurized dairy products, uncooked deli meats, melons, and hummus. A documented small outbreak has occurred even with pasteurized milk.
  - The organism is able to grow at temperatures approaching 0°C.
  - It has a long incubation time.
  - Severe disease such as meningitis and sepsis is associated with those <60 years of age or immunocompromised.
  - Pregnant women have a higher risk of fetal loss.
- **_Vibrio_ spp.** infection is associated with the consumption of raw shellfish/fish (particularly _V. parahaemolyticus_) and those with severe liver disease.
- **_Bacillus cereus_** infection occurs in previously contaminated food maintained at warm temperatures, which permits the growth of bacteria.
  - The **diarrheal form** is associated with meat/vegetable consumption, has an incubation time of 8 to 16 hours, is due to the ingestion of spores, and causes diarrhea and abdominal pain.
  - The **emetic form** is classically associated with rice consumption, has a short incubation time of 1 to 6 hours, is due to a heat-stable toxin, and causes nausea and vomiting.
- **_Aeromonas_ spp.** and **_Plesiomonas shigelloides_** have also been implicated as etiologic agents of acute diarrhea. Both can also cause chronic diarrhea extraintestinal manifestations. And both seem to have a predilection to cause more significant disease in the immunocompromised.
- Other bacterial etiologies to consider, not discussed in detail here, include _Clostridium perfringens_ and botulism.

Clostridium difficile–Associated Disease

- *C. difficile*–associated disease (CDAD) is caused by **cytotoxin** production, resulting in the formation of **pseudomembranes** within the colon.
- Disease is usually associated with **prior antibiotic use** but more recently **community-acquired** *C. difficile* disease has been documented and may be increasing in frequency.[24]
  - Additional risk factors include recent hospitalization and institutionalized persons.
- Disease is usually recognized by the onset of diarrhea in the appropriate clinical setting.
  - It should be noted that associated constipation can be a rather ominous sign in that the patient may be developing **toxic megacolon and perforation** may be imminent.
- A new epidemic strain has been associated with increased morbidity and mortality and is associated with fluoroquinolone use.

Protozoal

- Patients at risk for *Gardia lamblia* include hikers and campers as well as day care attendees. Transmission is through contaminated water supplies or fecal/oral transmission. *G. lamblia* not uncommonly causes recurrent/chronic diarrhea.
- *Cryptosporidium* spp. infection presents clinically in advanced HIV-positive patients; however, it may cause self-limited disease in normal hosts.
- *Entamoeba histolytica* is a worldwide pathogen present in contaminated water.
  - It is rarely found in the United States. Transmission is through fecal/oral routes and can be seen as an etiology of traveler's diarrhea.
  - Disease is worse in pregnancy, immunosuppression, steroid use, and malignancy.
- Additional protozoal infections include the following:
  - *Cyclospora cayetanensis:* Outbreaks in the United States have been due to contaminated raspberries, lettuce, basil, and snow peas. It may also be acquired during foreign travel. It does not appear to transmit directly from person-to-person. In AIDS it may cause a prolonged diarrheal illness similar to that of *Cryptosporidium* spp. and *Isospora belli.*
  - **Isospora belli:** This infection is most frequently seen HIV-positive in men who have sex with men. It can cause chronic diarrhea, abdominal pain, malabsorption, and weight loss.
  - **Microsporidial organisms:** They may cause acute or sometimes chronic diarrhea in normal hosts. The incidence of microsporidiosis in HIV patients has declined with the advent of highly active antiretroviral therapy.

Diagnosis

- A rational and cautious approach is important to limit antimicrobial and procedural overuse.
- Specific diagnoses may not benefit individual patients but can have significant public health implications.
- Additional history including recent travel; exposure to potentially infectious persons; consumption of unsafe food such as raw meats, unpasteurized dairy products, or shellfish; drinking unfiltered water from lakes or streams; exposure to pets or farm animals, underlying illnesses such as HIV or irritable bowel disease; potential sexual exposures; and recent antimicrobial use.
- One should consider the potential etiologies of diarrheal illness. These can be divided into three categories:
  - **Community-acquired diarrhea:** these are diseases such as enterotoxigenic *E. coli* or traveler's diarrhea, *Shigella* spp., etc.
  - **Nosocomial diarrhea:** mostly CDAD in patients with recent hospitalization or antimicrobial use.

TABLE 3	Potential Indications for Stool Culture	
Age ≥65	Tenesmus	Neutropenia
Duration >1 day	Bloody stool	HIV
Recent antimicrobial use	Mucopurulent stool	Other comorbid illness
Fever	Positive fecal leukocyte	Institutionalized
Dehydration	testing	persons
Daycare attendances		Food handlers
(employees and children)		

- **Persistent diarrhea:** frequently parasitic in etiology or postinfective lactase deficiency.

Diagnostic Testing
- Reports suggest that the diagnostic yield of stool culture is approximately 5%. Patients with a history of bloody diarrhea have a higher rate of positive cultures.
- Patient characteristics in which diagnostic testing may be warranted are listed in Table 3.
- Additional testing may include complete blood counts and basic metabolic panels.
- Lactoferrin testing may be useful and its sensitivity is quite good.[25,27] A positive test is associated with inflammatory causes of diarrhea.
- Diagnosis of CDAD is made by finding a positive toxin assay on stool.
  - Culture can be misleading as the bacterium may be present in the absence of toxic disease.
  - Additional toxin testing is generally not needed as the toxin may persist beyond clinical improvement.
  - Hypoalbuminemia and leukemoid reactions have been seen with active disease.
- Rarely are additional diagnostic procedures warranted.
  - Disease lasting >7 days should prompt consideration of stool testing for ova and parasites.
  - Such testing should target specific risk factors such as ELISA testing for *G. lamblia* or *Cryptosporidium* spp. in campers, shiga-toxin testing in patients with signs of HUS, or mycobacterial cultures of blood or CMV testing in patients with advanced HIV.
  - One should also begin to consider evaluation for noninfectious processes.

Treatment

Rehydration
The initial assessment for treatment should begin with an assessment of the patient's hydration status.
- **Rehydration should be prompt.** For the majority of adult patients with **mild to moderate dehydration,** soups and juices are generally sufficient.
- For more **moderate to severe dehydration,** patients should be encouraged to consume oral rehydration solutions with glucose-based electrolyte solutions.
  - The World Health Organization and United Nations Children's Fund oral rehydration solution consists of the following: 2.6 g NaCl, 13.5 g glucose, 1.5 g KCl, and 2.9 g trisodium citrate all in 1 L of water (total osmolality 245 mOsm/kg).

- There are similar commercially available oral rehydration products (e.g., Pedialyte). These products contain sodium, potassium, and carbohydrate and have an appropriate osmolality (approximately 200 to 300 mOsm/kg).
- Common liquids like soft drinks, fruit juice, and sports drinks (e.g., Gatorade) are of high osmolality (mostly due to carbohydrate), have insufficient sodium, and are not recommended for oral rehydration therapy particularly in children with severe diarrhea/dehydration. The higher osmolality can actually worsen diarrhea. Soups typically contain too much sodium and may result in hypernatremia and should also be avoided in the setting of severe diarrhea/ dehydration.
- **Intravenous therapy** should be limited to those who are obtunded or unable to tolerate oral therapy given the risks of intravenous lines.

Empiric Treatment
- **The majority of disease lasts <1 day and is of viral etiology, making antimicrobial therapy of no benefit.**
- **Unnecessary harm can occur from misuse of antimicrobials,** including prolonged carriage of *Salmonella* spp., worsening HUS from induction of shiga-toxin production, or development of *C. difficile* colitis.
- **Empiric therapy with quinolones** (ciprofloxacin 500 mg PO twice daily for 3 to 5 days) is warranted for traveler's diarrhea.
- Azithromycin (single dose of 1 g) is a reasonable second-line agent.
- **Loperamide** is an antimotility agent that is not systemically absorbed. It can often limit the symptoms of acute diarrhea but it **should not be used during disease caused by known or suspected invasive organisms (i.e., bloody diarrhea).** Complications of loperamide therapy include worsening of HUS and toxic megacolon.
- Nonpharmacologic means are of varying benefit.
  - Strict hand-washing for exposed and infected persons is imperative in limiting the spread of disease.
  - The BRAT (bananas, rice, applesauce, toast) diet is of no proven benefit.
  - Dairy avoidance is important given the potential for transient lactase deficiency.

Specific Therapy
Viral
- For **rotavirus** and **norovirus** supportive therapy alone is indicated.
- Antibiotic therapy is of no value.

Bacterial
- For **_E. coli_** antimicrobial therapy is generally not indicated except in traveler's diarrhea. Some reports suggest that antibiotics may worsen HUS by increased phage production of shiga-toxin.
- Antibiotic treatment for nontyphoidal **_Salmonella_ spp.** in generally not indicated as it prolongs the carrier state.
  - In several patient groups, treatment should be considered because of the risk of dissemination (Table 4). Treatment is with **trimethoprim-sulfamethoxazole (TMP-SMX) or fluoroquinolones** for 5 to 7 days.
- Treatment for **_Shigella_ spp.** is generally with **fluoroquinolones** (e.g., ciprofloxacin 500 mg PO bid for 5 days). **TMP-SMX** (160 mg/800 mg PO bid for 5 days) can be appropriate second-line therapy but resistance to this agent is increasing.
- **C. jejuni** infections are usually relatively mild and self-limited; therefore, antibiotic therapy is generally not indicated. However, treatment (e.g., azithromycin) should be considered for those who have or are at risk for severe disease (e.g., elderly, pregnant, immunocompromised).

TABLE 4	Indication for Treatment of Salmonella Infection

Age >50
Cancer
Hemoglobinopathies
HIV
Transplant patients
Patients with joint prosthesis
Vascular grafts
Valvular heart disease
Prolonged corticosteroids

- *Y. enterocolitica* infections usually resolve spontaneously and antibiotic treatment is most often unwarranted. If treatment is felt to be indicated for severe diarrhea, doxycycline can be used. Complicated/septicemic disease requires a combination of IV antibiotics.
- Parenteral therapy with ampicillin and gentamicin is indicated if **listeriosis** is suspected.
- Treatment of severe **noncholera *Vibrio* spp.** is with **ciprofloxacin.**
- Treatment of *B. cereus*–induced diarrhea is not necessary.
- Most cases of *Aeromonas* **spp.** and *P. shigelloides* diarrhea are self-limited. If warranted, **fluoroquinolones** or **TMP-SMX** are reasonable treatments.

Clostridium difficile–Associated Disease

- Treatment of CDAD involves **removal of the offending antimicrobial** if at all possible.
- Metronidazole has been considered the first-line agent for many years but oral vancomycin is the only drug approved by the Food and Drug Administration.
  - **Metronidazole is preferred as the agent** and is inexpensive, no known resistance has developed, and there are no fears of generating stool colonization with vancomycin-resistant enterococcus).[24,27] The latter fear is a subject of controversy.
  - Metronidazole is dosed 500 mg PO tid.
  - Oral vancomycin is not absorbed; it should be dosed no higher than 250 mg PO qid.
  - Duration of therapy for nonsevere disease is 14 days.
- **Probiotics are of no proven benefit** in treatment or prevention of CDAD. Bacteremia has resulted from the use of probiotics, so their routine use cannot be recommended.
- Additional experimental therapies include use of immune globulin, fecal transplant, and *Saccharomyces boulardii.*
- **Relapsing disease** is becoming more common and consultation with a specialist may be necessary.
  - Retreatment with metronidazole is indicated for the first relapse (nonsevere).

Protozoal

- *G. lamblia* is effectively treated with **metronidazole** 500 mg PO three times daily for 5 days.
- There is no effective antibiotic treatment for *Cryptosporidium* **spp.** Treatment in HIV-positive patients consists of immune reconstitution with highly active antiretroviral therapy.
- *E. histolytica* is treated with **metronidazole** 500 to 750 mg PO tid for 7 to 10 days **followed by iodoquinol** 650 mg tid for 21 days **or paromomycin** 25 to 30 mg/kg/day for 7 days. The first phase of treatment eliminates the invading trophozoites and the second luminal cysts.

- **_C. cayetanensis_** and **_I. belli_** are treated with **TMP-SMX.**
- **Microsporidia** can be treated with **albendazole** when necessary.

SKIN AND SOFT TISSUE INFECTIONS

- Managing these infections is quite simple in healthy patients but in patients with comorbidities such as diabetes, vascular disease, or patients with prosthetic materials (e.g., joint replacement), limb-threatening lesions can arise without proper early and aggressive therapy.
- Providers must also maintain a high index of suspicion for severe processes such as compartment syndrome or necrotizing fasciitis as their initial presentation can be quite benign.
- A wide variety of additional pathogens not discussed here can cause cutaneous infections. They must be suspected on the basis of history and include diseases such as anthrax, tularemia, cat-scratch disease, plague, VZV, fungal infections, erysipeloid, and nontuberculous mycobacteria.

Cellulitis and Erysipelas

General Principles

- These terms refer to cutaneous infections without underlying sources of infection such as abscesses, septic arthritis, or osteomyelitis.
- **Erysipelas** refers to infections of the dermis, whereas **cellulitis** refers to deeper processes involving the underlying cutaneous structures. In practice, **distinguishing between these entities is of minimal benefit.**[28]
- Erysipelas is usually caused by Group A β-hemolytic streptococci (e.g., _S. pyogenes_); Groups C and G have also been implicated. Group B Strep and _S. aureus_ can cause erysipelas as well.
  - This entity classically involves the face but is now recognized to be most common on the lower extremities.
  - It has sharply demarcated and indurated edges, its clinical hallmark.
- Cellulitis generally lacks sharp demarcated borders but is caused by the same pathogenic organisms as erysipelas.
- Traumatic breaks in the skin frequently serve as the nidus of infection.
- Diabetes, peripheral vascular disease, obesity, and eczema often predispose to infection.
- Obvious sources of infection are not frequently found.

Diagnosis

- Diagnosis is based on clinical presentation.
- The history may suggest alternative pathogens:
  - **_Pasteurella_ spp.:** dog or cat bite (see below).
  - **_V. vulnificus_:** exposure of the wound to fish/shellfish and/or estuarine water; those with chronic disease, particularly alcoholism, liver disease, and hemochromatosis.
  - **_Capnocytophaga canimorsus_:** dog or cat bite; asplenia; underlying liver disease (see below).
  - Polymicrobial including aerobes and anaerobes: human bite (see below).
- Patients with uncomplicated disease lack fever and have localized examination findings such as regional lymphadenopathy, local warmth and tenderness, and edema, which may present as peau d'orange.

- Vesicles and bullae may also form.
- When petechiae or other systemic findings are present (e.g., fever, hypotension), more serious infections may be present.
- Blood cultures are rarely positive and cutaneous punch biopsy provides minimal diagnostic information.
- Plain radiographs may help diagnose underlying osteomyelitis, whereas ultrasound is useful in diagnosing abscesses.
- Magnetic resonance imaging (MRI) and computerized tomography (CT) are rarely indicated for uncomplicated infections.
- Neutropenia may predispose persons to cutaneous infections with gram-negative organisms and fungi.
- Gout, VZV, or allergic dermatitis may be confused with typical cellulitis.

Treatment

- Underlying factors such as tinea pedis or other skin abnormalities may serve as a nidus for infection and should be treated. Routine skin care can help prevent recurrences.
- Elevation of the affected extremity aids in healing and remains a cornerstone of treatment.
- Agents such as **dicloxacillin** and **cephalexin** are appropriate for uncomplicated disease without concern for drug resistance. Five days of treatment is as effective as 10 days.[29]
- The treatment of alternative organisms (as above) may necessitate other antibiotic choices.
- Corticosteroids have shown some benefit, especially at reducing transient worsening after beginning antimicrobial therapy. However, their routine use is not recommended.

Community-Acquired Methicillin-Resistant *S. Aureus*

General Principles

- Cutaneous infections with community-acquired Methicillin-resistant *S. aureus* (CA-MRSA) are a growing trend.[30] They are a very common cause of skin infection presenting to the emergency department.
- The isolate typically carries a resistance pattern separate from that of hospital-acquired MRSA, usually being susceptible to TMP-SMX, clindamycin, doxycycline, and quinolones.
  - It has been associated with the Panton-Valentine leukocidin, a virulence factor thought to interfere with neutrophil function.[31]
- Risk associations include prior MRSA infection, household contacts with MRSA, men having sex with men, soldiers, Native Americans, Pacific Islanders, intravenous drug users, children, participating in contact sports, obesity, skin trauma, obesity, and body shaving.

Diagnosis

- The presentation of CA-MRSA infection can range from cellulitis to abscesses to necrotizing fasciitis.
- Patients sometimes present with the notion of an antecedent spider or insect bite. In reality, this was the initial infection.

- The organism can also cause necrotizing pneumonia, osteomyelitis, endocarditis, and sepsis.

Treatment

- Topical therapy can be used to treat impetigo (see Impetigo below) but mupirocin resistance may be a concern.
- **First-line oral agents include clindamycin 300 mg PO tid or TMP-SMX or doxycycline 200 mg PO bid.**
  - Double strength (DS) tablets contain 160 mg of TMP and patients should receive 10 mg/kg/day of TMP in divided doses (e.g., in a 70 kg person, two DS tablets PO bid should be sufficient; one should not exceed 2 DS tablets tid).
  - **TMP-SMX does not cover streptococcal species.**
  - Clindamycin resistance in CA-MRSA has been increasing.
- Parenteral therapy is required for severe infections.
- Improved personal hygiene can often mitigate recurrences. This includes routine bathing and washing of clothes, bed linens, and towels.
- The role of eliminating MRSA carriage remains debatable.

Abscesses

- A cutaneous abscess is a dermal or subdermal collection of pus, which is typically polymicrobial. It presents as a tender fluctuant lesion with surrounding erythema.
- Related lesions include **furuncles and carbuncles.** These are abscesses that form at the site of hair follicles. Carbuncles are simply coalesced furuncles.
- Moist heat without antibiotics is sufficient treatment for small lesions. Larger lesions require **incision and drainage** but antibiotic therapy likewise is not necessary for lesions <5 cm.
- For large lesions or recurrent disease, antibiotics are indicated in addition to drainage.
- Clindamycin 300 mg PO tid has become common treatment in the era of increased prevalence of CA-MRSA.

Impetigo

- Impetigo is a superficial skin infection seen throughout the world, usually in summer months, and frequently occurs in children.
- It is a superficial infection caused by **β-hemolytic streptococci and *S. aureus.***
- Poor hygiene generally contributes to disease.
- It occurs on all areas of the body, but typically on the face and extremities, where trauma is more common.
- Lesions may be bullous or nonbullous, single or multiple, and typically drain clear brown to yellow fluid.
- **Topical therapy with mupirocin is equally as efficacious as oral therapy** but one must be mindful of resistance to mupirocin.
- **When indicated, oral clindamycin is the first-line agent.**
- Complications of impetigo are uncommon, but there have been reports of poststreptococcal glomerulonephritis.
- For unknown reasons, rheumatic heart disease has not been documented as a complication.

Necrotizing Fasciitis

- This relatively rare infection can result in mortality or severe morbidity.
- Pathophysiologically, it develops after innocuous trauma, providing a nidus for infection to spread along fascial planes. It spreads rapidly and underlying tissues feel quite firm, especially proximal to externally involved tissues.
- **Systemic findings and failure to respond to initial antimicrobial therapy are clues to the diagnosis.** Findings of petechiae and pain out of proportion to examination findings are also common.
- **Clinical suspicion is extremely important;** however, diagnosis is based on surgical findings. When the diagnosis of necrotizing fasciitis is suspected, urgent surgical consultation is imperative.
- Given its complexity and need for prolonged inpatient care, full discussion of the management of this entity is beyond the scope of this chapter.

Bites

Dog and Cat Bites

- Bites from dogs and cats **typically become infected.** Risk factors for infection include presentation >8 hours after the event and deep puncture wounds.
- Complications include abscess, septic arthritis, osteomyelitis, and tenosynovitis. These are most commonly associated with puncture wounds.
- **Typical organisms** include *S. aureus,* streptococcal species, *Pasteurella multocida, Eikenella corrodens,* and anaerobes.
  - Capnocytophaga species can cause severe disease, mostly in immunosuppressed patients.
- Initial wound management with irrigation and debridement is essential and examination for deeper structural injury is important.[32]
  - Primary closure is generally contraindicated.
  - Scarring and disfigurement related to facial wounds may, however, necessitate primary closure.
- **Amoxicillin/clavulanate 875 mg PO bid is the first-line oral treatment.**
  - Treatment should be given empirically for 7 to 10 days, as **85% of wounds harbor pathogens** even after appropriate initial management.
  - For more serious wounds, admission and parenteral ampicillin/sulbactam should be given. Second-line therapy includes ciprofloxacin with clindamycin.
- Tetanus immunizations should be up-to-date.
- When there is **concern for rabies,** it is essential to give rabies immune globulin and rabies immunization. Consultation with local public health authorities can help guide management in these instances.

Bat Exposure

- Generally, patients bitten by a bat require prophylaxis from rabies consisting of rabies immune globulin and immunization.
- In endemic areas when a bat is found in a room where a person has been sleeping, rabies immune globulin and immunization should be given as many patients will not recall nor will they have evidence of a bite wound.
- Wounds from bats generally do not require empiric antimicrobial prophylaxis.

Spider Bites

- Spider bites are frequently overdiagnosed but should be in the differential of localized erythematous lesions.[33]
- Black widow (*Latrodectus mactans* and *L. Hesperus*) are most common in California and brown recluse (*Loxosceles reclusa*) are common in southeast and south central United States; both can cause significant lesions.
- **Black widow** spiders are identified by their red or orange markings on their ventral abdomen.
  - Severe disease can manifest as shock, seizure, respiratory distress, or muscle spasms. Abdominal rigidity without tenderness may be present.
  - Treatment is supportive and tetanus immunization should be up- to-date.
- **Brown recluse** spiders are identified by their violin-shaped markings on their dorsal surface.
  - The lesion is typically quite painful and may have central clearing.
  - Fever, nausea, vomiting, thrombocytopenia, and hemolysis can be seen with loxoscelism.
  - Severe tissue necrosis can develop requiring surgical intervention. Treatment is largely supportive but may include the use of antihistamines.

Human Bites

- The general management of human bites is similar to that of dog and cat bites.
- Clenched fist injuries can often result in tenosynovitis.
- *E. corrodens* is more common with human bite but usually oral flora is the predominate organism.
- Empiric therapy should be given after a human bite and **amoxicillin/clavulanate** would be the first-line agent.
- If the biter had trauma with bloody lesions in his or her mouth at the time of the bite, one should consider transmission of hepatitis B, hepatitis C, syphilis, and HIV. Postexposure prophylaxis for HIV is rarely indicated in this situation.

FUNGAL INFECTIONS

Superficial Fungal Infections

- The most common infection in this classification is **tinea versicolor** caused by *Malassezia* spp. The infection involves the stratum corneum.[34]
- Microscopic examination of skin scrapings treated with potassium hydroxide can provide the diagnosis. Other diagnostic considerations include vitiligo and pityriasis alba.
- **Topical treatments with selenium sulfide** (2.5% applied for 7 days and then on days 1 and 3 of a given month for 6 months total) **or antifungals** such as ketoconazole (2%) can be used and are the safest treatment options.
  - Oral therapy with itraconazole (200 mg daily for 5 to 7 days) or fluconazole (400 mg for one dose) may be needed at times but one should be mindful of side effects.
- **Piedra** is an infection of the hair shaft caused by *Piedraia hortae* ("black piedra") and *Trichosporon* spp. ("white piedra").
  - It causes soft nodules to form on the hair itself.
  - The best treatment for this lesion is shaving the affected area. Topical antifungals are of benefit when shaving is not an option.

Tinea and Onychomycosis

- Tinea infections and onychomycosis are the most common cutaneous fungal infections. These are frequently caused by **dermatophytes** (*Trichophyton* spp.). By themselves, they rarely cause severe disease but they can serve as the nidus for more severe infections.
- Tinea infections are named by their location and include tinea pedis ("athlete's foot"), tinea cruris ("jock itch"), tinea capitis ("scalp ringworm"), tinea corporis ("ringworm"), tinea faciei, tinea barbae, and tinea unguium (i.e., onychomycosis).
  - They present as areas of mild inflammation with pain and itching.
  - The margin of the infection is usually the area of most intense inflammation and central clearing is frequently seen.
  - Tinea pedis usually starts in the interdigital spaces and may spread to the dorsum or lateral aspect of the foot. The skin may crack and become macerated.
  - **Onychomycosis** is a common dermatophyte infection of the nails. The nails become thickened and discolored (white, yellow, or brown).
- Visualization of fungi on microscopic examination of skin scrapings can generally provide the diagnosis.
  - Ultraviolet light can help identify infected hairs for further evaluation.
  - Fungal culture can also be useful.
- Treatment of tinea and onychomycosis is discussed in detail in Chapter 39.

Sporotrichosis

- Sporotrichosis is a subcutaneous infection caused by *Sporothrix schenckii* and presents as a nodular, pustular skin lesion.
- It is found in decaying plant matter and infections are frequently linked to gardening.
- Ulcers may or may not be painful. Lymphatics are involved causing streaking, regional lymph node swelling, and secondary ulcerations.
- Pulmonary disease is a rare manifestation.
- Diagnosis is made by visualization on skin biopsy and culture.
- Although the lesions are rarely life threatening, treatment is usually indicated.
- **Oral itraconazole** (200 mg solution daily for 3 to 6 months) has largely replaced potassium iodide (1 to 2 drops three times daily for 3 to 6 months) as the treatment of choice.
- Pulmonary disease should be treated more aggressively because of its progressive nature.

Candidal Infections

- *Candida* spp. are normally present in the gastrointestinal tract. They are frequently recovered from bladder catheters, sputum, skin, and the female genital tract.
- Isolation of these organisms does not necessarily represent true infection.
- Pathological infections caused by *Candida* spp. can range from cutaneous to severe systemic disease.
- This discussion will focus only on frequently encountered outpatient infections.

Candiduria

- Candiduria is frequently observed but **rarely clinically significant.**
- Prior antibiotic use and genitourinary (GU) tract manipulation are risk factors for candiduria.

- **Treatment can be quite difficult and should be undertaken only in those with specific indications.** Without treatment, healthy patients generally clear their candiduria.
- Patients who should be treated are symptomatic patients (e.g., dysuria), neutropenic patients, transplant patients, and those undergoing GU tract manipulations.
- One should be mindful that candiduria can be a harbinger of disseminated disease in more severely ill patients.[35]
- **Fluconazole** 200 mg daily for 7 to 14 days will reduce the duration of candiduria. **Amphotericin B** may be needed in some instances.
- **Echinocandins do not penetrate the GU tract and should not be used.**

Oral Candidiasis

- Thrush is frequently seen in immunosuppressed patients, patients with diabetes, patients treated with antibiotics and inhaled corticosteroids, and children.
- It presents as curdlike patches on the tongue and buccal mucosa. Lesions can be scraped off leaving an erythematous lesion that may bleed.
- Esophageal disease may occur independently of oral disease and presents as severe odynophagia.
- Culture may be needed at times and can be misleading; clinical inspection is generally sufficient for diagnosis.
- Treatment with topical therapy such as **clotrimazole** troches (10 mg five times daily) and **nystatin** (4 to 6 mL of 100,000 units/mL qid) is generally effective.
- Oral **fluconazole** (100 mg daily for 7 to 14 days) may be needed for recurrent disease and is usually indicated at higher doses (200 to 400 mg daily) for esophageal disease.

Candidal Vaginitis

- Candidal vaginitis is a common infection occurring in patients with diabetes, with recent antibiotic use, and in pregnancy.
- Oral contraceptives may also increase the risk of colonization and cessation of oral contraceptives may be needed to cure recurrent cases.
- Patients present with dysuria, vaginal discharge, and erythema of the external genitalia.
- Visualization of yeast on a wet preparation of vaginal fluid aids in diagnosis.
- **Topical therapy** (e.g., nystatin, miconazole, clotrimazole, terconazole) is sufficient for uncomplicated disease.
- **Fluconazole** 150 mg for one dose is also an approved therapy but can be more expensive. Many patients will find it to be much more convenient.

Histoplasmosis

General Principles

- Histoplasmosis, caused by *Histoplasma capsulatum,* occurs worldwide, but in the United States infection is mostly seen in the Ohio and Mississippi River valleys.[36]
- Acute infection usually resolves within 1 month and patients recover in full with calcified nodules seen in the lungs on radiography.
- Acute infection can disseminate and complications may arise such as fibrosing mediastinitis, arthritis and arthralgias, hepatic involvement, and erythema nodosum.
- Clinical resolution appears to depend on cell-mediated immunity.

Diagnosis

- Diagnosis can be made by histopathologic visualization, growth in culture, or by high titers on complement fixation assays.

- Detection of antigenuria is useful primarily in disseminated disease and in patients with AIDS.

Treatment

- Treatment is usually not needed for mild to moderate disease.
- Persistent symptoms may require treatment, which can be accomplished with **itraconazole** 200 mg solution tid for 3 days and then once daily for 6 to 12 weeks.
- Severe disease requires initial treatment with **amphotericin B.**
- Chronic cavitary disease requires prolonged treatment with itraconazole and monitoring of drug levels.

Blastomycosis

General Principles

- Blastomycosis is caused by the dimorphic fungus *Blastomyces dermatitidis.*[37]
- It is commonly found in the southeast and south central United States as well as the Great Lakes region and territories around the St. Lawrence River.
- Patients acquire infection via inhalation of conidia from their natural environment.
- Acute infection mimics influenza or pneumonia.
- It can likewise present in an indolent fashion, being confused with TB or malignancy due to its ability to form mass like lesions.
- Extrapulmonary sites of infection include bone, skin, and the GU tract.
- Cutaneous involvement may be the only sign of infection, which consists of verrucous raised lesion on the upper extremities or face.

Diagnosis

- Diagnosis is based on isolation of the fungus in culture from a biopsy specimen.
- A presumptive diagnosis can be made on histopathological findings, revealing the classic **broad-based budding yeast.**
- Serologic testing is unreliable and plays a supportive role.

Treatment

- Treatment has reduced the mortality associated with blastomycosis from >90% to <10%.
- Mild to moderate disease can be treated with **itraconazole** (200 to 400 mg PO daily for a minimum of 2 months). Most patients require at least 6 months of therapy.
- Severe disease requires prolonged treatment with **amphotericin B,** which can be changed to itraconazole after the patient has improved.
- Given difficulties with absorption of itraconazole, one should consider monitoring drug levels.
- The oral solution has better absorption than tablets, which need to be taken with food or after drinking an acidic beverage.

Coccidioidomycosis

General Principles

- Coccidioidomycosis, otherwise known as "valley fever," is caused by *Coccidioides immitis* or *C. posadasii.*
- Infection is endemic to the southwestern region of the United States but is found elsewhere in the world as well.[38]

- Patients present 1 to 3 weeks after exposure with an acute illness indistinguishable from bacterial pneumonia that resolves spontaneously; however, some patients may experience prolonged fatigue.
- Patients with acute self-limited disease may have symptoms quite similar to a URI.
- Chronic disease or lung nodules may result in a minority of patients.
- Complications include dissemination to the central nervous system (CNS), skin, and bone. Patients may also have a rash similar to erythema multiforme or erythema nodosum.
- Latent infections and reactivation can occur in immunosuppressed patients.

Diagnosis

- Travel history aids in making a diagnosis in patients from nonendemic areas.
- Diagnosis is made by **culture** of the organism from a pulmonary sample.
- The microbiology laboratory should be notified if one is attempting to recover coccidioidomycoses through culture as this pathogen is a "select agent" per the CDC.
- **Serological testing** is quite helpful in making the diagnosis as well, being more reliable than serologies for other fungal infections.
- Chest radiographs can reveal multiple nodules with hilar adenopathy.

Treatment

- Acute infection in otherwise healthy individuals does not necessarily require treatment.
- Patients with immunosuppression, diabetes, or underlying cardiopulmonary disease should receive treatment.
  - **Itraconazole or fluconazole** at doses of 200 to 400 mg daily for 3 to 6 months should suffice.
  - For severe disease or disease in pregnancy, **amphotericin B** is the treatment of choice.

Cryptococcosis

General Principles

- Cryptococcosis is caused by *Cryptococcus neoformans,* a yeast distributed throughout the world in soil.[39]
- Various other species exist but rarely cause disease in humans.
- Infection begins with inhalation of spores.
- Pulmonary infection presents as cough, fever, dyspnea, and multiple nodular lung densities.
- Pregnant women can have a more complicated course with pulmonary disease.
- *C. neoformans* has a propensity to spread to the CNS.
- Meningitis commonly occurs and all patients with pulmonary disease should have a lumbar puncture performed to evaluate for CNS disease.
- Patients with CNS disease can present in various forms, but generally all patients complain of severe headache.
- Immunosuppression is an important risk factor for disseminated disease.

Diagnosis

- Diagnosis is made by **culture** or positive **cryptococcal antigen** titer on the serum or cerebral spinal fluid.
- These tests have largely replaced India ink preparations to identify encapsulated yeast.

- Patients who undergo lumbar puncture should have the opening pressure documented and it should not be reduced by >50% so as to avoid developing intracranial hypotension.

Treatment

- Treatment for pulmonary disease is with **fluconazole** 200 to 400 mg daily for 6 to 12 months. Itraconazole would be a second-line agent.
- Treatment of disseminated cryptococcal disease should be conducted with the aid of a specialist.
  - First-line treatment is with **amphotericin B and flucytosine** with subsequent prolonged induction therapy and long-term suppressive therapy with fluconazole.

TUBERCULOSIS

Active Tuberculosis

General Principles

- Renewed interest in TB control has arisen in light of the increasing prevalence of multidrug (MDR-TB) and the emergence of extensively drug-resistant tuberculosis (XDR-TB).
- TB is a systemic disease caused by *Mycobacterium tuberculosis.*
- Pulmonary disease is the most frequent clinical presentation but other sites such as lymphadenitis, GU disease, osteomyelitis, meningitis, peritonitis, pericarditis, and miliary dissemination may occur.
- TB is more common among debilitated and otherwise immunocompromised patients (e.g., alcoholics and patients with AIDS).
- The prevalence of TB is highest amongst immigrants from Asia, Africa, the Pacific Islands, and Latin America.

Diagnosis

- Diagnosis is established by **nucleic acid amplification** or by **culture** of the organism from sputum, sterile fluids, urine, or tissue.
- Appropriate response to therapy is another means of diagnosis in culture-negative disease.
- All positive cultures should be submitted for sensitivity testing.
- Sputum samples should be obtained on three separate days from morning samples.
- Gastric aspirates may be obtained from children who are too young to produce sputum.
- Positive smears for acid-fast bacilli are indicative of disease but one must confirm disease by nucleic acid amplification or culture methods.
- Hospitalized patients should be placed in respiratory isolation until the concern for disease has abated.
- Patients need not be hospitalized to evaluate for active TB so long as they are reliable, have an adequate home environment, and are compliant with wearing an N95 mask.

Treatment

- Treatment should be undertaken with the guidance of an expert and may include hospitalization to initiate therapy, patient education, and respiratory isolation.
- Treatment guidelines are available through the American Thoracic Society (www.thoracic.org) and the Infectious Diseases Society of America (www.idsociety.org).

- The local health department should be notified of all cases of TB so that contacts can be identified and arrangements for directly observed therapy (DOT) can be made.
- **Initial multidrug therapy is a cornerstone of therapy** given the emergence of drug resistance, and extended therapy is necessary because of the prolonged generation time of mycobacteria (>20 hours).
- Initial therapy includes **isoniazid** (INH) at 5 mg/kg/day (maximum 300 mg daily), **rifampin** at 10 mg/kg/day (maximum 600 mg daily), **pyrazinamide** at 15 to 20 mg/kg/day (maximum 2 g daily), and **ethambutol** at 15 to 20 mg/kg/day.
  - To minimize toxicities, supplemental pyridoxine should be provided (10 to 50 mg daily). Intermittent therapy can be given after 2 to 8 weeks of initial therapy.
  - Once susceptibility results are known and the patient has completed 8 weeks of initial therapy, therapy can be simplified to INH and rifampin if no resistance to these agents is present.
  - DOT is strongly encouraged for all patients and intermittent therapy should only be given by DOT.
  - Response to therapy should be monitored by following sputum samples every 2 weeks until culture is negative.
  - The standard treatment course is 6 months. Patients with cavitary disease who have a positive culture at 2 months of therapy should receive 9 months of treatment.
- Treatment of MDR-TB and XDR-TB requires a TB expert.
- Extrapulmonary disease can be treated in generally the same manner as pulmonary disease but requires therapy for 1 year in the case of TB meningitis or bone disease.
- Corticosteroid therapy may be required in life-threatening complications such as meningitis and pericarditis.
- Immunosuppressed patients should be treated with the same regimen but may also require prolonged therapy.
  - HIV-positive patients require treatment under the supervision of an expert in the field of HIV and TB coinfection given the complexity of the disease and drug interactions.

Latent Tuberculosis

Screening

- Screening for latent TB infection is done by tuberculin skin testing (PPD, also known as the Mantoux test) or by interferon-gamma release assays.
- A positive PPD or interferon-gamma release assays without active disease is indicative of latent TB infection (LTBI).
- The current approach to screening emphasizes targeted tuberculin testing among persons at highest risk for recent LTBI or with clinical conditions that increase the risk for TB.
  - These groups are most likely to benefit from treatment regardless of age. Testing is discouraged among persons at lower risk for TB.[40]
- **Criteria for a positive PPD are as follows**[41]:
  - **Five-millimeter induration:** patients with HIV infection, contacts of a known TB case, patients with chest radiographs that are typical for TB, and patients with organ transplants or other immunosuppressed patients (receiving the equivalent of ≥15 mg of prednisone daily for 1 month or more).

- **Ten-millimeter induration:** recent (≤5 years) immigrants from endemic areas, injection drug users, residents and employees of high-risk congregate settings (homeless shelters, prisons, nursing homes, hospitals, other long-term facilities for the elderly and persons with AIDS), mycobacteriology laboratory personnel, patients with chronic medical illnesses (e.g., silicosis, diabetes, end-stage renal disease, leukemia/lymphoma, malabsorption, low body weight), and children <4 years of age or infants, children, and adolescents exposed to adults at high risk.
- **Fifteen-millimeter induration:** individuals who are not in a high-prevalence group (and therefore who should not have been tested).

Treatment of Latent Tuberculosis Infection

Treatment of LTBI is with INH 5 mg/kg/day (maximum 300 mg) with pyridoxine (10 to 50 mg daily) for **9 months** in all persons **regardless of age** who:
- Develop a PPD test conversion (10-mm increase) within 2 years of a previously negative PPD.
- Have a positive PPD and are at high risk of developing active disease including the following:
  - Recent immigrants (within 5 years) from high-prevalence countries
  - Parenteral drug abusers
  - Patients with silicosis, diabetes mellitus, HIV/AIDS, or end-stage renal disease
  - Individuals with hematologic, lymphoreticular, or head and neck or lung malignancy
  - Conditions associated with rapid weight loss or chronic malnutrition
  - Patients who are receiving chronic immunosuppressive therapy equivalent to 15 mg prednisone daily.
  - Patients with a 5-mm reaction and are household members or close contacts of patients with active disease.
- Contacts with high risk for TB but a negative PPD, particularly children, should also be treated, but treatment can be stopped if a repeat PPD at 10 weeks is negative.
- Untreated contacts with a nonreactive PPD should have a repeat PDD after 10 weeks.
- All patients should be informed that they should discontinue INH and seek medical care if anorexia or nausea develops.
- No >1 month's worth of medication should be dispensed at a time.
- Monthly monitoring for signs and symptoms of disease is indicated for all patients who are prescribed INH.
- For persons with risk factors for hepatotoxicity (e.g., underlying liver disease, daily alcohol use, HIV, pregnancy or postpartum, or use of other potentially hepatotoxic drugs), monthly monitoring of the transaminases is indicated, with discontinuation of INH for elevations greater than three times the upper limit of normal if associated with symptoms and five times the upper limit of normal if asymptomatic.
- Alternative therapies include the following:
  - Weekly INH 900 mg twice weekly by DOT
  - Rifampin 600 mg daily for 4 months being mindful of drug interactions.
  - The combination of rifampin and pyrazinamide for 2 months is no longer recommended because of the risk of serious hepatotoxicity.
- Treatment of LTBI after MDR-TB and XDR-TB exposure is a complex issue and should be undertaken with the guidance of a TB expert. Options range from treatment with alternative agents for 6 to 12 months to observation for low-risk patients.

TICK-BORNE DISEASE

- Common tick-borne diseases in the United States include **ehrlichiosis, anaplasmosis, Lyme disease, Rocky Mountain spotted fever (RMSF), and babesiosis.** Each is endemic in various geographical regions based on tick distribution.
- **Knowledge of disease distribution and patient travel history to endemic areas is important to diagnosis.**
- When identified early, they have relatively minimal complications; however, when the diagnosis is delayed, serious complications and death may develop.[42]
- Other diseases transmitted by ticks within the United States include the following:
  - **Colorado tick fever:** a Coltivirus infection transmitted by the wood tick *Dermacentor andersoni.*
  - **Tick-borne relapsing fever:** *Borrelia* spp. infection transmitted by *Ornithodoros* spp. ticks.
  - **Tularemia:** acquisition of *Francisella tularensis* via ticks is just one of many means of inoculation and it is thought to be the most common way Americans contract the disease.
  - **Tick paralysis:** caused by tick salivary neurotoxins rather than by transmission of a microbial infection. Many tick species have been implicated.
- **Southern tick-associated rash illness** is an entity that can strongly resemble Lyme disease but typically occurs in areas where Lyme disease is uncommon. While presently **unproven,** many presume the cause to be *Borrelia lonestari* transmitted by the Lone Star tick, *Amblyomma americanum.* In spite of the name, it also occurs in the Mid-Atlantic states and the Midwest. There is currently no diagnostic test.
- Tick-borne diseases peak in the spring through fall but can occur any time during the year.

Lyme Disease

General Principles

- Lyme disease is caused by *B. burgdorferi.* There are additional pathogenic species in other parts of the world.
- Lyme disease was first identified in Connecticut in the 1970s and pockets of infection have been seen **throughout the northeastern United States as well as north central states** (mainly Wisconsin).
- It is transmitted by the tick *Ixodes scapularis.* Rodents and deer provide additional animal reservoirs.
- The acute form is most common but some patients may develop more chronic disease in untreated.
- The post-Lyme disease syndrome consists of chronic/recurrent subjective constitutional symptoms (e.g., fatigue, malaise, headache, arthralgia, myalgias, and poor concentration) after appropriately treated Lyme disease. It is not felt to be a manifestation of persistent infection.[43]

Diagnosis

- Diagnosis of acute disease centers on clinical presentation with appropriate tick exposures.
  - **Many patients do not recall a specific tick bite;** therefore, known tick bites are not necessary for making the diagnosis.

- **Acute forms** of the disease are characterized by a rash (**erythema chronicum migrans, ECM**) occurring 7 to 10 days after tick exposure.
  - Classically, this rash has central clearing; however, this may not always be seen.
  - In addition to the ECM rash, patients may develop fevers, constitutional symptoms, and adenopathy.
  - If left untreated, complications may include facial nerve paralysis, myocardial involvement, and arthritis.
- **Chronic forms** (i.e., not previously treated) of disease may present as heart block, chronic oligoarthritis, subacute encephalopathy, or axonal polyneuropathy.
- **ELISA antibody testing is an appropriate test for those with a potentially compatible clinical picture but false-positives are frequent.** Serology should not be used as a "screening test" in unselected populations.
  - **Positive ELISA must be confirmed by Western blot analysis.**
  - Serology alone should not be the sole means of diagnosis.
  - At the time of presentation with ECM many patients will be seronegative only later developing manifesting an appropriate immunologic response, at the time of early-disseminated disease.
  - Early antibiotic treatment may prevent seroconversion.
- Culture is rarely indicated.

Treatment

- **First-line treatment of acute disease is with doxycycline** (100 mg PO twice daily) for 14 days to prevent development of late manifestations of disease and allow more rapid resolution of disease.[42]
- Doxycycline has the added advantage of effectively treating *Anaplasma phagocytophilum* (see below).
- Alternative agents include amoxicillin and cefuroxime.
- Some patients may initially experience a Jarisch-Herxheimer reaction.
- Those with meningitis and/or carditis require more aggressive treatment.
- For untreated chronic Lyme disease, 28 days of doxycycline should be adequate therapy.
- Much controversy exists over the management and treatment of post-Lyme disease syndromes. Antibiotics do not appear to be beneficial.[43]

Rocky Mountain Spotted Fever

General Principles

- RMSF fever is caused by *Rickettsia rickettsii*.
- It was originally isolated from the northern regions of the Rocky Mountains in the United States; however, **disease is most prevalent in the Atlantic coastal states and south central United States.**
- It is transmitted by the dog tick *Dermacentor variabilis*.[42]
- Disease begins 5 to 7 days after tick exposure.

Diagnosis

- Diagnosis rests largely on the clinical syndrome.
- Patients present with rash and fever.
  - **The rash begins typically on the 3rd to 5th day of symptoms as a maculopapular eruption (then becomes petechial), on the extremities often involving the palms and soles, and progresses toward the trunk.**

- Patients can present with marked constitutional symptoms (e.g., fever, malaise, fatigue, arthralgia, myalgia, headache, anorexia, nausea, and emesis) before the rash develops.
- A minority of patients never develop the characteristic rash (i.e., "spotless").
- A history of tick exposure in this setting is sufficient to initiate treatment.
- Left untreated, patients can develop severe disease with meningeal involvement, respiratory failure, and renal dysfunction.
- **Acute and convalescent serologies** can confirm the diagnosis.
- Direct immunofluorescence of skin lesions can aid in diagnosis.
- Additional laboratory abnormalities may include elevated transaminases, leukopenia, and thrombocytopenia. All may be seen in ehrlichiosis and anaplasmosis adding further difficulty in differentiation.
- PCR techniques are under development.

Treatment

- Early treatment (often before the rash develops) reduces overall mortality.
- **Doxycycline** (100 mg bid) should be initiated promptly when disease is suspected.
- Patients severely ill with RMSF require hospital admission.

Ehrlichiosis and Anaplasmosis

General Principles

- Human granulocytic **anaplasmosis** is caused by **A. phagocytophilum** and is transmitted by *Ixodes* spp. It is commonly found in the northeastern parts of the United States. It is more common than ehrlichiosis.
- Human monocytic **ehrlichiosis** is caused by **Ehrlichia chaffeensis** and is transmitted by the Lone Star tick, *Amblyomma americanum*. Human monocytic ehrlichiosis occurs in the south central, southeastern, and Mid-Atlantic states. A few cases have been reported elsewhere.
- Rare cases of human granulocytic ehrlichiosis due to *E. ewingii* have been reported, mostly in immunocompromised (e.g., HIV) patients.
- More severe infection appears to occur in the immunocompromised patients.
- Coinfection with anaplasmosis and Lyme disease can occur.[43]
- Disease caused by these two agents is relatively similar and only recently have further distinctions between the two processes become known.

Diagnosis

- There is a wide spectrum of illness, including subclinical infection.
- Symptomatic patients present with a nonspecific febrile illness (e.g., malaise, fatigue, myalgias, and headache) after tick exposure.
- **Rash is much less common than with RMSF,** particularly so with human granulocytic anaplasmosis.
- Neurologic symptoms and signs are also possible.
- Severe complications include seizure, coma, renal failure, cardiopulmonary failure, and clinical picture similar to the systemic inflammatory response syndrome.
- **Common laboratory findings include thrombocytopenia, leukopenia, and elevated transaminases**—all possible in RMSF as well.
- Diagnosis is made by **acute and convalescent serologies.**
- **PCR** testing is available with good sensitivity and specificity when obtained prior to administration of antimicrobial therapy.

- As these organisms are typically found within macrophages, a peripheral smear showing intracellular morulae may be seen, aiding in the diagnosis.

Treatment
- The mainstay of treatment is **doxycycline** 100 mg bid for 10 days, which is also effective for the frequent alternative diagnosis of RMSF and possible coexistent Lyme disease.
- Patients should rapidly respond to therapy.
- Rifampin therapy (300 mg PO twice daily) can be used as an alternative in less severe anaplasmosis; however, one must be mindful of coinfection with babesiosis or Lyme disease as rifampin will not treat these.[43]

Babesiosis

General Principles
- Babesiosis, a malarialike illness, is caused by the intraerythrocytic parasite, *Babesia microti,* and is found in the northeastern United States. It is transmitted by *I. scapularis.*
- Blood transfusion is also a possible means of infection.
- Cases have been identified elsewhere within the United States. Interestingly, disease in Europe occurs in asplenic patients, whereas infection in the United States usually occurs in patients with intact spleens, although severe disease can result in asplenic patients from the United States.[42,43]
- The majority of infections in immunocompetent hosts are probably asymptomatic.
- Severe disease can occur in immunosuppressed patients and asplenic patients.
- Possible coinfection with Lyme disease and ehrlichiosis should be considered.

Diagnosis
- In symptomatic patients fever, malaise, and headache begin 1 week after tick exposure.
- Severe hemolytic anemia, renal failure, and hypotension can develop in some patients.
- Hepatosplenomegaly may occur.
- Laboratory findings include those compatible with hemolysis (e.g., anemia, abnormal red cell morphology, elevated lactic dehydrogenase, and decreased haptoglobin), thrombocytopenia, elevated transaminases, and hyperbilirubinemia.
- Diagnosis can be made by identification of ring forms on blood smear.
- Serological assays can be of benefit.

Treatment
- First-line therapy is with **atovaquone** (750 mg PO every 12 hours) **plus azithromycin** (500 to 1,000 mg on day 1 and then 250 mg PO daily) **or clindamycin** (300 to 600 mg every 8 hours) for 7 to 10 days.[42,43]
- Severe disease should be treated with quinine plus clindamycin. Close monitoring for side effects from quinine, including cinchonism, is necessary.

FEVER OF UNKNOWN ORIGIN

- Petersdorf and Beeson[44] classically defined fever of unknown origin (FUO) in their landmark 1961 article.
  - Temperature must be >38.3°C on several occasions over a period >3 weeks with a diagnosis remaining uncertain after 1 week of hospitalization.

- Given the changes in delivery of medical care, the requirement for hospitalization has become less stringent.
- Finding the correct diagnosis in these situations can be challenging and it is of utmost importance to **avoid excessive and unnecessary testing as well as empiric antimicrobial therapy.** Both of these errors can be misleading and cause increased morbidity for the patient.
  - **So long as the patient is not acutely ill, there is no need to rush to empiric therapy.** Reassurance should be provided to the patient.
- Case series suggest >200 potential causes. A systematic approach to evaluate for more common causes of FUO is important and an algorithm has been proposed by Mourad et al.[45]
- Commonly, disease has been classified into three categories.

Malignancy

- Of the many potential malignant causes of fever, lymphoma is probably the most common.
- Leukemia and renal cell carcinoma are also commonly implicated.
- For this reason, CT scanning of the chest, abdomen, and pelvis may be of benefit.
- In addition, bone marrow biopsy can be considered.

Connective Tissue Diseases/Vasculitis

- Multiple various autoimmune diseases have been implicated in causing FUO.
- Rheumatoid arthritis and systemic lupus erythematosus are common causes and frequently screening with tests for antinuclear antibodies and rheumatoid factor may be indicated.
- Results of CT scanning may provide clues to accessible lesions for biopsy as well.

Infectious

- The list of potential infections is quite lengthy.
- TB should be ruled out early in the evaluation.
- Subacute endocarditis is another frequent cause.
- Blood cultures should be obtained in sterile fashion on multiple occasions while the patient is free of all antimicrobials.
- Echocardiogram can be useful in evaluating for cardiac vegetations.

Other

- Frequently, a medication that the patient is already taking may be the cause of fever.
- Any nonessential medications should be discontinued.
- Blood clots are another frequent cause of fever and Doppler ultrasounds of the lower extremities may be helpful.

IMMUNOSUPPRESSION

- The topic of infections in a non-HIV infected patient with immunocompromise is quite complex and cannot be covered in its entirety in the scope of this chapter.
- This section aims to give a brief overview of common infections in this population as well as when to suspect immunodeficiencies in adult patients.
- Many patients who have undergone transplantation (solid organ or bone marrow) remain under close supervision of the transplant team. This is especially true in the

highly vulnerable and complex posttransplantation period, which can last up to 1 year after transplant.
- Much disease is managed by or with the help of specialists. Severe disease can develop quickly and care frequently requires an inpatient setting.

Antitumor Necrosis Factor Agents

- Immune modulating therapy has become commonplace in control of various autoimmune processes.
- Tumor necrosis factor (TNF) is a major cytokine in the control of disease but its misdirection is thought to be involved in the pathophysiology of inflammatory disorders.
- TNF seems to exert its effect by activating natural killer cells and CD8+ lymphocytes.
- Using a loose definition of a serious infection as any infection requiring antimicrobial therapy or hospitalization, Bongartz et al[46] found an odds ratio of 2.0 favoring serious infections in patients receiving anti-TNF agents compared with placebo.
- The most concerning infection in patients receiving anti-TNF agents is that of reactivating TB.
  - Patients should have PPD testing performed before initiating therapy with anti-TNF agents.
  - Should they have a PPD ≥5 mm, therapy for latent infection (after active infection has been ruled out) should be initiated before starting anti-TNF therapy.
  - There is no need to delay anti-TNF therapy until treatment of latent infection has been completed.

Primary Immunodeficiencies

- One of the more challenging diagnoses for clinicians is that of primary immunodeficiencies. These relatively common processes tend to have obscure presentations and are frequently overlooked as potential underlying disease states. In addition, their complexity and various forms are difficult to fully comprehend.
- Often times, simple treatments such as monthly intravenous immune globulin can reduce the number of infections that patients endure.[47]

Deficiencies in B Cell Function and Antibody Production

- These conditions are relatively common.
- Patients typically present with recurrent sinopulmonary disease.
- Other presenting features include sarcoidlike illness, recurrent viral meningitis, autoimmune cytopenias, bronchiectasis, and chronic enteropathy.
- Recurrent infections with encapsulated organisms (e.g., streptococci) are another clue.
- Primary B cell dysfunction may be a cause of failure to respond to vaccines.
- **Common variable immunodeficiency** is perhaps the most important primary immune deficiency of adults and its etiology is based on various defects in B cell differentiation and varying degrees of T cell dysfunction.
- Other diseases in this class of deficiency include **IgA deficiency** (also quite common), hyper-IgM syndrome, Good's syndrome, and individual IgG subclass deficiencies. The latter conditions tend to be relatively asymptomatic.
- When suspected, a simple screen of immunoglobulin levels can be helpful in identifying underlying processes.

- Additional testing of immune globulin subsets or specific vaccine responses can further delineate the diagnosis.
- Treatment by monthly intravenous immune globulin injections can reduce the number of recurrent infections.

Complement Deficiencies

- Complement deficiencies are somewhat common and can present in adulthood.
- Patients present with recurrent or severe neisserial infections or a lupuslike illness.
- C1 esterase deficiency is otherwise known as hereditary angioedema.
- Mannose-binding lectin deficiency, another component of complement, becomes apparent in various predisposing situations such as patients with HIV, common variable immunodeficiency, and postchemotherapy.
- Screening for these processes can be simply accomplished by testing total complement levels. More detailed testing may be necessary to uncover the exact deficiency.

Other Immunodeficiencies

- Adults can present with primary deficiencies commonly uncovered in childhood such as adenine deaminase deficiency, Job's syndrome (hyper-IgE syndrome), chronic granulomatous disease, and leukocyte adhesion defects.
- The presentation of these processes is quite diverse.
- Recurrent pyogenic abscesses can be one clue.
- Opportunistic infections may lead to additional testing as well in HIV-negative patients.
- Testing of lymphocyte and neutrophil function may be necessary as defects in cytokine production or oxidative bursts can be easily identified and can uncover the deficiency.
- Age should not be an absolute factor in ruling out such diseases.
- Recurrent mycobacterial infections or Salmonella infections may lead one to suspect a deficiency in interferon-γ. This group of genetic disorders is quite rare.

REFERENCES

1. Avorn J, Solomon DH. Cultural and economic factors that (mis)shape antibiotic use: the nonpharmacologic basis of therapeutics. *Ann Intern Med* 2000;133:128–135.
2. Piccirillo JF. Acute bacterial sinusitis. *N Engl J Med* 2004;351:902–910.
3. Snow V, Mottur-Pilson C, Hickner JM. Principles of appropriate antibiotic use for acute sinusitis in adults. *Ann Intern Med* 2001;134:495–497.
4. Fokkens W, Lund V, Bachert C, et al. EAACI position paper on rhinosinusitis and nasal polyps executive summary. *Allergy* 2005;60:583–601.
5. Hamilos D. Chronic sinusitis. *J Allergy Clin Immunol* 2000;106:213–227.
6. Ah-See KW, Evans AS. Sinusitis and its management. *BMJ* 2007;334:358–361.
7. Bisno AL, Gerber MA, Gwaltney JM Jr, et al. Practice guidelines for the diagnosis and management of group a streptococcal pharyngitis. *Clin Infect Dis* 2002;35:113–125.
8. Pichichero ME. Group A beta-hemolytic streptococcal infections. *Pediatr Rev* 1998;19:291–302.
9. Wenzel RP, Fowler III AA. Acute bronchitis. *N Engl J Med* 2006;355:2125–2130.
10. Centers for Disease Control and Prevention (CDC). Pertussis—United States, 2001–2003. *MMWR Morb Mortal Wkly Rep* 2005;54:1283–1286.
11. Couch RB. Prevention and treatment of influenza. *N Engl J Med* 2000;343:1778–1787.
12. Call SA, Vollenweider MA, Hornung CA, et al. Does this patient have influenza? *JAMA* 2005;293:987–997.
13. Advisory Committee on Immunization Practices, Smith NM, Bresee JS, Shay DK, et al. Prevention and control of influenza: recommendations of the Advisory Committee on Immunization Practices (ACIP). *MMWR Recomm Rep* 2006;55:1–42.

14. Mandell LA, Wunderink RG, Anqueto A, et al. Infectious Diseases Society of America/American Thoracic Society consensus guidelines on the management of community-acquired pneumonia in adults. *Clin Infect Dis* 2007;44:S27–S72.

15. Fine MJ, Auble TE, Yealy DM, et al. A prediction rule to identify low-risk patients with community-acquired pneumonia. *N Engl J Med* 1997;336:243–250.

16. Auwaerter PG. Infectious mononucleosis: return to play. *Clin Sports Med* 2004;23:485–497.

17. Kimberlin DW, Whitley RJ. Varicella-zoster vaccine for the prevention of herpes zoster. *N Engl J Med* 2007;356:1338–1343.

18. Dworkin RH, Johnson RW, Breuer J, et al. Recommendations for the management of herpes zoster. *Clin Infect Dis* 2007;44:S1–S26.

19. Oxman MN, Levin MJ, Johnson GR, et al. Shingles Prevention Study Group. A vaccine to prevent herpes zoster and postherpetic neuralgia in older adults. *N Engl J Med* 2005;352:2271–2284.

20. Harpaz R, Ortega-Sanchez IR, Seward JF. Advisory Committee on Immunization Practices (ACIP) Centers for Disease Control and Prevention (CDC). Prevention of herpes zoster: recommendations of the Advisory Committee on Immunization Practices (ACIP). *MMWR Recomm Rep* 2008;57:1–30.

21. Hill DR, Ericsson CD, Pearson RD, et al. The practice of travel medicine: guidelines by the Infectious Diseases Society of America. *Clin Infect Dis* 2006;43:1499–1539.

22. Griffith KS, Lewis LS, Mali S, Parise ME. Treatment of malaria in the United States. *JAMA* 2007;297:2264–2277.

23. Vugia D, Cronquist A, Hadler J, et al. Preliminary FoodNet data on the incidence of infection with pathogens transmitted commonly through food—10 States, 2006. *MMWR Mob Mortal Wkly Rep* 2007;56:336–339.

24. Bartlett JG. Narrative review: the new epidemic of Clostridium difficile-associated enteric disease. *Ann Intern Med* 2006;145:758–764.

25. Guerrant RL, Van Gilder T, Steiner TS, et al. Practice guidelines for the management of infectious diarrhea. *Clin Infect Dis* 2001;32:331–351.

26. Lew JF, Glass, RI, Gangarosa RE, et al. Diarrheal deaths in the United States, 1979 through 1987: a special problem for the elderly. *JAMA* 1991;265:3280–3284.

27. Thielman NM, Guerrant RL. Acute infectious diarrhea. *N Engl J Med* 2004;350:38–47.

28. Stevens DL, Bisno AL, Chambers HF, et al. Practice guidelines for the diagnosis and management of skin and soft-tissue infections. *Clin Infect Dis* 2005;41:1373–1406.

29. Hepburn MJ, Dooley DP, Skidmore PJ, et al. Comparison of short-course (5 days) and standard (10 days) treatment for uncomplicated cellulitis. *Arch Intern Med* 2004;164:1669–1674.

30. Moran GJ, Krishnadasan A, Gorwitz RJ, et al. Methicillin resistant S. aureus infections among patients in the emergency department. *N Engl J Med* 2006;355:666–674.

31. Daum RS. Skin and soft-tissue infections caused by methicillin-resistant Staphylococcus aureus. *N Engl J Med* 2007;357:380–390.

32. Fleisher GR. The management of bite wounds. *N Engl J Med* 1999;340:138–140.

33. Vetter RS, Bush SP. The diagnosis of brown recluse spider bite is overused for dermonecrotic wounds of uncertain etiology. *Ann Emerg Med* 2002;39:544–546.

34. Schwartz RA. Superficial fungal infections. *Lancet* 2004;364:1173–1182.

35. Pappas PG, Rex JH, Sobel JD, et al. Guidelines for treatment of candidiasis. *Clin Infect Dis* 2004;38:161–189.

36. Wheat LJ, Freifeld AG, Kleiman MB, et al. Clinical practice guidelines for the management of patients with histoplasmosis: 2007 update by the Infectious Diseases Society of America. *Clin Infect Dis* 2007;45:807–825.

37. Chapman SW, Brasher RW Jr, Campbell GD Jr, et al. Practice guidelines for the management of patients with blastomycosis. *Clin Infect Dis* 2000;30:679–683.

38. Galgiani JN, Ampel NM, Blair JE, et al. Coccidioidomycosis. *Clin Infect Dis* 2005;41:1217–1223.

39. Saag MS, Graybill RJ, Larsen RA, et al. Practice guidelines for the management of cryptococcal disease. *Clin Infect Dis* 2000;30:710–718.

40. Blumberg HM, Leonard MK Jr, Jasmer RM. Update on the treatment of tuberculosis and latent tuberculosis infection. *JAMA* 2005;293:2776–2784.

41. Targeted tuberculin testing and treatment of latent tuberculosis infection. American Thoracic Society. *MMWR Recomm Rep* 2000;49:1–51.

42. Spach DH, Liles WC, Campbell GL, et al. Tick-borne diseases in the United States. *N Engl J Med* 1993;329:936–947.

43. Wormser GP, Dattwyler RJ, Shapiro ED, et al. The clinical assessment, treatment, and prevention of Lyme disease, human granulocytic anaplasmosis, and babesiosis: clinical practice guidelines by the Infectious Diseases Society of America. *Clin Infect Dis* 2006;43:1089–1134.

44. Petersdorf RG, Beeson P. Fever of unexplained origin: report on 100 cases. *Medicine* 1961;40:1–30.

45. Mourad O, Palda V, Detsky AS. A comprehensive evidence-based approach to fever of unknown origin. *Arch Intern Med* 2003;163:545–551.

46. Bongartz T, Sutton AJ, Sweeting MJ, et al. Anti-TNF antibody therapy in rheumatoid arthritis and the risk of serious infections and malignancies. *JAMA* 2006;295:2275–2285.

47. Riminton DS, Limaye S. Primary immunodeficiency diseases in adulthood. *Int Med J* 2004;34:348–354.

23 Human Immunodeficiency Virus Infection and Sexually Transmitted Diseases

Hilary E. L. Reno and E. Turner Overton

HIV INFECTION AND AIDS

General Principles

- Human immunodeficiency virus (HIV) type 1 is a human retrovirus that infects T-lymphocytes and other cells that bear the CD4 surface marker. Infection leads to lymphopenia, CD4 lymphocyte deficiency and dysfunction, impaired cell-mediated immune response, and polyclonal B-cell activation with impaired B-cell responses to new antigens.
- This immune derangement gives rise to the acquired immunodeficiency syndrome (AIDS), which is characterized by opportunistic infections and unusual malignancies.
- Transmission is primarily by sexual and parenteral routes.
- Major risk groups therefore include sexual contacts of infected persons, intravenous (IV) drug users, and children born to HIV-infected mothers.
- Because management of HIV-infected patients is a complex and rapidly evolving field, **this viral infection is best managed in close coordination with an expert.** The information presented here is not intended as a substitute for expert care. Excellent sources of information for physicians who wish to familiarize themselves with HIV care include aidsinfo.nih.gov and hivinsite.ucsf.edu.

Diagnosis

- Patients with HIV infection may present acutely near the time of seroconversion or at a late stage with an AIDS-defining complication.
- Initial assessment of patients should be targeted to the determination of the degree of immunodeficiency with particular attention to the need for initiation of antiretroviral therapy and of prophylactic therapy against opportunistic infections.

Primary HIV Infection

- The **acute retroviral syndrome** often presents as a mononucleosislike syndrome with fever as the most common presenting symptom in >75% of patients.
- Other common symptoms include headache, rash, fatigue, and lymphadenopathy.
- Initial infection with HIV type 1 less commonly presents with neurologic manifestations such as aseptic meningitis, Guillain-Barré syndrome, spinal vacuolar myelopathy, peripheral neuropathy, and subacute encephalitis.
- As many as 90% of patients who are acutely infected with HIV experience at least some symptoms of the acute retroviral syndrome and can thus be identified as candidates for early therapy.

- Acute HIV infection is often not recognized in the primary care setting, however, because of the nonspecific nature of the symptoms. Maintaining a high index of suspicion and knowing the appropriate testing modality are critical for diagnosis at this time period. **Routine HIV tests are antibody assays and are often negative or nonreactive in this early phase while circulating viral RNA is extremely high.**

Initial Assessment

- For persons who are chronically infected, many patients are asymptomatic at the time of diagnosis.
- In some, recurrent oral candidiasis, lymphadenopathy, weight loss, fevers, night sweats, and chronic diarrhea may develop. History and physical examination should focus on such complications.
- Abnormal laboratory findings may include anemia, thrombocytopenia, leukopenia, hypertriglyceridemia, low high-density lipoprotein cholesterol levels, and elevated immunoglobulin levels.
- **The most important initial laboratory tests are measurement of the CD4 T-lymphocyte count** (normal range for adults is 600 to 1,500 cells/mm^3) **and HIV RNA viral load.**
- Given that HIV drug resistance is transmitted as much as 20% of the time, an **HIV genotype** should also be performed at baseline to evaluate for critical mutations.
- As HIV is a sexually transmitted disease, it is important to **evaluate for other sexually transmitted diseases** (STDs) including gonorrhea, Chlamydia, syphilis, and the viral hepatitides.
- It is also important to have **baseline blood counts, urinalysis, metabolic parameters, and lipid values** to monitor for complications of HIV and for possible medication toxicities.
- Finally, all HIV-infected persons should have a **baseline and yearly PPD** to screen for tuberculosis.

Treatment

Antiretrovirals

- Treatment of HIV includes specific antiretroviral therapy as well as prevention and treatment of opportunistic infections.[1]
- **Patients who should be started on antiretroviral therapy include the following:**
  - Patients with a history of an AIDS defining illness regardless of CD4 count or viral load.
  - Symptomatic patients with any CD4 count.
  - Asymptomatic patients with CD4 <200 cells/mm^3.
- Patients who should be offered treatment include asymptomatic patients with CD4 count of 201 to 350 cells/mm^3.
- Most authorities would defer treatment to asymptomatic patients with CD4 >350 cells/mm^3 but may offer treatment if the viral load is >100,000 copies.
- Treatment in other patients may be deferred with close follow-up.
- It is imperative to send a baseline genotype test to assist in selection of antiretroviral drugs as 1/5 of naïve patients will have resistance to at least one agent at baseline.
- **Typical highly active antiretroviral therapy (HAART) regimens** for initial therapy consist of a triple drug combination: nonnucleoside reverse transcriptase inhibitors or protease inhibitors **plus** a pair of nucleoside reverse transcriptase inhibitors.
- Choice and use of these agents are beyond the scope of this manual. However, the primary care physician who is treating patients with HIV disease, in conjunction

| TABLE 1 | Typical HAART Regimens |

One of the following NNRTI or PI
Efavirenz (NNRTI)
Fosamprenavir (PI) plus ritonavir (PI)[a]
Lopinavir (PI) plus ritonavir (PI)[a]
Atazanavir (PI) plus ritonavir (PI)[a]

With one of the following pairs of NRTI
Tenofovir plus emtricitabine
Abacavir plus lamivudine
Zidovudine plus lamivudine

[a]The addition of ritonavir is used to boost the level of the PI it is given with.
HAART, highly active antiretroviral therapy; NNRTI, nonnucleoside reverse transcriptase inhibitor; NRTI, nucleoside reverse transcriptase inhibitor; PI, protease inhibitor.
Modified from Panel on Clinical Practices for the Treatment of HIV Infection. Guidelines for the use of antiretroviral agents in HIV-1-infected adults and adolescents. 2006;1–139.

with an HIV expert, should familiarize himself or herself with the toxicities of these agents and drug-drug interactions to avoid them (Table 1).

Prophylactic Measures

- Prophylactic treatment against various organisms is recommended for HIV-infected patients, largely influenced by the CD4 count.[2]
- **Prophylaxis against pneumocystis pneumonia (PCP)** is indicated when the CD4 count is <200 cells/mm^3, when the percent of CD4 lymphocytes is <20% of the total lymphocyte count, or if the patient has thrush regardless of CD4 count. Appropriate regimens are trimethoprim-sulfamethoxazole (TMP-SMZ) one double strength tablet daily or dapsone, 100 mg daily.
- **Prophylaxis against toxoplasmosis** (TMP-SMX for PCP is adequate) is indicated when the CD4 count is <100 cells/mm^3.
- For patients with CD4 counts of <50 cells/mm^3, weekly azithromycin (1,200 mg) should be given as prophylaxis against infection with ***Mycobacterium avium* complex** (MAC).
- For patients with CD4 counts <50 cells/mm^3, eye examinations should be conducted to evaluate for **cytomegalovirus (CMV) retinitis.**
- If immune reconstitution with HAART occurs with sustained CD4 counts of >200 cells/mm^3, PCP and MAC prophylaxis can be discontinued.
- **Immunizations** such as annual influenza vaccine, pneumococcal vaccine, and, for hepatitis B virus (HBV)-seronegative patients, HBV vaccine should also be offered, although immunologic response with CD4 counts <200 cells/mm^3 may be poor.[3]
- HIV is an STD and therefore the Centers for Disease Control and Prevention (CDC) recommends **annual screening for other STDs** including gonorrhea, Chlamydia, and syphilis.
- Female patients with HIV should receive **screening for cervical cancer** with pap smears at least annually.
- **Because TB is an important complication of HIV infection, screening is warranted at the time of initial assessment.** Patients often become anergic as the degree of immune deficiency

progresses. Chest radiography should be performed as an alternative diagnostic procedure.

Complications

Viral Infections

Cytomegalovirus Reactivation

- CMV reactivation is common in patients with advanced AIDS (CD4 <100 cells/mm^3).
- Manifestations include viremia with fever and constitutional symptoms, chorioretinitis, esophagitis, gastritis, enterocolitis, pancreatitis, acalculous cholecystitis, bone marrow suppression, necrotizing adrenalitis, and upper and lower respiratory tract infections.
- End organ disease is seen most often when CD4 cell counts are <50 cells/mm^3.
- **Ganciclovir,** 5 mg/kg IV, or **valganciclovir,** 900 mg PO every 12 hours, is effective induction therapy for chorioretinitis and gastrointestinal (GI) disease but is associated with significant hematologic toxicity.[2]
  - Relapse after discontinuation of the drug is common, usually necessitating maintenance therapy until sustained immune reconstitution occurs with CD4 counts of >100 cells/mm^3 for 6 months.
  - It is imperative to monitor blood cell counts while on therapy and discontinuation of zidovudine or other immunosuppressive agents may be required when severe neutropenia develops.
  - Concomitant granulocyte colony-stimulating factor can be used as a possible means of ameliorating ganciclovir myelotoxicity.
- Patients with retinitis who are intolerant of systemic ganciclovir may benefit from intravitreal administration of the drug by an experienced ophthalmologist.
- Foscarnet is indicated for patients who have a documented ganciclovir-resistant CMV strain or who are failing ganciclovir therapy.

Other Herpesviridae

- **Herpes simplex virus-2** (HSV-2), but not HSV-1, has been identified more commonly in HIV-infected persons than in HIV negative individuals.
  - HSV-2 likely facilitates the transmission of HIV by providing a portal of entry (i.e., the genital ulcer) and by increasing HIV viral shedding in the genital tract.
  - Coinfection with HSV-2 has also been found to speed the progression of HIV to AIDS.
- HSV infection has been associated with esophagitis, proctitis, pulmonary disease, and large, atypical, persistent cutaneous ulcerations.
  - **IV acyclovir** is usually effective for these problems but relapses are frequent and persons may require chronic HSV suppression.[2]
- **Varicella-zoster virus** (VZV) may cause typical dermatomal lesions or may disseminate. Recurrent disease, meningoencephalitis, and cranial neuritis have been reported.
  - **Acyclovir,** 800 mg 5 times/day, or **famciclovir,** 500 mg tid, is the treatment of choice.
- Evidence of **Epstein-Barr virus** (EBV) infection is common in patients with AIDS, particularly oral hairy leukoplakia, a benign condition on the lateral aspect of the tongue.
  - Oral **acyclovir** may be effective but should be reserved for symptomatic cases.
  - EBV is also associated with CNS lymphomas in persons with advanced AIDS (generally CD4 count <50 cells/mm^3). In the face of immunodeficiency, EBV leads to this malignant clonal expansion of B cells.
  - Effective therapy for these EBV-related malignancies includes HAART.

JC Virus

- JC virus is a papovavirus that is associated with **progressive multifocal leukoencephalopathy.**
- Progressive multifocal leukoencephalopathy is characterized by progressive neurologic deficits including altered mental status, visual loss, weakness, and abnormalities of gait. The presenting symptoms depend on the location of the lesions.
- Nonenhancing hypodense lesions are seen on computerized tomography (CT) of the brain, but magnetic resonance imaging (MRI) is more sensitive and often reveals multifocal areas of white matter demyelinating lesions that do not conform to cerebrovascular territories.
- Polymerase chain reaction testing of cerebrospinal fluid (CSF) is often positive for JC virus.
- No effective therapy has been identified but the course may be significantly altered by HAART.[2]

Human Papillomavirus

- Human papillomavirus (HPV) causes a wide spectrum of disease in HIV-infected patients from transient infection to **anogenital warts and squamous cell cancers.**
- HIV-infected women have an increase of 5% to 10% in **cervical intraepithelial neoplasia** over non-HIV infected women. Risk of more advanced cervical cancer increases with lower CD4 counts.
- Likewise, **anal intraepithelial neoplasia** is more common in HIV-infected men.
- Lesions are usually asymptomatic though patients may experience pain or spotting from cervical, vaginal, or anal lesions.
- Therefore, pelvic examinations and cervical pap smears are recommended every 6 months in HIV-infected women.
- The role of anal pap smears in HIV-infected patients, especially men who have sex with men (MSM), is under investigation.
- Benign condylomata may contain areas of atypia and biopsy should be considered earlier in HIV-infected patients.

Bacterial Infections

Bacterial infections are common in patients with AIDS and often recur or follow an atypical or aggressive course despite adequate therapy.

Bacterial Pneumonia

- Bacterial pneumonias occur with increased frequency and are a common cause of morbidity.
- Pneumonias are usually due to *Streptococcus pneumoniae, Staphylococcus aureus,* or *Haemophilus influenzae.*
- Pneumonia due to gram-negative enteric organisms occurs in advanced HIV disease.
- Chest radiographs may reveal typical lobar pneumonia, but diffuse interstitial infiltrates similar to PCP have been reported.
- These infections usually respond to specific antibiotic therapy, but relapses are not uncommon.

Syphilis

- The natural history of syphilis may be altered by HIV infection.
- Reactivation of previously treated disease, active disease with negative serology, asymptomatic neurosyphilis, and relapse after standard therapy have all been reported. The optimal management of syphilis in this setting remains unclear.

- **Current guidelines suggest at least yearly screening for syphilis in HIV-infected persons.**
- Lumbar puncture is reserved for seropositive patients with neurologic symptoms. There are also data to support performing lumbar puncture in HIV-infected persons with a rapid plasma reagin (RPR) titer >1:32.
- Up to 20% of HIV-infected persons will remain "serofast" after successful treatment of syphilis; serum RPR or venereal disease research laboratory remains reactive at a low titer, generally <1:8. The clinical relevance of this in unclear, but a fourfold rise in titer above this "serofast" baseline is indicative of reinfection or reactivation.

Bacterial Diarrhea

- Bacterial diarrheas due to **Salmonella** spp., **Campylobacter** spp., and **Shigella** spp. are more common in HIV patients particularly MSM.
- Nontyphoidal salmonellae (especially *S. typhimurium*) are associated with invasive disease that often recurs or persists despite appropriate antibiotics.
  - Preferred treatment is with **ciprofloxacin** for 7 to 14 days for diarrhea or 4 to 6 weeks for bacteremia. Initial IV therapy should be followed by long-term oral suppressive therapy based on susceptibility testing; even then, relapse may occur as soon as therapy is discontinued.
- Campylobacter diarrhea is more severe in immune-compromised patients.
  - Treatment is with ciprofloxacin but resistance is increasing.
- Shigellosis causes fever and bloody diarrhea.
  - Treatment is with ciprofloxacin or TMP-SMX.

Mycobacterial Infections

Tuberculosis

- TB can occur at any CD4 cell count but extrapulmonary manifestations occur with increased frequency in patients with lower CD4 counts.
- In the developing world, TB is the most prominent AIDS-defining illness with often catastrophic consequences.
- In the developed world, TB is most commonly diagnosed in substance abusers, immigrants from high-prevalence countries, and the urban poor.
- Atypical radiographic patterns and extrapulmonary disease are quite common; apical cavitary disease is uncommon in advanced HIV disease.
- See Chapter 22 regarding the treatment of TB.
- After ruling out active disease, isoniazid for 9 months should be considered in any HIV-positive patient with a reactive (>5-mm induration) PPD skin test. Pyrazinamide plus rifampin for 2 months is an alternative, although there are significant drug interactions with HIV medications and rifampin.

Mycobacterium avium Complex

- MAC is one of the most frequently occurring opportunistic pathogens in patients with advanced AIDS. This ubiquitous opportunistic organism causes disseminated disease and occurs almost always in patients with CD4 cell counts <50 cells/mm^3.
- Generalized infection and GI disease are the most common manifestations.
- The organism can be cultured from blood, bone marrow, and tissue from the GI tract.
- Treatment with clarithromycin, ethambutol, and rifabutin is often effective.[2]
- For patients with CD4 counts <50 cells/mm^3, MAC prophylaxis therapy should be initiated with either azithromycin, 1,200 mg, once a week or clarithromycin, 500 mg PO twice a day.

Fungal Infections

Candidiasis
- Persistent oral, esophageal, and vaginal infections are common but dissemination is rare in the absence of other risk factors such as IV catheters.
- The severity and frequency of mucocutaneous candidiasis increase with declining immune function.
- **Oral thrush** is effectively treated with topical therapy, **clotrimazole** troches PO five times per day for 14 days.[2]
- **Esophagitis** should be treated with **fluconazole** (200 mg one time followed by 100 mg PO daily for 14 days; higher doses up to 400 mg daily may be required in some patients).
- **Vaginal candidiasis** can be treated with **fluconazole,** 150 mg PO one time.
- Frequently recurring thrush can be prevented with fluconazole, 100 mg PO daily.

Cryptococcosis
- *Cryptococcus neoformans* is the most common cause of fungal CNS disease in patients with AIDS.
- Symptoms may be mild and, therefore, **the threshold for performing a lumbar puncture should be low.**
- In addition to routine CSF chemistries (cell count, cryptococcal antigen, and culture) the CSF opening pressure should be measured to assess the possibility of intracranial hypertension as a complication.
- Lumbar puncture results include elevated opening pressure, lymphocyte predominant pleocytosis, and low glucose. However, normal CSF parameters occur in as many as 25% of AIDS patients with cryptococcal meningitis, so a **cryptococcal antigen should be sent for all AIDS patients in whom a lumbar puncture is performed.**
- Repeat lumbar puncture is indicated for clinical deterioration and is required to relieve increased opening pressure.
- Initial treatment is with IV **amphotericin B and flucytosine** for 2 weeks, followed by **fluconazole,** 400 mg daily for 8 to 10 weeks.[2]
- Following acute treatment, **maintenance therapy** is required with fluconazole, 200 mg daily until CD4 count is >200.
- Response is usually monitored clinically and is generally slow.

Histoplasmosis
- *Histoplasma capsulatum* is an important pathogen in patients with AIDS from endemic areas and may cause disseminated disease and septicemia. The organism's endemic area is broad including the Ohio and Mississippi river valleys in the United States, Central and South America, and part of southern Europe, Africa, eastern Asia, and Australia.
- Diagnosis is made by sending a **urine *H. capsulatum* antigen,** although the organisms can be cultured from blood and bone marrow as well.
- Pancytopenia may result from bone marrow involvement.
- Treatment includes a 12-week induction phase with subsequent long-term maintenance phase to complete 1 year of therapy.
- A cumulative dose of **amphotericin B,** 1.5 to 2.0 g is given initially for severely ill patients. For patients who are intolerant of amphotericin B, liposomal amphotericin B (Ambisome) can be considered. **Itraconazole** is effective for induction in milder disease. Itraconazole is also used for the maintenance phase.[2]
- Therapy can be discontinued after patients have sustained immune reconstitution.

Coccidioidomycosis

- *Coccidioides* spp. Infections also occur in patients with AIDS from endemic areas (southwestern United States and northern Mexico).
- The typical uncomplicated primary infection in immunocompetent hosts takes the form of a self-limited acute pneumonia (known as Valley Fever).
- Immunocompromise increases the risk of more severe and disseminated disease.
- Extensive pulmonary disease with extrapulmonary spread is common in AIDS patients.
- Coccidioidal meningitis and lymph node involvement may also occur.
- **Fluconazole,** 400 mg daily is appropriate for the treatment. Amphotericin B may be used as an alternative therapy.[2]
- Lifelong maintenance is required after treatment for coccidioidal meningitis.

Pneumocystis Pneumonia

- *Pneumocystis jiroveci* pneumonia remains the most common opportunistic infection in patients with AIDS and a leading cause of morbidity and mortality.
- Presenting symptoms include progressive dyspnea, fever, and cough.
  - Early disease may have a subtle presentation and a normal chest radiograph.
  - Extrapulmonary disease has been described, particularly in patients who receive aerosolized pentamidine for prophylaxis.
- **The treatment of choice for PCP is TMP-SMZ,** 5 mg/25 mg/kg PO or IV every 6 to 8 hours for 21 days.[2]
  - Anemia or rashes may occur in patients with AIDS who are treated with TMP-SMZ but may not require a change in therapy.[4]
  - For patients who do not tolerate TMP-SMX, **dapsone-trimethoprim** or **clindamycin-primaquine** can also be used for moderate disease.
  - **Pentamidine,** 4 mg/kg infused over 2 hours IV daily for 21 days, is additional option.
- In patients with well-documented PCP and moderate to severe disease (arterial oxygen pressure <75 torr on room air), prevention of respiratory failure and survival benefit have been demonstrated with **adjunctive use of steroids.**[5]
  - Prednisone (or equivalent parenteral methylprednisolone if the patient is unable to take oral medication), 40 mg PO bid for 5 days, followed by 40 mg PO daily for 5 days, followed by 20 mg PO daily for the duration of anti-Pneumocystis therapy is recommended. This limits inflammation leading to adult respiratory distress syndrome (ARDS).
- For persons with CD4 counts <200 cells/mm^3 or who have had PCP, prophylaxis should be given preferably with daily TMP-SMX or alternatively with dapsone.

Protozoal Infections

Toxoplasmosis

- *Toxoplasma gondii* typically presents in HIV-infected patients with CD4 counts <100 cells/mm^3.
- It represents reactivated disease and presents as encephalitis with headache, confusion, fever, and focal neurologic findings. Extracerebral toxoplasmosis has also been reported.
- Multiple CNS lesions may be found on brain imaging.
- Treatment with **sulfadiazine,** 25 mg/kg PO every 6 hours (or TMP-SMZ, 5 mg/25 mg/kg PO or IV q6–8h), plus **pyrimethamine,** 100 to 150 mg PO on day 1 and then 50 to 75 mg PO qd, often results in improvement, but **indefinite therapy is needed to prevent relapse.**[2]
  - Folinic acid, 5 to 10 mg PO daily, can be added to minimize hematologic toxicity.

- For patients who are intolerant of sulfonamides, clindamycin, 600 mg PO qid, can be substituted.
- The incidence of toxoplasmosis has decreased with the use of TMP-SMX prophylaxis for PCP. Persons with CD4 cell counts <100 cells/mm³ should receive prophylaxis for toxoplasmosis if not already on TMP-SMX.

Cryptosporidiosis

- *Cryptosporidium* spp. are an important global cause of human diarrheal illness and may cause severe and prolonged infections in patients with AIDS.
- Diagnosis is by microscopy, immunoassay, and PCR.
- **No therapy has proved to be effective** for cryptosporidiosis though HAART with improvement of CD4 count to >100 cells/mm³ generally results in resolution of diarrhea.[2]

Isosporiasis

- *Isospora belli* infection is most frequently seen HIV-positive in MSM.
- Symptoms include diarrhea, abdominal pain, malabsorption, and weight loss. Eosinophilia may be present.
- Acid-fast staining or other specific staining techniques are required for diagnosis.
- Treatment is with TMP-SMZ, 160 mg/800 mg PO qid for 10 days and then bid for 3 weeks. Relapses are not uncommon. Shorter courses of TMP-SMZ therapy followed by prophylaxis with pyrimethamine-sulfadoxine may also be effective.

Cyclosporiasis

- *Cyclospora cayetanensis* infection is acquired from contaminated water and fresh produce. Outbreaks in the United States have been due to contaminated raspberries, lettuce, basil, and snow peas. It may also be acquired during foreign travel. It does not appear to transmit directly from person-to-person.
- In AIDS it may cause a prolonged diarrheal illness similar to that of *Cryptosporidium* spp. and *I. belli.*
- Diagnosis is similar to *I. belli.*
- Treatment for HIV-infected patients consists of TMP-SMZ, 160 mg/800 mg PO qid for 10 days and then one tablet three times a week.

Neoplasms

- Neoplasms associated with AIDS include **non-Hodgkin lymphomas** and **Kaposi sarcoma. Primary CNS lymphomas** are common and may be multicentric. The treatment of these conditions is beyond the scope of this manual.
- Women should receive annual screening for **cervical cancer.** In addition, there is growing literature on the need for anal screening in both men and women.
- In the current HAART era, non-AIDS–associated malignancies are becoming more common, including lung cancer, other hematologic malignancies, and hepatocellular carcinoma.

SEXUALLY TRANSMITTED DISEASES

- A standardized, thorough evaluation including a complete history is important in the diagnosis of clinical syndromes.
- History should include the presence or absence of genital drainage or discharge; dysuria; sores or other lesions on or near the genitalia; the presence of warts, growths, or bumps on or near the genitalia; any rash; testicular pain or discomfort;

abdominal, rectal, or pelvic pain; and the presence of any oral or pharyngeal symptoms.
- Sexual history should include whether the patient has sex with men or women, or both; number of partners in the past year; sites of exposure (vaginal, penile, oral, rectal); condom use; known contact with STDs; any drug allergies; and, for women, menstrual history and pregnancy.
- Barrier methods should be encouraged.
- Physical examination must be compete and include the lower abdomen, palpation of inguinal area for lymphadenopathy, thorough external genitalia examination, and appropriate pelvic examination for women and visual examination of the urethra in men.

Urethritis and Cervicitis Syndromes

Symptoms in men generally include purulent urethral discharge and dysuria, although some patients may be asymptomatic. Vaginal discharge occurs, but many women are asymptomatic.

Gonorrhea

Diagnosis
- Gonorrhea typically causes urethritis in men and cervicitis in women.
- Diagnosis of infection is via Gram stain evaluation showing gram-negative diplococci within WBCs in urethral, endocervical, or anal samples; culture for *Neisseria gonorrhoeae* from urethral, endocervical, anal or pharyngeal samples; or use of nucleic acid amplification testing of urethral or endocervical samples.
- Pharyngeal gonorrhea can be documented only by a positive pharyngeal culture for *N. gonorrhoeae* because there are nonpathogenic *Neisseria* spp. that colonize the oropharynx.
- The patient's sex partners should be evaluated.

Treatment
- Recommended antigonococcal agents are **single doses of ceftriaxone (125 mg IM)** or cefixime (400 mg PO, not recommended for pharyngeal infection).[6]
- **Quinolones are no longer recommended** for the treatment of gonorrhea secondary to increased resistance.[7]
- Spectinomycin, 2 g IM, is an alternative therapy (not recommended for pharyngeal infection) but is not available in the United States.
- **Recommended concomitant therapy for *Chlamydia trachomatis*** is single-dose azithromycin (1 g PO) or doxycycline (100 mg PO bid for 7 days).
- Where the results of diagnostic probe tests are not promptly available, empiric therapy for *N. gonorrhea* and *C. trachomatis* is encouraged.
- Patients with disseminated gonococcal infection should be referred for hospital admission for IV antibiotics. The diagnostic evaluation often includes cultures of blood, mucosal sites, skin lesions, and joint aspirates.

Chlamydia

Diagnosis
- *C. trachomatis* is a major cause of urethritis/cervicitis.
- Diagnosis of chlamydia should include a urethral or endocervical genetic probe test (Pace2 or Gen-Probe) or direct fluorescent antibody test that is positive for

C. trachomatis (Micro Trak); urethral or endocervical culture positive for *C. trachomatis* (not generally available); or a DNA amplification test such as polymerase chain reaction or ligase chain reaction performed on urine or an endocervical or urethral specimen.

Treatment
- Treatment may be initiated before confirmatory testing results are available.
- **Treatment is single-dose azithromycin (1 g PO) or doxycycline (100 mg PO bid for 7 days).**[6]

Nongonococcal Urethritis and Mucopurulent Cervicitis

- Nongonococcal urethritis (NGU) and mucopurulent cervicitis (MPC) mimic infection with *N. gonorrhoeae*, and most cases are negative on testing for *C. trachomatis*.
- Other organisms that may cause NGU or MPC may include *Mycoplasma genitalium, Mycoplasma hominis, Ureaplasma urealyticum*, or *Trichomonas vaginalis* and occasionally HSV.
- Treatment should be initiated for NGU or MPC if two of the following are present:
  - There is a history of discharge or dysuria
  - There is purulent or mucopurulent discharge on examination
  - Gram stain shows >5 WBCs per high power field in men or >25 WBCs per high power field in women
- The recommended therapeutic approach is to provide adequate coverage for possible *C. trachomatis* infection and then treatment for *T. vaginalis* in patients who do not respond.
  - **Treatment for *C. trachomatis* is either single-dose azithromycin (1 g PO) or doxycycline (100 mg PO bid for 7 days).**
  - **Treatment of *T. vaginalis* is single-dose metronidazole (2 g PO).**[6]
- All sex partners should be evaluated and treated as indicated.

Vaginitis and Vaginosis Syndromes

- **Bacterial vaginosis** is a clinical syndrome of malodorous vaginal discharge possibly with pruritus. Diagnosis and treatment is discussed in Chapter 37.
- **Trichomoniasis** is an STD caused by the parasite *T. vaginalis*. It may be a cause of NGU in men and a profuse, purulent vaginal discharge in women. Further diagnosis and treatment is discussed in Chapter 37.
- **Vulvovaginal candidiasis** ("yeast infection") is suggested by the presence of vulvovaginal soreness, dyspareunia, vulvar pruritus, external dysuria, and thick or "cheesy" vaginal secretions.
  - Speculum examination may reveal candidal plaques that are adherent to the vaginal mucosa, with erythema or edema of the introitus.
  - In contrast to bacterial vaginosis and trichomoniasis, the vaginal pH in vulvovaginal candidiasis is usually <4.5.
  - The diagnosis can be made by inspection of the typical vaginal lesions or by observation of fungal elements (budding yeast and pseudohyphae) in a KOH preparation.
  - Treatment is usually indicated if clinical features are present, even if yeast is not seen on microscopic examination. A positive culture may be misleading because 10% to 20% of women normally have yeast in the vagina.
  - **Treatment is with single-dose fluconazole (150 mg PO) or intravaginal azole cream or suppository such as clotrimazole or miconazole.**

Genital Ulcer Syndromes

Syphilis

General Principles

- Syphilis is a systemic infection caused by *Treponema pallidum.*
- **Primary syphilis** is characterized by one or more painless, superficial ulcerations (chancres). These lesions are seen in the genital, anorectal, or pharyngeal sites.
  - A chancre typically has raised, sharply demarcated borders; a red, smooth, non-tender base; and scanty serous secretions.
  - Regional lymphadenopathy may be present.
  - The average time between exposure and chancre development is 3 weeks.
  - Spontaneous resolution of lesions generally occurs in 3 to 6 weeks, even without treatment.
- **The rash of secondary syphilis:**
  - Macular, maculopapular, or papular, typically involving the palms, soles, and flexor areas of the extremities.
  - The trunk, back, shoulders, abdomen, and face are commonly involved, and mucous patches may develop.
  - The average time from exposure to onset of secondary symptoms is 6 weeks.
- **Latent syphilis** is diagnosed serologically in the absence of primary or secondary symptoms.
  - Early disease (<1 year) is differentiated from late disease (>1 year) for treatment purposes.
  - If a negative serology within the past year cannot be documented, the patient should be treated for late latent disease.
- **Tertiary syphilis** is rare.
  - It may be manifest as mucocutaneous/osseous lesions (gummas), cardiovascular lesions (aortitis), or neurologic involvement (neurosyphilis).
  - Whereas neurosyphilis is generally a late complication, syphilitic meningitis may occur within the first few weeks of infection or at any time thereafter.

Diagnosis

- The classic diagnosis of syphilis is dark-field microscopy of lesion exudate, but this is seldom available and is quite insensitive.
- **Rapid plasma reagin (RPR) or the venereal disease research laboratory (VDRL) blood tests** are often reactive within 1 to 2 weeks of onset of the chancre but up to 30% may have negative RPR at the time of initial examination (chancre present).
- Also, false-positive tests occur in a variety of conditions (e.g., systemic lupus erythematosus, pregnancy).
- Confirmative testing by fluorescent treponemal antibody absorption or *T. pallidum* particle agglutination is necessary.

Treatment

- Treatment of adults with syphilis has become highly standardized.[6,8]
- **For all stages of syphilis, penicillin is the treatment of choice.**
- For pregnant patients with a history of penicillin allergy, penicillin skin testing and desensitization are recommended, because alternative medications do not treat the fetus.
- **For primary, secondary, and early latent infection (<1 year duration):**
  - **Single-dose benzathine penicillin G** (2.4 million units IM) is recommended.

- Alternatives include doxycycline (100 mg PO bid for 14 days), tetracycline (500 mg PO qid for 14 days), erythromycin (500 mg PO for 14 days, less effective), or ceftriaxone (250 mg IM qd for 8 to 10 days, less effective).
- **For the treatment of adults with late syphilis (>1 year duration—except neurosyphilis):**
  - **Benzathine penicillin G** (2.4 million units IM weekly for 3 weeks) is recommended.
  - Alternatives are tetracycline (500 mg PO qid for 28 days) or doxycycline (100 mg PO bid for 28 days).
- **For neurosyphilis:**
  - **Aqueous penicillin G** (18 to 24 million units daily IV, 3 to 4 million units every 4 hours for 14 days) is followed by a single dose of benzathine penicillin G (2.4 million units IM at the completion of IV therapy).
  - A recommended alternative regimen is procaine penicillin (2.4 million units IM daily) plus probenecid (500 mg PO qid for 10 to 14 days) followed by a single dose of benzathine penicillin G (2.4 million units IM) at the completion of IV therapy.
  - No data support the use of ceftriaxone, 1 to 2 g IV daily.
- **Follow-up care is recommended for all patients.**
  - **For early syphilis:**
    - Clinical examination and repeat serology at 6 and 12 months.
    - The RPR should show a fourfold decrease in titer within 6 months of treatment.
    - One must consider treatment failure or reinfection if symptoms persist or recur or if nontreponemal titer increases fourfold.
  - **For late syphilis:**
    - Repeat serologies at 6, 12, and 24 months.
    - Evaluate for neurosyphilis if the nontreponemal titer increases fourfold, if initially high titer ≥1:32 fails to fall fourfold in 12 to 24 months, or if signs or symptoms of neurosyphilis develop.
  - **For neurosyphilis:**
    - Repeat serologies at 3, 6, 12, and 24 months and follow up lumbar puncture at 6-month intervals until the cell count is normal.
    - Retreatment should be considered if cell count has not decreased at 6 months or CSF is not entirely normal at 2 years.
  - **For syphilis at any stage in HIV-positive patients:**
    - Follow-up with clinical examination should be performed in 1 week and repeat serology in 3, 6, 9, 12, and 24 months and then yearly, even if RPR becomes negative.

Herpes

General Principles
- HSV types 1 and 2 typically produce **painful grouped vesicles** on or near the genitalia. Over several days the lesions evolve into shallow ulcers, which generally heal within 1 to 2 weeks.
- HSV-1 and HSV-2 can be sexually transmitted, but most genital infections are caused by HSV-2.
- Virtually any genital ulcer may be herpetic regardless of clinical characteristics.

Diagnosis
Clinical Presentation
- Most patients with genital HSV are asymptomatic or have mild or nonspecific symptoms.

- The clinical courses of acute first-episode genital herpes among patients with HSV-1 and HSV-2 infections are similar. Virologic typing can be important because HSV-1 recurs less frequently than HSV-2.
- The first episode of genital herpes in patients who have had prior HSV-1 infection is associated with less severe systemic symptoms and faster healing than primary genital herpes.
- Clinical diagnosis relies on detection of grouped, tender vesicular or pustular lesions on an erythematous base. Lymphadenopathy, fever, headache, myalgias, urethritis, or cervicitis is variably present.
- Extragenital lesions of HSV commonly develop during the course of primary genital herpes.
  - Additional lesions may be located in the buttock, groin, or thigh areas.
  - CNS involvement may be manifested as aseptic meningitis, transverse myelitis, or sacral radiculopathy. This can result in episodes of spinal or meningeal symptoms that recur over many years (Mollaret meningitis).
  - These complications occur more commonly in women than in men.
- Recurrences usually cause fewer lesions and less frequent occurrence of systemic symptoms.
- Reactivation of HSV-2 infection shows a steady but gradual decrease in recurrence rates over time.

Diagnostic Testing
- Laboratory diagnosis should rely mainly on **HSV culture,** which should be included in the diagnostic workup of all genital ulcers.
- The sensitivity of the culture depends greatly on how the specimen is obtained and handled.
- Vesicular fluid is rich in virus and should be submitted whenever possible.
  - Unopened vesicles can be aspirated with a tuberculin syringe.
  - Alternatively, the lesion can be unroofed with a scalpel blade and the vesicular fluid soaked up with a cotton, rayon, or Dacron swab.
  - Calcium alginate swabs should not be used because this is inhibitory to HSV.
- HSV PCR is a more sensitive method for diagnosis and is available for samples from genital lesions, CSF, and ocular fluid.

Treatment
- Treatment of genital HSV can be with several effective agents[6]:
  - Acyclovir, 400 mg PO tid for 7 to 10 days
  - Famciclovir, 250 mg PO tid for 7 to 10 days
  - Valacyclovir, 1 g PO bid for 7 to 10 days
  - Early treatment usually reduces the symptomatic interval and may result in accelerated healing.
- **Suppressive therapy** may be recommended for patients with recurrent symptomatic infection:
  - Acyclovir, 400 mg PO bid
  - Famciclovir, 250 mg PO bid
  - Valacyclovir, 250 to 500 mg PO bid or 1 g PO daily
  - Suppressive therapy with antiviral agents may not show benefit until 4 to 6 months of treatment.
  - In many patients it may only shorten the symptomatic periods by 1 to 2 days.
  - Suppressive therapy is recommended for 1 year, after which the need for continued therapy should be reassessed.

- **Patients should be counseled that mild episodes may recur and that they will remain infectious even though they are receiving therapy.**
- Routine STD evaluation is recommended for all sex partners.

Chancroid

General Principles
- Chancroid is caused by infection with *Haemophilus ducreyi*.
- Chancroid is worldwide in distribution but rare in the United States outside the endemic areas in New York City and the Gulf Coast states, where 90% of cases are in non-Caucasian uncircumcised men. Prostitute contact is common.
- The incubation period is usually 5 to 7 days.

Diagnosis
- The typical lesions are **painful, nonindurated, excavated genital ulcers with undermined borders.**
- Tender, enlarged inguinal lymph nodes are often present.
- Fever and other systemic symptoms are generally absent.
- Laboratory diagnosis relies on culture or Gram stain from a lymph node aspirate.
  - Techniques for culture are only 50% to 75% sensitive.
  - A positive culture provides a definite diagnosis, whereas a smear of aspirated pus showing typical, small gram-negative bacilli provides only a presumptive diagnosis.
  - Gram stain of ulcer exudate may be misleading and is not recommended.
- Simultaneous workup for syphilis, HSV, and HIV is recommended. **It is essential to exclude syphilis in all cases of suspected chancroid.**

Treatment
- Treatment is single-dose **azithromycin** (1 g PO), single-dose **ceftriaxone** (250 mg IM), ciprofloxacin (500 mg PO bid for 3 days), or erythromycin base (500 mg PO qid for 7 days).[6]
- The patient should be reexamined in 2 to 3 days and then weekly until healed.

Lymphogranuloma Venereum

General Principles
- Lymphogranuloma venereum is caused by *C. trachomatis* serovars L1, L2, or L3, which predominantly infect the lymphatic tissue.
- Historically, this infection has occurred in underdeveloped tropical and subtropical areas, hence the alternative name tropical/climatic bubo (among others).
- Outbreaks have now occurred in Europe and the United States and mostly affected MSM.
- HIV-positivity appears to be a significant risk factor.
- Inoculation may occur via the genital (inguinal syndrome), rectal (anorectal syndrome), or rarely the pharyngeal mucosa (pharyngeal syndrome).
- The primary stage consists of an ulcer followed by the secondary lymphangitic/lymphadenitis stage.

Diagnosis
- The primary ulcerative stage is often unnoticed.
- The inguinal syndrome produces tender inguinal lymphadenopathy and even buboes, which may spontaneously rupture.
- The anorectal syndrome results in proctitis and inflammation of the surrounding lymphatic tissue.
- Diagnosis is largely clinical.

- Type-specific chlamydial serology is not available but type-specific PCR testing of lesion swab or bubo aspiration may be performed by the CDC.
- Chlamydial serology, though not type specific, may be suggestive if the titer is high, although acute and convalescent sera are preferred.

Treatment
- **Recommended treatment is doxycycline** (100 mg PO bid for 3 weeks) or erythromycin base (500 mg PO qid for 3 weeks).[6]
- Azithromycin in multiple doses >2 to 3 weeks may be effective, but clinical data are lacking.
- Sex partners during the 30 days before onset of symptoms should undergo routine STD examination, including chlamydia cultures and serology.

Granuloma Inguinale

General Principles
- Granuloma inguinale (also known as donovanosis, with reference to characteristic intracellular inclusions called Donovan bodies) is a progressive ulcerative condition caused by the intracellular gram-negative bacterium *Klebsiella granulomatis* (formerly known as *Calymmatobacterium granulomatis* or *Donovania granulomatis*).
- It is endemic to India, Papua New Guinea, southern Africa, and central Australia. Rare cases are reported in the United States via foreign travel.

Diagnosis
- **Painless, beefy-red ulcers** are typical, without lymphadenopathy. There are various classical presentations.
- Laboratory diagnosis relies on a tissue crush preparation or biopsy showing classic bipolar-staining Donovan bodies. The organism cannot be grown in standard culture media.

Treatment
- Treatment is **doxycycline** (100 mg PO bid for 3 weeks) or **TMP-SMZ** (160 mg/ 800 mg PO bid for 3 weeks).[6] Alternatives included ciprofloxacin (750 mg PO bid for 3 weeks), azithromycin (1,000 mg once per week for 3 weeks), or erythromycin base (500 mg PO qid for 3 weeks).
- In general, therapy should be continued until all lesions have completely healed.
- An aminoglycoside (e.g., gentamicin, 5 mg/kg IV daily) should be added if lesions do not respond after the first few days of oral therapy.

Exophytic Processes

Human Papillomavirus

General Principles
- HPV can result in a wide variety of epithelial manifestations including common, plantar, flat/juvenile warts.
- Anogenital warts (condylomata acuminata) are also caused by HPV and some have been linked epidemiologically to cervical, vaginal, vulvar, penile, and anal intraepithelial neoplasia and invasive squamous cell carcinoma.
- Serotypes 16 and 18 are associated with approximately 70% of all cervical cancers.[9] Other subtypes with a high malignant potential include 26, 31, 33, 35, 39, 45, 51, 52, 53, 56, 58, 59, 66, 68, 73, and 82.[10]

Diagnosis

- The diagnosis of anogenital warts is usually made by inspection, which reveals typical **flesh-colored "cauliflower" or wartlike masses,** usually involving the external genitalia, perineum, or perianal area.
- Coalescent lesions can become fairly large.
- The lesions are typically otherwise asymptomatic but minor complaints such as pruritus may be present.
- The differential diagnosis includes molluscum contagiosum or condyloma lata (secondary syphilis).
- A weak acetic acid solution (3% to 5%) can be used to highlight exophytic warts on the skin surface. The lesions turn white as the solution dries (do not apply to mucous membranes).
- A dermatologic consultation may be desirable for evaluation and biopsy of a lesion.
- Routine STD evaluation of all sex partners is recommended, including cervical cytology for female partners of infected men.

Treatment

- The treatment of warts is typically with application of liquid nitrogen, podophyllin, or trichloroacetic acid.
- **Liquid nitrogen** (cryotherapy) is applied by a 10- to 15-second spray followed by a thaw and a single repeat application.
- **Trichloroacetic acid,** 80% to 90%, is very caustic and physically destroys the lesions after repeated applications. It may be used during pregnancy.
- **Podophyllin,** 10% to 25% in tincture of benzoin, is applied once or twice a week and washed off 1 to 4 hours after each application. Podophyllotoxin is an antimitotic agent.
- Home therapy with podophyllin or imiquimod can also be tried.
- **Surgical removal** of warts may be necessary for extensive disease.
- There is now a prophylactic quadrivalent vaccine for serotypes 16 and 18 (the serotypes associated with 70% of cervical cancer) and serotypes 6 and 11 (the serotypes associated with 90% of anogenital warts).
- The vaccine is currently indicated for women aged 13 to 26 years. There is ongoing research to gain approval for men and a broader age range.

Molluscum Contagiosum

General Principles

- Molluscum contagiosum is a benign papular lesion caused by the molluscum contagiosum virus (a poxvirus), of which there are four types, MCV-1 to MCV-4.
- It can be transmitted sexually or nonsexually through close physical contact and is more common in children.
- HIV positivity is a significant risk factor.
- In healthy patients, it is a self-limited infection and lesions usually resolve spontaneously.
- In HIV-positive patients the lesions may be more widespread and larger.

Diagnosis

- Typical lesions are firm, small (1- to 5-mm diameter), **fleshy papules that are often umbilicated.**
- A firm white "pearl" is sometimes expressed on compression, followed by bleeding from the lesion.
- Very similar skin lesions may occur with disseminated *C. neoformans* or less commonly by *H. capsulatum.*

- Standard histology (molluscum bodies) or electron microscopy (visualization of poxvirus particles) can be used for a specific diagnosis.

Treatment
- Successful treatment of lesions may be with liquid nitrogen or trichloroacetic acid in the same fashion as described for warts.
- For those with concomitant HIV infection, more aggressive treatment and referral to a dermatologist may be appropriate. However, resolution usually occurs with treatment of the underlying HIV disease and immune reconstitution.

Systemic Sexually Transmitted Disease Syndromes

Pelvic Inflammatory Disease
General Principles
- Pelvic inflammatory disease (PID) occurs in women and is caused by upper genital tract infection. It is quite common.
- *N. gonorrhoeae* and *C. trachomatis* are the most common, although polymicrobial pelvic abscess disease is also common.
- Severe cases may present as tubo-ovarian abscess or perihepatitis.
- Most cases occur proximate to the menses.
- Risk factors include multiple sexual partners who are at greatest risk, aged 15 to 25 years, and prior PID.

Diagnosis
- PID is characterized by lower abdominal/pelvic pain, adnexal/cervical motion tenderness, and systemic signs and symptoms of infection.
- The patient's complaints may also include dyspareunia, vaginal discharge, and menorrhagia or metrorrhagia.
- The differential diagnosis is long and includes acute appendicitis, ectopic pregnancy, septic abortion, and ovarian torsion.
- All patients with PID should be tested for pregnancy and HIV. Urinalysis, fecal occult blood testing, and blood counts may be of value.
- In cases of *N. gonorrhoeae* PID, gram-negative intracellular diplococci may be seen but sensitivity is poor.
- Sonographic evidence of PID can also be seen but, again, sensitivity is poor.

Treatment
- Some patients with PID require hospitalization for IV antibiotics and possible surgical intervention.
- Treatment regimens use coverage for *N. gonorrhoeae* and *C. trachomatis* but many of these infections are polymicrobial, containing anaerobes such as *Bacteroides* spp.
- CDC guidelines for hospital admission should be reviewed prior to consideration of outpatient treatment.[6] They are as follows:
  - Surgical emergencies cannot be excluded
  - The patient is pregnant
  - Outpatient therapy has failed
  - The patient is unable to follow or tolerate outpatient treatment
  - The illness is severe, with nausea, vomiting, and high fever
  - Tubo-ovarian abscess is strongly suspected
  - The patient is immunocompromised

- Hospitalized patients should be treated for at least 2 weeks with IV or PO antibiotics, or both.
- **Outpatient treatment** should be one of the following: single-dose **ceftriaxone** (250 mg IM) **plus doxycycline** (100 mg PO bid for 14 days) **with or without metronidazole** (500 mg PO bid for 14 days).[6]
- **Quinolones are no longer recommended** for the treatment of gonorrhea secondary to increased resistance.[7]
- The patient should be advised to have an intrauterine device removed if present, abstain from sexual intercourse for 2 weeks, and comply with bed rest for 1 to 3 days or until pain is significantly improved.
- A follow-up examination within 72 hours is essential to ensure that an adequate response to therapy has occurred.
- All sex partners within the past 3 months should be examined.

Hepatitis B Virus
- Refer to Chapter 26 for a detailed discussion of hepatitis B.
- Hepatitis B can be transmitted sexually, parenterally, or from mother to child during pregnancy.
- Epidemiologic studies suggest that in the United States, 40% to 60% of cases of HBV infection are sexually transmitted.
- Patients with this sexually transmitted infection complain of nonspecific symptoms associated with hepatitis: malaise, fever, loss of appetite, abdominal pain, nausea, vomiting, jaundice, dark urine, arthralgias, or polyarthritis, but up to 50% may be asymptomatic.
- The physical examination may detect right upper quadrant abdominal tenderness, hepatic enlargement, or scleral or cutaneous jaundice.
- Laboratory diagnostic studies should include serologic testing for HBV, including hepatitis B surface antigen.
- Other useful diagnostic tests include hepatitis A immunoglobulin M, hepatitis C virus–enzyme–linked immunosorbent assay test, complete blood count, and liver function tests.
- **HBV is the only STD for which a 90% effective vaccine is available.**
- Treatment for acute HBV is supportive. Adequate fluid intake should be encouraged, as well as bed rest and abstinence from sexual contact until symptoms subside.
- A routine STD evaluation including HBV serology is recommended for all sex partners.

REFERENCES

1. Panel on Clinical Practices for the Treatment of HIV Infection. Guidelines for the use of antiretroviral agents in HIV-1-infected adults and adolescents. 2006;1–139. http://www.aidsinfo.nih.gov/Guidelines/. Accessed December 9, 2009.
2. Kaplan JE, Benson C, Holmes KH, et al; Centers for Disease Control and Prevention (CDC); National Institutes of Health; HIV Medicine Association of the Infectious Diseases Society of America. Guidelines for prevention and treatment of opportunistic infections in HIV-infected adults and adolescents: recommendations from CDC, the National Institutes of Health, and the HIV Medicine Association of the Infectious Diseases Society of America. *MMWR Recomm Rep* 2009;58:1–207.
3. Overton ET. An overview of vaccinations in HIV. *Curr HIV/AIDS Rep* 2007;4:105–113.
4. Sattler FR, Cowan R, Nielsen DM, Ruskin J. Trimethoprim-sulfamethoxazole compared with pentamidine for treatment of Pneumocystis carinii pneumonia in the acquired immunodeficiency syndrome. A prospective, noncrossover study. *Ann Intern Med* 1998;109:280–287.

5. Bozzette SA, Sattler FR, Chiu J, et al. A controlled trial of early adjunctive treatment with corticosteroids for Pneumocystis carinii pneumonia in the acquired immunodeficiency syndrome. California Collaborative Treatment Group. *N Engl J Med* 1990;323:1451–1457.

6. Centers for Disease Control and Prevention, Workowski KA, Berman SM. Sexually transmitted diseases treatment guidelines, 2006. *MMWR Recomm Rep* 2006;55:1–94.

7. Centers for Disease Control and Prevention (CDC). Update to CDC's sexually transmitted diseases treatment guidelines, 2006: fluoroquinolones no longer recommended for treatment of gonococcal infections. *MMWR Morb Mortal Wkly Rep* 2007;56:332–336.

8. Stoner BP. Current controversies in the management of adult syphilis. *Clin Infect Dis* 2007;44:S130–S146.

9. Schiffman M, Castle PE, Jeronimo J, et al. Human papillomavirus and cervical cancer. *Lancet* 2007;370:890–907.

10. Muñoz N, Bosch FX, de Sanjosé S, et al. International Agency for Research on Cancer Multicenter Cervical Cancer Study Group. Epidemiologic classification of human papillomavirus types associated with cervical cancer. *N Engl J Med* 2003;348:518–527.

Common Gastrointestinal Complaints

Babac Vahabzadeh and Dayna S. Early

DYSPHAGIA AND ODYNOPHAGIA

General Principles

- Swallowing apparatus consists of the pharynx, cricopharyngeus (upper esophageal sphincter), body of the esophagus, and lower esophageal sphincter.
- Dysphagia is a sense of difficulty with the passage of food from the pharynx to the stomach.
  - This should be distinguished from **globus,** which is a subjective feeling of fullness in the throat not related to eating.
- **Odynophagia** is the presence of pain on swallowing that may or may not accompany dysphagia.
- Dysphagia can be divided into oropharyngeal or esophageal dysphagia. These groups can be further subdivided into mechanical causes or neuromuscular causes.

Diagnosis

Clinical Presentation

History
Onset
- Progressive difficulty in swallowing solid foods, whereas liquids pass with ease, indicates mechanical obstructive cause such as malignancy or benign stricture.
- Dysphagia involving solids and liquids is consistent with esophageal motor dysfunction, such as achalasia or diffuse esophageal spasm, but can be seen in advanced obstruction.
- Intermittent dysphagia for solids, usually meat or bread, can result from mucosal abnormality of the lower esophagus known as Schatzki ring.[1]
- Hoarseness preceding dysphagia usually is of laryngeal origin; however, when it follows, the onset of dysphagia involvement of the recurrent laryngeal nerve by cancer should be considered.

Location
- Symptoms located in the lower part of the sternum are most likely due to abnormality in the distal esophagus. Otherwise, subjective localization of dysphagia is infrequently helpful.
- Hiccups can reflect a lesion in the distal esophagus caused by diaphragmatic irritation, or gastric or esophageal distention from aerophagia.

Characteristics
- Unintended weight loss may suggest carcinoma, particularly in those with heavy tobacco and alcohol use, and those with long-standing acid reflux.

- Tracheobronchial aspiration may occur in those with tracheoesophageal fistula, brainstem neuromuscular diseases, achalasia, or severe gastroesophageal reflux.
- Previous chronic heartburn associated with dysphagia is usually present in peptic strictures. These individuals may describe chronic antacid use.
- Chest pain may occur in those with severe reflux, accounting for half of the non-cardiac chest pain.[2]
- Odynophagia is frequently related to esophageal infections or pill ulcers.

Physical Examination
- Oral pharyngeal examination looking for evidence of thrush or lesions of pemphigus or epidermolysis bullosa.
- Examination of the neck may reveal structural defects such as thyromegaly, spinal deformity, and neck masses.
- Skin examination is important for features of collagen vascular disease including scleroderma or CREST syndrome (Calcinosis, Raynaud phenomenon, Esophageal dysmotility, Sclerodactyly, and Telangiectasias), which is associated with dysphagia and impaired peristalsis.

Differential Diagnosis
- Infections including candidal, herpetic, or other viral esophagitis must be considered in patients who describe odynophagia, are debilitated, or immunosuppressed.
- The differential diagnosis/causes of dysphagia are presented in Table 1.
- Acute **odynophagia** can be secondary to esophagitis or ulcers from pills such as tetracycline, potassium tablets, bisphosphonates, ferrous sulfate, quinidine, and nonsteroidal anti-inflammatory agents (NSAIDs).

Diagnostic Testing
- When esophageal dysphagia is suspected, **endoscopy** is the initial test to visualize the mucosa directly with biopsy of suspicious lesions.
- **Barium swallow** can be used in cases with high risk for sedation, patient anxiety, and anticoagulation concerns to identify structural defects.
- **Modified barium swallow** is used to evaluate real-time swallowing mechanisms to identify oropharyngeal dysmotility and aspiration.
- **Laryngoscopy** can identify oropharyngeal lesions.
- **Esophageal manometry** is the test of choice when esophageal motor disease is suspected.

Treatment

- Gastroesophageal reflux disease should be treated with **proton pump inhibitors.**[4]
- Esophageal strictures or rings can be treated with endoscopy by **bougienage** (the passage of dilators with or without guidewire assistance) or balloon dilators.
- Achalasia can be treated with the following:
  - **Pneumatic dilatation** via fluoroscopic and endoscopic visualization.
  - Heller **myotomy** (surgical procedure that dissects the smooth muscle of the hypertensive lower esophageal sphincter).
  - **Botulinum toxin** injection can be used for those at high risk for other interventions.
- Odynophagia may be treated symptomatically with opioid analgesic agents or topical viscous lidocaine.
  - Pill ulcers are generally self-limited.
  - Infectious causes of odynophagia should be treated with appropriate antimicrobials.

TABLE 1	Causes of Dysphagia	
Location	**Mechanism**	**Causes**
Esophageal	Mechanical	Peptic stricture
		Previous radiation therapy resulting in stricture
		Other strictures
		Schatzki ring
		Webs
		Cancer
		Erosive esophagitis
		Extrinsic compression (e.g., mediastinal tumor, thoracic aortic aneurysm, left atrial enlargement)
		Foreign body
Esophageal	Neuromuscular	Achalasia
		Diffuse esophageal spasm
		Nutcracker esophagus
		Scleroderma
Oropharyngeal	Mechanical	Oropharyngeal tumors
		Zenker diverticulum
		Postsurgical or postradiation change
		External compression (e.g., goiter, cervical osteophytes, cervical esophageal rings/webs)
		Decreased saliva/dry mouth
Oropharyngeal	Neuromuscular[3]	Cerebrovascular accident
		Cricopharyngeal achalasia
		Parkinson disease
		Multiple sclerosis
		Myasthenia gravis
		Amyotrophic lateral sclerosis
		Polymyositis/dermatomyositis
		Other neuromuscular disorders

NAUSEA AND VOMITING

General Principles

- Nausea and vomiting are nonspecific symptoms.
- History should focus on associated symptoms that may narrow the differential diagnosis.

Diagnosis

Clinical Presentation

History

Onset

- The initial evaluation should determine the duration and severity of symptoms.

- Presence of diarrhea may indicate an infectious gastroenteritis.
- Association with certain triggers including smells, tastes, emotional or physical stress, headaches, and abdominal pain.

Location
- If abdominal pain is the main symptom, refer to the "Abdominal Pain" section of this chapter for the differential diagnosis.
- Nausea and/or vomiting associated with right upper quadrant (RUQ) or epigastric pain could be secondary to biliary colic, pancreatitis, cholecystitis, peptic ulcer disease, or acute viral hepatitis.
- Initial periumbilical pain that relocates to the right lower quadrant accompanied by nausea and vomiting may be due to appendicitis.
- Left lower quadrant pain in the presence of vomiting may be secondary to diverticulitis.
- Flank pain along with fever and vomiting may indicate pyelonephritis.

Characteristics
- Occurrence soon after meals can be a result of gastric outlet obstruction.
- Vomiting that is delayed after meals and consists of partially digested food or food consumed several hours earlier may indicate gastroparesis (particularly in diabetics) as well as intestinal obstruction.
- Vomiting undigested food is seen with Zenker diverticulum (pharyngoesophageal diverticulum) and achalasia, which are also associated with severe halitosis.

Physical Examination
- Evaluate for orthostatic hypotension defined by fall of systolic blood pressure of 20 mm Hg or 10 mm Hg diastolic with positional change, which may be present in persistent emesis due to volume depletion.
- Decreased skin turgor or dry mucous membranes are signs of significant fluid losses.
- Severe halitosis may be associated with intestinal obstruction, gastroparesis, gastrocolic fistula, bacterial overgrowth, achalasia, and Zenker diverticulum.
- Oral examination may reveal poor dentition and enamel erosion in those with eating disorders such as bulimia.
- Auscultation of the abdomen to distinguish the presence or absence of bowel sounds.
- High-pitched noises may suggest small bowel obstruction while succussion splash (the movement of gastric fluid within the stomach heard on auscultation) is sometimes noted in gastric outlet obstruction or gastroparesis.
- Palpation to find areas of tenderness, abdominal masses, or Murphy sign.

Differential Diagnosis
The differential diagnosis of nausea and vomiting is extensive and is presented in Table 2.

Diagnostic Testing
Laboratories
- Serum chemistries evaluating electrolytes, bilirubin, amylase, lipase, alkaline phosphatase, and transaminases.
  - Evaluation specifically for hyponatremia and azotemia as these may cause nausea and vomiting.
  - Hyponatremia and hyperkalemia can be seen in adrenal insufficiency. Check AM cortisol if adrenal insufficiency is suspected.

| TABLE 2 | Causes of Nausea and Vomiting |

Gastrointestinal
Gastroenteritis
Toxin mediated (e.g.,
 Staphylococcus aureus,
 Bacillus cereus)
Viral (e.g., rotaviruses,
 enteric adenovirus,
 Norwalk agent)
Gut obstruction (essentially
 any cause, any level)
Esophageal webs/
 rings/achalasia/cancer
Gastric cancer/
 gastroparesis/pyloric
 stenosis/outlet
 obstruction
Intestinal cancer
Adhesions
Intussusception
Hernia
Volvulus
Zenker diverticulum
 (regurgitation)
Gastroesophageal reflux
 disease (regurgitation)
Peptic ulcer disease
Appendicitis
Ileus
Colonic
 pseudoobstruction
Inflammatory bowel
 disease
Toxic megacolon
Eosinophilic
 gastroenteritis
Constipation
Hepatitis
Passive hepatic congestion
 resulting from congestive
 heart failure
Cholecystitis/
 choledocholithiasis
Pancreatitis
Pancreatic cancer
Peritonitis
Mesenteric ischemia

Central nervous system
Increased intracranial
 pressure (any cause)
Tumor
Hemorrhage/infarct/
 associated edema (e.g.,
 cerebellar, brainstem)
Cerebral vein and dural
 sinus thrombosis
Pseudotumor cerebri
Meningitis/encephalitis
Hydrocephalus (congenital,
 acquired, and many
 causes)
Migraine headache
Seizure disorders

Labyrinthine disorders
Motion sickness
Vestibular neuronitis
Acute labyrinthitis

Endocrine disorders
Diabetic ketoacidosis
Adrenal insufficiency
Hypercalcemia/
 hyperparathy roidism

Functional
Nonulcer dyspepsia
Irritable bowel syndrome
Cyclic vomiting syndrome

Psychiatric disorders
Eating disorders
Somatization disorder
Depressive disorders
Anxiety disorders
Rumination syndrome

Medications/toxins
Chemotherapeutic
 agents
Nonsteroidal
 anti-inflammatory
 agents (NSAIDs)
Opiate analgesics
Colchicine
Antibiotics (e.g.,
 erythromycin,
 metronidazole,
 sulfa drugs, and
 tetracycline)
Cardiovascular drugs
 (e.g., β-blockers,
 calcium channel
 blockers, diuretics,
 digoxin)
Central nervous system
 agents (e.g.,
 antidepressants,
 benzodiazepines,
 medications for
 Parkinson disease,
 anticonvulsants)
Estrogen replacement
 or hormone therapy
General anesthetics
Other drugs (e.g.,
 theophylline, iron,
 and many others)
Ethanol
Many poisons
Narcotic withdrawal

Other
Pregnancy
Hyperemesis gravidarum
Pyelonephritis
Nephrolithiasis
Myocardial infarction
Uremia
Acute glaucoma
Radiation therapy
Acute intermittent
 porphyria

Modified from Quigley EM, Hasler WL, Prkman HP. AGA technical review on nausea and vomiting.
Gastroenterology 2001;120:263–286.

- Complete blood cell count (CBC) evaluating for leukocytosis indicating acute inflammation or infection as well as anemia indicating possible blood loss within the gastrointestinal (GI) tract.
- Pregnancy test should be obtained in women of childbearing age.

Imaging
- If nausea and vomiting is associated with pain, an **obstructive series** consisting of three views (upright, supine, and lateral decubitus plain films) is important in searching for intestinal obstruction, air fluid levels, bowel gas pattern, and free air.
- Upper GI **endoscopy** can detect mechanical sources of nausea and emesis. If negative, consider a small bowel follow-through.
- Radionuclide **gastric-emptying scan** and manometry can evaluate for motility disorders.
- **Computerized tomography (CT)** may be obtained to evaluate for intra-abdominal processes, such as pancreatitis or appendicitis.
- CT scan or magnetic resonance imaging (MRI) of the brain may be pertinent if an intracranial process is suspected.

Treatment

- Identify and treat underlying process; however, antiemetic agents may temporarily alleviate symptoms.
  - Prochlorperazine starting at 5 to 10 mg PO tid/qid or 25 mg suppositories every 12 hours.
  - Promethazine starting at 12.5 to 25 mg PO every 4 to 6 hours or 25 mg suppositories every 4 to 6 hours.
  - Also refer to Chapter 32 for a more detailed discussion of antiemetic therapy.
- Prokinetic medication such as metoclopramide is usually started at 10 mg PO/IM/IV 1 hour before meal and at bedtime.
  - Mechanical obstruction must be **excluded before** using prokinetics.
  - **Metoclopramide should not be used for prolonged periods and/or in high doses,** particularly in the elderly, because of the risk of drug-induce tardive dyskinesia.
- A number of serotonin receptor inhibitors, such as ondansetron, or antagonists of substance P/neurokinin 1 receptors, such as aprepitant, are frequently used in nausea and emesis related to chemotherapy.
- Indications for hospitalization include the following:
  - Clinical evidence of severe volume depletion with benefit from intravenous fluids.
  - Electrolyte derangements that may need careful correction.
  - Patients at extremes of age, those with diabetes and/or accompanying debilitating illnesses that may require more than outpatient treatment.

DYSPEPSIA

General Principles

- Persistent or recurrent discomfort or pain located in the upper abdominal area.
- Can be accompanied by bloating, heartburn, nausea, and food intolerance.
- Symptoms can be generalized broadly into two categories:
  - **Peptic ulcer disease.**
  - **Nonulcer dyspepsia.**

Diagnosis

Clinical Presentation
History
Onset
- Pain in the preprandial state or nocturnal pain that results in awakening several hours after ingestion of food is suspicious for peptic ulcer disease.
- Similar pain that is relieved by food is indicative of a duodenal ulcer.

Location
- Pain radiating to the back and somewhat improved on leaning forward is consistent with pancreatitis, perforated peptic ulcer, or leaking abdominal aneurysm.
- Pain referred to the right scapula may originate in the gallbladder or from any process that result in diaphragmatic irritation.
- Constipation, diarrhea, tenesmus, or nonspecific lower abdominal discomfort in association with upper abdominal complaints may be due to irritable bowel disease.

Characteristics
- Early satiety can result from ulcers at the gastric outlet or infiltrating tumors creating reduced gastric wall compliance.
- Fear of eating because of subsequent abdominal pain should be concerning for mesenteric ischemia or intestinal angina particularly in those with cardiovascular disease or elderly.
- History of peptic ulcer disease, gastric surgery, cigarette smoking, or alcohol use are risk factors for the development of dyspepsia.
- Early satiety, recurrent vomiting, or bloating that is not accompanied by visible distention or pain could indicate dysmotility.
- Aerophagia is excess swallowing of air that results in fullness, belching, or reflux-like symptoms relieved by repetitive belching. Aerophagia is usually psychiatric in origin.

Red Flags
- Concerning signs and symptoms associated with dyspepsia include the following:
  - Weight loss.
  - GI bleeding.
  - Recurrent vomiting.
  - Dysphagia.
  - NSAID use.
  - Neoplasia (more common in older patients).

Physical Examination
- Abdominal tenderness to palpation may be seen in peptic ulcer disease and pancreaticobiliary disorders.
- RUQ tenderness increased with palpation upon inspiration (Murphy sign) indicates cholecystitis.
- Evaluation for peritoneal signs such as guarding and rebound tenderness, which is the discomfort induced by movement of an irritated peritoneum during the release of pressure from palpation.
- Jaundice may suggest a hepatic or biliary process.
- Examination for blood in stool.

Diagnostic Testing

Laboratory Testing

CBC looking for anemia if bleeding ulcers are suspected as well as leukocytosis indicating possible intra-abdominal infection.

Diagnostic Procedures

- **Endoscopy** of the upper GI tract is indicated for those with alarm symptoms and for whom trials of acid-suppressing medications are inadequate.[5]
- ***Helicobacter pylori* testing** is appropriate if mucosal abnormalities, such as peptic ulcers, erosive gastropathy, or duodenitis, are detected.
- **Upper GI** barium x-rays are reserved for patients who cannot undergo endoscopy.
- Gastroparesis can be demonstrated by **gastric-emptying scintigraphy** but is usually suspected clinically.
- Transabdominal **ultrasound** can be used to evaluate for liver and biliary tract abnormalities.

Treatment

- Peptic ulcer disease should be managed with acid suppression.
  - **Documentation of healing is recommended for gastric ulcer.**[6]
  - ***H. pylori* should be eradicated if positive.**
- Nonulcer dyspepsia may not respond to specific treatment but may improve with acid suppression or tricyclic antidepressants.
  - In those with alarm symptoms, upper endoscopy is warranted.[7]
- **Reflux should be treated symptomatically** with regularly scheduled proton pump inhibitors as well as weight reduction, dietary changes, and elevation of the head of bed.[4]
- Dysmotility-like dyspepsia may benefit from prokinetic agents such as metoclopramide. Metoclopramide should not be used for prolonged periods and/or in high doses, particularly in the elderly, because of the risk of drug-induce tardive dyskinesia.

ABDOMINAL PAIN

General Principles

- **One of the most valuable diagnostic tools in evaluating the patient with abdominal pain is the history.**
- Location and features of pain is useful in narrowing the differential diagnosis to an organ (i.e., hepatobiliary, gastric, and intestinal) as well as to a cause (i.e., inflammation, obstruction, ischemia, and neurogenic).

Diagnosis

Clinical Presentation

History

Onset

- The initial evaluation should focus on the chronology of events and determine the duration of symptoms, whether acute (Table 3)[8] or chronic (Table 4).
- The first consideration for a patient with acute pain is whether they can be evaluated in an outpatient setting or whether an emergency room is more appropriate.

TABLE 3	Common Causes of Acute Abdominal Pain by Location

Right upper quadrant
Acute cholecystitis, cholangitis,
  choledocholithiasis
Acute hepatitis
Budd-Chiari syndrome
Congestive heart failure with hepatic
  congestion
Hepatic abscess
Hepatic cancer
Acute sickle hepatic crisis
Subdiaphragmatic abscess
Fitz-Hugh-Curtis syndrome
Myocardial infarction, pericarditis
Pneumonia

Left upper quadrant
Gastritis, gastric ulcer
Splenic infarct/rupture/abscess
Splenic flexure ischemia
Acute pancreatitis
Myocardial infarction, pericarditis
Pneumonia

Right lower quadrant
Appendicitis
Infective terminal ileitis/mesenteric adenitis
Infectious colitis
Inflammatory bowel disease
Inguinal hernia
Acute pancreatitis
Ectopic pregnancy
Rupture ovarian cyst
Salpingitis
Pelvic inflammatory disease
Renal disorders
Right ureteric calculus
Pyelonephritis
Bladder distension
Testicular torsion
Pyogenic sacroiliitis

Left lower quadrant
Acute diverticulitis
Infectious colitis
Inflammatory bowel disease
Inguinal hernia
Acute pancreatitis
Ectopic pregnancy
Rupture ovarian cyst
Salpingitis
Pelvic inflammatory disease
Renal disorders
Left ureteric calculus
Pyelonephritis
Bladder distention
Testicular torsion
Pyogenic sacroiliitis

Central abdominal pain
Gastroenteritis, gastritis
Peptic ulcer disease/gastroesophageal
  reflux disease
Small bowel obstruction
Mesenteric ischemia
Acute pancreatitis
Myocardial infarction, pericarditis
Aortic dissection/ruptured aortic
  aneurysm
Pneumonia

Diffuse abdominal pain
Perforated ulcer (gastric or duodenal)
Appendicitis
Small bowel obstruction
Diverticulitis
Inflammatory bowel disease
Toxic megacolon
Mesenteric ischemia
Hemorrhagic pancreatitis
Acute infectious peritonitis
Spontaneous bacterial peritonitis
Diabetic ketoacidosis
Acute noninfectious peritonitis
Familial Mediterranean fever
Sickle cell crisis

Modified from Yamada T, Alpers DH, Laine L, et al. Textbook of gastroenterology. 3rd Ed.
New York: Lippincott Williams & Wilkins, 1999:804.

TABLE 4	Causes of Chronic Abdominal Pain

Pancreaticobiliary disease
Sphincter of Oddi dysfunction/biliary
 dyskinesia
Chronic pancreatitis (particularly with
 chronic alcohol use)

Inflammatory disease
Inflammatory bowel disease
Celiac disease (often with diarrhea)
Familial Mediterranean fever
Eosinophilic gastrointestinal disorders
Hereditary angioedema/C1 inhibitor
 deficiency/dysfunction

Infectious disease
Liver abscess
Schistosomiasis
Chronic Giardiasis
Whipple disease (often with diarrhea)

Motility disorders
Gastroparesis
Constipation

Intermittent obstructive disease
Internal or abdominal wall hernia
Crohn disease
Adhesions
Intussusception

Other gastrointestinal
Peptic ulcer disease
Gastroesophageal reflux disease (GERD)
Drug-induced dyspepsia

Vascular disease
Intestinal ischemia (postprandial)
Superior mesenteric artery syndrome
Celiac artery compression syndrome
 (postprandial)
Polyarteritis nodosa and other forms of
 vasculitis

Neoplastic
Gastric cancer
Hepatic cancer
Pancreaticobiliary neoplasm
Colon cancer

Metabolic
Lactose intolerance
Adrenal insufficiency
Heavy metal (lead) poisoning
Acute intermittent porphyria

Neurologic disease
Abdominal migraine
Abdominal epilepsy
Radiculopathy (diabetes,
 spinal cord compression/
 fractures)
Abdominal cutaneous nerve
 entrapment syndrome
Postherpetic neuralgia

Musculoskeletal
Myofascial abdominal wall pain
 (trigger points)
Painful rib syndrome

Functional bowel disease
Irritable bowel syndrome
Nonulcer dyspepsia

Gynecologic disease
Endometriosis (often related to
 menstrual cycle)
Dysmenorrhea (related to
 menstrual cycle)
Mittelschmerz (related to
 menstrual cycle)
Uterine fibroids
Ovarian cysts
Ovarian cancer
Somatization disorder

Location
- Some causes of abdominal pain can be well localized, particularly if they result from inflammation in the parietal peritoneum (Table 3).
- Substernal chest pressure or pain can be indicative of esophageal disorders. This can result in pain that radiates to the neck, jaw, arms, and back and may mimic cardiac angina.

- Epigastric discomfort may be secondary to a process affecting the stomach, duodenum, and pancreas, while stretching of the liver capsule or gallbladder distention can result in RUQ pain.
- Small bowel obstruction or inflammation (i.e., appendicitis) localizes to the periumbilical area, and colonic pain is less well localized to the lower abdomen.
- Abdominal disease causing inflammation under the diaphragm can produce referred pain in the shoulder.
- Non-GI abdominal pain can result from the following:
  - Urinary tract disease (i.e., cystitis, pyelonephritis, obstructive uropathy, and nephrolithiasis) manifested by dysuria or hematuria can cause pain in the flanks or suprapubic area as well as significant abdominal discomfort.
  - Pleural, pulmonary, or pericardial etiologies causing upper abdominal pain.
  - Gynecologic etiology, which must be considered in women with lower abdominal symptoms (Tables 3 and 4).

Characteristics

- Qualities such as sharp, tearing, and cutting may indicate an acute process, whereas descriptors such as gnawing, burning, dull, or boring point toward a chronic process.
- Colic describes episodic pain with a waxing and waning intensity.
- Certain movements can generate abdominal pain due to musculoskeletal disorders or nerve root compression, and pain worse while supine may indicate pancreatic disease.
- Postprandial pain may indicate a process such as cholecystitis, pancreatitis, or gastric ulcers. In contrast, pain from duodenal ulcers generally improves with food ingestion.
- Intestinal angina may be associated with a fear of eating due to pain resulting in weight loss and seen more commonly in older persons with mesenteric ischemia.
- Nausea and emesis are nonspecific symptoms and can frequently occur because of non-GI causes.
- Diarrhea associated with nausea and emesis may lead to the discovery of an infectious source.
- Hiccups can result from distention of the esophagus or stomach or irritation of the diaphragm.

Bowel Habits

- Patients should be questioned about changes in bowel movements and stool caliber and volume.
- Constipation can result in diffuse abdominal discomfort, while diarrhea can be accompanied by cramping.
- Patients with alternating complaints of diarrhea and constipation may have irritable bowel disease.
- GI bleeding raises concern for ulcers, infections, or ischemia.
  - Melena (dark, tarry stool) usually signals an upper GI source, although it can occur during right-sided colonic bleeding or small bowel bleeding.
  - Hematochezia (bright red blood from the rectum) usually reflects a colonic source but sometimes presents during massive upper bleeding.

Miscellaneous History

- Menstrual cycles, irregularity, or abnormalities in bleeding may generate abdominal pain or worsening of underlying GI disorders.
  - Symptoms of inflammatory bowel disease or irritable bowel syndrome can clearly worsen during and around the time of menses.
  - Pain that follows a close pattern of menstrual cycles may be due to underlying endometriosis.

- Psychiatric causes should be considered in patients with underlying depression and anxiety, after organic causes are eliminated.

Red Flags

Signs and symptoms especially concerning are as follows:
- Pain that awakens the patient from sleep.
- Fever.
- Prolonged severe pain of more than several hours' duration.
- Persistent emesis.
- Changes in patterns or location.
- Significant alterations in appetite or mental status.
- Unintentional weight loss.
- GI bleeding.

Physical Examination
- Inspection and assessment for signs of systemic illness including the following:
  - Cachexia.
  - Pallor.
  - Severity of distress.
  - Presence of ascites, masses, prior surgical procedures, or other abnormalities.
  - Presence of cutaneous findings, known as stigmata of liver disease, may indicate underlying cirrhosis.
- Auscultation for presence or absence of bowel sounds.
  - High-pitched sounds may indicate bowel obstruction, whereas absence of sounds may be a feature of ileus or peritonitis.
- Percussion:
  - Tympanic percussion can indicate gas-filled or dilated loops of bowel.
  - Dullness may indicate a mass or ascites, particularly if percussed in the flanks.
  - Dullness below the left costal margin may indicate splenomegaly, while normal liver spans are usually 6 to 12 cm in the right midclavicular line and 4 to 8 cm in the midsternal line.
- Palpation:
  - Palpation for the detection of hepatomegaly or splenomegaly.
  - Palpation should be performed searching for masses or tenderness in a particular location indicating a visceral source.
  - Murphy sign is palpable tenderness in the RUQ, which induces a midinspiratory pause in breathing and is indicative of cholecystitis.
- Mesenteric ischemia classically presents with pain that is out of proportion to findings on physical examination.
- Signs worrisome for surgical abdomen include the following:
  - Guarding and peritoneal signs (rebound tenderness or a rigid abdomen).
  - Fever.
  - Murphy sign.
  - Iliopsoas sign (hyperextension of right hip causing abdominal pain associated with appendicitis or terminal ileal disease).
  - Absent or high-pitched bowel sounds.

Diagnostic Testing

Laboratories
- CBC, looking for the following:
  - Leukocytosis suggesting acute inflammatory response.

- Anemia, which can indicate GI bleeding.
- Thrombocytopenia suggesting liver disease.
- Serum chemistries evaluating electrolytes, bilirubin, amylase, lipase, alkaline phosphatase, and transaminases.
- Urinalysis to assess hydration, proteinuria, infection, and renal disease.

Imaging
- **Plain films** (obstructive series) are easy, inexpensive, and low risk.
  - Can detect obstruction or perforation (free air under the diaphragm).
  - However, when there is no real concern for obstruction or perforation, plain films are rarely diagnostic.
- **Ultrasound** to evaluate for organomegaly, masses, or biliary tract disease.
- **CT scan** may be more sensitive in detecting intra-abdominal processes.

DIARRHEA

General Principles

- Subjective increase in the frequency of stools as well as liquid consistency.
- Stool quantity that exceeds 200 g/24-hour period.
- Acute diarrhea is that which has been present for <2 to 3 weeks, whereas chronic diarrhea exceeds this time frame.

Diagnosis

Clinical Presentation

History
Onset
- Relation to eating can be important in determining if the diarrhea is due to osmotic or secretory cause, as the latter does not improve with fasting (Table 5).
- Nighttime diarrhea could indicate organic causes including infectious, secretory, inflammatory, or diabetic diarrhea.
- Functional diarrhea such as irritable bowel syndrome tends not to disturb the patient during sleep.

Characteristics
- Ascertain if the patient has had recent travel or contact with others at work, home, or otherwise who have similar symptoms.
- Blood, mucus, or pus in the stool and/or fever may indicate an invasive bacterial pathogen.
- Localized abdominal pain to the lower quadrants or rectum in the presence of bleeding, tenesmus, and weight loss are features of inflammatory bowel disease.
  - Pain is more commonly associated with Crohn disease than ulcerative colitis.
  - Nonspecific diffuse pain or discomfort may be reported with irritable bowel syndrome.
- Tenesmus is the sense of incomplete rectal evacuation accompanied by pain, cramping, and involuntary straining with a similar sensation resulting from proctitis or other inflammatory processes affecting the rectum.
- Patients with steatorrhea (fat malabsorption) often describe light-colored loose stools that are difficult to flush and stick to the toilet bowl.
  - Fatty food intolerance may be observed in disorders of pancreatic exocrine insufficiency.

TABLE 5	Causes of Chronic Diarrhea

Osmotic/Malabsorptive Diarrhea	Secretory Diarrhea	Inflammatory Diarrhea
Causes		
Ingestion of unabsorbed solutes	Hormonal	Crohn disease
Lactose intolerance	VIPoma	Ulcerative colitis (multifactorial)
Medications (e.g., sorbitol, antacids, magnesium laxatives)	Watery diarrhea-hypokalemia-achlorhydria (WDHA) syndrome	Eosinophilic gastroenteritis
Maldigestion	Zollinger-Ellison (gastrinoma)	Intestinal ischemia
Chronic intestinal ischemia	Carcinoid	
Short-bowel syndrome/ bacterial overgrowth	Bile salt malabsorption	
Gastrocolic fistula	Pancreatic cholera	
Mucosal transport defects/ mucosal disease	Collagen vascular disease	
Celiac sprue	Intestinal lymphoma	
Whipple disease		
Acrodermatitis enteropathica		
Lymphatic obstruction		
Chronic pancreatitis		
Signs and symptoms		
Moderate volume of stool	Voluminous stool	Moderate amount of stool (possibly with blood and mucus)
Improved with fasting	Little change with fasting	Little change with fasting
Weight loss	Nighttime symptoms	Weight loss
Signs of nutrient deficiency		Extraintestinal manifestations (arthritis, erythema nodosum, ocular signs)
Diagnosis		
Increased osmolar gap (measured osmolality is 100 mOsm greater than twice the sum of stool cations [K and Na])	Stool osmolality approximates serum osmolality 24-hour stool quantity >1 L	Colonoscopy with mucosal biopsy
Sometimes acidic stool pH	Usually neutral stool pH	Upper endoscopy
Fecal fat >7–10 g/ 24 hours (in steatorrhea)	VIP, vasoactive intestinal polypeptide	Angiography

- Nighttime visual impairment and bone pain may be associated with fat-soluble vitamin malabsorption of vitamins A and D, respectively.
- Frequent small volumes of stool output with urgency suggest distal colorectal pathology, whereas larger volumes with less frequency may be noted in small bowel or proximal colonic disorders.

Physical Examination
- Dehydration should be assessed:
  - Orthostatic hypotension and pulse changes.
  - Poor skin turgor.
  - Dry mucous membranes.
- Cutaneous findings of systemic diseases may be present including the following:
  - Dermatitis herpetiformis which is an intensely pruritic rash of grouped lesions found on the scalp, buttocks, and extensor surface associated with celiac sprue.
  - Acrodermatitis enteropathica, characterized by a maculopapular erythema of the extremities and perineum along with alopecia, sometimes seen in those with zinc and other mineral deficiencies.

Differential Diagnosis

- Sugar substitutes and sugar-free candy or chewing gum containing sorbitol, mannitol, or olestra are a common cause of diarrhea.
- Antibiotic use within the preceding 8 weeks is a predisposing factor for *Clostridium difficile*–associated pseudomembranous colitis.[9]
- Acute diarrhea is usually infectious:
  - Viruses such as Norovirus in adults and older children; rotavirus in young children.
  - Enterotoxigenic bacteria such as *Escherichia coli* (traveler's diarrhea), *Bacillus cereus*, *Clostridium perfringens*, and *Staphylococcus aureus*.
  - Enteropathic agents, which can be invasive, include *Campylobacter*, *Salmonella*, *Shigella*, and certain species of *Yersinia*.
  - Protozoa including *Giardia* species, which can be acquired from spring water consumption during camping and travel as well as amebiasis being common in similar travelers and homosexual men.
- Bloody diarrhea may be secondary to the following:
  - Invasive infections particularly *Campylobacter* and *Shigella*.
  - Acute onset of watery diarrhea that becomes bloody within 24 to 48 hours and is accompanied by fever suggests hemorrhagic colitis caused by *E. coli* O157:H7.
  - Inflammatory bowel disease.
  - Drug-induced colitis.
  - Older individuals with superior mesenteric artery or vein thrombosis.
  - Ischemic colitis particularly in those with previous episode of hypotension.
- Diverticular diarrhea can have features of left lower quadrant discomfort, rectal urgency, pain with defecation, and tenesmus and fever.
- Fecal impaction may paradoxically cause diarrhea in the elderly or in those who consume opioid pain medications with small liquid stool leakage around an impacted hard stool.
- Several categories of chronic diarrhea exist including osmotic, secretory, malabsorptive, and inflammatory (Table 5).
- Dumping syndrome is the voluminous diarrhea shortly after eating, commonly seen in postgastrectomy states. Within a few hours, some may experience the latent phase characterized by weakness, lightheadedness, flushing, and hypoglycemia due to reactive insulin release.

- Irritable bowel syndrome can be characterized by alternating features of diarrhea and constipation and abdominal pain, and frequently coexists with depression or anxiety.
- Diabetic diarrhea occurs in those with poorly controlled and/or long-standing diabetes and usually coexists with other signs of peripheral neuropathy.
- Factitious diarrhea is the surreptitious use of laxatives resulting in severe watery diarrhea, nausea, vomiting, and weight loss.
  - The majority of these individuals are women <30 years of age who have eating disorders or middle-aged women with extensive medical histories who have secondary gains from being chronically ill.[10]
- Significant intestinal resection, particularly segments of the ileum that exceed 100 cm, can result in malabsorption and a bile acid-induced diarrhea.[11]

Diagnostic Testing

Laboratories
- Electrolytes, blood urea nitrogen, and creatinine can assist in identifying severity of dehydration or metabolic acidosis.
- CBC to assess for anemia or leukocytosis.
- Thyroid-stimulating hormone (TSH) level in those with chronic diarrhea.
- Presence of immunoglobulin A (IgA) anti-tissue transglutaminase antibody is highly sensitive and specific for celiac sprue.[12,13]
  - About 10% of celiac sprue patients have selective IgA deficiency, so total IgA levels should be checked as well.
- Stool should be examined for the following:
  - Ova, parasites, and culture.
  - *C. difficile* toxin.
  - Fecal leukocytes, which are nonspecific but indicate inflammatory cause.
  - Stool electrolytes and osmolality to calculate osmotic gap.
  - Sudan staining of stool for fat. If abnormal, obtain 24-hour stool specimen for fat and volume.

Diagnostic Procedures
- **Sigmoidoscopy** workup with biopsies for infectious and inflammatory colitis can be a useful tool for those who have had diarrhea for >1 week.
  - If initially negative or if colitis is present, a full colonoscopy may become necessary to determine the extent of involvement.
- **Upper endoscopy with small bowel biopsies** can be performed in chronic diarrhea to identify celiac sprue histologically.
  - Alternatively, serologic testing can be performed, and upper endoscopy is performed only if serology is abnormal.

Treatment

- **Oral rehydration** with noncaffeinated and nonalcoholic products is preferred, but intravenous fluid administration may be necessary.
- **Antidiarrheal medications** include the following:
  - Kaolin and pectin-containing agents (Kaopectate) may add bulk to stool.
  - Bismuth subsalicylate has antisecretory, antimicrobial, and anti-inflammatory properties.
  - Loperamide (Imodium) initially given as 4 mg dose followed by 2 mg capsules with a maximum of 8 mg/day.

- Diphenoxylate plus atropine (Lomotil) can be given as 5 mg initially and then 2.5 mg after each loose stool to a maximum of 20 mg/day.
- Tincture of opium (0.6 mL every 4 hours).
- Belladonna/opium (1 suppository every 12 hours).
- Codeine (30 to 60 mg PO every 4 hours).
- **All of these agents impair intestinal motility and should be avoided in bacterial infectious states, as they may delay clearance of the organism.**
- **Anticholinergic agents** such as atropine and hyoscyamine products are useful to some, particularly with cramping that accompanies diarrhea.
- **Bulk-forming substances** such as psyllium and methylcellulose may ameliorate functional diarrhea.
- **Cholestyramine** can improve refractory diarrhea of malabsorption or bile acid-induced diarrhea, which can occur as a result of distal small bowel resections.
- **Antibiotics are not required for most acute infectious diarrhea** as it is usually self-limited.
  - Severe traveler's diarrhea that presents as dysentery with bloody stools with/without fever may require antibiotics (discussed in Chapter 22).

CONSTIPATION

General Principles

- Constipation is the subjective feeling of infrequency or difficulty in passing stools.
- The frequency of bowel movements may decrease with age.
- Absolute inability to pass stools can be referred to as obstipation.

Diagnosis

Clinical Presentation

History

Onset
- Recent significant alterations in bowel habits without previous problems should alert the clinician to search for organic causes.
- Intermittent constipation may be due to medications, dietary habits, or functional bowel disease.
- Symptoms that do not relent should be investigated for serious illness such as an obstructive state secondary to a mass.
- Patients with a rectal mass may sometimes describe a gradual reduction of stool caliber.

Characteristics
- Constipation in association with pain could indicate either inflammatory or obstructive causes such as the following:
  - Diverticulitis (left lower quadrant pain).
  - Anal fissures (anorectal pain).
  - Inflammatory colitis (diffuse pain).
  - Thrombosed external hemorrhoids (anal pain).
  - Cancer.
- Cramping abdominal pain associated with bloating relieved by defecation may indicate irritable bowel syndrome if organic pathology has been excluded.
- Digital manipulation either through the vagina or the rectum may be described by the patient as a routine practice to induce bowel movements.

Physical Examination
- Abdominal examination evaluating for distention, tenderness, and masses.
- Tympanic distention may indicate ileus or varying degrees of obstruction.
- Perineal and rectal examination to identify external deformities, such as rectal prolapse and hemorrhoids.
- Digital examination of the rectum assessing for fissures, distal fixed stenosis, masses, or fecal impaction as well as to test perineal sensation, rectal sphincter tone, and reflexes.

Differential Diagnosis
- Medications including opiate pain products, calcium channel blockers, anticholinergic agents, iron supplements, and laxatives in setting of overuse.
- Constipation that accompanies urinary incontinence, particularly in postmenopausal women, could indicate the following:
  - Abnormal pelvic floor relaxation.
  - Rectocele.
  - Cystoceles.
- Inadequate intake of fiber or fluid (6 to 8 glasses daily).
- Colonic inertia.
- Constipation—predominant irritable bowel syndrome.
- Colorectal neoplasia.
- Stricture (postoperative, diverticular, and radiation).
- Hypothyroidism.
- Neurologic/autonomic dysfunction (e.g., diabetes, Parkinson disease, Hirschsprung disease).

Diagnostic Testing
Laboratories
- Serum electrolytes, particularly low potassium, magnesium, and abnormally low or high calcium levels, may become clinically significant.
- Thyroid studies to evaluate for hypothyroidism.
- Hyperglycemia may identify diabetics who may have delayed transit time.

Diagnostic Procedures
- New onset or progressive constipation (especially in those >50 years of age), **colonoscopy** is essential to evaluate for colon cancer or strictures.
  - Melanosis coli, a dark pigmentation that is most often seen in the distal colon, can be seen on colonoscopy in patients who use excess laxatives.
- **Barium enema** may be helpful when combined with flexible sigmoidoscopy to exclude obstructive colonic process.
- **Obstructive series and abdominal CT** may evaluate for obstruction and megacolon (grossly dilated colon with significant abdominal distention).
- **Proctoscopy** may be useful to identify rectal pathology such as hemorrhoids, fissures, and masses.
- **Anorectal manometry** can be used to determine anorectal dysfunction.

Treatment

- Treatment here presumes that serious etiologies have been excluded.
- For **mild** symptoms:

- Increased fiber and fluid intake increases stool bulk and intestinal motility, which is generally only effective for mild constipation or constipation alternating with diarrhea.
- Most individuals with mild constipation are able to achieve a positive response with 20 to 30 g of daily fiber supplementation.[14]
- Behavioral changes include the creation of regular schedule for defecation.
- Bulk-forming laxatives including the following:
  - Psyllium (e.g., Metamucil, 1 tsp in liquid or packet with liquid PO bid-qid).
  - Methylcellulose (e.g., Citrucel, 1 tbsp in 8 oz water qd-tid).
  - Polysaccharide derivatives (e.g., FiberCon, 1 g qid prn; 500-, 625-, and 1,000-mg tablets accompanied by 4 to 6 glasses of water).
- Stool softeners including docusate (100 mg PO bid) can be used along with bulk-forming therapy for maintenance.[15]
- For **moderate** symptoms:
  - Hyperosmolar agents including the following:
    - Polyethylene glycol (17 g PO qd), well tolerated and now available over the counter.
    - Lactulose (15 to 30 g PO every 2 to 3 hours prn) can cause bloating, which may be limiting.
  - Emollient laxatives including the following:
    - Mineral oil (15 to 45 mL PO every 6 to 8 hours) should be used with caution because of the risk of aspiration and lipid pneumonia.
  - Saline laxatives including the following:
    - Magnesium citrate (200 mL PO qid).
    - Fleet phospho soda if no contraindications.
- For **severe** symptoms:
  - Stimulant laxatives including the following:
    - Castor oil (15 to 60 mL qd).
    - Cascara (1 tsp PO bid).
    - Senna (2 tsp PO bid).
    - Bisacodyl (10 to 15 mg PO qd-bid).
    - Lubiprostone (e.g., Amitiza, 24 mcg PO bid).
    - Colchicine (0.6 mg PO bid). It is important to remember, however, that the margin between therapeutic and toxic is rather narrow with this drug.
  - Enemas including the following:
    - Saline enemas (120 to 240 mL).
    - Tap water enemas (500 to 1,000 mL).
    - Oil-retention enemas such as cottonseed with docusate.
- **Routine long-term use of laxatives should be avoided** except for fiber supplements, hyperosmolar agents, and stool softeners, which have an adequate safety profile.
- Surgical treatment reserved for rectal deformities, intestinal obstruction and masses, resuspension of rectal intussusception, or prolapse and pelvic floor disorders.

ANORECTAL COMPLAINTS

General Principles

- In the anus, the dentate line (mucocutaneous junction) divides the sensory (anus) and nonsensory (rectum) regions.
- The varied presentation of anorectal complaints in the ambulatory setting can often provide ample information to guide the identification of a specific etiology.

Diagnosis

Clinical Presentation

History
- Evaluation for anal pruritus, pain with defecation, bleeding, and fever.
- Association with underlying constipation, inflammatory bowel disease, or other medical illness.
- Evaluation of bowel habits, incontinence, and rectal pain changing with position.

Physical Examination
- Simple visual inspection after spreading the buttocks can often identify a tear, lesion, or fluctuant mass with purulence.
- Digital examination of the rectum for impacted stool, anal sphincter tone, blood, fissure, or mass.
- A lateral or anterior fissure found on examination may suggest Crohn disease, proctitis, leukemia, syphilis, tuberculosis, or carcinoma. Posterior fissures are often benign and self-limited.

Differential Diagnosis
- **External hemorrhoids** (form below dentate line) manifesting as anal pruritus and sometimes pain, the most exquisite pain and bleeding occur with thrombosis of an external hemorrhoid.
- **Internal hemorrhoids** (form above dentate line) may produce mild discomfort, but significant pain is seen primarily in prolapse and strangulation.
  - Bleeding from internal hemorrhoids is usually minimal, bright red in color, and found on the outside of stool or on toilet paper.
- **Anal fissure** is a linear tear of the tissue or sphincter as a result of passage of hard stool found in the anal canal and is often associated with pain and rectal bleeding.
- **Perirectal fistula** characterized as a chronic purulent, foul-smelling discharge from the rectum, or small opening in the perineum is found with Crohn disease.
  - Perirectal abscess should raise suspicion for Crohn disease or immunosuppression.
- **Rectal prolapse** manifesting as extrusion of the rectum during defecation and may need manual reduction by the patient. This is often seen in women and may be associated with urinary symptoms.
- **Rectosigmoid intussusception** presenting with hematochezia and pain.
- **Proctalgia fugax** is a condition found in young adults characterized by sudden brief episodes of severe rectal pain occurring along the midline. Symptoms are typically mild and are a result of levator ani musculature spasm.
- **Fecal incontinence** with episodes of rectal urgency and fecal soiling of garments.
- **Pruritus ani** is the itching sensation of the anus or perianal skin.
  - It is a possible manifestation of residual fecal material, hemorrhoids, rectal fistula, anal fissures, malignancy, psoriasis, or ingestion of certain foods.
  - Infections may cause these symptoms such as pinworms, scabies, pubic lice, and certain sexually transmitted diseases.

Diagnostic Testing
- **Anoscopy** generally used to evaluate for anal fissures with 90% of lesions found at the posterior midline.
- Direct visualization via **sigmoidoscopy or colonoscopy** to evaluate for hemorrhoids, perirectal fistula, intussusception, malignancy, or inflammatory bowel disease.

- Perineal sensory disturbances, identifiable by nerve conduction studies, can be a sign of low back injury or degenerative disk disease with nerve damage.
- Endoscopic ultrasound can assess the sphincter for mechanical disruption.

Treatment

- Increased **dietary fiber,** resulting in softer bulky stools and less straining, as well as **stool softeners, analgesic suppositories, warm sitz baths** given two to three times a day can alleviate most anorectal pains.[16]
- Topical nitroglycerin or injection with botulinum toxin has achieved temporary relaxation of sphincter tone to permit healing with anal fissures.[17]
- Antibiotics such as ciprofloxacin and metronidazole may aid in healing of perirectal fistulas, with alternative medical therapy available if related to Crohn disease.
- Pelvic floor muscle strengthening with biofeedback can be used in appropriate patients.
- Patients with proctalgia fugax benefit from reassurance and symptomatic relief with local heat and massage.
- Pruritus ani benefits from treatment including the following:
  - Antimicrobial therapy for specific organism, if indicated.
  - Oral antihistamines for nocturnal symptoms.
  - Short-term topical treatment with hydrocortisone cream 1% (not to exceed 2 weeks' duration) or zinc oxide ointment.
- Surgical interventions may be needed for the following:
  - Persistent symptomatic hemorrhoids for endoscopic band ligation or hemorrhoidectomy.
  - Chronic anal fissures requiring anal sphincterotomy.
  - Excision and drainage of perirectal fistulas.
  - Incision and drainage of perirectal abscesses.
  - Reduction of rectal prolapse or frequent partial prolapse.
  - Refractory fecal incontinence.

APPROACH TO ABNORMAL LIVER CHEMISTRIES

General Principles

- Laboratory evaluation, imperfect and incomplete by itself, must be integrated with the clinical history, physical examination, and setting. A full discussion of liver diseases is presented in Chapter 26.
- Liver tests abnormalities can be very generally grouped into those that indicate the following:
  - **Hepatocellular disease** (aspartate aminotransferase [AST] and alanine aminotransferase [ALT] elevated more than bilirubin and alkaline phosphatase).
  - **Cholestatic disease** (bilirubin zand alkaline phosphatase elevated more than AST and ALT).

Diagnosis

Clinical Presentation
History
Location
- The constellation of RUQ pain, fever, and jaundice is known as Charcot triad and can be the presentation of cholecystitis.

- The addition of mental status alteration and hypotension to this triad is known as Reynolds pentad and can indicate ascending cholangitis.
- Pain in the mid-abdomen that radiates to the back may be present in pancreatitis.

Characteristics

- Evaluate for nonspecific symptom including nausea, vomiting, chills, fevers, anorexia, and weight loss.
- Fatigue alone is frequently reported as the primary presenting symptom by many individuals with liver disease.
- Dark urine is noted by many patients earlier than jaundice and is an indication of increased urobilinogen.
- Exposure to viruses should be ascertained, particularly hepatitis and questions regarding blood transfusion history, intravenous drug use, and sexual contacts as well as travel to areas endemic for hepatitis.
- Presence of pruritus, which is usually generalized and present in almost all cases of jaundice that exceeds 3 to 4 weeks.
- Acute onset may indicate hemolysis or biliary tract obstruction.
- Painless jaundice should raise suspicion for pancreaticobiliary disorders, as neoplasms of the pancreatic head may result in extrahepatic biliary obstruction.
- Abdominal pain may reflect stretching of the liver capsule or a space-occupying lesion.
- Congestive heart failure and passive hepatic congestion can account for up to 10% of all jaundice in those >60 years of age.[18]
- RUQ pain and fever with jaundice should raise the possibility of cholangitis.
  - Rapid intense RUQ pain may imply choledocholithiasis, particularly in those with prior cholelithiasis or cholecystectomy.

Physical Examination

- Evaluate for **stigmata of chronic liver** disease such as parotid gland enlargement, spider angiomas (most commonly found on the trunk), palmar erythema, Dupuytren contractures (fibrous contractures of the palmar fascia), gynecomastia, hepatomegaly or small liver size, splenomegaly, caput medusa, testicular atrophy, and ascites.
- **Fever** can be found in acute and chronic illness and may be suggestive of infection.
- **Hepatomegaly** >15 cm in span can be found in passive congestion, malignant or fatty infiltration, or other infiltrative disorders.
- **Splenomegaly** is found in patients with portal hypertension and cirrhosis, and may also be found in those with hemolysis and a vast array of hematologic disorders and malignancies.
- **Murphy sign** (RUQ tenderness palpated during inspiration) may indicate cholecystitis.
- **Ascites** may be present in cirrhosis of various causes and intra-abdominal malignancy as well as congestive heart failure and pancreatitis.
- **Palpable distended gallbladder** without tenderness (Courvoisier sign) is commonly found in pancreaticobiliary malignancy with obstruction.
- Cutaneous findings include xanthomas, which may be seen in chronic cholestasis of primary biliary cirrhosis.
- Gray-bronze discoloration of the skin may suggest hemochromatosis with hepatic involvement.
- Urticaria may be a sign of acute hepatitis B infection.

Differential Diagnosis

The differential diagnosis for abnormal liver tests is presented in Table 6.

TABLE 6	Causes of Abnormal Liver Tests

Hepatocellular Disease

Dugs/toxins

Acetaminophen, with the use of as little as 4 g/day in an individual with prior liver disease can result in hepatocyte damage

Herbal agents

Vitamin A

NSAIDs[19]

Propylthiouracil

Antidepressants (e.g., duloxetine, sertraline, phenelzine)

General anesthetics

Antimicrobials (e.g., sulfonamides, erythromycin, isoniazid, antifungals)

Anticonvulsants (e.g., phenytoin, carbamazepine)

Many others (particularly with idiosyncratic drug reactions)

Certain occupational exposures can result in hepatotoxicity with exposure to chemicals such as arsenic in many industrial settings and in organic gardening as well as insecticides for agricultural workers

Alcohol use

Daily consumption that exceeds 80 g (72 oz beer, 9 oz liquor, or 30 oz wine) for 10–15 years can lead to cirrhosis in men, while lower levels possibly 20–40 g/day for women.

Hepatitis

Viral (A, B, C, D, E, Ebstein-Barr virus, cytomegalovirus)

Autoimmune hepatitis

Other

Hemochromatosis

Wilson disease

α-1-Antitrypsin deficiency

Shock liver

Cholestatic Disease

Intrahepatic causes

Viral hepatitis

Alcoholic liver disease

Drugs

Antimicrobials (nitrofurantoin, floxins, macrolides, amoxicillin-clavulanic acid and other penicillin-based antibiotics)

Anabolic steroids

Oral contraceptives

Sulfonyureas

Phenothiazines (e.g., chlorpromazine, prochlorperazine)

Malignancy such as hepatocellular carcinoma, lymphoma or other masses

Sepsis

Abscesses

Pregnancy

Primary biliary cirrhosis

Primary sclerosing cholangitis

Sarcoidosis

Amyloidosis

Pregnancy

Total parenteral nutrition

Extrahepatic causes

Choledocholithiasis

Cholangiocarcinoma

Pancreatitis

Pancreatic cancer or pseudocyst

Papillary stenosis

Primary sclerosing cholangitis

NSAIDs, nonsteroidal anti-inflammatory agents.

Diagnostic Testing

Laboratories

Evaluate for hemolysis with a CBC, peripheral blood smear, elevated reticulocyte count, lactate dehydrogenase, and reduced haptoglobin as well as predominantly indirect hyperbilirubinemia.

Bilirubin

- Impaired excretion of bilirubin results in an increase in the conjugated form, and clinical icterus presents if the total bilirubin level exceeds 2.5 mg/dL.
- Bilirubin elevation can be prolonged despite convalescence of the acute illness because of its binding to albumin.
- An isolated indirect hyperbilirubinemia that does not exceed 5 mg/dL with normal transaminases and no indications of hemolysis may be the result of a benign familial disorder known as Gilbert syndrome, and the hyperbilirubinemia may occur during states of fasting and physiologic stress.

Prothrombin Time

- Measure of the liver's synthetic function.
- Vitamin K-dependent factors of coagulations II, VII, IX, and X are reflected by this test and normal value is dependent on intact synthesis and absorption of intestinal vitamin K.
- Cirrhosis, hepatitis, and cholestatic syndromes may have prolonged values and as a result serves as a useful prognosticator in patients with cirrhosis.

Albumin

- Another measure of the liver's synthetic function.
- Half-life of 20 days, making it better indicator of chronic rather than acute liver process.
- Low levels may be present in some patients with poor nutrition.
- Levels do not often correlate accurately, however, and should not be used as a primary assessment of a patient's nutritional status.
- Loss of this protein can occur through the GI tract or kidneys.
- Dilutional effect should also be considered in volume overload states, normal pregnancy, and in acute or chronic inflammatory states.

Aminotransferases

- AST can be released into the blood from numerous tissues, including liver, cardiac and skeletal muscle, kidney, and brain.
- ALT is more specific to the liver, and serum levels rise with hepatocyte death.
- Highest elevations, in the thousands, seen in viral hepatitis and toxin- or ischemia-induced hepatic injury.
- Elevation of AST and ALT in a ≥2:1 ratio, high-serum γ-glutamyl transpeptidase (GGT), and an elevated mean corpuscular volume of red cells can be highly suspicious for alcoholic liver disease.
- Injury from alcohol almost never results in elevations that exceed 10-fold of the normal values.

Alkaline Phosphatase

- Elevated serum levels can arise from processes that affect the liver, skeletal system, intestines, placenta, kidneys, and leukocytes.
- GGT levels can differentiate between biliary and other sources of alkaline phosphatase.
- Largest increases are seen in cholestatic syndromes, intrahepatic, and extrahepatic biliary ductal obstruction.

- Markedly increased levels without associated liver disease are sometimes seen in congestive heart failure, bone diseases, and Hodgkin lymphoma.

Others
- Antimitochondrial antibody (AMA) indicating primary biliary cirrhosis.
- Antismooth-muscle antibody (ASMA) and antinuclear antibody and immunoglobulins indicating autoimmune hepatitis.
- Iron studies for hemochromatosis.
- Viral hepatitis panel.
- α-Fetoprotein (AFP) for hepatocellular malignancy.[20]

Diagnostic Procedures
- **Ultrasound** should be used initially for the rapid evaluation of the biliary system.
  - Sensitivity is 95% for detection of cholelithiasis and acute cholecystitis and identifying ductal dilation.
- **CT scan** should be obtained for distinction between stones, tumors, and stricture as well as liver parenchyma examination.
- **Endoscopic retrograde cholangiopancreatography (ERCP)** is most useful in diagnosing and treating obstructive jaundice in setting of choledocholithiasis, cholangitis, intra- and extrahepatic strictures, and pancreatic ductal disease. **Magnetic resonance cholangiopancreatography (MRCP)** is also useful diagnostically but has no therapeutic use.
- **Liver biopsy** is helpful in diagnosing the etiology of liver disease in those with abnormal enzymes for >6 months and if obstruction is excluded.
- If ascites is present, **paracentesis** with initial studies including the following:
  - Cell count to rule out infection.
  - Serum-ascites albumin gradient (SAAG, the difference between serum and ascites albumin measurements), values of >1.1 indicate portal hypertension.
  - Cytology to evaluate for malignancy.

Treatment

Treatment depends on the underlying illness. See Chapter 26 for specific management.

REFERENCES

1. Jalil S, Castell DO. Schatzki's ring: a benign cause of dysphagia in adults. *J Clin Gastroenterol* 2002;35:295–298.
2. Hewson EG, Sinclair JW, Dalton CB et al. Twenty-four-hour esophageal pH monitoring: The most useful test for evaluating noncardiac chest pain. *Am J Med 1991*;90:576–583.
3. Domenech E, Kelly J. Swallowing Disorders. *Med Clin North Am* 1999;83:97–113.
4. DeVault KR, Castell DO. Updated guidelines for diagnosis and treatment of gastroesophageal reflux disease. *Am J Gastroenterol* 2005;100:190–200.
5. Talley NJ, Vakil NB, Moayyedi P. American Gastroenterological Association technical review on the evaluation of dyspepsia. *Gastroenterology* 2005;129:1756–1780.
6. Cohen J, Safdi MA, Deal SE, et al. ASGE/ACG Taskforce on Quality in Endoscopy. Quality indicators for esophagogastroduodenoscopy. *Am J Gastroenterol* 2006;101:886–891.
7. Fisher RS, Parkman HP. Management of nonulcer dyspepsia. *N Engl J Med* 1998;339:1376–1381.
8. Yamada T, Alpers DH, Laine L, et al. Textbook of Gastroenterology. 3rd Ed. New York: Lippincott Williams & Wilkins, 1999:804.
9. Hurley BW, Nguyen CC. The spectrum of pseudomembranous enterocolitis and antibiotic-associated diarrhea. *Arch Intern Med* 2002;162:2177–2184.

10. Ewe K, Karbach U. Factitious diarrhoea. *Clin Gastroenterol* 1986;15:723–740.
11. Potter GD. Bile acid diarrhea. *Dig Dis* 1998;16:118–124.
12. Carroccio A, Vitale G, Di Prima L, et al. Comparison of anti-transglutaminase ELISAs and an anti-endomysial antibody assay in the diagnosis of celiac disease: a prospective study. *Clin Chem* 2002;48:1546–1550.
13. Rostom A, Dubé C, Cranney A, et al. The diagnostic accuracy of serologic tests for celiac disease: a systematic review. *Gastroenterology* 2005;128:S38–S46.
14. Soffer EE. Constipation: an approach to diagnosis, treatment, referral. *Cleve Clin J Med* 1999;66(1):41–46.
15. Schiller LR. Clinical pharmacology and use of laxatives and lavage solutions. *J Clin Gastroenterol* 1999;28(1):11–18.
16. Hager T. Anal fissure. *Ther Umsch* 1997;54:190–192.
17. Dhawan S, Chopra S. Nonsurgical approaches for the treatment of anal fissures. *Am J Gastroenterol* 2007;102:1312–1321.
18. Qureshi WA. Intrahepatic cholestatic syndromes: pathogenesis, clinical features and management. *Dig Dis* 1999;17:49–59.
19. Zimmerman HJ. Update of hepatotoxicity due to classes of drugs in common clinical use: non-steroidal drugs, anti-inflammatory drugs, antibiotics, antihypertensives, and cardiac and psychotropic agents. *Semin Liver Dis* 1990;10(4):322–338.
20. Frank BB. Clinical evaluation of jaundice. A guideline of the Patient Care Committee of the American Gastroenterological Association. *JAMA* 1989;262:3031–3034.

Gastroesophageal Reflux Disease

C. Prakash Gyawali

General Principles

- Gastroesophageal reflux disease (GERD) is a condition characterized by symptoms or tissue damage from reflux of gastric contents into the esophagus or beyond.
- Population surveys indicate that GERD is very common, with 10% to 20% of the general population reporting at least weekly symptoms.[1,2]

Pathophysiology

- There are several barriers to reflux of gastric contents into the esophagus.[3,4]
  - Resting tone in the lower esophageal sphincter (LES) keeps the gastroesophageal junction closed in between swallows.
  - The diaphragmatic crura, normally aligned with the LES, pinch the gastroesophageal junction during inspiration to prevent reflux when intrathoracic pressure is negative relative to the atmosphere.
  - Any refluxed material is promptly returned back into the stomach by secondary peristaltic waves initiated by local esophageal neural reflexes.
  - Residual acidic material in the mucosa is neutralized by saliva, which is alkaline.
- Despite these measures, physiologic reflux occurs in most individuals, typically after meals.
- Inappropriate transient LES relaxation is the most frequent mechanism of reflux, in health and in patients with GERD.[3,4]
  - The LES is designed to relax immediately at the initiation of a swallow.
  - A transient LES relaxation is said to occur inappropriately when the LES relaxes in between swallows.
  - Several triggers, including a full stomach and the presence of a hiatus hernia, may precipitate frequent transient LES relaxations, which in turn can lead to reflux of gastric contents into the esophagus.
- Low tone in the LES is seen in approximately a quarter of reflux patients, wherein the barrier to gastroesophageal reflux is weak.[3,4]
  - A prototype condition associated with extremely low LES tone is scleroderma esophagus, where fibrosis of the esophageal smooth muscle leads to near absent tone in the LES, and hypomotility or aperistalsis in the esophageal body.
  - Certain medications and food items that can lower LES tone are listed below:
    - Anticholinergics.
    - Smooth muscle relaxants.
    - Caffeine.
    - Theophylline.
    - Alcohol.
    - Fatty or greasy foods.

- A hiatus hernia results when the diaphragmatic crura are not snug against the gastroesophageal junction, allowing a pouch of stomach to prolapse proximal to the crura.[3,4]
  - The typical axial hiatus hernia slides up and down through the diaphragmatic hiatus. The presence of a hiatus hernia disrupts the physiologic barrier to gastroesophageal reflux by several mechanisms.
    - First, the anatomic integrity of the barrier formed by close alignment of the diaphragmatic crura and the closed LES is lost.
    - A pouch of gastric mucosa is now above the level of the diaphragmatic pinch, which can serve as a reservoir for gastric (acidic) secretions that can easily reflux when the patient lays supine.
    - Finally, local neural reflexes may be affected by the presence of the hiatus hernia, allowing for a higher frequency of inappropriate LES relaxations.
  - The larger the hiatus hernia, the higher the likelihood for reflux.
  - However, **not every patient with a hiatus hernia has GERD, and not every patient with GERD has a hiatus hernia.**

Diagnosis

Clinical Presentation

Typical Presentation

Heartburn is the most frequent reflux symptom, described by patients as a burning sensation retrosternally or in the epigastrium.[4]
- The discomfort may radiate upward to the neck, to the shoulders, or even to the back.
- Acid reflux can occur often in the postprandial state but can sometimes occur at night and awaken the patient from sleep.
- Eating or taking an antacid promptly relieves the symptom by neutralizing refluxed acid.
- Heartburn may be associated with regurgitation of a sour, bitter liquid with an acidic taste.
- Bending over, laying supine, and wearing tight garments over the abdomen may provoke both heartburn and regurgitation in some instances.
- Mucosal inflammation in the esophagus from acid reflux can also prompt the sensation of dysphagia in some patients, which may improve with acid suppressive therapy.
- **Heartburn and regurgitation are considered typical reflux symptoms.**

Atypical Presentations

Over the past few decades, several atypical reflux symptoms have been identified. It is important to recognize atypical symptoms, as they may occur even when typical symptoms are absent.[5]
- The most significant atypical symptom is **chest pain,** important because chest pain may indicate concomitant cardiac disease. Conversely, cardiac disease needs careful exclusion before chest pain is attributed to GERD in appropriate age groups. In older patients, both GERD and coronary artery disease can coexist. Despite documenting correlation of reflux with chest pain, many patients continue to worry about cardiac disease, making noncardiac chest pain an important cause for health care expenditure.
- **Wheezing and asthma** have also been linked to reflux, especially adult-onset symptoms in the absence of an allergic component. There are two mechanisms by which reflux can result in asthma:
  - Regurgitation of gastric contents to the pharynx and tracheal microaspiration.
  - Triggering of a reflex bronchospasm in susceptible individuals by smaller amounts of acid in the distal esophagus.

- When correlation between bronchospastic symptoms and reflux exists, adequate management of GERD can lead to better treatment outcomes. Other pulmonary symptoms and disorders linked to reflux include cough, interstitial fibrosis, and aspiration pneumonia.
- Other supraesophageal manifestations of reflux disease include hoarseness, throat clearing, dental erosions, and posterior laryngitis. Dyspeptic symptoms, nausea, and back pain may also have etiologic links to GERD in certain situations.

Differential Diagnosis

Eosinophilic Esophagitis

- Eosinophilic esophagitis is a condition characterized by eosinophil infiltration of the esophageal mucosa and submucosa, leading to mucosal inflammation, fibrosis, and luminal narrowing.[6,7]
- It is seen most often in young men.
- Presenting manifestations can be perceptive, such as heartburn and chest pain, or obstructive, such as dysphagia and recurrent food bolus impactions.
- Upon endoscopic evaluation, the esophageal lumen may be narrowed with a corrugated trachea-like appearance; linear furrows, erosions, and exudates can also be seen.
- Mucosal biopsies typically demonstrate >20 eosinophils/high power field.
- **Topical steroids** (e.g., fluticasone inhaler, sprayed to the back of the throat and swallowed, two puffs twice a day) are now considered first-line treatments; montelukast and cromolyn have also been used with variable success.
- Cautious dilation can be considered for dysphagia resistant to topical steroid therapy.

Infectious Esophagitis

- **Candida esophagitis** is the most frequent infectious esophagitis seen in immunocompromised individuals.[8]
  - Other risk factors include esophageal stasis (strictures, achalasia, and neoplasia), antibiotic use, steroid use, diabetes, and malnutrition.
  - Endoscopic evaluation reveals whitish exudates, and plaques in the esophagus and fungal hyphae can be seen on cytology.
  - If an immunocompromised patient has esophageal symptoms (dysphagia and odynophagia) and oropharyngeal thrush is encountered, empiric therapy with **fluconazole** (100 mg daily for 14 days) or **nystatin** (100,000 units/mL, 5 mL tid for 14 to 21 days) can be empirically initiated, reserving endoscopy for refractory symptoms.
- **Herpes esophagitis** can occur in both immunocompetent and immunocompromised hosts.[8]
  - A history of cold sores is frequently elicited.
  - Patients present with severe odynophagia, resulting in food aversion.
  - Endoscopic evaluation may reveal grouped vesicles or ulcers, biopsies from which may reveal intracytoplasmic inclusions.
  - Therapy consists of **acyclovir** for 10 to 14 days.
- **Cytomegalovirus esophagitis** is only seen in immunocompromised hosts, typically after solid organ transplants and in advanced AIDS with low CD4 counts.[8]
  - Endoscopy typically reveals deep ulcers, and biopsies demonstrate typical intranuclear inclusions.

Pill Esophagitis

- Pill esophagitis is usually seen in conjunction with esophageal stasis, strictures, and hypomotility disorders.[9]

- Presentation may include heartburn, chest pain, and odynophagia.
- Frequent locations for pill esophagitis are the levels of the aortic arch and the LES.
- Usual culprits include quinidine, tetracycline, doxycycline, nonsteroidal anti-inflammatory drugs, and alendronate.

Functional Heartburn and Chest Pain
- Perceptive esophageal symptoms similar to that seen with GERD can be encountered in patients with visceral hyperalgesia.[10]
- Symptoms may overlap with nonerosive reflux disease, functional heartburn, and functional chest pain.

Diagnostic Testing
Proton Pump Inhibitor Trial
- **The most convenient and cost-effective approach for diagnosis of GERD is by initiating a therapeutic trial of proton pump inhibitor (PPI) therapy.**[11]
- This approach has been studied using omeprazole (40 mg before breakfast and 20 mg before supper) for 1 week in patients with typical symptoms.
- Symptom resolution predicts good diagnostic accuracy with a sensitivity of 78% and specificity of 54% in meta-analyses.[12]
- Patients with atypical symptoms require double doses of PPIs and longer-therapeutic trials, as long as 1 month for atypical chest pain and 3 to 6 months for supraesophageal symptoms.[5]

Endoscopy
- Endoscopy is performed frequently in patients with reflux symptoms.[13]
- However, esophagitis is visualized in only 50% to 60% of GERD patients with typical symptoms if endoscopy is performed prior to initiation of antireflux therapy; the number goes down to <10% if adequate antireflux therapy has already been initiated.[13,14]
- The frequency of finding visible esophagitis is lower in patients with atypical symptoms (30% for asthma, 15% to 20% for atypical chest pain, and ≤15% for laryngeal symptoms) even under ideal circumstances.
- Therefore, the best use of endoscopy is to evaluate for complications and to **screen for Barrett esophagus**.[11,13]
- Patients with **alarm symptoms** (dysphagia, weight loss, anemia, and family history of esophageal cancer), with a long history of reflux symptoms (>5 years), older patients (>45 years), or those failing to respond adequately to antisecretory therapy are offered endoscopy, typically performed after the patient has been taking a PPI for 8 to 12 weeks. The purpose of the procedure is, therefore, to evaluate for ongoing erosive esophagitis, alternate causes of esophagitis (e.g., eosinophilic esophagitis, and infectious esophagitis), strictures, Barrett esophagus, and esophageal neoplasia).

Ambulatory pH Monitoring
- Ambulatory pH monitoring is considered the **gold standard for quantifying esophageal acid exposure**.[11,15]
  - The test is not used to diagnose GERD but rather to confirm its presence in patients referred for antireflux surgery, patients with atypical symptoms, and patients not responding to seemingly adequate antireflux measures.
  - Ambulatory pH monitoring allows not just measurement of acid exposure time, but also provides correlation of symptoms and reflux events.

- There are two techniques of pH monitoring:
  - **Catheter-based monitoring** with one or two pH sensors.
  - **Wireless monitoring,** where a pH sensor capsule is temporarily attached to the esophageal mucosa and communicates with a receiver worn by the patient.
- The test is performed off antireflux therapy (off PPIs for a week, H_2 receptor blockers for 3 days, and antacids for 24 hours) when quantification of acid exposure is desired or when correlation between symptoms and reflux events is sought.
- Testing on twice a day PPI therapy allows assessment of adequacy of treatment in patients with persisting symptoms despite therapy. This latter indication may be taken over by the use of esophageal impedance-pH testing as described below.
- Ambulatory pH monitoring only measures acidic elements in the refluxate, but impedance monitoring assesses for all refluxed elements regardless of the pH of the refluxate.[15,16]
  - Impedance is measured by passing minute electrical currents through pairs of electrodes implanted on a catheter, changes in the resistance to flow of current indicating movement of liquid refluxate or air (e.g., belch), and direction of movement of the change indicating swallows or reflux events.
  - Impedance catheters typically have a pH sensor for distal esophageal pH measurement. Impedance-pH monitoring is an attractive option for patients with ongoing symptoms despite antireflux therapy, especially if symptoms are regurgitation predominant.

Esophageal Manometry
- Esophageal manometry contributes little to the diagnosis of GERD but may define pathophysiologic mechanisms in patients with impaired esophageal peristalsis or low LES resting tone.[11,15,17]
- It is performed most often **prior to antireflux surgery** to assess adequacy of esophageal peristaltic performance and to exclude potentially confounding diagnoses such as achalasia.
- Esophageal manometry also identifies the location of the LES for placement of catheter-based pH and impedance-pH probes.

Barium Esophagogram
- Barium contrast esophagograms provide accurate anatomic information and delineate even subtle strictures or narrowings.
- Barium studies are **not accurate in initial diagnosis of GERD** and should not be used for this indication.[13,18]

Other Diagnostic Procedures
Other specialized esophageal investigative studies used in the research setting include the Bernstein test, balloon distension studies, esophageal planimetry, high-definition ultrasound, and transit time measurements.

Treatment

Medications
Acidic gastric contents are corrosive to the esophageal mucosa; therefore, the basis of pharmacologic treatment is to reduce gastric acidity to render the refluxate less corrosive.

Proton Pump Inhibitors
- **The standard of acid suppressive therapy is the PPI.**[11,19]

TABLE 1	Typical Doses of Antisecretory Medication for GERD
Drug	**Dosage**
Proton pump inhibitors	
Esomeprazole (Nexium)	20–40 mg daily/bid
Lansoprazole (Prevacid)	15–30 mg daily/bid
Omeprazole (Prilosec, generic)	20–40 mg daily/bid
Omeprazole with $NaHCO_3$ (Zegerid)	20–40 mg daily/bid
Pantoprazole (Protonix)	40 mg daily/bid
Rabeprazole (Aciphex)	20 mg daily/bid
Histamine$_2$ receptor antagonists	
Cimetidine (Tagamet, generic)	200–400 mg bid
Famotidine (Pepcid, generic)	20–40 mg bid
Ranitidine (Zantac, generic)	150–300 mg bid

- PPIs are administered 30 to 60 minutes before a meal to allow the agent to circulate in the blood stream when the proton pumps are activated by a meal.
- The PPIs then bind to the proton pump and render them inactive, thereby lowering gastric acidity for 12 to 18 hours.
- For continued efficacy, these agents have to be administered daily, prior to breakfast if used once a day, and additionally prior to supper if used twice a day.
- PPIs are remarkably safe, minor side effects include abdominal pain and diarrhea. Fundic gland polyps may develop in some patients on long-term acid suppression.[20] Concern for rare side effects arises from prolonged continued use, but reports are limited and long-term studies continue to establish overall safety of these agents.[21]
- These rare side effects include small intestinal bacterial overgrowth, *Clostridium difficile* colitis, vitamin B_{12} malabsorption, and calcium malabsorption leading to osteopenia and hip fractures in susceptible individuals.[22–24]
- Commonly available PPIs are listed in Table 1.

Histamine$_2$ Receptor Antagonists
- H$_2$ receptor antagonists also lower gastric acid secretion and may be effective in patients with intermittent or mild symptoms.
- H$_2$ receptor antagonists have been used in addition to PPI therapy in patients with nocturnal breakthrough symptoms.
- These agents may be **subject to tachyphylaxis,** which may affect continued efficacy.
- Side effects include drug interactions and rarely thrombocytopenia and confusion.

Promotility Agents
- **There are no effective promotility agents appropriate for management of GERD symptoms currently in the market.**[11]
- Metoclopramide is sometimes prescribed to enhance gastric emptying but is associated with frequent side effects, including irritability and extrapyramidal dysfunction. Benefit has not been systematically demonstrated.
- Cisapride, a 5-HT$_4$ receptor agonist, has been noted to augment esophageal peristalsis and at one time was evaluated as an adjunctive agent to antisecretory therapy. However, the potential for cardiac rhythm disturbances makes this agent unsuitable for routine use, and it has been removed from the U.S. general market.

- Baclofen may reduce the frequency of transient inappropriate LES relaxations but is associated with frequent side effects including sedation. Efforts are ongoing to identify a baclofen-like agent with a favorable side effect profile.

Lifestyle Modification

- Lifestyle modification measures make physiologic sense but are **not considered adequate in themselves for management of symptomatic reflux disease.** Rather, these measures are recommended in conjunction with pharmacologic therapy.[11]
- These measures include the following:
  - Avoid large meals.
  - Avoid eating 2 to 3 hours before lying down.
  - Avoid foods and beverages that can decrease the lower-esophageal sphincter pressure (e.g., chocolate, peppermint, caffeine, and alcohol).
  - Individual patients should avoid foods that worsen their symptoms—common examples include acidic foods, spicy foods, and fatty foods, but this is not necessarily consistent from patient to patient.
  - Avoid tight-fitting garments.
  - Lose weight.
  - Elevate the head of the bed (placement of 4 to 6 in blocks underneath the legs of the bed is preferred to propping the head up with pillows).
  - Quit smoking and stop alcohol use.

Surgical Management

- Antireflux surgery performed by an experienced surgeon is an alternate option to pharmacologic management in patients with well-documented GERD.[11]
- Patients with large hiatus hernias, low LES resting tone, and regurgitation predominant symptoms appear to benefit most from this approach.
- Good to excellent results can be expected in patients who respond to PPI therapy, especially when there is good symptom-reflux correlation on ambulatory pH monitoring.
- It is estimated that the cost of antireflux surgery compares with that of pharmacologic therapy in approximately 10 years.
- Breakthrough reflux symptoms may develop in some, especially after 5 to 10 years and supplemental antisecretory therapy may be required.

Complications

Mucosal Erosion/Strictures

- Mucosal erosions are seen in the esophagus in approximately 60% of patients with typical reflux symptoms prior to initiation of antireflux therapy.
- In 10% to 15% patients, these erosions can be circumferential and associated with ulcerations.
- Healing of ulcerated areas can lead to luminal narrowing and **stricture formation.**

Barrett Esophagus

- In genetically susceptible individuals, acid reflux can trigger a change in the distal esophageal mucosal lining from the normal squamous cell lining to incomplete intestinal metaplasia, termed Barrett esophagus.[11,25]
- This is characterized visually as a change in color from normal pearly white to salmon pink, either in a circumferential fashion or as slivers of changed mucosa extending proximally from the gastroesophageal junction, also called "tongues."

- Barrett esophagus is seen most frequently in middle-aged Caucasian males who are obese and who smoke and consume alcohol.[26]
- The overall prevalence of Barrett esophagus is thought to be about 5% to 15% in the GERD population and about 1% to 2% in the general population.[26,27]
- The significance of Barrett esophagus is the **small but real risk of progression to high-grade dysplasia and esophageal adenocarcinoma.**
- The incidence of esophageal adenocarcinoma has been rising over the past few decades and has overtaken squamous cell cancer as the most frequent esophageal cancer in Caucasian males.
- Although Barrett esophagus is asymptomatic, erosive disease and adenocarcinoma both can lead to symptoms of dysphagia, anemia, and rarely weight loss, making these **alarm symptoms** necessitating endoscopic evaluation of the esophagus.

Extraesophageal Complications

- Extraesophageal complications of GERD include laryngitis, tracheal stenosis, interstitial pneumonitis, aspiration pneumonia, dental erosions, worsening of asthma, and chronic cough.
- It is not completely clear if reflux of gastric contents can contribute to laryngeal cancer.

Management of Complications

Esophageal Strictures

- Esophageal strictures result from chronic esophageal injury related to acid reflux.
- When dysphagia results, esophageal dilation is frequently needed.[28]
- Dilation can be performed with through-the-scope endoscopic balloons or bougies, either passed blindly (Maloney dilators) or over a guide wire (Savary dilators).
- Continued acid suppression with a PPI may delay recurrence of peptic esophageal strictures.
- Refractory strictures that recur within short intervals may benefit from steroid injection into the rents created by dilation, which may prolong intervals between dilations.

Barrett Esophagus

- Characterized by the transformation of squamous mucosa to specialized intestinal type columnar mucosa.[25]
- Most authorities agree that patients with established Barrett esophagus should undergo surveillance endoscopy with biopsies every 1 to 3 years to assess for dysplastic changes that are suggestive of degeneration toward malignancy.[25]
- Any degree of dysplasia requires confirmation by an expert pathologist.
- If **high-grade dysplasia** is encountered, intervention is needed:
  - Esophagectomy remains an option but is not the only therapy available.
  - Endoscopic options include photodynamic therapy, radiofrequency ablation, endoscopic mucosal resection, endoscopic thermal, and cryotherapy.
  - Any mucosal irregularity, including nodularity or ulceration, requires intense biopsy and endoscopic mucosal resection if possible, to exclude adenocarcinoma. Endoscopic ultrasound may help further characterize mucosal nodules.
  - When high-grade dysplasia is unifocal, repeat surveillance after 3 months of aggressive PPI therapy can be an option, as mucosal inflammation can rarely lead to histopathologic findings mimicking dysplasia. The risk of development of adenocarcinoma is 30% with high-grade dysplasia.

- **Low-grade dysplasia** is monitored with more frequent endoscopic biopsy surveillance, typically every 6 months initially, which can subsequently be extended to every 12 months in the absence of progression.
- All patients with Barrett esophagus are maintained on PPI therapy, mainly to heal esophagitis proximal to the Barrett segment, and also because Barrett esophagus is an accurate indicator of high acid exposure times.

REFERENCES

1. Dent J, El-Serag HB, Wallander MA, Johansson S. Epidemiology of gastroesophageal reflux disease: a systematic review. *Gut* 2005;54:710–717.
2. Locke GR III, Talley NJ, Fett SL, et al. Prevalence and clinical spectrum of gastro-esophageal reflux: a population based study in Olmstead County, Minnesota. *Gastroenterology* 1997;112:1448–1456.
3. Galmiche JP, Janssens J. The pathophysiology of gastro-oesophageal reflux disease: an overview. *Scand J Gastroenterol Suppl* 1995;211:7–18.
4. Richter JE. Gastroesophageal reflux disease. In: Yamada T, Alpers DH, Kaplowitz N, Laine L, et al. eds. Textbook of Gastroenterology, 4th Ed. Philadelphia, PA: Lippincott Williams & Wilkins, 2003:1196–1224.
5. Richter JE. Extraesophageal presentations of gastroesophageal reflux disease: an overview. *Am J Gastroenterol* 2000;95:S1–S3.
6. Katzka DA. Eosinophilic esophagitis. *Curr Opin Gastroenterol* 2006;22:429–432.
7. Dellon E, Aderogu A, Woosley JT, et al. Variability in diagnostic criteria for eosinophilic esophagitis: a systematic review. *Am J Gastroenterol* 2007;102:2300–2313.
8. Wilcox CM. Esophageal infections and disorders associated with acquired immunodeficiency syndrome. In: Yamada T, Alpers DH, Kaplowitz N, et al., eds. Textbook of Gastroenterology. 4th Ed. Philadelphia, PA: Lippincott Williams &Wilkins 2003:1225–1237.
9. Winstead NS, Bulat R. Pill esophagitis. *Curr Treat Options Gastroenterol.* 2004;7:71–76.
10. Gyawali CP, Clouse RE. Approach to dysphagia, odynophagia and noncardiac chest pain. In: Yamada T, Alpers DH, Kalloo AN, et al., eds. Principles of Clinical Gastroenterology. Hoboken, NJ: Wiley-Blackwell, 2008:62–83.
11. DeVault KR, Castell DO. Updated guidelines for the diagnosis and treatment of gastroesophageal reflux disease. *Am J Gastroenterol* 2005;100:190–200.
12. Numans ME, Lau J, de Wit NJ, et al. Short-term treatment with proton-pump inhibitors as a test for gastroesophageal reflux disease: a meta-analysis of diagnostic test characteristics. *Ann Intern Med* 2004;140:518–527.
13. Lichtenstein DR, Cash BD, Davila R, et al. Role of endoscopy in the management of gastroesophageal reflux disease. *Gastrointest Endosc* 2007;66:219–224.
14. Pilotto A, Franceschi M, Leandro G, et al. Long-term clinical outcome of elderly patients with reflux esophagitis: a six-month to three-year follow-up study. *Am J Ther* 2002;9:295–300.
15. Hirano I, Richter JE. ACG practice guidelines: Esophageal reflux testing. *Am J Gastroenterol* 2007;102:668–685.
16. Sifrim D, Holloway R, Silny J, et al. Acid, nonacid, and gas reflux in patients with gastroesophageal reflux disease during ambulatory 24-hour pH-impedance recordings. *Gastroenterology* 2001;120:1588–1598.
17. Kahrilas PJ, Quigley EM. Clinical esophageal pH recording: a technical review for practice guideline development. *Gastroenterology* 1996;110:1982–1996.
18. Johnston BT, Troshinsky MB, Castell JA, et al. Comparison of barium radiology with esophageal pH monitoring in the diagnosis of gastroesophageal reflux disease. *Am J Gastroenterol* 1996;91:1181–1185.
19. Miner P, Katz PO, Chen Y, Sostek M. Gastric acid control with esomeprazole, lansoprazole, omeprazole, pantoprazole, and rabeprazole: a five way crossover study. *Am J Gastroenterol* 2003;98:2616–2620.

20. Jalving M, Koornstra JJ, Wesseling J, et al. Increased risk for fundic gland polyps during long term proton pump inhibitor therapy. *Aliment Pharmacol Ther* 2006;24:1341–1349.
21. Klinkenberg-Knol E, Nelis F, Dent J, et al. Long-term omeprazole treatment in resistant gastroesophageal reflux disease. *Gastroenterology* 2000;118:661–669.
22. Howden CW. Vitamin B12 levels during prolonged treatment with proton pump inhibitors. *J Clin Gastroenterol* 2000;30:29–33.
23. Dial S, Delanye JAC, Barkun AN, Suissa S. Use of gastric acid-suppressive agents and the risk of community acquired Clostridium difficile-associated disease. *JAMA* 2005;294:2989–2995.
24. Yang Y-X, Lewis JD, Epstein S, Metz DC. Long-term proton pump inhibitor therapy and risk of hip fracture. *JAMA* 2006;296:2947–2953.
25. Wang KK, Sampliner RE. Updated guidelines 2008 for the diagnosis, surveillance and therapy of Barrett's esophagus. *Am J Gastroenterol* 2008;103:788–797.
26. Westhoff B, Brotze S, Weston A, et al. The frequency of Barrett's esophagus in high-risk patients with chronic GERD. *Gastrointest Endosc* 2005;61:226–231.
27. Ronkainen J, Aro P, Storskrubb T, et al. Prevalence of Barrett's esophagus in the general population: an endoscopic study. *Gastroenterology* 2005;129:1825–1831.
28. Spechler SJ. AGA technical review on treatment of patients with dysphagia caused by benign disorders of the distal esophagus. *Gastroenterology* 1999;117(1):233–254.

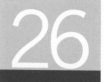

26 Hepatobiliary Diseases

Amanda Camp and Kevin M. Korenblat

GENERAL CONSIDERATIONS OF LIVER DISEASES

Assessment of Liver Function and Laboratory Testing

- The term liver function test is frequently used to refer to any serum measurement that relates to the liver. This is misleading, as liver function need not be compromised for some of these tests to be abnormal. Blood tests, including the serum albumin, bilirubin, and measurement of prothrombin time (PT), provide an assessment of the actual metabolic function of the liver. In contrast, the aminotransferases (aspartate aminotransferase [AST] and alanine aminotransferase [ALT]) often reflect necroinflammatory activity in the liver.
- The evaluation of a patient for suspected liver disease involves two steps:
  - **Assessment of the type of liver injury.**
  - **Assessment of the liver's degree of functional impairment.**
- These steps involve both blood tests and clinical evaluation by history and physical examination. Once liver disease is suspected, it is often useful to segregate the disease into one of three categories:
  - **Hepatocellular:** A primary hepatocyte injury.
  - **Cholestatic:** A disruption of canalicular activity, bilirubin metabolism, or the delivery of bile to the duodenum.
  - **Mixed** hepatocellular and cholestatic features.
- Early in the course of liver disease, this differentiation is often diagnostically and therapeutically helpful. In more advanced liver disease, regardless of the cause of liver disease, distinctions become blurred and clinical consequences overlap.
- These tests and implications are listed in Table 1.[1]

Serum Aminotransferases

- These tests include AST and ALT. Both can be elevated among patients with hepatocellular injury and, perhaps less markedly so, among patients with cholestatic liver disease.
- ALT is relatively specific for liver disease.
- AST can be elevated in various liver and extrahepatic (muscle, blood cells, and cardiac) injuries.

Cholestatic Markers

- Serum **alkaline phosphatase** is the most readily available marker of cholestatic liver injury. Unfortunately, the alkaline phosphatase is not specific for biliary processes—it can also be elevated in pregnancy, bone diseases, and, less often, intestinal disease.
- Serum levels of **5′-nucleotidase** and γ-glutamyltransferase **(GGT)** are supplemental tests that, if elevated, suggest a hepatic or biliary tree source of an elevated alkaline

TABLE 1	Characteristic Patterns of Liver Test Abnormalities[a]			
Test	Hepatocellular Injury	Cholestatic Injury	Cirrhosis with Hepatic Insufficiency	Hemolysis or Gilbert Syndrome	Bone Disease
Albumin	Normal, low	Normal, low	Low, very low	Normal	Normal
ALT and AST	Modest-to-marked elevation	Normal or mild-to-modest elevation	Normal, modest elevation	Normal	Normal
Bilirubin	Normal to high total and direct	High total and direct, may be normal	Normal, high total and direct	High total, normal direct	Normal
Alkaline phosphatase	Mild-to-modest elevation	Modest-to-marked elevation	Mild, modest elevation	Normal	Elevated
5'-Nucleotidase or GGT	Normal-to-modest elevation	Modest-to-marked elevation	Mild, modest elevation	Normal	Normal
Prothrombin time	Normal-to-marked prolongation	Normal-to-marked prolongation	Mild-to-marked prolongation	Normal	Normal
Platelet count	Normal	Normal	Low	Normal	Normal

ALT, alanine aminotransferase; AST, aspartate aminotransferase; GGT, γ-glutamyltransferase.
[a]Although helpful, overlap of patterns prevents laboratory tests alone from being diagnostic.

phosphatase. Heat fractionation can also segregate hepatobiliary from bone origin of alkaline phosphatase. The GGT is frequently reported in many metabolic panels; however, many processes including medications can result in elevations of GGT independent of elevations in alkaline phosphatase.

Liver Synthetic Function

- **Albumin** is a serum glycoprotein that is synthesized by the liver. It serves as a carrier protein and is a means by which intravascular oncotic pressure is maintained. Although the serum albumin can be low in liver disease, it can also be low in protein-losing enteropathies, nephrotic syndrome, and almost any severe acute or chronic illness.
- **Bilirubin** is the end product of the catabolism of heme, the prosthetic moiety of hemoglobin, myoglobin, and other hemoproteins. Bilirubin exists in two distinct forms:
  - **Unconjugated (indirect) bilirubin** has not been processed by the liver. Unconjugated hyperbilirubinemia is the result of any process that increases bilirubin production, decreases bilirubin clearance, or results in both processes acting in concert. Hemolysis and increased ineffective erythropoiesis are the most common causes of increased bilirubin production. Inherited disorders of glucuronosyltransferase activity (e.g., Gilbert syndrome, Crigler-Najjar syndrome) can also cause indirect hyperbilirubinemia.
  - **Conjugated (direct) bilirubin** has been processed by the liver and is thus rendered soluble. It is excreted into the bile canaliculi and passes via the biliary tree into the proximal duodenum. From there it is either excreted into the stool or undergoes enterohepatic circulation after deconjugation and conversion into **urobilinogens** by the enteric bacteria.
- **PT** is often abnormal with liver or biliary disease. Two major causes are as follows:
  - Primary hepatic insufficiency of production of clotting factors.
  - Deficiency in fat-soluble vitamins (including vitamin K) due to severe cholestasis. For these patients without other liver failure, the parenteral administration of vitamin K can correct the coagulopathy.
- **Complete blood cell count** may also provide information that is helpful in gaining insight regarding the chronicity and nature of any liver disease. Patients with advanced liver disease may have portal hypertension and associated hypersplenism. This can be manifested as leukopenia and thrombocytopenia. Although these abnormalities are not specific for liver disease, they can provide useful adjuncts in selected situations.

Cirrhosis

- Cirrhosis is a histologic condition of the liver that is defined by extensive **bridging fibrosis** and the formation of **regenerative nodules.**
- Many patients with histologic changes of cirrhosis have normal liver function due to the impressive reserve capacity of the liver.
- Once complications develop, the patient is stated to have "decompensated cirrhosis." The management of common complications of cirrhosis is described below.
- Most patients who experience these complications should be managed in conjunction with an experienced hepatologist, as liver transplantation should be a consideration in the care of these individuals.

Gastroesophageal Varices

- Gastroesophageal varices are the result of portal hypertension. Shunting of blood results in dilated blood venous passages (characteristically in the distal esophagus and proximal stomach) under increased pressures.

- The annual incidence of variceal hemorrhage is at least 20%. The mortality from variceal bleeds has decreased over time with improved management approaches, such as endoscopic banding, but the mortality rate remains high.
- **Screening for varices is recommended in cirrhotics,** particularly in those with thrombocytopenia as this is a marker of significant portal hypertension.[2]
- If small varices are present, no therapy is indicated, but repeated screening is recommended in 1- to 2-year intervals for detection of progression.
- If medium-to-large varices are present, lifelong therapy with **nonselective β-blockers,** such as propranolol and nadolol, **decreases the risk of variceal bleeding.**
- Patients with an established history of variceal hemorrhage should be evaluated for long-term management that might include endoscopic obliteration of varices or vascular shunting procedures.

Ascites

- Ascites is the accumulation of fluid within the peritoneal cavity, most commonly resulting from decompensated liver disease.
- Initial evaluation of ascites should include serologic tests of liver function and diagnostic paracentesis.
  - All patients in whom the diagnosis of **spontaneous bacterial peritonitis** is considered should be treated with empiric antibiotics and underg **diagnostic paracentesis.** These patients likely require hospitalization.
  - Diagnostic evaluation of the peritoneal fluid should include a cell count and differential, gram stain and culture, and albumin.
  - Other tests that may be considered in certain circumstances include lactic dehydrogenase, cytology, and glucose.
  - The fluid should be evaluated to calculate a **serum ascites albumin gradient (SAAG).**
    - The SAAG is calculated by subtracting the ascites albumin concentration (g/dL) from the serum albumin concentration (g/dL).
    - Ascites that forms as a consequence of portal hypertension has a SAAG >1.1 g/dL.
- **Sodium restriction** (<2 g/day) and diuretics, typically spironolactone (recommended starting dose 100 mg PO qd, with a maximal dose of 400 mg PO qd) and furosemide (recommended starting dose 40 mg PO qd, with a maximal dose of 160 mg PO qd), are used for the initial management of ascites. **Care must be taken to avoid renal failure and electrolyte abnormalities.**[3]
- Ascites is considered refractory when fluid continues to accumulate despite maximal diuretics or the patient is unable to tolerate diuretic therapy.
  - Refractory ascites may require treatment with large volume paracentesis or transjugular intrahepatic portosystemic shunt (TIPS).
  - These patients should also be considered for possible liver transplantation.

Portosystemic (Hepatic) Encephalopathy

- Portosystemic encephalopathy (PSE) is a central neurologic dysfunction that probably results from disordered clearance of neurotransmitters and gut-derived toxins.
- Initial manifestations can be subclinical and detected only by electroencephalography or neuropsychiatric testing. More advanced manifestations can include sleep pattern disturbances and confusion. In severe cases, patients may become unresponsive.
- Seizures should not be considered a routine complication of hepatic encephalopathy. They are sometimes seen with cerebral edema as an unusual and extreme complication of PSE, but other diagnoses need to be considered.

- Physical examination findings commonly include asterixis, hyperreflexia, and an abnormal mental status examination. Following shunting procedures for varices or ascites, patients face a 20% risk of new or worsening encephalopathy.
- The initial management of PSE is the **elimination of medications,** such as opiates and sedatives that may further contribute to an altered mental status. After this, **lactulose** can be administered and titrated to produce two to five soft bowel movements daily (usual starting dosage for lactulose is 30 mL PO bid). Lactulose is a nonabsorbable disaccharide that alters the colonic flora and leads to the fecal excretion of amines and ammonia.
- **Nonabsorbed oral antibiotics** (neomycin 500 mg PO bid-qid or rifaximin 400 mg PO tid) can also be used to alter bacterial flora and treat PSE.

Cholestasis

- Cholestasis is often noted in liver failure and may lead to fat-soluble vitamin deficiency, bone disease, jaundice, and pruritus.
- Cirrhotic patients should be monitored for **fat-soluble vitamin deficiency,** and, if present, appropriate supplements should be provided.
- **Pruritus** from cholestasis can be quite disabling. Management options include the use of antihistamines, soothing lotions, and cool showers with pat drying of the skin to avoid excessive drying. Further first-line medical options include the use of cholestyramine resin 4 g PO bid-qid, ursodeoxycholic acid 13 to 15 mg/kg/day, or naltrexone 50 mg qd-bid.

Hepatocellular Carcinoma

- Hepatocellular carcinoma (HCC) is an increasing common complication of chronic liver disease. The 2003 United States Cancer Statistics (USCS) showed that liver and intrahepatobiliary tumors have risen to be the ninth leading cause of cancer death in the United States.
- The biggest risk lies among patients with cirrhosis from hepatitis B, hepatitis C, hemochromatosis, and alcohol abuse.
- Symptoms of HCC are nonspecific and may reflect worsening of other manifestations of cirrhosis.
- Practice guidelines recommend that all subjects at risk for HCC be screened by semiannual liver ultrasound.
- Screening techniques can also include quantitative measurements of serum α-fetoprotein and cross-sectional imaging techniques (triple-phase abdominal contrast CT scan or abdominal magnetic resonance imaging [MRI]).
- Full details on the current guidelines on recommendations for screening can be found on the website of the American Association for the Study of Liver Disease (AASLD) at http://www.aasld.org (last accessed December 14, 2009).
- The finding of a solid, hypervascular liver mass in a cirrhotic patient who has an α-fetoprotein of >200 ng/mL is virtually diagnostic of HCC.
- The treatment of HCC is individualized. Potential treatment options include surgical resection, radiofrequency ablation, transarterial chemoembolization, percutaneous alcohol injection, liver transplantation, and systemic chemotherapy.

Risk Assessment

- Surgery, especially with general anesthesia, exposes cirrhotic patients to increased risk for mortality or hepatic decompensation (e.g., ascites, PSE, and bleeding).
- If possible, for patients with acute hepatitis, surgery should be avoided.

TABLE 2	Child-Pugh Classification		

	Points		
	1	**2**	**3**
Encephalopathy	None	Asterixis/hyperreflexia or controlled with medical therapy	Obtundation or coma
Ascites	None	Medically controlled	Refractory to medical management
Bilirubin (mg/dL)	1–2	2.1–3.0	>3
Albumin (g/dL)	>3.4	2.8–3.4	<2.8
Prothrombin time (second prolonged)	<4	4–6	>6

Grade A: 5–6 points; Grade B: 7–9 points; Grade C: ≥10 points.

Estimated Surgical Risk with General Anesthesia		
	Chance of Decompensation	**Liver-Related Mortality**
Grade A	10%–15%	0%–10%
Grade B	20%–50%	4%–30%
Grade C	Almost 100%	20%–75%

From CF Gholson, JM Provenza, BR Bacon. Hepatologic considerations in patients with a parenchymal liver disease undergoing surgery. *Am J Gastroenterol* 1990;85:487, with permission.

- The extent of risk for patients with chronic liver disease is typically based on Child-Pugh grading of liver disease as outlined in Table 2.
- In addition, intra-abdominal varices, coagulopathy, and thrombocytopenia may contribute to bleeding risks.[4]

Model for End Stage Liver Disease
- This model was initially developed to assess the 3-month mortality in end stage liver disease (ESLD) patients undergoing TIPS. Its use has since been broadened to encompass various aspects of liver disease.
- The initial model was calculated using international normalized ratio (INR), bilirubin, and creatinine.
- A modified version of the model for end stage liver disease (MELD) is currently utilized by the United Network for Organ Sharing (UNOS) as part of the evaluation for liver transplantation.

$$\text{MELD} = 3.8(\text{Ln } S_{Bili}) + 11.2(\text{Ln INR}) + 9.6(\text{Ln } S_{Cr}) + 6.4$$

where S_{Bili}, serum bilirubin in mg/dL; INR, international normalized ratio; S_{Cr}, serum creatinine in mg/dL; and Ln, natural logarithm.
- MELD emerged as an ideal scoring system of liver disease severity.
- Initial studies of predictive ability revealed that waiting list mortality was directly proportional to the MELD score at the time of listing.
- Mortality was 1.9% for patients with MELD score of <9, and 71.3% for patients with a MELD score of ≥40.5.[5]

- The MELD score has prognostic value in several clinical settings outside of the liver transplantation, including predicting mortality associated with the following:
  - Alcoholic hepatitis
  - Hepatorenal syndrome
  - Acute liver failure
  - Sepsis in cirrhosis
  - Surgical procedures in chronic liver disease patients
  - TIPS procedure
- The current model and its specific uses can be accessed at http://www.mayoclinic.org/meld/mayomodel6.html (last accessed December 14, 2009).

VIRAL LIVER DISEASE

Hepatitis A

General Considerations
- Hepatitis A is caused by an RNA virus (picornavirus).
- It is spread from person to person via a **fecal-oral route.**
- In infected patients, an acute hepatitis develops that can vary from mild to very severe. **There is no chronic form of hepatitis A.**
- The morbidity and mortality (case-fatality rate) of infection are increased with an increased age of onset.

Diagnosis
- Characteristic manifestations of hepatitis A include elevated serum transaminases, fever, nausea/vomiting, abdominal pain, and jaundice.
- The diagnosis is based on finding immunoglobulin M (IgM) antibodies to hepatitis A capsid protein. This test is typically ordered as HAV Ab-IgM.
- Findings of a positive HAV Ab-IgG or total, in the absence of an acute hepatitis, suggest immunity to hepatitis A rather than an acute infection.

Treatment
- Patients can usually be treated supportively on an outpatient basis, but hospitalization may be required for those who are unable to maintain hydration. **Preparations for emergency liver transplantation should be considered for patients in whom acute liver failure develops.**
- For nonimmune patients who are exposed to hepatitis A, immunoprophylaxis is available in the form of hepatitis A immune globulin (0.2 mL/kg). The immune globulin should be given to those who are exposed to the virus within a 2-week window.
- Postexposure protection with hepatitis A vaccine administration given within 14 days of exposure has also been shown to not be inferior to the standard therapy of immune globulin. This may be an acceptable alternative in select patient populations.[6]
- Vaccination is also recommended for high-risk populations (residents of high-risk population centers, men who have sex with men, residents and staff of institutions that serve the mentally handicapped, and restaurant workers).

Hepatitis B

General Considerations
- The causative virus of hepatitis B is a DNA virus (hepadnavirus).

- In the United States, the virus is most commonly transmitted through **injection drug use and sexual contact.** In Asia, vertical transmission continues to be a major public health problem.[7]
- Hepatitis B can cause both acute and chronic hepatitis.
  - **Acute hepatitis:** In most cases, the outcome of acute infection is recovery with the development of anti-HBs (hepatitis B surface antibody), the central neutralizing antibody to hepatitis B virus (HBV). Less commonly, acute infection can result in acute liver failure.
  - **Chronic hepatitis:** Chronic viral activity can lead to cirrhosis and HCC. The risk of chronic disease is <5% when the infection is acquired in adulthood and >90% when the infection is acquired during infancy, very early childhood, or in immunosuppressed subjects.

Diagnosis

The diagnosis of hepatitis B is based on a variety of serologic markers that assess disease activity and the immune response. These markers are listed in Table 3.

Hepatitis B Surface Antigen
- Hepatitis B surface antigen (HBsAg) is the protein that forms the outer coat of the viral nucleocapsid.
- HBsAg usually (but not invariably) disappears with the production of anti-HBs if the infection is cleared. The persistence of HBsAg for 6 months beyond initial infection is diagnostic of chronic infection.

Hepatitis B Surface Antibody
- The development of anti-HBs occurs with the clearance of a natural HBV infection.
- The presence of anti-HBs may also indicate prior exposure to or vaccination against hepatitis B.

Hepatitis B Core Antibody
- Hepatitis B core antibody (anti-HBc) reflects antibodies to the nucleocapsid core proteins and can be either IgG or IgM. Frequently these antibodies are measured as either IgM alone or both (IgM and IgG).
- A reactive anti-HBc (IgM) most commonly reflects acute hepatitis B infection.
- Anti-HBc (IgG) is the most durable marker of exposure to HBV and can be present even after serum levels of anti-HBs have declined to below assay detection thresholds.

Hepatitis B e Antigen and Antihepatitis B e Antibody
- Hepatitis B e antigen (HBeAg) is the hallmark of chronic active viral replication.
- Patients who are positive for HBeAg are believed to have active viral replication and are capable of transmitting the virus.
- Loss of HBe antigen with gain of anti-HBe typically occurs with the resolution of acute infection or transformation to the inactive carrier state in chronically infected subjects.
- In a subset of individuals of chronic hepatitis B, active viral replication can be ongoing despite the absence of HBe antigen. These individuals harbor mutations in the precore or basal core promoter.

Hepatitis B DNA
- Serum hepatitis B DNA (HBV-DNA) is measured by polymerase chain reaction (PCR) assays.

TABLE 3	Serologic Testing for Hepatitis B							
	HBsAg	Anti-HBs	Anti-HBc (IgM)	Anti-HBc Total	HBeAg	Anti-HBe	HBV-DNA PCR	ALT/AST
Acute infection	Positive	Negative	Positive	Positive	Positive	Negative	Positive	Markedly elevated
Recovery from acute infection	Negative	Positive	Negative	Positive	Negative	Positive	Undetectable	Normal
Immunity from vaccination	Negative	Positive	Negative	Negative	Negative	Negative	Undetectable	Normal
Chronic infection								
HBeAg+	Positive	Negative	Negative	Positive	Positive	Negative	>20,000 IU/mL	Modestly elevated or normal
HBeAg–	Positive	Negative	Negative	Positive	Negative	Negative	>2,000 IU/mL	
Inactive carrier state								
HBeAg+	Positive	Negative	Negative	Positive	Positive	Negative	<20,000 IU/mL	Normal
HBeAg–	Positive	Negative	Negative	Positive	Negative	Positive	<2,000 IU/mL	

ALT, alanine aminotransferase; AST, aspartate aminotransferase; anti-HBc, hepatitis B core antibody; HBeAg, hepatitis B e antigen; anti-HBs, hepatitis B surface antibody; HBsAg, hepatitis B surface antigen; HBV, hepatitis B virus; PCR, polymerase chain reaction.

- Real-time PCR assays can achieve detection thresholds as low as 5 to 10 IU/mL and as high as 8 to 9 10 IU/mL.
- The quantification of HBV DNA is an essential component to the clinical evaluation of HBV infection and response to antiviral therapy.

Treatment

- The treatment options for chronic hepatitis B include a rapidly growing list of oral nucleoside and nucleotide inhibitors and injectable pegylated interferon.
- Current guidelines for the treatment of hepatitis B and available treatment options are available at http://www.aasld.org.

Hepatitis C

General Considerations

- Hepatitis C is caused by an RNA virus and is transmitted **primarily by parenteral exposure.**
- Common modes of transmission include the receipt of blood products prior to the introduction of antibody screening in 1992, intravenous illicit drug use, and intranasal cocaine use.
- The risk for both sexual transmission among monogamous couple and vertical transmission is low, though the risk may be enhanced in the setting of coinfection with the human immunodeficiency virus (HIV).

Diagnosis

- The diagnosis of chronic hepatitis C requires a high index of suspicion. Patients with risk factors for hepatitis C should be tested by hepatitis C antibody test, as should all patients with unexplained serum transaminase abnormalities or liver insufficiency.
- The nonspecific manifestations of chronic hepatitis C include the following:
  - Fatigue
  - Myalgias
  - Arthralgias
- A small group of patients may have associated extrahepatic manifestations, such as cryoglobulinemia, glomerulonephritis, porphyria cutanea tarda, or lichen planus.[8]

Laboratories
- Initial testing for hepatitis C involves testing for antibodies to hepatitis C virus (anti-HCV).
- If anti-HCV testing is reactive, the direct detection of HCV RNA by PCR and HCV genotyping should be undertaken. In only rare instances is anti-HCV a false negative.
- Information from these tests may be useful in predicting the course of HCV infection and the chances for successful therapy against HCV.
- Patients with genotypes other than 1 and 4, low viral loads, and less advanced fibrosis by biopsy have the best chance for a good outcome with therapy.[9]

Treatment

The treatment of HCV should be divided into conservative measures and specific antiviral therapies.

Conservative Measures
- **Discontinuation of alcohol.** The synergistic effect of liver damage with Hepatitis C and alcohol is well known. Patients should be advised that abstinence is the best approach to avoid accelerating their disease.
- **Vaccination:** Hepatitis A and B can follow an especially virulent course among patients who are coinfected with chronic hepatitis C. Patients should be screened for immunity and offered vaccination if necessary.
- **Screening:** Patients with cirrhosis from hepatitis C should be screened for hepatocellular cancer. Current treatment guidelines recommend that this be accomplished with semiannual ultrasound.

Pegylated Interferon and Ribavirin
- All present therapies against hepatitis C involve the subcutaneous administration of interferon.
- Interferons have immunomodulatory and antiviral effects.
- Interferon-based therapies are plagued by **adverse side effects** and poor response rates, and for those patients who do respond, there is a high risk for viral relapse when therapy is discontinued.[10]
- Side effects to interferon include pain at the injection site, fever, myalgias, worsening or unmasking of psychiatric disorders, thyroid abnormalities, bone marrow suppression, and worsening or unmasking of autoimmune processes.
- The most effective forms of interferon in current use are pegylated and typically administered on a weekly basis.
- Contraindications to interferon include decompensated liver disease, leukopenia, thrombocytopenia, and uncontrolled psychiatric disease.
- Ribavirin is an antiviral agent that, when used in combination with interferon, can increase the chances of a sustained response.
- **There is no role for ribavirin monotherapy** to treat chronic hepatitis C.[11]
- Ribavirin's side effects include hemolysis, nonproductive cough, and rash.
- The current first-line therapy for chronic HCV infection is a weekly injection of pegylated interferon and daily ribavirin.

METABOLIC LIVER DISEASE

Nonalcoholic Fatty Liver Disease

General Considerations
- Nonalcoholic fatty liver disease (NAFLD) is an increasingly common metabolic disorder of the liver strongly associated with insulin resistance, the metabolic syndrome, and its cardiometabolic complications.
- The disorder can range from the benign accumulation of triglyceride in hepatocytes (benign steatosis) to the nonalcoholic steatohepatitis (NASH) characterized by steatosis with varying degrees of necroinflammation.

Diagnosis
- Usually NAFLD is asymptomatic, being detected only by the finding of elevated aminotransferases. **In those with NASH, the disease may progress to cirrhosis.**
- Before NAFLD is diagnosed, other forms of liver disease (especially hepatitis C, hepatitis B, Wilson disease, and alcohol-induced liver disease) must be excluded.

- The diagnosis of NAFLD is also supported by the presence of other manifestations of the metabolic syndrome, including obesity, hyperlipidemia, and diabetes mellitus, though none of these are required.
- Imaging studies, including ultrasound, CT, and MRI, may suggest steatosis but do not allow assessment for the presence of inflammation.

Treatment

- In morbidly obese subjects, bariatric surgery has been shown to improve NAFLD.
- Although there are no established guidelines for the treatment of NAFLD, prudent recommendations include weight loss, control of dyslipidemia, and control of diabetes.
- Cessation of medications associated with NAFLD (amiodarone, corticosteroids, and total parenteral nutrition) should also be considered.

Alcohol-Induced Liver Disease

General Considerations

- The sensitivity of the liver to damage from heavy alcohol consumption varies widely. This is typified by the fact that among patients with chronic heavy alcohol consumption, the development of cirrhosis is not inevitable. **Only 10% to 20% progress to cirrhosis.**[12]
- **Alcoholic hepatitis** is characterized by steatosis and necroinflammatory changes within the liver.
  - Characteristically, the serum AST is elevated more substantially than the ALT; however, this pattern is not a foolproof means of establishing the diagnosis.
  - More severe cases of alcoholic hepatitis may be associated with fever, abdominal pain, jaundice, and complications of liver failure or portal hypertension.
- **Alcoholic cirrhosis** is typically micronodular and results from chronic alcohol consumption.

Diagnosis

- The diagnosis of alcoholic liver disease is based on a thorough history and physical examination, although the reports of alcohol consumption are notoriously inaccurate.
- Other causes of hepatic injury should be excluded. Alcohol may also be potentiating damage caused by another underlying disease process such as a viral hepatitis.
- The severity of alcohol-related hepatitis can be estimated from the Madden discriminant function (DF).[13]

$$DF = (4.6 \times [\text{measured PT} - \text{control PT}]) + \text{bilirubin (mg/dL)}$$

A DF of >32 is considered severe alcohol-related hepatitis and is associated with a high 30-day mortality rate.

Treatment

- For patients with a DF of <32, alcohol abstinence, good nutrition, and supportive care are sufficient treatment.
- For severe disease (DF ≥ 32), treatment options include corticosteroids and pentoxifylline.
- Individual studies and meta-analyses of trials of **corticosteroids** for alcoholic hepatitis have resulted in conflicting results.
  - Currently, corticosteroids (prednisolone 40 mg daily × 30 days) should be considered in subjects with alcoholic hepatitis and a DF of >32 or encephalopathy.[12]

- Even with treatment, mortality rates of at least 40% exist, and at least seven patients need to be treated to prevent one death.
- The efficacy and safety of corticosteroids has not been studied in patients with gastrointestinal bleeding, active infection, or pancreatitis.
- Treatment with **pentoxifylline** 400 mg PO tid was the subject of one study and resulted in a reduction in the 30-day mortality rate.[14] The improvement was attributed to a reduction in hepatorenal syndrome in treated patients.

AUTOIMMUNE LIVER DISEASE

Autoimmune Hepatitis

General Considerations

- Autoimmune hepatitis (AIH) is an idiopathic disorder characterized by immune-mediated necroinflammatory liver injury.
- There are two basic types: Classic **type 1,** which is associated with ANA (antinuclear antibodies) and/or ASMA (antismooth muscle antibodies), and **type 2,** which is associated with anti-LKM-1 (liver/kidney/microsome) and/or ALC-1 (liver cytosol antigen) antibodies. AIH displays a 4:1 female-male predominance.
- All types show a strong female preponderance, approximately 4:1.
- Immunosuppression therapies can be successful in preventing the progression to liver failure and improving liver function among patients who have active inflammation.
- The mortality of untreated AIH probably exceeds 50% in 5 years.

Diagnosis

Clinical Presentation

- The diagnosis of AIH is based on epidemiologic factors, laboratory findings, and liver biopsy.
- **Other forms of liver disease must be excluded** (especially chronic viral infection).
- Some patients are essentially asymptomatic while others have a chronic fluctuating course.
- Those who are symptomatic often have constitutional/nonspecific complaints, such as fatigue, malaise, anorexia, abdominal pain, nausea, and small joint arthralgias.
- Other patients present with an acute hepatitis picture, sometimes fulminant, and some have evidence of liver failure (jaundice, ascites, and portal hypertension) at the time of diagnosis.
- AIH is not uncommonly associated with extrahepatic autoimmune processes (e.g., arthritis, autoimmune hemolytic anemia, celiac disease, glomerulonephritis, "idiopathic" thrombocytopenic purpura, lichen planus, thyroid disease, ulcerative colitis, uveitis, and others).

Diagnostic Testing

Laboratories

- Elevated serum transaminases are characteristic.
- Hypergammaglobulinemia is common. The IgG can be >1.5 times the upper limit of normal.
- As noted above, type 1 AIH is associated with ANA and/or ASMA and type 2 with anti-LKM-1 and/or ALC-1 antibodies.
- Occasionally, patients with ANA and/or ASMA will also have antimitochondrial antibodies (AMA).

Diagnostic Procedures

- **Liver biopsy** findings typically include piecemeal necrosis with an inflammatory infiltrate of which plasma cells are a noticeable component.
- Eosinophils and giant cells are sometimes seen.
- Minority can also have bile duct changes.
- Cirrhosis can develop.

Treatment

- Treatment is generally felt to be indicated in those with transaminases of >10 times the upper limit of normal, those with transaminases of >5 times the upper limit of normal and serum immunoglobulin ≥2 times normal, and those with biopsy findings of bridging necrosis or multiacinar necrosis.
- The goals of treatment include biochemical normalization and histologic remission.
- Patients who have evidence of liver failure (jaundice, ascites, and portal hypertension) at the time of diagnosis often improve with treatment, and therefore these features should not discourage treatment if there is evidence of active necroinflammatory activity (as manifest by biopsy or blood tests).
- Treatment regimens include those that use **steroids** both as monotherapy and as steroid-sparring therapies.
- The **steroid-sparring regiments** typically use **azathioprine** for maintenance of remission following tapering doses of steroids for induction of remission.
- Current recommendations for the treatment of AIH are summarized on the AASLD website at http://www.aasld.org.
- If remission is achieved and sustained with immunomodulatory therapy, survival is 90% at 10 years. Even responding patients who have cirrhosis at the time of diagnosis can expect this survival rate.[15]

Primary Biliary Cirrhosis

General Considerations

- Primary biliary cirrhosis (PBC) is an idiopathic disorder characterized by microscopic intrahepatic bile duct inflammation.
- Progressive inflammation of the interlobular bile ducts leads to progressive ductopenia. The resultant cholestasis can slowly lead to fibrosis, then cirrhosis, and eventually ESLD in some patients; however, the course of PBC is highly variable.
- The disease is more commonly seen in women.
- It is also commonly associated with other autoimmune phenomena including Sjögren syndrome, scleroderma, and rheumatoid arthritis.
- Hypothyroidism, hyperlipidemia, and osteopenia have also been noted to be more frequent in patients with PBC.[16]

Diagnosis

- Up to 50% to 60% of patients are asymptomatic at the time of diagnosis. In its earliest form, patients may be noted to have only isolated laboratory abnormalities (usually a **cholestatic picture** with elevated alkaline phosphatase).
- As the disease progresses, symptoms and laboratory findings of more marked cholestasis usually develop within 2 to 4 years. The main symptoms that progress over this time period include fatigue and pruritis.[15]
- The diagnosis is suggested by the presence of **AMA,** which is present in 95% of patients with PBC, as well as elevated serum IgM antibodies.

- ANA is present in about 50% of patients.
- Hyperlipidemia can be marked.
- Characteristic liver biopsy findings in early (Stage 1) disease include marked **periductal inflammation** (florid bile duct lesion). In Stage 2, the number of bile ducts is decreased and inflammation extends beyond the portal triads. Stage 3 brings fibrosis between adjacent portal triads. Cirrhosis with regenerative nodules appears in Stage 4.

Treatment

- **Ursodeoxycholic acid** (13 to 15 mg/kg/day) has been the only drug that has been universally accepted as clinically worthwhile.
- Ursodeoxycholic acid has been shown to improve liver function test abnormalities and liver biopsy appearance and, most important, to slow down the progression of the disease, particularly in patients with mild disease.
- Current management is reviewed by the AASLD at http://www.aasld.org.

Primary Sclerosing Cholangitis

General Considerations

- Primary sclerosing cholangitis (PSC) is another idiopathic inflammatory disorder of the bile ducts. Unlike PBC, it affects intra- and extrahepatic medium and large biliary ducts.
- The disease most often affects men (7:3 when compared with women).
- PSC is **associated with superimposed inflammatory bowel disease** (usually ulcerative colitis) in 85% of patients. However, only 2.5% to 7.5% of patients with inflammatory bowel disease will develop PSC.[17]
- The inflammation of PBC leads to **bile duct structuring,** which ultimately cause the clinical consequences.
- Over the course of an average of 9 to 17 years from diagnosis, patients are at risk for the development of **cirrhosis.**
- This time period may also be punctuated by episodes of **infectious cholangitis.**
- Over the course of the disease, there is a 9% to 15% incidence of **cholangiocarcinoma.**

Diagnosis

Clinical Presentation

- Many patients are asymptomatic at the time of diagnosis.
- PSC should be considered in those with inflammatory bowel disease who also have an elevated alkaline phosphatase level.
- The clinical progression of PSC is unpredictable, but most patients have insidious progression to cirrhosis and ESLD.
- As with PBC, pruritus and fatigue are common but nonspecific symptoms.
- Charcot triad (fever, jaundice, and right upper quadrant pain) should raise the possibility of ascending cholangitis.
- Steatorrhea with vitamin deficiencies may develop due to decreased conjugated bile acid excretion.
- Those with cirrhosis have typical findings (e.g., ascites, varices, splenomegaly).

Diagnostic Testing

Laboratories

- Liver test usually show a cholestatic picture with alkaline phosphatase elevation more prominent than transaminases elevation.

- Bilirubin levels are variable, and persistent jaundice does not usually develop until later stages.
- Test results of hepatic synthetic function are usually normal until later stages.
- Similar to PBC, elevated immunoglobulin levels can be seen.
- There is no autoantibody specific for PSC, though autoantibodies are often present (e.g., perinuclear antineutrophil cytoplasmic antibody, ANA, ASMA, rheumatoid factor, and others).
- AMAs are generally absent.

Imaging
- **Cholangiography** (usually endoscopic retrograde cholangiopancreatography [ERCP]) is the gold standard test. It will show the intra- and extrahepatic strictures and irregularities of the bile ducts.
- Newer radiographic studies such as magnetic resonance cholangiopancreatography (MRCP) are also useful diagnostic tools.

Diagnostic Procedures
- **Liver biopsy** may be suggestive but is not usually diagnostic.
- The most characteristic lesion is fibrotic "onion skinning" of the small bile ducts.
- Nonspecific findings include a paucity of normal bile ducts with fibrosis and inflammation at the portal triad, similar to PBC.

Treatment

- No specific drug treatments have been shown to slow down or alter the disease progression; however, recent studies of high-dose ursodeoxycholic acid (15 to 20 mg/kg) have shown promise.[17]
- Treatment of inflammatory bowel disease (even colectomy in ulcerative colitis patients) does not eliminate the risk for the development of PSC.
- Management of patients with PSC includes conservative treatment of cholestasis, antibiotic therapy for episodes of cholangitis, and ERCP dilation of strictures or placement of stents to treat mechanical obstruction.
- For appropriate patients with liver failure and severe cholestasis that cannot be managed medically or endoscopically, or with recurrent episodes of bacterial cholangitis, liver transplantation is recommended.[18] PSC can recur after transplantation.
- Patients with concomitant ulcerative colitis must be carefully screened for colon cancer.

DRUG-INDUCED LIVER INJURY

- The incidence of drug-induced liver injury has been reported between 1 in 10,000 and 1 in 100,000. This is likely an underrepresentation due to lack of reporting of clinically insignificant reactions as well as lack of routine monitoring.
- Many drugs have been associated with hepatotoxicity (see Table 6 of Chapter 24).
- Commonly accepted definitions for liver injury are as follows:
  - ALT level of more than three times the upper limit of normal.
  - Alkaline phosphatase level of more than two times the upper limit of normal.
  - Total bilirubin level of more than two times the upper limit of normal if associated with any elevation of the ALT or the alkaline phosphatase.
- Toxicity may be seen as **dose related** (i.e., acetaminophen) or more commonly **idiosyncratic** with injury occurring independent of dose or duration.
- Presentations range from asymptomatic elevations of liver test (hepatocellular and/or static patterns) to fulminant hepatic failure.

- Jaundice development with drug injury is a particularly foreboding sign with a case fatality rate of 10% to 50%. This is known as "Hy's law" after the hepatopathologist Hyman Zimmerman.
- The cornerstone of treatment for a drug-induced hepatic injury involves **stopping the offending agent** and, when applicable, instituting **drug-specific therapy.**[19]

Acetaminophen Hepatotoxicity

General Principles

- Acetaminophen (otherwise known as paracetamol) is a safe and effective analgesic and antipyretic if consumed at the recommended dose of <4 g/day. However, it is the most common cause of acute hepatic failure in the United States.[20]
- The toxicity with acetaminophen is **dose dependent.** Overdose is defined as >150 mg/kg in children and >10 to 15 g in adults. Toxicity can actually occur at doses <10 g.
- Toxicity is due to the metabolism of acetaminophen to toxic *N*-acetyl-p-benzoquinone imine (NAPQI) by cytochromes P450-1A2/2A6/2E1/3A4 (2E1 being the most significant). At usual doses, NAPQI is quickly detoxified by conjugation with glutathione.
- **The role of ethanol in acetaminophen hepatotoxicity is unclear.** Theoretically, in chronic drinkers, glutathione stores can be reduced and cytochrome P450-2E1 can be induced. It would appear that in chronic ethanol abusers, a picture of more chronic acetaminophen-induced liver toxicity can develop.
- Genetic polymorphisms of P450 may contribute to the variability of acetaminophen toxicity.
- Hepatotoxicity is also increased in the setting of underlying liver disease.

Diagnosis

Clinical Presentation

- Patients may present asymptomatically, and symptoms of toxicity may not develop until 1 to 2 days after ingestion. This fact may unfortunately delay effective treatment and belie the severe, even fatal, hepatoxicity that may develop.
- The initial symptoms are nonspecific and include anorexia, malaise, nausea, and vomiting. This is followed by right upper quadrant pain.
- Subsequently, hepatic failure develops, including jaundice, encephalopathy, and coagulopathy. Renal failure can also develop at this point, due to drug-induced acute tubular necrosis and dehydration.
- Gastroenteritis, choledocholithiasis/cholecystitis, pancreatitis, alcoholic hepatitis, viral hepatitis, Reye syndrome, shock liver, and other forms of drug/toxin hepatotoxicity (e.g., mushroom poisoning, alfatoxins, kava, arsenic) are important points on the **differential diagnosis.**

Diagnostic Testing

- Serum transaminases begin to rise sharply about 12 hours after ingestion. Peak levels occur at about 72 hours and are frequently >3,000 IU/L.
- Hepatic synthetic function declines as hepatotoxicity progresses (e.g., prolonged PT, hyperbilirubinemia, hypoalbuminemia, and hypoglycemia).
- Electrolyte disturbances, acidosis, and azotemia may occur.
- Patients should be screened for hypophosphatemia and treated.
- The **Rumack-Matthew nomogram** is used to predict the likelihood of hepatotoxicity given the serum level obtained and the time since consumption.[20]

- Treatment is indicated if the serum acetaminophen concentration falls in the area for concern for hepatic toxicity by the Rumack-Matthew nomogram (line connecting 150 mcg at 4 hours with 50 mcg at 12 hours).

Treatment

- Treatment involves the prompt administration of **N-acetylcysteine** (a glutathione precursor) to protect the liver against the toxic metabolites of acetaminophen.[20]
- Ideally, treatment should begin within 8 to 10 hours but may be beneficial up to 24 hours.
- N-acetylcysteine is given orally or intravenously.
  - Oral: Loading dose of 140 mg/kg followed by a maintenance dose of 70 mg/kg every 4 hours for a total of 17 doses over 72 hours.
  - Intravenous: Loading dose of 150 mg/kg IV in 5% dextrose over 15 minutes followed by a maintenance dose of 50 mg/kg over 4 hours followed by 100 mg/kg over 16 hours. Other IV dosage regimens have also been suggested.
- Patients who present late (>10 hours after ingestion) may benefit from longer treatment durations than those described above.
- Careful attention should be paid to detecting and correcting fluid, electrolyte, and acid-base abnormalities.
- If the patient progresses to liver failure despite these treatments, **liver transplantation** should be considered.[20]

METAL OVERLOAD DISEASE

Hereditary Hemochromatosis

General Considerations

- The underlying feature of hereditary hemochromatosis (HHC) is increased absorption of orally ingested iron from food. This excess iron deposited in the liver, heart, endocrine pancreas, and pituitary can lead to injury and dysfunction.
- Ninety percent of individuals with HHC have a homozygous recessive gene mutation in the HFE gene on chromosome 6. The disease is associated with homozygosity of the C282Y mutation and the compound heterozygous C282Y/H63D mutation.[21] **Penetrance is variable.**[22]
- Heterozygosity of the recessive gene is fairly common in the United States and western European Caucasian populations, approximately 10%; 0.30% to 0.5% are homozygotes.
- In the case of cirrhosis from hemochromatosis, patients are also at markedly increased risk for the development of HCC.

Diagnosis

Clinical Presentation

- The classic triad of cirrhosis, bronzing of the skin, and diabetes is quite rare due to early detection of the HHC by routine blood tests. Patients with early hemochromatosis are usually asymptomatic.
- As the disease progresses, constitutive symptoms including fatigue and more specific symptoms of arthritis, heart failure, diabetes, loss of libido, and liver failure may develop.
- Cutaneous iron deposition can lead to bronzing of the skin, especially in sun-exposed regions.[22,23]

Diagnostic Testing

Laboratories

- The utility and cost-effectiveness of large-scale population screening has yet to be clearly determined.[22,24]
- There is also no clear consensus regarding first-degree relatives of those with hemochromatosis; however, it can be done with fasting transferrin saturation/ferritin and/or HFE gene testing.
- Phenotypic screening tests include fasting transferrin saturation and ferritin.[25]
  - **Transferrin saturation:** $\geq 50\%$ in women and $\geq 60\%$ in men or $> 55\%$ for both. Some suggest that $> 45\%$ for both for greater sensitivity but less specificity.
  - **Ferritin:** > 200 ng/mL for women and > 300 ng/mL for men, in the absence of inflammation. Ferritin of $> 1,000$ ng/mL have a greater risk of developing cirrhosis.[26]

Imaging

- CT and MRI can both be used to detect deposition of iron in the liver and heart.
- Accurate measurements of hepatic iron concentration can be made using superconducting quantum interference device (SQUID) but, of course, this in not widely available.[27]

Diagnostic Procedures

- Indications for liver biopsy include the following:
  - Age > 40 years.
  - Ferritin of $> 1,000$ ng/mL.
  - Elevated transaminases.
- Liver biopsy is also performed in select populations, including the less common genetic mutations (approximately 10% of patients). This can assist in confirming the diagnosis by measurement of the hepatic iron index and evaluation of the pattern of iron deposition in the liver.[28,29]

Treatment

- Treatment is weekly phlebotomy (500 mL blood) until the ferritin is < 50 mg/L.
- If the hemoglobin level falls to < 10 g/dL, phlebotomy frequency should be decreased to every other week.
- Once the goal ferritin is achieved, maintenance phlebotomy is offered every 3 to 4 months.
- Screening first-degree relatives of affected individuals is also recommended (see above).
- Further details on the guidelines for management of HHC can be found at http://www.aasld.org.

Wilson Disease

General Considerations

- Wilson disease is a rare autosomal recessive disease of copper overload.
- A gene defect in ATP7B on chromosome 13 leads to decreased hepatocyte excretion of copper into bile. The copper accumulates and eventually reaches levels toxic to hepatocytes and also leaks into the serum and causes systemic symptoms.
- The classic organs involved are liver, cornea, brain, and kidney.
- It affects approximately 1 in 30,000 to 1 in 100,000 individuals and can lead to acute and chronic liver failure and neuropsychiatric symptoms.

Diagnosis

- The clinical presentation is quite variable.

- It most frequently affects those aged 6 to 20 years old but can have a wide variety of clinical presentations including liver disease, neurologic symptoms, or psychiatric illness.
- Some may be diagnosed when asymptomatic elevations of liver tests are inadvertently discovered.
- Wilson disease can also present fulminantly with dramatic findings such as jaundice, coagulopathy, renal failure, and a Coombs-negative hemolytic anemia.
- Slit-lamp examination may show the classical Kayser-Fleisher rings.
- Transaminases are mildly to moderately elevated but do not accurately predict the severity of liver damage.
- The diagnosis is suggested by a low serum ceruloplasmin of <20 mg/dL (seen in 85% of patients) and elevated 24-hour urine copper level of >100 mcg/24 hours. Extremely low levels (<5 mg/mL) are strongly suggestive.[30]
- If these tests are abnormal, a liver biopsy should be pursued for definitive diagnosis to allow calculation of hepatic copper levels.

Treatment
- Chelation therapy is the standard of care.
- The typical agents utilized include D-penicillamine, triethylene tetramine dihydrochloride, or zinc.[30]
- With the fulminant presentation, consideration for liver transplantation is the only treatment option.
- Current guidelines are outlined on the AASLD website at http://www.aasld.org.

OUTPATIENT BILIARY AND PANCREATIC DISEASES

Cholelithiasis

General Considerations
- Cholesterol and pigment stones are the two principal chemical types of gallstones.
- Gallstone formation usually occurs in the gallbladder, which can provide a reservoir for bile stasis and for the precipitation of cholesterol or bilirubin calcium salts.
- Biliary sludge appears to be capable of producing biliary symptoms.

Cholesterol Stones
- Cholesterol stones account for **80% of the biliary stones** in developed Western nations.
- Risk factors for cholesterol stones include the following:
  - Female gender
  - Obesity
  - Northern European or Native American ancestry
  - History of estrogen therapy
- Factors that increase bile stasis, such as prolonged bowel rest, weight reduction, or some drugs (e.g., octreotide), also enhance the risk of cholesterol gallstone formation.

Pigment Stones
- Although less common than cholesterol stones, pigment stones are frequently responsible for biliary pathology.
- These stones are seen with hemolytic anemias, notably **sickle cell disease.**

Diagnosis
- Most gallstones are **asymptomatic;** however, complications from obstruction of the biliary tree may develop in 15% to 20%.

- **Uncomplicated biliary colic** is the most common manifestation and is characterized by prolonged periods (hours) of colicky right upper quadrant or epigastric pain that radiates to the shoulder and associated with nausea and emesis.
- More serious complications include ascending cholangitis and gallstone pancreatitis.
- **Ultrasound** is the most sensitive test for the detection of gallstones. Ultrasound does not always detect sludge or microlithiasis (i.e., very small stones). Endoscopic ultrasound may be more sensitive.
- CT is less sensitive, as many stones are the same density as bile.

Treatment
- Cholecystectomy is the treatment of choice to prevent recurrent symptoms or complications from symptomatic gallstones.
- Asymptomatic gallstones found incidentally on imaging do not require any treatment.
- Dissolution therapy with ursodeoxycholic acid may be minimally effective.[31,32]

Pancreatic Cancer

General Considerations
- Adenocarcinoma of the head or proximal portion of the pancreas is the most frequent cause of malignant biliary obstruction.
- Pancreatic cancer is the fourth leading cause of cancer death in the United States.
- The incidence is approximately 8 to 10 case per 100,000 person years. Unfortunately the mortality rate is essentially the same number.
- Risk factors include age >45, male, African-American, smoking, diabetes, chronic pancreatitis, and BRCA-2 mutations.

Diagnosis
- The classical symptom is painless jaundice, but many patients do have abdominal pain.
- Weight loss can be substantial.
- Contrast-enhanced CT scan frequently establishes the diagnosis. Endoscopic ultrasound is an increasingly used technique to provide a tissue diagnosis and assess for surgical resectability.

Treatment
- Ninety percent of patients with pancreatic cancer have local or distant tumor spread at the time of diagnosis.
- Most patients are elderly (the median age of diagnosis is in the eighth decade of life) and may have comorbid illnesses.
- In rare selective cases, a surgical resection may be possible, so an experienced biliary surgeon should evaluate patients before abandoning curative efforts.[33]

Chronic Pancreatitis

General Considerations
- Chronic pancreatitis is permanent morphologic and functional damage to the pancreas.
- Insufficiency can occur if >90% of pancreatic function is compromised.
- Causes include the following:
  - **Alcohol consumption:** Accounts for the cause in up to 60% to 70% of patients in westernized countries. On the other hand, most alcoholics never develop chronic pancreatitis.

- **Cystic fibrosis:** Because of improved survival of cystic fibrosis patients, a greater number are developing this more long-term complication.
- **Chronic/recurrent obstruction:** Stones, tumor, trauma, etc.
- **Autoimmune:** In association with lupus, Sjögren syndrome, and PBC, for example, or confined to the pancreas (associated with elevated IgG4 levels).
- **Hereditary:** Autosomal dominant and strongly associated with pancreatic cancer.
- **Idiopathic:** Some reports have up to 30% to 40% of patients with no known etiology.[34]
- **"Tropical" pancreatitis:** Occurs in India and other parts of the tropics, where it is a frequent cause of chronic pancreatitis. The cause is unknown.
- **Complications** of chronic pancreatitis include pseudocysts, pseudoaneurysms, bile duct obstruction, intestinal obstruction, ascites, and splenic vein thrombosis.

Diagnosis

- Chronic abdominal pain is classically described as upper abdominal pain that may radiate to the mid-back or scapula and increases after eating.
- Fat malabsorption with resulting steatorrhea results from the exocrine pancreatic insufficiency.
- Intermittent exacerbations of pain are characteristic and sometimes necessitate hospital admission.
- Glucose intolerance results when the insulin secretion of the pancreas is compromised.
- Diagnosis is mainly based on clinical grounds, but some complicated testing is available.
- Imaging with plain abdominal films will show pathognomonic calcifications in up to 30% of patients.
- ERCP is necessary for diagnosis in some patients; however, this is being done more often now with MRCP.

Treatment

- **Alcohol cessation** is very important.
- **Pancreatic enzyme supplementation** is the primary treatment, which alleviates steatorrhea and may decrease pain.
- As lipase is highly sensitive to acid deactivation, acid suppression and enteric-coated enzyme formulations, although costly, are important in management.
- Pain management can be a serious challenge.
- Endoscopic and surgical procedures that include pseudocyst drainage and pancreaticojejunostomy are potential approaches to the care of chronic pancreatitis.

REFERENCES

1. Kamath P. Clinical approach to the patient with abnormal liver test results. *Mayo Clin Proc* 1996;71:1089–1095.
2. Bosch J, Abraldes J, Groszmann R. Current management of portal hypertension. *J Hepatol* 2003;38:S54–S68.
3. Runyon BA. Treatment of patients with cirrhosis and ascites. *Semin Liver Dis* 1997;17: 249–260.
4. Gholson C, Provenza M, Bacon B. Hepatologic considerations in patients with parenchymal liver disease. Undergoing surgery. *Am J Gastroenterol* 1990;85:487–496.
5. Wiesner R, Edwards E, Freeman R, et al. Model for end-stage liver disease (MELD) and allocation of donor livers. *Gastroenterology* 2003;124:91–96.
6. Victor J, Monto A, Surdine T, et al. Hepatitis A vaccine versus immune globulin for postexposure prophylaxis. *N Eng J Med* 2007;357:1685–1694.

7. Margolis H, Alter M, Hadler S. Hepatitis: evolving epidemiology and implications for control. *Semin Liver Dis* 1991;11:84–92.

8. Koff R, Dienstag J. Extrahepatic manifestations of hepatitis C and the association with alcoholic liver disease. *Semin Liver Dis* 1995;15:101–109.

9. Poynard T, Marcellin P, Lee S, et al. Randomized trial of interferon alpha-2b plus ribavirin for 48 weeks or for 24 weeks versus interferon alpha2 b plus placebo for 48 weeks for treatment of chronic infection with hepatitis C virus. *Lancet* 1998;352:1426–1432.

10. Poynard T, Leroy V, Cohard M, et al. Meta-analysis of interferon randomized trials in the treatment of viral hepatitis C: effects of dose and duration. *Hepatology* 1996;24:778–789.

11. McHutchinson J, Gordon S, Schiff E, et al. Interferon alpha-2b alone or in combination with ribavirin as initial treatment for chronic hepatitis C. *N Engl J Med* 1998;339:1485–1499.

12. McCullough A, O'Connor B. Alcoholic liver disease: proposed recommendations for the American College of Gastroenterology. *Am J Gastroenterol* 1998;93:2022–2036.

13. Maddrey W, Boitnott J, Bedine M, et al. Corticosteroid therapy of alcoholic hepatitis. *Gastroenterology* 1978;75:193–199.

14. Akrviasdis E, Butla R, Briggs W, et al. Pentoxifylline improves short-term survival in severe acute alcoholic hepatitis: a double-blind, placebo-controlled trial. *Gastroenterology* 2000; 119:1637–1648.

15. Roberts S, Therneau T, Czaja A. Prognosis of histological cirrhosis in type 1 autoimmune hepatitis. *Gastroenterology* 1996;110:848–857.

16. Kaplan M, Gershwin ME. Primary biliary cirrhosis. *N Eng J Med* 2005;353:1261–1273.

17. Levy C, Lindor K. Current Management of primary biliary cirrhosis and primary sclerosing cholangitis. *J Hepatol* 2003;38:S24–S37.

18. Lee Y, Kaplan M. Primary sclerosing cholangitis. *N Engl J Med* 1995;332:924–933.

19. Navarro V, Senior J. Drug-related hepatotoxicity. *N Engl J Med* 2006;354:731–739.

20. Larson A. Acetaminophen hepatotoxicity. *Clin Liver Dis* 2007;11:525–548.

21. Tavill A. Diagnosis and management of hemochromatosis. *Hepatology* 2001;33:1321–1328.

22. Whitlock EP, Garlitz BA, Harris EL, et al. Screening for hereditary hemochromatosis: a systematic review for the U.S. Preventive Services Task Force. *Ann Intern Med* 2006;145: 209–223.

23. Edwards C, Kushner J. Screening for hemochromatosis. *N Engl J Med* 1993;328: 1616–1620.

24. Phatak PD, Bonkovsky HL, Kowdley KV. Hereditary hemochromatosis: time for targeted screening. *Ann Intern Med* 2008;149:270–272.

25. Qaseem A, Aronson M, Fitterman N, et al.; Clinical Efficacy Assessment Subcommittee of the American College of Physicians. Screening for hereditary hemochromatosis: a clinical practice guideline from the American College of Physicians. *Ann Intern Med* 2005;143: 517–521.

26. Morrison ED, Brandhagen DJ, Phatak PD, et al. Serum ferritin level predicts advanced hepatic fibrosis among U.S. patients with phenotypic hemochromatosis. *Ann Intern Med* 2003;138:627–633.

27. Sheth S. SQUID biosusceptometry in the measurement of hepatic iron. *Pediatr Radiol* 2003;33:373–377.

28. Andrews N. Disorders of iron metabolism. *N Engl J Med* 1999;341:1986–1995.

29. Bacon B, Olynyk J, Brunt E, et al. HFE genotype in patients with hemochromatosis and other liver diseases. *Ann Intern Med* 1999;130:953–962.

30. Roberts EA, Schilsky ML; American Association for Study of Liver Diseases (AASLD). Diagnosis and treatment of Wilson disease: an update. *Hepatology* 2008;47:2089–2111.

31. Johnston D, Kaplan M. pathogenesis and treatment of gallstones. *N Engl J Med* 1993;328: 412–421.

32. Ransohoff D, Gracie W. Treatment of gallstones. *Ann Intern Med* 1993;119:606–619.

33. Schoeman MN, Huibregtse K. Pancreatic and ampullary carcinoma. *Gastrointest Endosc Clin N Am* 1995;5:217–236.

34. Steer M, Waxman I, Freedman S. Chronic pancreatitis. *N Engl J Med* 1995;332:1482–1490.

27 Inflammatory Bowel Disease

Christina Ha and Matthew A. Ciorba

General Principles

- Ulcerative colitis (UC) and Crohn disease (CD) are chronic inflammatory disorders of the gastrointestinal (GI) tract categorized under the spectrum of inflammatory bowel diseases (IBDs). The underlying etiology is currently unknown. Genetic, environmental, and autoimmune factors may all play a role.
- There is no specific test to diagnose IBD. Clinical history and physical examination in combination with objective findings from laboratory studies, radiology, endoscopy, and pathology suggest the diagnosis of an IBD.[1]
- The IBDs have a high enough prevalence that most primary care physicians are likely to encounter one of more IBD patients in their own practice; therefore, understanding the nomenclature, clinical features, and basic management of the IBD is important.
  - The primary care physician has a particularly important role in recognizing the initial disease presentation as well as identifying whether a patient's other symptoms or signs represent an IBD extraintestinal manifestation or flare.
  - Ultimately, patients with this multifaceted disease are best managed through collaboration between the astute primary care physician and a gastroenterologist who is well versed with the diseases.

Epidemiology

- Incidence rates of IBD follow a bimodal distribution with the majority of diagnoses occurring between the ages of 15 and 30 and a second smaller peak between the ages of 50 and 80.
- Incidence is higher in white Northern Europeans and North Americans.
- The prevalence of IBD in North Americans is
  - CD: 26 to 199/100,00
  - UC: 27 to 246/100,000
- **Risk factors** for IBD:
  - Patients who have first-degree relatives with IBD have an increased risk of having IBD themselves.
  - Current smokers have a lower risk of developing UC. Former smokers, however, have a 1.7-fold increased risk for UC than nonsmokers.
  - Smoking is associated with an increased risk of CD and increases the chance of disease recurrence.
  - Concomitant infections (intestinal and extraintestinal) can exacerbate IBD.

Ulcerative Colitis

- UC is defined by **mucosal** inflammation limited to the colon.

TABLE 1	Classifying Disease Extent in Ulcerative Colitis
Proctitis	Inflammation limited to the rectum
Distal colitis or proctosigmoiditis	Inflammation extending to the mid-sigmoid colon
Left-sided colitis	Inflammation extending to the sigmoid flexure
Extensive colitis	Inflammation extending beyond the splenic flexure but sparing the cecum
Pancolitis	Continuous inflammation from rectum to cecum
Backwash ileitis	Ileal inflammation in association with pancolitis

- Inflammatory changes most typically involve the distal rectum and extend proximally in a **circumferential and uninterrupted** distribution.
- The nomenclature for UC describes the extent of inflammation and is important when determining medical therapies for UC (Table 1).
- **Bloody diarrhea with associated rectal urgency and tenesmus** (the sense of incomplete defecation) **is the hallmark presentation of active UC.** Patients also commonly complain of passing mucus and pus with stools.
- Disease severity is characterized by patient symptoms[1]:
  - **Mild disease:** Less than four stools per day and no signs of systemic toxicity.
  - **Moderate disease:** Four to six stools per day and minimal signs of systemic toxicity.
  - **Severe disease:** More than six stools per day with signs of systemic toxicity (fever, tachycardia, anemia, and increased erythrocyte sedimentation rate).
  - **Fulminant disease:** >10 stools per day, continuous bleeding, abdominal tenderness or distention, and dilation on radiographic imaging.
  - The clinical manifestations of UC compared with those of CD are presented in Table 2.
- Patients with UC can develop **toxic megacolon** (which can also be caused by infectious colitis).
  - Potential precipitating factors include electrolyte abnormalities, opiates, and other drugs that can decrease motility.
  - Possibly life-threatening complications of toxic megacolon are perforation, hemorrhage, and sepsis.

Crohn Disease

- CD is characterized by **transmural** intestinal inflammation that can involve any part of the GI tract from the oropharynx to the anus.
- Inflammatory changes are usually **asymmetric and discontinuous** with skip areas showing normal tissue separating diseased intestinal segments.
- CD is often described by location with the ileum, colon, and ileo-colon most commonly involved. It is also classified by its behavior: penetrating (fistulae, abscesses), stricturing, inflammatory, or perianal disease.
- The manifestations of CD vary with the degree and segment of intestinal involvement.
  - Upper GI tract involvement may present as oral ulcers, gum pain, odynophagia, dysphagia, or even symptoms consistent with gastric outlet obstruction.
  - Small bowel and colonic symptoms include diarrhea, abdominal pain, weight loss, obstructive symptoms, and fever.
  - Gross rectal bleeding occurs but is less common in UC, and a small percentage of CD patients do not have diarrhea.

TABLE 2	Comparison of Crohn Disease and Ulcerative Colitis	
	Crohn Disease	**Ulcerative Colitis**
Scope of disease	Entire GI tract; ileum most common	Rectum and proximally
Clinically	Abdominal pain or mass, diarrhea, weight loss, vomiting, perianal disease	Rectal bleeding, diarrhea, passage of mucus, crampy pain, tenesmus
Endoscopy	Rectal sparing, skip lesions, aphthous ulcers, cobblestoning, linear ulceration	Rectal involvement, continuous, friability, loss of vascularity
Radiology	Small bowel and terminal ileal disease, segmental, strictures, fistulae	Colon disease, loss of haustra, continuous ulceration, no fistulae
Histology	Transmural disease, aphthous ulcers, noncaseating granulomas	Abnormal crypt architecture, superficial inflammation
Cigarette smoking	Increases risk of disease, recurrence rate, decreases time to surgery, and lessens therapeutic efficacy	Current smoking decreases risk

Modified from Paradowski TJ, Ciorba MA. Inflammatory bowel disease. In: Gyawali CP, ed. The Washington Manual Gastroenterology Subspecialty Consult. 2nd Ed. Philadelphia, PA: Lippincott Williams & Wilkins, 1999:129–139.

- Assessing disease severity is sometimes more difficult than with UC but is still important in CD. Symptoms of pain and diarrhea can sometimes be due to a separate, though many times concurrent, irritable bowel syndrome. A proposed classification system for CD includes[1]:
  - **Mild-moderate disease:** Outpatients able to tolerate oral intake without signs of dehydration, abdominal pain, systemic toxicity, or weight loss of >10%.
  - **Moderate-severe disease:** Patients who have failed therapy for mild-moderate disease or have abdominal pain, nausea/vomiting, and signs of systemic toxicity such as fevers, dehydration, anemia, or weight loss of >10%.
  - **Severe-fulminant disease:** Persistent symptoms despite corticosteroid use or patients with high fevers, cachexia, persistent vomiting, intestinal obstruction, surgical abdomen, or abscess formation.
  - **Remission:** Asymptomatic patients or those who have responded to medical or surgical intervention without evidence of residual/recurrent disease (not on steroids).
- Patients with CD can also develop **toxic megacolon.**

Extraintestinal Manifestations of IBD

IBD can be associated with extraintestinal manifestations.[2] Many, but not all, of these extraintestinal symptoms have increased activity associated with the colonic IBD activity.

Musculoskeletal
- Central arthropathies, including **ankylosing spondylitis** and **sacroiliitis,** are associated more commonly with CD than with UC. They tend to correlate poorly with IBD activity.

- **Pauciarticular peripheral arthritis** tends to flare with colonic inflammation. Joint involvement is usually asymmetric with the involvement of the larger joints (knees, hips, ankles, wrists, and elbows).
- **Polyarticular peripheral arthritis** is symmetric, involves smaller joints (fingers and toes) and is independent of IBD activity.
- **Osteoporosis** is increased in IBD patients presumably due to cumulative steroid use, malabsorption, low body weight, and relative hypogonadism related to disease activity. Guidelines suggest using dual energy x-ray absorptiometry (DEXA) testing to screen for osteoporosis in all postmenopausal women with IBD and those individuals who have received prolonged or frequent courses of corticosteroids. All patients with disease severe enough to require steroids at least once should take supplemental vitamin D (800 IU) daily along with 1,000 to 1,500 mg calcium supplementation.

Dermatologic
- **Erythema nodosum** (EN) is a painful, poorly demarcated, nodular lesion that tends to be bilateral but asymmetric. It is closely related to IBD activity, and treatment of the underlying disease results in improvement of EN lesions.
- **Pyoderma gangrenosum** (PG) is a debilitating skin disease characterized by irregular, blue-red ulcers with purulent necrotic bases. Lesions are usually found on the lower extremities, buttocks, abdomen, and face. PG can develop independently of IBD activity.
- **Aphthous ulcers** in the oropharynx are seen in 10% to 30% of patients with IBD.

Ocular
- **Episcleritis** is an inflammation of the episclera. Visual acuity is not affected and episodes tend to coincide with IBD flares.
- **Uveitis** is an inflammation of the interior of the eye and may affect visual acuity. It does not always coincide with disease activity and tends to be more chronic in duration. Acute episodes may cause permanent ocular damage; therefore, prompt diagnosis and steroid treatment are important.

Hepatobiliary
- **Gallstones** may develop in patients with CD due to malabsorption of bile salts in the ileum.
- **Primary sclerosing cholangitis** (PSC) is more commonly associated with UC than CD and is a chronic inflammatory disease of the bile ducts (refer to Chapter 26). Endoscopic retrograde cholangiopancreatography (ERCP) or magnetic resonance cholangiopancreatography (MRCP) reveals strictures of intrahepatic and extrahepatic ducts. Patients with PSC have an increased risk of developing cholangiocarcinoma.

Vascular
Thromboembolism is increased in patients with IBD and can be a major source of mortality.

Renal
- **Nephrolithiasis** can occur in patients with CD.
- Oxalate stones and hyperoxaluria are common and related to fat malabsorption, which increases the amount of dietary oxalate available for absorption in the colon.

Diagnosis

Clinical Presentation

History

- Obtaining a thorough history is the first step in the clinical diagnosis of IBD as well as defining disease severity.
- Questions should focus on relevant features of IBD: abdominal symptoms, systemic signs of toxicity, family history of IBD, medication history, smoking history, and the presence of extraintestinal manifestations.
- The principle historic features of UC are bloody diarrhea with associated rectal urgency and tenesmus. Patients also commonly complain of passing mucus and pus with stools. These symptoms usually begin gradually, but some present with fulminant symptoms.
- The symptomatology of CD is much more variable. Chronic fatigue, diarrhea (sometimes with blood), abdominal pain, weight loss, and fever are typical.

Physical Examination

- The vital signs can imply systemic toxicity by the presence of fever, hypotension, and tachycardia.
- A careful abdominal examination is important. High pitched or absent bowel sounds may suggest obstruction.
- Peritoneal signs (rebound, guarding, and rigid abdomen) is concerning for intestinal perforation.
- A palpable right lower quadrant mass is sometimes felt in patients with CD, suggestive of ileal inflammation or abscess.
- A careful rectal and perianal examination is important. Skin tags, fistulae, and anal fissures suggest CD. Rectal exam may often be painful due to the severity of inflammation or presence of fissures. Occult or overt GI bleeding is often present during flares.
- With toxic megacolon, the transverse colon typically is dilated for >5 to 6 cm and the abdomen is distended, painful, and tender. Patients can, as the name implies, appear quite toxic (e.g., fever, hypotension, and tachycardia). Steroids may mask some of these signs.
- Ocular, skin, and musculoskeletal exams may reveal extraintestinal manifestations of IBD.

Differential Diagnosis

The differential diagnosis of IBD is extensive including infections, neoplasias, ischemia, and other inflammatory conditions that can present with similar symptoms as IBD and must be ruled out first (Table 3).

Diagnostic Testing

Laboratories

- There is currently no specific laboratory test for IBD; however, several autoantibodies have been detected in IBD patients including perinuclear antineutrophil cytoplasmic antibody (P-ANCA) and anti-*Saccharomyces cerevisiae* antibodies.
- Initial evaluation of patients with IBD or suspected IBD should include a complete blood cell count (CBC) to evaluate for anemia and leukocytosis.
- A comprehensive metabolic panel is useful to evaluate for metabolic derangements due to disease activity and prior to initiating specific therapies for IBD.
- Elevations in the erythrocyte sedimentation rate and C-reactive protein may suggest active disease.

TABLE 3	Differential Diagnosis for IBD	

Infectious Etiologies

Bacterial	Mycobacterial	Viral
Salmonella spp.	Tuberculosis	Cytomegalovirus
Shigella spp.	*Mycobacterium*	Herpes simplex
Toxigenic *Escherichia coli*	*avium*	HIV

	Parasitic	Fungal
Campylobacter spp.	Amebiasis	Histoplasmosis
Yersinia spp.	*Isospora belli*	Candidiasis
Clostridium difficile	*Trichuris trichura*	Aspergillosis
Gonorrhea	Hookworm	
Chlamydia trachomatis	*Strongyloidiasis*	

Noninfectious Etiologies

Inflammatory	Medications	Neoplasias
Appendicitis	NSAIDs	Lymphomas
Diverticulitis	Chemotherapy	Carcinomas
Microscopic colitis		(colon, small
Ischemic colitis		bowel)
Radiation enteritis		
Behçet disease		

HIV, human immunodeficiency virus; IBD, inflammatory bowel disease; NSAID, nonsteroidal anti-inflammatory drug.
Modified from Paradowski TJ, Ciorba MA. Inflammatory bowel disease. In: Gyawali CP, ed. The Washington Manual Gastroenterology Subspecialty Consult. 2nd Ed. Philadelphia, PA: Lippincott Williams & Wilkins, 1999:129–139.

- Stool studies (*Clostridium difficile* toxin, culture, ova, and parasites) are important to look for infectious etiologies that may mimic IBD.

Imaging
- For patients presenting with systemic toxicity and significant abdominal complaints, a plain abdominal radiography is often useful to look for dilated loops of bowel, toxic megacolon, or free air.
- Imaging studies such as small bowel follow-through, computerized tomography, and magnetic resonance enterography (MRE) are frequently ordered to look for strictures, abscesses, and fistulae.

Diagnostic Procedures
- The role of endoscopy is to determine location, extent, and severity of disease.
- Endoscopic features can often aid in distinguishing CD from UC.
- In addition, biopsies are obtained for histological examination.
- Histology in UC shows inflammation confined to the mucosa and superficial submucosa. The crypt architecture is distorted and there may be basal lymphoid aggregations and plasma cells.

- The inflammation in CD is transmural with crypt abscesses and noncaseating granulomas. Intervening areas without inflammation are common.

Treatment

Medications

- The general principles of medical management of CD and UC are the induction and maintenance of remission.[3,4]
- The location of the disease activity and the nature of extraintestinal problems should be noted, and therapy should be appropriately targeted to maximize benefit while minimizing the chances of drug toxicity.
- Superimposed infections should be ruled out prior to initiating immunosuppressant or immunomodulator therapy.
- Treatment of toxic megacolon consists of complete bowel rest, correction of dehydration and electrolyte abnormalities, discontinuation of all drugs that can reduce motility, and high-dose steroids. Surgery may be necessary for those unresponsive to medical management or for those with perforation or severe hemorrhage.

Antibiotics

- Antibiotics such as **ciprofloxacin** and **metronidazole** are occasionally used to treat perianal, fistulizing, or mildly active CD.
- Antibiotics are often initiated in the setting of systemic toxicity, as bacterial translocation may occur during fulminant disease such as toxic megacolon.
- The long-term safety profile of chronic metronidazole therapy is poorly understood and monitoring for neurologic toxicities (e.g., peripheral neuropathy) is important.
- Both antibiotics should be used sparingly during pregnancy, especially during the first trimester.

Aminosalicylates

- 5-Aminosalicylates (5-ASA) drugs are often the first-line therapies to treat patients with **mild-to-moderate IBD.**
- Various formulations of 5-ASA compounds are available and are generally well tolerated. **Mesalamine** (e.g., Asacol, Pentasa, Aprisio, and Lialda) and **balsalazide** (Colazal) are the formulations available in the United States.
- Patients with proctitis or left-sided colitis may benefit from the addition of 5-ASA suppositories or enemas.
- Adverse effects include headache, diarrhea, and abdominal pain. These drugs should also be used with caution in patients with salicylate or sulfa allergies but are safe to use during pregnancy.
- Sulfasalazine is the prodrug of 5-ASAs.
  - It is effective particularly in treating patients with colonic disease and an associated peripheral arthropathy.
  - Its use is dose limited by the **sulpha moiety** but remains an effective and less expensive alternative for many patients.

Corticosteroids

- While undesirable in both side effect profiles and their **inability to maintain remission,** steroids are **commonly used to induce remission** in moderate-to-severe IBD or for patients who continue to have active disease despite other therapies such as 5-ASA.

- An increase in frequency of their use or prolonged period of usage generally signals the need for an immunomodulatory drug to be initiated (see later).
- >50% of patients become steroid dependent (i.e., symptoms flare with decreased doses or upon discontinuing steroids) or steroid resistant (i.e., symptoms persist despite high doses of steroids).
- Topical and systemic preparations are used, but systemic therapy should be used sparingly and with caution if infectious etiologies for disease flare have not been excluded.
- Steroids are ineffective as maintenance therapy and lead to significant side effects including metabolic, psychiatric, ocular, GI, and osseous side effects.
- If therapeutic effect is seen, the clinician should pursue a slow taper over 2 to 3 months to attempt to discontinue use. A more rapid taper typically leads to recurrence.

Immunomodulators

- Immunomodulators such as **6-mercaptopurine (6-MP)** and its prodrug **azathioprine (AZA)** are widely used in the management of IBD. These medications are used to **maintain steroid-free disease remission;** therapeutic effect can take up to 3 to 6 months of continued use.
- These drugs are especially used to treat patients who have recurrent disease flares or who are unable to be weaned from steroids without recurrent flares.
- Adverse effects of 6-MP and AZA include **bone marrow suppression;** therefore, the patient's CBC should be followed frequently initially and then at least every 3 months after the patient has reached their goal dose.
- Some gastroenterologists may check thiopurine methyltransferase activity or genetics prior to the initiation of immunomodulator therapy to stratify at-risk patients for bone marrow suppression.
- 6-Thioguanine levels (6-TG) are sometimes checked during the course of treatment with 6-MP or AZA to assess for adequate therapeutic levels of the medications.
- A common idiosyncratic effect of these drugs is **pancreatitis.** If pancreatitis develops, the drug should be immediately discontinued. Repeat challenge with either 6-MP or AZA is contraindicated.
- Other immunosuppressant drugs, including **methotrexate** (for CD) and **cyclosporine** (in UC), have been used successfully to manage moderate-to-severe IBD.
- The use of these drugs during **pregnancy** remains controversial. No prospective study has evaluated this question and retrospective studies show conflicting results. It is generally considered that recurrence of disease activity leads to more complications than continuation of 6-MP or AZA. Ultimately the decision on whether or not to continue these drugs must fall between the patient and her treating physicians.

Tumor Necrosis Factor Alpha Antagonists

- Tumor necrosis factor alpha antagonists (anti-TNF-α) are used **for moderate-to-severe or steroid-dependent disease.**
- Infliximab, adalimumab, and certolizumab pegol are FDA-approved anti-TNF-α therapies for CD. Infliximab is also approved for the therapy of UC.
- They are administered as a series of induction therapies with maintenance doses given at interval time periods after induction.
- Prior to starting treatment, a PPD skin test and chest radiograph are often obtained because of the risk of reactivation of latent tuberculosis.
- Adverse effects include acute and delayed infusion reactions, injection site reactions, infections, and a possible increased risk for lymphomas.

Surgical Management

- Indications for surgery are severe GI hemorrhage, toxic megacolon/perforation, medically refractory disease, recurrent/persistent obstructions, significant fistulizing disease, or abscesses.
- **Total colectomy is potentially curative for UC.** Surgery for CD involves limited resection of diseased segments.
- UC patients with colonic carcinoma, high-grade dysplasia, or multifocal low-grade dysplasia found during surveillance colonoscopy should also be referred for total colectomy.

Postoperative Complications

- Postcolectomy many patients opt to have an ileal pouch created in lieu of a permanent ostomy. **Pouchitis** occurs in up to 50% of patients—typical symptoms include increased stool frequency, abdominal cramping, rectal urgency, rectal bleeding, incontinence, and fever.
  - Antibiotics, ciprofloxacin or metronidazole, and steroid or 5-ASA enemas/suppositories are commonly used for treatment.
  - Recurrent or refractory pouchitis may represent misdiagnosed CD. Pouch excision is required in approximately 5% of patients.
  - Cuffitis is an inflammation due to a short "cuff" of retained rectal mucosa and is treated with topical steroid or 5-ASA suppositories.
- **Postoperative recurrence of CD is common.** Smoking has been associated with an accelerated time to disease recurrence postoperatively in CD patients.

Treatment of Extraintestinal Manifestations of IBD

- Treatments for ankylosing spondylitis and sacroiliitis include analgesics, methotrexate, or anti-TNF therapy for severe cases (Chapter 28).
- Treatment of the underlying colitis tends to improve pauciarticular peripheral arthritis.
- The course of polyarticular peripheral arthritis is more protracted, occasionally requiring immunosuppressants for treatment.
- Young patients diagnosed with osteoporosis will benefit from seeing an osteoporosis specialist prior to initiation of a bisphosphonate (Chapter 37).
- Treatment of the underlying disease results in improvement of EN lesions.
- PG calls for aggressive local wound care and systemic steroids are often required.
- Aphthous ulcers tend to resolve with disease remission.
- Treatment of episcleritis consists of controlling the underlying disease flare as well as topical corticosteroids.
- Topical steroids are the primary treatment for uveitis.
- Treatment of PSC includes endoscopic dilation of symptomatic strictures. Patients with severe disease may ultimately require liver transplantation (refer to Chapter 26).
- Inpatients should be given thromboembolism prophylaxis with heparin products unless severe bleeding is present. Avoidance of prolonged immobilization, indwelling catheters, and control of disease activity are also important.

Cancer Surveillance

- Patients with IBD have an increased risk of developing colorectal cancer. The risk is even higher if a family history of colon cancer is present.
- Cancer risk is related to duration (after 10 years), extent (much greater risk with pancolitis as opposed to proctitis), and severity of disease (based on histology).

- The current recommendation is to begin colorectal cancer screening after 8 to 10 years of IBD. Surveillance colonoscopies should be performed every 1 to 2 years.
- Patients with high-grade dysplasia or multifocal low-grade dysplasia seen on colon biopsies should be referred to a colorectal surgeon.
- Patients with an ileal pouch should undergo flexible sigmoidoscopy with biopsies every other year.

REFERENCES

1. Baumgart DC, Sandborn WJ. Inflammatory bowel disease: clinical aspects and established and evolving therapies. *Lancet* 2007;369:1641–1657.
2. Rothfuss KS, Stange EF, Herrlinger KR. Extraintestinal manifestations and complications in inflammatory bowel diseases. *World J Gastroenterol* 2006;12:4819–4831.
3. Lichtenstein GR, Abreu MT, Cohen R, Tremaine W; American Gastroenterological Association. American Gastroenterological Association Institute medical position statement on corticosteroids, immunomodulators, and infliximab in inflammatory bowel disease. *Gastroenterology* 2006;130:935–939.
4. Kornbluth A, Sachar DB. Ulcerative colitis practice guidelines in adults (update): American College of Gastroenterology, Practice Parameters Committee. *Am J Gastroenterol* 2004;99:1371–1385.

28 Rheumatologic Diseases

J. Chad Byrd and Richard D. Brasington

APPROACH TO THE PATIENT WITH PAINFUL JOINTS

General Principles

- **Initial evaluation** of patient with painful joints is carried out to rule out emergent versus nonemergent causes of arthritis.
- While early diagnosis and treatment of most causes of arthritis is important to ensure the best possible outcome, infectious causes of arthritis such as septic arthritis and endocarditis require emergent evaluation and treatment.
- A logical approach to the evaluation of painful joints includes separating into the number of joints involved including **monoarticular** arthritis versus **polyarticular** arthritis.

Diagnosis

An algorithmic approach to the diagnosis of monoarticular and polyarticular arthritis is presented in Figures 1 and 2, respectively.[1]

Clinical Presentation

History

- Characteristic **inflammatory symptoms** include swelling, warmth, redness, morning stiffness, stiffness after inactivity (the so-called gelling phenomenon), and sometimes fever.
- **Mechanical symptoms** include pain with activity that is relieved with rest, minimal morning stiffness, joint locking or "giving out," and lack of swelling or heat.
- **Location** of pain can help provide clues.
  - History of **preceding injury** might suggest degenerative arthritis of the joint, whereas the classic presentation of podagra with inflammation of the first metatarsophalangeal (MTP) joint suggests gout.
  - Osteoarthritis (OA) tends to affect the first carpometacarpal joint in the hand and the large weight-bearing joints.
  - Multiple pain complaints and diffuse tender points suggest a chronic pain syndrome such as fibromyalgia or depression.

Physical Examination

- **Gait:** Observing the patient walking away, turning, and walking back can help localize the source of pain.
- **Hand:** Have the patient make a fist and inspect the dorsum of the hand; observe supination; and inspect the palm of the hands. Look carefully at each of the joints and palpate the metacarpophalangeal joints for swelling or tenderness.

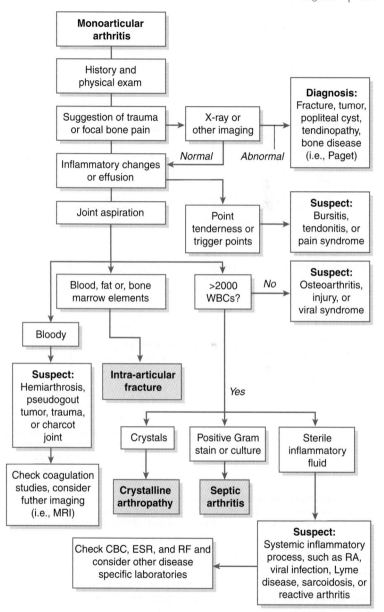

Figure 1. Evaluation of monoarticular arthritis. CBC, complete blood cell count; ESR, erythrocyte sedimentation rate; RA, rheumatoid arthritis; RF, rheumatoid factor; WBC, white blood cells. (Modified from Guidelines for the initial evaluation of the adult patient with acute musculoskeletal symptoms. American College of Rheumatology Ad Hoc Committee on Clinical Guidelines. *Arthritis Rheum* 1996;39:1–8.)

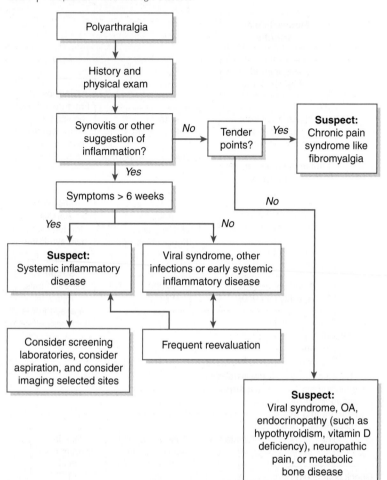

Figure 2. Evaluation of polyarthralgia. OA, osteoarthritis. (Modified from Guidelines for the initial evaluation of the adult patient with acute musculoskeletal symptoms. American College of Rheumatology Ad Hoc Committee on Clinical Guidelines. *Arthritis Rheum* 1996;39:1–8.)

- **Shoulder:** Ask the patient to put both hands together above the head and observe any abnormal movement of the scapula; put both hands behind the head; and put both hands behind the back (normally the thumb tip can reach the tip of the scapula).
- **Cervical spine:** Have the patient touch the tip of the chin to chest, look up, and look over each shoulder.
- **Lower spine:** Ask the patient to bend forward to touch the toes without bending the knees and observe movement of the lumbar spine (normally there should be reversal of lordosis with flexion of the lumbar spine).
- **Hip:** The FABER maneuver (flexion-abduction-external rotation) is performed by having the patient put the heel on the contralateral knee, with the examiner then

pressing down on the medial knee, putting the hip into external rotation. The important aspect here is where pain is elicited.

- Pain in the groin is indicative of hip joint pathology, but pain may also be elicited from the sacroiliac joint and the lateral aspect of the hip from the trochanteric bursa.
- **Knee:** The patient should be able to straighten the knee fully and flex it so that the heel almost touches the buttocks. Look for symmetry and effusions. The patella can be held in place with one hand and should have little give normally. In the presence of an effusion, the joint becomes ballotable (ballottement test).
- **Ankle:** One should look for limitations in flexion and extension and inversion and eversion.

Diagnostic Testing

Laboratories

- Few rheumatology tests are designed to serve as an independent diagnostic tool and test results must always be interpreted in a clinical context.
- **Erythrocyte sedimentation rate** (ESR): The ESR is a **very nonspecific** indicator of inflammation and is often elevated in inflammatory conditions.
  - Anemia, kidney disease (especially proteinuria), and aging can all elevate the ESR in the absence of inflammation.
- **C-reactive protein** (CRP): CRP is an acute phase reactant and component of the innate immune system; levels rise rapidly with inflammation and infection and fall quickly as inflammation resolves.
  - Unlike the ESR, the CRP is not influenced by anemia and abnormal erythrocytes.
  - Today, most laboratories perform a high sensitive assay for the presence of CRP that can identify minute increases in this protein.
- **Rheumatoid factor** (RF): RF is elevated in approximately 80% of patients with rheumatoid arthritis (RA), but this test result can also be elevated in Sjögren syndrome, sarcoidosis, chronic infections, and other conditions where immune complexes are formed.
  - The RF is an immune complex of immunoglobulin (Ig) M that binds to the Fc portion of IgG.
- **Antineutrophil cytoplasmic antibody** (ANCA): ANCA detects antibodies in a patient's serum against neutrophils and is reported as either a cytoplasmic pattern (c-ANCA) or a perinuclear pattern (p-ANCA).
  - If either of these is detected, the presence of antibodies for the disease-specific antigens (proteinase-3 for c-ANCA and myeloperoxidase for p-ANCA) can be ascertained by an enzyme-linked immunosorbent assay (ELISA).
  - Antibodies against **proteinase-3 (c-ANCA) are specific for Wegener granulomatosis,** but antibodies against myeloperoxidase is less specific and are seen in conditions such as microscopic polyarteritis and polyarteritis nodosa and Goodpasture syndrome (in up to 30% of patients).
- **Antinuclear antibody** (ANA): The ANA test detects antibodies in patient's serum that bind to nuclear antigens.
  - It is a **very sensitive test** for patients with systemic lupus erythematosus (SLE) (sensitivity >95%) and may be abnormal in many other autoimmune diseases such as scleroderma, Sjögren syndrome, and polymyositis (PM). Yet, because the specificity of the ANA is low, a positive ANA result alone is seldom useful.
- **Extractable nuclear antigens:** This test encompasses a panel of saline-soluble nuclear antigens that include Smith (Sm), Ro-Sjögren syndrome (SS)-A, SS-B, and ribonuclear protein antigens.

- **Anti-Scl-70 antibodies:** Directed against topoisomerase I and is associated with diffuse scleroderma.
- **Anticentromere antibodies:** Directed against 70/13-kDa proteins making up the centromere complex and are associated with limited scleroderma.
- **Anti-Jo-1 antibodies:** Directed against histidyl tRNA synthetase and associated with myositis with interstitial lung disease and arthritis.
- Table 1 presents an overview of the various autoantibodies and their disease associations.[2]

Synovial Fluid Evaluation
- Obtaining synovial fluid from a patient with undiagnosed arthritis, particularly monoarticular arthritis, can be very beneficial.
- The synovial fluid is often characterized by a number of cells (especially polymorphonuclear leukocytes [PMNs]), viscosity, and color.
- The status of Gram stain plus culture and the presence or absence of crystals can confirm the diagnosis (Table 2).

Imaging
- Radiographic changes are common, even in early forms of arthritis.
- The distribution, appearance, severity, and other features of the radiography can help limit the differential diagnosis (Table 3).

OSTEOARTHRITIS

General Principles

- The usual joints that are involved in primary OA are lower cervical spine, lower lumbar spine, first carpometacarpal joint of the thumb, proximal interphalangeal joints (Bouchard nodes), distal interphalangeal (DIP) joints (Heberden nodes), hip, knee, and first MTP joint.
- Primary OA is rarely seen in the following locations and, if present here, should raise the suspicion for secondary causes (trauma, inflammatory arthritis, etc.): shoulders, elbows, and wrists.

Diagnosis

- **History** consists of mechanical pain (i.e., pain that is worse with activity and relieved with rest). Morning stiffness may be present but usually lasts for <30 to 60 minutes.
- **Examination** reveals reduced range of motion, mild swelling, and bony hypertrophy. Small-to-moderate effusions may be present in the knee. Crepitus may be observed with range of motion examination.
- **Laboratory tests** are noncontributory except to rule out other causes of arthritis. Synovial fluid if drawn tends to have <2,000 cells/mm^3.
- **Radiographic** findings are indicated in Table 3.

Treatment

Guidelines for the treatment of OA have been published by the American College of Rheumatology (ACR).[3]

TABLE 1   Autoantibodies and Disease Associations

Disease	ANA	Pattern	RF	dsDNA	Sm	SS-A/Ro	SS-B/La	Scl-70	Centromere	Jo-1	RNP
Systemic lupus erythematosus	>95%	P, H, S, N	20	50–70	30	35	15	0	0	0	30–50
Rheumatoid arthritis	15–35	H	80–85	<5	0	10	5	0	0	0	10
Sjögren syndrome	>90	H, S	75	<5	0	55	40	0	0	0	15
Diffuse scleroderma	>90	S, N, H	25–33	0	0	5	1	40	<5	0	30
Limited scleroderma	>90	S, N, H, C	25–33	0	0	5	1	<15	60–80	0	30
Polymyositis and dermatomyositis	75–95		33	0	0	0	0	0	0	20–30	0
Mixed connective tissue disease	>95%	S, H	0	0	0	<5	<5	0	0	0	100

C, centromere; H, homogenous or diffuse; P, peripheral or rim; N, nucleolar; S, speckled.
Modified from Klippel JH, ed. Primer on the Rheumatic Diseases. 12th Ed. Atlanta, GA: Arthritis Foundation, 2001.

TABLE 2	Classification of Synovial Fluid		
Type of Fluid	Special Features	Leukocytes/mm^3	Example Conditions
Normal	Clear, colorless, viscous	<200	Healthy adult
Noninflammatory	Clear, yellow, viscous	200–2,000	Osteoarthritis, trauma
Inflammatory	Cloudy, yellow, decreased viscosity	2,000–100,000	Rheumatoid arthritis, crystalline arthropathy, seronegative arthritis, etc.
Septic	Purulent, markedly decreased viscosity	Usually >50,000 (>95% PMNs)	Septic arthritis

Medications

- **Acetaminophen** at doses of 1,000 mg qid is often helpful and may be as beneficial as nonsteroidal anti-inflammatory drugs (NSAIDs) for some patients. **Maximum total daily dose should not exceed 2,000 mg in those with significant liver disease.**
- **NSAIDs** including those that are selective inhibitors of cyclooxygenase-2 (COX-2) are commonly prescribed and have been specifically demonstrated to relieve the signs and symptoms of OA. It may require a trial of several of these agents to find the most efficacious agent in this class. Major toxicities include but are not limited to the following:
  - **Gastrointestinal (GI) toxicity,** particularly if certain risk factors are present (i.e., age ≥65, use of oral steroids/anticoagulants, and history of ulcer disease/GI bleeding).[3] The use of celecoxib or a proton pump inhibitor along with a nonselective NSAID may dramatically reduce this risk.[4]
  - **Nephrotoxicity** and nephrogenic sodium retention.
  - **Cardiovascular risks**—recent placebo-controlled trials have demonstrated an increased risk of thrombotic cardiovascular events such as myocardial infarction and strokes with COX-2 selective NSAIDs.[5] It is possible that this cardiovascular risk extends to all NSAIDs.
- **Glucosamine and chondroitin** have both been used to treat OA and may be beneficial for some patients.[6]
- **Topical capsaicin and lidocaine** can improve symptoms particularly if few joints are involved.
- Analgesics such as tramadol and opiates are sometimes indicated. With chronic opiate use, tolerance typically develops, requiring progressively higher doses.

Joint Injections

Intra-articular Steroids
- Intra-articular steroids have been used for the treatment of OA since the 1950s and are routinely performed by general practitioners. Their use should be limited to those with training in the procedure.

TABLE 3	Radiographic Changes by Disease				
	Osteoarthritis	Rheumatoid Arthritis	Seronegative Spondyloarthropathy	Gout	Septic Arthritis
Alignment	Affected late	Affected late	Affected late	Typically not affected	Can be altered early
Distribution	Hips, knees, ankles, and the CMC PIP, DIP, of hands	Symmetric MCP, MTP, wrists	SI joint involvement and lower spine	First MTP classic, but all joints possible	Knees, ankles, but all joints possible
Erosions	None (except in erosive OA)	Symmetric, marginal and 50% of patients have them at 2 years	Can occur and are marginal and at sites of tendon insert	"Mouse bite" erosions with "overhanging edges" and a "punched out" appearance	Loss of cortical line and a destructive process
Periarticular osteoporosis	Absent	Present	Absent	Absent	Often present
Joint space	Narrowed	Narrowed in affected joints	Narrowed in affected joints	Preserved	May be narrowed
Special features	Extra bone formation with osteophytes is common; subchondral sclerosis	Feet may be affected prior to hands	Ankylosis of the spine with enthesitis and syndesmophytes	Erosions tend to occur late and in patients with tophaceous gout	May have no changes at all in mild disease

CMC, carpometacarpal; DIP, distal interphalangeal; MCP, metacarpophalangeal; MTP, metatarsophalangeal; OA, osteoarthritis; PIP, proximal interphalangeal; SI, sacroiliac.

- Available steroid preparations include triamcinolone hexacetonide (fluorinated), triamcinolone acetonide (fluorinated), methylprednisolone acetate (nonfluorinated), and dexamethasone.
- **Dose varies on location** and no controlled studies to guide therapy. General guidelines are as follows:
  - Large joint (knee and shoulder), 40 to 80 mg (1 to 2 mL).
  - Medium joint (wrist, ankle, and elbow), 30 mg.
  - Small spaces (metacarpophalangeal and proximal interphalangeal joints, tendon sheaths), 10 mg.
- **Precautions:**
  - Do not inject through cellulitis or psoriatic skin lesion.
  - **Do not inject the same joint more than three to four times a year.**
  - Infections can occur but are rare occurring in only 6 of >100,000 procedures in one classic series.[7]
  - Steroid-induced crystalline arthritis can occur because the steroid preparations involve crystalline glucocorticoid. The reactions usually occur within 24 hours after injection and last 2 to 3 days similar to gout, while septic arthritis from an injection tends to occur >48 hours after the injection.

Hyperviscosity Therapy
- Hyperviscosity treatment includes the intra-articular injection of hyaluronic acid derivatives. Two available preparations include hylan G-F 20 (2 mL intra-articular weekly for 3 doses or 6 mL once) and sodium hyaluronate (2 mL intra-articular weekly for 3 to 5 doses).
- Early studies have shown efficacy equal to naproxen in the treatment of OA, but a large meta-analysis of several studies have shown little benefit.[8] It is possible that a subset of patients may have benefited and this therapy can be considered in patients with early disease.
- Iatrogenic joint infection, postinjection inflammation (pseudoseptic reaction), and aspiration proven pseudogout can complicate hyaluronate injections.

Nonpharmacologic Measures
- Weight loss
- Use of a cane or walker
- Braces and other orthotics
- Exercise with and without formal physical therapy. Muscle strength surrounding an affected joint can help stabilize the joint, relieve pain, and help prevent progression of degeneration.
- Acupuncture

Surgery
- Orthopedic consultation should be considered for patients who are surgical candidates.
- The timing of surgery is a complicated decision but is primarily based on the severity of the patient's symptoms.

RHEUMATOID ARTHRITIS

General Principles
- Rheumatoid arthritis, the prototypical inflammatory arthritis, affects approximately 1% of the population and accounts for a significant degree of morbidity in affected patients.

- RA is a chronic, polyarticular inflammatory arthritis with a symmetric distribution that affects the hands and feet.
- The etiology is still not well understood, but identification and characterization of biologic mediators of the inflammatory response associated with RA has led to the development of new treatments.[9]

Diagnosis

The ACR has specified seven criteria associated with RA of which four are required for diagnosis (Table 4).[10] These criteria help outline the symptoms at presentation, but all may not be present in the early course of the disease.

Extra-articular Manifestations

- **Pulmonary:** RA can cause several types of abnormalities in pulmonary function, such as isolated rheumatoid lung nodules, interstitial lung disease with pulmonary infiltrates, and/or progression to fibrosis.
- **Felty syndrome** is a syndrome of seropositive RA, neutropenia, and splenomegaly. It usually occurs in patients with long-standing severe disease and can result in increased risk of infection and is often a poor prognostic indicator.
- **Ocular:** The eye can be affected in many ways. Scleritis with a painful red eye that may lead to a thinning of the sclera (scleromalacia) is an indication of severe refractory disease and often requires aggressive treatment both systemically and topically.
- **Vasculitis:** Rheumatoid vasculitis can affect any blood vessel, but the most common manifestation is distal arteritis ranging from nail fold infarcts to gangrene of the fingertips.
- **Cardiovascular risk:** Chronic inflammation may play a role in the pathophysiology of atherosclerosis.
  - Patients with chronic inflammatory conditions have been shown to be at increased risk of macrovascular complications such as stroke and myocardial infarction.
  - Indeed, the same is true for RA, and aggressive therapy targeting reducing cardiovascular risks is an important aspect of RA management.[11]

TABLE 4	ACR Criteria for the Classification of Acute Rheumatoid Arthritis

At least four of seven criteria required with 1–4 present at least 6 weeks:
1. Morning stiffness lasting at least 1 hour
2. Soft-tissue swelling or fluid in at least three joint areas simultaneously
3. At least one area swollen in a wrist, MCP, or PIP joint
4. Symmetric arthritis
5. Rheumatoid nodules
6. Abnormal amounts of serum rheumatoid factor
7. Erosions or bony decalcification on radiographs of the hand and wrist

ACR, American College of Rheumatology; MCP, metacarpophalangeal; PIP proximal interphalangeal.
Modified from Arnett FC, Edwothy SM, Bloch DA, et al. *Arthritis Rheum* 1988;31:315–324.

Diagnostic Testing

Laboratory Evaluation
- See the "General Principles" section above regarding RF, ESR, and CRP.
- **Anticyclic citrullinated peptide (anti-CCP) antibodies:**
  - Anti-CCP antibodies recognize a posttranslational modification of proteins (a conversion of arginine to citrulline) that is thought to occur in the synovium of patient with RA.
  - The assay is now routinely performed, has a higher specificity for the diagnosis, and may be predictive of progressive of joint disease.[12]
- CBC, CMP, and hepatitis panel (to rule out hepatitis C as a cause of a positive RF result and arthralgias and avoid using hepatotoxic medications in patients with chronic viral hepatitis).

Imaging
- Classical findings on plain radiography include soft tissue swelling, joint space loss, periarticular osteoporosis, and erosions (which eventually develop in the large majority of patients).
- Baseline chest radiography is warranted given the possibility of pulmonary involvement.

Treatment

The following aspects of RA management can be achieved in primary care: establish the diagnosis early, document baseline activity, educate the patient, consider NSAIDs therapy, refer for physical/occupational therapy, and initiate disease-modifying therapy within 3 months (e.g., corticosteroids, hydroxychloroquine, sulfasalazine, or methotrexate [MTX]). Patients should be reassessed frequently and referred to a rheumatologist if the response is inadequate.[13] **Early treatment with disease-modifying antirheumatic drugs (DMARDs) has the potential to retard the progression of disease.**

Medications

NSAIDs
Most patients with RA benefit symptomatically from the use of NSAIDs, but they **do not prevent the progression** of bone and cartilage damage.

Classic Disease-Modifying Antirheumatic Drugs
Glucocorticoids
- Glucocorticoids (especially prednisone) in low doses are extremely effective for promptly reducing the symptoms of RA and can be considered to help patients recover their previous functional status.
- Unfortunately, short courses of oral corticosteroids produce only interim benefit and chronic therapy is often required to maintain symptom management and to prevent progression of disease.
- Corticosteroids are particularly helpful in treating patients with a high burden of disease. It is also useful in patients who are titrating the dose or awaiting clinical response from a slow-acting DMARD.
- Side effects of corticosteroids are many and include hyperglycemia, adrenal insufficiency, osteopenia, and avascular necrosis. If a dose equivalent to ≥ 5 mg of prednisone is to be used for longer than 3 months, then a bisphosphonate should be used unless contraindicated to prevent bone loss.[14]

- **Intra-articular steroids** are particularly useful in patients with a flare of RA in a monoarticular or oligoarticular pattern.

Hydroxychloroquine
- Hydroxychloroquine is indicated for moderate RA.
- It is effective at doses of 400 mg PO daily but is contraindicated in patients with renal or hepatic insufficiency.
- The risk of macular toxicity is extremely unusual at these doses and rarely occurs before 5 years of treatment. Nonetheless, an ophthalmologist should perform a baseline examination and monitor the patient at least annually on this medication.

Sulfasalazine
- Sulfasalazine is also indicated for moderate RA and in those who are poor candidates for MTX therapy.
- It should be initiated at 500 mg PO bid and gradually increased to 1,000 to 1,500 mg PO bid.
- GI intolerance is common and may be lessen with an enteric-coated preparation.
- It is contraindicated in those allergic to sulfa antibiotics and those with glucose-6-phosphate dehydrogenase deficiency. Severe/fatal skin reactions have occurred.
- Monitoring of liver tests and blood counts is required.

Methotrexate
- MTX is **generally considered to be the DMARD of choice** for most RA patients. The usual maintenance dose is 7.5 to 20 mg/week orally.
- If MTX is at least partially effective, it should be continued as other agents are added.
- Common side effects include stomatitis, nausea, diarrhea, and thinning of the hair. It is teratogenic.
- Supplementation with folic acid at doses of 1 to 3 mg PO daily can reduce side effects, although efficacy may be somewhat attenuated.
- Serious adverse reactions include hepatotoxicity, lung toxicity, and bone marrow suppression.
- **MTX should only be prescribed by those experienced in its use** and careful monitoring of liver tests and blood counts is required.

Leflunomide
- Leflunomide is a pyrimidine synthesis inhibitor that has been shown to have efficacy comparable with that of MTX in the treatment of RA. It may also be used in combination with MTX in patients with an inadequate response to MTX alone and who are not candidates for other treatments.
- Common side effects include diarrhea, nausea, and alopecia. It is teratogenic.
- Monitoring of liver tests and blood counts is required due to the risk of hepatotoxicity and bone marrow suppression. **Leflunomide should only be proscribed by those experienced in its use.**

Biologics
- **Etanercept** (Enbrel) is a genetically engineered human fusion protein consisting of both the soluble tumor necrosis factor (TNF) receptor and the Fc component for IgG.
- **Infliximab** (Remicade) **and adalimumab** (Humira) are monoclonal antibodies against TNF-α (chimeric and humanized, respectively).
- **Anakinra** (Kineret) is a recombinant interleukin-1 (IL-1) receptor antagonist.
- **Abatacept** (Orencia) is a selective costimulation modulator (inhibitor) and a fusion protein consisting of an Ig fused to the CTLA4 extracellular domain. Studies have shown it to be efficacious in patients who have failed prior treatment with anti-TNF therapy.[15]

- **Rituximab** (Rituxan) is a chimeric monoclonal antibody against CD20 and results in the destruction of B cells. This agent has been shown to be efficacious in patients with inadequate responses to TNF inhibitors, and is FDA approved in this setting.[16]
- All of these biologic agents have been used in rheumatoid arthritis. The specifics of such therapy are beyond the scope of this chapter.
- As one would expect, significant side effects and adverse events can occur (e.g., infection/TB, drug-induced lupus, worsened heart failure, and demyelinating syndromes).

Combination Therapy
- Combination regimens of multiple DMARDs or DMARDs plus biologic agents may be particularly effective in RA.[9] **Such combined therapy should only be done in conjunction with a rheumatologist.**
- Consensus among rheumatologists suggests that MTX should be part of every combination, if tolerated.

Other Nonpharmacologic Therapies
- **Occupational therapy** usually focuses on the hand and wrist and can help patients with splinting, work simplification, activities of daily living, and assistive devices.
- **Physical therapy** assists in stretching and strengthening exercises for large joints such as the shoulder and knee, gait evaluation, and fitting with crutches and canes.
- Moderate exercise is appropriate for all patients and can help to reduce stiffness and maintain joint range of motion.
- In general, an exercise program should not produce pain for >2 hours after its completion.

Surgical Management
- Orthopedic surgery to correct hand deformities and replace large joints such as the hip, knee, and shoulder may benefit patients with advanced disease.
- Total joint arthroplasty to replace the knee or hip should also be considered when pain cannot be controlled adequately with medications.
- The decision to pursue joint replacement in younger patients may be complicated by the likelihood that individuals may outlive their prosthetic joints, necessitating future surgery.

INFECTIOUS ARTHRITIS AND SEPTIC BURSITIS

General Principles

- Infectious arthritis is generally categorized into gonococcal and nongonococcal infection.
- The usual presentation is with fever and acute monoarticular arthritis, although multiple joints may be affected by hematogenous spread of pathogens.
- **Nongonococcal** infectious arthritis in adults tends to occur in patients with previous joint damage or compromised host defenses.
  - Nongonococcal septic arthritis is caused most often by *Staphylococcus aureus* (60%) and *Streptococcus* spp.
  - Gram-negative organisms are less common, except with IV drug abuse, neutropenia, concomitant urinary tract infection, and with prosthetic joints.
- **Gonococcal arthritis** is more common than nongonococcal septic arthritis and is the most common cause of monoarticular arthritis in patients between the age of 20 and 30.[17]

- The clinical spectrum of disease often includes migratory or additive polyarthralgias, followed by tenosynovitis or arthritis of the wrist, ankle, or knee and asymptomatic dermatitis on the extremities or trunk.
- **Nonbacterial infectious** arthritis is common with many viral infections, especially hepatitis B, rubella, mumps, infectious mononucleosis, parvovirus, enterovirus, adenovirus, and HIV.
  - Hepatitis C infection is associated with the formation of cryoglubulinemia, which can present as a polyarticular inflammatory arthritis with glomerulonephritis, cutaneous vasculitis, and mononeuritis multiplex.
- Septic bursitis, usually involving the olecranon or prepatellar bursa, can be differentiated from septic arthritis by localized, fluctuant superficial swelling and by relatively painless joint motion (particularly extension).
  - Most patients have a history of previous trauma to the area or an occupational predisposition (e.g., "housemaid's knee," "writer's elbow").
  - *S. aureus* is the most common pathogen.

Diagnosis

- Joint fluid examination, including Gram stain of a centrifuged pellet, and culture are **mandatory to make a diagnosis and to guide management.**
- A joint fluid leukocyte count is useful diagnostically and as a baseline for serial studies to evaluate response to treatment.
- Cultures of blood and other possible extraarticular sites of infection should also be obtained.
- In contrast to nongonococcal septic arthritis, Gram staining of synovial fluid and cultures of blood or synovial fluid often is negative.

Treatment

- Hospitalization is indicated to ensure drug compliance and careful monitoring of the clinical response.
- IV antimicrobials provide good serum and synovial fluid drug concentrations. **Oral antimicrobials are not appropriate as initial therapy,** and there is no role for intra-articular antibiotic therapy.
- Repeated arthrocenteses should be performed daily or as often as necessary to prevent reaccumulation of fluid and monitor response to therapy.
- General supportive measures include splinting of the joint, which may help to relieve pain. However, prolonged immobilization can result in joint stiffness.

Medications

- An NSAID or selective COX-2 inhibitor is often useful to reduce pain and to increase joint mobility but should not be used until response to antimicrobial therapy has been demonstrated by symptomatic and laboratory improvement.
- **Initial therapy is based on the clinical situation and a carefully performed Gram stain,** which reveals the organism in approximately 50% of patients.[18]
  - With a positive Gram stain result, antibiotic coverage can be focused accordingly.
  - With a nondiagnostic Gram stain, antibiotics should be chosen to cover *S. aureus* and *Streptococcus* spp. and *Neisseria gonorrhoeae* in otherwise healthy patients, whereas broad-spectrum antibiotics are appropriate in immunosuppressed patients.

- IV antimicrobials usually are given for at least 2 weeks, followed by 1 to 2 weeks of oral antimicrobials, with the course of therapy tailored to the patient's response. Infections disease consultation can be helpful for treatment.
- Treatment for gonococcal arthritis is begun with an IV antibiotic for the first 1 to 3 days, generally ceftriaxone, 1 g daily, or ceftizoxime, 1 g every 8 hours.
  - Response to IV antibiotics is usually noted within the first 24 to 36 hours of treatment.
  - After initial clinical improvement, therapy is continued with an oral antibiotic to complete 7 to 10 days of treatment.
  - Ciprofloxacin, 500 mg bid, or amoxicillin clavulanate, 500 to 875 mg bid, can be used, although increasing resistance to fluoroquinolones is increasing and decision regarding treatment should be based on regional guidelines.[19]
- These viral arthritides are generally self-limited, lasting for <6 weeks, and respond well to a conservative regimen of rest and NSAIDs.
- Septic bursitis should be treated with aspiration, which can be repeated if fluid reaccumulates.
  - Oral antibiotics and outpatient management are usually appropriate, and surgical drainage is rarely indicated.

Surgical Management

Surgical drainage or arthroscopic lavage and drainage are indicated for the following:
- A septic hip, which cannot be easily accessed by arthrocentesis.
- Joints in which the anatomy, large amounts of tissue debris, or loculation of pus prevent adequate needle drainage.
- Septic arthritis with coexistent osteomyelitis.
- Joints that do not respond in 4 to 6 days to appropriate therapy and repeated arthrocenteses.
- Prosthetic joint infection.

CRYSTALLINE ARTHRITIS

- Deposition of microcrystals in joints and periarticular tissues results in gout, pseudogout, and basic calcium phosphate (BCP) disease.[20]
- A definitive diagnosis of gout or pseudogout is made by finding intracellular crystals in joint fluid examined with a compensated polarized light microscope.
  - **Urate crystals,** which are diagnostic of gout, are needle shaped and strongly negatively birefringent.
  - **Calcium pyrophosphate dihydrate crystals** seen in pseudogout are pleomorphic and weakly positively birefringent.
  - Hydroxyapatite complexes and BCP complexes can be identified only by electron microscopy, mass spectroscopy, or alizarin red staining, none of which are readily available to the clinician.

GOUT

General Principles

- Gout is caused by the accumulation of excess amounts of uric acid in the body, leading to deposition of monosodium urate crystals when levels exceed solubility.

- Gout can produce four distinct clinical syndromes:
  - Acute gouty arthritis
  - Chronic tophaceous gout
  - Urate nephropathy
  - Urate nephrolithiasis
- All complications of gout result from hyperuricemia. **In 90% of cases, this occurs as a result of underexcretion of urate,** with overproduction accounting for the remainder.
- Risk factors include male sex,[21] hypertension, hyperlipidemia, obesity, renal dysfunction, alcohol, dehydration, and drugs (e.g., low-dose salicylates, diuretics, ethambutol, pyrazinamide, levodopa, cyclosporine, and tacrolimus).

Diagnosis

Clinical Presentation

- Acute gouty arthritis presents with acute pain and swelling, usually of a single joint.
- Commonly affected joints include the great toe MTP joint (podagra), ankle, knee, and wrist.
- Episodes often occur at night and frequently accompany acute medical illnesses, postsurgical periods, dehydration, fasting, or heavy alcohol consumption.
- Pain may be severe, and immediate medical attention to provide pain relief is essential.
- Periarticular involvement is rare at presentation but may occur in long-standing cases.
- Intense periarticular inflammation with desquamation of skin may give the appearance of cellulitis.

Diagnostic Testing

- Gout is diagnosed by polarized microscopy of synovial fluid demonstrating bright, negatively birefringent, and needle-shaped crystals (often found within a PMN).
- Cell counts of synovial aspirates are usually consistent with an inflammatory arthritis (white cells in the tens of thousands, mostly PMNs).
- Aspiration of superficial tophi with a 25-gauge needle can also provide diagnostic material.

Treatment

NSAIDs

- **NSAIDs are particularly effective and are the treatment of choice for acute gout.**
- They should be started in maximal doses and tapered over several days once the gouty flare has subsided.
- A common high-dose NSAID regimen is indomethacin, 50 mg PO qid given for several days until relief is obtained, followed by 50 mg tid for 2 to 3 days, 50 mg bid for 2 to 3 days, 50 mg/day for a few days, and then discontinuation.
- Naproxen, ibuprofen, sulindac, and other NSAIDs are also effective and are generally better tolerated than high-dose indomethacin.

Colchicine

- Oral colchicine as a treatment for acute gout is poorly tolerated because of diarrhea and abdominal cramping, and **the dose should be reduced in patients with renal and hepatic impairment.**

- The use of colchicine at >0.6 mg PO bid is safe only in patients with normal renal and hepatic function. **Once diarrhea develops, it should be stopped.**
- The traditional dose of colchicine every hour is obsolete and should not be used.
- IV colchicine avoids GI toxicity but may cause **severe myelosuppression and should not be used because of several deaths with IV colchicine in patients with renal insufficiency.**[22]

Glucocorticoids

- Oral steroids can be used when other therapies are contraindicated.
  - Prednisone initiated at 60 mg/day and tapered rapidly can provide adequate symptomatic relief while avoiding toxicities of long-term steroid use.
- Intra-articular aspiration and corticosteroid injection is appropriate for large joints such as knees and ankles and an excellent choice for patients who are not good candidates for NSAIDs.
  - Because the knee joint often has a tense effusion, aspiration of as much fluid as possible can bring immediate relief, followed by injection of 1 to 2 mL corticosteroid with an equal volume of 1% lidocaine. A volume of 1 mL is appropriate for the ankle.

Prophylactic Treatment

- Prophylactic treatment is advisable when patients have recurrent attacks several times per year.
- **Colchicine,** 0.6 mg once or twice daily, may be effective, as may low-dose NSAIDs such as indomethacin, 25 mg bid, or naproxen, 250 mg bid. In patients with multiple recurrent attacks, uric acid–lowering therapy may be beneficial.
- **Allopurinol,** a xanthine oxidase inhibitor, reduces uric acid production and is much easier to administer than probenecid.
  - Allopurinol is indicated for recurrent attacks that are not controlled with colchicine or NSAIDs.
  - Other indications for allopurinol include the presence of tophi, renal stones, and severe hyperuricemia (>13 mg/dL).
  - **Asymptomatic hyperuricemia should not be treated with allopurinol.**
  - A starting dose of 100 to 150 mg/day can be increased after 2 to 4 weeks to 300 mg/day. Sometimes higher doses (400 to 600 mg/day) are required to bring the serum uric acid down to a target level of approximately <6 mg/dL.
  - Allopurinol should not be started during an acute attack as it may cause a severe flare of the disease in other joints.
    - Administration of prophylactic colchicine or low-dose NSAIDs before initiation of uric acid–lowering therapy may prevent the gouty attacks that sometimes accompany the initiation of allopurinol treatment.
    - It is not necessary to discontinue its use if a gout attack occurs after it is started.
  - This medication is usually well tolerated, although elevated liver test and a **severe hypersensitivity syndrome** can occur. The latter is more common with renal insufficiency and diuretic use.
- **Probenecid** prevents tubular reabsorption of uric acid and can be used to enhance urinary excretion of uric acid provided that the baseline 24-hour urinary uric acid is ≤600 mg.
  - If the 24 hour uric acid is >600 mg, increasing the urinary excretion of uric acid may precipitate uric acid kidney stones
  - Probenecid can be initiated at 500 mg PO daily and increased as needed, not exceeding 3,000 mg in three divided doses.
  - Normal renal function is necessary for probenecid to be effective.

- Salicylates antagonize the effect of probenecid, and even low-dose aspirin can negate its effect.
- **Diet:** A 12-year study of 730 patients with gout suggested that high levels of meat and seafood in the diet is associated with an increased risk of gout, whereas dairy products may be protective. The level of purine-rich vegetables and total protein intake was not associated with an increased risk of gout.[23]

PSEUDOGOUT

- Pseudogout is caused by deposition of **calcium pyrophosphate crystals** and tends to occur more often in elderly individuals.
- It may be precipitated by surgery and has been associated with hypothyroidism, hyperparathyroidism, diabetes, and hemochromatosis and these diagnoses should be considered.
- Like gout, pseudogout tends to cause monoarticular attacks, **especially in the knee.**
- Symmetric involvement of the hands may mimic RA.
- Periarticular inflammation can be severe, mimicking cellulitis.
- Polarized microscopy of synovial fluid reveals **rhomboid-shaped crystals that are positively birefringent.**
- Radiographic studies may demonstrate chondrocalcinosis (especially knee, wrist, and symphysis pubis) but alone are not diagnostic of pseudogout.
- Treatment is the same as for gout, except that there is no role for allopurinol or probenecid. Joint aspiration, alone or with steroid injection, often provides immediate relief of pain

APATITE DEPOSITION DISEASE

- Apatite deposition disease may present with periarthritis or tendonitis, particularly in the elderly and patients with chronic renal failure.
- An episodic oligoarthritis may also occur and apatite disease should be suspected when no crystals are present in the synovial fluid.
- Erosive arthritis may be seen, particularly in the shoulder (Milwaukee shoulder, a syndrome of large shoulder effusion, rotator cuff pathology, and the presence of BCP crystals in synovial fluid).
- The treatment of apatite disease is similar to that of pseudogout, except that recent studies suggest that early intervention and washing out the joint may help prevent progression of the disease.[24]
- Referral to orthopedic surgery may be required.

SYSTEMIC LUPUS ERYTHEMATOSUS

General Principles

- SLE is a multisystem autoimmune disease of unknown etiology that commonly occurs in women of childbearing age. There is clearly a genetic predisposition.
- Manifestations of SLE are protean, and organ systems involved may include skin, heart, lungs, nervous system, kidneys, hematopoietic system, and joints.
- African-Americans and Mexican Hispanics have a worse prognosis.
- SLE can occur in the elderly but when it does, it is usually milder.

TABLE 5	ACR Systemic Lupus Erythematosus Classification Criteria Definitions

Criteria	Description
Malar rash	Fixed erythema, flat or raised, sparing the nasolabial folds
Discoid rash	Raised patches, adherent keratotic scaling, follicular plugging; older lesions may cause scarring
Photosensitivity	Skin rash from sunlight
Oral or nasopharyngeal ulcers	Usually painless
Arthritis	Nonerosive, inflammatory in two or more peripheral joints
Serositis	Pleuritis or pericarditis
Renal disorder	Persistent proteinuria or cellular casts
Neurologic disorder	Seizures or psychosis
Hematologic	Hemolytic anemia, leukopenia ($<4,000/mm^3$), lymphopenia ($<1,500/mm^3$), or thrombocytopenia ($<100,00/mm^3$)
Immunologic disorder	Antibodies to dsDNA or Antibodies to Sm or Antiphospholipid antibodies: IgG/IgM antibodies or positive lupus anticoagulant test results or false-positive serologic test results for syphilis
Antinuclear antibodies	Present

ACR, American College of Rheumatology; dsDNA, double-stranded (native) deoxyribonucleic acid; Sm, Smith nuclear antigen.
Modified from Tan EM, Cohen AS, Fries JF, et al. *Arthritis Rheum* 1982;25:1271–1277.

Diagnosis

Clinical Presentation

- The ACR has proposed 11 criteria for the diagnosis of SLE (Table 5).[25]
- For research purposes, a diagnosis requires that at least four of them be present at some point through the course of the disease.
- These criteria may be useful in clinical practice to guide history and physical examinations of putative SLE patients, but a **clinical diagnosis of SLE does not require satisfying the four criteria.**[25]

Diagnostic Testing

- The **ANA is highly sensitive** and is detectable in virtually all patients with SLE.
  - Therefore, **a negative ANA result is useful to exclude SLE;** however, a positive ANA test result alone is of little significance.
  - Regardless of how high the titer, an isolated positive ANA test result is not diagnostic of SLE or any related disease.
- **Antibodies to double-stranded DNA are very specific** for SLE, especially when present at high titers.
  - Several techniques are available for measuring these antibodies. Two of the more common are the *Crithidia luciliae* fluorescent slide test and the ELISA test.

- High levels of anti-DNA antibody can correlate with disease activity, especially with lupus nephritis. Therefore, quantitative anti-DNA titers are sometimes useful in monitoring disease flares and response to treatment.
- **Anti-Sm** is part of a panel of antibodies to extractable nuclear antigens. Although **very specific** for SLE, it is detectable in a minority of patients.
- **Serum complement measures, C3 and C4,** are sometimes abnormal in active SLE, especially in the setting of nephritis, and may rise and fall with disease activity.
- **Antiphospholipid antibodies** are important in diagnosing the **antiphospholipid syndrome (APS),** characterized by fetal loss, venous and arterial thromboses, CNS events, and thrombocytopenia.[26]
  - Diagnosis of antiphospholipid syndrome is relevant, as the treatment may necessitate lifelong anticoagulation.
  - Anticardiolipin antibody is measured by ELISA. IgG antibodies in significant titer are more predictive of clinical events than is IgM or IgA.
  - **False-positive Venereal Disease Research Laboratory test (VDRL) or rapid plasma regain (RPR)** is a laboratory artifact. The fluorescent treponemal antibody absorption test should be negative, although a low-titer "beaded" pattern is sometimes observed.
  - **The lupus "anticoagulant"** (LAC) is not specific for lupus and promotes coagulation.
    - The activated thromboplastin time assay is prolonged.
    - A positive LAC is a more predictive test for clinical events due to antiphospholipid antibody than due to anticardiolipin antibody or VDRL.

Treatment

- Treatment for SLE is dependent on the clinical scenario. The level of aggressiveness in treatment should match the severity of disease.
- For patients without life- or organ-threatening disease, initiation of conservative therapy is appropriate for mild symptoms. Such treatments include the following:
  - Sunscreen and sun avoidance for patients with photosensitivity.
  - Topical steroids for isolated skin lesions.
  - Maintenance of adequate hydration.
  - Hydroxychloroquine for arthralgias and fatigue.
- More severe cases of SLE may require more aggressive therapy. In general, prednisone in moderate (15 to 30 mg/day) or higher (40 to 60 mg/day) doses is usually the first-line therapy for a moderate-to-severe lupus flare. Steroid-sparing therapies are frequently needed when flares are recurrent. Such therapies include the following:
  - Mycophenolate mofetil
  - Azathioprine
  - To a lesser extent MTX or leflunomide
  - Cyclophosphamide for life-threatening disease.
  - Investigational new therapies such as B-cell depletion with anti-CD20 antibodies (rituximab) and immunoablation with or without stem cell transplantation for refractory disease.

Symptom-Specific Treatments

- **Arthritis** often responds to NSAIDs, although they must be used with caution in patients with decreased renal function. The addition of prednisone in low doses (5 to 10 mg/day) may be necessary. Long-term treatment with hydroxychloroquine often helps control arthritis (see the "Rheumatoid Arthritis" section).

- **Rashes** may respond to topical corticosteroids (fluorinated topical steroids on the face should be avoided because of the risk of subcutaneous atrophy). If topical agents are not effective, systemic corticosteroids may be needed. Hydroxychloroquine is often beneficial in the long-term management of rash and may help to reduce the need for corticosteroids.
- **Oral ulcers** can be treated with dental paste that contains benzocaine (Orabase B) or triamcinolone (Kenalog in Orabase) or an over-the-counter anesthetic oral rinse (e.g., Ulcer Ease).
- Mild cases of **pleuritis and pericarditis** sometimes respond to NSAIDs, whereas more severe cases require corticosteroids.
- The treatment of **renal disease** is complicated.[27]
  - For most serious renal lesions, periodic monthly cyclophosphamide is administered, although mycophenolate mofetil is being used more frequently as first-line therapy.
  - High doses of corticosteroids, administered either orally or intravenously, are also commonly used in the acute setting as cyclophosphamide and mycophenolate mofetil may take weeks to reach peak efficacy.
- For **hematologic problems,** such as hemolytic anemia, severe leukopenia, or thrombocytopenia, corticosteroids in moderate-to-high doses are required.
- **Neuropsychiatric disease** is difficult to assess because there is no laboratory test or physical finding that can unequivocally support the diagnosis of lupus affecting the central nervous system. The diagnosis is based on clinical factors and is a diagnosis of exclusion. Aggressive treatment with high-dose steroids may be necessary to help control symptoms of neuropsychiatric lupus.

SERONEGATIVE SPONDYLOARTHROPATHIES

General Principles

- The spondyloarthropathies are a group of articular disorders characterized by involvement of the axial skeleton and negative test results for RF.[28]
- These disorders include ankylosing spondylitis, reactive arthritis, psoriatic arthritis, and arthritis associated with inflammatory bowel disease.

Classic Syndromes

- **Ankylosing spondylitis,** the prototype of the spondyloarthropathies, is diagnosed in men much more commonly than in women, partly because the spine symptoms in women tend to be more subtle. Acute iritis produces severe eye pain and blurred vision and requires urgent referral to an ophthalmologist.
- **Reactive arthritis** occurs after infectious syndromes such as nongonococcal urethritis or infectious diarrhea with *Shigella* spp., *Salmonella* spp., or *Yersinia enterocolitica.* A reactive arthritis syndrome of urethritis, arthritis, and conjunctivitis was previously referred to as Reiter syndrome.
- **Psoriatic arthritis** has five basic presentations: spinal predominance, polyarticular small joint involvement (negative for RF), oligoarticular asymmetric large joint involvement, DIP joint predominance, and the rare arthritis mutilans with telescoping digits. In general, the severity of joint disease does not parallel that of the skin disease, except for the DIP pattern, which correlates with nail abnormalities.
- **Ulcerative colitis and Crohn disease** may be accompanied by inflammatory arthritis of two types. The peripheral joint variety tends to parallel the activity of the bowel

disease, whereas the spondylotic pattern typically has an independent course of the bowel disease.

Diagnosis

Clinical Presentation

History
- The characteristic history is that of **inflammatory back pain.** Five distinguishing symptoms include gradual onset, onset before the age of 40 years, morning stiffness, improvement with mild exercise, and duration of >3 months.
- When **peripheral joint involvement** is present, it is typically asymmetric and oligoarticular, generally in the lower extremities.
- Inflammation generally occurs where tendons insert on bone **(enthesopathy)** and produces "sausage digits" of individual fingers and toes (dactylitis), plantar fasciitis, and Achilles tendinitis.
- Nonarticular symptoms may include aphthous stomatitis, ocular inflammation such as conjunctivitis and iritis, and aortic dilatation.

Physical Examination
- **Spine motion** may be simply assessed by having the patient bend forward with the knees extended and measuring the distance between the fingertips and floor (recognizing that hamstring tightness reduces the range of motion).
- **Peripheral joints** should be checked for diffuse fusiform swelling of fingers and toes (sausage digits or dactylitis) and asymmetric swelling of large joints, especially the knees and ankles.
- **Ocular findings** in ankylosing spondylitis and reactive arthritis include redness and a pupil that reacts asymmetrically (synechiae), indicating previous episodes of ocular inflammation.
- **Skin findings** in psoriasis are usually obvious, but the following areas should be specifically examined to look for subtle changes: the scalp, external auditory canal, umbilicus, and intergluteal cleft. It may be difficult to distinguish the skin findings of reactive arthritis from those of psoriasis.

Diagnostic Testing
- The **RF** is by definition negative and the **ESR** is inconsistently elevated.
- Although the **human leukocyte antigen B27** is present in >90% of Caucasians with ankylosing spondylitis, its frequency is lower in other ethnic groups and in other spondyloarthropathies. It is present in approximately 8% to 10% of normal Caucasians.
- **Radiographs** to look for sacroiliitis include an anteroposterior view of the pelvis, sometimes supplemented by modified Ferguson views of the sacroiliac joints (taken with a 30-degree cephalad angle).
  - Definite radiographic changes take years to develop.
  - MRI of the sacroiliac joints enables diagnosis of early disease.
  - Radiographs of peripheral joints show periostitis.

Treatment

- **Physical therapy** to improve and maintain spinal motion is extremely important.
- **NSAIDs** are the mainstay of symptomatic treatment. High doses are generally required (e.g., indomethacin, 50 mg qid; naproxen, 500 mg tid).

- **Sulfasalazine** is efficacious in some patients for whom NSAIDs do not provide adequate relief (see the "Rheumatoid Arthritis" section).
- MTX has a well-established role in treating psoriatic arthritis and is sometimes effective for peripheral joint problems in the other spondylotic disorders. Patients with psoriasis have an increased risk of fibrosis and cirrhosis from MTX and should undergo liver biopsy at cumulative dose intervals of 2.5 to 3.0 g.
- The **TNF blockers** have been shown to be effective in providing symptomatic relief of disease in ankylosing spondylitis and psoriatic arthritis, and have been the first agents shown to delay progression of radiographic progression of the axial skeleton in these diseases.[29]

SCLERODERMA

General Principles

- The etiology of scleroderma is a poorly understood process that leads to pathologic changes of small-vessel vasculopathy (distinct from vasculitis), fibrosis, and proliferation of myofibroblasts in affected organs.
- The two major forms of this disease are diffuse scleroderma and limited scleroderma (known as the **CREST syndrome** which stands for **C**alcinosis, **R**aynaud phenomenon, **E**sophageal dysmotility, **S**clerodactyly, and **T**elangiectasias). The disease is characterized by fibrosis of skin and internal organs, especially the lungs, heart, kidneys, and GI tract.

Diagnosis

Clinical Presentation
- The diagnosis of scleroderma rests on the history and physical examination.
- Skin findings on physical examination are key to the diagnosis:
  - Patients with diffuse as well as limited disease may have sclerodactyly.
  - In diffuse disease, skin in the upper arms may also be involved, as well as loss of facial wrinkles and perioral fibrosis.

Raynaud Phenomenon
- Raynaud phenomenon is present in almost all patients with scleroderma but may be associated with other connective tissue diseases as well.
- The classic history is one of the triphasic skin color change: pallor (vasospasm) followed by cyanosis (desaturation of tissue hemoglobin) followed by rubor (reactive hyperemia). Many patients note only two of these changes.
- Cold temperatures, tobacco smoke, stress, and certain medications may provoke symptoms.
- The nail fold capillaries can be visualized by coating the cuticle with a thin layer of clear surgical lubricant and looking through an ophthalmoscope set at +40. Dilatation or dropout of nail fold capillaries increases the likelihood that Raynaud phenomenon will evolve into a systemic rheumatic disease.[30]

Diagnostic Testing
- ANA is present in most patients.
- **Anticentromere antibody** is a special subset of ANA, with a finely speckled pattern, and is seen in the majority of patients with limited disease.

- **Anti-Scl 70** is an antibody to topoisomerase that is quite specific for diffuse disease but is found in a minority of patients. This antibody is associated with interstitial lung disease and scleroderma renal crisis.

Treatment

- Treatment is largely supportive and organ system specific because there is no treatment that clearly alters the long-term course of this disease.
- The most important aspect of treatment of **Raynaud phenomenon** is protecting the hands from cold temperatures. Covering the head during cold weather is essential, because much of the core body heat can be lost through the head, leading to lower body temperature in the extremities.
  - Various vasodilating calcium channel blockers (especially dihydropyridines such as nifedipine or amlodipine) help reduce recurrence and severity of symptoms.
  - Sildenafil and bosentan are not FDA approved for this indication but may be effective in refractory cases.[31]
- Azotemia, proteinuria, and a microangiopathic hemolytic anemia can develop in patients with **scleroderma renal crisis.** Hypertension must be managed aggressively, and the angiotensin-converting enzyme inhibitors are the drugs of choice primarily for their renoprotective properties. Their use has resulted in a decrease in the mortality in scleroderma, such that pulmonary disease is now the leading cause of death in these patients.
- **GI complications:**
  - **Gastroesophageal reflux** can be treated with proton pump inhibitors or high-dose histamine-2 receptor blockers. Surgery to correct reflux should be avoided in these patients because of coexisting motility disorders.
  - **Esophageal strictures** sometime require mechanical dilatation.
  - **Malabsorption** due to bacterial overgrowth can be treated with broad-spectrum antibiotics.
- Limited data indicate that cyclophosphamide therapy can reduce the progression of **interstitial lung disease,** although reduction in mortality has not been demonstrated.[32]
- Many patients with systemic sclerosis may develop complications of **pulmonary hypertension.**
  - Recent advances have been made in the treatment of pulmonary hypertension associated with scleroderma and include the use of drugs such as sildenafil, bosentan, and other prostacyclin analogues.[33,34]
- **Coronary artery vasospasm** can cause angina that may be responsive to calcium channel blockers.

SJÖGREN SYNDROME

General Principles

- Sjögren syndrome is a multisystem autoimmune disease characterized by dysfunction of exocrine glands.
- It may occur as a primary disorder or secondary to other rheumatic diseases, such as RA, SLE, scleroderma, or inflammatory myopathy.

Diagnosis

Clinical Presentation

History
- History is notable for the sicca symptoms of dry eyes and dry mouth.
- Parotid gland swelling may occur, and occasionally patients have symptoms of pancreatic insufficiency with diarrhea and malabsorption.
- Symptoms of vaginal dryness may be present in women.

Physical Examination
- It often shows a diminished corneal light reflex and reduced tear meniscus.
- Oral examination reveals a diminished or absent sublingual salivary pool, and the tongue and buccal mucosa may appear dry.
- The major salivary glands commonly are enlarged.
- Inflammatory arthritis and cutaneous vasculitis may also be associated with Sjögren syndrome.
- In addition, patients with Sjögren syndrome often have symptoms of Raynaud phenomenon.
- Enlargement of lymph nodes, liver, or spleen raises the suspicion of lymphoma or other causes of secondary Sjögren syndrome.

Diagnostic Testing
- Laboratory tests associated with Sjögren syndrome include serum tests of systemic autoimmunity, including ANA, RF, or the presence of SSA (anti-Ro) or SSB (anti-La) antibodies.
- Lymphocytic infiltration on biopsy of minor salivary glands from the inner surface of the lower lip helps support the diagnosis of Sjögren syndrome.

Treatment

- Artificial tears are helpful for **dry eye symptoms** and can be self-administered as needed.
  - Optic cyclosporine has been shown to decrease symptoms of ocular dryness but should be monitored by an ophthamalogist.[35]
  - For more severe cases, an ophthalmologist can accomplish temporary or permanent occlusion of the lacrimal puncta.
- Treatment of **dry mouth symptoms** is more challenging but important to reduce discomfort and the incidence of dental caries.
  - Conservative measures, such as increased oral water intake and chewing sugarless gum, can provide symptomatic relief.
  - Oral pilocarpine, 5 mg qid, or cevimeline, 30 mg tid, has been shown to increase saliva production and improve symptoms of oral dryness.
  - Various saliva substitutes are available over the counter but may be poorly tolerated.
- Hydroxychloroquine (see the "Rheumatoid Arthritis" section above) is sometimes prescribed for various manifestations of Sjögren syndrome.
- Immunosuppressive agents, such as cyclophosphamide, may be required for systemic vasculitis that affects major organs such as nerves.

VASCULITIS

General Principles

- The clinical manifestations of vasculitis are protean. Fever, weight loss, mononeuropathy, rash, arthritis, abdominal pain, sinusitis, pulmonary hemorrhage, and glomerulonephritis are among the many presenting symptoms.
- Physical manifestations tend to be nonspecific, but skin lesions such as palpable purpura, livido reticularis, and digital gangrene are suspicious for vasculitis.
- Wrist drop or foot drop is suggestive of mononeuropathy, another important clue to the presence of systemic vasculitis.

Diagnosis

Specific Vasculitic Syndromes

- **Polyarteritis nodosa** exhibits many of the above symptoms but typically presents with hypertension, glomerulonephritis, abdominal pain, and mononeuropathy (commonly wrist drop or foot drop). Onset may be gradual or sudden, and patients are systemically ill.
- **Giant cell arteritis** (GCA) presents with headache, visual disturbance, tongue and jaw claudication, and scalp tenderness. This is often associated with polymyalgia rheumatica (PMR).
- **Takayasu arteritis** affects the aorta and its branches. It occurs most commonly in young Asian women and is often detected by asymmetric pulses or blood pressure measurements. Other symptoms include headache, arm claudication, visual changes, and arthralgias.
- **Wegener granulomatosis** presents with the classic triad of upper-airway disease (sinusitis), lower-airway disease (pulmonary hemorrhage), and glomerulonephritis. Limited Wegener granulomatosis occurs without renal involvement.
- **Churg-Strauss vasculitis** is classically associated with severe asthma and systemic eosinophilia. Peripheral neuropathy, mononeuritis, pulmonary, and cutaneous involvement are common.
- **Cutaneous vasculitis** may be common to all subtypes of vasculitis and commonly presents with palpable purpura, usually in dependent areas of the lower extremities. Although often associated with systemic diseases, vasculitis may be limited to the skin.
- **Cryoglobulinemia,** frequently associated with hepatitis C, can present with purpura, arthritis, and glomerulonephritis.
- **Secondary vasculitis:** Vasculitis may also occur secondary to other rheumatic diseases, such as RA and SLE, and should be suspected when symptoms include cutaneous vasculitis, peripheral neuropathies, or mesenteric ischemia.

Diagnostic Testing

- Laboratory findings are nonspecific but anemia, elevated ESR, and urinalysis abnormalities (proteinuria, hematuria, and cellular casts) are often seen.
- c-ANCA that truly represents antibody to proteinase-3 is specific for Wegener granulomatosis.
- Biopsy of affected tissues, such as skin, muscle, artery, and nerve, can be valuable in establishing the diagnosis.

- The gastrocnemius muscle and sural nerve are the common sources of diagnostic material.
- Renal biopsy findings tend to be nonspecific (crescentic glomerulonephritis with negative immunofluorescence) and rarely include vasculitis.

Treatment

- Treatment depends on the specific diagnosis.
- **High-dose corticosteroids** (prednisone at 1 mg/kg/day) are usually effective, especially in the short term.
- **Cyclophosphamide** can also be used, either in a daily oral dose of 1 to 2 mg/kg/day or a monthly IV dose of 0.5 to 1.0 g/m^2.
- Vasculitis that is limited to the skin does not require potent immunosuppressive treatment, and therapies such as MTX, azathioprine, or even colchicine may be effective.

POLYMYALGIA RHEUMATICA AND GIANT CELL ARTERITIS

General Principles

- PMR and GCA represent a continuum of disease. A patient may have one or both diagnoses, and they can develop in either order.
- PMR and GCA occur after the age of 50 years, and the incidence increases with age.

Diagnosis

Clinical Presentation

History
- The classic history for PMR is morning stiffness, worse in the neck, shoulder, and pelvic girdle region.
- The patient may complain of the inability to roll over in bed at night.
- GCA presents with headache, tongue or jaw claudication, scalp tenderness, and vision loss (typically amaurosis fugax).
- Systemic symptoms such as fever and weight loss may also occur in GCA.

Physical examination
- Physical examination of patients with PMR is most notable for a profound inability to abduct and elevate the shoulders in most cases.
- Synovitis, if present, should be minimal.
- Although an uncommon finding, in GCA, a tender, nodular superficial temporal artery with reduced or absent pulse strongly suggests the diagnosis.

Diagnostic Testing
- **Virtually all patients with PMR or GCA have an elevated ESR.**
  - The high sensitivity of this test makes PMR/GCA unlikely with a normal ESR.
  - CRP may also be elevated.
- A temporal artery **biopsy** should be performed in all patients in whom GCA is suspected.
  - The pathologic findings of granulomatous inflammation with giant cells and fragmentation of the internal elastic lamina confirm the diagnosis.

- Because the temporal artery biopsy does not have 100% sensitivity, the diagnosis may rarely be made despite a negative biopsy when the clinical presentation is convincing.

Treatment

- Treatment for PMR is oriented toward relieving discomfort and improving quality of life.
  - Although NSAIDs occasionally are effective for PMR, most patients require prednisone in doses of 10 to 15 mg/day for relief.
  - Failure of the patient to improve dramatically and rapidly with low-dose corticosteroids should lead to reconsideration of the diagnosis of PMR.
  - Treatment can be tapered over approximately 1 year, although some patients require longer treatment.
- **GCA must be treated aggressively as a systemic vasculitis.**
  - For suspicion of GCA, **high-dose prednisone must be initiated immediately** at approximately 60 mg daily to prevent the complication of irreversible vision loss.
  - Treatment **should not be delayed until a temporal artery biopsy** can be performed, because the diagnostic findings on biopsy can still be demonstrated several days after corticosteroid therapy has been started. Furthermore, patients may develop blindness during the first few days of therapy.
  - The dose of prednisone can be tapered slowly over several months, provided that the patient remains asymptomatic.
  - MTX may be an effective steroid-sparing agent in some patients, although the evidence is conflicting.

POLYMYOSITIS AND DERMATOMYOSITIS

General Principles

- PM and dermatomyositis (DM) are similar yet distinct conditions. Both are idiopathic inflammatory myopathies.
- DM is associated with skin manifestations but PM is not.
- Proximal myopathy is characteristic of both, but DM may sometimes occur without myositis.
- There does appear to be an association with malignancy in a minority of patients, more so with DM.

Diagnosis

Clinical Presentation

History
- The cardinal feature of myositis is **proximal muscle weakness** without pain.
  - Typically, patients notice difficulty in getting out of a car, chair, or bathtub; climbing stairs; or using their arms above the head.
  - Distal muscle strength should be normal except in inclusion body myositis, which tends to occur in older individuals.
- **Dysphagia** with nasal regurgitation may occur if there is weakness of the striated muscle of the upper esophagus.

- **Dyspnea** due to interstitial lung disease and joint pain from inflammatory arthritis may occur, especially in the antisynthetase syndrome (PM with anti-Jo-1 antibody).

Physical Examination
- The examination should focus on evidence of proximal muscle weakness, a sensitive test of which is the ability to raise the head from the supine position.
  - Standing up from a chair with the arms folded across the chest and rising from a deep squat are other good tests for proximal weakness.
- Patients with DM have typical skin findings such as a heliotrope rash on the eyelids, Gottron papules on the knuckles, and nail fold capillary abnormalities.
- Mechanic's hands are classically associated with the "antisynthetase syndrome."

Diagnostic Testing
- Laboratory studies should include serum **muscle enzymes,** especially creatine phosphokinase (CK), which is elevated in virtually all cases of inflammatory myopathy.
  - Elevations of aspartate aminotransferase (AST) and aldolase may occur but are less specific for muscle injury.
  - Myositis-associated antibodies (such as anti-Jo-1, anti-MI-2, and anti-SRP) are primarily important for classifying diseases in research but sometimes can be helpful in atypical cases.
- Most patients should undergo **electromyography** (EMG) to look for the classic myopathic findings of fibrillations, positive sharp waves, and low-amplitude polyphasic motor unit potentials.
- **Muscle biopsy** can be done on the contralateral side, corresponding to the most abnormal area on the EMG.
  - The biceps, deltoid, and vastus medialis are the muscles that are easily biopsied.
  - MRI has recently been shown to help in identifying affected muscles to aid in directing biopsy.

Treatment

- Treatment involves **high doses of corticosteroids,** either 1 mg/kg/day prednisone orally or pulse doses of methylprednisolone.
  - Sustained high doses for several months are usually required to control disease activity.
  - Normalization of CK levels precedes improvement in muscle strength by several weeks.
  - After several months of treatment, it is usually possible to taper the dose of prednisone, often to an every-other-day regimen.
- Patients whose disease cannot be controlled with corticosteroids can be treated with MTX or azathioprine as steroid-sparing agents.
- IV immunoglobulins can be beneficial, particularly in the short-term.
- Newer approaches to therapy include using immunomodulators such as mycophenolate, tacrolimus, cyclosporine, and rituximab as steroid-sparing agents.

FIBROMYALGIA

General Principles

- Fibromyalgia is a common cause of musculoskeletal pain. It can be described as a soft-tissue amplification syndrome, in which patients experience diffuse musculoskeletal pain.

- Recent data with functional MRI indicates that pain input is processed differently in the brain in fibromyalgia patients, compared with controls.[36]

Diagnosis

- **History suggestive** of fibromyalgia includes diffuse nonarticular pain; sleep disturbance resulting in nonrestorative sleep and fatigue; and accompanying symptoms such as headache, irritable bowel syndrome, paresthesias, depression, and vasomotor symptoms in the hands and feet.
- **Physical examination** is notable for tenderness to palpation in at least 11 of 18 predetermined tender points. Although the tender points were included in the initial ACR Classification Criteria for Fibromyalgia, opinion is divided as to whether tender points must be present to make the diagnosis.
- **Laboratory** studies are normal.

Treatment

- Treatment has three primary goals: improve sleep, relieve pain, and enhance physical conditioning.
- Nonhabit-forming medications that aid in sleep include tricyclic antidepressants (e.g., amitriptyline, 10 to 50 mg qHS), trazodone (25 to 100 mg qHS), and cyclobenzaprine (10 to 20 mg qHS).
- Antidepressant medications (such as venlafaxine and duloxetine) may also be beneficial. Duloxetine has been shown to be effective in reducing pain in fibromyalgia, regardless of whether depression is present.
- Pregabalin recently became the first drug approved by the FDA for the treatment of fibromyalgia and shows promise.
- NSAIDs and other analgesics may bring some relief of pain but **opiates typically require escalating doses to control symptoms and are problematic in the chronic treatment of fibromyalgia.**
- An aerobic exercise program is essential and can be supplemented by stretching exercises.
- Cognitive behavior programs when available are also effective.

REFERENCES

1. Guidelines for the initial evaluation of the adult patient with acute musculoskeletal symptoms. American College of Rheumatology Ad Hoc Committee on Clinical Guidelines. *Arthritis Rheum* 1996;39:1–8.
2. Klippel JH, ed. Primer on the Rheumatic Diseases. 12th Ed. Atlanta, GA: Arthritis Foundation, 2001.
3. Recommendations for the medical management of osteoarthritis of the hip and knee: 2000 update. American College of Rheumatology Subcommittee on Osteoarthritis Guidelines. *Arthritis Rheum* 2000;43:1905–1915.
4. Goldstein JL, Howard KB, Walton SM, et al. *Clin Gastroenterol Hepatol* 2006;4:1337–1345.
5. Stacy ZA, Dobesh PP, Trujillo TC. Cardiovascular risks of cyclooxygenase inhibition. *Pharmacotherapy* 2006;26:919–938.
6. Clegg DO, Reda DJ, Harris CL, et al., Glucosamine, chondroitin sulfate, and the two in combination for painful knee osteoarthritis. *N Engl J Med* 2006;354:795–808.
7. Holander JL. 9 Years of Experience with Steroid Therapy, Using Intra-Articular Administration. *Hospital (Rio J)* 1963;64:491–495.

8. Lo GH, LaValley M, McAlindon T, Felson DT. Intra-articular hyaluronic acid in treatment of knee osteoarthritis: a meta-analysis. *JAMA* 2003;290:3115–3121.

9. O'Dell JR. Therapeutic strategies for rheumatoid arthritis. *N Engl J Med* 2004;350: 2591–2602.

10. Arnett FC, Edworthy SM, Bloch DA, et al. The American Rheumatism Association 1987 revised criteria for the classification of rheumatoid arthritis. *Arthritis Rheum* 1988;31:315–324.

11. Wolfe F, Freundlich B, Straus WL. Increase in cardiovascular and cerebrovascular disease prevalence in rheumatoid arthritis. *J Rheumatol* 2003;30:36–40.

12. Nishimura K, Sugiyama D, Kogata Y, et al. Meta-analysis: diagnostic accuracy of anti-cyclic citrullinated peptide antibody and rheumatoid factor for rheumatoid arthritis. *Ann Intern Med* 2007;146:797–808.

13. Guidelines for the management of rheumatoid arthritis: 2002 Update. American College of Rheumatology Subcommittee on Rheumatoid Arthritis Guidelines. *Arthritis Rheum* 2002;46:328–346.

14. Recommendations for the prevention and treatment of glucocorticoid-induced osteoporosis: 2001 update. American College of Rheumatology Ad Hoc Committee on Glucocorticoid-Induced Osteoporosis. *Arthritis Rheum* 2001;44:1496–1503.

15. Genovese MC, Becker JC, Schiff M, et al. Abatacept for rheumatoid arthritis refractory to tumor necrosis factor alpha inhibition. *N Engl J Med* 2005;353:1114–1123.

16. Edwards JC, Szczepanski L, Szechinski J, et al. Efficacy of B-cell-targeted therapy with rituximab in patients with rheumatoid arthritis. *N Engl J Med* 2004;350:2572–2581.

17. O'Brien JP, Goldenberg DL, Rice PA. Disseminated gonococcal infection: a prospective analysis of 49 patients and a review of pathophysiology and immune mechanisms. *Medicine (Baltimore)* 1983;62:395–406.

18. Pinals RS. Polyarthritis and fever. *N Engl J Med* 1994;330:769–774.

19. Centers for Disease Control and Prevention (CDC). Update to CDC's sexually transmitted diseases treatment guidelines, 2006: fluoroquinolones no longer recommended for treatment of gonococcal infections. *MMWR Morb Mortal Wkly Rep* 2007;56:332–336.

20. Wise CM. Crystal-associated arthritis in the elderly. *Rheum Dis Clin North Am* 2007;33:33–55.

21. Kashyap AS, Kashyap S. Hormone replacement therapy and serum uric acid. *Lancet* 1999;354:1643–1644.

22. Bonnel RA, Villalba ML, Karwoski CB, Beitz J. Deaths associated with inappropriate intravenous colchicine administration. *J Emerg Med* 2002;22:385–387.

23. Choi HK, Atkinson K, Karlson EW, et al. Purine-rich foods, dairy and protein intake, and the risk of gout in men. *N Engl J Med* 2004;350:1093–1103.

24. Epis O, Caporali R, Scirè CA, et al. Efficacy of tidal irrigation in Milwaukee shoulder syndrome. *J Rheumatol* 2007;34:1545–1550.

25. Tan EM, Cohen AS, Fries JF, et al. The 1982 revised criteria for the classification of systemic lupus erythematosus. *Arthritis Rheum* 1982;25:1271–1277.

26. Wilson WA, Gharavi AE, Koike T, et al. International consensus statement on preliminary classification criteria for definite antiphospholipid syndrome: report of an international workshop. *Arthritis Rheum* 1999;42:1309–1311.

27. Weening JJ, D'Agati VD, Schwartz MM, et al. The classification of glomerulonephritis in systemic lupus erythematosus revisited. *Kidney Int* 2004;65:521–530.

28. Dougados M, van der Linden S, Juhlin R, et al. The European Spondylarthropathy Study Group preliminary criteria for the classification of spondylarthropathy. *Arthritis Rheum* 1991;34:1218–1227.

29. Baraliakos X, Listing J, Rudwaleit M, et al. Radiographic progression in patients with ankylosing spondylitis after 2 years of treatment with the tumour necrosis factor α antibody infliximab. *Ann Rheum Dis* 2005;64:1462–1466.

30. Spencer-Green G. Outcomes in primary Raynaud phenomenon: a meta-analysis of the frequency, rates, and predictors of transition to secondary diseases. *Arch Intern Med* 1998;158:595–600.

31. Heymann WR. Sildenafil for the treatment of Raynaud's phenomenon. *J Am Acad Dermatol* 2006;55:501–502.

32. Tashkin DP, Elashoff R, Clements PJ, et al. Cyclophosphamide versus placebo in scleroderma lung disease. *N Engl J Med* 2006;354:2655–2666.
33. Highland KB, Garin MC, Brown KK. The spectrum of scleroderma lung disease. *Semin Respir Crit Care Med* 2007;28:418–429.
34. Badesch DB, Tapson VF, McGoon MD, et al. Continuous intravenous epoprostenol for pulmonary hypertension due to the scleroderma spectrum of disease: a randomized, controlled trial. *Ann Intern Med* 2000;132:425–434.
35. Thanou-Stavraki A, James JA. Primary Sjögren syndrome: current and prospective therapies. *Semin Arthritis Rheum* 2008;37:273–292.
36. Nebel MB, Gracely RH. Neuroimaging of fibromyalgia. *Rheum Dis Clin North Am* 2009; 35:313–327.

29 Musculoskeletal Complaints

Thomas M. De Fer

NECK PAIN

General Principles

- Neck pain is an extremely common symptom, but most episodes are short lived and seldom require medical care.
- Those patients who come to medical attention generally need only conservative treatment.
- With conservative therapy, more than half of the patients have improvement in neck pain within 2 to 4 weeks, and the majority is asymptomatic by 2 to 3 months.

Etiology/Pathogenesis

- By far, most neck pain is not serious and is musculoskeletal-biomechanical in origin, caused by minor trauma or age-related changes in the cervical spine. A much smaller number of patients have serious systemic diseases that affect the neck or referred pain.
- **Strain/sprain/spasm** of the paracervical musculature is an especially common cause of acute nonspecific neck pain, particularly in younger patients. It may develop after a prolonged period in an awkward position, sudden jarring neck movement related to minor trauma, or activities that require new, unusual, or repetitive neck movements.
- **Acute flexion-hyperextension neck injury (whiplash)** occurs most commonly after a rear-end car collision.
  - For unclear reasons, whiplash tends to respond less well to therapy than do typical cervical sprains. After 12 months, 15% to 20% of patients remain symptomatic, with 5% severely affected.[1]
  - Facet (zygapophyseal) joint pain has been suggested to be the most common cause for chronic neck pain after whiplash. Imaging tests are unrevealing. Fluoroscopically guided, controlled diagnostic blocks of the painful joint may establish the diagnosis.
- **Osteoarthritis/spondylosis:** Degenerative cervical spine changes generally begin in the fourth decade of life.
  - Disk degeneration can result in posterior and lateral bulging.
  - Osteoarthritis develops in the zygapophyseal synovial joints. Osteophyte formation may occur, originating from the vertebral body, facet joints, and neural foramina margins. Occasionally, there is segmental instability or subluxation. This entire process is referred to as cervical spondylosis, and it is thought to be a common cause of chronic mechanical neck pain in older individuals.
  - Encroachment on the neural foramina and spinal canal may result in radiculopathy or cervical myelopathy.

- **Degenerative cervical disk disease** increases with age and may result in neck pain with or without radiculopathy. Acute cervical disk herniations may also cause neck pain or radiculopathy, or both.
- **Cervical radiculopathy** may be caused by multiple processes, most commonly acute disk herniation, chronic disk degeneration, and cervical spondylosis.
  - Radiculopathy is occasionally caused by a more serious condition such as malignancy or infection.
  - Thoracic outlet syndrome, brachial plexus disorders, and upper-extremity peripheral nerve compression syndromes may mimic radicular symptoms.
- **Serious or systemic causes** of neck pain and/or radiculopathy are much less common and include vertebral osteomyelitis, epidural abscess, discitis, meningitis, rheumatoid arthritis (RA), spondyloarthropathies, polymyalgia rheumatica, fibromyalgia, and primary or metastatic tumors. Cervical fractures are generally the result of significant trauma and may or may not present with neurologic symptoms. Osteoporotic fractures of the cervical spine are unusual.
- **Other structures in the neck** may produce pain, such as thyroiditis, pharyngitis, retropharyngeal or peritonsillar abscess, and carotodynia.
- **Referred pain** to the neck may be the result of headaches, shoulder disorders, angina, esophageal disorders, and vascular dissection.

Diagnosis

- In most patients, a thorough but focused history and physical examination is the primary diagnostic tool.
- An important goal is to detect symptoms and signs that suggest a potentially serious condition or a neurologic urgency.
- In the absence of such findings, special diagnostic tests are generally not indicated.

Clinical Presentation

History

- The history should focus on the mode of onset, nature, and location of the pain.
- A history of trauma is important. Patients should also be asked about activities that may have preceded the pain (e.g., prolonged neck extension or flexion, twisting, new physical activity, sport, or job).
- Neck pain often does not develop until 12 to 24 hours after such activity.
- Acute neck pain that is unrelated to trauma suggests cervical strain or disk herniation (that may or may not be associated with radicular symptoms).
- Chronic neck pain with intermittent acute exacerbations (sometimes with radiculopathy) is often due to cervical spondylosis.
- Mechanical neck pain is typically exacerbated by movement and relieved by rest.
- Morning stiffness may be present in patients with an inflammatory arthropathy.
- Neurologic symptoms are a vital component of the history.
  - **Radiculopathy** may involve single, multiple, or bilateral roots. Sensory changes are usually more pronounced than motor symptoms. Patients may also complain of paresthesias that radiate from the neck into the arm. Weakness is the primary symptom of motor involvement. Extensive paralysis only occurs with multiple root involvement.
  - Symptoms of cervical **myelopathy** (due to severe cervical spondylosis) generally develop slowly and intermittently. Patients complain of upper- and lower-extremity weakness and sensory changes. Spastic paraparesis of the legs and loss of sphincter control may eventually develop.

- In patients with RA, neck pain may indicate impending neurologic compromise. Forward subluxation of C1 can compress the spinal cord, resulting in sudden motor and sensory deficits at multiple levels.
- Symptoms or history suggestive of a serious etiology, such as malignancy or infection, should be carefully sought (e.g., fever, weight loss, very severe pain, pain unrelieved by rest, a history of cancer, long-term corticosteroid use, and IV drug use).

Physical Examination
- The physical examination should include the entire cervical spine and surrounding areas (e.g., shoulders and head) and an appropriate neurologic examination.
- The range of motion (ROM) of the neck normally decreases with age.
  - Lateral flexion of the neck may worsen radiculopathy symptoms, as may vertical pressure on the head **(Spurling maneuver).**
  - **Lhermitte sign,** electric shock sensation down the spine into the arms and legs with spine extension, may be seen in cervical myelopathy/cord compression.
- Localized tenderness of the cervical spine and "spasm" of the paraspinal musculature may be present. The sensitivity and specificity of severe bony tenderness for fracture are unknown.
- When the patient has neurologic complaints, a thorough **neurologic examination** is necessary.
  - Not all patients with radiculopathy have demonstrable findings on examination.
  - Cervical radiculopathy has characteristic sensory changes and motor weakness (Table 1).
  - Motor weakness in the upper and lower extremities, spasticity, hyperreflexia, clonus, Babinski sign, and reduced sphincter tone are consistent with cervical myelopathy.

Diagnostic Testing
Plain Radiography
- Plain radiography of the cervical spine should be used judiciously in patients with nonspecific mechanical neck pain.
- Use of plain radiographs in evaluating neck pain has two important limitations:
  - First, **cervical spondylosis is extremely common in asymptomatic individuals** and increases with age.

TABLE 1	Features of Cervical Radiculopathy		
Nerve Root	Area of Sensory Change	Motor Weakness	Reflex
C5	Upper lateral arm	Shoulder abduction	Biceps and brachioradialis
C6	Lower lateral forearm into thumb and index finger	Forearm supinators and pronators	Biceps and brachioradialis
C7	Dorsal and palmar surface of forearm into middle finger	Triceps and wrist extension flexion	Triceps
C8	Medial forearm into ring and little fingers	Intrinsic hand muscles	

- Second, plain radiographs are of **very limited value in assessing nerve root or spinal cord compression.**
- Nonetheless, plain films should generally be done in patients with radiculopathy to evaluate for serious bony abnormalities.
- Plain cervical spine films are warranted when a serious disorder is suspected or in cases that are related to significant trauma.
- If plain films are unrevealing but strong suspicion still exists, other imaging studies, such as computed tomography (CT) or magnetic resonance imaging (MRI), should be done.

CT and MRI
- CT or MRI is recommended when tumor, infection, fracture, or other space-occupying lesion is strongly suggested by the clinical findings or in the setting of serious neurologic signs and symptoms.
- In the absence of severe or progressive neurologic symptoms, it is generally not necessary to do a CT or MRI for patients with typical radiculopathy.
  - Many patients with cervical radiculopathy have substantial improvement in a few weeks.
  - If symptoms have not improved with several months of conservative management and the patient is an appropriate potential candidate for surgery, CT or MRI may be useful.

Electrodiagnostic Testing
- Electrodiagnostic tests are usually not indicated in individuals with obvious radiculopathy.
- They are probably most useful when the cause of upper-extremity pain is unclear or surgery is being considered.

Treatment

- Simple conservative therapy is appropriate for the majority of patients with nonspecific mechanical neck pain. In most cases, the pain improves in several weeks.
- **Modest activity restriction** is generally believed to be appropriate.
  - Patients should avoid activities that worsen their neck pain.
  - Bed rest is not indicated, and patients should be encouraged to continue most daily activities.
  - Soft cervical collars are also frequently recommended and may reduce symptoms in some patients. These collars are not particularly effective at reducing neck motion but may serve as a reminder to the patient to limit movements that can increase pain. Rigid cervical collars should not be prescribed by the untrained.
- **Pharmacotherapy** with **acetaminophen, nonsteroidal anti-inflammatory drugs (NSAIDs)** may provide relief for nonspecific mechanical neck pain. **Opiate analgesics** may be an effective time-limited option for patients with acute severe neck pain. Some patients may find **muscle relaxants** effective, but sedation is a common side effect. Supportive data are limited for all of these medications.[2]
- **Neck mobilization and manipulation** do not appear to be effective on their own but may be of benefit as part of a multimodal treatment strategy plus exercise.[3]
- **Stretching and strengthening exercises** of the cervical and shoulder/thoracic area may be effective for acute and chronic mechanical neck disorders.[4]
- There is very limited data regarding **electrotherapy and electromagnetic therapy** that a definitive statement of their effectiveness is not possible.[5]

- Simple application of **local heat or ice** is an option for symptomatic relief.
- Limited evidence suggests that **myofascial trigger point injections** with lidocaine may be effective.[2]
- **Acupuncture** appears to be moderately effective for chronic neck pain.[6]
- **Traction** has unclear efficacy for neck pain with or without radiculopathy due to the lack of high-quality data.[7]
- The benefit of **massage** is unknown.[8]
- **Surgery** has no role in the relief of neck pain secondary to cervical spondylosis in the absence of significant persistent neurologic involvement.
- **Whiplash** does not seem to respond as well to conservative treatments, but they are frequently used and their effectiveness is unclear.[9]
  - For patients with chronic cervical zygapophyseal joint pain after whiplash confirmed with double-blind placebo-controlled local anesthesia, percutaneous radiofrequency neurotomy may provide lasting relief.[10,11]
  - A small study suggests that the acute treatment with high-dose methylprednisolone may be beneficial in preventing extensive sick leave after whiplash.[2,12]
- **Neck pain with radiculopathy** is generally treated in a manner similar to that of nonspecific mechanical neck pain.
  - Patients with prolonged severe radicular symptoms may benefit from surgical decompression. Those who are agreeable to surgery and are medically appropriate surgical candidates can be referred to a neurosurgeon.
  - Patients with persistent radicular pain secondary to cervical spondylosis may respond to fluoroscopically guided therapeutic selective nerve root block.[13]
- **Myelopathy** often requires surgical treatment and is best managed in conjunction with a neurosurgeon, neurologist, or both.

LOW BACK PAIN

General Principles

Epidemiology

- Low back pain (LBP) is an exceedingly common complaint, with a lifetime incidence of >70%.
- Patients present along a wide spectrum of pain and disability, which unfortunately often does not correlate well with the seriousness of the underlying etiology.
- The medical and societal costs are enormous (up to $50 billion a year), with the majority due to a small percentage of patients with temporary or permanent disability.
- There is an epidemiological association between LBP and **obesity.** Whether or not losing weight reduces LBP is a largely unanswered question.
- There is also an association with **smoking** but true cause and effect are unknown.[14-16]

Etiology

- Many of the etiologies of LBP are presented in Table 2.
- The distribution of diagnoses varies somewhat among populations and degree of chronicity.
  - Regardless, the large majority of cases are due to mechanical causes with lumbar sprain/strain probably accounting for the biggest proportion (about 70%).
  - The pathologic corollary to sprain/strain is unknown and the concept of skeletal muscle "spasm" is not universally accepted.

TABLE 2	Etiologies of Low Back Pain

Mechanical or Activity Related	Medical Conditions of the Spine
Lumbosacral myofascial strain, strain, "spasm"	**Rheumatologic**
Degenerative changes of the vertebrae, disks, facet joints (spondylosis)	Spondyloarthropathies (e.g., ankylosing spondylitis, psoriatic arthritis, reactive arthritis, inflammatory bowel disease related)
Herniated intervertebral disk[a]	Rheumatoid arthritis
Lumbar spinal stenosis[a]	
Discogenic low back pain[b]	**Neoplastic**
Facet joint syndrome[b]	Primary tumors
Sacroiliac joint dysfunction without sacroiliitis/ spondyloarthropathy[b]	Metastatic disease (e.g., multiple myeloma, lymphoma, carcinoma)
Osteoporotic compression fracture	**Infectious**
Traumatic fractures	Discitis
Other anatomical/congenital abnormalities	Epidural abscess
Spondylolisthesis	Vertebral osteomyelitis
Kyphosis	**Metabolic**
Scoliosis	Paget disease

Referred Pain

Vascular
Abdominal aortic aneurysm
Aortic dissection

Genitourinary
Nephrolithiasis
Pyelonephritis
Pelvic inflammatory disease
Endometriosis
Prostatitis

Gastrointestinal
Cholecystitis
Pancreatitis
Peptic ulcer disease

[a]Often associated with neurogenic leg pain.
[b]Validity of the diagnosis, method of precise diagnosis, and optimal unique management not universally accepted.
Modified from Deyo RA, Weinstein JN. Low back pain. *N Engl J Med* 2001;26:153–159.

- Ultimately, in approximately 85% of cases, a specific diagnosis cannot be made, so-called **nonspecific musculoskeletal (or idiopathic) LBP.** Medical LBP specialists and surgeons will see a higher percentage of specific pathologies.[17]
- **Spondylosis** is a generalized degenerative change of the spine, including disk degeneration, with disk space narrowing and osteoarthritic changes of the facet joints.

Spondylosis is just as common in asymptomatic as in symptomatic individuals. In general, LBP patients with spondylosis have the same prognosis as those without spondylosis.

- **Spondylolisthesis** is the forward movement of the body of one of the lower lumbar vertebrae on the vertebra below it or on the sacrum.
  - Minor degrees of spondylolisthesis are fairly common and usually asymptomatic. Individuals with LBP that is presumed to be secondary to spondylolisthesis usually follow a similar course as those with nonspecific LBP.
  - When the slippage is severe, it may cause back pain and radiculopathy.
- **Lumbar disk herniation** is common and increases with age.
  - Of disk herniations, 95% occur at the L4-L5 or L5-S1 levels.
  - Disk herniation may result in LBP, sciatica, or both. However, disk herniations may also be totally asymptomatic.
  - Large midline disk herniations occasionally cause the cauda equina syndrome.
- **Spinal stenosis** is usually caused by hypertrophy of the ligamentum flavum and facet joints, resulting in narrowing of the spinal canal, often at multiple levels.
  - This narrowing may result in entrapment of nerve roots, with resultant symptoms in the legs.
  - **Pseudoclaudication** or neurogenic claudication is characterized by back pain and pain and numbness of the lower extremities that worsen with walking and extension of the spine.
- Several reputed conditions are not universally accepted as valid diagnoses, including **discogenic LBP,**[18] **facet joint syndrome,**[19] and **sacroiliac joint dysfunction** (without sacroiliitis or spondyloarthropathy).[20,21] None has sufficiently distinct historical or physical findings allowing for certain diagnosis by this method. All are reportedly substantiated by injection into the potentially pathogenic area—contrast under pressure for discogenic LBP and local anesthetic/steroid for facet joint syndrome and sacroiliac joint dysfunction. **Gold standard tests are lacking.** These diagnoses are made frequently by some clinicians and rarely or never by others. Their exact incidence and prevalence is unknown. Potentially effective and unique therapies are being investigated but none has been clearly shown to be effective in randomized controlled trials.
- A very small number of patients have serious systemic diseases that affect the spine or have referred pain.

Diagnosis

- In the vast majority of patients, the primary diagnostic tool is a careful but focused history and physical examination searching for **"red flags"** that suggest a potentially serious underlying condition or a neurologic urgency (Table 3).[22]
- In primary care, individual "red flags" may have a very high false-positive rate.[23]
- Though initially designed with reference to acute LBP, it has some face validity with regard to chronic LBP.
- In the absence of red flags, special diagnostic tests are rarely indicated during the first month of pain.

Clinical Presentation

History

- Symptoms and historical features potentially suggestive of **malignancy** include current or prior malignancies, breast mass, smoking, family history of cancer, and systemic symptoms (e.g., weight loss, night sweats, fever, and decreased appetite).

TABLE 3	Red Flags of Low Back Pain

Age >50 years
History of cancer
Unexplained weight loss
Chronic steroid use
Pain duration >1 month
Pain unresponsive to treatment for 1 month
Pain unrelieved or worsened by rest
IV drug use
Urinary tract or other infection
Fever
Bladder dysfunction
Saddle anesthesia
Unilateral or bilateral major motor weakness
Significant trauma relative to age
Rapidly progressive severe radiculopathy

Modified from Bigos S, Bowyer O, Braen G, et al. Acute Low Back Problems in Adults. Clinical Practice Guideline no. 14. AHCPR publication 95-0642. Rockville, MD: Agency for Health Care Policy and Research, December 1994.

- Symptoms and historical features potentially suggestive of **infection** include HIV, chronic use of steroids or other immunosuppressants, history of IV drug abuse, hemodialysis, osteomyelitis/abscess, endocarditis, fever, chills, and sweats.
- Those that suggest **fracture** include female sex, trauma relative to age, age >70 years, and prolonged steroid use.[23]
- Symptoms compatible with **cauda equina syndrome** include bowel and/or bladder dysfunction, saddle anesthesia, bilateral lower extremity sciatica, sensory changes, and/or weakness.
- Pain worst with standing is typical of lumbar **spinal stenosis,** while pain worst with sitting or flexing the spine suggests **disk herniation.**
- Associated leg pain with standing and ambulation may represent spinal stenosis–related **pseudoclaudication.** True claudication generally does not occur just with standing. Some patients with spinal stenosis will have leg pain only. Flexion of the spine may improve the symptoms. The discomfort typically lasts longer after walking than it does in true vascular claudication.
- **Sciatica** is most specifically defined as pain radiating down the posterolateral leg below the knee. The sensitivity of the symptom of sciatica, defined as pain radiating into the buttocks and down the leg below the knee, is sufficiently high (0.95) that its absence makes a clinically significant disk herniation unlikely.[24]
- Coughing, sneezing, and valsalva can worsen sciatica secondary to disk herniation.
- Questions about personal or family history of spondyloarthropathies and RA may suggest these as potential causes. Morning stiffness may also provide a clue to these diagnoses.

Psychosocial History
- All patients should be asked about their occupational history, including current employment and exactly what kinds of physical activities are involved.

- There does not appear to be a relationship between leisure time sport or exercises, sitting, and prolonged standing/walking and LBP. Evidence is conflicting regarding home repair, gardening, whole-body vibration, nursing tasks, heavy physical work, and working with the trunk in a bent/twisted position.[25]
- Low job satisfaction and insufficient social support in the workplace are associated with the development of new-onset LBP.[26]
- Psychological distress, depressed mood, and somatization play a role in the development of chronic LBP.[27]
- Fear-avoidance-type behaviors may also contribute to the development of chronic LBP and disability. Interventions that break the cycle of fear and avoidance might be of benefit.[28–30]
- The "yellow flags" of acute back pain may help identify those patients at risk for chronicity[31]:
  - Belief that back pain is harmful or potentially severely disabling.
  - Fear-avoidance behavior and reduced the activity levels.
  - Tendency to low mood and withdrawal from social interaction.
  - Expectation that passive treatments rather than active participation will help.

Physical Examination
- Look for fever and tachycardia as potential clues to infection or inflammatory arthropathy.
- ROM, kyphosis, scoliosis, costovertebral angle tenderness, surgical scars, and spinal/paravertebral tenderness/spasm. Unfortunately, assessments of ROM and tenderness/spasm are not particularly very reproducible and do not have high values for sensitivity or specificity.[24]
- A thorough joint exam may reveal evidence of synovitis.
- A rectal exam may reveal prostatitis or a prostate mass.
- Decreased perianal sensation or rectal tone is worrisome for spinal neurologic involvement.
- **Straight leg raise** (SLR) testing may be performed with the patient supine or sitting up; considered positive if reproduction or worsening of sciatic pain occurs at <60°. The ipsilateral SLR has a high sensitivity (0.85) and low specificity (0.52), while the contralateral (crossed) SLR has a high specificity (0.84) and low sensitivity (0.30) (Table 4).[32]

TABLE 4	Neurologic Examination for Sciatica
Test	**Comment**
Knee reflex	Upper lumbar disk herniation
Ankle reflex	Disk herniation usually L5-S1
Ankle dorsiflexion	Disk herniation usually L4-L5
Great toe dorsiflexion	Disk herniation either L4-5 or L5-S1
Pinprick medial foot	Suggests L4 compression
Pinprick dorsal foot	Suggests L5 compression
Pinprick lateral foot	Suggests S1 compression
Straight leg raise	Positive if leg pain at <60° (sensitivity 0.85, specificity 0.52)
Crossed straight leg raise	Positive if pain in contralateral leg (sensitivity 0.30, specificity 0.84)

- An abbreviated **neurologic examination** can be done in most patients without neurologic symptoms (Table 4).
- When neurologic symptoms other than sciatica are present, a complete neurologic examination is warranted. Patients with the **cauda equina syndrome** typically have saddle anesthesia, bilateral radicular findings, and decreased anal sphincter tone.
- Often referred to as "Waddell signs" or "nonorganic signs," the presence of three or more behavioral responses to being examined suggests that the patient does not have only a straightforward physical problem.[33] These signs, however, do not exclude organic causes or specifically detect "secondary gain and/or malingering.[34]
  - Superficial tenderness.
  - Nonanatomic tenderness.
  - Pain on axial loading of the skull.
  - Pain on passive rotation of the shoulders and pelvis.
  - Sitting and supine straight leg raising discrepancy.
  - Regional weakness.
  - Regional sensory change.
  - Inconsistent "overreaction" to examination (e.g., tremor, sweating, collapse, exaggerated verbalizing, inappropriate sighing, guarding, bracing, rubbing, insistence on standing or changing position, and questionable use of walking aids or equipment).

Diagnostic Testing

Assuming there are no red flags present, it is reasonable to hold off any imaging or laboratory tests for the first month because the majority of patients will be significantly improved during that period of time with or without intervention.

Laboratories

- The use of laboratory tests should be judicious and guided by the history and physical examination.
- The large majority of patients will not need any laboratory tests specifically for the purpose of elucidating the cause of LBP.
- If the history and physical examination suggest the possibility of serious diagnoses (e.g., malignancy, infection, rheumatologic, and conditions that can cause referred LBP), appropriate laboratory tests should be done.
- Some have advocated the erythrocyte sedimentation rate (ESR) as a nonspecific screening test for potentially serious and related conditions.[35]

Imaging
Plain Radiographs

- Plain lumbosacral films correlate poorly with the presence of LBP. Many patients without back pain have degenerative changes, and many patients with back pain will have no or nondiagnostic radiographic abnormalities.
- Degenerative changes increase with age and are extremely common in the elderly. Therefore, when degenerative changes are present, it is very difficult to know if they are causative.
- Plain films cannot detect disk herniation, spinal stenosis, or nerve root impingement and may not clearly show evidence of infection or malignancy.
- In the final analysis, plain films will often be nondiagnostic and generally do not detect abnormalities not already suggested by the history and physical examination. Nonetheless, when red flags are present, plain films are reasonable.[36]

- In patients with very chronic LBP, the red flag of duration of >1 month should not be interpreted as a mandate for plain films.
- Of course, clinical judgment may override these general guidelines at any time.
- One study suggests that while patients may be more "satisfied" when plain films are done, short-term pain and other clinical outcomes are not improved.[37]

CT and MRI
- The obvious advantages of CT and MRI over plain films are much clearer delineation of bony and soft tissue abnormalities.
  - Both are capable of disclosing disk herniation, spinal stenosis, nerve root and spinal cord compression, malignancy, fractures, and infection.
  - On the other hand, they also detect more nondiagnostic degenerative changes.[38–40]
  - Degenerative findings on MRI are poorly predictive of the subsequent development of LBP.[41,42]
  - This does not mean that such findings cannot be the cause of LBP in some patients.[43,44]
- When there is serious consideration of malignancy, infection, cauda equina syndrome, fracture undiagnosed by plain films, spinal cord compression, or severe radiculopathy, CT or MRI is indicated. CT or MRI should also be considered in patients with prolonged (>1 month) moderate-to-severe radicular symptoms who would be reasonable surgical candidates (from a medical point of view) and who are open to the possibility of surgical treatment.[36]

Other Diagnostic Tests
- **Myelography and CT-myelography** are generally only indicated in special situations for preoperative planning in consultation with a surgeon.
- **Bone scintigraphy** is rarely needed in the diagnostic evaluation of patients with LBP. Bone scans may have a high yield for spinal metastases in patients with a known history of cancer. However, when they are positive, other diagnostic tests are usually required (i.e., CT or MRI).
- **Electrophysiologic tests** are usually not indicated in individuals with obvious radiculopathy or in those with only LBP. These tests appear to be most useful in the diagnostic evaluation of patients with leg pain when the diagnosis is unclear.

Treatment

- In the absence of red flags, treatment for most patients with acute nonspecific LBP can be simple and conservative.
- Most patients improve in approximately 1 month with or without treatment.
- Pain that has persisted without improvement for more than a month should be re-evaluated.
- The goals of treatment are to reduce pain, increase mobility, return to functioning at home, return to work, and prevent the development of chronic pain and disability.

Nonpharmacologic Therapies
- **Education:** The overall good prognosis of acute LBP should be stressed but not oversold. Although acute LBP may rapidly and completely resolve, it certainly does not always do so, and recurrences are common. Patients should be encouraged to notify the physician if symptoms change significantly. Intensive education may reduce pain.[45]
- In the occupational setting, **back school** appears to be effective for reducing pain and improving function.[46]

- **Bed rest** may actually delay recovery and potentially contribute to the development of chronic back pain. Patients with acute nonspecific LBP should be advised to continue ordinary activities as much as possible. Patients with sciatica also should be encouraged to go about daily activities as much as tolerated.[47]
- **Activity restriction:** It is reasonable to advise the patient to limit temporarily activities that are known to increase mechanical stress on the spine, including prolonged unsupported standing, heavy lifting, and bending or twisting the back while lifting.
- **Physical therapy (PT, trunk-strengthening exercises)** has not been clearly shown to be beneficial in acute LBP. However, exercise therapy is somewhat effective.[48,49]
- **Local heat or cold** may be efficacious and are relatively low cost with minimal risk of side effects, particularly low level heat wraps.[50] Patients should be warned against sleeping with heating pads and placing ice in direct contact with the skin due to the potential for burns and frostbite.
- **Massage** might be beneficial for subacute or chronic LBP, but it can be relatively expensive.[51,52]
- **Spinal manipulation** (chiropractic) continues to engender controversy. Multiple reviews and meta-analyses have been published with somewhat differing conclusions. Though not precisely clear, the preponderance of data suggests that spinal manipulation is minimally to moderately superior to sham manipulation/ineffective therapies and is at least as effective as other conservative therapies for acute and chronic LBP.[49,52,53] The occurrence of adverse outcomes appears to be very rare.
- Data regarding the utility of **acupuncture** are contradictory, but it may be effective for those with chronic LBP.[52,54,55]
- Data support the use of **cognitive-behavior therapies** for subacute and chronic LBP.[49,56]
- **Multidisciplinary biopsychosocial therapy** attempts to address all aspects of LBP, involving physicians, psychologists, physical/occupational therapists, and social workers. It requires the patient to take part in a substantial amount of active therapies (>100 hours) that incorporate the concept of functional restoration. Though expensive and not widely available, it has been shown to be effective for chronic LBP.[57]
- **Lumbar supports** do not appear to be useful for preventing LBP, and their role in treatment is unclear.[58]
- **Traction** as a single therapy is ineffective for LBP with or without sciatica.[59]
- Data do not support the use of **transcutaneous electrical nerve stimulation (TENS)** for LBP.[60]
- Data regarding **therapeutic insoles** are severely limited. They do not appear to prevent back pain in relatively young, highly active populations. Efficacy in treating LBP is unknown.[61]
- **Nonsurgical spinal decompressive therapy** (e.g., Vax-D) is of unproven benefit.[62]
- Data regarding **low-level laser therapy** are insufficient to draw conclusions.[63]

Medications

- **Acetaminophen** is a reasonable first-line choice for the treatment of acute and chronic LBP.[64]
- **NSAIDs** are more effective than placebo in patients with acute nonspecific LBP.[64,65]
- **Tramadol** (50 to 100 mg qid) is a reasonable alternative for patients who fail to respond to or who cannot take nonselective or selective NSAIDs, but side effects are common (e.g., nausea, constipation, and drowsiness).
- **Muscle relaxants** have been shown to be superior to placebo for acute LBP.[64,66,67] The concept of muscle "spasm" is ill defined and these drugs do not relax skeletal muscles.

Their exact mechanism of action is unknown. There is insufficient evidence to suggest that one muscle relaxant is better than the others. Many patients will experience significant sedation.

- **Opiates** may be considered as a time-limited option for severe acute LBP.
  - The use of opiates in chronic LBP continues to be controversial, and it is not clear whether they improve functioning (as opposed to pain).
  - Notwithstanding, chronic LBP is a very common nonmalignant reason for prescribing ongoing narcotics.
  - Long-term narcotic use for LBP is associated with increased rates of substance-abuse disorders and aberrant medication-taking behaviors.[68]
- **Antidepressants** may be useful in patients with chronic LBP with or without depression, though reviews have come to contradictory conclusions.[64,69]
  - Antidepressants that inhibit the uptake of norepinephrine (tricyclics) seem to produce moderate symptomatic benefit.
  - Based on limited evidence, pure serotonin reuptake inhibitors (SSRIs) do not appear to be effective.
  - Venlafaxine and duloxetine are SSRIs that also inhibit the uptake of norepinephrine—there is limited evidence to suggest that both may be effective for other chronic pain conditions.
  - Antidepressants are not indicated solely for the treatment of acute LBP.
  - Potential risks of therapy should be carefully considered especially in the elderly.
- **Anticonvulsants** are increasingly being used to modulate chronic LBP. Some supportive evidence is beginning to emerge, particularly regarding topiramate and gabapentin (for sciatica).[70,71]

Injection Therapies

- Injection therapies have been tried in multiple different areas of the spine, including the facet joints, the epidural space, and soft tissue (trigger points, acupuncture points, or ligaments). Corticosteroids, local anesthetics, and saline have all been used.
- **Trigger point injections** are done fairly frequently. The theory of trigger points as a cause or perpetuator of LBP is controversial at best. Evidence is insufficient to recommend for or against their use in either acute or chronic LBP.[72]
- **Facet joint injections** have been advocated for the treatment of the "facet joint syndrome." The syndrome is diagnosed clinically in patients with lumbar pain that improves with the injection of corticosteroid or local anesthetic into or near the facet joints. The efficacy of such treatment is unclear but can be considered in selected patients with chronic LBP in whom more conservative treatment has failed.[72]
- **Epidural steroid injections** have been recommended for subacute or chronic LBP with and without sciatica. Results from multiple studies have been conflicting. Epidural steroids can be considered for patients in whom conservative therapy has failed.[72]
- **Prolotherapy** (proliferative injection therapy), the injection of an irritant solution intended to strengthen weakened lumbosacral ligaments), does not appear to be an effective sole treatment for chronic LBP.[73]
- The efficacy of **sacroiliac joint injections** is unknown.

Other Modalities

- Radiofrequency denervation may be effective of facet joint syndrome.[11]
- Likewise, intradiscal radiofrequency thermocoagulation might be useful for discogenic LBP, but data are very limited.[74]

Surgical Management

- There is good evidence that **surgical discectomy** provides effective relief of sciatica for properly selected patients.[75–77]
  - The primary benefit of discectomy appears to be the more rapid relief of symptoms in those individuals in whom conservative therapy has failed.
  - Whether there is a significant difference in long-term outcomes is less clear.[78]
- Similarly, surgery for appropriately selected patients with lumbar **spinal stenosis** is effective, but the effect diminishes over time.[76,79,80]
- Surgical intervention for **spinal stenosis with spondylolisthesis** may also be effective.[81]
- Surgical treatment for **degenerative lumbar spondylosis** is especially controversial. Surgical treatments may include decompression, spinal fusion, or both. The data available are limited, sometimes of poor quality, and conflicting and often focus on technical rather than patient-centered outcomes. The most recent review concluded that for nonradicular back pain associated with degenerative changes, spinal fusion is no more effective than intensive rehabilitation but more beneficial compared with standard nonsurgical therapies.[76]

SHOULDER PAIN

General Principles

- The **glenohumeral (GH) joint** is very shallow and is the most commonly dislocated joint.
- The **rotator cuff** supports the GH joint and consists of the tendons of four muscles: supraspinatus, infraspinatus, teres minor, and subscapularis.
  - The tendons of these muscles blend with the shoulder joint capsule and insert on the greater and lesser tuberosities of the humeral head.
  - The rotator cuff muscles assist in internal and external rotation and depress the humeral head during shoulder elevation.
  - This action holds the humeral head down, minimizing impingement on the acromion process and the intervening tissues.
- The **subacromial bursa** lies deep to the deltoid muscle and superficial to the insertion point of the supraspinatus tendon.
- The long head of the biceps originates from the **glenoid labrum.** The **biceps tendon** passes out of the GH joint through the bicipital groove.
- Patients with acute shoulder problems have a better prognosis than those with chronic shoulder pain.[82]

Etiology

- **The shoulder impingement syndrome causes the majority of painful nontraumatic shoulder problems.** It is due to mechanical impingement of the rotator cuff structures by the humeral head against the subacromial structures. This is related to a continuum of inflammation, degeneration, and attrition of the rotator cuff structures, especially the supraspinatus tendon. As a result, the rotator cuff fails to prevent upward migration of the humeral head during shoulder elevation. Several interrelated conditions are involved in the impingement syndrome; all may occur simultaneously.
  - **Rotator cuff tendonitis** refers to a spectrum of changes that affect the tendons of the rotator cuff, particularly the supraspinatus. Acute inflammation with hemorrhage and edema can occur secondary to trauma or overuse, particularly in younger

patients. Acute rotator cuff tendonitis is sometimes associated with calcification of the supraspinatus and biceps tendons (so-called **calcific tendonitis**). The pain of calcific tendonitis can be severe and may lead to a **"frozen shoulder."** With aging, the tendons undergo degenerative changes and attenuation related to chronic inflammation and repeated mechanical insults.[83]

- **Rotator cuff tears** can occur suddenly secondary to falling on an outstretched arm or with lifting a heavy object. Tears can also occur more indolently in older patients with attrition of the rotator cuff or with a chronic inflammatory condition such as RA or the "Milwaukee shoulder" (progressive, destructive shoulder arthropathy associated with bloody shoulder effusions and the deposition of basic calcium phosphate crystals).

- **Subacromial bursitis and bicipital tendonitis** may accompany rotator cuff tendonitis. In fact, it is often difficult to distinguish these entities, as they frequently occur simultaneously. Occasionally, the proximal biceps tendon **ruptures.**

- **Adhesive capsulitis (frozen shoulder)** may complicate any painful shoulder condition and has been associated with myocardial infarction, diabetes mellitus, apical lung cancer, cervical disk disease, metastatic lesions, and thyroid disease. However, such clinical associations are often lacking. The precise pathophysiology of adhesive capsulitis is not entirely clear but appears to involve initial hypervascular synovitis and subsequent fibrosis. What triggers this process is unknown.[84] It is not unusual for frozen shoulder to develop subsequently in the contralateral shoulder.

- **Osteoarthritis** does not commonly occur as a primary process in the GH joint, with two exceptions: (1) rapidly progressive osteoarthritis of the shoulder in elderly women and (2) the Milwaukee shoulder. Secondary osteoarthritis may occur as a result of RA, trauma, repetitive manual labor, calcium pyrophosphate deposition disease, and long-standing rotator cuff tears (cuff-tear/rotator arthropathy).

- **Shoulder instability and dislocation:** The shoulder joint is inherently unstable and the most commonly dislocated joint. Acute GH dislocation occurs most frequently in young active adults after a fall on an outstretched arm and results in anterior displacement of the humeral head. Recurrent dislocation is not unusual, with subsequent episodes requiring less force. Some patients have a chronic syndrome of GH instability with subluxation. This is often seen in athletes such as baseball pitchers.

- **Inflammatory arthropathies** such as RA and lupus can affect the GH joint.

- **Crystalline arthropathies** occasionally occur in the shoulder, such as the above-mentioned "Milwaukee shoulder" (hydroxyapatite crystals) and pseudogout/ pyrophosphate arthropathy (calcium pyrophosphate dihydrate crystals). Gout is relatively rare.

- The **acromioclavicular joint** can also be painful due to sprain/separation and arthritic changes.

Diagnosis

Clinical Presentation

History

- Intrinsic shoulder pain is typically worse at night and aggravated by lying on the affected shoulder.
- Motion of the shoulder generally increases the discomfort, particularly full forward-flexed elevation and abduction to 90°.
- A history of recent trauma, new physical activity (e.g., repetitive overhead arm motion), and prior dislocation are important.

- Patients with shoulder instability may complain that the shoulder has a disconcerting "going out" sensation.
- **Impingement syndrome** patients may have a history of repetitive overhead arm motion. Pain tends to be focal and anterior, occurring at night or when the patient is lying on the shoulder. Activities such as throwing, working with arms overhead, and swimming aggravate the pain.
- **Adhesive capsulitis** is most common in women in the fifth and sixth decades of life. The key historical feature is a painful and significant reduction in ROM. The onset can be fairly acute or chronic. As the condition progresses, pain subsides, but the limitation of ROM may become quite severe. After months of symptoms, some patients have a slow progressive improvement in ROM.
- Individuals with **GH instability** complain of a chronic feeling of the shoulder "going out" with certain activities and sometimes pain. A history of significant trauma (usually related to sports) and pain is elicited from patients with acute **GH dislocation** and **acromioclavicular separation.**

Physical Examination

- **Physical examination** of the shoulder should include observation, palpation of the bony and soft tissues, assessment of passive and active ROM, strength testing, and certain provocative tests.
- Normal **abduction** of the internally rotated (palm-down) shoulder is approximately 120° and externally rotated (palm-up) shoulder is 180°.
- Normal **elevation** (forward flexion) of the shoulder is 180°, **extension** 40°, and **internal and external rotation** 90°.
- If active ROM is limited, passive ROM should be carefully tested.
- Marked loss of both active and passive ROM is consistent with adhesive capsulitis.
- **Crepitus** during ROM may be appreciated with osteoarthritis.
- **Cross-chest abduction** (touch the opposite shoulder) tests internal rotation and adduction.
- The **Apley scratch test** evaluates external rotation and abduction from above (scratch between the scapulae from above) or internal rotation and adduction from below.
- Patients with acute **anterior dislocation** have a loss of the shoulder's normally rounded appearance. The acromion process becomes the most lateral structure. A prominence of the humeral head is present anterior and inferior to the glenoid. ROM is painfully restricted. Patients with acute dislocation should have a detailed neurovascular examination, specifically the motor and sensory innervation of the axillary nerve.

Impingement Tests

- The **impingement sign** is elicited by passive forward flexion of the arm by the physician. Passive abduction to 90° with internal rotation also causes pain.
- The **apprehension sign** is elicited by having the patient point straight ahead with the shoulder in flexion; when the examiner exerts downward pressure on the upper arm, the patient's apprehension is evident due to impingement of the supraspinatus tendon.
- **Neer impingement sign:** With the patient in the seated position, elbow extended, forearm pronated (humerus internally rotated), passively elevate (forward flex) the GH joint with the examiner's hand distal to the elbow while the other stabilizes the posterior aspect of the shoulder. Pain indicates a positive sign, especially near the end for the ROM. Sensitivity and specificity are estimated to be 0.79 and 0.53, respectively.[85]
- **Hawkins impingement sign:** With patient sitting or standing, grasp the arm at the elbow and wrist, flex the elbow and shoulder to 90°, then passively internally rotate

the shoulder. Pain, particularly at the end of the ROM, is a positive test—sensitivity 0.79 and specificity 0.59.[85]

- **Yocoum test** consists of having the patient place the palm on the affected side on the opposite shoulder and then to raise the elbow without elevating the shoulder. Pain is indicative of impingement—sensitivity 0.79 and specificity 0.40.[86]
- The **drop arm sign** to demonstrate a rotator cuff tear is performed by assisting the patient in abducting and elevating the shoulder. When the examiner withdraws support of the upper arm, the patient is unable to hold the arm up if there is a complete tear of the rotator cuff.
- The **supraspinatus liftoff test** demonstrates evidence of less advanced rotator cuff disease. The patient places the hand of the affected side on the small of the back, with the palm oriented posteriorly, and pushes against resistance. Normally, the patient should be able to push the examiner's hand away from the back. Weakness indicates rotator cuff disease.

Shoulder Instability Tests
- Anterior instability is most common and is suggested by pain with the **anterior apprehension test.**
  - With the shoulder initially at 90° of abduction and neutral rotation, the arm is externally rotated (as in a throwing position), and the examiner applies slight anteriorly directed pressure from behind.
  - The patient's discomfort is apparent through verbal and nonverbal cues.
  - If the apprehension is significantly decreased by the application of posteriorly directed force during external rotation, this is a **relocation sign.**
  - Impingement produces an apprehension sign, but it is not significantly altered by relocation.
- **The posterior apprehension test** is performed by having the patient flex the elbow and elevate the internally rotated shoulder to 90° (hand on opposite shoulder). Posterior force is then applied to the elbow, and apprehension is apparent.

Other Specific Tests
- **Yergason sign** produces pain and tenderness over the bicipital groove with resisted supination of the forearm while the elbow is flexed and held at the side. Passive extension of the shoulder may also reproduce the pain of bicipital tendonitis.
- **Speed test** is thought to identify tendonitis/inflammation of the biceps tendon-superior labral complex. The patient flexes the shoulder against resistance with the elbow extended and the forearm supinated. Pain is noted along the long head of the biceps brachii tendon. Estimated sensitivity and specificity for superior labral tears are 0.32 and 0.61, repectively.[85]
- Rupture of the biceps tendon is evident as the **"Popeye sign,"** a mass of contracted muscle midway between the shoulder and the elbow.

Diagnostic Testing

Plain Radiographs
- Plain radiographs are not necessary or appropriate in the initial evaluation of every patient with shoulder pain, especially if the history and physical examination suggest impingement.
- Nonetheless, they are frequently done and are often nondiagnostic.
- Anteroposterior (AP) views of the GH joint in internal and external rotation and an axillary view are typically done.

- Arthritis of the GH and acromioclavicular joints and calcification of the rotator cuff tendons can be visualized. Osteoarthritis is indicated by joint space narrowing and, in more advanced cases, flattening of the humeral head, subchondral cysts, and marginal osteophytes.
- Detection of shoulder dislocation may require special views.
- Plain films should be obtained in patients who do not appear to be responding to conservative treatment for impingement syndrome.
  - The primary value of a radiograph in this situation is to assess the degree of impingement, based on the vertical distance between the inferior aspect of the acromion and the superior aspect of the humeral head.
  - Normally, the width of a ballpoint pen should "fit" in between the acromion and the humeral head.
  - Narrowing of this space suggests that the patient has chronic rotator cuff disease, in which case response to conservative treatment may be inadequate.
- Diffuse osteopenia is sometimes seen with adhesive capsulitis.

Other Imaging

- **MRI,** or, in some centers, a diagnostic **ultrasound,** can assess the degree of supraspinatus tendon pathology.
- If the tendon is significantly narrowed or partially or completely torn, the patient should be referred to an orthopedist who is experienced in shoulder surgery.

Treatment

Impingement Syndrome

- Treatment goals are to reduce pain and improve shoulder function and ROM.
- The optimal management of impingement syndrome is unclear.
- Methodologically strong trials are limited, and, therefore, it is difficult to provide evidence-based recommendations.
- The individual entities can be difficult to distinguish clinically, often coexist, and can overlap with other shoulder disorders.
- They are usually self-limited, and conservative treatments are generally sufficient. Some cases, however, are resistant to treatment, and recurrences can occur.
- **Relative rest of the shoulder** is reasonable. Patients should avoid activities and movements that aggravate the pain but must not stop moving the shoulder all together.
- **Gentle ROM exercises** are usually recommended to maintain ROM and avoid adhesive capsulitis. Pendulum exercises are easy for patients to do at home and consist of flexing at the waist 90°, supporting the upper body on a low table, and loosely swinging the arm like a pendulum against gravity. The arc of movement is slowly increased over time.
- Referral to **PT** for careful strengthening of the shoulder muscles may be beneficial.[87]
- Evidence is insufficient to clearly support the use of **physiotherapy modalities** (e.g., ultrasound, laser, heat, cold, manipulation, and electrotherapy).[87]
- Application of **heat or ice** may be comforting.
- **NSAIDs** are probably effective for the pain of impingement syndrome.
- **Local corticosteroid injections** (subacromial bursa and rotator cuff region) are also frequently done, but their effectiveness remains unclear.[88–90] Methylprednisolone acetate, 40 mg, is a typical dose. Repeated injections should be avoided. Potential complications of steroid injections include infections, skin atrophy, and tendon

weakening and rupture. Steroid injections may be inadvisable for patients with more than small rotator cuff tears.

- **Referral to an orthopedist** who is experienced in shoulder surgery is appropriate for patients who are potentially accepting of surgery and who have prolonged pain and limitation of function. Early referral should be considered for all patients with moderate-to-large rotator cuff tears.

Other Conditions

- Treatment for **adhesive capsulitis** is generally noninvasive including PT and NSAIDs.
  - Many patients will have resolution over 1 to 2 years.
  - **Corticosteroid injections** directly into the GH joint (usually done under fluoroscopy) may be of some benefit, particularly early in the course. Oral steroids may also provide short-term relief (<6 weeks).[91]
  - Arthroscopic capsular release is sometimes recommended for recalcitrant cases.
- **Osteoarthritis** treatment is also generally conservative, including NSAIDs and PT. Patients with advanced cases may require a total shoulder arthroplasty for pain relief.
- Treatment of **acute shoulder dislocation** is best handled by immediate orthopedic consultation.
- Patients with **chronic GH instability** are treated conservatively with a program of PT and avoiding activities that provoke subluxation. Surgery may be indicated for some young patients and for those with continued intolerable symptoms.

ELBOW PAIN

General Principles

- Elbow pain is a fairly common complaint in the ambulatory setting. In general, only one of a few conditions is causative.
- **Lateral epicondylitis or tendinosis (tennis elbow)** is the most common cause of elbow pain. The condition is caused by chronic overuse of the wrist extensors and supinators that originate from the lateral epicondyle. This results in repetitive microtears and angiofibroblastic degeneration or tendinosis of the origins of these muscles. No significant degree of inflammatory reaction appears to occur.[92]
- **Medial epicondylitis or tendinosis (golfer's elbow)** is very similar to but less common than lateral epicondylitis. It involves overuse and degenerative changes of the tendinous origins of the wrist flexor/pronator muscles at the medial epicondyle.
- **Ulnar nerve entrapment (cubital tunnel syndrome)** results from compression of the ulnar nerve as it passes behind the medial epicondyle through the cubital tunnel, where it is very superficial. Direct pressure, repetitive elbow bending, prolonged elbow flexion, elbow arthritis, diabetes, and certain occupations and activities have all been associated with the condition. A firm direct blow to this area produces the familiar "funny bone" sensation.
- **Olecranon bursitis (student's elbow)** is a common condition that results from acute inflammation of the olecranon bursa. This bursa does not connect with the synovial cavity of the elbow. The cause may be infectious or noninfectious. The most common infectious agent is *Staphylococcus aureus*. Common noninfectious causes include repetitive trauma, gout, pseudogout, and RA. It can be difficult to differentiate an infectious from a noninfectious inflammatory bursitis.

Diagnosis

Clinical Presentation

History

- Patients usually complain of pain but may also report stiffness or swelling, or both.
- A history of acute trauma is important and may suggest fracture, dislocation, or tendon rupture.
- Repetitive overuse is a major cause of elbow pain, and patients should be asked about recreational and occupational activities.
- The specific location of the pain may be the key to proper diagnosis.
- A history of weakness and sensory changes should also be sought.
- Patients with **lateral epicondylitis** complain of lateral elbow pain that worsens with certain activities, usually related to sports (e.g., racquet sports) or other repetitive uses that involve wrist extension and power gripping (e.g., carpentry or lifting with the palm facing down). Symptoms may develop acutely or more slowly. A direct blow to the outside of the elbow can also trigger lateral epicondylitis. Tenderness over the lateral elbow may be reported.
- Patients with **medical epicondylitis** also complain of pain and tenderness but over the medial epicondyle that is worsened by certain activities. It too is often related to sports (golf and throwing activities) and work.
- With **ulnar nerve entrapment,** patients complain of medial elbow pain and sensory changes (numbness and paresthesias) in the ulnar nerve distribution, particularly the fourth and fifth digits. The symptoms may be worse at night. Weakness is sometimes reported.
- **Olecranon bursitis** typically presents with tender painful swelling of the posterior elbow that may develop acutely or more slowly. A history of trauma should be sought.

Physical Examination

- The elbow examination should include inspection, palpation, ROM, and neurologic assessment.
- The point of maximal tenderness should be determined if possible.
- The normal range of extension and flexion is 0° to 140°. Normal supination and pronation are 80° each way.
- The neck, shoulder, and wrist should be examined to evaluate for referred pain.
- With **lateral epicondylitis,** examination of the elbow reveals maximal tenderness over the lateral epicondyle. Resisted wrist extension with the elbow extended often reproduces the pain.
- With **medial epicondylitis,** the tenderness expectedly increases over the medial epicondyle. The pain may be reproduced by resisted wrist flexion.
- **Ulnar entrapment** findings include sensory changes and weakness in the ulnar nerve distribution. Light touch and pinprick sensation are decreased in the ring and little fingers. Tapping the ulnar nerve where it passes behind the medical epicondyle causes pain along the inner elbow and paresthesias in the fourth and fifth digits **(Tinel sign).** Full elbow flexion can produce a similar result **(elbow flexion test).** Reduced grip strength and intrinsic hand muscle weakness may be present. With prolonged nerve compression, atrophy of the intrinsic muscles may be seen.
- With **bursitis,** the exam is most notable for an obvious swelling (goose egg) of the olecranon bursa, which may be quite large. **Infectious and noninfectious causes may be indistinguishable on examination.** Both can present with erythema, tenderness, and warmth. Marked findings are more likely to be traumatic or infectious in origin. Chronic or recurrent bursitis may be nontender.

Diagnostic Testing

- **Plain radiographs** of the elbow typically include the AP and lateral views.
  - In many cases, plain films are nondiagnostic (e.g., lateral and medial epicondylitis).
  - They should probably be done in all patients with significant acute trauma to evaluate for dislocation and fracture.
  - With ulnar nerve entrapment, they are generally unnecessary unless a bony abnormality causing nerve compression is suspected.
  - Special views are sometimes taken to evaluate the olecranon fossa and radial head.
- **CT and MRI** are occasionally indicated for better delineation of the bony and soft tissues.
- **Nerve conduction studies and electromyography** may be useful when the diagnosis of ulnar nerve entrapment is uncertain or surgery is being considered.
- When the olecranon bursa is acutely swollen, **aspiration** of the bursal fluid should be done to evaluate for infection. The fluid should be sent for Gram stain, culture, cell count, and crystal examination. Synovial fluid cell counts in infectious bursitis are generally lower (several thousand cells/mL) than in septic arthritis. The bursal fluid may be obviously bloody in cases of trauma.

Treatment

- Treatment of **lateral epicondylitis** is usually conservative.
  - **Relative rest** (i.e., initially avoiding the activities that cause pain) and NSAIDs are probably useful.
  - A **compressive strap** worn just below the elbow (tennis elbow splint) might be useful but data are contradictory.[93]
  - Some patients find local application of ice comforting.
  - Proper racquet size and backhand technique may also be of value.
  - **Local corticosteroid injection** (e.g., 40 mg methylprednisolone) is an often-recommended alternative for patients who fail to respond to simple measures. It is generally believed to be effective, at least in the short term.[94]
  - Multiple other treatments are available but their effectiveness is uncertain.[93]
  - Surgery is rarely necessary.
- Treatment of **medial epicondylitis** is similar to that of lateral epicondylitis. Local corticosteroid injection may be effective in the short term for those who do not respond to more conservative therapy.
- Treatment of **ulnar nerve entrapment** is also usually conservative.
  - The elbow should be kept straight as much as possible. A **splint** can be worn at night to prevent flexion of the elbow during sleep.
  - If possible, the patient's work environment should be altered to prevent further compression. A cushioning **elbow pad** can be worn to protect the nerve during work.
  - A trial of **NSAIDs** is reasonable for pain.
  - Surgery may be necessary for patients with recalcitrant symptoms.
- Aspiration of the olecranon bursa is not only diagnostic but also therapeutic for **olecranon bursitis.**
  - Fluid reaccumulation is not unusual in noninfectious cases, and repeat aspiration may be necessary. A **compression dressing** can be applied to help prevent recurrence, and an elbow pad can be used to prevent trauma.
  - **NSAIDs** are frequently given.
  - **Injection of 20 mg methylprednisolone** into the bursa may also reduce recurrence in patients with nonseptic olecranon bursitis.[95] Corticosteroid injection is contraindicated in infectious bursitis.

- Empiric **antibiotic treatment** (e.g., dicloxacillin or a cephalosporin) should be given when infection is suspected pending culture results. Daily aspiration is usually necessary for septic bursitis.

WRIST AND HAND PAIN

General Principles

- Wrist and hand complaints are common in primary care. Because of their obvious functional importance, careful diagnosis and treatment are particularly important.
- **Stenosing tenosynovitis** is an inflammation and thickening of tendons, sheaths, and synovium in the hand, sometimes with nodular enlargement of the tendon. It is frequently related to repetitive overuse, particularly those activities that involve gripping.
  - **Trigger finger or thumb** is caused by stenosing tenosynovitis of the flexor tendons of the fingers and thumb.
  - **de Quervain tenosynovitis** is a very similar condition that affects the tendons and sheaths of the abductor pollicis longus and the extensor pollicis brevis.
  - **Dupuytren contracture** is a fibroproliferative disorder that results in painless thickening and nodularity of the palmar aponeurosis. The flexor tendons of the hand are not primarily involved. The fibrosis of the palmar fascia draws the fingers (most commonly the ring and little finger) into flexion at the MCP joint. The condition generally affects men >40 years and appears to have a strong genetic component. It is also associated with diabetes, alcoholism, repetitive trauma, and seizure disorders.
- **Carpal tunnel syndrome** (CTS) is the most frequently occurring entrapment neuropathy.
  - It results from compression of the median nerve as it passes through the carpal tunnel.
  - It is most common in middle-aged women and usually affects the dominant hand.
  - CTS is known to occur with increased frequency in patients with diabetes, amyloidosis, renal failure on hemodialysis, RA and other arthropathies of the wrist, pregnancy, hypothyroidism, and previous wrist trauma. It is often related to repetitive overuse of the hands and wrists.
- **Ulnar nerve entrapment** can occasionally occur at the wrist as the nerve passes through the canal of Guyon. It may be caused by repetitive trauma (e.g., operating a jackhammer, using the hand as a hammer, and resting the ulnar side of the wrist and hand on the edge of a desk or keyboard) or a space-occupying lesion (e.g., ganglion or lipoma).
- **Arthritic conditions** of the wrist and hand are common. **RA** characteristically involves the wrist, metacarpophalangeal (MCP), and proximal interphalangeal joints. The erosive synovitis causes pain, stiffness, deformity, and loss of functionality. **Osteoarthritis** typically involves the distal interphalangeal and carpometacarpal joints (especially of the thumb). See Chapter 28 for a full discussion of the management of these conditions.
- **Infectious causes** of hand/finger pain include **paronychia and felons.** The latter are a more serious infection of the entire distal pulp of the fingertip. The most common organism is *S. aureus.* They are generally caused by a puncture wound to the thumb or index finger.
- **Subungual hematoma** is a very common traumatic cause of finger pain.

Diagnosis

Clinical Presentation

History

- With **trigger finger/thumb,** digit extension is limited when the affected tendon catches on the pulley at the base of the digit. This results in pain with use, and the affected digit can become painfully stuck in flexion. The finger may need to be forcibly extended with the other hand, often with a painful and audible pop.
- Patients with **de Quervain tenosynovitis** complain of pain, tenderness, and swelling on the radial side of the wrist in the region of the anatomic snuffbox. Ulnar deviation of the wrist and movement of the thumb exacerbate the pain, and a "squeaking" or "creaking" sensation may be described.
- Affected patients with **Dupuytren contracture** complain of painless nodules in the palm, an inability to extend the fingers fully, and difficulty in picking up large objects.
- Patients with **CTS** usually complain of an aching pain in the wrist and hand, which may radiate up the forearm. Intermittent paresthesias and numbness in the median nerve distribution (palmar surface of the thumb, index, long, and radial side of the ring fingers) are typical.
  - Less-than-classic descriptions of the location of discomfort are not unusual.
  - Symptoms are frequently worse at night and with overuse of the hands.
  - The patient may describe "shaking out" the hand to improve the symptoms (the "flick sign"). The sensitivity and specificity is low, however.[96]
  - Weakness, clumsiness, and a tendency to drop objects may also be reported.
  - Patients should be questioned about trauma, work-related duties, hobbies, and activities.

Physical Examination

- Palpation at the distal palmar crease in **trigger finger** may reveal a thickened tendon sheath or a tender nodule, or both, usually overlying the MCP joint of the affected finger.
- **Finkelstein sign** is diagnostic for **de Quervain tenosynovitis.** The patient makes a fist enclosing the thumb; if this does not produce pain, the examiner forces the wrist into ulnar deviation as an additional stress. Focal tenderness is usually present over the radial styloid.
- With **Dupuytren contracture,** examination reveals painless thickening and nodularity of the palmar fascia with flexion deformity of one or more fingers.
- In **CTS,** the examination classically reveals decreased sensation (hypalgesia) in the median nerve distribution, weakness of thumb abduction, and **Tinel and Phalen signs.**
  - In Phalen maneuver, the wrists are held in unforced flexion for 30 to 60 seconds. Reproduction or worsening of the symptoms constitutes a positive sign.
  - Tinel sign is the development of paresthesias in the median nerve distribution when the median nerve is tapped at the distal wrist crease.
  - When compared with electrodiagnostic testing, however, Tinel and Phalen signs may have little diagnostic value.[97]
  - Thenar atrophy can occur with long-standing CTS.

Diagnostic Testing

- **Radiographs** of the hands and wrists may provide diagnostic information, particularly if arthritis is suspected.
  - However, definitive changes may not be apparent until the disease has been present for an extended period of time.
  - In cases of significant trauma, plain films are usually mandatory.

- **Electrodiagnostic testing** (median nerve conduction) is generally thought to be the gold standard for CTS, but false positives and false negatives do occur. Such testing should be considered only when the diagnosis is uncertain or surgical treatment is being considered or in cases of work-related compensation.

Treatment

- Treatment of **trigger finger** initially consists of splitting the MCP joint in extension and a short course of NSAIDs. Corticosteroid injection (methylprednisolone, 15 to 20 mg) with lidocaine into the flexor digital tendon sheath can also be effective.[98] Recurrence is common, and surgical release may be required.
- **de Quervain tenosynovitis** treated with a short opponens splint is therapeutic, supplemented by NSAIDs. Refractory cases may respond to corticosteroid injection (methylprednisolone, 20 to 30 mg) with lidocaine.[99] Surgical release is sometimes required.
- Apart from gently stretching the fingers, there is no known effective conservative treatment for **Dupuytren contracture.** Surgical treatment can be considered for the severely affected, but recurrences are common.
- Treatment for **CTS** is likewise initially conservative.
  - Symptoms often improve with a simple **cock-up wrist splint** (worn primarily at night) and a course of **NSAIDs.**[100]
  - Work-related **ergonomic modifications** should be undertaken if necessary.
  - If these simple measures fail, the patient can be referred for a single **corticosteroid injection** (40 mg methylprednisolone) with lidocaine (10 mg) into the area close to the carpal tunnel, which may be more effective for up to 4 weeks.[101]
  - Definitive treatment entails **surgical release,** a simple outpatient procedure in which the flexor retinaculum is incised, relieving the pressure on the median nerve. Surgery is very effective in treating CTS, provided that the diagnosis has been confirmed electrodiagnostically and is more effective than splinting.[102]

HIP PAIN

General Principles

- Hip pain has many potential causes but only a few are common.
- Pain may emanate from the hip joint, periarticular soft tissues, pelvic bones, and sacroiliac joint or be referred from another location (usually the lumbosacral spine).
- **Osteoarthritis** of the hip joint is very common and increases with age. It is characterized by loss of the articular cartilage of the joint. Predisposing factors include childhood hip disorders, leg-length anomalies, and work that involves heavy lifting and carrying. The diagnosis and treatment of osteoarthritis is discussed in Chapter 28.
- **Trochanteric bursitis** is another common cause of hip pain. It can occur in association with iliotibial band syndrome, hip joint pathology, previous hip surgery, leg-length discrepancy, and mechanical back pain.
- **Avascular necrosis (osteonecrosis, AVN)** is the death of a variable amount of trabecular bone in the femoral head.
  - The precise pathophysiology is not known, but it is unusual in the absence of known risk factors, which include corticosteroid treatment (especially in those

with lupus), alcoholism, trauma or prior fracture, RA, sickle cell disease, myeloproliferative disorders, and radiation.

- A high index of suspicion should be maintained in patients with these risk factors. The condition may be bilateral.
- Severe AVN can cause collapse to the femoral head.
- **Meralgia paresthetica** is an entrapment neuropathy caused by compression of the lateral femoral cutaneous nerve. It may be related to one or more factors, including obesity, pregnancy, diabetes, wearing tight garments around the waist (e.g., pantyhose, tool belts), local surgery, trauma, repetitive hip extension (joggers, cheerleaders who do splits frequently), and, rarely, intrapelvic masses.
- **Hip fractures** are particularly common in elderly women and usually occur at the femoral neck or the intertrochanteric area. They are associated with a high morbidity and mortality. Age, Caucasian race, female sex, osteoporosis, and falls are common predisposing factors.

Diagnosis

Clinical Presentation

History

- Patients typically complain of painful limited ROM and difficulty in ambulating.
- The location of the pain can be the key to proper diagnosis.
  - True hip joint pain usually affects the groin and radiates to the buttock. Bearing weight worsens the pain.
  - Buttock pain alone without groin pain is likely to originate in the low back, sacroiliac joint, or ischial tuberosity.
  - Lateral proximal thigh pain suggests trochanteric bursitis.
  - Anteriolateral thigh pain suggests lateral femoral cutaneous nerve entrapment.
  - Pain that radiates down the posterior thigh is frequently due to lumbosacral radiculopathy.
- Patients with chronic progressive disease have increasing difficulty in ambulating and performing the activities of daily living.
- Patients with **trochanteric bursitis** complain of lateral hip pain that may radiate down the leg. The pain is worse with exercise and at night, especially when the patient lies on the affected side. Some patients complain of a limp.
- **AVN** pain tends to come on suddenly and can be severe, but the onset can be more gradual. A few patients may be asymptomatic. The pain is typically in the groin radiating to the buttocks and is increased with weight bearing.
- **Meralgia paresthetica** is remarkable for pain, burning, and dysesthesia in the groin and anterolateral thigh. The discomfort may extend to the lateral knee. No motor symptoms occur.
- Most patients with **hip fracture** report a fall and subsequent inability to walk. They have pain in the groin that radiates to the buttocks. A few patients may be able to walk with assistance, but pain increases with weight bearing.

Physical Examination

- The patient should be observed **standing and walking.**
- A limp or expression of pain may be demonstrative of the patient's complaint.
- The **abductor lurch (Trendelenburg gait)** suggests intra-articular hip pathology. The patient shifts weight over the affected leg to unload weakened abductors.

- The **Trendelenburg test** should be done. Ask the standing patient to raise the knee on the unaffected side so that weight is borne on the affected side. Normally, the pelvis elevates on the raised-knee side. A drop in the pelvis on the raised-knee side suggests weakness of the hip abductors on the straight-knee (affected) side.
- **Patrick test, or the FABERE sign** (flexion-abduction-external rotation-extension), is performed by placing the supine patient's heel on the contralateral knee. The examiner then pushes the knee and thigh downward to put the hip into external rotation, producing pain in intrinsic hip disease.
- **Palpation** of the hip joint and surrounding area is done to elicit tenderness.
- **ROM** should be tested. Normal hip flexion is approximately 120°; normal internal rotation is 30° and external rotation 60°. Hip joint pathology tends to affect internal rotation most.
- **Strength** of the adductors, abductors, and flexors should be tested. The lumbar spine and the sacroiliac joints should be examined.
- The groin is examined, looking for evidence of an inguinal or femoral hernia.
- Local tenderness over the trochanteric prominence can be demonstrated with **trochanteric bursitis** and hip ROM should be unrestricted.
- With **AVN,** internal and external rotation of the hip is painful and sometimes reduced. The patient often has a limp.
- Examination in **meralgia paresthetica** usually reveals hypoesthesia or dysesthesia, or both, in the lateral femoral cutaneous nerve distribution. Examination of the hip is normal unless coexistent hip pathology is present.
- **Hip fracture** classically reveals an externally rotated, abducted, and foreshortened leg. Ecchymosis or hematoma formation may be present at the hip.

Diagnostic Testing

- **Plain radiographs,** when indicated, should include AP and lateral views of the hip and an AP view of the pelvis.
- **CT or MRI** is occasionally needed to evaluate the hip further (e.g., occult hip fractures and osteonecrosis).
- Films in **AVN** may show sclerosis of the femoral head. Collapse of the femoral head is seen in advanced cases. If initial radiographs are normal, an MRI should be considered because of its high sensitivity for this diagnosis.
- **Hip fractures** are usually obvious, but plain films are occasionally negative. A bone scan, CT scan, or MRI may be necessary for diagnosis.

Treatment

- **Trochanteric bursitis** is slow to respond to therapy but almost never becomes chronic.
  - **NSAIDs** often provide symptomatic relief, and **PT** for modalities and iliotibial band stretching can be helpful. Patients should be encouraged to continue with stretching exercises at home.
  - A **corticosteroid injection** (30 to 40 mg methylprednisolone) with local anesthetic (3 mL/1% lidocaine) into the greater trochanteric bursa usually brings at least temporary relief.[103,104]
  - Care should be taken to avoid a fluorinated corticosteroid preparation such as triamcinolone acetonide or hexacetonide, because these can result in atrophy of the skin and subcutaneous fat.
- Limited weight bearing with a cane or walker may be sufficient for some patient with **AVN,** but orthopedic consultation should always be obtained to evaluate the

need for surgical core decompression or total hip arthroplasty. If corticosteroid therapy remains necessary, efforts should be made to reduce the dose as much as possible.

- For **meralgia paresthetica,** treatment consists of eliminating the source of nerve compression or repetitive trauma. Weight loss in obese patients can be effective.
- Treatment of **hip fractures** is almost always surgical, and an orthopedic consultation is mandatory. A patient with an osteoporotic fracture should have bone density measured by dual x-ray absorptiometry as a baseline and should be started on medications to increase bone density and decrease the risk of subsequent fracture (Chapter 37).

KNEE PAIN

General Principles

- With normal use, the knee is subject to considerable wear and tear and is vulnerable to injury (often sports related). As such, knee pain is a common complaint.
- Degenerative disease, trauma, and inflammatory processes are the most frequent causes.

Etiology

- **Osteoarthritis** of the knee is an extremely common condition and an important source of disability.
  - Important associations include age, wear and tear, obesity, genetic factors, prior trauma (e.g., fractures, ligamentous injuries that cause instability, and meniscal damage), and prior knee surgery. Osteoarthritis may affect any or all of the three compartments of the knee (medial and lateral tibiofemoral, patellofemoral).
  - The medial compartment is the most commonly involved.
  - The diagnosis and treatment of osteoarthritis is discussed in Chapter 28.
- The **inflammatory conditions** can be divided into **noninfectious and infectious** causes.
  - Noninfectious causes include **RA, lupus, psoriatic arthritis, Reiter syndrome, gout, and pseudogout.**
  - The most common infectious causes are **gonococcal arthritis** (especially in sexually active young adults) and **S. aureus.** Extra-articular infections, previous damage to the joint, prosthetic joints, serious underlying chronic illness, immunosuppression, corticosteroid therapy, and IV drug use are predisposing factors for septic arthritis.
  - The treatment inflammatory arthropathies is discussed in Chapter 28.
- **Patellofemoral pain syndrome** (PFPS) is characterized by retropatellar or peripatellar pain and crepitation with certain activities.
  - The condition is ill defined and poorly understood, but nonetheless **anterior knee pain** of this type is very common and may become chronic and limit activity.
  - Multiple associations and predisposing factors have been proposed, including overuse/overloading, maltracking of the patella, patellar subluxation, obesity, malalignment of the knee-extensor mechanism, quadriceps weakness, and trauma. Many patients, however, have no such associations.
  - The relationship of PFPS to chondromalacia of the patella is controversial. PFPS can occur without chondromalacia, and patients with chondromalacia may have no symptoms.[105]
- **Ligamentous injuries** are generally seen after trauma in athletic young adults. These injuries comprise a spectrum from torn and stretched ligamentous fibers to complete tear or rupture. Collateral and cruciate ligament injuries can occur alone or together, with or without meniscal damage.

- **Meniscal tears** typically occur after a **twisting injury,** and the medial meniscus is much more commonly affected. This type of injury can occur in isolation or with a medial collateral or anterior cruciate ligament (ACL) tear, or both. Older individuals may experience a degenerative meniscal tear after minimal trauma.
- **Bursitis** can occur at several locations in the knee. Bursae are synovially lined and produce a small amount of fluid that decreases friction between adjacent structures. Chronic overuse, trauma, and friction can result in inflammation.
  - **Prepatellar bursitis** is usually caused by repeated trauma involving a lot of kneeling (e.g., "housemaid's knee" and "clergyman's knee").
  - The **pes anserine bursa** lies under the insertion of the hamstrings on the proximal medial tibia. It can become inflamed with overuse (e.g., walking or running) and in those with osteoarthritis of the knee.
- **Baker cyst** (popliteal cyst or semimembranosus-gastrocnemius bursitis) is a fluid-filled sac located in the popliteal fossa, usually on the medial side. It frequently connects with the joint cavity. It is often associated with knee effusions, posterior meniscal tears, and degenerative arthropathy.[106] It is also very common in RA.[107]
- **Iliotibial band friction syndrome** is a common overuse injury in runners and cyclists. Repetitive movement of a tight iliotibial over the lateral femoral condyle causes friction and pain, particularly with climbing stairs and running down hills.
- **Tibial tubercle apophysitis (Osgood-Schlatter disease)** generally presents in adolescents, with pain localized to the insertion of the patellar tendon at the tibial tubercle. It is often related to an ossicle of bone within the tibial tendon anterior to the tubercle. Pain usually resolves with time when the ossicle fuses with the underlying bone. Until that time, pain should limit athletic activity.

Diagnosis

Clinical Presentation

History
- Knee disorders usually present with one or more of the following: pain, stiffness, swelling, redness, warmth, tenderness, giving way, locking, and cracking.
- Acute knee pain is often traumatic, and the mechanism of injury should be detailed. An audible pop is sometimes heard. Subacute and chronic knee discomfort is also common.
- The possibility of septic arthritis (discussed in detail in Chapter 28) should always be considered with acute monoarticular arthritis of the knee.
- Patients should be carefully asked about exacerbating activities, sports, and prior episodes of trauma.
- A history of pain in the contralateral knee or other joints, or both, can be important.
- Inflammatory conditions characteristically present with a large effusion and morning stiffness that improves with activity.
- With mechanical causes, pain is typically worsened with activity and improved with rest.
- **PFPS** patients complain of anterior knee pain with activities such as going down steps or hills, squatting, running, jumping, and prolonged sitting (the "theater sign").
- **ACL tears** are usually caused by a significant **twisting injury.** A popping sensation may be described. Pain is immediate, quickly followed by the development of a large effusion, giving way, and great difficulty in walking.
- **Collateral ligament tears** usually follow an **abduction or adduction force** (medial or lateral collateral ligaments, respectively). These patients complain of pain, stiffness, and localized swelling. Most are able to ambulate after the injury.

- With **meniscal injuries,** patients usually report pain, swelling, and stiffness after a significant twisting injury. Pain may be referred to the popliteal area. Clicking, locking, or giving way may also be described. Most patients are able to walk after the injury.
- Many **Baker cysts** are asymptomatic, but swelling, tenderness, and fullness behind the knee may be reported. Very large cysts can cause significant pain and even neurovascular compromise because of the pressure on surrounding structures. Some cysts become symptomatic only when they rupture, producing redness, swelling, warmth, pain, and tenderness of the calf, which can be confused with a deep venous thrombosis.

Physical Examination
- Physical examination of the knee includes inspection, palpation, ROM, strength, and gait. Acute knee inflammation may make adequate examination difficult or impossible. Normal flexion of the knee is 135° and extension is 0°.
- The **bulge sign** can be used to detect **small knee effusions.**
  - The patient's knee is extended flat on the examination table.
  - Joint fluid is milked up into the suprapatellar pouch by moving the hand proximally along the medial side of the patella.
  - The fluid is then milked down into the medial knee by moving the hand from above the lateral side of the patella along the lateral knee and down to the tibia.
  - Excessive fluid creates a bulge medial to the patella.
- The **anterior drawer test** and **Lachman test** are used to test for **cruciate ligament instability.** Both knees should be tested for comparison.
  - The anterior drawer test is performed with the patient supine and the knee flexed to 90°. The tibia is grasped with both hands and pulled anteriorly.
  - Lachman test is performed with the supine patient's knee in 20° of flexion. The distal femur is stabilized with one hand while the other hand pulls the tibia forward.
  - Excessive anterior displacement of the tibia and a less than sharp end point suggest ACL damage.
  - Lachman test is generally believed to be the more sensitive test but the combination of both tests may be better still.[108,109]
- **Stability of the collateral ligaments** should be tested in 20° to 30° of flexion and full extension. One hand stabilizes the lateral side of the knee, while the other hand applies abduction force to the distal leg, or one hand stabilizes the medial side of the knee, while the other hand applies adduction force to the distal leg. Excessive motion, usually with pain, signifies medial or collateral ligament damage.
- **McMurray test** can be used to detect meniscal tears. With the supine patient's knee in full flexion, the knee is slowly extended as the tibia is rotated internally and externally. A palpable or audible pop, often with pain, suggests a meniscal tear. This test is insensitive but fairly specific.[109] Combining McMurray test with **joint line tenderness** may improve diagnostic ability.[108,110]
- The examination with **osteoarthritis** often reveals tenderness along the joint line, a small effusion, crepitus during knee motion, and sometimes palpable osteophytes. Patients with significant medial compartment disease often have a varus (bowleg) deformity when standing. Less commonly, a valgus (knock-knee) deformity may occur with lateral compartment disease.
- With **PFPS,** crepitus and malalignment of the patella with flexion and extension (patella tracks too far laterally) can sometimes be appreciated. Some quadriceps atrophy may also be present. A knee effusion is infrequently seen.

TABLE 5	Ottawa Knee Rules

Obtain radiographs when any of the following factors are present:
Age >55
Tenderness at head of fibula
Isolated tenderness of patella
Inability to flex knee to 90°

Modified from Stiell IG, Wells GA, Hoag RH, et al. Implementation of the Ottawa Knee Rule for the use of radiography in acute knee injuries. *JAMA* 1997;278:2075–2079.

- The **patellar compression test** supports the diagnosis. The examiner immobilizes the patella while the patient contracts the quadriceps muscle, pulling the patella proximally against the femoral condyles, reproducing the pain.
- The **prepatellar bursa** lies between the skin and the patella. It produces swelling directly above the patella. There may also be redness and warmth suggesting an infectious process.
- With **pes anserine bursitis,** pain occurs on the anteromedial aspect of the knee, and the area is exquisitely tender.
- A **Baker cyst** may be appreciated as a prominence in the medial aspect of the popliteal fossa. In the situation of a ruptured cyst, inflammation of the calf occurs, potentially simulating thrombophlebitis.

Diagnostic Testing

- **Plain radiographs** of the knee are frequently done as a part of the evaluation of knee pain, but they are not always necessary.
- If the history and physical examination suggest a periarticular problem, plain films are unlikely to be diagnostic and are generally unnecessary.
- When a significant mechanical articular problem is suggested by the history and physical examination, plain films may be helpful.
- The **Ottawa knee rules** can be used to determine which patients with acute knee injuries require knee films (Table 5).[109,111]
- Standard films include AP and lateral views, and standing films should be obtained if possible.
- Detection of some fractures by plain radiography may require special views.
- With **PFPS**, radiographs of the patella (Merchant view) may show malalignment of the patella but are usually normal.
- **Ligamentous and meniscal damage** cannot be diagnosed with plain films but can be done to evaluate for avulsion fractures.
- **MRI** detects meniscal tears but false positives can occur.
- Ultrasound can be used to visualize a **Baker cyst** and evaluate for thrombophlebitis of the leg. MRI can also be used to visualize a Baker cyst.

Treatment

- **Septic arthritis** demands swift and aggressive treatment to minimize joint destruction.
  - Unless there is an established diagnosis of noninfectious cause, strong consideration should be given to admission for empiric antibiotics until the synovial fluid cultures are negative.

- Definitive treatment of septic arthritis includes IV antibiotics (agent and duration determined by culture results), serial joint aspiration, and occasionally surgical drainage.
- For **PFPS,** relative rest, PT, acetaminophen, NSAIDs, and ice are reasonable treatment options for most patients. Quadriceps training is generally believed to be of potential value. Knee taping and knee braces are advocated by some. Surgery may be appropriate for a few patients (e.g., those with serious chondromalacia or marked patellar maltracking or subluxation).
- If **ligamentous injury** is suspected, referral to an orthopedist or sports medicine specialist should be obtained. Initial conservative treatment includes rest, ice, compression, elevation, NSAIDs, crutches, and a knee brace. More specific treatment and possible surgical intervention should be directed by the orthopedic consultant.
- Orthopedic consultation is reasonable for most patients with a **meniscal tear.** Many patients heal with conservative treatment, which includes rest, ice, compression, elevation, NSAIDs, and gradual return to activity. Surgery should be reserved for patients who continue to have pain or locking, or both. In the presence of osteoarthritis of the knee, surgical treatment for a torn meniscus may actually lead to an intensification of knee pain, necessitating a total knee arthroplasty.
- Patients with noninfectious **prepatellar bursitis** can be managed conservatively with avoidance of the inciting trauma, ice, and NSAIDs. When infection is likely or confirmed, antibiotic administration should be combined with daily aspiration of the bursa to be sure that the cell count falls and the Gram stain and culture become negative with treatment. Patients who are systemically ill should be admitted to the hospital for IV antibiotics. Surgical incision and drainage are rarely necessary.
- For **pes anserine bursitis,** conservative treatment with relative rest, ice, and NSAIDs is frequently helpful. Local corticosteroid injection may also be effective.
- Mild to moderately symptomatic unruptured **Baker cysts** can be treated with as-needed acetaminophen or NSAIDs. Some advocate knee joint aspiration (sometimes with corticosteroid injection) as effective treatment for more symptomatic individuals. Surgical treatment may be useful for a small number of patients. Ruptured cysts can be treated with relative rest, elevation, heat, and NSAIDs.

ANKLE AND FOOT DISORDERS

- Ankle and foot problems are frequently encountered in the ambulatory setting. They are often related to mechanical abnormalities or inappropriate footwear.
- The most common complaint is pain, and precise localization of the pain can be very important diagnostically.
- Medical history (e.g., diabetes mellitus, gout, RA, vascular disease, and neuropathy), exacerbating and alleviating factors, chronicity, association with trauma, athletic and work activities, and footwear may provide valuable clues.
- If possible, patients should be observed standing and walking with and without shoes. The shoes should be observed for type (e.g., severely pointed high heels) and unusual wear. ROM and inflammation of the joints should be assessed. Normal ankle dorsiflexion is 15° and plantar flexion is 55°. Normal heel inversion is 35° and eversion is 20°.
- One should take note of corns, calluses, ulcerations, and the appearance of the nails.
- Circulation and sensation should be evaluated.

ANKLE PAIN

General Principles

- **Ankle sprains** are one of the most common injuries encountered.
  - They are typically caused by inversion injuries and, therefore, usually involve the lateral ligaments.
  - The severity of sprains can range from minimal to quite severe.
  - Chronic ankle instability and recurrent injury after an ankle sprain is not uncommon.
- **Primary osteoarthritis of the tibiotalar (ankle) joint is rare,** but secondary osteoarthritis may develop after trauma or an inflammatory arthropathy such as RA.
- An ankle effusion suggests inflammatory arthritis, sarcoidosis, gout, or infection and should be aspirated to establish a diagnosis.

Diagnosis

- Ankle sprain patients usually report a trip or fall that results in forced inversion of the ankle. Eversion injuries do occur but are much less common.
- Swelling, tenderness, and painful ambulation are common. Some patients have severe pain and possibly an inability to walk.
- **Examination** is notable for swelling, tenderness, and sometimes ecchymosis over the lateral collateral ligaments (deltoid ligament for an eversion injury). Swelling may extend to involve the entire ankle. The medial and lateral malleoli should be palpated for tenderness. Discomfort with attempted manual inversion is obvious. Weight bearing may or may not be possible.
- **Plain radiographs** of the ankle are not always necessary and are often overused. The **Ottawa ankle rules** (Table 6) can be successfully used to determine when ankle films to evaluate for fracture are necessary.[112]

Treatment

- Treatment for most ankle sprains is conservative, consisting of rest, ice, compression, elevation, and NSAIDs. An air stirrup-type ankle brace can be used for added support. As tolerated, weight bearing is permissible, but some patients require crutches.
- When the patient can bear weight without pain, increased activity can begin. Continued use of an air stirrup brace should be encouraged.
- Organized PT for ankle strengthening after a sprain may be beneficial.

TABLE 6	Ottawa Ankle Rules

Obtain radiographs with any pain in the malleolar zone and if any of the following are present:
Bony tenderness at the posterior edge or tip of the lateral malleolus
Bony tenderness at the posterior edge or tip of the medial malleolus
Inability to bear weight immediately and in the emergency department

Modified from Stiell IG, McKnight RD, Greenberg GH, et al. Implementation of the Ottawa ankle rules. *JAMA* 1994;271:827–832.

- Severe sprains require more intensive treatment, and an orthopedic consultation should be obtained for these patients.
- Use of an ankle support (semirigid orthosis or air stirrup) during sporting activities can reduce the risk of a recurrent sprain.[113]

HEEL PAIN

General Principles

- **Plantar fasciitis** is the most common cause of plantar heel pain.
  - It is a painful inflammation of the insertion of the plantar fascia into the calcaneus.
  - Plantar fasciitis is more common with a pronated foot and a flattened longitudinal arch, obesity, and excessive walking.
  - Although it is usually an isolated problem, its presence may be a clue to a spondyloarthropathy such as Reiter syndrome.
- **Achilles tendonitis** is a painful inflammatory condition of the Achilles tendon at or just proximal to its insertion onto the calcaneus.
  - It usually affects young athletic individuals (e.g., runners and dancers).
  - In older patients, degenerative changes in the tendon may be causative.
  - Inflammation in this enthesis may also indicate a spondyloarthropathy, such as ankylosing spondylitis or Reiter syndrome.
  - Complete Achilles tendon rupture occasionally occurs.

Diagnosis

- With **plantar fasciitis,** patients complain of pain under the heel, particularly when first rising in the morning or after a period of non–weight bearing. Physical examination discloses point tenderness over the plantar fascia insertion and for a short distance along the fascia.
- **Achilles tendonitis** is notable for the insidious onset of pain in the Achilles tendon that is typically worsened by activity. Patients sometimes report a "squeaking" or "creaking" during plantar flexion. Physical examination may reveal thickening and tenderness of the Achilles tendon. A protuberant posterolateral bony process of the calcaneus may also be present. "Pump bumps" (localized soft tissue swelling) may occur where the shoe contacts the posterior heel.
- Radiographs are generally unnecessary for either condition. **The actual clinical significance of heel spurs is uncertain.** Those with them may not have plantar fasciitis and those with plantar fasciitis may not have them.

Treatment

- Treatment of **plantar fasciitis** is almost always conservative and consists of a cushioning heel insert (can be purchased over the counter), NSAIDs, ice, and Achilles and plantar-stretching exercises.
  - Conservative treatment may require several weeks to months to be significantly effective.
  - Dorsiflexion night splints may be effective for some patients.[114]
  - Local corticosteroid injections are sometimes used; however, there is only very limited quality evidence to support the use of this therapy.[114]

- Data regarding the efficacy of extracorporeal shock wave therapy are conflicting.
- A very few patients require more aggressive treatment and can be referred to a **podiatrist** or **orthopedic surgeon** if symptoms persist after prolonged conservative management.
- Treatment for **Achilles tendonitis** is also usually conservative and often includes relative rest, heel lifts, ice, stretching exercises, and NSAIDs.
  - Corticosteroid injections are contraindicated because of the increased risk of tendon rupture.
  - Patients who are unresponsive to conservative management may benefit from an orthopedic or sports medicine consultation.

MID- AND FOREFOOT PAIN

General Principles

- **Hallux valgus** is the most common great-toe malady and is characterized by the lateral movement of the first metatarsophalangeal (MTP) joint.
  - The medial head of the first metatarsal enlarges with bony hypertrophy, and the bursa over it becomes inflamed as a **"bunion."**
  - A marked female predominance is seen, probably because of constricting footwear; there may also be a hereditary predisposition.
  - A similar condition may affect the lateral foot and fifth MTP joint and lead to "bunionette" formation.
- **Hallux rigidus** entails pain and stiffness of the osteoarthritic first MTP, which must extend with each step. It usually affects older individuals.
- **Metatarsalgia** is a general term for pain under one or more of the metatarsal heads.
  - It typically occurs when the pronated forefoot spreads out, and the second, third, and fourth metatarsal heads begin to bear weight with resultant callus formation.
  - It may also be secondary to claw toe deformities (with distal migration of the plantar fat pad and subsequent exposure of the metatarsal heads) and cavus foot.
- **Morton neuroma** is characterized by pain in the web space between the third and fourth toes and is caused by compression on the interdigital nerve at this location.
- **Gout,** and less commonly **pseudogout,** can present as acute inflammation of the first MTP joint **(podagra).** Management of crystalline arthropathies is discussed in Chapter 28.
- **Stress fractures** (fatigue fractures) of the metatarsals occur as a result of repetitive overuse. They are common in runners and dancers, and a recent increase in the level of activity is common. The second and third metatarsals are most commonly affected.
- **Pes planus (flat feet)** per se is not always symptomatic, but chronically pronated feet often lead to pain and further deformity.
  - Flat feet may be related to multiple different foot problems, particularly **posterior tibial tendon dysfunction,** which is a common, but underdiagnosed, cause of ankle pain and foot deformity.
  - This is characterized by sudden or progressive loss of strength of the posterior tibialis tendon with secondary progressive **flatfoot deformity.**
  - The deformity is initially reversible but can become permanent.
  - Multiple etiologies are possible, including **avulsion/rupture** of the tendon (usually traumatic), **partial tendon tear** and elongation, and **tendonitis.**

Diagnosis

- With **hallux valgus,** patients complain of pain, swelling, and deformity that are aggravated by shoe wearing. Numbness over the medial aspect of the great toe may also be reported. Examination reveals medial deviation of the first metatarsal head and lateral deviation of the great toe phalanges. Impingement of the other toes is often present and the second toe may override the great toe. Bunion formation is frequent, and there may be ulceration of the overlying skin.
- Restricted dorsiflexion of the first MTP is characteristic of **hallux rigidus** on examination.
- **Metatarsalgia** pain is often concentrated at the second metatarsal head.
- Plantar pain and dysesthesia of the affected toes are typical of **Morton neuroma.** Walking and high-heeled, constrictive shoes worsen the symptoms. Squeezing the metatarsal heads may reproduce the discomfort.
- A **stress fracture** presents as sudden or gradual onset of pain occurs in the forefoot near the metatarsals, which can be tender.
- Plain radiographs can show the characteristic bony displacement of hallux valgus and typical osteoarthritic changes of hallux rigidus.
- Stress fractures are not detectable with plain radiographs during the first 2 weeks, but after that callus may be seen. A bone scan is positive within the first week. MRI can detect very early stress fractures but is not usually required.

Treatment

- A shoe with a wide toe box is critical for symptom relief of **hallux valgus,** sometimes supplemented by an insole. Surgical treatment may be appropriate in patients who are unresponsive to conservative measures.
- A sole stiffener, such as a steel shank, reduces motion of the MTP joint and therefore reduces pain of **hallux rigidus.** A rocker-bottom sole can be used; however, it produces a gait that is difficult to get used to. Surgical arthrodesis, without a prosthetic implant, may be effective if conservative measures fail.
- Relief from **metatarsalgia** can often be provided with a metatarsal pad, inserted into the shoe such that weight bearing occurs proximal to the metatarsal heads. In the presence of coexisting foot problems, such as pronation or osteoarthritis, it may be better to order a full-contact, custom-molded insole into which a metatarsal pad can be incorporated.
- Properly fitting footwear with low heels can reduce pain of **Morton neuroma.** A metatarsal pad may also be effective. Some authorities advocate local corticosteroid injection. Surgery may be effective for patients who are unresponsive to conservative treatment.
- **Stress fractures** call for conservative treatment: rest, ice, and NSAIDs. Stiff-soled shoes should be worn. Patients who do not respond may need immobilization.

REFERENCES

1. Bogduk N, Teasell R. Whiplash: the evidence for an organic etiology. *Arch Neurol* 2000;57:590–591.
2. Peloso P, Gross A, Haines T, et al.; Cervical Overview Group. Medicinal and injection therapies for mechanical neck disorders. *Cochrane Database Syst Rev* 2007;(3):CD000319.
3. Gross AR, Hoving JL, Haines TA, et al.; Cervical Overview Group. Manipulation and mobilisation for mechanical neck disorders. *Cochrane Database Syst Rev* 2004;(1): CD004249.

4. Kay TM, Gross A, Goldsmith C, et al.; Cervical Overview Group. Exercises for mechanical neck disorders. *Cochrane Database Syst Rev* 2005;(3):CD004250.
5. Kroeling P, Gross A, Houghton PE; Cervical Overview Group. Electrotherapy for neck disorders. *Cochrane Database Syst Rev* 2005;(2):CD004251.
6. Trinh KV, Graham N, Gross AR, et al.; Cervical Overview Group. Acupuncture for neck disorders. *Cochrane Database Syst Rev* 2006;3:CD004870.
7. Graham N, Gross A, Goldsmith CH, et al. Mechanical traction for neck pain with or without radiculopathy. *Cochrane Database Syst Rev* 2008;(3):CD006408.
8. Haraldsson BG, Gross AR, Myers CD, et al.; Cervical Overview Group. Massage for mechanical neck disorders. *Cochrane Database Syst Rev* 2006;3:CD004871.
9. Verhagen AP, Scholten-Peeters GG, van Wijngaarden S, et al. Conservative treatments for whiplash. *Cochrane Database Syst Rev* 2007;(2):CD003338.
10. Lord SM, Barnsley L, Wallis BJ, et al. Percutaneous radio-frequency neurotomy for chronic cervical zygapophyseal-joint pain. *N Engl J Med* 1996;335:1721–1726.
11. Niemisto L, Kalso E, Malmivaara A, et al. Radiofrequency denervation for neck and back pain. A systematic review of randomized controlled trials. *Cochrane Database Syst Rev* 2003;(1):CD004058.
12. Pettersson K, Toolanen G. High-dose methylprednisolone prevents extensive sick leave after whiplash injury. A prospective, randomized, double-blind study. *Spine (Phila Pa 1976)* 1998;23:984–989.
13. Slipman CW, Lipetz JS, Jackson HB, et al. Therapeutic selective nerve root block in the nonsurgical treatment of atraumatic cervical spondylotic radicular pain: a retrospective analysis with independent clinical review. *Arch Phys Med Rehabil* 2000;81:741–746.
14. Leboeuf-Yde C. Smoking and low back pain. A systematic literature review of 41 journal articles reporting 47 epidemiologic studies. *Spine (Phila Pa 1976)* 1999;24:1463–1470.
15. Goldberg MS, Scott SC, Mayo NE. A review of the association between cigarette smoking and the development of nonspecific back pain and related outcomes. *Spine (Phila Pa 1976)* 2000;25:995–1014.
16. Mikkonen P, Leino-Arjas P, Remes J, et al. Is smoking a risk factor for low back pain in adolescents? A prospective cohort study. *Spine (Phila Pa 1976)* 2008;33:527–532.
17. Deyo RA, Weinstein JN. Low back pain. *N Engl J Med* 2001;344:363–370.
18. Zhou Y, Abdi S. Diagnosis and minimally invasive treatment of lumbar discogenic pain—a review of the literature. *Clin J Pain* 2006;22:468–481.
19. Cohen SP, Raja SN. Pathogenesis, diagnosis, and treatment of lumbar zygapophysial (facet) joint pain. *Anesthesiology* 2007;106:591–614.
20. Cohen SP. Sacroiliac joint pain: a comprehensive review of anatomy, diagnosis, and treatment. *Anesth Analg* 2005;101:1440–1453.
21. Foley BS, Buschbacher RM. Sacroiliac joint pain: anatomy, biomechanics, diagnosis, and treatment. *Am J Phys Med Rehabil* 2006;85:997–1006.
22. Clinical Practice Guideline Number 14: Acute Low Back Problems in Adults: Assessment and Treatment. Rockville, MD: US Department of Health and Human Services, Agency for Healthcare Policy and Research; 1994. Publication 95–0643.
23. Henschke N, Maher CG, Refshauge KM, et al. Prevalence of and screening for serious spinal pathology in patients presenting to primary care settings with acute low back pain. *Arthritis Rheum* 2009;60:3072–3080.
24. Deyo RA, Rainville J, Kent DL. What can the history and physical examination tell us about low back pain. *JAMA* 1992;268:760–765.
25. Bakker EW, Verhagen AP, van Trijffel E, et al. Spinal mechanical load as a risk factor for low back pain: a systematic review of prospective cohort studies. *Spine (Phila Pa 1976)* 2009;34:E281–E293.
26. Hoogendoorn WE, van Poppel MN, Bongers PM, et al. Systematic review of psychosocial factors at work and private life as risk factors for back pain. *Spine (Phila Pa 1976)* 2000;25:2114–2125.
27. Pincus T, Burton AK, Vogel S, et al. A systematic review of psychological factors as predictors of chronicity/disability in prospective cohorts of low back pain. *Spine (Phila Pa 1976)* 2002;27:E109–E120.

28. Pincus T, Vlaeyen JW, Kendall NA, et al. Cognitive-behavioral therapy and psychosocial factors in low back pain: directions for the future. *Spine (Phila Pa 1976)* 2002;27: E133–E138.

29. Klenerman L, Slade PD, Stanley IM, et al. The prediction of chronicity in patients with an acute attack of low back pain in a general practice setting. *Spine (Phila Pa 1976)* 1995;20:478–484.

30. Pincus T, Vogel S, Burton AK, et al. Fear avoidance and prognosis in back pain: a systematic review and synthesis of current evidence. *Arthritis Rheum* 2006;54:3999–4010.

31. Kendall NAS, Linton SJ, Main CJ. Guide to Assessing Psychosocial Yellow Flags in Acute Low Back Pain: Risk Factors for Long-Term Disability and Work Loss. Wellington, NZ: ACC and The National Health Committee (www.acc.co.nz), 1997.

32. Vroomen PC, de Krom MC, Knottnerus JA. Diagnostic value of history and physical examination in patients suspect of sciatica due to disc herniation: a systematic review. *J Neurol* 1999;246:899 906.

33. Waddell G, McCulloch JA, Kummel E, Venner RM. Nonorganic physical signs in low-back pain. *Spine (Phila Pa 1976)* 1980;5:117–125.

34. Fishbain DA, Cutler RB, Rosomoff HL, Rosomoff RS. Is there a relationship between nonorganic physical findings (Waddell signs) and secondary gain/ malingering? *Clin J Pain* 2004;20:399–408.

35. van den Hoogen HM, Koes BW, van Eijk JT, Bouter LM. On the accuracy of history, physical examination, and erythrocyte sedimentation rate in diagnosing low back pain in general practice. A criteria-based review of the literature. *Spine (Phila Pa 1976)* 1995;20:318–327.

36. Jarvik JG, Deyo RA. Diagnostic evaluation of low back pain with emphasis on imaging. *Ann Intern Med* 2002;137:586–597.

37. Kendrick D, Fielding K, Bentley E, et al. Radiography of the lumbar spine in primary care patients with low back pain: randomised controlled trial. *BMJ* 2001;322:400–405.

38. Wiesel SW, Tsourmas N, Feffer HL, et al. A study of computer-assisted tomography. I. The incidence of positive CAT scans in an asymptomatic group of patients. *Spine (Phila Pa 1976)* 1984;9:549–551.

39. Jensen MC, Brant-Zawadzki MN, Obuchowski N, et al. Magnetic resonance imaging of the lumbar spine in people without back pain. *N Engl J Med* 1994;331:69–73.

40. Jarvik JJ, Hollingworth W, Heagerty P, et al. The Longitudinal Assessment of Imaging and Disability of the Back LAIDBack Study: baseline data. *Spine (Phila Pa 1976)* 2001;26: 1158–1166.

41. Borenstein DG, O'Mara JW Jr, Boden SD, et al. The value of magnetic resonance imaging of the lumbar spine to predict low-back pain in asymptomatic subjects: a seven-year follow-up study. *J Bone Joint Surg Am* 2001;83–A:1306–1311.

42. Jarvik JG, Hollingworth W, Heagerty PJ, et al. Three-year incidence of low back pain in an initially asymptomatic cohort: clinical and imaging risk factors. *Spine (Phila Pa 1976)* 2005;30:1541–1548.

43. Cheung KM, Karppinen J, Chan D, et al. Prevalence and pattern of lumbar magnetic resonance imaging changes in a population study of one thousand forty-three individuals. *Spine (Phila Pa 1976)* 2009;34:934–940.

44. Kjaer P, Leboeuf-Yde C, Korsholm L, et al. Magnetic resonance imaging and low back pain in adults: a diagnostic imaging study of 40-year-old men and women. *Spine (Phila Pa 1976)* 2005;30:1173–1180.

45. Engers A, Jellema P, Wensing M, et al. Individual patient education for low back pain. *Cochrane Database Syst Rev* 2008;(1):CD004057.

46. Heymans MW, van Tulder MW, Esmail R, et al. Back schools for non-specific low-back pain. *Cochrane Database Syst Rev* 2004;(4):CD000261.

47. Hagen KB, Hilde G, Jamtvedt G, Winnem M. Bed rest for acute low-back pain and sciatica. *Cochrane Database Syst Rev* 2004;(4):CD001254.

48. Hayden JA, van Tulder MW, Malmivaara A, Koes BW. Exercise therapy for treatment of non-specific low back pain. *Cochrane Database Syst Rev* 2005;(3):CD000335.

49. Chou R, Huffman LH; American Pain Society; American College of Physicians. Non-pharmacologic therapies for acute and chronic low back pain: a review of the evidence for an American Pain Society/American College of Physicians clinical practice guideline. *Ann Intern Med* 2007;147:492–504.

50. French SD, Cameron M, Walker BF, et al. Superficial heat or cold for low back pain. *Cochrane Database Syst Rev* 2006;(1):CD004750.

51. Furlan AD, Imamura M, Dryden T, Irvin E. Massage for low-back pain. *Cochrane Database Syst Rev* 2008;(4):CD001929.

52. Cherkin DC, Sherman KJ, Deyo RA, Shekelle PG. A review of the evidence for the effectiveness, safety, and cost of acupuncture, massage therapy, and spinal manipulation for back pain. *Ann Intern Med* 2003;138:898–906.

53. Assendelft WJ, Morton SC, Yu EI, et al. Spinal manipulative therapy for low back pain. *Cochrane Database Syst Rev* 2004;(1):CD000447.

54. Furlan AD, van Tulder MW, Cherkin DC, et al. Acupuncture and dry-needling for low back pain. *Cochrane Database Syst Rev* 2005 Jan 25;(1):CD001351.

55. Cherkin DC, Sherman KJ, Avins AL, et al. A randomized trial comparing acupuncture, simulated acupuncture, and usual care for chronic low back pain. *Arch Intern Med* 2009;169:858–866.

56. Ostelo RW, van Tulder MW, Vlaeyen JW, et al. Behavioural treatment for chronic low-back pain. *Cochrane Database Syst Rev* 2005 Jan 25;(1):CD002014.

57. Karjalainen K, Malmivaara A, van Tulder M, et al. Multidisciplinary biopsychosocial rehabilitation for subacute low back pain among working age adults. *Cochrane Database Syst Rev* 2003;(2):CD002193.

58. van Duijvenbode IC, Jellema P, van Poppel MN, van Tulder MW. Lumbar supports for prevention and treatment of low back pain. *Cochrane Database Syst Rev* 2008;(2): CD001823.

59. Clarke JA, van Tulder MW, Blomberg SE, et al. Traction for low-back pain with or without sciatica. *Cochrane Database Syst Rev* 2007;(2):CD003010.

60. Khadilkar A, Odebiyi DO, Brosseau L, Wells GA. Transcutaneous electrical nerve stimulation (TENS) versus placebo for chronic low-back pain. *Cochrane Database Syst Rev* 2008;(4):CD003008.

61. Sahar T, Cohen MJ, Ne'eman V, et al. Insoles for prevention and treatment of back pain. *Cochrane Database Syst Rev* 2007;(4):CD005275.

62. Macario A, Pergolizzi JV. Systematic literature review of spinal decompression via motorized traction for chronic discogenic low back pain. *Pain Pract* 2006;6:171–178.

63. Yousefi-Nooraie R, Schonstein E, Heidari K, et al. Low level laser therapy for nonspecific low-back pain. *Cochrane Database Syst Rev* 2008;(2):CD005107.

64. Chou R, Huffman LH; American Pain Society; American College of Physicians. Medications for acute and chronic low back pain: a review of the evidence for an American Pain Society/American College of Physicians clinical practice guideline. *Ann Intern Med* 2007;147:505–514.

65. Roelofs PD, Deyo RA, Koes BW, et al. Non-steroidal anti-inflammatory drugs for low back pain. *Cochrane Database Syst Rev* 2008;(1):CD000396.

66. Browning R, Jackson JL, O'Malley PG. Cyclobenzaprine and back pain: a meta-analysis. *Arch Intern Med* 2001;161:1613–1620.

67. van Tulder MW, Touray T, Furlan AD, et al. Muscle relaxants for non-specific low back pain. *Cochrane Database Syst Rev* 2003;(2):CD004252.

68. Martell BA, O'Connor PG, Kerns RD, et al. Systematic review: opioid treatment for chronic back pain: prevalence, efficacy, and association with addiction. *Ann Intern Med* 2007;146:116–127.

69. Urquhart DM, Hoving JL, Assendelft WW, et al. Antidepressants for non-specific low back pain. *Cochrane Database Syst Rev* 2008;(1):CD001703.

70. Muehlbacher M, Nickel MK, Kettler C, et al. Topiramate in treatment of patients with chronic low back pain: a randomized, double-blind, placebo-controlled study. *Clin J Pain* 2006;22:526–531.

71. Yaksi A, Ozgönenel L, Ozgönenel B. The efficiency of gabapentin therapy in patients with lumbar spinal stenosis. *Spine (Phila Pa 1976)* 2007;32:939–942.

72. Staal JB, de Bie R, de Vet HC, et al. Injection therapy for subacute and chronic low-back pain. *Cochrane Database Syst Rev* 2008;(3):CD001824.

73. Dagenais S, Yelland MJ, Del Mar C, Schoene ML. Prolotherapy injections for chronic low-back pain. *Cochrane Database Syst Rev* 2007;(2):CD004059.

74. Helm S, Hayek SM, Benyamin RM, Manchikanti L. Systematic review of the effectiveness of thermal annular procedures in treating discogenic low back pain. *Pain Physician* 2009;12:207–232.

75. Gibson JN, Waddell G. Surgical interventions for lumbar disc prolapse. *Cochrane Database Syst Rev* 2007;(2):CD001350.

76. Chou R, Baisden J, Carragee EJ, et al. Surgery for low back pain: a review of the evidence for an American Pain Society Clinical Practice Guideline. *Spine (Phila Pa 1976)* 2009;34: 1094–1109.

77. Weinstein JN, Lurie JD, Tosteson TD, et al. Surgical vs nonoperative treatment for lumbar disk herniation: the Spine Patient Outcomes Research Trial (SPORT) observational cohort. *JAMA* 2006;296:2451–2459.

78. Atlas SJ, Keller RB, Wu YA, et al. Long-term outcomes of surgical and nonsurgical management of sciatica secondary to a lumbar disc herniation: 10 year results from the maine lumbar spine study. *Spine (Phila Pa 1976)* 2005;30:927–935.

79. Atlas SJ, Keller RB, Wu YA, et al. Long-term outcomes of surgical and nonsurgical management of lumbar spinal stenosis: 8 to 10 year results from the maine lumbar spine study. *Spine (Phila Pa 1976)* 2005;30:936–943.

80. Weinstein JN, Tosteson TD, Lurie JD, et al.; SPORT Investigators. Surgical versus non-surgical therapy for lumbar spinal stenosis. *N Engl J Med* 2008;358:794–810.

81. Weinstein JN, Lurie JD, Tosteson TD, et al. Surgical versus nonsurgical treatment for lumbar degenerative spondylolisthesis. *N Engl J Med* 2007;356:2257–2270.

82. Reilingh ML, Kuijpers T, Tanja-Harfterkamp AM, van der Windt DA. Course and prognosis of shoulder symptoms in general practice. *Rheumatology (Oxford)* 2008;47: 724–730.

83. Hurt G, Baker CL Jr. Calcific tendinitis of the shoulder. *Orthop Clin North Am* 2003;34: 567–575.

84. Hannafin JA, Chiaia TA. Adhesive capsulitis. A treatment approach. *Clin Orthop Relat Res* 2000 Mar;(372):95–109.

85. Hegedus EJ, Goode A, Campbell S, et al. Physical examination tests of the shoulder: a systematic review with meta-analysis of individual tests. *Br J Sports Med* 2008;42:80–92.

86. Silva L, Andréu JL, Muñoz P, et al. Accuracy of physical examination in subacromial impingement syndrome. *Rheumatology (Oxford)* 2008;47:679–683.

87. Green S, Buchbinder R, Hetrick S. Physiotherapy interventions for shoulder pain. *Cochrane Database Syst Rev* 2003;(2):CD004258.

88. Buchbinder R, Green S, Youd JM. Corticosteroid injections for shoulder pain. *Cochrane Database Syst Rev* 2003;(1):CD004016.

89. Arroll B, Goodyear-Smith F. Corticosteroid injections for painful shoulder: a meta-analysis. *Br J Gen Pract* 2005;55:224–228.

90. Koester MC, Dunn WR, Kuhn JE, Spindler KP. The efficacy of subacromial corticosteroid injection in the treatment of rotator cuff disease: a systematic review. *J Am Acad Orthop Surg* 2007;15:3–11.

91. Buchbinder R, Green S, Youd JM, Johnston RV. Oral steroids for adhesive capsulitis. *Cochrane Database Syst Rev* 2006;(4):CD006189.

92. Kraushaar BS, Nirschl RP. Tendinosis of the elbow (tennis elbow). Clinical features and findings of histological, immunohistochemical, and electron microscopy studies. *J Bone Joint Surg Am* 1999;81:259–278.

93. Bisset L, Paungmali A, Vicenzino B, Beller E. A systematic review and meta-analysis of clinical trials on physical interventions for lateral epicondylalgia. *Br J Sports Med* 2005;39: 411–422.

94. Smidt N, Assendelft WJ, van der Windt DA, et al. Corticosteroid injections for lateral epicondylitis: a systematic review. *Pain* 2002;96:23–40.

95. Smith DL, McAfee JH, Lucas LM, et al. Treatment of nonseptic olecranon bursitis. A controlled, blinded prospective trial. *Arch Intern Med* 1989;149:2527–2530.

96. Hansen PA, Micklesen P, Robinson LR. Clinical utility of the flick maneuver in diagnosing carpal tunnel syndrome. *Am J Phys Med Rehabil* 2004;83:363–367.

97. D'Arcy CA, McGee S. The rational clinical examination. Does this patient have carpal tunnel syndrome? *JAMA* 2000;283:3110–3117.

98. Peters-Veluthamaningal C, van der Windt DA, Winters JC, Meyboom-de Jong B. Corticosteroid injection for trigger finger in adults. *Cochrane Database Syst Rev* 2009;(1): CD005617.

99. Peters-Veluthamaningal C, van der Windt DA, Winters JC, Meyboom-de Jong B. Corticosteroid injection for de Quervain's tenosynovitis. *Cochrane Database Syst Rev* 2009;(3): CD005616.

100. O'Connor D, Marshall S, Massy-Westropp N. Non-surgical treatment (other than steroid injection) for carpal tunnel syndrome. *Cochrane Database Syst Rev* 2003;(1): CD003219.

101. Marshall S, Tardif G, Ashworth N. Local corticosteroid injection for carpal tunnel syndrome. *Cochrane Database Syst Rev* 2007 Apr 18;(2):CD001554.

102. Verdugo RJ, Salinas RA, Castillo JL, Cea JG. Surgical versus non-surgical treatment for carpal tunnel syndrome. *Cochrane Database Syst Rev* 2008;(4):CD001552.

103. Shbeeb MI, O'Duffy JD, Michet CJ Jr, et al. Evaluation of glucocorticosteroid injection for the treatment of trochanteric bursitis. *J Rheumatol* 1996;23:2104–2106.

104. Williams BS, Cohen SP. Greater trochanteric pain syndrome: a review of anatomy, diagnosis and treatment. *Anesth Analg* 2009;108:1662–1670.

105. Kannus P, Natri A, Paakkala T, Järvinen M. An outcome study of chronic patellofemoral pain syndrome. Seven-year follow-up of patients in a randomized, controlled trial. *J Bone Joint Surg A*m 1999;81:355–363.

106. Miller TT, Staron RB, Koenigsberg T, et al. MR imaging of Baker cysts: association with internal derangement, effusion, and degenerative arthropathy. *Radiology* 1996;201: 247–250.

107. Andonopoulos AP, Yarmenitis S, Sfountouris H, et al. Baker's cyst in rheumatoid arthritis: an ultrasonographic study with a high resolution technique. *Clin Exp Rheumatol* 1995;13:633–636.

108. Solomon DH, Simel DL, Bates DW, et al. The rational clinical examination. Does this patient have a torn meniscus or ligament of the knee? Value of the physical examination. *JAMA* 2001;286:1610–1620.

109. Jackson JL, O'Malley PG, Kroenke K. Evaluation of acute knee pain in primary care. *Ann Intern Med* 2003;139:575–588.

110. Eren OT. The accuracy of joint line tenderness by physical examination in the diagnosis of meniscal tears. *Arthroscopy* 2003;19:850–854.

111. Stiell IG, Wells GA, Hoag RH, et al. Implementation of the Ottawa Knee Rule for the use of radiography in acute knee injuries. *JAMA* 1997;278:2075–2079.

112. Stiell IG, McKnight RD, Greenberg GH, et al. Implementation of the Ottawa ankle rules. *JAMA* 1994;271:827–832.

113. Handoll HH, Rowe BH, Quinn KM, de Bie R. Interventions for preventing ankle ligament injuries. *Cochrane Database Syst Rev* 2001;(3):CD000018.

114. Crawford F, Thomson C. Interventions for treating plantar heel pain. *Cochrane Database Syst Rev* 2003;(3):CD000416.

30 Hematologic Diseases

Reshma Rangwala and Morey A. Blinder

ANEMIA

Initial Approach to Anemia

General Principles

- Anemia is defined as a decrease in circulating red blood cell (RBC) mass; the usual criteria being hemoglobin (Hgb) <12 g/dL or hematocrit (Hct) <36% in women and Hgb <14 g/dL or Hct <41% in men.
- A systematic approach to anemia is best at narrowing down the diagnosis and guiding the subsequent diagnostic workup.
- Anemia can be broadly classified into three etiologic groups: **blood loss (acute or chronic), decreased RBC production, and increased RBC destruction (hemolysis).**

Diagnosis

Clinical Presentation
- As with any other medical condition, the history and physical examination play key roles in approaching anemia.
- Based on symptoms, one can often discern time line (acute, subacute, or chronic), severity, and possibly the underlying etiology.
- Patients may be asymptomatic, but patients with an Hgb <7 g/dL will usually have symptoms.
- The clinical presentation of anemia can be accompanied by a variety of signs and symptoms depending on the severity of the anemia, its chronicity, and its pace of development.
- Common signs of anemia including pallor, tachycardia, hypotension, dizziness, tinnitus, headaches, loss of concentration, fatigue, and weakness occasionally occur. Atrophic glossitis, angular cheilosis, koilonychias (spoon nails), and brittle nails also occur. Reduced exercise tolerance, dyspnea on exertion, and congestive heart failure (CHF) are seen in more severe anemia. High output CHF and shock may be seen in the most severe forms.
- Adaptive compensatory mechanisms can mask many signs or symptoms of anemia that have an insidious onset and/or are present over a prolonged period of time.
- In contrast to chronic anemia, patients with abrupt onset of anemia tolerate diminished red cell mass poorly. The anemia may be relatively mild (i.e., Hct >30%), but the patient may have symptoms of fatigue, malaise, dizziness, syncope, or angina. Acute blood loss most commonly occurs in the gastrointestinal (GI) tract (gastritis due to alcohol or nonsteroidal anti-inflammatory drugs, diverticulosis, or peptic or gastric ulcer disease) and may be accompanied by epigastric symptoms, nausea and vomiting, or diarrhea.

Laboratories
- The complete blood cell count measures white blood cells (WBC), Hgb, Hct, platelets, and the red cell indices.

- The Hgb measures the concentration of Hgb in blood as expressed in g/dL, whereas the Hct is the percentage of space that the RBC occupies in the blood. Remember that the Hgb and Hct are unreliable indicators of red cell mass in the setting of rapid shifts of intravascular volume (i.e., an acute bleed).
- The most useful red cell indices include the **mean corpuscular volume (MCV), red cell distribution width (RDW), and mean cell Hgb concentration (MCHC).**
- MCV is the mean size of the red cells and the normal range is 80 to 100 fL. RBCs can be classified as **microcytic if the MCV is <80 fL, macrocytic when >100 fL, and normocytic when 80 to 100 fL.**
- RDW is a reflection of the variability in the size of the red cells and is proportional to the standard deviation of the MCV. **An elevated RDW indicates an increased variability in RBC size.**
- MCHC describes the concentration of Hgb in each cell and an elevated level is often indicative of spherocytes or a hemoglobinopathy.
- The **reticulocyte count** measures the percentage of immature red cells in the blood and reflects the bone marrow's (BM) response to anemia (i.e., a normal BM response is to increase the production of red cells in anemia so that the observed reticulocyte count increases).
  - A nascent RBC circulates for about 120 days, and the BM is constantly replenishing the bloodstream with new RBCs, with the normal reticulocyte count being approximately 1%.
  - In the setting of anemia or blood loss, the BM should increase its production of RBC in proportion to loss of RBC, and thus a 1% reticulocyte count in the setting of anemia is inappropriate.
  - The **reticulocyte index (RI)** is calculated as % reticulocytes × actual Hct/normal Hct and is important in determining whether a patient's BM is responding appropriately to the level of anemia.
  - In normal individuals, RI 1.0 to 2.0 is acceptable; however, **RI <2 with anemia indicates decreased production of RBCs (hypoproliferative anemia). RI >2 with anemia may indicate hemolysis or loss of RBCs** leading to increased compensatory production of reticulocytes **(hyperproliferative anemia).**
- The **peripheral smear** is a necessary part of the initial hematologic evaluation. RBC shape, size, the presence of inclusions, and orientation of cells in relation to each other are important factors to look for in a smear. RBCs can appear in many abnormal forms, such as acanthocytes, schistocytes, spherocytes, or teardrop cells and abnormal orientation such as Rouleaux formation.
- A **BM biopsy** may be indicated in cases of normocytic anemias with a low reticulocyte without an identifiable cause or anemia associated with other cytopenias. The biopsy may confirm myelophthisic process (i.e., presence of teardrop or fragmented cells, normoblasts, or immature WBCs on peripheral blood smear) in the setting of pancytopenias.

HYPOPROLIFERATIVE ANEMIA

Microcytic Anemia

General Principles
- **Iron deficiency** is the most common cause of anemia in the ambulatory setting.
- Menstrual blood loss or pregnancy is the most common etiology.

- In the absence of menstrual bleeding, GI blood loss is the presumed etiology in most patients, and the appropriate radiographic and endoscopic procedures should be pursued to identify a source and exclude occult malignancy.
- Other causes of microcytic anemia include sideroblastic anemia, lead poisoning, thalassemia, and anemia of chronic disease (ACD) which more typically presents as a normocytic anemia.

Diagnosis

Clinical Presentation
- Patients may present with fatigue or malaise, which is related to the importance of iron in cellular metabolism and its role in oxygen delivery, as well as pica. Iron deficiency has also been increasingly associated with restless leg syndrome.
- A careful history relating to menstrual frequency and duration as well as GI blood loss (melena, hematochezia, hematemesis) is essential.
- Diseases of the stomach and proximal small intestine (e.g., *Helicobacter pylori* infection, achlorhydria, celiac disease, and bariatric surgery) often lead to impaired iron absorption.

Laboratories
- The laboratory evaluation depends in part on patient demographics.
- With adequate follow-up, a microcytic anemia in a menstruating female needs only a baseline Hgb/Hct that is repeated 2 to 4 months after initiation of oral iron therapy.
- Postmenopausal women and men require more detailed evaluation, including evaluation of potential RBC losses, commonly via the GI tract (e.g., peptic ulcer disease, colon carcinoma) or, rarely, the urinary tract (e.g., paroxysmal nocturnal hemoglobinuria).
- Because evaluating these patients may require considerable expense and effort, laboratory studies are necessary to document iron deficiency before further evaluation.
- **Ferritin** is the primary storage form for iron in the liver and BM and is the best surrogate marker of iron stores.
  - A ferritin level of <10 ng/mL in women or 20 ng/mL in men is a specific marker of low iron stores.
  - Ferritin is an acute-phase reactant, so normal levels may be seen in inflammatory states despite low iron stores. **A serum ferritin of >200 ng/mL generally excludes an iron deficiency;** however, in renal dialysis patients, a functional iron deficiency may be seen with a ferritin up to 500 ng/mL.
- **Iron, transferrin, and transferrin saturation** are often used to diagnose iron deficiency anemia but are not as reliable as ferritin for the diagnosis.
  - In this setting, serum iron declines to <50 mg/dL once iron stores are exhausted.
  - Transferrin increases linearly to approximately 400 mg/dL once patients are in negative iron balance, so that **transferrin saturation falls below 16% only when iron stores are exhausted.**
- A **BM biopsy** that shows absent staining for iron is the definitive test for establishing iron deficiency and is helpful when the serum tests fail to confirm the diagnosis.

Treatment

Oral Iron Therapy
- In stable patients with mild symptoms, this consists of **ferrous sulfate,** 325 mg PO, one to three times/day.
  - Iron is best absorbed on an empty stomach, and between 3 mg and 10 mg elemental iron can be absorbed daily.

- Oral iron ingestion may induce a number of GI side effects, including epigastric distress, bloating, and constipation; as a result, noncompliance is a common problem. These side effects can be decreased by initially administering the drug with meals or once per day and increasing the dose as tolerated. Concomitant treatment with a stool softener can also alleviate these symptoms.
- Administration of vitamin C along with the iron improves absorption by maintaining the iron in the reduced state.

Parenteral Iron Therapy
- Parenteral iron therapy may be useful in patients with:
  - Poor absorption (e.g., inflammatory bowel disease, malabsorption).
  - Very high iron requirements that cannot be met with oral supplementation (e.g., ongoing bleeding).
  - Intolerance to oral preparations.
- The total amount of iron necessary to replete the deficiency can be estimated by a formula using the starting Hgb level; however, in practice, parenteral iron is often infused to a dose of 1 to 1.2 g.
- **Iron dextran:**
  - IV iron dextran therapy (INFeD, Dexferrum) can be complicated by serious side effects including **anaphylaxis;** therefore, an IV **test dose** of 25 mg in 50 mL of normal saline should be administered over 5 to 10 minutes. Methylprednisolone, diphenhydramine, and 1:1,000 epinephrine 1-mg ampule (for subcutaneous administration) should be immediately available at all times during the infusion.
  - Delayed reactions to IV iron, such as arthralgia, myalgia, fever, pruritus, and lymphadenopathy may be seen within 3 days of therapy and usually resolve spontaneously or with nonsteroidal anti-inflammatory drugs.
- **Alternatives to iron dextran** include sodium ferric gluconate (Ferrlecit) and iron sucrose (Venofer).
  - The side effect profile for these preparations appears to be better than that of iron dextran with less hypersensitivity infusion reactions.
  - **However, they cannot be used to replenish the entire iron deficit with a single infusion.**
  - The recommended dosage of sodium ferric gluconate is 125 mg diluted in 100 mL of normal saline infused IV over 1 hour or as a **slow** IV push over 10 minutes (12.5 mg/min). This can be repeated weekly until circulating iron (to a normal Hct) and storage iron (1 to 3 g) are replenished.
  - Iron sucrose is administered as a 100 to 200 mg IV push or up to 400 mg over a 2.5-hour IV infusion.

Macrocytic/Megaloblastic Anemia

General Principles
- Megaloblastic anemia is a term used to describe disorders of impaired DNA synthesis in hematopoietic cells that affect all proliferating cells. Almost all cases are due to folic acid or vitamin B_{12} deficiency.
- **Folate deficiency** arises from a negative folate balance arising from malnutrition, malabsorption, or increased requirement (pregnancy, hemolytic anemia).
  - Patients on slimming diets, alcoholics, the elderly, and psychiatric patients are particularly at risk for nutritional folate deficiency.

- **Pregnancy and lactation** require higher (three- to fourfold) daily folate needs and are commonly associated with megaloblastic changes in maternal hematopoietic cells, leading to a dimorphic (combined folate and iron deficiency) anemia.
- Folate malabsorption can also be seen in celiac disease.
- **Drugs** that can interfere with folate absorption include ethanol, trimethoprim, pyrimethamine, diphenylhydantoin, barbiturates, and sulfasalazine.
- Patients who are undergoing dialysis require enhanced folate intake because of folate losses.
- Patients with hemolytic anemia, particularly sickle cell anemia, require increased folate for accelerated erythropoiesis and can present with aplastic crisis (rapidly falling RBC counts) with folate deficiency.
- **Vitamin B$_{12}$ deficiency** occurs insidiously over $\geq$3 years, because daily vitamin B$_{12}$ requirements are 1 to 3 μg, whereas total body stores are 1 to 3 mg.
  - Because multivitamins now contain folic acid, the hematologic manifestations of vitamin B$_{12}$ deficiency may be obscured, leading solely to neurologic presentations.
  - Causes of vitamin B$_{12}$ deficiency include partial (up to 20% of patients within 8 years of surgery) or total gastrectomy and pernicious anemia (PA). Older patients with gastric atrophy may develop a vitamin B$_{12}$ deficiency in which vitamin B$_{12}$ absorption is impaired.
  - PA occurs in individuals who are >40 years (mean onset, age 60 years). Up to 30% of patients have a positive family history. PA is associated with other autoimmune disorders (Graves disease 30%, Hashimoto's thyroiditis 11%, and Addison disease 5% to 10%). Of patients with PA, 90% have antiparietal cell IgG antibodies and 60% have anti-intrinsic factor antibodies.

Diagnosis

Clinical Presentation

- Folate deficient patients present with sleep deprivation, fatigue, and manifestations of depression, irritability, or forgetfulness.
- By the time anemia due to vitamin B$_{12}$ is clinically manifest, neurologic manifestations including peripheral neuropathy, paresthesias, lethargy, hypotonia, and seizures are common.
- **Physical examination** may indicate poor nutrition, pigmentation of skin creases and nail beds, or glossitis. Jaundice or splenomegaly may indicate ineffective and extramedullary hematopoiesis. Vitamin B$_{12}$ deficiency may cause decreased vibratory and positional sense, ataxia, paresthesias, confusion, and dementia. Neurologic complications may occur even in the absence of anemia and may not fully resolve despite adequate treatment. **Folic acid deficiency does not result in neurologic disease.**

Laboratories

- A macrocytic anemia is usually present and leukopenia and thrombocytopenia may occur.
- The peripheral smear may show anisocytosis, poikilocytosis, and macro-ovalocytes; hypersegmented neutrophils (containing $\geq$5 nuclear lobes) are common.
- Lactic dehydrogenase (LDH) and indirect bilirubin are typically elevated, reflecting ineffective erythropoiesis and premature destruction of RBCs.
- **Serum vitamin B$_{12}$ and RBC folate levels** should be measured.
- RBC folate is a more accurate indicator of body folate stores than serum folate, particularly if measured after folate therapy or improved nutrition has been initiated.

- **Serum methylmalonic acid and homocysteine** may be useful when the vitamin B_{12} or folate level is equivocal. Serum methylmalonic acid and homocysteine are elevated in vitamin B_{12} deficiency; only homocysteine is elevated in folate deficiency.
- A **Schilling test** may be useful in the diagnosis of PA due to vitamin B_{12} deficiency but rarely affects the therapeutic approach. Therefore, it is rarely done anymore.
- Detecting **antibodies to intrinsic factor** is specific for the diagnosis of PA.
- BM **biopsy** may be necessary to rule out a myelodysplastic syndrome or acute leukemia since these disorders may present with findings similar to those of megaloblastic anemia.

Treatment
- Treatment is directed toward replacing the deficient factor.
- Potassium supplementation may be necessary when treatment is initiated to avoid potentially serious arrhythmias due to hypokalemia induced by enhanced hematopoiesis.
- Reticulocytosis should begin within 1 week of therapy, followed by a rising Hgb over 6 to 8 weeks.
- Coexisting iron deficiency is present in one third of patients and is a common cause for an incomplete response to therapy.
- Folic acid, 1 mg PO daily, is given until the deficiency is corrected. High doses of folic acid (5 mg PO daily) may be needed in patients with malabsorption syndromes.
- Vitamin B_{12} deficiency is corrected by administering **cyanocobalamin.** Unless the patient is severely ill (decompensated CHF due to anemia, advanced neurologic dysfunction), treatment with full doses of cyanocobalamin (1 mg/day IM) should await the laboratory diagnosis.
- After 1 week of daily therapy, 1 mg/week should be given for 4 weeks and then 1 mg/month for life.
- Patients who decline or cannot take parenteral therapy can be prescribed oral tablets or syrup at 50 µg/day for life.

Normocytic Anemia

The causes of hypoproliferative (i.e., low RI) normocytic anemias include malignancies and other BM infiltrative diseases, stem cell disorders (e.g., myelodysplasia), some endocrine disorders, anemia of chronic renal insufficiency, and ACD. The latter two are quite common.

Anemia of Chronic Renal Insufficiency

General Principles
Anemia of chronic renal insufficiency is attributed primarily to decreased endogenous erythropoietin (Epo) production and may occur as the creatinine clearance declines below 50 mL/minute. Other causes including iron deficiency may contribute to the etiology. This topic is also discussed in Chapter 20.

Diagnosis
- Laboratory evaluation reveals a normal MCV in 85% of the cases.
- The Hct is usually 20% to 30%.

- If the patient's creatinine is >1.8 mg/dL, the primary cause of the anemia can be assumed to be Epo deficiency and/or iron deficiency, and an Epo level is unnecessary.
- Iron deficiency should be evaluated in patients who are undergoing dialysis because of chronic blood loss via ferritin and transferrin saturation. Oral iron supplementation is not effective in chronic kidney disease, so parenteral iron to maintain a ferritin >500 ng/mL is recommended.[1]

Treatment

- Treatment has been revolutionized by erythropoiesis-stimulating agents (ESA) including epoetin alfa and darbepoetin alfa.
- Therapy is initiated in predialysis patients who are symptomatic.
- Objective benefits of reversing the anemia include enhanced exercise capacity, improved cognitive function, elimination of RBC transfusions, and reduction of iron overload. Subjective benefits include increased energy, enhanced appetite, better sleep patterns, and improved sexual activity.
- Administration of ESAs can be IV (hemodialysis patients) or SC (predialysis or peritoneal dialysis patients). In dialysis and predialysis patients with chronic kidney disease, **the target Hgb should be between 11 and 12 g/dL and should not exceed 13 g/dL.** An Hgb and Hct should be measured at least monthly while receiving an ESA. Dose adjustments should be made to maintain the target Hgb.
- Adverse reactions to ESAs: targeting higher Hgb levels and/or exposure to high doses of ESAs is associated with a greater risk of cardiovascular complications and mortality. In addition, a higher Hct from ESAs increases the risk of stroke, CHF, and deep vein thrombosis.[2]
- **Suboptimal responses to ESA therapy** are a common phenomenon due to iron deficiency, inflammation, bleeding, infection, malignancy, malnutrition, and aluminum toxicity.
  - Because anemia is a powerful determinant of life expectancy in patients on chronic dialysis, intravenous iron administration has become standard therapy in many individuals who receive ESA therapy and has also been shown to reduce the ESA dosage that is required to correct anemia.
  - A ferritin and transferrin saturation should be tested at least monthly during the initiation of ESA therapy with a goal ferritin of >200 ng/mL and a transferrin saturation >20% in dialysis-dependent patients and a ferritin of >100 ng/mL and a transferrin saturation >20% in predialysis or peritoneal dialysis patients.
  - Iron therapy is of unlikely benefit if the ferritin is >500 ng/mL.
  - Secondary hyperparathyroidism that causes BM fibrosis and relative ESA resistance may also occur.

Anemia of Chronic Disease

General Principles

- ACD often develops in patients with long-standing inflammatory diseases, malignancy, autoimmune disorders, and chronic infection.
- The etiology seems to be multifactorial with defective iron mobilization during erythropoiesis, inflammatory cytokine-mediated suppression of erythropoiesis, and impaired Epo response to anemia; all play a role.
- ACD is also a common complication of therapy for the underlying disease (e.g., chemotherapy for malignancy, zidovudine for HIV infection).

Diagnosis

- **At present no laboratory test is diagnostic** for the ACD.
- A normocytic, normochromic anemia is typical.
- Iron studies may be similar in patients with iron deficiency and are difficult to interpret.
- Clinical responses to iron therapy can be seen in patients with ferritin levels of up to 100 ng/mL.
- A BM evaluation for storage iron may be necessary to rule out an absolute iron deficiency accompanying an ACD.

Treatment

- Therapy for ACD is directed at the underlying disease and at eliminating exacerbating factors such as nutritional deficiencies and marrow-suppressive drugs.
- ESA therapy should be considered if the patient is transfusion dependent or has symptomatic anemia. The risks of ESA therapy include cardiovascular and arterial and venous thromboembolic events and hypertension.
- Transfusion should be considered for patients with Hct levels of <24% or if they are symptomatic.

Anemia in Patients with Cancer

The role of ESAs in patients receiving chemotherapy has come under question. Recent studies indicate that ESA may potentiate cancer growth and decrease disease-free survival. In addition, ESAs have not shown to significantly reduce the need for RBC transfusions in patients not receiving chemotherapy nor did they increase quality of life. ESA therapy should be considered in transfusion-dependent patients with a target Hgb of 11 to 12 g/dL.[3–7]

Aplastic Anemia

Aplastic anemia is an acquired disorder of hematopoietic stem cells, presenting in people of all ages not only as anemia but also as pancytopenia. Most cases are idiopathic but in approximately one third of patients a history of drug exposure (Table 1)[8] or viral infection (e.g., hepatitis, Epstein-Barr virus, cytomegalovirus) is demonstrated. Therapy is supportive, with early referral to a tertiary care center for possible immunosuppressive therapy and/or stem cell transplantation is recommended. Transfusions should be minimized and, when administered, should be leuko-depleted and from nonfamily members.

Myelodysplastic Syndrome

- **Myelodysplastic syndrome (MDS)** is an acquired, clonal disorder that precedes the onset of acute leukemia, sometimes for many years.
- Several classifications are available and are based on findings on the peripheral smear, cytogenetics, and BM biopsy: (1) refractory anemia, (2) refractory anemia with ringed sideroblasts, (3) refractory anemia with excess blasts, (4) 5q- syndrome, and (5) chronic myelomonocytic leukemia.
- MDS usually occurs in the elderly, and a history of environmental exposure to chemicals (benzene), radiation, or prior chemotherapy with alkylating agents is sometimes present.

TABLE 1 Drugs That Can Induce RBC Disorders

Sideroblastic Anemia	Aplastic Anemia[a]	Hemolytic Episode in G6PD Deficiency	Immune Hemolytic Anemia			
			Autoantibody	Hapten	Immune Complex[b]	
Chloramphenicol	Acetazolamide	Dapsone	α-Methyldopa	Akfluor 25%	Amphotericin B	
Cycloserine	Antineoplastic drugs	Furazolidone	Cephalosporins	Cephalosporins	Antazoline	
Ethanol	Carbamazepine	Methylene blue	Diclofenac	Penicillins	Cephalosporins	
Isoniazid	Chloramphenicol	Nalidixic acid	Ibuprofen	Tetracycline	Chlorpropamide	
Pyrazinamide	Gold salts	Nitrofurantoin	Interferon-alpha	Tolbutamide	Diclofenac	
	Hydantoins	Phenazopyridine	L-Dopa		Diethylstilbestrol	
	Penicillamine	Primaquine	Mefenamic acid		Doxepin	
	Phenylbutazone	Sulfacetamide	Procainamide		Hydrochlorothiazide	
	Quinacrine	Sulfamethoxazole	Teniposide		Isoniazid	
		Sulfanilamide	Thioridazine		p-Aminosalicylic acid	
		Sulfapyridine	Tolmetin		Probenecid	
					Quinidine	
					Quinine	
					Rifampin	
					Sulfonamides	
					Thiopental	
					Tolmetin	

Note: Data compiled from multiple sources. Agents listed are available in the United States.
[a] Drugs with >30 cases reported; many other drugs rarely are associated with aplastic anemia and are considered low risk.
[b] Some sources list mechanisms for many of these drugs as unknown.
G6PD, glucose-6-phosphate dehydrogenase.
From Blinder M, Field J. Anemia and Transfusion Therapy. In: Cooper DH, Krainik AJ, Lubner SJ, Reno HEL (eds). The Washington Manual of Medical Therapeutics, 32nd Ed. Philadelphia, PA: Lippincott Williams & Wilkins, 2007:548–571, with permission.

- Presentations range from mild cytopenias without symptoms to severe pancytopenia.
- Prognosis is stratified into low, intermediate, and high-risk patients on the basis of cytopenia, cytogenetics, and the presence of blasts.
- Progression to marrow failure or acute leukemia commonly occurs.
- **Anemia is the predominant manifestation and may be normocytic or macrocytic.** Leukopenia and thrombocytopenia may also occur. The diagnosis is established by demonstrating abnormal hematopoietic cells in the BM.
- Therapy is based in part upon prognosis at diagnosis. Low-risk MDS is treated primarily with supportive therapies including blood transfusion which may result in clinically significant iron overload (see "Thalassemia" section). Intermediate and high-risk MDS can be treated with azacytidine and decitabine. Referral to a hematologist-oncologist is recommended.

ANEMIAS ASSOCIATED WITH INCREASED RED BLOOD CELL DESTRUCTION

- If the presentation is within 5 days of an acute onset, the only abnormal laboratory value may be decreased Hgb and Hct.
- An **elevated reticulocyte response** occurs in 3 to 5 days, which is indicative of an appropriate erythropoietic response.
- **LDH and bilirubin are increased** in most patients reflecting an increase in RBC turnover.
- **Serum haptoglobin is decreased** with hemolysis because of clearance of intravascular Hgb.
- With severe hemolysis, free Hgb can be measured in the plasma, and hemosiderin can also be detected in the urine with more chronic hemolysis.
- Examination of the peripheral smear is an important clue to detect hemolysis and may help define the cause. Intravascular hemolysis may reveal **red cell fragmentation** (schistocytes, helmet cells), whereas **spherocytes** indicate extravascular, immune-mediated hemolysis.
- Polychromasia and nucleated RBCs can be seen with intense hemolysis and increased erythropoiesis.
- Evaluation for hemolysis includes the direct Coombs test (direct antibody testing) for the presence of antibody attached to red cells; the indirect Coombs test indicates the presence of free antibody in the plasma.

Sickle Cell Disease

General Principles

- The sickle cell diseases are a group of hereditary Hgb disorders in which the Hgb undergoes sickle shape transformation under conditions of deoxygenation.
- The most common are homozygous sickle cell anemia (Hgb SS) or other heterozygous conditions (Hgb SC, Hgb S-beta thalassemia).
- Newborn screening programs for hemoglobinopathies now identify most patients in infancy.
- **Sickle cell trait** is present in 2.5 million people in the United States, occurring in 8% of African Americans.
- No hematologic findings are associated with sickle cell trait, which is a benign hereditary condition. Nevertheless, some risks have been reported in patients with

sickle cell trait, including high-altitude hypoxia leading to splenic infarction, cerebrovascular complications, and basic training of military recruits associated with increased incidence of sudden death related to extreme exertion and dehydration.

- The National Institutes of Health provides useful guidelines for sickle cell disease (http://www.nhlbi.nih.gov/health/prof/blood/sickle/sc_mngt.pdf, last accessed December 15, 2009).[9]

Diagnosis

Clinical Presentation

- Clinical manifestations are variable but generally relate to complications from chronic hemolysis and/or vascular occlusion.
  - Vaso-occlusive complications include pain crises, avascular necrosis, priapism, and acute chest syndrome.
  - Hemolytic complications include pulmonary hypertension, cholelithiasis, and leg ulcers. Strokes and renal medullary infarctions are complications of both.
- Delayed growth and development occur in the pediatric years.
- **Acute intermittent complications** account for much of the care provided to these patients and include:
- **Acute painful episodes ("sickle cell crisis")**
  - Vaso-occlusive pain crises are the most common manifestation of sickle cell disease. Pain is typically in the long bones, back, chest, and abdomen. These crises are precipitated by stress, including vasoreactivity of the microvascular system along with dehydration or infection, or both, and generally last for 2 to 6 days.
  - Although each individual tends to have a consistent pattern of presentation, wide variability is found among patients. Patient-specific factors related to the ability to cope with stress and chronic illness may also contribute to the clinical variability.
  - Some patients have mild disease with rare painful episodes and may be characterized by higher Hgb F levels. Nevertheless, these patients are at still at risk of all of the complications of the disease.
- **Acute chest syndrome** occurs when hypoxia (<90% oxygen saturation) leads to increased intravascular sickling and irreversible occlusion of the microvasculature (predominantly pulmonary) circulation. Patients with lung pathology, such as pneumonia, are particularly at risk.
- **Aplastic "crisis"** presents with a sudden decrease in Hgb level. The RI is inappropriately low, reflecting suppression of erythropoiesis. The most common etiology in pediatric patients is infection with parvovirus B19; folate deficiency should also be suspected because of the chronic increased requirements for erythropoiesis.
- **Priapism:** often presents in adolescence and may persist into adulthood.
- **Cerebrovascular events:** stroke may occur at any age but is most common in children <10 years of age and is usually caused by cerebral infarction.
- **Infections** in adults typically occur in tissues that are susceptible to vaso-occlusive infarcts (bone, kidney, lung). *Staphylococcus* spp., *Salmonella* spp., and enteric organisms are the most common. Pneumonia is most likely to be caused by *Mycoplasma pneumoniae, Staphylococcus aureus,* or *Haemophilus influenzae* and must be distinguished from acute chest syndrome.
- **Renal medullary infarction** results in chronic polyuria due to impaired urinary concentration, leading to a chronic risk of dehydration.
- **Renal tubular defects** caused by sickling in the anoxic hyperosmolar environment of the renal medulla may lead to isosthenuria (inability to concentrate urine) and

hematuria in both sickle cell trait and disease. These conditions predispose patients to dehydration, which increases the risk of vaso-occlusive events.
- **Cholelithiasis** is present in >80% of patients, primarily due to bilirubin stones.
- **Osteonecrosis** of the femoral heads occurs in up to 50% of patients and is a cause of severe pain in adults.
- **Leg ulceration** occurring at the ankle is often chronic and recurring.
- **Pregnancy** in a sickle cell patient should be considered high risk and is associated with increased spontaneous abortions or premature delivery, along with increased vaso-occlusive crises.

Laboratories
- Hgb electrophoresis or high-pressure liquid chromatography is used to diagnose hemoglobinopathies and distinguishes homozygous sickle cell disease (Hgb SS) from other abnormal Hgbs.
- The mean Hgb in Hgb SS disease is about 8 g/dL (range 5 to 10 g/dL). The MCV may be slightly elevated because of reticulocytosis but is low in Hgb S-beta thalassemia.
- Leukocytosis (10,000 to 20,000/mm^3) and thrombocytosis (>450,000/mm^3) are common due to enhanced stimulation of the marrow compartment and autosplenectomy.
- Peripheral smear shows sickle-shaped RBCs, target cells (particularly in Hgb SC and Hgb S-beta thalassemia), and Howell-Jolly bodies, indicative of functional asplenism.
- The degree of anemia and reticulocytosis is generally milder in Hgb SC disease.

Treatment

Acute Vaso-Occlusive Complications
- Outpatient management of **acute painful episodes** consists of rehydration (oral fluids, 3 to 4 L/day), evaluation for and management of infections, analgesia, and, if needed, antipyretic and empiric antibiotic therapy.
  - **Morphine** (0.3 to 0.6 mg/kg PO every 4 hours) is the drug of choice for moderate to severe pain.
  - Outpatient pain management is a complex problem that may require multidisciplinary approaches, including social services, psychiatric consultation, and pain service, to optimize the use of opiate medications.
  - Transfusion therapy has no role in the treatment of uncomplicated vaso-occlusive crises.
  - **Indications for hospitalization** include inability to ingest adequate oral fluids, requirement for parenteral opioids or antibiotics, a declining Hgb level associated with inadequate erythropoiesis, or hypoxia.
  - **Hydroxyurea** therapy (15 to 35 mg/kg PO daily) has been shown to increase levels of Hgb F and significantly decreases the frequency of vaso-occlusive crises and acute chest syndrome in adults with sickle cell disease.
- Individuals with suspected **acute chest syndrome** require immediate hospitalization and aggressive transfusion therapy, including red cell exchange. The presentation of acute chest syndrome is clinically indistinguishable from pneumonia, thus empiric broad-spectrum antibiotics should be administered.
- **Priapism** is initially treated with hydration and analgesia. Persistent erections for >24 hours may require transfusion therapy or surgical drainage.

Prevention and Health Maintenance
- **Dehydration and hypoxia** should be avoided because they may precipitate or exacerbate irreversible sickling.

- **Folic acid,** 1 mg PO daily, is generally administered to all patients with sickle cell disease because of chronic hemolysis.
- **Antimicrobial prophylaxis** with penicillin VK, 125 mg PO bid up to age 3 years and then 250 mg PO bid until 5 years, is effective in reducing the risk of infection. Patients who are allergic to penicillin should receive erythromycin, 10 mg/kg PO bid. In most patients, antimicrobial prophylaxis should be discontinued after 5 years of age to decrease the risk of resistant organisms.[10]
- **Immunizations** against the usual childhood illnesses should be given to children with sickle cell disease, including hepatitis B vaccine. After 2 years of age, a polyvalent pneumococcal vaccine should be administered. Yearly influenza vaccine is recommended.
- **Ophthalmologic examinations** are recommended yearly in adults because of the high incidence of proliferative retinopathy, which leads to vitreous hemorrhage and retinal detachment.
- **Surgery and anesthesia.** Local and regional anesthesia can be used without special precautions. With general anesthesia, measures to avoid volume depletion, hypoxia, and hypernatremia are crucial. For major surgery, RBC transfusions to increase the Hgb concentration to 10 g/dL seem to be as effective as more aggressive regimens in most circumstances.[11]

Complications of Chronic Hemolysis
- Patients with suspected **aplastic crisis** require hospitalization. Therapy includes folic acid, 5 mg/day, as well as RBC transfusions.
- **Cholelithiasis** may lead to acute cholecystitis or biliary colic. Acute cholecystitis should be treated medically with antibiotics and cholecystectomy should be performed when the attack subsides. Elective cholecystectomy for asymptomatic gallstones is controversial.

Chronic Organ Damage
- Treatment of osteonecrosis consists of local heat, analgesics, and avoidance of weight bearing. Hip and shoulder arthroplasty may be effective in decreasing symptoms and improving function.
- In those with a history of stroke, long-term transfusions to maintain the Hgb S concentration at <50% for at least 5 years reduce the incidence of recurrence.
- **Leg ulcers** should be treated with rest, leg elevation, and intensive local care. Wet to dry dressings should be applied three to four times per day. A zinc oxide-impregnated bandage (Unna boot), changed weekly for 3 to 4 weeks, can be used for nonhealing or more extensive ulcers.

Thalassemia

General Principles
- The **thalassemia syndromes** are inherited disorders characterized by reduced Hgb synthesis associated with mutations in either the α- or β-chain of the molecule.
- Affected individuals are of Mediterranean, Middle Eastern, Indian, African, or Asian descent.
- **Beta-thalassemia** results in a decreased production of β-globin and a resultant excess of α-globin, forming insoluble alpha tetramers and leading to ineffective erythropoiesis.
  - **Thalassemia minor (trait)** occurs with one gene abnormality with variable amounts of β-chain underproduction. Patients are asymptomatic and present with microcytic, hypochromic RBCs and Hgb levels >10 g/dL.

- **Thalassemia intermedia** occurs with dysfunction in both β-globin genes, so that the anemia is more severe (Hgb 7 to 10 g/dL).
- **Thalassemia major** (Cooley anemia) is caused by severe abnormalities of both genes and requires lifelong transfusion support.
- **Alpha thalassemia** occurs with a deletion of one or more of the four α-globin genes leading to a β-globin gene excess.
  - Mild microcytosis and mild hypochromic anemia (Hgb >10 g/dL) are seen with loss of one or two genes, whereas **Hgb H disease** (deletion of three α-globin genes) results in splenomegaly and hemolytic anemia.
  - Treatment of Hgb H disease rarely requires transfusion or splenectomy, but oxidant drugs similar to those that exacerbate glucose-6-phosphate dehydrogenase deficiency should be avoided because increased hemolysis may occur (Table 1).
  - Hydrops fetalis occurs with the loss of all four α-globin genes and is incompatible with life.

Diagnosis

Clinical Presentation
- A family history of microcytic anemia or microcytosis is helpful.
- Splenomegaly may be the only physical manifestation.

Laboratories
- Microcytic hypochromic RBCs are seen, along with poikilocytosis and nucleated RBCs.
- Hgb electrophoresis is diagnostic for beta-thalassemia showing an increased percentage of Hgb A_2 and Hgb F.
- **Silent carries with a single α-chain loss have an essentially normal electrophoresis.** Those with Hgb H disease (loss of three loci) have increased Hgb H (β-tetramers). The diagnosis is made by α-globin gene analysis.

Treatment
- Those with thalassemia trait require no specific treatment.
- In patients with more severe forms of the disease, RBC transfusions to maintain a Hgb of 9 to 10 g/dL are needed to prevent the skeletal deformities that result from accelerated erythropoiesis.
- Transfusion-dependent anemia often results in iron overload. Chelation therapy with deferasirox 20 to 30 mg/kg PO everyday is indicated to limit hepatic, cardiac, and endocrine damage.[12] Chelation therapy should be continued until ferritins <1,000 μg/L is maintained. Side effects of deferasirox include mild to moderate GI disturbances and skin rash.
- Hydroxyurea 15 to 35 mg/kg/day may benefit some patients with beta-thalassemia.
- Splenectomy should be considered in patients with accelerated (>2 units/month) transfusion requirements.
- Stem marrow transplant should be considered in young patients with thalassemia major who have human leukocyte antigen–identical related donors.

Red Cell Enzyme Deficiencies

General Principles
- The most common hereditary enzyme deficiency is glucose-6-phosphate dehydrogenase deficiency, a sex-linked disorder that typically affects men.

- RBCs that are deficient in this enzyme are more susceptible to hemolysis via oxidant stress, triggered by infections or drug exposure (Table 1), leading **to chronic or episodic hemolysis.**

Diagnosis

Clinical Presentation
- A mild form of the disease is seen in approximately 10% of African-American men and the anemia is often precipitated by infection, fever, or some medications.
- A more severe form is the Mediterranean variant, in which hemolysis is precipitated when susceptible individuals ingest fava beans and present with fatigue, jaundice, and bilirubinuria.

Laboratories
- The peripheral smear shows "bite cells," and special stains can show Heinz bodies (representing denatured Hgb) within RBCs.
- Diagnosis is made by demonstrating reduced levels of the enzyme. Because older senescent cells with lower enzyme levels hemolyze first during an acute hemolytic episode, a younger population of RBCs may result in a falsely elevated (normal) enzyme level so that the diagnosis may have to await recovery from the hemolytic episode.

Treatment

- Acute hemolytic episodes are largely intravascular and self-limited. Therapy, including hydration and transfusion, is therefore supportive.
- Identification and removal of oxidant stresses such as drugs are paramount.

Autoimmune Hemolytic Anemia

General Principles
- **Autoimmune hemolytic anemia (AIHA)** is caused by antibodies to RBCs, leading to a shortened RBC life span.
- The diagnosis rests on the detection of RBC-bound antibody by a direct antibody test (DAT).
- "Warm" AIHA refers to IgG antibodies that react best at 37°C, whereas in "cold" AIHA, antibodies (usually IgM) are most reactive at lower temperatures.
  - **Warm-antibody AIHA** may be idiopathic or associated with an underlying malignancy (lymphoma, chronic lymphocytic leukemia), collagen vascular disorder, or drugs (Table 1).
  - **Cold-antibody AIHA** is associated with episodic cold-induced hemolysis, resulting in cyanosis of the ears, nose, fingers, and toes precipitated by the cold. Cold agglutinin disease is the most common syndrome. It may be chronic and associated with a B-cell neoplasm (lymphoma, chronic lymphocytic leukemia, Waldenström macroglobulinemia) or acute and caused by an infection (*Mycoplasma* spp., mononucleosis).

Diagnosis
Clinical Presentation
- Mild cases of warm-antibody AIHA may present with a stable anemia and reticulocytosis. In fulminant cases with an RBC life span of <5 days, the anemia can be severe and the compensatory erythropoiesis inadequate, with a presentation of a

rapidly declining Hgb, fever, chest pain, and dyspnea. Jaundice, icterus, and dark urine reflect elevated indirect bilirubin from Hgb degradation.

- In cold-antibody AIHA, severe acute hemolysis may be triggered by exposure to cold ambient temperatures in some patients, so that avoiding the cold is of the utmost importance. The disease is otherwise generally characterized by mild anemia with intermittent exacerbations.

Laboratories

- Laboratory evaluation of warm-antibody AIHA shows a positive DAT for IgG, with 80% of patients having antibodies detectable in the serum (positive indirect Coombs test). Plasma haptoglobin is decreased, LDH is increased, and the peripheral smear shows spherocytes.
- The cold agglutinin is a monoclonal IgM antibody. IgM and C3 are present on the RBC, but the DAT identifies only the presence of C3. IgG is negative on the DAT. The anemia is often mild and stable because serum complement inhibitors (C3 inactivator) limit complement activation on the RBC membrane. Plasmapheresis is often helpful in the acute setting.

Treatment

- Therapy for warm-antibody AIHA is directed at identifying and treating any underlying cause. Steroid therapy (prednisone, 1 to 2 mg/kg/day), splenectomy, and rituximab for patients with refractory disease are used to decrease the immune clearance of RBC.
- Cold avoidance and additional evaluation to identify and treat any underlying malignancy are key for cold-antibody AIHA. Steroids and splenectomy are not effective in the treatment of IgM-mediated disease.

Drug-Induced Hemolytic Anemia

- **Drug-induced hemolytic anemia** is caused by one of three different mechanisms. Treatment consists of discontinuing the offending agent. Medications that are known to cause these effects are listed in Table 1.
- **Drug-induced autoantibodies** present similarly to warm AIHA. The DAT is positive for IgG. α-methyldopa is the prototype.
- **Haptens** form when a drug (usually an antimicrobial) coats RBC membranes, forming a new antigenic determinant. If antibodies against the drug are present and the patient receives the drug (particularly at high doses), a DAT-positive hemolytic anemia may result.
- **Immune complexes** occur in most cases of drug-induced hemolysis. IgM (occasionally IgG) antibodies may develop against a drug and form a drug-antibody complex that adheres to the RBCs. Because the antibody is usually IgM, the DAT is positive only for C3.

Microangiopathic Hemolytic Anemia

- Microangiopathic hemolytic anemia (MAHA) is a morphologic classification in which fragmented RBCs (schistocytes) are seen on peripheral blood smear. It is not a specific diagnosis but suggests a limited differential diagnosis.
- Processes that cause RBC fragmentation and hemolysis include disseminated intravascular coagulation (DIC), thrombotic thrombocytopenic purpura (TTP), hemolytic-uremic syndrome (HUS), malignant hypertension, the preeclampsia/eclampsia

syndromes, vasculitis, adenocarcinoma, malfunctioning heart valves, and improper use of blood warmers. DIC, TTP, and HUS are discussed in Chapter 9.
- The cause of RBC damage appears to be endothelial damage, fibrin deposition, and platelet aggregation in the small blood vessels.
- Therapy is directed at the underlying process that is causing hemolysis.

OTHER RED BLOOD CELL DISORDERS

Polycythemia Vera

General Principles
Polycythemia vera is a myeloproliferative disorder characterized by an unregulated proliferation of all hematopoietic elements but presents primarily with an increased RBC mass.

Diagnosis
Clinical Presentation
- Patients have a variety of symptoms, including weight loss (secondary to hypermetabolism), weakness, gout, pruritus, and central nervous system (CNS) symptoms (headaches, dizziness).
- Physical examination may reveal hypertension, splenomegaly, and a ruddy complexion.
- Clinical factors that could cause secondary polycythemia, particularly hypoxemia from chronic lung disease, sleep apnea, or right-to-left shunts, need to be considered.

Laboratories
- Leukocytosis and thrombocytosis occur in the majority of patients.
- RBC morphology may reflect iron deficiency due to chronic, occult GI hemorrhage, and secondary thrombocytosis may be seen. Iron replacement is occasionally observed before the elevated RBC mass becomes apparent.
- Jak-2 mutations have a 94% sensitivity in the detection of polycythemia vera.[13]
- Epo levels are decreased or at the low end of normal.
- A direct measurement of RBC mass ([51]chromium labeling) may be needed to document absolute polycythemia and rule out pseudopolycythemia but does not distinguish between polycythemia vera and secondary polycythemia.

Treatment
- Initial management of polycythemia vera is with phlebotomy. Maintenance therapy is with intermittent phlebotomy or hydroxyurea titrated to an Hct <45%.
- Nevertheless, thrombotic events are characteristic and account for the most common cause of death in patients who are managed by phlebotomy alone. Addition of low-dose aspirin (81 to 100 mg daily) can reduce these risks.[14]

WHITE BLOOD CELL DISORDERS

Leukocytosis

General Principles
- Leukocytosis is an elevation in the absolute WBC count (>10,000/mm^3).
- An elevated WBC count typically reflects the normal response of BM to an infectious or inflammatory process, steroid, β-agonist or lithium therapy, splenectomy, and stress, and usually causes an **absolute neutrophilia**.

- Occasionally, leukocytosis is due to a primary BM abnormality in WBC production, maturation, or death (apoptosis) related to a leukemia or myeloproliferative disorders and can affect any cell in the leukocyte lineage.
- An excessive WBC response (i.e., >50,000/mm³) associated with a cause outside the BM is termed a **"leukemoid reaction"** which can be either reactive or malignant in origin.
- Lymphocytosis is less commonly encountered and is associated with a viral infection, medication effect, or leukemia.

Diagnosis
Clinical Presentation
History
- Patients with leukocytosis can present with a wide variety of nonspecific symptoms including fevers, chills, fatigue, and malaise.
- Weight loss is a concerning finding for an underlying malignancy.
- A careful history including the temporal nature of the symptoms, specific infectious symptomatology, and a detailed medication history should be elicited.
- In addition, patients with circulating immature WBCs including blasts or those with extreme leukocytosis may present with signs and symptoms of stasis such as CNS and visual disturbances.

Physical Examination
- The physical examination should be directed toward identification of an infectious process.
- Lymphocytosis secondary to chronic lymphocytic leukemia, however, will often present with splenomegaly and lymphadenopathy.
- Patients with chronic myelogenous leukemia present with leukocytosis and splenomegaly; they will rarely present with lymphadenopathy.
- Clinical findings associated with thrombocytopenia or anemia may also occur.

Laboratories
- A complete blood count with peripheral smear is necessary for the evaluation of WBC disorders.
- The presence of blasts on a peripheral smear is concerning for an acute leukemia and warrants emergent evaluation.
- Unexplained neutrophilia should be assessed with a BCR-abl molecular study for the diagnosis of chronic myelogenous leukemia.
- Acute leukemia may also have an associated elevation in LDH and uric acid from the high cell turnover.
- If a malignant etiology is suspected, a BM biopsy, cytogenetics, and flow cytometry often establish the diagnosis.

Treatment
- A number of patients with a neutrophilia will have an infectious or inflammatory etiology and treatment should be directed at the underlying cause.
- Medications implicated in leukocytosis such as corticosteroids should be considered as an etiology.
- The treatment of acute and chronic leukemia requires expertise in hematology-oncology that is beyond the scope of this chapter.

Leukopenia

- Leukopenia is a reduction in the WBC count ($<3,500$ cells/mm^3).
- It can occur in response to infection, inflammation, malignancy, drugs, environmental exposure to heavy metals or radiation, and vitamin deficiencies, with a majority due to medications such as chemotherapeutic or immunosuppressive drugs; the latter are usually dose-dependent effects.
- Idiosyncratic leukopenia can occur secondary to numerous medications and should be suspected when developing shortly after starting a new agent.
- A severe neutropenia with an absolute neutrophil count (<500/mm^3) increases the risk of a life-threatening bacterial infection. If patients develop a neutropenic fever, immediate treatment with broad-spectrum antibiotics should be instituted.
- Growth factor support should be considered in patients with chronic neutropenia and ongoing infections until the neutropenia resolves.

MONOCLONAL GAMMOPATHIES

Monoclonal Gammopathy of Unknown Significance

- Monoclonal gammopathy of unknown significance (MGUS) refers to the presence of a monoclonal protein ("M protein") in the absence of related organ failure and a known related disease, such as multiple myeloma or amyloidosis.
- Most patients identified with a monoclonal gammopathy are classified as having MGUS, whereas the others are diagnosed with a malignant lymphoproliferative disorder including multiple myeloma, amyloidosis, Waldenström macroglobulinemia, lymphoma, or chronic lymphocytic leukemia.
- Monoclonal gammopathies are commonly found on serum protein electrophoresis; most of the gammopathies are identified as IgG but gammopathies in all immunoglobulin classes have been identified.
- The incidence of MGUS increases with age; 3% of persons >70 years of age have an MGUS.
- Characteristics of MGUS include a monoclonal gammopathy <3 g/dL and no evidence of organ damage (e.g., anemia, hypercalcemia, renal insufficiency, or plasmacytoma). A BM examination must show $<10\%$ plasma cells in patients with MGUS. The presence of any of these abnormalities or significant amounts of monoclonal immunoglobulin in the urine suggests a more serious lymphoproliferative disorder.
- MGUS **evolves into a more serious lymphoproliferative malignancy** at a rate of about 1% per year and the risk continues for a long term. Most of these malignancies are multiple myeloma. Therefore, it is recommended that patients with MGUS should be followed indefinitely.
  - Three risk factors for progression have been identified: Non-IgG gammopathy (IgM or IgA), abnormal serum free light-chain ratio (κ/λ ratio), and initial gammopathy concentration of >1.5 g/dL each increase the risk of progressing and the presence of all three confers the highest risk of 58% at 20 years.[15]

Multiple Myeloma

- Multiple myeloma is a lymphoproliferative disorder associated with a monoclonal gammopathy that can present with an unexpected skeletal fracture (long bone or vertebral

body), renal failure (due to Bence Jones proteinuria), hematologic abnormalities (anemia, neutropenia, thrombocytopenia), hypercalcemia, or a combination of these.
- The diagnosis is usually established by a BM examination with the presence of plasma cells >30% in the marrow.
- Treatment with pulse corticosteroids in combination with other chemotherapy (melphalan, thalidomide, lenalidomide, or bortezomib) is usually successful in achieving a response.

Waldenström Macroglobulinemia

- Waldenström macroglobulinemia is an uncommon IgM monoclonal disorder also known as lymphoplasmacytic lymphoma, characterized by mild hematologic abnormalities and accompanied by tissue infiltration including lymphadenopathy, splenomegaly, or hepatomegaly. Because of its high molecular weight and concentration, IgM gammopathy can lead to hyperviscosity (CNS, visual, cardiac) manifestations.
- Treatment with chemotherapy is usually successful in achieving a response.
- Patients with complications of viscosity often benefit from treatment with plasmapheresis to decrease the IgM concentration.

Amyloidosis

- Primary (amyloid light chain [AL]) amyloidosis is an infiltrative disorder due to monoclonal light-chain deposition in various tissues most often involving the kidney (renal failure, nephrotic syndrome), heart (nonischemic cardiomyopathy), peripheral nervous system (neuropathy), and GI tract/liver (macroglossia, diarrhea, nausea, vomiting). Unexplained findings in any of these organ systems should prompt evaluation for amyloidosis.
- An M protein in urine or serum is found in >90% of patients helping establish the diagnosis. Biopsy of an affected organ or BM is often done; diagnosis is made by identification of amyloid protein in the biopsy tissue.
- Treatment of amyloidosis is difficult and progressive organ failure is frequent.
- Cardiac involvement with amyloidosis has a particularly poor prognosis with a median survival of <1 year.

REFERENCES

1. Van Wyck DB, Roppolo M, Martinez CO, et al; for the United States Iron Sucrose (Venofer) Clinical Trials Group. A randomized, controlled trial comparing IV iron sucrose to oral iron in anemic patients with nondialysis-dependent CKD. *Kidney Int* 2005;68: 2846–2856.
2. Singh AK, Szczech L, Tang KL, et al; CHOIR Investigators. Correction of anemia with epoetin alfa in chronic kidney disease. *N Engl J Med* 2006;355:2085–2098.
3. Leyland-Jones B; BEST Investigators and Study Group. Breast cancer trial with erythropoietin terminated unexpectedly. *Lancet Oncol* 2003;4:459–460.
4. Henke M, Laszig R, Rübe C, et al. Erythropoietin to treat head and neck cancer patients with anaemia undergoing radiotherapy: randomised, double-blind, placebo-controlled trial. *Lancet* 2003;362:1255–1260.
5. Leyland-Jones B, Semiglazov V, Pawlicki M, et al. Maintaining normal hemoglobin levels with epoetin alfa in mainly nonanemic patients with metastatic breast cancer receiving first-line chemotherapy: a survival study. *J Clin Oncol* 2005;23:5960–5972.

6. Grote T, Yeilding AL, Castillo R, et al. Efficacy and safety analysis of epoetin alfa in patients with small-cell lung cancer: a randomized, double-blind, placebo-controlled trial. *J Clin Oncol* 2005;23:9377–9386.

7. Wright JR, Ung YC, Julian JA, et al. Randomized, double-blind, placebo-controlled trial of erythropoietin in non-small-cell lung cancer with disease-related anemia. *J Clin Oncol* 2007;25:1027–1032.

8. Blinder M, Field J. Anemia and Transfusion Therapy. In: Cooper DH, Krainik AJ, Lubner SJ, Reno HEL (eds). The Washington Manual of Medical Therapeutics, 32nd Ed. Philadelphia, PA: Lippincott Williams & Wilkins, 2007:548–571.

9. The Management of Sickle Cell Disease. Division of Blood Diseases and Resources. National Heart, Lung, and Blood Institute. Washington DC: National Institutes of Health, 2002. NIH Publication No. 02–2117.

10. Falletta JM, Woods GM, Verter JI, et al. Discontinuing penicillin prophylaxis in children with sickle cell anemia. Prophylactic Penicillin Study II. *J Pediatr* 1995;127:685–690.

11. Vichinsky EP, Haberkern CM, Neumayr L, et al. A comparison of conservative and aggressive transfusion regimens in the perioperative management of sickle cell disease. The Preoperative Transfusion in Sickle Cell Disease Study Group. *N Engl J Med* 1995;333:206–213.

12. *Oncologist* 2009;14(5):489.

13. Rapado I, Albizua E, Ayala R, et al. Validity test study of JAK2 V617F and allele burden quantification in the diagnosis of myeloproliferative diseases. *Ann Hematol* 2008;87:741–749.

14. Landolfi R, Marchioli R, Kutti J, et al; European Collaboration on Low-Dose Aspirin in Polycythemia Vera Investigators. Efficacy and safety of low-dose aspirin in polycythemia vera. *N Engl J Med* 2004;350:114–124.

15. Rajkumar SV, Kyle RA, Therneau TM, et al. Serum free light chain ratio is and independent risk factor for progression in monoclonal gammopathy of undetermined significance. *Blood* 2005;106:812–817.

31 Care of the Cancer Patient

Maria Q. Baggstrom

General Principles

- Before treatment of a cancer patient is initiated, all patients should have a diagnosis of cancer based on tissue pathology, and, if possible, a clinical, biochemical, or radiographic marker of disease should be identified to assess the results of therapy.
- **Stage** is a clinical or pathologic assessment of tumor spread. The major role of staging is to define the optimal therapy and prognosis in subsets of patients. Treatment plans are generally determined by the stage of the tumor. The role of local therapies, surgery, and radiation is determined by regional spread of disease. The role of systemic therapy, or chemotherapy, is also dependent on the stage of the tumor. In general, the probability of survival correlates well with tumor stage.
- The **grade** of a tumor defines its retention of characteristics compared to the cell of origin. It is designated as low, moderate, or high as the tissue loses its normal appearance. Although grade is important in determining prognosis for many tumors, it is not used as commonly as stage in d efining treatment plans.
- **Performance status** is a gauge of a patient's overall functional status. Two scales are commonly used: the Karnofsky performance status scale and the Eastern Cooperative Oncology Group performance status scale (Table 1). Performance status is an essential component of the evaluation of cancer patients, as it helps predict response to treatment, duration of response, and survival. For most solid tumors, patients with poor performance status are unlikely to derive significant benefit from systemic chemotherapy. However, patients with tumors that respond dramatically to chemotherapy may benefit from this treatment, even if they have poor performance status.
- Cancers are broadly characterized as "liquid" or "solid" malignancies.
  - **Leukemias and lymphomas comprise the "liquid" group.** The treatment of liquid tumors is usually chemotherapy or radiation therapy, or both.
  - **The "solid" tumors include tumors that arise from any solid organ or tissue.** Solid tumors are treated with surgery, radiation therapy, chemotherapy, or some combination of these modalities.
- **Chemotherapy** is administered in several different settings. Specific mechanisms of action and toxicities will be discussed in detail below.
  - **Induction** chemotherapy is used to achieve a complete remission.
  - **Consolidation** chemotherapy is administered to patients who initially respond to treatment.
  - **Maintenance** therapy refers to low-dose, outpatient treatment used to prolong remissions; its use has proved effective in a few malignancies.
  - **Adjuvant** chemotherapy is given after complete surgical or radiologic eradication of a primary malignancy to eliminate any unmeasurable metastatic disease.

TABLE 1	Performance Status		
Karnofsky Performance Status Scale		**ECOG Performance Status Scale**	
%	**Definition**	**Grade**	**Definition**
100	Normal; no complaints; no symptoms of disease	0	Fully active, able to carry on all predisease activity without restriction
90	Able to carry on normal activity; minor signs or symptoms of disease	1	Restricted in physically strenuous activity but ambulatory and able to carry out work of a light or sedentary nature
80	Normal activity with effort; some signs or symptoms of disease		
70	Able to care for self; unable to carry on normal activity or to do active work	2	Ambulatory and capable of all self-care but unable to carry out any work activities; up and about >50% of waking hours
60	Requires occasional care for most needs	3	Capable of only limited self-care; confined to bed or chair; >50% of waking hours
50	Requires considerable assistance and frequent medical care		
40	Disabled; requires special care and assistance	4	Completely disabled; cannot carry on any self-care; totally confined to bed or chair
30	Severely disabled; hospitalization is indicated, although death is not imminent		
20	Very sick; hospitalization necessary; active supportive treatment necessary		
10	Moribund; fatal process progressing rapidly		
0	Dead		

ECOG, Eastern Cooperative Oncology Group.
From Naughton M. Medical management of malignant disease. In: Cooper DH, ed. The Washington Manual of Medical Therapeutics. 32nd Ed. Philadelphia, PA: Lippincott Williams & Wilkins, 2007:572–599, with permission.

- **Neoadjuvant** chemotherapy is given in the presence of local disease, before planned local therapy.
- Survival data are often reported in terms of median survival and 5-year survival and cause confusion among patients with newly diagnosed malignancies; these data must be conveyed to the patient with caution by the treating oncologist who can help interpret these data.
  - **Median survival** equates to the period of time during which 50% of studied subjects are alive and 50% are dead.
  - **Five-year survival** means the percentage of patients studied who are alive at 5 years.

Diagnosis

Breast Cancer

- Breast cancer develops in approximately 11% of women during their lifetime in the United States.
- A breast lump in a premenopausal woman is less likely to be cancerous than a breast lump in a postmenopausal woman.
- In a younger woman, a mass should be observed for 1 month to identify any cyclic changes that suggest benign disease.
- If the mass is still present, bilateral mammography should be performed. The accuracy of mammography to diagnose cancer in pre-and postmenopausal women is approximately 90%. **Nevertheless, a woman with a clinically suspicious lump and negative mammograms should undergo biopsy.**

Cancer of Unknown Primary Site

- Approximately 5% of cancer patients present with symptoms of metastatic disease but no primary tumor site is identifiable on physical examination, routine laboratory studies, or chest radiography.
- The histopathologic cell type and the site of the metastasis should direct a search for the primary lesion.
- Immunohistochemical stains may identify specific tissue antigens that help define the origin of the tumor and guide subsequent therapy.

Cervical Adenopathy

- This suggests cancer of the lung, breast, head and neck, or lymphoma.
- Initial evaluation usually includes panendoscopy (nasendoscopy, laryngopharyngoscopy, bronchoscopy, and esophagoscopy) and biopsy of any suspicious lesion before excision of the lymph node.
- If squamous cell carcinoma is identified, the patient is presumed to have primary head and neck cancer and radiation therapy may be curative.

Midline Mass in the Mediastinum or Retroperitoneum

- In both sexes, a midline mass in the mediastinum or retroperitoneum may be an extragonadal germ cell cancer.
- Elevations in AFP or β-HCG (human chorionic gonadotropin) further suggest this diagnosis.
- This neoplasm is potentially curable.

Lymphoma

- Lymphoma is usually diagnosed by biopsy of an enlarged lymph node.
- Staging of Hodgkin disease and non-Hodgkin lymphoma is organized into four categories.
  - **Stage I** is disease localized to a single lymph node or group.
  - **Stage II** is disease involving more than one lymph node group but confined to one side of the diaphragm.
  - **Stage III** is disease in the lymph nodes or the spleen and occurs on both sides of the diaphragm.
  - **Stage IV** is disease involving the liver, lung, skin, or bone marrow.
- **B symptoms** include fever above 38.5°C, night sweats that require a change in clothes, or a 10% weight loss over 6 months. These symptoms suggest bulky disease and a worse prognosis.

- **Hodgkin disease** usually presents with cervical adenopathy and spreads in a predictable manner along lymph node groups.
- **Non-Hodgkin lymphoma** is classified as low, intermediate, or high grade based on the histologic type.
  - Staging evaluation is the same as for Hodgkin disease, but non-Hodgkin lymphoma has a less predictable pattern of spread.
  - Advanced-stage disease (Stage III or IV) is very common and can usually be diagnosed by computed tomography (CT) scan or bone marrow biopsy; exploratory laparotomy and lymphangiography are rarely necessary.

Leukemia

Acute Leukemias

- Patients may present with manifestations of cytopenias, including fatigue and dyspnea (anemia), cutaneous or mucosal hemorrhage (thrombocytopenia), and fever/infection (neutropenia).
- Patients may also present with leukemic infiltration of organs, manifested as lymphadenopathy, splenomegaly (more common in acute lymphocytic leukemia), gingival hyperplasia, and skin nodules (more common in acute myeloid leukemia).
- Leukemic **blasts** are usually present in the blood.
- **Bone marrow aspiration/biopsy** is performed to establish the diagnosis and often shows nearly complete replacement by blasts.
- **Flow cytometry and cytogenetics** must be performed on the bone marrow aspirate for classification and to provide prognostic information.

Chronic Leukemias

- **Chronic lymphocytic leukemia** (CLL) usually presents with lymphocytosis, lymphadenopathy, and splenomegaly. Malignant cells resemble mature lymphocytes.
- **Chronic myelogenous leukemia** (CML) presents with leukocytosis and a left shift, as well as splenomegaly.
  - Thrombocytosis, basophilia, and eosinophilia are also common.
  - The diagnosis of CML is confirmed by demonstration of the **Philadelphia chromosome (t9:22),** which results in production of a hybrid protein (bcr-abl).
- **Hairy cell leukemia** represents only 2% to 3% of all adult leukemias.
  - Clinical presentation includes splenomegaly, pancytopenia, and infection.
  - Patients are at increased risk for bacterial, viral, and fungal infections and have a unique susceptibility to atypical mycobacterial infections.
  - Bone marrow biopsy reveals infiltration by cells that have prominent cytoplasmic projections (thus the name).

Multiple Myeloma

- Multiple myeloma (MM) is a malignant plasma cell disorder that is usually accompanied by a **serum or urine paraprotein,** or both.
- Presenting manifestations may include hypercalcemia, anemia, lytic bone lesions with bone pain, and acute renal failure.
- The initial evaluation should include a radiographic bone survey, bone marrow aspiration and biopsy, serum and urine protein electrophoresis, β2-microglobulin, and quantitative immunoglobulins.

Treatment

General Principles of Chemotherapy

- **The advice of an oncologist and precise adherence to a treatment plan are mandatory because of the low therapeutic index of chemotherapeutic agents.** Specific agents are included in Table 2.
- The dosage of chemotherapy is usually based on body surface area; for some agents, dosage is determined by body weight and should be adjusted when changes in body weight occur.
- An assessment of the patient disease status, determination of side effects from the previous treatment, and a complete blood count should be obtained before each cycle of chemotherapy.
- Drug dosages usually must be adjusted for the following conditions:
  - Neutropenia
  - Thrombocytopenia
  - Stomatitis
  - Diarrhea
  - Limited metabolic capacity for the drug

Route of Administration

Oral Drug Administration
- May be accompanied by nausea and vomiting and may require antiemetic therapy.
- For some agents, oral absorption is erratic and parenteral administration is preferred.

IV Drug Administration
- Should be performed by experienced personnel.
- Care should be taken to ensure free flow of fluid to the vein and adequate blood return should be verified before instillation of chemotherapy.
- Infusions should be through a large-caliber, upper extremity vein. When possible, veins of the antecubital fossa, wrist, dorsum of the hand, and arm ipsilateral to an axillary lymph node dissection should be avoided.
- In patients with poor peripheral venous access or those who require many doses of chemotherapy, indwelling venous catheter devices should be considered.

Intrathecal Chemotherapy
- Intrathecal (IT) chemotherapy is administered for the treatment of meningeal carcinomatosis or as central nervous system (CNS) prophylaxis.
- Side effects include acute arachnoiditis, subacute motor dysfunction, and progressive neurologic deterioration (leukoencephalopathy).
- Impaired cognitive function and leukoencephalopathy occur more often when IT chemotherapy is combined with whole-brain radiation.

Intracavitary Instillation
- May be useful in some circumstances.
- Some chemotherapeutic agents can be instilled directly into the pleural or peritoneal spaces.
- Systemic toxicities can be observed if the agent is systemically absorbed.

Intra-arterial Chemotherapy
- Is advocated as a method of achieving high drug concentrations at specific tumor sites.

TABLE 2	Chemotherapeutic Medications

Drugs	Toxicities
Antimetabolites	
Ara-C	Myelosuppression, GI toxicity, conjunctivitis, cerebellar ataxia, pancreatitis, hepatitis
5-FU	Myelosuppression, stomatitis, diarrhea, cerebellar ataxia, chest pain, hand-foot syndrome
Methotrexate	Mucositis, prolonged reabsorption in patients with effusions, interstitial pneumonitis, hepatitis, renal failure
6-Mercaptopurine	Decreased metabolism in patients taking allopurinol, hepatic cholestasis
Cladribine (2-chlorode-oxyadenosine	Myelosuppression
Gemcitabine	Fever, edema, flu-like symptoms, rash, pneumonitis
Alkylating agents	
Busulfan	Interstitial pneumonitis, gynecomastia, reversible Addison-like syndrome
Chlorambucil	Myelosuppression
Cyclophosphamide	Hemorrhagic cystitis, hemorrhagic myocarditis
Dacarbazine	Flu-like syndrome, fever, myalgias, facial flushing, malaise, elevations of hepatic enzymes
Ifosfamide	Hemorrhagic cystitis, neurologic toxicity, including seizures
Mechlorethamine (nitrogen mustard)	Skin irritant, drug rash
Melphalan	Idiosyncratic interstitial pneumonitis
Nitrosoureas (carmustine [BCNU] and lomustine [CCNU])	Myelosuppression, giddiness, flushing, phlebitis
Temozolomide	Nausea, vomiting, teratogenicity
Thiotepa	Myelosuppression
Antitumor antibiotics	
Anthracyclines (daunorubicin, doxorubicin, mitoxantrone, idarubicin)	Cardiomyopathy, bone marrow suppression, mucositis
Bleomycin	Severe allergic reactions with hypotension, interstitial pneumonitis
Mitomycin-C	Delayed myelosuppression, hemolytic-uremic syndrome
2-Deoxycoformycin (pentostatin)	Myelosuppression

(*continued*)

| TABLE 2 | Chemotherapeutic Medications (*Continued*) |

Drugs | **Toxicities**

Plant alkaloids

Drugs	Toxicities
Vincristine	Dose-limiting neuropathy, SIADH, Raynaud phenomenon
Vinblastine	Myelosuppression, myalgias, obstipation, transient hepatitis
Etoposide (VP-16)	Myelosuppression
Teniposide (VM-26)	Myelosuppression, hypersensitivity reactions, alopecia, hypotension
Paclitaxel	Anaphylactoid reactions, myelosuppression, arthralgias, neuropathy, arrhythmias
Docetaxel	Third-space fluid collections
Navelbine	Pain at IV injection site

Platinum-containing agents

Drugs	Toxicities
Cisplatin	Severe nausea and vomiting, neurotoxicity, renal toxicity, hypomagnesemia, ototoxicity
Carboplatin	Myelosuppression, neurotoxicity, ototoxicity, nephrotoxicity
Oxaliplatin	Sensory neuropathy

Other agents

Drugs	Toxicities
Hydroxyurea	Myelosuppression
L-asparaginase	Allergic or anaphylactoid reactions, hemorrhagic pancreatitis, hepatic failure, encephalopathy
Procarbazine	Monoamine oxidase inhibitor, disufiramlike effect
Topotecan	Myelosuppression
Irinotecan	Severe diarrhea

Hormonal agents

Drugs	Toxicities
Tamoxifen and raloxifene	Hormone flare (bone pain, erythema, hypercalcemia), endometrial cancer, deep vein thrombosis
Aromatase inhibitors (anastrazole, letrozole, exemestane)	Hot flashes, night sweats
Progestational agents (megestrol acetate and medroxy-progesterone)	Weight gain, fluid retention, hot flashes, vaginal bleeding with discontinuation of therapy
Antiandrogens (flutamide and bicalutamide)	Nausea, vomiting, gynecomastia, breast tenderness

Targeted therapies

Drugs	Toxicities
Trastuzumab	Cardiomyopathy
Rituximab	Chills, fever, rare hypersensitivity reactions
Alemtuzumab	Immunodeficiency and opportunistic infections
Bevacizumab	Hypertension, proteinuria, serious bleeding or clotting events, gastrointestinal perforations

(*continued*)

TABLE 2	Chemotherapeutic Medications (*Continued*)
Drugs	**Toxicities**
Cetuximab	Infusion reactions, rash, diarrhea
Panitumumab	Infusion reactions, rash, diarrhea
Gemtuzumab	Nausea, fever, myelosuppression, tumor lysis, hypersensitivity reaction
Ibritumomab and iodine 131 tositumomab	Myelosuppression
Imatinib	Edema, nausea, rash, musculoskeletal pain, congestive heart failure
Erlotinib	Rash, diarrhea
Sunitinib	Hypertension, fatigue, asthenia, diarrhea, hand-foot syndrome, hypothyroidism
Sorafenib	Hypertension, skin rash, diarrhea, hand-foot syndrome
Nonspecific immunotherapy	
Interferon-α	Nausea, vomiting, flu-like symptoms, headache
Aldesleukin (interleukin-2)	Fluid overload, hypotension, prerenal azotemia, elevation of liver enzymes
Chemopreventive agents	
Retinoids	Dry skin, cheilitis, hyperlipidemia, elevation of transaminases

BCNU, bis-chloronitrosourea or carmustine; CCNU, lomustine; GI, gastrointestinal; SIADH, syndrome of inappropriate antidiuretic hormone.

- Although it is of theoretical advantage, there are no absolute indications for chemotherapy administered by this route.

Therapy of Selected Solid Tumors

Breast Cancer
- **Surgical options:** treatment is focused on local control and the risk of systemic spread.
  - Local control with **tylectomy** (lumpectomy and axillary lymph node dissection) is as effective as a modified radical mastectomy. An axillary lymph node dissection should be included because it provides prognostic information and is of therapeutic value.
  - **Sentinel lymph node mapping** and dissection allow many women to be spared full axillary dissection. In this procedure, blue dye, a radiotracer, or both are injected around the tumor bed. The lymph node(s) that pick up the dye/tracer are excised. If no cancer cells are seen in these lymph nodes, further axillary dissection can be avoided.
- **Radiation therapy** is indicated for patients treated with tylectomy and for some individuals with axillary lymph node involvement. It can also be used for palliation of painful or obstructing metastatic lesions.
- **Systemic therapy** is given for two reasons in the treatment of breast cancer:
  - **Adjuvant therapy** is given to a woman who has had surgery to completely remove her tumor to reduce recurrence risk.

- **Palliative therapy** is given to women with metastatic breast cancer to slow the progression of their disease and to extend their lives.
- **Hormone therapy** is used for women with estrogen receptor (ER)–positive and/or progesterone receptor–positive disease.
- **Trastuzumab** (Herceptin) is appropriate for women with **her-2-neu–positive** breast cancer.
- **Anthracycline-based chemotherapy** is potentially useful in all subtypes.

Adjuvant Therapy

- **The presence or absence of axillary lymph node metastases is the most important prognostic factor in breast cancer. All women with axillary nodal involvement should receive adjuvant therapy.**
- Women with node-negative breast cancer should also be considered for adjuvant therapy if the tumor is >1 cm, is ER-negative, or has overexpression of her-2.
- Chemotherapy should be considered in patients who are premenopausal, have cancers that are ER negative, or overexpress her-2.
- **Tamoxifen,** 20 mg PO daily for 5 years, is recommended for all ER-positive breast cancers in premenopausal women.[1]
- In postmenopausal women, the **aromatase inhibitors** anastrozole, letrozole, and exemestane have generally replaced tamoxifen for adjuvant hormone therapy.
- **Trastuzumab** has been found to be effective in the adjuvant treatment of women with her-2-neu–positive disease.[2]

Metastatic Disease

- Menopausal status, hormone receptor status, her-2-neu expression, and sites of metastatic disease dictate initial treatment.
- ER-negative breast cancer, lymphangitic lung disease, and liver metastasis seldom respond to hormonal manipulation and should be treated with chemotherapy.
- ER-positive disease is treated with hormonal manipulation.
  - Premenopausal women are initially treated with tamoxifen and a luteinizing hormone–releasing hormone (LHRH) agonist; postmenopausal women should receive a hormonal agent such as tamoxifen or an aromatase inhibitor. If the disease responds to hormonal therapy, subsequent disease progression may respond to other hormonal agents.
  - Chemotherapy should be considered if there is no response to initial hormonal therapy or if progression occurs during subsequent hormonal manipulations.
- In her-2-overexpressing cancers, the addition of **trastuzumab** to first-line chemotherapy produced an improvement in survival compared to chemotherapy alone.[3]
- In women with more than one osteolytic metastasis, the monthly administration of zoledronic acid, 4 mg IV, produces an improvement in quality of life, greater response to therapy, fewer extravertebral fractures, and possibly a prolongation in survival.[4]

Inflammatory and Unresectable Cancers

- Inflammatory breast cancer manifests as "peau d'orange" changes or erythema involving more than one third of the chest wall.
- Because of the high likelihood of metastases at diagnosis, these patients and those with inoperable primary breast cancers are initially treated with chemotherapy.
- Subsequently, surgery and radiation therapies are used for maximal local control.

Lung Cancer

- Lung cancer is the most common cause of cancer death in the United States and is the most preventable given its relationship to cigarette smoking.
- Treatment is based on the histology and stage of the disease.

Small-Cell Lung Cancer
- Small-cell lung cancer (SCLC) is often responsible for a variety of paraneoplastic syndromes in addition to local symptoms.
- It is treated according to whether disease is limited (confined to one hemithorax and ipsilateral regional lymph nodes) or extensive stage.
  - For **limited disease,** combination chemotherapy and radiation therapy result in an 85% to 90% response rate, a median survival of 12 to 18 months, and a cure in 5% to 15% of patients.
  - With **extensive disease,** the median survival is 8 to 9 months, and cures are rare.
- For patients who achieve a complete remission with chemotherapy, **prophylactic whole-brain radiation therapy** has been shown to decrease the risk of central CNS metastases.[5]
- Radiation therapy to the chest as consolidation therapy may improve survival in limited disease but is not recommended in extensive disease except for palliation of local symptoms.

Non–Small-Cell Lung Cancer
- **Whenever possible, surgical resection should be attempted for non–small-cell lung cancer (NSCLC) because it affords the best chance of cure.**
- Survival rates after resection of NSCLC are improved using adjuvant chemotherapy with or without radiation therapy.
- For unresectable disease confined to the lung and regional lymph nodes, radiation therapy in combination with chemotherapy is the conventional treatment.
- In patients with metastatic disease, cisplatin-based combination chemotherapy may modestly improve survival.
- Bevacizumab, a monoclonal antibody that targets vascular endothelial growth factor, has been approved for the treatment of metastatic NSCLC.
- Erlotinib, a tyrosine kinase inhibitor targeting epidermal growth factor receptor, is also approved for NSCLC.

Gastrointestinal Malignancies
Esophageal Cancers
- Esophageal cancers are either squamous cell (associated with cigarette smoking and alcohol use) or adenocarcinoma (arising in Barrett's esophagus).
- Surgical resection of the esophagus is recommended in small primary tumors and in selected patients after chemoradiation.
- Local control of unresectable cancers can be achieved with combined chemotherapy and radiation therapy.[6]
- Palliation of obstructive symptoms can be accomplished by radiation therapy, dilation, prosthetic tube placement, or laser therapy.

Gastric Cancer
- Gastric cancer is usually adenocarcinoma and can be cured with surgery in the rare patient with localized disease.
- Adjuvant chemotherapy and concurrent radiation have been shown to improve outcomes in surgically resected gastric cancer.[7]
- Locally advanced but unresectable cancers may benefit from concomitant chemotherapy and radiation therapy.
- Chemotherapy may offer palliation for metastatic disease.

Colon and Rectal Adenocarcinomas
- These cancers are primarily treated by surgical resection.

- In all patients who are undergoing surgical resection of colon or rectal cancer, a preoperative **carcinoembryonic antigen** level should be measured and followed. A persistently elevated or increasing level may indicate residual or recurrent tumor.
- A prolonged survival in patients with colon cancer and regional lymph node involvement is seen with administration of postoperative **5-fluorouracil** (5-FU) and **levamisole** for 12 months or 5-FU and leucovorin (LV) for 6 months.[8]
- The addition of **oxaliplatin** to the traditional 5-FU and LV improves risk reduction in Stages II and III colon cancer.[9]
- Rectal cancer that arises below the peritoneal reflection commonly recurs locally after surgery alone; postoperative radiation therapy and 5-FU are recommended.
- A number of chemotherapy agents are available for the treatment of metastatic colorectal cancer. These include 5-FU, irinotecan, capecitabine, and oxaliplatin. In metastatic disease, the addition of irinotecan to 5-FU/LV produces a higher likelihood of response and possible survival advantage.[10]
- Three **monoclonal antibodies** have been approved for the treatment of metastatic colon cancer. Bevacizumab targets vascular endothelial growth factor. Both cetuximab and panitumumab target epidermal growth factor receptor.
- Selected patients with metastases confined to the liver may be candidates for liver resection.[11]

Anal Cancer

- **Chemotherapy with concurrent radiation therapy** appears to result in a higher cure rate than surgical resection and usually preserves the anal sphincter and fecal continence.[12]
- Surgical resection should be used only as salvage therapy.

Genitourinary Malignancies
Bladder Cancer

- In the United States, blander cancer usually presents as **transitional cell carcinoma.** A variety of chemical carcinogens, including those in cigarette smoke, have been implicated.
- **Unifocal** tumors confined to the mucosa should be managed with cystoscopy and transurethral resection or fulguration, repeated at approximately 3-month intervals.
- **Multifocal** mucosal disease is treated with intravesicular bacillus Calmette-Guérin, thiotepa, or mitomycin-C.
- **Locally invasive** cancers should be resected.
- Adjuvant chemotherapy improves survival when regional lymph node involvement is confirmed in the cystectomy specimen.
- In metastatic or recurrent disease, the highest response rates are seen with cisplatin-containing regimens.

Prostate Cancer

- Prostate cancer is the most common cancer in men besides nonmelanoma skin cancer.
- Prostate-specific antigen is useful as a marker for recurrence, bulk of disease, and response to therapy and may detect asymptomatic early-stage disease.
- **Local control** of the primary lesion can be achieved with either prostatectomy or radiation therapy.
- In patients with **metastatic disease,** bilateral orchiectomy and luteinizing hormone–releasing hormone analogs with or without an antiandrogen produce tumor regression in approximately 85% of patients for a median of 18 to 24 months.
  - Disease that has relapsed after hormonal therapy may respond to withdrawal of that antiandrogen.[13]

- Anthracyclines, taxanes, vinblastine, and estramustine may be of palliative value in hormone-refractory disease.
- Anemia and bone pain dominate the advanced phases of this disease and are best relieved with transfusions, growth factors, and palliative radiation therapy.

Renal Cell Cancer
- Renal cell cancer is treated by **surgical resection,** which may be curative if disease is localized; no effective adjuvant therapy is available.
- Chemotherapy, interferon-α, and interleukin-2 have reported response rates of 15% to 30%.
- Two new agents, sunitinib and sorafanib, have been approved for the treatment of metastatic renal cell cancer. Both agents are multitargeted tyrosine kinase inhibitors and appear more active and better tolerated than previously available agents.

Testicular Cancer
- It is considered one of the most curable malignancies and should be treated aggressively.
- A patient suspected of having cancer of the testis should have tissue obtained only through an inguinal orchiectomy because a transscrotal incision facilitates tumor spread to the inguinal lymph nodes.
- The initial evaluation should include serum **α-fetoprotein** and **β-human chorionic gonadotropin** levels and a CT scan of the abdomen and pelvis.
- Most patients with **seminoma** should be treated with radiation therapy.
- In **nonseminomatous germ cell cancer,** a retroperitoneal lymph node dissection should be performed for staging, except in the instance of bulky abdominal disease or pulmonary metastasis.
  - If **microscopic disease** is identified at surgery, two alternatives are acceptable: two cycles of postoperative chemotherapy or observation until relapse occurs followed by institution of chemotherapy.
  - With **gross metastatic disease,** cisplatin-based chemotherapy is curative for most germ cell cancers. If tumor markers normalize after chemotherapy but a radiographic mass persists, exploratory surgery should be performed. The lesion proves to be residual cancer in approximately one third of the patients. Patients with residual cancer should receive additional chemotherapy.[14]

Gynecologic Malignancies
Cervical Cancer
- The recognized risk factors are multiparity, multiple sexual partners, and infection with **human papillomavirus.**
- **Carcinoma in situ** and superficial disease can be treated by endocervical cone biopsy.
- **Microinvasive disease** is treated with an abdominal hysterectomy.
- **Advanced local disease** (invasion of the cervix or local extension) is initially treated with surgery or radiation therapy, or both. The addition of chemotherapy to radiation therapy postoperatively is associated with improved survival.[15]
- Inoperable cancer can be controlled with radiation therapy; metastatic disease is treated with cisplatin-based chemotherapy.
- A **vaccine for human papillomavirus** has recently been approved and is being administered to young women in hopes of reducing the rates of cervical carcinoma.

Ovarian Cancer
- Ovarian cancer is primarily a disease of postmenopausal women.
- Because symptoms are uncommon with localized disease, most patients present with advanced local disease, malignant ascites, or peritoneal metastases.

- **Surgical staging** and treatment include an abdominal hysterectomy, bilateral oophorectomy, lymph node sampling, omentectomy, peritoneal cytology, and removal of all gross tumor.
  - If the tumor is localized to the ovary, the surgery may be curative and further treatment is not routinely recommended. However, if microscopic foci of cancer are identified, chemotherapy is administered postoperatively.
- The serum marker **CA-125,** although not specific, is elevated in >80% of women with epithelial ovarian cancer and is a sensitive indicator of response.
- After a response is achieved, a **"second-look laparotomy"** is performed to restage and remove residual tumor.
  - Approximately one third of the patients who are in pathologic complete remission after a second-look laparotomy are cured.
  - Those patients who have residual cancer should receive additional chemotherapy.

Endometrial Cancer
- The risks include obesity, nulliparity, polycystic ovaries, and the use of unopposed estrogens (including tamoxifen).
- Patients generally present with vaginal bleeding.
- **Surgery and radiation therapy are often curative.**

Head and Neck Cancer
- Head and neck cancer is usually a squamous cell cancer.
- It may arise in a variety of sites, each of which has a different natural history.
- Early lesions can be cured with surgery, radiation therapy, or both.
- Despite aggressive surgical and radiation therapy, approximately 65% of patients with head and neck cancer have uncontrolled local disease.
- The addition of chemotherapy to radiation therapy improves the survival in patients with nasopharyngeal cancers and selected patients with other primary disease sites.[16]

Malignant Melanoma
- This should be considered in any changing or enlarging nevus, and suspicious lesions should be removed by **excisional biopsy.** Subsequently, a wide local excision is performed to remove possible vertical and radial spread of tumor.
- Deeper invasion is associated with a worse prognosis.
- **High-dose interferon** prolongs the survival of selected high-risk resected patients.[17]
- Systemic disease may respond to dacarbazine, interferon-α, or interleukin-2 in 10% to 30% of patients.

Sarcomas
- Sarcomas are tumors arising from mesenchymal tissue and occur most commonly in soft tissue or bone.
- Initial evaluation should include a CT scan of the chest, as hematogenous spread to the lungs is common.

Soft Tissue Sarcoma
- Prognosis is primarily determined by tumor grade and not by the cell of origin.
- **Surgical resection** should be performed when feasible and may be curative.
- In low-grade tumors, local and regional recurrence is most common, and **adjuvant radiation therapy** may be of benefit.
- High-grade tumors often recur systemically but no advantage to the routine use of adjuvant chemotherapy has been demonstrated.

- In **metastatic disease,** doxorubicin, ifosfamide, and dacarbazine produce responses in 40% to 55% of patients.

Osteogenic Sarcoma
- Osteogenic sarcoma treated with surgical resection followed by adjuvant chemotherapy for 1 year.
- Treatment of isolated pulmonary metastasis by surgical resection is associated with long-term survival.

Kaposi Sarcoma
- In an immunocompetent patient, Kaposi sarcoma is generally a low-grade lesion of the lower extremities that is readily treated with **local radiation therapy or vinblastine.**
- When Kaposi sarcoma complicates organ transplantation or AIDS, it is more aggressive and may arise in visceral sites.
- **Liposomal doxorubicin** alone is as effective as combination chemotherapy for palliation.[18]

Therapy of Selected Hematologic Malignancies
Lymphoma
Hodgkin Disease
- **Treatment is based on the presenting stage of the disease;** the cell type is relatively unimportant in the natural history and prognosis.
- Initial staging evaluation includes a CT scan of the chest, abdomen, and pelvis, and bilateral bone marrow biopsies to determine the clinical stage of the disease.
- Exploratory laparotomy with splenectomy and liver biopsy is performed only if the findings will change the disease stage and treatment.
- **Stages I and IIA** are treated with radiation therapy or a combination of chemotherapy and radiation.
- **Stage IIIA** disease can be treated either by radiation therapy or by chemotherapy.
- All **Stage IV** patients should receive combination chemotherapy.
- When **B symptoms** are present, chemotherapy is recommended regardless of the stage.

Non-Hodgkin Lymphoma
- Low-grade lymphoma:
  - It often involves the bone marrow at diagnosis but the disease has an indolent course.
  - Because this tumor is **not curable with standard chemotherapy,** treatment can be delayed until the patient is symptomatic ("watch and wait").
  - **Radiation therapy** or an alkylating agent (e.g., cyclophosphamide) can be used to ameliorate symptoms.
  - Radiation therapy may produce a long-term complete remission in Stage I or II disease.
  - **Rituximab** produces an objective response in approximately 50% of patients with follicular lymphoma without the usual toxicities of chemotherapy.
- Intermediate-grade lymphoma:
  - This has a more aggressive course, usually does not involve the bone marrow at diagnosis, and **can be cured with chemotherapy.**
  - Complete response rates exceed 80%.
  - Features associated with a lower likelihood of cure include an elevated lactate dehydrogenase level, stage III/IV disease, age >60 years, more than one extranodal site, and poor performance status.
- High-grade lymphoma:
  - This subtype includes Burkitt's and lymphoblastic lymphoma.

- They are **most aggressive subtypes** and have a high frequency of CNS and bone marrow involvement.
- Cerebrospinal fluid (CSF) cytology should be included as part of the initial evaluation.
- Combination chemotherapy is the mainstay of treatment and should include CNS prophylaxis if the CSF is cytologically free of tumor.
- If tumor cells are seen in the CSF, additional therapy may be indicated.
- Prophylaxis to prevent **tumor lysis syndrome** should be initiated before induction chemotherapy.

Leukemia

Acute Leukemias

- Acute myeloid leukemia:
  - Acute myeloid leukemia constitutes approximately 80% of adult acute leukemia.
  - Approximately 50% to 80% of patients achieve complete remission with **induction chemotherapy** that includes cytarabine (cytosine arabinoside [ara-C]) and daunorubicin.
  - **Consolidation therapy** is given with at least one additional cycle of chemotherapy, which is typically ara-C at a dose of 10 to 30 times that is used for induction (high-dose ara-C). High-dose ara-C consolidation results in cure in approximately 30% to 40% of patients <60 years of age.
  - Pretreatment factors associated with a low (<10%) chance for cure include the following:
    - Preceding myelodysplastic syndrome
    - Prior exposure to radiation, benzene, or chemotherapy
    - Adverse cytogenetic abnormalities
  - For these high-risk patients, **allogeneic stem cell transplant** in first remission increases the likelihood of cure.
- Acute promyelocytic leukemia:
  - Acute promyelocytic leukemia is characterized by a chromosomal translocation (t[15;17]) that results in a hybrid protein (pml-rar).
  - Treatment with oral **tretinoin** (all-trans retinoic acid) results in complete remission in >90% of patients.
  - After consolidation chemotherapy, approximately 75% of patients are cured.
- Acute lymphocytic leukemia:
  - With only 25% of all cases of acute lymphocytic leukemia occurring in patients >15 years of age, it is typically a disease of childhood.
  - For adults, **induction and consolidation** involve treatment with multiple chemotherapeutic agents over a period of approximately 6 months followed by at least 18 months of lower-dose **maintenance** chemotherapy.
  - To prevent CNS relapse, patients receive **IT chemotherapy** and either cranial radiation or CNS penetrating chemotherapy.
  - Approximately 60% to 80% of adults achieve complete remission, with about 30% to 40% being cured. Increasing age, higher white blood cell count, and longer time to remission are associated with reduced survival.
    - Cytogenetics are crucial in determining prognosis and **allogeneic stem cell transplantation** during the first remission should be considered in patients with a poor prognosis.

Chronic Leukemias

- Chronic lymphocytic leukemia:
  - Treatment of CLL is similar to that for low-grade lymphoma except that **fludara-bine** appears to be more active than alkylating agents.
  - Median survival is approximately 6 to 8 years.
  - Anemia and thrombocytopenia are associated with shortened survival.
  - As in low-grade lymphoma, patients are treated for control of symptoms or cytopenias.
  - Because CLL is accompanied by immunodeficiency, life-threatening infections may occur. Therefore, febrile patients must be evaluated carefully.
  - **Immune hemolytic anemia or immune thrombocytopenia** may develop as complications of CLL. Treatment of these conditions is with **glucocorticoids** (e.g., prednisone, 1 mg/kg PO daily) or chemotherapy, or both.
  - CLL may transform to an intermediate or high-grade lymphoma **(Richter trans-formation).**
- Chronic myelogenous leukemia:
  - During the stable phase of the CML, leukocytosis, thrombocytosis, and splenomegaly can be controlled for several years with **oral hydroxyurea,** and most patients are asymptomatic.
  - **Acute leukemic transformation (blast phase)** is inevitable and unpredictable, with a median time to transformation of 5 to 7 years. Blast phase is highly resistant to treatment and is usually fatal.
  - For younger patients (40 to 50 years of age) with HLA-identical siblings, **allo-geneic stem cell transplantation** performed in stable phase within 1 year of diagnosis is the treatment of choice, resulting in a 50% to 70% likelihood of cure.
  - For older patients and for those without an HLA-identical sibling, options include unrelated donor transplant or therapy with interferon-α. The latter agent delays blast phase in some patients.
  - **Imatinib** is an orally administered medication designed specifically to inhibit the bcr-abl tyrosine kinase.
    - Because imatinib is more active and has far less toxicities than does interferon, it is currently the first-line therapy for this disease.
    - Even blast-phase CML or Philadelphia chromosome–positive acute leukemia may respond to imatinib. Responses in this setting are generally of relatively short duration.
- Hairy-cell leukemia:
  - For hairy cell leukemia a single 7-day course of **chlorodeoxyadenosine** (cladribine) produces remission in >90% of patients.
  - Although this drug is not curative, 5-year progression-free survival exceeds 50%.

Multiple Myeloma

- Treatment of MM generally includes a combination of an oral alkylating agent (i.e., melphalan) and prednisone or vincristine/doxorubicin/dexamethasone.
- Local radiation therapy can be used to relieve painful bone lesions, and zoledronic acid, 4 mg IV every month, decreases skeletal complications.
- **Thalidomide,** an immunomodulatory agent, has been shown to be effective in MM.
  - Because thalidomide can cause severe fetal malformations, prescribing this medication requires participation in a prescriber program.
  - Combinations of dexamethasone and thalidomide are also active in the treatment of MM.

- **Bortezomib** (Velcade), a proteasome inhibitor that degrades ubiquitinated proteins, has recently been approved for the treatment of MM that has progressed despite two previous treatments. Toxicities of bortezomib are primarily thrombocytopenia and neuropathy.
- After induction chemotherapy, consolidation with high-dose therapy and **autologous stem cell transplant** improves survival.

Complications

Complications Related to Tumor

Brain Metastasis
- Patients with parenchymal brain metastasis may present with headache, mental status changes, weakness, or focal neurologic deficits. Papilledema is observed in only 25% of patients.
- In individuals with malignancy, a CT scan of the head showing one or more round, contrast-enhancing lesions surrounded by edema is usually sufficient for the diagnosis.
- If cancer has not been diagnosed previously, tissue should be obtained from the brain lesion or a more accessible site before radiation therapy is initiated.
- Therapy with **dexamethasone**, 10 mg IV or PO, should be initiated to decrease cerebral edema and should be continued at a dosage of 4 to 6 mg PO every 6 hours throughout the course of **radiation therapy**, or longer if symptoms related to edema persist.
- Subsequent therapy depends on the number and location of the brain lesions as well as the prognosis of the underlying cancer.
- Patients with a chemotherapy-responsive neoplasm and a solitary accessible lesion should be considered for surgical resection.
- **All patients who have not received prior radiation therapy should be given whole-brain radiation therapy.**
- **Meningeal carcinomatosis** should be suspected in a cancer patient with headache or cranial neuropathies.
  - This pattern of spread is most often seen with lung or breast cancer, melanoma, or lymphoma.
  - The diagnosis is confirmed by cytology of the CSF.
  - A CT scan of the head should be performed to rule out parenchymal metastases or hydrocephalus before a lumbar puncture is performed.
  - Local radiation therapy or IT chemotherapy may provide temporary relief of symptoms.
  - Meningeal lymphoma may respond to IV ara-C.[19]

Spinal Cord Compression
- Spinal cord compression is most commonly caused by hematogenous spread of cancer to the vertebral bodies followed by expansion into the spinal canal or ischemia of the spinal cord.
- The most common malignancies causing spinal cord compression are breast, lung, and prostate cancer, but the diagnosis should be considered in any patient with cancer who complains of back pain.
- **Treatment involves urgent neurosurgical and radiation oncology consultation in addition to high-dose corticosteroid therapy.**
- **Magnetic resonance imaging** is the imaging modality of choice to assess for acute cord compression.

Superior Vena Cava Obstruction
- Is most commonly caused by cancers that arise in or spread to the mediastinum, such as lymphoma or lung cancer.
- The compressed superior vena cava leads to swelling of the face or trunk, chest pain, cough, and shortness of breath.
- Dilated superficial veins of the chest, neck, or sublingual area suggest an engorged collateral circulation.
- The presence of a mass on chest radiograph or CT scan usually confirms the diagnosis.
- A mediastinal mass may compromise the airway.
- If the histologic origin of the obstruction is unknown, tissue can be obtained for diagnosis via bronchoscopy or mediastinoscopy.
- Therapy is directed at the underlying disease.
- **Chemotherapy** should be administered through a vein that is not obstructed by the lesion.
- Neoplasms that are not responsive to chemotherapy are treated with **radiation therapy.**[20]

Malignant Effusions
Malignant Pericardial Effusions
- Most malignant pericardial effusions commonly result from cancer of the breast or lung.
- Initial presentations range from dyspnea to acute cardiovascular collapse from cardiac tamponade requiring emergency pericardiocentesis.
- After cardiovascular stabilization, some patients may improve with treatment if the tumor is chemotherapy sensitive.
- When the pericardial effusion is a complication of uncontrolled disease, palliation can be achieved by **pericardiocentesis** with sclerosis.
- The effusion should be completely drained, followed by instillation of 30 to 60 mg bleomycin through the drainage catheter, which is subsequently clamped for 10 minutes and then withdrawn.
- Subxiphoid **pericardiotomy** can be performed in patients whose effusions do not respond to other treatment.

Malignant Pleural Effusions
- Malignant pleural effusions develop as a result of pleural invasion by tumor or obstruction of lymphatic drainage.
- When systemic control is impossible and reaccumulation of fluid occurs rapidly after drainage, removal of the fluid followed by instillation of a **sclerosing agent** into the pleural space is recommended.
- Resistant effusions can be controlled with **pleurectomy** or placement of an **indwelling pleural catheter,** which can drain pleural fluid as needed.

Malignant Ascites
- Is most commonly caused by peritoneal carcinomatosis and is best controlled by systemic chemotherapy.
- Therapeutic paracenteses can provide symptomatic relief.
- Intraperitoneal instillation of chemotherapy has been used but is not routinely recommended.

Bone Metastases
- Bone metastases result in spontaneous (pathologic) fractures.
- Prophylactic surgical pinning and radiation therapy may be indicated.

- Bisphosphonates may also protect against skeletal complications from myeloma and breast cancer.[21]

Paraneoplastic Syndromes

- Are complications of malignancy not directly caused by a tumor mass effect and are presumed to be mediated by either secreted tumor products or the development of autoantibodies.
- Paraneoplastic syndromes can affect virtually every organ system, and in most cases, successful treatment of the underlying malignancy eliminates these effects.

Metabolic Complications

- **Hypercalcemia** is the most common metabolic complication in malignancy and can cause mental status changes, gastrointestinal (GI) discomfort, arrhythmias, and constipation.
- The **syndrome of inappropriate antidiuretic hormone** (SIADH) should be considered in a patient with euvolemic cancer patient with unexplained hyponatremia.
  - Although a variety of neoplasms have been described in association with SIADH, **SCLC** is most often responsible.
- **Cancer anorexia and cachexia:**
  - Refer to the clinical syndrome of anorexia, distortion of taste perception, and loss of muscle mass.[21]
  - The asthenic appearance of patients is more often related to tumor type than to tumor burden.
  - **Megestrol acetate,** 160 mg PO daily, has been used as an appetite stimulant and results in weight gain in some patients.[22]
  - Other appetite stimulants include corticosteroids, cannabinoids, and promotility agents such as metoclopramide.

Neuromuscular Complications

- **Dermatomyositis,** more often than polymyositis, has been associated with a variety of malignancies, including NSCLC and colon, ovarian, and prostate cancers.
  - In some patients, successful treatment of the underlying malignancy has resulted in resolution of the symptoms.
  - An exhaustive search for a malignancy is not recommended because a primary malignancy is found in <20% of patients.[23]
- **Lambert-Eaton myasthenic syndrome** is characterized by proximal muscle weakness, decreased or absent deep tendon reflexes, and autonomic dysfunction.
  - Electromyography using high-frequency nerve stimulation may show posttetanic potentiation.
  - **SCLC** is most often associated with this syndrome, and effective chemotherapy may result in improvement.
  - Worsening symptoms have been reported with the use of calcium channel antagonists; these agents are contraindicated in this syndrome.[24]

Hematologic Complications

- Although cytopenias occur more often as a complication of treatment or marrow involvement with cancer, elevated counts may be explained by paraneoplastic syndromes.
- **Erythrocytosis** is a rare complication of hepatoma, renal cell cancer, and benign tumors of the kidney, uterus, and cerebellum.
  - Debulking the tumor with surgery or radiation therapy generally results in resolution of the erythrocytosis.
  - Occasionally, therapeutic phlebotomy is indicated.

- **Granulocytosis (leukemoid reaction)** in the absence of infection occurs in cancer that arises in the stomach, lung, pancreas, brain, and lymphoma. Because the neutrophils are mature and seldom exceed $100,000/mm^3$, complications are rare and intervention is generally unnecessary.
- **Thrombocytosis** in patients with cancer may be caused by splenectomy, iron deficiency, acute hemorrhage, or inflammation; treatment is usually not necessary.

Thromboembolic Complications
- Mucin-secreting adenocarcinomas of the GI tract and lung cancer have been associated with a **"hypercoagulable state,"** resulting in recurrent venous and arterial thromboembolism.
- **Nonbacterial thrombotic (marantic) endocarditis,** usually involving the mitral valve, may also occur.
- Heparin anticoagulation or low–molecular-weight heparin should be instituted, as well as treatment of the underlying cancer.
- Long-term warfarin with a target international normalized ratio of 2 to 3 or daily low–molecular-weight heparin is recommended to prevent subsequent thrombi.[25]

Glomerular Injury
- Glomerular injury has been observed as a paraneoplastic syndrome.
- **Minimal change disease** is often associated with lymphoma, especially Hodgkin disease.
- **Membranous glomerulonephritis** is more often seen with solid tumors.
- The process can be reversed with treatment of the underlying cancer.

Clubbing and Hypertrophic Osteoarthropathy
- This includes polyarthritis and periostitis of long bones.
- Most often observed in NSCLC but are also seen with lesions that are metastatic to the mediastinum.
- Some improvement in the osteoarthropathy can be achieved with nonsteroidal anti-inflammatory drugs but definitive therapy requires treatment of the underlying malignancy.

Fever
- Fever may accompany lymphoma, renal cell cancer, and hepatic metastasis.
- Once an infectious etiology for the fever has been excluded, nonsteroidal anti-inflammatory drugs (e.g., ibuprofen, 400 mg PO every 6 hours, or indomethacin, 25 to 50 mg PO tid) may provide symptomatic relief.

Complications Related to Treatment
- Cancer treatments can cause serious or life-threatening toxicity.
- The most common and predictable toxicities are to the rapidly proliferating cells of hematopoietic and mucosal tissue.
- Because repair of these tissues cannot be accelerated, palliation during the healing process is the primary goal.

Complications of Radiation Therapy
- Toxicity is related to the location of the therapy, total dose delivered, and rates of delivery.
- Large-dose fractions of radiation are associated with greater toxicity to the normal tissues encompassed in the radiation field.
- **Acute toxicity:**
  - Develops within the first 3 months of therapy and is characterized by an inflammatory reaction in the tissue receiving radiation.

- Such toxicity may respond to anti-inflammatory agents such as glucocorticoids.
- Local irritations or burns in the treatment field generally resolve with time.
- Close observation and treatment of any infections and palliation of symptoms such as pain, dysphagia, dysuria, or diarrhea (depending on the site of treatment) are the mainstays of supportive care until healing has occurred.
- **Subacute toxicity:**
  - Between 3 and 6 months of therapy and chronic toxicity after 6 months are less amenable to therapy, as fibrosis and scarring are present.
  - Daily amifostine before head and neck radiation therapy decreases the incidence of xerostomia.[26]

Tumor Lysis Syndrome
- Tumor lysis syndrome occurs in patients with rapidly proliferating neoplasms that are highly sensitive to chemotherapy.
- Rapid tumor cell death releases intracellular contents and causes **hyperkalemia, hyperphosphatemia, and hyperuricemia.**
- Although reported in the treatment of a variety of malignancies, it is usually associated with **high-grade non-Hodgkin lymphoma and acute leukemia.**
- The diagnosis of tumor lysis syndrome is based on susceptibility, clinical suspicion, and close monitoring of laboratory data in patients at risk. Rapidly progressive hyperkalemia, hyperphosphatemia, and hyperuricemia as well as acutely worsening renal failure are the hallmarks.
- **Prophylaxis and pretreatment** are paramount in preventing tumor lysis syndrome.
- During induction chemotherapy, prophylactic measures should include the following:
  - **Allopurinol,** 300 to 600 mg PO daily, and aggressive IV volume expansion (e.g., 3,000 mL/m²/day).
  - The addition of **sodium bicarbonate,** 50 mEq/1,000 mL IV fluid, to alkalinize the urine above a pH of 7 may prevent uric acid nephropathy and acute renal failure. When hyperphosphatemia accompanies hyperuricemia, urine alkalinization should be avoided because calcium phosphate precipitation may result in renal failure.
- **Rasburicase** is a recombinant urate oxidase enzyme that catalyzes the oxidation of uric acid into allantoin, a soluble metabolite. It can be used prophylactically or in the treatment of hyperuricemia. It can be administered as a daily dose of 0.15 to 0.20 mg/kg/day for up to 5 days.
- Despite these preventive measures, **hemodialysis** may be needed for hyperkalemia, hyperphosphatemia, acute renal failure, or fluid overload.

Hematologic Complications
Myelosuppression and Febrile Neutropenia
- A febrile neutropenic patient should be **presumed to be infected** and must be evaluated and treated promptly.
  - The risk of infection increases dramatically with neutropenia (defined as an absolute neutrophil count of <500/mm³) and is directly related to the duration of the neutropenia.
  - Fever is defined as a single core temperature reading of >38.3°C or two readings of >38.0°C spanning 1 hour.
  - Other clinical signs of infection must be considered because the inflammatory response may be muted in the absence of neutrophils.
- A complete physical examination should be performed to locate potential sites of infection, with particular attention to indwelling catheter sites, sinuses, and the oral

and perirectal areas. Digital rectal examination should be avoided to prevent bacterial translocation.

- Laboratory studies/imaging should include the following:
  - Cultures of blood, urine, stool, sputum, and other foci that are susceptible to bacterial infections (e.g., fluid collections) should be collected.
  - A chest radiograph should be obtained to check for infection.
- Neutropenic patients should be maintained in **modified reverse isolation.**
  - Those who enter the room should wash their hands thoroughly with antiseptic soap or an alcohol-based hand-cleaning solution.
  - Visitors with colds should wear a mask and those with fevers should not enter.
  - Because of the risk of fungal infection, live plants should not be allowed in the room.
- **Antimicrobial therapy:**
  - **Empiric treatment should be initiated immediately after cultures are obtained.**
  - **Low-risk patients** can be discharged on an oral broad-spectrum agent such as a fluoroquinolone or trimethoprim/sulfamethoxazole. Characteristics of low-risk patients are afebrile after institution of antibiotics, negative cultures, and anticipated to recover from myelosuppression in <1 week.
  - Standard therapy, in the absence of a known source, should provide broad coverage for gram-negative bacilli (including *Pseudomonas aeruginosa*) and gram-positive cocci (including α-hemolytic *Streptococcus spp.*).
  - In choosing a regimen, local susceptibility patterns should also be considered.
  - Initial therapy may consist of combination therapy with an aminoglycoside and semisynthetic penicillin or a fourth generation cephalosporin as a single agent.
  - **Antimicrobials are continued until the neutrophil count is >500/mm^3.**
  - **Vancomycin** should not be included in initial empiric regimens unless the patient is clinically unstable or has had a recent oxacillin-resistant *Staphylococcus aureus* infection.
  - Persistent fever, in the absence of other data, does not warrant an empiric change in the antibacterial therapy.
  - Empiric antifungal therapy with **amphotericin B** (starting at 0.5 mg/kg and advanced to 1.0 mg/kg daily) should be added if the fever continues for longer than 72 hours.
  - Additional agents should be tailored to the culture data or clinical picture.
  - Coverage against *S. epidermidis*, *Clostridium difficile*, or anaerobic infections is commonly necessary based on physical examination findings and suspected foci of infection.
- **Growth factors:**
  - Growth factors include many cytokines that may ameliorate the myelosuppression associated with cytotoxic chemotherapy. They act on hematopoietic cells, stimulating proliferation, differentiation, commitment, and some functional activation.
  - Because they can increase myelosuppression, **they should not be given within 24 hours of chemotherapy or radiation.**
  - **G-CSF,** given at an initial dose of 5 μg/kg SC/day or IV beginning the day after the last dose of cytotoxic chemotherapy, may reduce the incidence of febrile neutropenic events.
    - Blood counts should be monitored twice a week during therapy.
    - Bone pain is a common toxicity that can be managed with nonopiate analgesics.
    - A pegylated form of G-CSF is now available, allowing for single-dose/cycle administration at a dose of 6 mg.

- **GM-CSF,** given subcutaneously at a dose of 250 μg/m^2/day beginning the day after the last dose of cytotoxic chemotherapy, shortens the period of neutropenia after stem cell transplant.

Anemia

- Anemia is a common side effect of multiple chemotherapeutic agents. Symptoms include fatigue, dyspnea, or lethargy.
- RBC transfusions are indicated for patients who have symptoms of anemia, active bleeding, or a hemoglobin concentration below 7 to 8 g/dL. Because of anecdotal reports of graft-versus-host disease (GVHD) associated with transfusions, radiation of all blood products is generally recommended for immunosuppressed marrow transplant patients.
- **Recombinant erythropoietin** given at a starting dose of 150 units/kg SC three times a week has been shown to improve anemia and decrease transfusion requirements in cancer patients, particularly those in whom the anemia is predominantly caused by cytotoxic chemotherapy.[27]
  - Hematocrit should be monitored weekly during therapy and the dosage should be adjusted accordingly.
- **Darbepoetin alfa** is a recombinant erythropoietin with a longer half-life.
  - It is indicated for the treatment of chemotherapy-induced anemia in patients with solid tumors and can be dosed every 2 weeks.[28]

Thrombocytopenia

- Thrombocytopenia is another common side effect of chemotherapeutic agents toxic to the bone marrow. Symptoms include easy bruising and bleeding, including epistaxis and gingival bleeding.
- Thrombocytopenia <10,000/mm^3 which is the result of chemotherapy should be treated with platelet transfusions to minimize the risk of spontaneous hemorrhage.
- Interleukin-11 was approved to reduce the duration and severity of thrombocytopenia after chemotherapy. However, limited efficacy and significant toxicity (fluid retention and atrial arrhythmias) have limited its use.
- When prolonged thrombocytopenia is anticipated, histocompatibility testing should be performed before therapy so that HLA-matched single-donor platelets can be provided when alloimmunization makes the patient refractory to random-donor platelets.

Gastrointestinal Complications
Stomatitis

- The severity of stomatitis ranges from mild (oral discomfort) to severe (ulceration, impaired oral intake, and hemorrhage).
- It is commonly the dose-limiting toxicity of methotrexate and 5-FU but can be the unpleasant consequence of many chemotherapeutic agents.
- Toxicity is more severe with simultaneous administration of radiation therapy.
- Healing generally occurs within 7 to 10 days of the development of symptoms.
- For mild cases of stomatitis, **oral rinses** (chlorhexidine, 15 to 30 mL swish and spit tid, or the combination of equal parts diphenhydramine elixir, saline, and 3% hydrogen peroxide) may provide relief. Polyvinylpyrrolidone-sodium hyaluronate gel can also be used.
- **Palifermin,** a keratinocyte growth factor analog, has been approved for use in chemotherapy-induced stomatitis.[29]
- In severe cases, IV morphine is appropriate.
- IV fluids should be used to supplement oral intake as needed.

- Patients with moderate or severe stomatitis may develop aspiration. Precautions should include elevation of the head of the bed and availability of a handheld suction apparatus.
- In severe or prolonged episodes, superinfection with Candida or herpes simplex is possible and requires appropriate diagnosis and antimicrobial intervention.

Diarrhea
- In this context, diarrhea is the result of cytotoxicity to proliferating cells of the intestinal mucosa.
- In some cases of diarrhea, IV fluids are necessary to avoid intravascular volume depletion.
- The use of oral opioid agents as antidiarrheals is commonly limited by abdominal cramping.
- Severe diarrhea associated with 5-FU and LV has been reported to respond to octreotide, 150 to 500 µg SC tid.

TABLE 3	Recommendations for Antiemetic Therapy

Dopamine antagonists
Phenothiazines
Prochlorperazine, 5–10 mg PO or IV q4–6 hours (maximum IV dose, 40 mg/day) or 25 mg per rectum q4–6 hours
Chlorpromazine, 10 mg PO q4–6 hours

Butyrophenones
Droperidol, 1–5 mg IV q4–6 hours

Benzamides
Trimethobenzamide, 100 mg PO or IM q4–6 hours
Metoclopramide[a], 2–3 mg/kg IV before chemotherapy and q2 hours for three doses

Serotonin 5-HT$_3$ receptor antagonists
Granisetron, 1 mg IV or 2 mg PO 15 minutes before chemotherapy
Palonosetron, 0.25 mg IV 15–30 minutes before chemotherapy
Ondansetron, 8–32 mg IV 15–30 minutes before chemotherapy or 24 mg PO or 8 mg PO tid
Dolasetron, 100 mg IV or PO 30 minutes before chemotherapy

Antihistaminic
Diphenhydramine, 50 mg PO or IV q4–6 hours

Anxiolytic
Lorazepam, 1–2 mg PO or IV tid to qid

Glucocorticoid
Dexamethasone, 10–30 mg IV before chemotherapy

NK1 Antagonist
Aprepitant 125 mg PO day 1, 80 mg PO daily days 2 and 3 (in conjunction with corticosteroids/serotonin antagonists)

[a]Metoclopramide is also a 5-HT$_4$ agonist and also a central and vagal 5-HT$_3$ antagonist.

- Diarrhea, sometimes severe, is a common side effect of the topoisomerase 1 inhibitor irinotecan and can be treated with loperamide, 4 mg PO and then 2 mg every 2 hours while awake and 4 mg every 4 hours during the night.

Nausea and Vomiting

It can develop in varying degrees and frequency. Suggestions for antiemetic agent(s) are listed in Table 3.

Other Specific Complications

- **Interstitial pneumonitis** may develop as a dose-related, cumulative toxicity or as an idiosyncratic reaction.
- The implicated agent should be discontinued.
- The institution of glucocorticoids (e.g., prednisone, 1 mg/kg PO daily or equivalent) may be of some benefit. The long-term outcome, however, is unpredictable.
- **Hemorrhagic cystitis** may develop with either **cyclophosphamide or ifosfamide.**
- Hemorrhagic cystitis is best anticipated and treated with prophylactic **mesna** at a dosage of at least 0.6 mg mesna to 1 mg ifosfamide.
- Treatment consists of continuous bladder irrigation with isotonic saline and should continue until the hematuria resolves.

REFERENCES

1. Goldhirsch A, Glick JH, Gelber RD, et al. Meeting highlights: International Consensus Panel on the Treatment of Primary Breast Cancer. *J Natl Cancer Inst* 1998;90:1601–1608.
2. Piccart-Gebhart MJ, Procter M, Leyland-Jones B, et al. Trastuzumab after adjuvant chemotherapy in HER2-positive breast cancer. *N Engl J Med* 2005;353:1659–1672.
3. Slamon DJ, Leyland-Jones B, Shak S, et al. Use of chemotherapy plus a monoclonal antibody against HER2 for metastatic breast cancer that overexpresses HER2. *N Engl J Med* 2001;344:783–792.
4. Rosen LS, Gordon D, Kaminski M. Zoledronic acid versus pamidronate in the treatment of skeletal metastases in patients with breast cancer or osteolytic lesions of multiple myeloma: a phase III, double-blind, comparative trial. *Cancer J* 2001;7:377–387.
5. Auperin A, Arriagada R, Pignon JP, et al. Prophylactic cranial irradiation for patients with small-cell lung cancer in complete remission. Prophylactic Cranial Irradiation Overview Collaborative Group. *N Engl J Med* 1999;341:476–784.
6. Walsh TN, Noonan N, Hollywood D, et al. A comparison of multimodal therapy and surgery for esophageal adenocarcinoma. *N Engl J Med* 1996;335:462–467.
7. Macdonald JS, Smalley SR, Benedetti J, et al. Chemoradiotherapy after surgery compared with surgery alone for adenocarcinoma of the stomach or gastroesophageal junction. *N Engl J Med* 2001;345:725–730.
8. Moertel CG, Fleming TR, Macdonald JS, et al. Fluorouracil plus levamisole as effective adjuvant therapy after resection of stage III colon carcinoma: a final report. *Ann Intern Med* 1995;122:321–326.
9. Andre T, Boni C, Mounedji-Boudiaf L, et al. Oxaliplatin, fluorouracil, and leucovorin as adjuvant treatment for colon cancer. *N Engl J Med* 2004;350:2343–2351.
10. Saltz LB, Cox JV, Blanke C, et al. Irinotecan plus fluorouracil and leucovorin for metastatic colorectal cancer. Irinotecan Study Group. *N Engl J Med* 2000;343:905–914.
11. Fong Y, Cohen AM, Fortner JG, et al. Liver resection for colorectal metastases. *J Clin Oncol* 1997;15:938–946.
12. Martenson JA, Lipsitz SR, Lefkopoulou M, et al. Results of combined modality therapy for patients with anal cancer (E7283). An Eastern Cooperative Oncology Group study. *Cancer* 1995;76:1731–1736.
13. Kelly WK, Slovin S, Scher HI. Steroid hormone withdrawal syndromes. Pathophysiology and clinical significance. *Urol Clin North Am* 1997;24:421–431.

14. Einhorn LH. Treatment of testicular cancer: a new and improved model. *J Clin Oncol* 1990;8:1777–1781.

15. Keys HM, Bundy BN, Stehman FB. Cisplatin, radiation, and adjuvant hysterectomy compared with radiation and adjuvant hysterectomy for bulky stage IB cervical carcinoma. *N Engl J Med* 1999;340:1154–1161.

16. Calais G, Alfonsi M, Bardet E, et al. Randomized trial of radiation therapy versus concomitant chemotherapy and radiation therapy for advanced-stage oropharynx carcinoma. *J Natl Cancer Inst* 1999;91:2081–2086.

17. Kirkwood JM, Strawderman MH, Ernstoff MS, et al. Interferon alfa-2b adjuvant therapy of high-risk resected cutaneous melanoma: the Eastern Cooperative Oncology Group Trial EST 1684. *J Clin Oncol* 1996;14(1):7–17.

18. Gill PS, Wernz J, Scadden DT, et al. Randomized phase III trial of liposomal daunorubicin versus doxorubicin, bleomycin, and vincristine in AIDS-related Kaposi's sarcoma. *J Clin Oncol* 1996;14:2353–2364.

19. Glantz MJ, LaFollette S, Jaeckle KA, et al. Randomized trial of a slow-release versus a standard formulation of cytarabine for the intrathecal treatment of lymphomatous meningitis. *J Clin Oncol* 1999;17:3110–3116.

20. Ahmann FR. A reassessment of the clinical implications of the superior vena caval syndrome. *J Clin Oncol* 1984;2(8):961–969.

21. Berenson JR, Lichtenstein A, Porter L, et al. Efficacy of pamidronate in reducing skeletal events in patients with advanced multiple myeloma. Myeloma Aredia Study Group. *N Engl J Med* 1996;334:488–493.

22. Tisdale MJ. Biology of cachexia. *J Natl Cancer Inst* 1997;89:1763–1773.

23. Sigurgeirsson B, Lindelof B, Edhag O, et al. Risk of cancer in patients with dermatomyositis or polymyositis. A population-based study. *N Engl J Med* 1992;326:363–367.

24. McEvoy KM, Windebank AJ, Daube JR, et al. 3,4-Diaminopyridine in the treatment of Lambert-Eaton myasthenic syndrome. *N Engl J Med* 1989;321:1567–1571.

25. Gould MK, Dembitzer AD, Doyle RL. Low-molecular-weight heparins compared with unfractionated heparin for treatment of acute deep venous thrombosis. A meta-analysis of randomized, controlled trials. *Ann Intern Med* 1999;130:800–809.

26. Kemp G, Rose P, Lurain J, et al. Amifostine pretreatment for protection against cyclophosphamide-induced and cisplatin-induced toxicities: results of a randomized control trial in patients with advanced ovarian cancer. *J Clin Oncol* 1996;14:2101–2112.

27. Crawford J. Recombinant human erythropoietin in cancer-related anemia. Review of clinical evidence. *Oncology (Williston Park)* 2002;16(9 Suppl 10):41–53.

28. Mirtsching B, Charu V, Vadhan-Raj S, et al. Every 2-week darbepoeitin alfa is comparable to rHuEPO in treating chemotherapy induced anemia. *Oncology* 2002;16(10 Suppl 11): 31–36.

29. Hueber AJ, Leipe J, Roesler W. Palifermin as treatment in dose-intense conventional polychemotherapy induced mucositis. *Haematologica* 2006;91(8 Suppl):ECR32.

32 Palliative Care and Hospice Medicine
Nadia Khoury and Maria C. Dans

General Principles

Over the course of the past century, how and where Americans die has changed greatly. Life expectancy has increased, and many people live for years with diseases that once heralded a rapid death. As the technology of medicine has advanced, its focus has shifted toward cure and away from symptom control. The process of dying has lengthened, and it has moved from homes to healthcare facilities. Although our ability to treat many diseases has improved, this evolution has created a new set of problems for patients, their families, and healthcare providers. The palliative care and hospice movements aim to use the advancements of modern medicine not only to lengthen life but also to relieve suffering and to enhance quality of life.

Definition
- The World Health Organization defines palliative care as "the active total care of patients . . . Control of pain, of other symptoms, and of psychological, social, and spiritual problems . . . [in order to provide] . . . the best quality of life for patients and their families."[1]
- The National Consensus Project for Quality Palliative Care has broadened the definition:
  - The goal of palliative care is to prevent and relieve suffering and to support the best possible quality of life for patients and their families, regardless of the stage of the disease or the need for other therapies.
  - Palliative care is both a philosophy of care and an organized, highly structured system for delivering care.
  - Palliative care expands traditional disease-model medical treatments to include the goals of enhancing quality of life for patient and family, optimizing function, helping with decision making, and providing opportunities for personal growth.[2]
- In summary, palliative care attempts to alleviate suffering associated with chronic life-limiting illnesses, whether or not these illnesses are terminal.

Epidemiology
- Over the past century, the most common causes of death in the United States have undergone a shift toward chronicity (i.e., congestive heart disease vs. acute myocardial infarction and chronic obstructive pulmonary disease vs. pneumonia).[3,4]
- As the technological aspects of medicine have advanced, dying has been viewed more as a failure of therapy and less as a natural part of human existence. The emphasis on diagnosis and cure has supplanted suffering and symptomatic distress as intrinsically worthy targets of therapy.
- Many people are very debilitated during the time before their death; increasingly, the care they need is provided not at home, but in institutions (Table 1).[5]

TABLE 1	Percentage of Deaths by Location in the United States[a]

Location of Death	Percentage
Hospital	57% (16% of these in emergency departments)
Residence	20%
Nursing home	17%
Other	6% (including those dead on arrival to hospital)

[a]Based on 1992 U.S. vital statistic data published by the Institute of Medicine in 1997. Modified from Committee on Care at the End of Life, Institute of Medicine, Field MJ, Cassel CK, eds. Approaching Death: Improving Care at the End of Life. Washington, DC: National Academy Press, 1997.

- In 2007, 38.8% of Americans died on hospice (a gradual increase from 11% in 1995). The median length of stay was 20 days; approximately 30% of people died within 7 days of initiation of hospice care.[6]
- Along with the shift toward institutional care at the end of life, there has been a dramatic increase in the cost of this care.
  - In 1992, the cost of care provided during the last 6 months of life was estimated at $44.9 billion annually (1992).[7]
  - Much of this care is subsidized by the federal government. Medicare and Medicaid were not designed for care of the dying but provide approximately 50% of the funding.[8]
  - The rest of the financial burden falls mainly upon patients and their families, with up to 30% of families impoverished by a family member's death.[9]
- The modern hospice movement, and subsequently the specialty of palliative care developed in response to these changes.
  - Saint Christopher's Hospice opened in London, UK, in 1967, and the first inpatient hospices were introduced in North America in the 1970s.
  - The Omnibus Budget Act of 1983 created the Medicare Hospice Benefit. It changed the concept of hospice in the United States by emphasizing that care be provided at home rather than at inpatient facilities.
  - The subspecialty of palliative care grew out of the modern hospice movement in the 1980s to address the needs of people with serious illness who might still be pursuing curative treatment. In 2006, the American Board of Medical Specialties approved the creation of Hospice and Palliative Medicine as an official subspecialty of 10 participating specialty boards (Anesthesiology, Emergency Medicine, Family Medicine, Internal Medicine, Pediatrics, Physical Medicine and Rehabilitation, Psychiatry and Neurology, Radiology, Surgery, and Obstetrics and Gynecology). Also in 2006, the Accreditation Council for Graduate Medical Education (ACGME) began the process of establishing standards for the creation of ACGME-accredited fellowships in Hospice and Palliative Medicine.

Diagnosis

Palliative care and hospice services involve a multidisciplinary approach to address patient suffering.

Appropriate Timing
Appropriate timing for palliative care and hospice interventions is presented in Figure 1.[10]

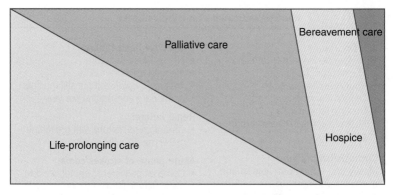

Time from terminal diagnosis ⟶

Figure 1. Palliative and hospice care in the course of illness. (From Hallenbeck J. Stanford University Faculty Development Center End-of-Life Curriculum, 2007. www.growthhouse.org/stanford/, with permission.)

- Palliative care does not exclude the continuation of life-prolonging treatment but rather complements curative therapy by helping clarify goals of care and improving symptomatic control.
- Hospice has a defined end point based on Medicare guidelines: eligibility requires a diagnosis considered terminal and a life expectancy of <6 months. Hospice eligibility may be renewed for patients living beyond 6 months who wish to continue the program.

Indications for Palliative and Hospice Care

While palliative care consults may be considered at any point during the course of a person's disease, national guidelines have been established to assist providers with determining **when to consider hospice** for specific life-limiting noncancer conditions.[11] These are detailed in Table 2.

Venues for Palliative Care and Hospice Interventions

- Palliative care and hospice care may be provided in either inpatient or outpatient settings.
- In the outpatient setting, palliative care may be performed:
  - By the primary care provider or treating specialists themselves based on the precepts of palliative care described below and
  - In a palliative care subspecialty clinic by a board-certified palliative care provider and a multidisciplinary group that may involve social workers, chaplains, nurses, and therapists.
- Outpatient hospice care can be arranged by a physician by contacting a local hospice organization that serves the patient's residential area. Admission to hospice does not require a "do not resuscitate" order and can be concurrent to other therapies.

Goal of Palliative Care

The goals of palliative care are addressed with input from a multidisciplinary team to improve quality of life for both patient and family in the remaining time a patient has. These aims include:

TABLE 2	Possible Indications for Hospice Care

COPD:
- Oxygen dependent or unresponsive to bronchodilators
- Poor exercise capacity
- Unintentional weight loss
- Resting tachycardia
- Multiple acute care admissions per year

Cirrhosis/liver failure:
Mostly bed-bound with at least one of multiple comorbidities:
- Recurrent variceal bleeding
- Encephalopathy
- Refractory ascites
- Hepatorenal syndrome
- History of spontaneous bacterial peritonitis

Dementia:
- Bed-bound and unable to communicate verbally or ambulate without assistance.
- Progressive weight loss
- Fecal or urinary incontinence
- Presence of recurrent medical complications such as infections, dysphagia, or weight loss that require frequent acute care admissions

Congestive heart failure:
- NYHA Class IV failure
- Ejection fraction <20%
- Treatment optimized but still multiple acute care admissions per year

Renal failure:
- Chronic renal failure with creatinine >8.0 mg/dL, off dialysis.

Acute phase of strokes/coma:
- Coma or persistent vegetative state secondary to stroke beyond 3 days' duration.
- Coma with any four of the following on day 3 of coma:
  - Abnormal brain stem response
  - Absent verbal response
  - Absent withdrawal response to pain
  - Serum creatinine >1.5 mg/dL
  - Age >70

Chronic phase of strokes/coma:
Clear-cut predictors are not well established but may include:
- Poor functional or nutritional status
- Weight loss
- Significant dementia
- Serum albumin <2.5 mg/dL
- Recurrent medical complications requiring frequent acute care admissions.

COPD, chronic obstructive pulmonary disease; NYHA, New York Heart Association.
Modified from Medical Guidelines for Determining Prognosis in Selected Non-Cancer Diseases. *Hosp J* 1996;11:47–63.

- Clarifying patient, family, and care team goals, preferences, and choices.
- Providing holistic care of patient and family.
- Providing aggressive control of bothersome symptoms.

Assessing the Experience of the Suffering Patient

- Traditional medical practice views symptoms and signs as evidence of disease. This evidence should disappear once the appropriate diagnosis is made and therapeutic measures initiated.
- The palliative care approach complements traditional models by emphasizing that symptoms themselves are appropriate targets for therapy. It uses the clues that the disease process provides to understand and treat the symptoms.
- Symptoms have both physical and psychological components.
  - **Physical aspects** may be local (e.g., what is causing pain) or central (e.g., how pain is sensed) components.

- **Psychological components** include affective (how an illness is emotionally experienced), cognitive (what patients understand about their illness), and spiritual (how symptoms are organized by patients into a framework that allows them to understand their illness).

Treatment

The principles of palliative care can assist in:
- Assessing and controlling bothersome symptoms such as pain, nausea, and dyspnea.
- Sharing bad news.
- Clarifying patient, family, and healthcare provider goals.
- Identifying additional stakeholders.
- Facilitating discussions to align the goals of care with the treatment plan.

Steps to Sharing Bad News

- Many physicians have minimal formal training in sharing bad news during their preclinical years and few watch more experienced physicians model such conversations during their clinical rotations.[12]
- Discussions of bad news frequently involve raw emotion. They are difficult even under the best of circumstances and can be both personally and professionally challenging. Done skillfully, however, they can help patients, families, and healthcare providers move through difficult situations in a productive manner.
- Traditionally, effective communication has been viewed as something that physicians-in-training absorb through experience as a function of natural aptitude and not as a set of teachable skills. More recent authors have emphasized that, regardless of affinity, there are several key steps to facilitating conversations about bad news.[13]
  - **Preparation** is extremely important and includes:
    - Understanding the medical condition and implications of available therapies and preparing resources if barriers exist.
    - Arranging an in-person meeting (if possible) to share the news, along with having a support person available.
    - Finding a quiet place and adequate time to sit and talk with minimal distractions. Turning beepers/cell phones to vibrate and instructing support staff not to interrupt, or when possible, including support staff who have a relationship with the patient may be helpful.
  - Next, **making a connection** with the person hearing the news is important. This begins with introductions of all parties involved, followed by an assessment of their immediate needs, comfort, and their understanding of the situation.
  - **Sharing the news** involves speaking slowly using clear and unambiguous language, prefacing the news with a statement such as "I unfortunately have some bad news," and giving the news briefly.
  - After delivering the news, **watch and listen to the reaction.** Frequently, a direct question about what the patient or family is thinking may prompt useful dialogue. Respond with brief, simple answers, and recognize that the emotional impact of the bad news may restrict the quantity of information that can be delivered. Follow-up is essential. If the recipient of the bad news is alone, ask whether someone should be called to provide additional support.
  - Finally, **transition to follow up** by establishing a concrete plan for a future meeting to address additional questions. If a referral is necessary, identify whom that provider will be and how he or she will be contacted. Close the meeting with a **statement of concern and commitment to help.**

- It may be helpful after difficult discussions to debrief with other members of the healthcare team—pay attention to your feelings and needs as the provider who shares the bad news.

Goals of Care Discussions

Once the initial shock of bad news has subsided, it is important to establish clear goals for care in order to develop a rational therapeutic plan. One algorithm for addressing goals of care discussions is the GOOD acronym, developed as part of the Stanford End of Life Curriculum.[14]

Goals
- Before the discussion begins, it is essential to identify the stakeholders and assess what they understand of the current situation. The patient and his/her family are obvious stakeholders, but there are frequently many other people as well, including healthcare providers or members of the community.
- "Big picture goals" about the "who, what, when, and where" of living should be identified first because they provide the context. In addition, most "big picture" goals reveal underlying values that must be understood before moving onto specific aims.

Options
- Next, specific options are discussed by listing them and then narrowing them down by the requests of the involved stakeholders.
- Providers have an important role in discussing the benefits and burdens of the options available.
- The provider helps stakeholders understand the possible outcomes with available options.
- Values of the stakeholders are again important because they help assign the relative importance of each outcome state.

Opinion
- Offer your opinion in a neutral manner, incorporating earlier data elucidated about patient and family views, clinician goals, benefits and burdens of care, probabilities of outcomes, and the values of the stakeholders involved.
- Many patients are, in fact, interested to know what their caregivers' opinions are.

Document
- Finally, write a note that includes key information from the meeting including the names and relationships of the participants, decisions regarding the "big picture goals," the immediate care plan, and the care plan in the event of discussed scenarios.
- Also, include an assessment of the decision-making process and whether it makes sense in light of the "big-picture goals."

Addressing Artificial Nutrition Support

- Many clinicians recommend for or against artificial nutrition on the basis of cultural or personal biases (fear of starving the patient, etc.) rather than medical evidence. A review of the published literature indicates the following:
  - Artificial nutrition can improve survival in acute catabolic states such as sepsis or in highly functional patients with advanced proximal gastrointestinal cancer, and in those with amyotrophic lateral sclerosis who desire nutrition.[15]
  - Tube feeding does not reduce the risk of aspiration pneumonia.[16,17]
  - Tube feeding does not prolong life in those with advanced cancer or dementia.[18]

- Tube feeding may not improve quality of life and can decrease quality of life by depriving a patient of the pleasure of eating.[19]
- Most actively dying patients do not complain of hunger or thirst, though dry mouth is prevalent.[20]
- Knowing these facts and sharing them with involved stakeholders may ease decision making about enteral feeding.
- It can also be helpful to differentiate between the provision of artificial nutrition and the acts of eating or feeding. Most people enjoy eating and feeding a loved one who is sick can be a significant and pleasant nurturing activity for both patient and family.
- As with other options in the care of those with life-limiting illness, addressing patient and family concerns about artificial nutrition must take place in the larger context of a goals-of-care discussion.
- It is important to validate family members' concerns, especially in terms of their intent as those who love and care for the patient. Reframing the concerns in light of the goals of care and acknowledging the difficulty of the situation and the commitment of all concerned to the patient's well-being may help families make informed decisions regarding artificial nutrition.

Assessing and Controlling Nonpain Symptoms

Nausea and Vomiting

- Nausea and vomiting arise from the emetic center in the medulla, which receives input from the gastrointestinal tract, the chemoreceptor trigger zone, the vestibular apparatus, and the cerebral cortex.
- Causes of nausea and vomiting may arise from multiple sources including the following:
  - Derangement of the gastrointestinal tract through dysmotility, obstruction, or compression (e.g., hepatomegaly causing "squashed stomach" and early satiety).
  - Infection or inflammation of the body or more specifically, the gastrointestinal tract.
  - Effects of medications that are sensed as toxins in the chemoreceptor trigger zone.
  - Vestibular components.
  - Cognitive and affective components (e.g., environmental clues, underlying depression or anxiety) that impact the cerebral cortex.
- The widely available antiemetics act on receptors that are important in the signaling in the emetic center in the medulla and include H_1 histamine, D_2 dopamine, and muscarinic cholinergic receptors (Table 3).[21]
- Other agents used primarily in cancer and chemotherapy-related nausea include steroids, marijuana/dronabinol, and the antidepressant mirtazapine ($5\text{-}HT_3$ and $5\text{-}HT_2$ blockade).
- Because of their particular receptor activity, these drugs may be specifically helpful for nausea caused by the mechanisms previously discussed (Table 4).[22]

Dyspnea

- Dyspnea is the experience of shortness of breath.
- The sensation of dyspnea is due to an imbalance between the perceived need to breathe and the perceived ability to breathe.
- Oxygen saturation is a poor identifier of those with dyspnea.
- Dyspnea has a large affective component, most commonly panic and fear.
- **Opioids** are the best-studied medicines in the treatment of dyspnea though the mechanism is not well understood. It is likely not due to inhibition of respiratory drive as most commonly thought but rather due to inhibition of sensation of respiratory

TABLE 3	Pharmacologic Activity of Antiemetic Agents
Agent	**Pharmacologic Activity**
Scopolamine (Transderm Scop)	Anticholinergic >>> antihistaminic = dopamine-antagonist
Dimenhydrinate (Dramamine)	Antihistaminic >> anticholinergic > dopamine-antagonist
Promethazine (Phenergan)	Antihistaminic > anticholinergic = dopamine-antagonist
Prochlorperazine (Compazine)	Dopamine-antagonist >> antihistaminic = anticholinergic > 5-HT$_3$-antagonist
Chlorpromazine (Thorazine)	Dopamine-antagonist = antihistamine >> cholinergic > 5-HT$_3$-antagonist
Droperidol (Inapsine)	Dopamine-antagonist >>> antihistaminic = 5-HT$_3$-antagonist
Haloperidol (Haldol)	Dopamine-antagonist >>> antihistaminic
Metoclopramide (Reglan)	Dopamine-antagonist > 5-HT$_3$-antagonist
Ondansetron (Zofran)	5-HT$_3$-antagonist
Mirtazapine (Remeron)	5-HT$_2$- and 5-HT$_3$-antagonist > antihistaminic > anticholinergic

Modified from Brunton LL, Lazo JS, Parker KL, eds. Goodman & Gilman's the Pharmacological Basis of Therapeutics. 11th Ed. New York, NY: McGraw-Hill, 2006.

muscle fatigue thereby limiting the perception that the body cannot meet the need to breathe.[14]

- **Benzodiazepines** are useful in relieving anxiety and pain related to dyspnea but are otherwise not helpful.
- Oxygen can also reduce dyspnea, especially in those who are hypoxic, by yet unexplained mechanisms that can include decreased airway resistance.[23]

TABLE 4	Antiemetics for Specific Causes	
Cause of Nausea	**Receptors Involved**	**Useful Drugs**
V Vestibular	H$_1$ histaminic M cholinergic	Scopolamine, promethazine
O Obstruction from constipation	H$_1$ histaminic M cholinergic ?5-HT$_3$ serotonergic	Senna products, ?mirtazapine
M Dysmotility of the upper GI tract	H$_1$ histaminic M cholinergic ?5-HT$_3$ serotonergic	Metoclopramide
I Infection, inflammation	H$_1$ histaminic M cholinergic	Promethazine, prochlorperazine
T Toxins, such as opioids	D$_2$ dopaminergic ?5-HT$_3$ serotonergic	Prochlorperazine, haloperidol, ondansetron

Modified from Hallenbeck J. Fast Fact and Concept #5: Causes of Nausea and Vomiting. 2nd Ed. End-of-Life/Palliative Education Resource Center, 2005. www.eperc.mcw.edu.

Referral

Referral may be considered to other subspecialties such as pain management (for invasive palliative anesthesia such as nerve or spinal blocks), radiation oncology (for palliative radiation therapy to improve pain), chaplaincy (for spiritual or existential distress), or psychiatry (for more complicated anxiety, depression, or associated psychosis).

Monitoring/Follow-Up

The use of a palliative care approach involves a multidisciplinary effort to support patients and families in clarifying and achieving their goals. This may involve frequent follow-up with various members of the team, including nurses to facilitate patient care and coach families in new ways to nurture; physicians to develop and coordinate a medical plan for symptom control; social workers to provide grief counseling and address complex psychosocial issues; and chaplains to address spiritual aspects of end-of-life care.

Additional Resources

The following is a list of Web sites that physicians may find helpful to learn more about the palliative care movement and hospice and also to learn about important resources for their patients:

1. Growth House, http://www.growthhouse.org, run by the Inter-Institutional Collaborating Network on End-of-Life Care.
2. End-of-Life/Palliative Education Resource Center, http://www.eperc.mcw.edu, run by the Medical College of Wisconsin, provides among other resources, a series of handouts, or Fast Facts, on important palliative care topics for the practicing physician caring for patients facing life-limiting illnesses.
3. The American Academy of Hospice and Palliative Medicine, http://www.aahpm.org.
4. The National Hospice and Palliative Care Organization, http://www. nhpco.org, including a search link for hospice and palliative care providers.
5. The Center to Advance Palliative Care, http://www.capc.org.

REFERENCES

1. Doyle DG, Hanks GWG, MacDonald N, eds. Oxford Textbook of Palliative Medicine. 2nd Ed. Oxford, UK: Oxford University Press, 1998:3.
2. National Consensus Project for Quality Palliative Care (2009). Clinical Practice Guidelines for Quality Palliative Care. 2nd Ed. http://www.nationalconsensusproject.org. Accessed December 16, 2009.
3. Brim OG Jr, Friedman HE, Levine S, Scotch NA, eds. The Dying Patient. New York, NY: Russell Sage Foundation, 1970.
4. Anderson RN. Deaths: leading causes for 1999. *Natl Vital Stat Rep* 2001;49:1–87.
5. Committee on Care at the End of Life, Institute of Medicine, MJ Field, Cassel CK, eds. Approaching Death: Improving Care at the End of Life. Washington, DC: National Academy Press, 1997.
6. NHPCO Facts and Figures: Hospice Care in America. Alexandria, VA: National Hospice and Palliative Care Organization, 2008.
7. Cohen SB, Carlson BL, Potter DEB. Health Care Expenditures in the Last Six Months of Life. *Health Policy Rev (American Statistical Association Section on Health Policy)* 1995;1:1–13.

8. Gornick M, Warren JL, Eggers PW, et al. Thirty years of Medicare: impact on the covered population. *Health Care Financ Rev* 1996;18:179–237.

9. Covinsky KE, Landefeld CS, Teno J, et al. Is economic hardship on the families of the seriously ill associated with patient and surrogate care preferences? *Arch Intern Med* 1996;156: 1737–1741.

10. Hallenbeck J. Stanford University Faculty Development Center End-of-Life Curriculum, 2007. www.growthhouse.org/stanford/

11. Medical guidelines for determining prognosis in selected non-cancer diseases. *Hosp J* 1996;11:47–63.

12. American Association of Medical Colleges. The Increasing Need for End of Life and Palliative Care Education. Contemporary Issues in Medical Education. Washington, DC, 1999.

13. Buckman R. How to Break Bad News. Baltimore, MD: Johns Hopkins University Press, 1992.

14. Hallenback J. Palliative Care Perspectives. Oxford, UK: Oxford University Press, 1993.

15. Gibson S, Wenig BL. Percutaneous endoscopic gastrostomy in the management of head and neck carcinoma. *Laryngoscope* 1992;102:977–980.

16. Nakajoh K, Nakagawa T, Sekizawa K, et al. Relation between incidence of pneumonia and protective reflexes in post-stroke patients with oral or tube feeding. *J Intern Med* 2000;247: 39–42.

17. Croghan J, Burke EM, Caplan S, Denman S. Pilot study of 12-month outcomes of nursing home patients with aspiration on videofluoroscopy. *Dysphagia* 1994;9:141–146.

18. Meier DE, Ahronheim JC, Morris J, et al. High short-term mortality in hospitalized patients with advanced dementia: lack of benefit of tube feeding. *Arch Intern Med* 2001;161:594–599.

19. Callahan CM, Haag KM, Weinberger M, et al. Outcomes of percutaneous endoscopic gastrostomy among older adults in a community setting. *J Am Geriatr Soc* 2000;48: 1048–1054.

20. Conill C, Verger E, Henríquez I, et al. Symptom prevalence in the last week of life. *J Pain Symptom Manage* 1997;14:328–331.

21. Brunton LL, Lazo JS, Parker KL, eds. Goodman & Gilman's the Pharmacological Basis of Therapeutics. 11th Ed. New York, NY: McGraw-Hill, 2006.

22. Hallenbeck J. Fast Fact and Concept #5: Causes of Nausea and Vomiting. 2nd Ed. End-of-Life/Palliative Education Resource Center, 2005. www.eperc.mcw.edu. Accessed December 16, 2009.

23. Libby D, Briscoe WA, King TK. Relief of hypoxia-related bronchoconstriction by breathing 30 percent oxygen. *Am Rev Respir Dis* 1981;123:171–175.

Pain Management
Amy Sheldahl and Maria C. Dans

General Principles

- Pain is one of the most common complaints evaluated by physicians. It is the presenting symptom of a myriad of medical conditions. Some of these conditions are curable, but in many cases the role of the physician is not to cure the disease but to control the pain associated with it.
- Historically, treatment of pain has been limited by fears of addiction and dependence as well as societal conventions on the role of pain in character development and the dying process. Pain therapy has evolved as physicians have come to view treatment of pain as an essential component of patient care—a task as important as treatment of the disease itself.
- This chapter will discuss general principles of pain management. While many of these concepts have been developed for the treatment of chronic cancer pain, they can be applied to patients experiencing pain associated with many other disease states.

Definition

The International Society for the Study of Pain defines pain as "an unpleasant sensory and emotional experience, associated with actual or potential tissue damage, or described in terms of such damage."[1] Pain is extremely subjective by nature, so a more clinically accessible definition might be that "pain is whatever the patient says it is."

Classification

Classification of pain into subsets based on mechanism and time course can guide therapy. Pain in a given patient often falls into several of these categories; all relevant categories should be addressed for adequate treatment.

Acute Pain
- Acute pain is associated with a recent, often reversible etiology.
- Examples include joint injuries, postoperative pain, and pain associated with acute infection.

Chronic Pain
- Chronic pain results from irreversible or not easily reversible etiologies.
- Examples include pain due to malignancy, some forms of low back pain, and severe degenerative joint disease.

Nociceptive Pain
- Nociceptive pain is classically associated with acute pain and injury. Tissue damage via mechanical, chemical, or thermal processes triggers activation of nociceptive pain fibers.
- Pain is usually described as sharp, gnawing, or aching. It is usually well localized and often worse with movement.

Neuropathic Pain
- Neuropathic pain (also referred to as neurogenic pain) is due to nerve injury in the central or peripheral nervous system. All pain is modulated by central pain processing pathways; in neuropathic pain, there is frequently an abnormality caused by tissue damage or disease in the processing pathways that contributes to the ongoing pain.
- Pain is usually described as burning or stinging, and may be accompanied by numbness, tingling, allodynia, or hyperalgesia.

Visceral Pain
- Visceral pain is due to stretching, crushing, or ischemia of organs supplied by visceral nerve fibers.
- Pain is often difficult to describe and may by expressed as squeezing, cramping, dull, or aching. This pain is poorly localized and may be referred to a cutaneous dermatome supplied by the same nerve roots.

Epidemiology
- Low back pain accounts for one fifth of visits to medical clinics.[2]
- Up to 75% of patients with advanced cancer report being in pain.[3]
- Up to 50% of patients with cancer or their surrogates reported moderate to severe pain in last 3 days of life.[4]
- Cancer pain is more likely to be poorly controlled in the elderly (age >70), minorities, and patients with a good functional status.[5]

Pathophysiology
- Painful stimuli activate nociceptors in the skin, joints, organs, and other tissues. Nerves transmit these signals to the central nervous system.
- Synaptic transmission and central pain processing pathways modulate the transmission of pain signals, and pain is ultimately experienced via the central nervous system.
- Pain may be due to injury at any level of the pain pathway, including tissue damage that stimulates nociceptors, injury to nerves that carry or modulate pain signals, and damage to central nervous system neurons involved in pain processing.

Diagnosis

The patient's history is the key diagnostic tool for guiding diagnosis and therapy.

Clinical Presentation
History
A thorough history is paramount for the accurate diagnosis and eventual treatment of pain. A history should include the information regarding the patient's pain as presented in Table 1.

Physical Examination
- Physical examination can aid in diagnosing some causes of acute pain, such as joint injury or infection.
- The physician should also assess for signs of a source of chronic pain, such as cancer or neuropathy.
- All patients should be assessed for signs of hemodynamic instability, peritonitis, or other causes of acute pain, which require emergent evaluation for stabilization.

TABLE 1	Pain History

• **Location**	• **Associated symptoms**
• **Radiation**	○ Dyspnea
• **Quality**	○ Nausea/vomiting
○ Somatic	○ Diaphoresis
○ Visceral	• **Psychological state**
○ Neuropathic	○ Spiritual distress
• **Longitudinal course**	○ History of mood disorder
○ Acute	○ History of substance abuse
○ Chronic	• **Impact of pain on the patient's**
○ Breakthrough	**daily functioning**
○ Episodic	○ Self-care
○ Diurnal variation	○ Work
• **Aggravating/alleviating factors**	○ Hobbies
○ Prior therapies and their efficacies	• **Severity, multiple scales available**
○ Specific triggering activities	○ Numerical scale: 0–10
○ Positional component	○ Visual analogue scale
	○ Faces scale by Wong-Baker for patients with limited cognition

- Acute pain is typically accompanied by physical signs such as tachycardia, diaphoresis, hypertension, and obvious physical discomfort. Patients with chronic pain often have few physical signs of pain.
- Pain may exist without physical manifestations.

Diagnostic Testing

- **No diagnostic test is available to provide objective assessment of pain.**
- Diagnostic testing is indicated when the history and physical examination point toward sources of pain which may be amenable to curative treatment.
- Additional testing is sometimes indicated for pain, which may require specialized interventions such as surgery, although a discussion of this topic is beyond the scope of this text.

Treatment

- A thorough history, physical examination, and diagnostic tests as indicated should identify potentially curable causes of pain. If treatable causes of pain are discovered, pain control should be pursued along with curative therapy.
- When no curable cause of pain is found, therapy should proceed with a combination of nonpharmacologic treatments, medications, and possibly targeted procedures, if applicable.
- All interventions and therapies should be tailored to meet the needs of each patient. **Complete relief of pain may not be possible;** satisfactory control of pain, however, may allow participation in important activities or other specific goals of the patient.

Historical Perspective—WHO Pain Ladder

- The World Health Organization (WHO) pain ladder, developed in 1982, was the result of a public health initiative designed to provide a framework to improve pain control for patients with cancer worldwide. In its simple algorithm, treatment of pain is addressed in three steps. If pain persists at a given step, treatment is advanced to the next step. All steps recommend the use of adjuvant therapy, if indicated.

- **Step 1 (Mild pain):** Nonopioid analgesic such as acetaminophen or nonsteroidal anti-inflammatory drugs (NSAIDs).
- **Step 2 (Moderate pain):** Weak opioid $+/-$ nonopioid analgesic
- **Step 3 (Severe pain):** Strong opioid $+/-$ nonopioid analgesic
- The WHO ladder helped change attitudes toward pain management and heightened physician awareness of the importance of pain management.
- When the WHO ladder is used, addiction and tolerance are unlikely to be clinical problem.[6]
- While most patients can achieve improved pain relief using this algorithm, **the WHO ladder does have limitations.**
  - It does not include an assessment step.
  - It does not take into account targeted therapy for neuropathic pain.
  - It does not allow for nonpharmacologic strategies.
  - While it is common practice to follow the WHO ladder's recommendation to combine NSAIDs with opioids, there is no evidence base to support a clinical difference in pain relief when opioids are given in combination with NSAIDs as compared with either drug alone.[7]

Basic Pain Management Principles

- For acute self-limited pain, short-acting agents can be used as needed.
  - Analgesics may be used before engaging in activities that provoke pain, for example, dressing changes, physical therapy.
- **For chronic pain, adequate analgesia is best obtained with a combination of long-acting basal pain medication and doses of short-acting medications as needed** for breakthrough pain.
  - Breakthrough doses should be 5% to 15% of total daily dose.
  - Basal dose should be increased in patients requiring >2 to 3 breakthrough doses per day.
  - Dose escalation for inadequate pain control should increase the 24-hour dose by 30% to 50%.
- While neuropathic pain is responsive to opioid therapy, adjuvant therapy with antidepressants or anticonvulsants may confer additional benefit in these patients.[8]
- Start with the lowest effective dose of medication and titrate up as needed.
- Be careful to avoid acetaminophen overdose when using opioid/acetaminophen combination pills.

Medications

Nonopioid Analgesics

Nonsteroidal Anti-Inflammatory Drugs

- NSAIDs exert antipyretic, analgesic, and anti-inflammatory effects via inhibition of cyclooxygenase isoenzymes (COX1 and/or COX2 depending on the agent), which leads to decreased production of thromboxane and prostaglandins via the arachidonic acid pathway.
- NSAIDs are effective for mild pain, especially pain with an inflammatory component.
- Most NSAIDs have an analgesic **ceiling effect**—a dose above which analgesia does not increase.
- These drugs are relatively contraindicated in patients with renal insufficiency or with a history of peptic ulcer disease.

TABLE 2	Commonly Used Nonsteroidal Anti-Inflammatory Drugs	
Drug	**Dose**	**Forms**
Aspirin	325–650 mg PO q4–6 hours Ceiling effect on analgesia at 1,000 mg/day	Tablets/caplets Buffered caplets Enteric coated Chewable Gum (Aspergum) Rectal suppository
Ibuprofen	200–800 mg PO 3–4 times/day	Tablets/caplets
Diclofenac	100–150 mg/day in 2–3 divided doses	Immediate or extended release tablet Gel for topical use with osteoarthritis (Voltaren Gel) Transdermal patch (Flector)
Naproxen	250–500 mg q12 hours Ceiling effect on analgesia at 1,000 mg/day	Tablet Suspension
Celecoxib	100–200 mg q12–24 hours	Tablet
Indomethacin	20–50 mg PO tid	Short-acting or extended release tablets Suppository Suspension

- Adverse effects of NSAIDs include gastrointestinal tract bleeding via gastritis or ulcer formation, platelet dysfunction, and renal insufficiency. Aspirin may precipitate bronchospasm in patients with severe asthma.
- Gastrointestinal side effects may be reduced by using proton pump inhibitors or H_2 blockers to suppress gastric acid production.
- Details regarding commonly used NSIADs are presented in Table 2.

Acetaminophen
- Acetaminophen exerts analgesic and antipyretic effects. Its exact mechanism of action is poorly understood.
- Analgesic dosing is 325 to 650 mg PO every 4 to 6 hours or 1 g 3 to 4 times per day. **Maximum daily dose should not exceed 4 g/day for patients with normal hepatic function; patients with liver disease should not take >2 g/day. The recommended maximum dose for patients >70 years of age is 3 g/day.**
- An analgesic ceiling effect likely occurs at doses of 1 g.[9]
- Acetaminophen is available in tablet, liquid, and suppository forms.
- The major adverse effect of acetaminophen is liver toxicity, ranging from mild transaminitis to fulminant hepatic failure. Patients with underlying liver disease or heavy alcohol use can experience liver damage at lower doses.

Opioids
- Opioids exert analgesic effects via opioid receptors in both the central nervous system and the spinal cord to alter pain perception.
- Unlike other classes of analgesics, there is **no analgesic ceiling effect** with increasing doses of opioids.

- Opioids offer flexibility in dosing routes that can be customized to a patient's needs.
- Doses can be given via oral, transdermal, sublingual, intravenous, rectal, subcutaneous, intrathecal, intraventricular, buccal, and epidural routes.
- Refer to Table 3 for commonly prescribed opioids and dosing.[10]

Opioid Selection

Data comparing opioid efficacy are limited, and the results are largely equivocal. Opioid selection may be based on desired route of administration, availability, and individual patient tolerance for a given drug.

- **Tramadol:**
  - Tramadol is both an opioid agonist and a centrally acting nonopioid analgesic that acts on pain processing pathways.
  - Dosing is 50 to 100 mg PO every 4 to 6 hours. Maximum daily dose is 400 mg/day.
  - Side effects include flushing, headache, dizziness, insomnia, somnolence, nausea, vomiting, constipation, dyspepsia, and pruritus. Dose titration starting with 25 mg and gradually increasing can improve tolerance.
  - Tramadol is **metabolized by the liver and excreted largely by the kidneys.** It is not dialyzable. **It has an active metabolite that can lower the seizure threshold,** particularly when taken in combination with some antidepressant medications. It should not be used in patients with known seizure disorders.
- **Codeine:**
  - Codeine is an opioid prodrug with modest antitussive effects.
  - To exert analgesic effect it must be converted to morphine via hepatic metabolism. However, **at least 10% of the U.S. population lacks the appropriate enzyme for codeine metabolism.** In these patients, codeine will provide analgesia similar to acetaminophen, but with higher rates of constipation.
- **Oxycodone:**
  - While a single meta-analysis found pain control to be slightly better with morphine than with oxycodone, dry mouth and drowsiness were less prevalent with oxycodone.[11]
  - Oxycodone has no renally cleared active metabolites.
- **Morphine:**
  - Morphine is often a first-line opioid given its safety profile, ease of use, availability, and physician experience with its use.
  - An **active metabolite** of morphine can accumulate in renal insufficiency, so alternate opioids may be considered in renal insufficiency.
- **Methadone:**
  - Methadone is an opioid agonist as well as an N-methyl-D-aspartic acid antagonist, producing analgesia with additional adjuvant effects for neuropathic pain.
  - The half-life of methadone is relatively long and varies significantly between patients. **The duration of methadone's analgesic effect is much shorter than its half-life.**
  - Methadone interacts with many common medications, resulting in further **pharmacokinetic variability.**
  - Methadone has similar efficacy to morphine for cancer pain with similar side effects in short-term studies. However, in long-term studies, methadone side effects were more pronounced.[12] In addition, recent data suggest an increase in mortality in patients using methadone, and the Food and Drug Administration (FDA) has urged caution and careful titration of methadone in pain therapy.[13]
  - Methadone can be a very useful drug for chronic pain, but it is best prescribed by physicians experienced in its use. Close follow-up during dose titration is essential.

| TABLE 3 | Commonly Prescribed Opioids[a] |

Drug	Generic or Trade Name(s) and Formulations	Recommended Dosing Interval
Morphine		
Short-acting	Morphine sulfate immediate release tablet: 15, 30 mg	q2–4 hours[b]
	Morphine sulfate solution: 10 mg/5 mL, 20 mg/5 mL, 20 mg/mL	q2–4 hours[c]
	Roxanol solution: 20 mg/mL, 100 mg/5 mL	q4 hours
	Morphine sulfate suppository: 5, 10, 20, 30 mg	q4 hours
Extended release	Morphine sulfate extended release tablet: 15, 30, 60, 100, 200 mg	q8–12 hours
	Avinza: 30, 60, 90, 120 mg	q24 hours
	Kadian: 10, 20, 30, 50, 60, 80, 100, 200 mg	q12–24 hours
	MS Contin: 15, 30, 60, 100, 200 mg	q8–12 hours
	Oramorph SR: 15, 30, 60, 100 mg	q8–12 hours
Oxycodone		
Immediate release	Oxycodone tablet: 5, 10, 15, 20, 30 mg	q4–6 hours
	OxyIR: 5 mg	q4 hours
	ETH-Oxydose solution: 20 mg/mL (berry flavor)	q4 hours
	OxyFast solution: 20 mg/mL	q4 hours
Sustained release	Oxycodone extended release tablet: 10, 20, 40, 80 mg	q12 hours
	OxyContin: 10, 15, 20, 30, 40, 60, 80, 160 mg	q12 hours
Hydromorphone		
Tablet	Hydromorphone: 2, 4, 8 mg	q3–4 hours
	Dilaudid: 2, 4, 8 mg	q3–4 hours
Suppository	Hydromorphone suppository: 3 mg	q6–8 hours
	Dilaudid: 3 mg	q6–8 hours
Liquid	Dilaudid: 1 mg/mL	q3–4 hours
Fentanyl		
Transdermal	Fentanyl: 12[d], 25, 50, 75, 100 μg/hr	q72 hours
	Duragesic: 12[d], 25, 50, 75, 100 μg/hr	q72 hours
Transmucosal	Actiq: 200, 400, 600, 800, 1,200, 1,600 mg (berry flavored, also known as fentanyl lollipop)	May repeat 1× after initial dose if pain persists; Maximum 4 units/day

[a]Opioids are generally administered intravenously only in the hospital setting, although occasionally they are given subcutaneously in the outpatient setting. This usually occurs in a home hospice setting, and dosing is equivalent to intravenous dosing. Intravenous administration of opioids will not be discussed in this outpatient care manual.
[b]Peak serum concentration of most short-acting oral morphine preparations occurs after 1 hour. Short-acting doses can be given as frequently as every 2 hours without stacking/overlapping doses. While relatively stable pain is appropriately treated with breakthrough doses every 4 hours as needed, out-of-control pain can be addressed by dosing short-acting opioids every 2 hours.
[c]Initial dosing of short-acting oral morphine for opioid naïve patients is 5 to 10 mg every 4 hours as needed. For an opioid naïve patient starting oral morphine, solution should be used, as short-acting tablets are only available in 15 and 30 mg formulations.
[d]Duragesic and fentanyl 12 μg/hr patches actually supply 12.5 μg/hr.
Drug information from: Lexi-comp Online Drug Database. 2009. http://www.crlonline.com/crlsql/servlet/crlonline. Accessed May 27, 2009.

- **Hydromorphone:**
  - Available data suggest no significant difference in analgesia or side effects between hydromorphone and other opioids.[14]
  - Hydromorphone has no renally cleared active metabolites.
- **Fentanyl:**
  - While initial studies suggested decreased rates of constipation with fentanyl as compared with other opioids, a more recent study suggested no difference in constipation rates when fentanyl was compared with morphine and methadone.[15,16]
  - Transdermal fentanyl is best used for stable pain syndromes.
  - Fentanyl patch absorption requires skin adhesion and is unpredictable in patients with fever or diaphoresis.
- **Meperidine:**
  - Meperidine is **NOT recommended** for treatment of pain because of limited efficacy and a very short duration of analgesia with significant euphoria.
  - Its active metabolite **normeperidine accumulates in renal failure and can lower the seizure threshold.**
- **Propoxyphene:**
  - A recent FDA advisory committee has **recommended AGAINST the use of propoxyphene for treatment of pain** given concerns regarding limited efficacy and possible safety issues.
- **Opioid combination pills** with acetaminophen or ibuprofen are available in a wide variety of doses, but dose titration is limited by the maximum daily dose of acetaminophen or ibuprofen. Commonly prescribed combination pills are presented in Table 4.
- Considerations for patients unable or unwilling to take oral analgesics:
  - Transdermal fentanyl is useful if pain is stable.
  - **Extended release formulations of any oral opioids must not be chewed or crushed.** Special coatings on the tablets or granules slow the medication's release; destroying the integrity of the coating can result in potentially fatal overdose.
  - Kadian (morphine sulfate extended release) comes in a capsule that can be opened. The granules must not be crushed but may be sprinkled in water and administered via gastrostomy tube ($\geq$16 French).
  - Liquid formulations of short-acting opioid formulations can be given at scheduled intervals to provide basal analgesia. For example, 10 mg liquid morphine sulfate every 6 hours as basal medication, with 5 mg liquid morphine every 4 hours as needed for breakthrough pain.

Conversion between Opioids
- Use caution when converting between opioids as equianalgesic doses are approximations only (refer to Table 5).
  1. Calculate the 24-hour dose of the current drug.
  2. Convert this drug to the equivalent dose of the desired new drug with the following equation:

$$\left(\begin{array}{c} \text{24-hour dose of} \\ \text{current drug} \end{array} \right) \times \left(\frac{\begin{array}{c} \text{New drug equianalgesic} \\ \text{equivalent} \end{array}}{\begin{array}{c} \text{Current drug equianalgesic} \\ \text{equivalent} \end{array}} \right) = \text{New drug 24-hour dose}$$

  3. Give only 50% of the calculated new drug equivalent dose to account for incomplete cross-tolerance between opioids.

TABLE 4	Opioid Combination Preparations	
Drug	**Generic or Trade Name(s) and Formulations**	**Recommended Dosing Interval**
Oxycodone + APAP	Dosage in mg oxycodone/mg APAP	q6 hours
Tablets	Oxycodone/APAP: 5/325, 7.5/325, 7.5/500, 10/325, 10/650	
	Endocet: 5/325, 7.5/325, 7.5/500, 10/325, 10/650	
	Magnacet: 2.5/400, 5/400, 7.5/400, 10/400	
	Percocet: 2.5/325, 5/325, 7.5/500, 10/650	
	Primalev: 2.5/300, 5/300, 7.5/300, 10/300	
	Roxicet: 5/500	
	Tylox: 5/500	
Solution	Roxicet: 5/325 per 5 mL	q6 hours
Hydrocodone + APAP	Dosage in mg hydrocodone/mg APAP	
Tablet	Hydrocodone/APAP: 2.5/325, 2.5/500, 5/325, 5/500, 5/650, 7.5/325, 7.5/500, 7.5/650, 7.5/750, 10/325, 10/500, 10/650, 10/660	q4–6 hours
	Lortab: 5/500, 7.5/500, 10/500	
	Norco: 5/325, 7.5/325, 10/325	
	Vicodin: 5/500, 7.5/750 ES, 10/660 HP	
Elixir	Hydrocodone: 7.5/500 per 15 mL	q4–6 hours
	Lortab: 7.5/500 per 15 mL	
Hydrocodone + ibuprofen	Dosage in mg hydrocodone/mg ibuprofen	
Tablet	Hydrocodone/ibuprofen: 7.5/200	q4–6 hours
	Vicoprofen: 7.5/200	

APAP, acetaminophen; ES, extra strength; HP, high potency.

TABLE 5	Equianalgesic Opioid Doses
Drugs	**Equianalgesic Dose**
Morphine PO	30 mg
Morphine IV	10 mg
Oxycodone	20 mg
Hydrocodone	30 mg
Hydromorphone PO	7.5 mg
Hydromorphone IV	1.5 mg

Drug information from Lexi-comp Online Drug Database. 2009. http://www.crlonline.com/crlsql/servlet/crlonline. Accessed January 13, 2010.

4. Divide the calculated new 24-hour dose by the number of doses planned per day. For example, divide by 2 for twice daily OxyContin or by 4 for doses of oxycodone given every 6 hours.
5. If using a basal dose of analgesic, calculate breakthrough doses of the new drug as 5% to 15% of the total daily dose, given at a frequency based on drug half-life.

- Ensure that the patient has adequate doses of breakthrough analgesia available when converting between opioids.
- The basal analgesic dose is intentionally reduced during opioid conversion to avoid risks of oversedation and respiratory depression with incomplete opioid cross-tolerance. This means that a patient's pain may initially be undertreated with the new basal dose.
- Short-acting opioids can be given as frequently as every 2 hours for breakthrough pain during opioid transitions to avoid pain crises in the setting of lowered basal analgesia.
- Patients requiring >2 to 3 doses of breakthrough pain medication may require an increase in their basal dose.
- **Conversion to/from fentanyl:**
  - Use Table 6 when converting between fentanyl transdermal patches and oral morphine.
  - Increase the dose of fentanyl patch on the basis of the amount of daily breakthrough opioid required.
  - Do not titrate patch dose more frequently than every 3 days.
  - Patches may not be cut. The lowest dose fentanyl patch is 12.5 μg/hr.
  - **Converting to the fentanyl patch:** The fentanyl patch takes 8 to 12 hours to reach peak effect, so place the patch at the same time as the last dose of oral long-acting medication is given.
  - **Discontinuing the fentanyl patch:** Remove the patch and 1 to 2 hours later start the new extended release opioid.
  - Short-acting oral opioids can be used as needed every 2 hours for breakthrough pain during transitions to and from fentanyl patches.

Adjuvant Drugs for Opioid Side Effects
Constipation

- Both pain relief and constipation are related to steady-state levels of opioids. All patients on opioids are at risk for constipation, and this side effect tends to worsen with increasing doses.
- All patients on chronic opioids should be on a **stool softener** plus a **stimulant laxative.**

TABLE 6	Oral Morphine/Transdermal Fentanyl Conversions
24-hour PO Morphine Dose	**Transdermal Fentanyl Equivalent**
60 mg	25 μg/hr
120 mg	50 μg/hr
180 mg	75 μg/hr
240 mg	100 μg/hr
300 mg	125 μg/hr
360 mg	150 μg/hr
420 mg	175 μg/hr
480 mg	200 μg/hr

- Docusate/sennosides tablets (50 mg/8.6 mg) provide convenient combined dosing of a detergent stool softener (docusate sodium) and a stimulant laxative (sennosides). Begin dosing at one tablet PO twice daily and titrate up as needed to a maximum of four tablets bid.
- It may be less expensive for the patient if docusate and sennosides are prescribed separately.
- Lactulose 10 to 30 g/day (15 to 30 mL) can be added and titrated up to 60 mL/day if needed.
- Polyethylene glycol is an osmotic agent that may also be added. Dosing is 17 g (about one heaping tablespoon) dissolved into 4 to 8 oz of water once daily. This agent has not been FDA approved for long-term use.
- Titrate the daily bowel regimen up if no bowel movement occurs for 2 to 3 days.
- If refractory constipation develops, rule out complete or partial bowel obstruction before advancing therapy.
- PO **naloxone** can also be helpful for refractory opioid-induced constipation.
  - Dose is 0.4 mg PO every 2 to 4 hours as needed.
  - There is almost no systemic absorption of PO naloxone, so oral dosing will not interfere with pain control.
- Subcutaneous **methylnaltrexone** is useful for patients with advanced illness and opioid-induced constipation who cannot tolerate oral therapy. It is contraindicated in patients with partial or complete bowel obstruction. Dosing varies with patient weight.

Sedation
- Sedation is common with opioids but tolerance develops over time.
- If sedation persists consider decreasing the basal opioid dose and using increased breakthrough doses when needed.
- Switching opioids may help if sedation is refractory.

Nausea
- There are two forms of nausea associated with opioids, early and late.
- **Early onset nausea** occurs within 15 to 30 minutes of drug administration, is related to changes in serum drug concentration, and is more common with intravenous opioids.
  - This type of nausea responds well to serotonin antagonists such as ondansetron 4 to 8 mg PO/IV or dopamine antagonists such as low-dose haloperidol (dose may be as low as 0.5 to 1 mg PO/IV, this use of haloperidol is not FDA approved).
- **Nausea that occurs later** in opioid therapy is usually due to insufficient treatment of constipation. This form of nausea responds to improved bowel regimen.

Respiratory Depression
- Respiratory depression can occur with opioids, although tolerance develops over time to this side effect.
- Respiratory depression is related to changes in serum concentration of opioids and is therefore less common with oral than intravenous formations.
- Dosage should be started low and titrated up carefully in opioid naïve patients.
- IV naloxone can be used for life-threatening respiratory depression.

Pruritus
- Pruritus occurs with opioid use due to opioid-induced histamine release.
- This side effect is classically associated with morphine and may be less pronounced with other opioids such as hydromorphone or oxycodone.
- Antihistamines can be used as needed.
- Tolerance usually develops, but if persistent, consider switching opioids.

Adjuvants for Neuropathic Pain

Antidepressants

- One third of patients with neuropathic pain achieve moderate or better pain relief with adjuvant therapy with **tricyclic antidepressants** (TCAs). Venlafaxine has similar efficacy to TCAs for treatment of neuropathic pain. However, one fifth of patients in these studies taking antidepressants for pain discontinued them due to side effects.[17]
- **Selective serotonin reuptake inhibitors** are better tolerated than TCAs but current data are limited regarding their efficacy in treatment of neuropathic pain.
- Duloxetine has also been approved by the FDA for diabetic neuropathy.

Anticonvulsants

- **Gabapentin** is effective for diabetic neuropathy and for postherpetic neuralgia.
  - Starting dose is generally 300 mg at bedtime. This may be titrated up to a maximum of 3,600 mg/day, given in divided doses every 8 hours.
  - Maximum dose is lower in patients with renal insufficiency.
  - Most patients will require at least 900 to 1,500 mg/day to achieve pain control.
  - Gabapentin can cause sedation, but this effect usually attenuates after 3 to 5 days.
- **Pregabalin** is a newer anticonvulsant, with a mechanism of action, efficacy, and range of adverse effects similar to gabapentin.
  - Dose range is 100 to 600 mg/day divided into 2 or 3 doses.
- **Carbamazepine** has some efficacy in neuropathic pain such as trigeminal neuralgia and diabetic neuropathy. **Oxcarbazepine** is a related agent that may have less risk of toxicity.
- **Dilantin** has some efficacy for diabetic neuropathy.
- There is no evidence to support anticonvulsant therapy for acute pain.[18]

Other Adjuvants

- **Local anesthetics** such as lidocaine patches may be effective for some localized pain due to strains and sprains or tumor invasion of tissue.
- **Steroids** are useful for patients with severe bone pain or pain due to spinal cord compression.
- **Benzodiazepines and selective serotonin/norepinephrine reuptake inhibitors** may decrease anxiety and thus help patients cope with chronic pain.
- **Neuroleptics** cannot be recommended or discouraged for adjuvant pain therapy on the basis of current available data.[19]

Other Nonpharmacologic Therapies

- Psychotherapy, cognitive behavioral therapy, mindfulness, and counseling can be useful adjuncts for patients with chronic pain.
- Physical and occupational therapy can help some patients increase functionality and independence.
- Acupuncture has also been used with success as a therapy in cancer-related pain.
- Massage may be helpful for some patients.
- Radiation therapy is indicated for pain from boney metastases.
- Transcutaneous electrical nerve stimulation is available for pain therapy, although there is currently insufficient data to support transcutaneous electrical nerve stimulation for acute, chronic, or cancer pain.[20–22]

Referral

- If pain cannot be adequately controlled, referral to a pain specialist should be considered for more advanced medical management or specialized procedures.

- A full discussion of procedural interventions for pain syndromes is beyond the scope of this chapter.
- Available techniques include steroid injections, neurolytic blocks, and surgical procedures such as rhizotomy, chordotomy, and implantation of intrathecal or intraventricular opioid delivery systems.

Monitoring/Follow-Up

- Treatment of pain is an iterative process; one of its most important components is close follow-up and frequent reevaluation of the therapeutic plan.
- If pain is not controlled, appropriate adjustments to the patient's regimen should be made.

REFERENCES

1. Pain terms: a list with definitions and notes on usage. Recommended by the IASP Subcommittee on Taxonomy. *Pain* 1979;6:249.
2. Hart LG, Deyo RA, Cherkin DC. Physician office visits for low back pain. Frequency, clinical evaluation, and treatment patterns from a U.S. national survey. *Spine* 1995;20:11–19.
3. Riechelmann RP, Krzyzanowska MK, O'Carroll A, Zimmermann C. Symptom and medication profiles among cancer patients attending a palliative care clinic. *Support Care Cancer* 2007;15:1407–1412.
4. Teno JM, Hakim RB, Knaus WA, et al. Preferences for cardiopulmonary resuscitation: physician-patient agreement and hospital resource use. The SUPPORT Investigators. *J Gen Intern Med* 1995;10:179–186.
5. Cleeland CS, Gonin R, Hatfield AK, et al. Pain and its treatment in outpatients with metastatic cancer. *N Engl J Med* 1994;330:592–596.
6. Azevedo São Leão Ferreira K, Kimura M, Teixeira MJ. The WHO analgesic ladder for cancer pain control, twenty years of use. How much pain relief does one get from using it? *Support Care Cancer* 2006;14:1086–1093.
7. McNicol ED, Strassels S, Goudas L, et al. NSAIDS or paracetamol, alone or combined with opioids, for cancer pain. *Cochrane Database Syst Rev* 2005;(1):CD005180.
8. Eisenberg E, McNicol E, Carr DB. Opioids for neuropathic pain. *Cochrane Database Syst Rev* 2006;3:CD006146.
9. Skoglund LA, Skjelbred P, Fyllingen G. Analgesic efficacy of acetaminophen 1000 mg, acetaminophen 2000 mg, and the combination of acetaminophen 1000 mg and codeine phosphate 60 mg versus placebo in acute postoperative pain. *Pharmacotherapy* 1991;11: 364–369.
10. Lexi-comp Online Drug Database. 2009. http://www.crlonline.com/crlsql/servlet/crlonline. Accessed May 27, 2009.
11. Reid CM, Martin RM, Sterne JA, et al. Oxycodone for cancer-related pain: meta-analysis of randomized controlled trials. *Arch Intern Med* 2006;166:837–843.
12. Nicholson AB. Methadone for cancer pain. *Cochrane Database Syst Rev* 2007;(4): CD003971.
13. FDA. Methadone Hydrochloride Information-FDA ALERT [11/2006]: Death, Narcotic Overdose, and Serious Cardiac Arrhythmias. http://www.fda.gov/CDER/drug/infopage/methadone/default.htm. Published April 2009. Accessed May 27, 2009.
14. Quigley C, Wiffen P. A systematic review of hydromorphone in acute and chronic pain. *J Pain Symptom Manage* 2003;25:169–178.
15. Ahmedzai S, Brooks D. Transdermal fentanyl versus sustained-release oral morphine in cancer pain: preference, efficacy, and quality of life. *J Pain Symptom Manage* 1997;13:254–261.
16. Mercadante S, Porzio G, Ferrera P, et al. Sustained-release oral morphine versus transdermal fentanyl and oral methadone in cancer pain management. *Eur J Pain* 2008;12:1040–1046.

17. Saarto T, Wiffen PJ. Antidepressants for neuropathic pain. *Cochrane Database Syst Rev* 2007;(4):CD005454.
18. Wiffen P, Collins S, McQuay H, et al. Anticonvulsant drugs for acute and chronic pain. *Cochrane Database Syst Rev* 2005;(3):CD001133.
19. Seidel S, Aigner M, Ossege M, Pernicka, et al. Antipsychotics for acute and chronic pain in adults. *Cochrane Database Sys Rev* 2008;(4):CD004844.
20. Nnoaham KE, Kumbang J. Transcutaneous electrical nerve stimulation (TENS) for chronic pain. *Cochrane Database Syst Rev* 2008;(3):CD003222.
21. Robb K, Oxberry SG, Bennett MI, et al. A Cochrane systematic review of transcutaneous electrical nerve stimulation for cancer pain. *J Pain Symptom Manage* 2009;37:746–753.
22. Walsh DM, Howe TE, Johnson MI, Sluka KA. Transcutaneous electrical nerve stimulation for acute pain. *Cochrane Database Syst Rev* 2009;(2):CD006142.

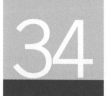

Geriatrics
Syed Khalid and David B. Carr

Primary care providers are frequently faced with an aging patient population in their practice. Many practitioners also work in hospital settings or skilled nursing centers that have an ever-increasing elderly population. Identifying and evaluating geriatric syndromes such as dementia and incontinence, addressing polypharmacy, preventing injury and disability, maintaining function, and discussing advance directives are just a few of the important priorities in providing appropriate care to older adults.

Preventing Disability and Maintaining Function

- The decision to screen for various diseases in the older adult is often complicated by limited life expectancy with advanced age, the presence of comorbid illness, the reluctance of the patient to undergo testing, and the paucity of literature that would demonstrate efficacy of screening in late life.
- However, it should be noted that **the average 85-year-old woman has a life expectancy well past 5 years,** which is often within the range of survival rates quoted for many cancer treatments.
- In addition, the common causes of morbidity and mortality in advanced age remain atherosclerosis, cancer, injury, dementia, infections, and adverse drug events.
- Thus, the decision to perform screening and health maintenance in the older adult should focus on a variety of health issues while remaining **individualized for each patient.**
- **Smoking cessation** has been found to be beneficial and bestow health benefits despite advanced age.
- **Primary prevention of hypercholesterolemia** in patients older than age 70 years is now less controversial and secondary prevention has been demonstrated to decrease rates of myocardial infarction and death in older adults.
- The benefits of **weight training and aerobic activity** in maintaining cognitive or physical health, or both, are well proven and these interventions should be discussed and encouraged with elderly patients.

Geriatric Syndromes

- Common geriatric syndromes or disorders in the outpatient setting that should be identified may include the following:
  - Dementia
  - Delirium
  - Depression
  - Falls
  - Urinary incontinence (UI)
  - Malnutrition

- Impotence
- Sensory deprivation
- Polypharmacy
- These conditions may be identified by the clinician, patient, and/or family. However, many of these syndromes are not identified or evaluated unless the primary care physician systematically screens for them.
- Clinicians should inquire about the presence of these syndromes with their older adult patients and caregivers during office visits.
- **Selected screening measures** should also be incorporated in yearly health examinations for patients >65 years of age. These may include the following:
  - Comprehensive medication reviews
  - Screening for hearing impairment (by questionnaire or hand-held audiometry) and visual impairment (Snellen eye chart or Rosenbaum pocket chart)
  - Identifying the presence or risk for falls or motor vehicle crashes
  - Screening for dementia (Table 1) and depression[1]

TABLE 1	Short Blessed Screening Test for Cognitive Impairment[1]				
Cognitive Screen	Maximum Error	Patient's # of Errors	Weighting Factor	Subscore
1. What year is it now?	1	_____	X 4	_____
2. What month is it now?	1	_____	X 3	_____
Repeat this phrase after me and remember it: John Brown, 42 Market Street, Chicago Number of trials to learning: _____				
3. About what time is it without looking at your watch? (within 1 hour) Response _____ Actual time _____	1	_____	X 3	_____
4. Count backward from 20 down to 1. Mark correctly sequenced numbers: 20 19 18 17 16 15 14 13 12 11 10 9 8 7 6 5 4 3 2 1	2[a]	_____	X 2	_____
5. Say the months of the year in reverse. Mark the correct months: D N O S A JL JU MY AP M F J	2[a]	_____	X 2	_____
6. Repeat the name and address I asked you to remember. Mark correct responses: John Brown, 42 Market Street, Chicago[b]	5	_____	X 2	_____
Total weighted error score[c]				_____

[a]Scoring: 0 = no errors; 1 = 1 error; 2 = ≥2 errors.
[b]An answer of either Market or Market Street is acceptable.
[c]A total weighted error score of ≥9 indicates a need for further assessment.

TABLE 2	Activities of Daily Living
Instrumental Activities of Daily Living	**Basic Activities of Daily Living**
Shopping	**D**ressing
Housework	**E**ating
Accounting	**A**mbulation
Food preparation	**T**oileting/incontinence
Transportation/driving	**H**ygiene/grooming

Modified from Fleming KC, Evans JM, Weber DC, Chutka DS. Practical functional assessment of elderly patients: a primary care approach. *Mayo Clin Proc* 1995;70;890–910.

- Discussing and documenting advance directives and identifying a surrogate decision maker
- In addition, many of these screens can serve as a baseline and can be repeated during future examinations to determine response to treatment.

Assessment of Function

- Many disorders come to the attention of the physician if they are impairing job performance or function at home.
- Diagnoses such as dementia require the new onset of functional impairment.
- Improvements in functional status are often used as a marker of treatment success.
- In addition, a review of the activities of daily living can assist in targeting additional assistance that may be needed at home.
- Thus, clinicians should be prepared to quickly assess and document the presence of functional impairment.
- Two mnemonics for basic and instrumental activities of daily living are listed in Table 2.[2]
- The presence of functional impairment due to any illness should be documented and monitored for further changes in function over time.

Geriatric Assessment

- Geriatric assessment is a holistic approach to patient care and focuses on the physical, functional, social, and psychological health of the individual along with providing assistance to caregivers.
- These assessments are typically performed in the outpatient or hospital setting by a geriatrician, gerontological nurse specialist, and/or social worker.
- The role of the social worker may include locating a chore worker to assist the caregiver, finding a durable power of attorney, providing financial information, assisting with Medicare or Medicaid eligibility, management of caregiver stress, counseling, referral to state and local area agencies on aging, addressing advance directives, or recommending relocation to assisted living or long-term care centers.
- Geriatric assessment can practically be performed in the outpatient setting by the primary care clinician in conjunction with a social worker or a gerontological case manager, who can be consulted in difficult cases.
- Geriatric evaluations should include the physical, functional, social, and psychological assessment of patients in the context of their current environment.

- These assessments can assist patients and their families regarding the myriad of issues that can affect the independence of frail older adults in the community.

DEMENTIA

General Principles

- Healthy older adults demonstrate an age-related reduction in working memory, where information must be stored or held while performing other cognitive activities. This in turn may correspond to frequent complaints by elderly persons concerning poor retrieval of names and limited capacity to keep several items in mind simultaneously.
- Age-associated deficits also have been reported for language, psychomotor speed, and visuospatial abilities.
- In healthy older persons, these changes typically do not interfere substantially with usual activities or social or occupational performance.
- The maintenance of functional ability in everyday activities is a major clinical feature that distinguishes cognitively healthy aging from dementia.
- The use of a brief cognitive screen may assist the primary care physician in identifying older adults with significant cognitive impairment (Table 1).

Diagnosis

- Dementia can be simply defined as a memory and cognitive disorder that impairs an individual's function and/or social relationships.
- **Diagnostic and Statistical Manual (DSM) IV criteria** for diagnosing a dementing illness include **memory impairment** (impaired ability to learn new information or to recall learned information) and at least one of the following:
  - **Agnosia** (failure to recognize or identify objects despite intact sensory function)
  - **Aphasia** (disturbance in language)
  - **Apraxia** (impaired ability to carry out motor activities despite intact motor function)
  - **Executive function disturbances** (abstract thinking, planning, organizing, sequencing)
  - In addition, the cognitive deficits must cause significant impairment in social or occupational functioning and represent a decline.
- The mnemonic **DEMENTIA**—**D** (drugs), **E** (emotional disorders), **M** (metabolic disorders), **E** (eye and ear disorders), **N** (nutritional deficiencies), **T** (tumor/trauma), **I** (infection), **A** (arteriosclerosis)—is often used to identify the presence of potentially treatable causes of cognitive decline.
- Diagnostic tests such as vitamin B_{12} and thyroid-stimulating hormone level may be justifiable in all patient evaluations.
- The decision to pursue a rapid plasma reagin, EEG, and/or a lumbar puncture in the evaluation of dementia should be individualized and based on the clinical index of suspicion as raised by history and physical examination.
- The indications for obtaining a brain-imaging study are listed in Table 3.[3]
  - In general, an MRI study is preferred when focal deficits are found on the neurologic examination. A CT scan without contrast may be appropriate for more chronic cases that have a nonfocal presentation, such as ruling out a subdural hematoma or assessing ventricular size when considering normal-pressure hydrocephalus.
  - The pretest probability of the disease should guide the test selection rather than using a "blanket" approach.

TABLE 3	Indications for Brain Imaging in the Diagnostic Workup of Dementia

Sudden onset of symptoms (e.g., 1–2 months)
Subacute course (e.g., <2 years)
Age <60 years
New focal neurologic symptoms/signs
Otherwise unexplainable neurologic symptoms (e.g., headaches, blurred vision, seizures)
Early onset of gait disorder/incontinence
Unusual or atypical cognitive symptoms or presentation (e.g., progressive aphasia)
History or current diagnosis of cancer
Use of anticoagulation
Head trauma/falls
Weight loss/depression

Modified from Patterson CJ, Gauthier S, Bergman H, et al. The recognition, assessment and management of dementing disorders: conclusions from the Canadian Consensus Conference on Dementia. *CMAJ* 1999;160:S1–S15.

DEMENTIA OF THE ALZHEIMER'S TYPE

General Principles

- Dementia of the Alzheimer's type (DAT) may affect as many as four million people in the United States.
- It is largely a disease of the elderly, increasing exponentially after 70 years of age to achieve prevalence rates up to 47% of those >85 years of age.
- Because the percentage of the population >80 years of age will double by 2010, the burden of DAT to society will increase to enormous proportions.

Diagnosis

- The clinical hallmark of DAT is the gradual onset and progression of memory loss and other cognitive functions.
- The diagnosis is greatly facilitated with information from a collateral source or caregiver that the cognitive changes represent a decline from a prior level of performance and are sufficient to interfere with everyday function.
- Short-term memory impairment is often manifested by repetition, misplacement of items, and missed appointments.
- Incomplete or absent recall of recent events increasingly occurs, and eventually remote memory is also impaired.
- Behavioral changes of passivity, lack of interest, and withdrawal are frequent.
- The initial changes are often subtle, and the diagnosis is frequently missed.
- Functional performance, however, declines, as evidenced by impaired driving, financial imprudence, and inability to produce a complete meal. Impairment of language, constructional ability, praxis, recognition, judgment, and abstraction can occur throughout the course of the illness.

- **Currently, no validated test is available for the diagnosis of DAT.** Rather than simply a diagnosis of exclusion, the characteristic onset and course of memory and other cognitive deficits increasingly make DAT a diagnosis of inclusion.
- Laboratory and neuroimaging procedures are usually obtained for screening for the presence of other diseases that can contribute to cognitive impairment.
- Apolipoprotein E genotype testing is currently recommended for only research purposes.

Treatment

Care of the patient with Alzheimer disease usually focuses on assisting the caregiver(s), drug treatment for the symptoms of cognitive impairment, and treatment of behavior.

Caregiver Stress

For any dementing illness, the patient and family should be informed of the disease, the extent to which it is treatable, the degree of disability, the prognosis, and the areas of cognition that are intact. The social and psychological needs of the caregiver should be assessed. Future changes regarding levels of care should be discussed. Referral to a geriatric assessment center, a geriatric case manager, local support services, and especially the Alzheimer's Association should be considered to assist the family. Legal issues, such as identifying a durable power of attorney, should be pursued along with a discussion of advance directives. Assisted living and nursing home placement may be appropriate during the course of the illness. Community aging services may be available to assist in the home.

Pharmacotherapy for Cognitive Impairment

Cholinesterase Inhibitors
- Various cholinesterase inhibitors can be initiated for the treatment of DAT in the early stages of the disease.
  - **Donepezil,** 5 mg PO qd for 1 month, and increase to 10 mg PO qd if tolerated
  - **Galantamine,** 4 mg PO bid for 1 month, and increase to 8 mg bid if tolerated
  - **Rivastigmine,** 6 to 12 mg/day with bid dosing after titrating up slowly from 3 mg bid
- The patient and family should be committed to **at least a 6-month to 1-year trial,** because it may take some time to determine efficacy.
- The beneficial cognitive effects of these agents are modest, and the intent is to **achieve cognitive stability** for 1 to 2 years and **not expect improvement in symptoms.**
- Some patients and family members desire to stay on the medication as long as there is no observed progression of symptoms.
- Side effects are infrequent and are related to excess cholinergic activity, such as anorexia, weight loss, diarrhea, nausea, vomiting, urinary frequency, muscle cramps, nightmares, and hypersalivation.

Vitamin E
- In one study, vitamin E appeared to delay the onset of disability and/or progression to placement in nursing homes.[4]
- Although the dose used for this study was 1,000 IU bid, a lower dose of vitamin E at 400 IU qd is recommended because of concerns of increased mortality with the use of higher doses.[5]

N-Methyl-D-Aspartic Acid Antagonists

- **Memantine** is the only currently available *N*-methyl-D-aspartic acid receptor antagonist and is approved as monotherapy for the treatment of moderate to severe DAT.[6]
- It may reduce functional and cognitive decline and has a very favorable side effect profile. Dose titration is recommended to minimize side effects.
- Adverse effects are rare but include constipation, headache, dizziness, and increased confusion.
- Combination therapy with both memantine and a cholinesterase inhibitor **appears to have additive benefits over monotherapy.**[7]

Treatment of Behavior

- Many behaviors in patients with dementia are difficult to manage. These may include wandering, anxiety, psychosis, delusions, disruptive vocalization, combativeness, or insomnia.
- The mnemonic **DRNO** (**D** [describe the behavior], **R** [reason for the behavior], **N** [nonpharmacologic approach], **O** [order medication as a last step]) may provide a useful systematic approach to address difficult behaviors in the DAT patient.
- The goal is to describe specifically the unwanted behavior and then to determine the possible reasons behind the behavior (e.g., pain, hunger, need for elimination).
- Nonpharmacologic approaches based on structuring the environment and behavioral interventions should be attempted first and are listed in Table 4.

Pharmacologic Treatment

- Medications are the last line of therapy and should be prescribed for short-term use (weeks to months).
- Pharmacologic agents that are recommended for use in demented patients depend on the primary behavioral problem.
- Psychotropic drugs for behavior should be used on an as-needed basis. Any routine use of these drugs should be short term with periodic trials to taper or discontinue their use.
  - **Insomnia:** trazodone, 50 mg PO qh, temazepam, 7.5 mg PO qhs, zolpidem, 5 mg PO qhs.

TABLE 4	Environmental and Behavioral Interventions for Managing Difficult Behaviors in Dementia

Educate about dementia and agitation
Talk to patients/distract attention
Identify specific precipitants to behavior
Experiment with targeted changes to schedule
Separate disruptive and noisy persons from quieter persons
Control door access; use safety latches to prevent egress
Provide reassurance and verbal efforts to calm
Reduce isolation
Encourage the joining of support groups
Provide a predictable routine for the patient
Structure the environment
Provide orienting stimuli
Provide bright enough daytime lighting
Use a night light in bedroom during sleep

- **Anxiety:** trazodone, 50 mg PO every 6 hours prn.
- **Acute psychosis:** haloperidol, 0.5 to 2.0 mg in divided doses, and risperidone, 0.25 to 2.0 mg in divided doses, may be used safely, **if given for a brief period of time.**
- Persons with dementia with Lewy bodies are particularly susceptible to the extrapyramidal side effects of antipsychotics and may develop severe Parkinsonism.
- Newer atypical or novel antipsychotic agents (e.g., olanzapine, quetiapine, aripiprazole, ziprasidone) are expensive and may be sedating but should be considered for short-term use in those individuals with concomitant extrapyramidal disease or long-term use since they have a lower incidence of tardive dyskinesia.

Antipsychotics
- Atypical or "novel" agents for psychosis have been widely embraced but recent studies have called into question their usefulness.[8]
- The indications for their use should be focused on cases of combativeness and/or frank psychosis (e.g., delusions and/or hallucinations). **We do not advocate their use for general agitation, depression, anxiety, or repetitive behaviors.** A detailed discussion of these drugs is beyond the scope of this chapter but the reader is referred to a recent excellent review.[9]
- For difficult cases, referral to a geropsychiatrist is advised.
- Atypical antipsychotic drugs are not without the **potential for side effects.** These agents may cause orthostasis, sedation, impaired balance, weight gain, and glucose intolerance.
- A large study of >37,000 older adults found an increased risk of mortality for those patients who used these drugs.[10]
  - In this study, conventional agents (e.g., haloperidol) had a higher dose-dependent risk.
  - Subsequent studies have also confirmed the increase in mortality and an increase in hospital admission rate.[11]
  - The specific types of deaths that have been implicated related to these drugs are from infections like pneumonia and heart failure and sudden death possibly from a prolonged QT syndrome, stroke, and falls with injuries.[12]
  - One of the mechanisms for morbidity and mortality may be increased thrombosis, including venous thromboembolism.
- It should be noted that the Food and Drug Administration has labeled these medications with a **black box warning.**
- These agents should be used with caution in persons with a history of cardiovascular and cerebrovascular disease.
- The American College of Neuropsychopharmacology recommends monitoring blood pressure, weight, and presence of extrapyramidal effects every 3 months and blood glucose and lipids every 3 to 6 months.[13]
- In many patients with dementia and behavioral disturbances, the risk/benefit ratio for prescribing these medications still warrants utilization of these drugs. **Each case should be individualized** and a specific determination made whether to initiate the medication or to taper and discontinue these agents.
- Until further data are available, the following are recommendations regarding antipsychotic drug use in persons with dementia.[14]
  - Efforts should be made to determine reversible and treatable causes for behavioral problems in persons with dementia (e.g., infections, drugs, pain control).
  - Attempts should be made to handle behavioral difficulties using nonpharmacologic methods.

- Cholinesterase inhibitors with or without memantine should be considered for behavioral symptoms and antidepressants should be considered when depressive or anxiety symptomatology is present.
- If an antipsychotic medication is to be initiated or continued, discussion with the patient and family should occur regarding the acceptability of these risks and this information should be documented in the patient's chart.
- Patients should routinely be monitored for hyperglycemia, weight gain, excessive sedation, orthostasis, and Parkinsonism.
- Any cardiac events, transient ischemic attacks or strokes, or pneumonia should trigger a reevaluation of the risk-benefit ratio.

VASCULAR DEMENTIA AND ATYPICAL DEMENTIAS

Vascular Dementia

- The diagnosis of vascular dementia (VD) may be difficult because there are no universally accepted criteria or consensus on the amount of infarcted brain volume at specific anatomic sites that are necessary to establish a dementing illness.
- In addition, most clinicopathologic studies indicate that it is more likely to have a diagnosis of DAT with vascular disease than to have an isolated VD alone.
- Nevertheless, focal areas of injury appear to be highly associated with the onset and development of DAT and the degree of periventricular white matter or small vessel disease appears to correlate with higher levels of cognitive impairment.[15,16]
- A clinical determination can usually be made as to whether focal or global cerebral insult was present on the basis of the patient's history and clinical examination.
- **Signs and symptoms of an ischemic VD** include abrupt onset, a stepwise deterioration, an early onset of gait or incontinence problems, emotional lability, somatic complaints, focal findings on clinical examination, and infarcts identified on brain-imaging studies.
- **Risk factors** include hypertension, atrial fibrillation, and advanced age.
- Currently there is **no treatment for the improvement of symptoms.**
- Management focuses on **prevention of additional brain injury** by modifying vascular risk factors such as cessation of smoking, control of diabetes and hypertension, daily aspirin use, and anticoagulation with warfarin, if not contraindicated for atrial fibrillation. Studies have indicated that mixed dementias (DAT and VD) appear to achieve the same degree of response to cholinesterase inhibitors, as the studies with DAT alone.

Atypical Dementia

A growing number of primary degenerative dementias are increasingly recognized but are beyond the scope of this chapter. In summary, dementias that are associated with extrapyramidal signs (diffuse Lewy body disease, progressive supranuclear palsy, cortical basal ganglionic degeneration); early onset of gait disorder or incontinence or both (normal-pressure hydrocephalus, VD); behavioral problems and/or primary language impairment (frontotemporal dementia); or a subacute course (Jakob-Creutzfeldt disease, viral encephalopathy) should be referred to a neurologist or dementia specialist for further evaluation.

PHARMACOTHERAPEUTICS IN THE OLDER PATIENT

Factors that Affect Drug Metabolism

- The duration that a particular drug exerts its effect in any patient is based on the volume of distribution (Vd) of the drug, the metabolism of the drug (hepatic function), the clearance (renal function), or a combination of factors, all of which can change with aging.
- The time for a drug to decline to one half of its concentration is known as the **drug's biologic half-life.**
- The half-life is directly proportional to the Vd and inversely proportional to the clearance.
- Vd is determined by the degree of plasma protein binding and by the patient's body composition.

Age-Related Changes in Drug Metabolism

Changes in Body Composition

- The **proportion of adipose tissue increases** with aging. This increase results in a larger Vd and longer half-life, and therefore **lipophilic medications** such as benzodiazepines have a longer duration of action.
- Total **body water decreases** by 15% in those >80 years of age. The Vd for **hydrophilic drugs,** such as lithium, cimetidine, and ethanol, is decreased, resulting in higher drug concentrations.
- Elderly persons have on average a **decreased lean body mass.** Digoxin, which binds to muscle adenosine triphosphatase, may have a decreased Vd, meaning that toxicity can occur at lower doses.
- The concentrations of plasma proteins such as **albumin** also tend to **decline in older adults.** This results in a reduced protein-bound form of many drugs and greater amount of free drug levels. Examples include digoxin, theophylline, phenytoin, and warfarin. Most drug level determinations measure total (protein-bound and free levels) drug concentrations. Thus, total drug levels may not accurately reflect drug activity.

Changes in Hepatic and Renal Metabolism

- In general, there is a decrease in the number of hepatocytes and liver mass with age.
- Drugs that have a large first-pass effect in the liver, such as β-blockers, nitrates, calcium channel blockers, and tricyclic antidepressants, may be effective at lower doses.
- Phase I (cytochrome P-450) oxidation declines on average with aging and doses of medications such as benzodiazepines should be reduced.
- Knowledge about cytochrome P-450 drug interactions has grown and should be reviewed by all prescribing clinicians.
- Medications that are primarily excreted by the kidney often need to be adjusted by estimating creatinine clearance by age and body weight (see Chapter 19). Examples such as aminoglycosides, digoxin, atenolol, vancomycin, lithium, acyclovir, and amantadine require dose reductions in older adults.

Changes in Pharmacodynamics

- End-organ responsiveness to a drug at the receptor level may be changed with age.

- Changes in receptor binding, a decrease in receptor number, or altered translation of a receptor-initiated cellular response into a biochemical reaction may be responsible.
- Consistent findings in the literature include the following:
  - A decreased response to β-blockers.
  - An increased sensitivity to benzodiazepines, opiates, warfarin, and anticholinergics
  - Thus, clinicians need to be aware that dose adjustments in these drugs may be necessary.

Steps in Preventing Polypharmacy and Drug Toxicity

Reducing Medications

- The initial step in assessing polypharmacy is to identify all prescription and over-the-counter drugs.
- Older adults may be treated by several physicians and obtain their medications at several pharmacies.
- The patient and, if necessary, a family member should **bring in all medications** each visit for review including over-the-counter medications and herbal products.
- All drugs should be recorded by generic name and **unnecessary medications should be discontinued.**
- The clinical indication should be identified for all drugs.
- The side effect profiles should be reviewed and safer medications should be substituted. Side effects may not be reported by patients, so obtaining a careful history focused on drug side effects is very important.

Starting New Medications

- Before a new drug is started, risk factors for adverse drug reactions, such as advanced age, liver or kidney disease, or use of multiple medications, should be identified.
- A review of the specific allergic reaction to any medications should be done and drugs that have cross-reactivity should be identified.
- It is imperative to make a firm diagnosis (e.g., DAT) before drug therapy is initiated.
- Attempts should be made to manage medical conditions (e.g., hypertension) without drugs when possible.
- The individual clinical status of each patient (e.g., chronic renal insufficiency) needs to be reviewed.
- The clinician should establish a therapeutic goal and an appropriate time frame for treatment duration.
- Generic medications are generally preferred for their lower cost; exceptions include warfarin, levothyroxine, anticonvulsants, and cyclosporine. The major issue with such medications is a narrow therapeutic index or significant variations that may occur when changing between a name brand and generic or between different generic suppliers. Pharmacies are not presently required to notify patients when the latter has occurred.
- Choosing a once-a-day drug, starting at a low dose, and titrating slowly are sound principles when adjusting medications.
- **Avoid treating side effects of one drug with more drugs** (e.g., treating edema from calcium channel blocker with furosemide).

Adherence

- The risk of medication errors increases dramatically with the number of medications taken by the patient.

- Several steps to improve adherence when ordering medications are suggested:
  - Drug regimens should be simple.
  - Use the same dosage schedule with other drugs and time their administration with a daily routine such as a meal.
  - Instruct relatives and caregivers on drug regimens and enlist others, such as home health nurses and pharmacists, to assist with appropriate delivery.
  - Be sure that the patient can afford the medication, has transportation to the pharmacy, and can open the container.
  - Encourage the use of aids, such as pillboxes, calendars, and an updated medication record.
  - Attempt to treat multiple problems with one medication.
- Reviewing the patients' knowledge of the reason they take each medication and inquiries about adverse drug reactions on each visit are essential aspects of successful prescribing.

Avoid Drugs with Anticholinergic Side Effects

- Medications with anticholinergic side effects can contribute to falls, cognitive impairment, and delirium in elderly patients and physician needs to be aware of the anticholinergic side effect potential of the drug.
- An anticholinergic risk scale (ARS) has recently been described estimating the extent to which an individual patient is at risk of anticholinergic side effects that may lead to cognitive impairment and delirium.[17]
  - Higher ARS scores have been associated with increased risk of anticholinergic adverse effects in elderly patients.
  - The ARS ranks medications for anticholinergic potential on a 3-point scale (0, no or low risk; 3, high anticholinergic potential); these are presented in Table 5.
- Some of the most commonly prescribed medications for the elderly have also been looked for in vitro anticholinergic activity and this information is presented in Table 6.[18]

FALLS

General Principles

- Injury is the fourth leading cause of death in the older adult population.
- Common causes of injuries include falls and motor vehicle crashes. Burns, accidental poisoning, smoke inhalation, and hypothermia in demented patients are not uncommon.
- These safety issues should be addressed for all older adults, with special attention paid to patients with DAT and their caregivers.
- Falls are important to identify and prevent in the elderly population.
- Osteoporosis should be considered and treated if identified. A family history of fracture or a patient history of fracture, falls, gait difficulties, or balance impairment should be discussed.
- In addition, a lower-extremity mobility screen such as the "up and go" test should be considered for older adults.[19] Focusing on lower-extremity muscle strength, gait, and balance tests appears to be a powerful predictor of disability in the older adult.[20]

TABLE 5	Anticholinergic Risk Scale	

3 Points	2 Points	1 Point
Amitriptyline (Elavil)	Amantadine	Carbidopa-levodopa
Atropine	(Symmetrel)	(Sinemet)
Benztropine (Cogentin)	Baclofen (Lioresal)	Entacapone (Comtan,
Carisoprodol (Soma)	Cetirizine (Zyrtec)	catechol-O-methyl
Chlorpheniramine	Cimetidine (Tagamet)	transferase inhibitor)
(Chlor-Trimeton)	Clozapine (Clozaril)	Haloperidol (Haldol)
Chlorpromazine (Thorazine)	Cyclobenzaprine	Methocarbamol
Cyproheptadine (Periactin)	(Flexeril)	(Robaxin)
Dicyclomine (Bentyl)	Desipramine	Metoclopramide
Diphenhydramine (Benadryl)	(Norpramine)	(Reglan)
Fluphenazine (Prolixin)	Loperamide	Mirtazapine
Hydroxyzine (Atarax/Vistaril)	(Imodium)	(Remeron)
Hyoscyamine (Levsin)	Loratadine (Claritin)	Paroxetine (Paxil)
Imipramine (Tofranil)	Nortriptyline (Pamelor)	Pramipexole (Mirapex)
Meclizine (Antivert)	Olanzapine (Zyprexa)	Quetiapine (Seroquel)
Oxybutynin (Ditropan)	Prochlorperazine	Ranitidine (Zantac)
Perphenazine (Trilafon)	(Compazine)	Risperidone
Promethazine (Phenergan)	Triprolidine	(Risperdal)
Thioridazine (Mellaril)	(antihistamine	Selegiline (Eldepryl)
Thiothixene (Navane)	component of	Trazodone (Desyrel)
Tizanidine (Zanaflex)	Actifed)	Ziprasidone (Geodon)
Trifluoperazine (Stelazine)	Tolterodine (Detrol)	

Modified from Rudolph JL, Salow MJ, Agelini MC, et al. The anticholinergic risk scale and anticholinergic adverse effects in older persons. *Arch Intern Med* 2008;168:508–513.

Risk Factors

- To prevent falls and subsequent injury a thorough review of the patient and environment is needed to target recommendations.[21,22]
- Common **intrinsic factors** for falls in older adults include the following:
  - Gait and balance disorders
  - Proximal muscle weakness
  - Dizziness
  - Sedating drugs
  - Postural hypotension
  - Visual impairment
- Common causes of these disorders include the following:
  - Dementia
  - Parkinson disease
  - Cerebrovascular accidents
  - Peripheral neuropathy
  - Alcohol use
  - Deconditioning
  - Arthritis
  - Cataracts
  - Glaucoma

TABLE 6	In Vitro Anticholinergic Activity[a] of the 24 Medications Most Commonly Prescribed to Elderly People in the United States[b]

Detectable Atropine-like Activity (Ranked from Highest to Lowest)	No Detectable Atropine-like Activity
Cimetidine	α-Methyldopa
Prednisolone	Atenolol
Theophylline	Diltiazem
Digoxin	Hydrochlorothiazide
Furosemide	Ibuprofen
Nifedipine	Insulin
Ranitidine	Metoprolol
Isosorbide dinitrate	Nitroglycerine
Warfarin	Propranolol
Dipyridamole	Salicylic acid
Codeine	Timolol
Hydrochlorothiazide/triamterene	
Captopril	

[a]At a concentration of 10 nmol/L.
[b]In 1990.
Modified from Tune L, Carr S, Hoag E, Cooper T. Anticholinergic effects of drugs commonly prescribed for the elderly: potential means of assessing risk of delirium. *Am J Psychiatry* 1992;149:1393–1394.

- Orthostatic hypotension from dehydration or drugs
- Foot abnormalities
- Psychotropic medications
- Many of these conditions are amenable to treatment or intervention.
- Syncope, seizures, vestibular dysfunction, acute illnesses, arrhythmia, subclavian steal, and carotid sinus hypersensitivity should be considered but are less common.
- **Extrinsic factors** are very common. A review of the household environment should include the following:
  - Improper lighting
  - Throw rugs
  - Uneven steps
  - Low-lying tables
- Grab bars for the bathroom are imperative when necessary.

Prevention

- A thorough search for intrinsic and extrinsic risk factors as described above is the first step in prevention.
- A home occupational therapy assessment can assist with management of extrinsic risk factors.
- Physical therapy is often helpful in gait and balance training, evaluation for an assistive device, and muscle strengthening when indicated.
- Identifying and treating the cause of postural hypotension and visual impairment are often necessary.

- There is growing interest in hip protectors to prevent hip fractures from falls. These devices may become readily available as more randomized controlled trials are completed.

Treatment

- A thorough examination of the older adult for occult fractures on presentation after a fall is mandatory.
- Plain films may be negative for a fracture in the initial evaluation of a geriatric patient who has a painful joint after falling.
- A high clinical index of suspicion for a nondisplaced fracture should be maintained.
- Common occult fractures that are missed on plain films include pelvic insufficiency and hip fractures.
- A low threshold should exist for obtaining a bone scan or MRI in patients who have persistent pain despite negative initial plain films.

MOTOR VEHICLE CRASHES

General Principles

- Driving concerns in the older adult may come to the attention of the primary care physician for several reasons.
- Patients may have insight into their driving skills and may question their own ability to drive safely.
- A concerned family member or friend may have observed unsafe driving behaviors.
- Finally, the department of motor vehicles may have raised some concerns and referred the individual to the physician for an evaluation of driving competency.

Diagnosis

- The initial assessment begins with the driving history.
- Inquiries about crashes, tickets, near misses, or becoming lost in previously familiar environments should be addressed to the patient and, if possible, a friend or family member.
- Information from a collateral source who has driven with the patient may be beneficial.
- A review of medications that have the potential to sedate the older driver should be sought, with efforts at drug reduction or substituting safer alternatives.
- A search for diseases that have the potential to increase crash risk should be pursued and may include dementia, psychiatric disorders, stroke, sleep apnea, arthritis, alcohol use, sensory deprivation, seizures, diabetes, or heart disease.
- Vision, hearing, attention, visuospatial skills, judgment, muscle strength, and flexibility should be assessed.
- The American Medical Association has recently recommended that office practitioners can adopt a brief set of office tests that may identify older adults who are at risk for driving problems.[23]
- Efforts should be made at stabilizing or improving these illnesses or physiologic variables when possible.
- Counseling older drivers to use safety restraints, refrain from drinking alcohol when driving, obey the speed limit, avoid cellular phones, and consider a refresher course

for driving such as the AARP Driver Safety Program (sponsored by the American Association of Retired Persons, http://www.aarp.org/family/housing/driver_safety_program/, last accessed December 18, 2009), is an important issue in motor vehicle crash prevention.

- Referral may be necessary if the primary care physician is unsure as to whether the patient is safe behind the wheel.
- Occupational therapists or **driving rehabilitation specialists** who have experience in assessing older drivers can be invaluable in the evaluation process with on-the-road tests or by recommending and implementing adaptive equipment.

Treatment

- In the event that the clinician makes a recommendation to stop driving, this information should be communicated in a professional and sensitive manner and documented in the medical record.
- It is helpful if alternate modes of transportation are discussed.
- Referral to a social worker or gerontological care manager may be useful in this situation.
- Patients may refuse to stop driving despite the advice of their physician or family, or both.
- DAT drivers may lack insight into their own safety risk. Therefore, removing the car from the premises, hiding the car keys, changing the locks, filing down the ignition key, or disabling the battery cables may be necessary.
- Letters can be written to the department of motor vehicles and may be ethically appropriate. Some states have laws that grant physicians civil immunity from reporting unsafe drivers or have mandatory reporting requirements. **Physicians should be aware of state and local requirements for reporting and obtain legal advice before breaching confidentiality.**

URINARY INCONTINENCE

General Principles

- UI, the complaint of involuntary leakage of urine, is a common problem for older adults.
- There are several **reversible causes** of UI including the following:
  - Infections
  - Delirium
  - Decreased mobility
  - Medication like diuretics
  - Polyuria due to other medical condition like diabetes mellitus.
- There are different **types of UI.**
  - **Urge** incontinence is part of the overactive bladder syndrome and is presumed to be due to uninhibited bladder contractions or detrusor overactivity.
  - **Stress** incontinence or stress leakage occurs when increases in intra-abdominal pressure overcome sphincter closure mechanisms in the absence of a bladder contraction. Stress UI is the most common cause of UI in younger women and the second most common cause in older women. It may occur in older men after transurethral or radical prostatectomy.

- **Mixed** incontinence is the most common type of UI in women. This is generally thought to represent the overlap of two mechanisms, detrusor overactivity and impaired urethral sphincter function.
- The term **"overflow incontinence"** has been used to describe the dribbling and/or continuous leakage associated with incomplete bladder emptying due to impaired detrusor contractility and/or bladder outlet obstruction. Leakage typically is in small volume, although its continual nature can lead to significant wetting.

Diagnosis

- Patients may be reluctant in discussing it with the physician, so all women who have had children, all patients at increased risk for UI (i.e., diabetes, neurologic disease), and all patients >65 years of age should be asked specifically about incontinence symptoms.
- Patients should be asked about symptoms compatible with a urinary tract infections (UTI) such as, dysuria/burning, frequency, urgency, foul-smelling urine, suprapubic pain, hematuria, back/flank pain, and fever.
- Vaginal symptoms (discharge, odor, dryness, pruritus, and dyspareunia) may suggest a gynecologic cause.
- **Urgency** is accepted as both a sensitive and specific symptom for detrusor overactivity, but published trials are lacking.
- Leakage with **stress** maneuvers (e.g., coughing, laughing, bending over, running, changing position) is highly sensitive for stress UI.
- With **overflow** incontinence there may be a weak urinary stream, dribbling, intermittency, hesitancy, frequency, and nocturia.
- A bladder diary with measured bladder volumes is helpful.
- Unless the history and/or other portion of the physical examination are highly suggestive of a specific cause, a genital and rectal examination should be done.
- A urinalysis should be done to evaluate for a UTI.
- The postvoid residual is elevated with overflow incontinence.
- Some patients will require referral to a urologist or urogynecologist for a more detailed evaluation (e.g., urodynamic testing, cystoscopy).

Treatment

Nonpharmacologic Therapies

- The first step in management is to **identify and/or treat reversible causes;** avoid caffeine, alcohol, excessive fluid intake, treat UTI, uncontrolled diabetes, and so forth.
- Up to two voiding per night is normal in older adults. Sleep disorders should be excluded.
- For nocturia, patients should **restrict fluid intake 4-hours before bedtime.**
- **Eliminate medications** causing or exacerbating UI, if possible.
- Nonpharmacological behavior interventions should be considered as the next step.
  - For stress and urge incontinence bladder retraining, regular voiding based on bladder diary and urgency control is recommended.
  - Pelvic muscle/Kegel exercises also help control UI.
  - For cognitively impaired population prompted toileting every 2 to 3 hours is recommended.
- Pessaries may be used in women with vaginal or uterine prolapse.

Medications

- Pharmacological treatment of UI is the subsequent step and is widely used for urge and mixed incontinence if behavioral therapy alone is not successful.
- **Anticholinergics** with antimuscarinic effects are the most frequently prescribed medications for urge incontinence. Commonly used agents include the following:
  - **Oxybutynin,** started at a low dose of 2.5 mg two 2 to 3 times daily up to 20 mg/day in divided doses.
  - **Tolterodine,** 1 to 2 mg twice a day (immediate release), 2 to 4 mg/day (extended release).
  - **Fesoterodine,** start 4 mg once daily, may increase to 8 mg once daily.
  - **Trospium** (immediate release) 20 mg twice daily but dose needs to be decreased to 20 mg once daily in elderly and with renal impairment.
  - Because of their anticholinergic actions patients need to be monitored for side effects (e.g., dry mouth, drowsiness, constipation, blurred vision, urinary retention).
- Agents like **solifenacin** and **darifenacin** are more selective for M-3 receptors that are found in the bladder and gastrointestinal tract but evidence for superior clinical efficacy and tolerability is not clear.
- **α-Adrenergic antagonists** (nonselective—terazosin and doxazosin; selective—tamsulosin, alfuzosin, and silodosin) can be used in men with overflow incontinence due to benign prostatic hypertrophy.
- **Topical estrogen** may be tried in postmenopausal women with atrophic vaginitis.

Surgical Management

- Avoid the use of catheters for chronic urinary retention, but they may be considered in the treatment of Stage III or IV pressure ulcers or when requested by patient or family for comfort measures.
- Surgical treatment is considered in stress UI when patients do not respond to medical treatment adequately.
- Surgical treatment of benign prostatic hypertrophy may also be indicated and effective but may result in postoperative incontinence due to prostatectomy itself.

PRESSURE ULCERS

General Principles

Classification

- **Stage 1:** Skin intact but with nonblanchable redness for >1 hour after relief of pressure.
- **Stage 2:** Blister or other break in the dermis with partial thickness loss of dermis, with or without infection.
- **Stage 3:** Full thickness tissue loss. Subcutaneous fat may be visible; destruction extends into muscle with or without infection. Undermining and tunneling may be present.
- **Stage 4:** Full thickness skin loss with involvement of bone, tendon, or joint, with or without infection. Often includes undermining and tunneling.

Risk Factors

- The most common causes of wounds in older adults are pressure and friction.

- Risk factors include the following:
  - Malnutrition
  - Immobility
  - Vascular insufficiency
  - Other systemic illnesses
- Moisture from urinary or fecal incontinence, friction (pulling the patient across bedsheets), and shearing forces (patients sliding down a bed with the head elevated) can combine to damage tissue further.
- Once the pressure on tissue exceeds intracapillary pressure (10 to 30 mm Hg), tissue ischemia can occur.

Prevention

- **Remove pressure** by frequent position changes, mobility and exercise, massage, and/or physical therapy.
- **Keeping the skin dry, preventing friction, and avoiding sheering forces** can assist in prevention and healing.
- **Topical creams and lubricants** can be helpful to treat dry skin, provide a skin barrier, and increase blood flow to the area with application.
- Excess moisture can also promote breakdown of the skin and it is necessary to **protect patients who are incontinent** from being exposed to urine.

Diagnosis

- The clinical diagnosis of pressure ulcers is relatively straightforward.
- The usual patient is elderly but they also occur in younger patients with significant neurologic impairment and/or severe illness.
- Typical locations include sacrum, ischial tuberosities, greater trochanters, lateral malleoli, and heels.
- The clinical staging is as described above.
- It is worth noting that essentially all pressure ulcers are colonized with bacteria. Clinically significant wound infection may be suggested by erythema, warmth, swelling, tenderness, and purulent discharge.
- More deep-seated infections may present with symptoms and signs of cellulitis, osteomyelitis, and sepsis.
- Available testing modalities for osteomyelitis include plain radiography (limited sensitivity and specificity), MRI (high sensitivity but low specificity), CT, and nuclear imaging (operating characteristics very dependent on the clinical situation).
- Alternative or potentially coexistent conditions include venous insufficiency ulcers, arterial/ischemic ulcers, and diabetic neuropathic ulcers.

Treatment

- Treatment of pressure ulcers depends on the stage and severity of the ulcer. Close monitoring of the pressure ulcer should be documented and may be facilitated by using one of the scales for healing ulcers.
- **Nutrition** is critical and calorie or protein supplements, or both, may be helpful adjuncts to promote healing of wounds.
- Recent data question the usefulness of vitamin C and zinc supplementation.
- Foley catheters should be avoided but may be necessary to prevent contamination of nonhealing wounds.

- Adequate pain control should be provided.
- Stage 1 ulcer is a warning that more serious lesions may follow, if appropriate preventive measures are not instituted in a timely fashion. Preventive measures should be reviewed and intensified in this setting.
- For Stage 2 and 3 wounds, dressings and gels, such as **hydrocolloids** (DuoDERM, Tegasorb) and **hydrogels** (IntraSite, SoloSite), that cover the wound bed and provide a surface on which epithelial cells can migrate are often helpful.
- **Wet-to-dry dressings** can be used for noninfected wounds. However, if not changed routinely, they simply remove migrating epithelial tissue and inhibit further healing.
- **Topical enzymatic débridement** agents with collagenase and/or **sharp mechanical débridement** can be used to remove black eschar, with the goal of promoting granulating tissue, which promotes healing.
- **Alginates** (Kaltostat) are very absorbent and can be helpful in exudative wounds.
- **Topical antibiotic creams** are generally not used for routine wound care unless the area is infected. Polysporin, silver sulfadiazine, or mupirocin (the latter for methicillin-resistant *Staphylococcus aureus*) can be helpful in reducing bacterial counts.
- **Systemic antibiotics** should be used in cellulitis, deep-seated infections, and/or sepsis.
- Osteomyelitis should be considered in nonhealing wounds that continue to drain or are exudative.
- Finally, **support mattresses** that use foam, air, or water can also assist in prevention or healing. Deep wounds into the muscle or bone (Stage IV) or multiple nonhealing wounds may benefit from an air-fluidized bed or low–air-loss bed. However, their cost and size may be prohibitive.
- **Consultation with a general or plastic surgeon** to assist in wound healing, which could include debridement or flap procedures, or both, to close the wound may be necessary.

MALNUTRITION

General Principles

- Weight loss and anorexia have a multitude of causes in the older adult and are often multifactorial. They include the following:
  - The use of "therapeutic diets," such as a salt-restricted or diabetic diet.
  - Cachexia from advanced end-organ disease (e.g., congestive heart failure, chronic obstructive pulmonary disease)
  - Malabsorption
  - Cancer
  - Thyroid disease
- Zinc deficiency, acute or chronic illnesses, alcoholism, medications, nonconducive environment, poor food preparation and presentation, and ethnic preferences may also contribute.
- Difficulty in feeding due to hand and upper-extremity disability, cognitive impairment, psychosis, oral or dental disease, or ill-fitting dentures is not uncommon.
- The mnemonic MEALS ON WHEELS may be helpful to the clinician in identifying reversible causes for protein-energy malnutrition (Table 7).[24]

TABLE 7	Reversible Causes for Protein-Energy Malnutrition

M: medications (e.g., antibiotics, antiarrhythmics, anticonvulsants, antineoplastics, colchicine, digoxin, NSAIDs, hormones, iron, laxatives, opiates, psychiatric drugs, and many others)

W: wandering, continuous pacing, and other dementia-related behaviors

E: emotional problems (e.g., depression, bereavement), elder abuse

H: hyperthyroidism, hypercalcemia, hypoadrenalism

A: anorexia tardive (i.e., anorexia nervosa in the elderly), alcoholism

E: enteric problems (e.g., achalasia, chronic constipation, GERD, malabsorption, PUD)

L: late-life paranoia/mania

E: eating problems (e.g., apraxia, lack of hand-feeding)

S: swallowing problems (e.g., dysphagia, odynophagia, apraxia, globus hystericus), stones (i.e., cholelithiasis)

L: low-cholesterol and low-sodium diets

O: oral problems (e.g., poor dentition, ill-fitting dentures)

S: shopping and meal preparation problems

N: no money, no friends, nosocomial infection

GERD, gastroesophageal reflux disease; NSAIDs, nonsteroidal anti-inflammatory drugs; PUD, peptic ulcer disease.
Modified from Morley J. Anorexia of aging: physiologic and pathologic. *Am J Clin Nutr* 1997;66:760–773.

Diagnosis

- A simple method of identifying protein-calorie under nutrition in the older adult is to follow serial weights. In general, weight loss is significant if there is a 5% loss of body weight in 1 month, 7.5% loss in 3 months, or 10% loss in a 6-month period of time.
- The clinician should not count weight loss that is due to diuresis or volume status.
- In the long-term care setting, frequent measurements of weight and early assessment by a dietician are appropriate.
- A more detailed general discussion of malnutrition may be found in Chapter 18.

Treatment

- If patients are unable to sustain themselves from a nutritional standpoint after reversible causes of weight loss have been identified and treated, input from a dietitian and the judicious use of nutritional supplements may be in order.
- Medications such as **tetrahydrocannabinol** and **megestrol** have been effective in promoting weight gain in certain conditions (e.g., AIDS and cancer) but there are limited data regarding their usefulness in the elderly.
- **Mirtazapine** can also stimulate appetite and cause weight gain.
- **Oxandrolone** (Oxandrin) is an anabolic steroid and can also be used in certain cases for weight gain. A course of therapy is about 2 to 4 weeks and can be used intermittently according to response of the patient.

- Of course, all medications to promote weight gain can have serious side effects and these must be very carefully considered in the context of the potential benefits.
- Despite these efforts, the use of artificial nutrition and hydration may need to be addressed.
- It is important that the risks and benefits of **tube feedings** (typically administered after pursuing surgical or percutaneous gastrostomy) are discussed with the patient or surrogate decision maker, or both.
  - Tube feedings can assist with providing adequate calories and are helpful in preventing dehydration.
  - Gastrostomy feeding tubes are typically helpful in cases in which there is anticipated functional improvement (e.g., cerebrovascular accident).
  - However, there is a paucity of data to indicate that gastrostomy feeding tubes prevent respiratory infection, improve morbidity, prevent pressure sores, or delay mortality in the patient with advanced DAT.[25]

ETHICS

Advance Directives

- Many physicians are well versed with the use of advance directives in the hospital setting.
- It is also imperative in the outpatient and long-term care setting that advance directives are discussed openly with the frail older adults and their family members.
- Many patients or surrogate family members, or both, desire to avoid cardiopulmonary resuscitation, intubation and/or ventilation, intensive care unit treatment, dialysis, or tube feedings on the basis of quality-of-life issues or futility of treatment.
- Even if questions such as code status cannot be decided before an acute event, it is of the utmost importance to identify a surrogate decision maker for the patient. Usually, a family member or friend can be identified who can assist in making difficult decisions.
- A legal document such as a durable power of attorney is preferred, because guardianship is often a lengthy process that is difficult to expedite.

Informed Consent and Decision-Making Capacity

- When discussing options or interventions with a patient, it is important to follow the steps of informed consent. This generally includes the nature and purpose of the test or procedure, the risk and benefits, the probable outcome of the intervention or refusal of the plan, and any additional alternatives to the diagnostic test or procedure.
- Decision-making capacity of the patient should be assessed, because many individuals have cognitive impairment or behavioral problems.
- Steps for assessing capacity include the ability to communicate choices, understand and retain relevant information, appreciate the situation and its consequences, and manipulate information rationally.[26,27]

Additional Resources

The American Geriatric Society
www.americangeriatrics.org (last accessed June 30, 2009)

Administration on Aging
www.aoa.gov (last accessed June 30, 2009)
Alzheimer's Disease Education and Referral Center
www.nia.nih.gov/Alzheimers/ (last accessed June 30, 2009)
Family Caregiver Alliance
www.caregiver.org (last accessed June 30, 2009)

REFERENCES

1. Katzman R, Brown T, Fuld P, et al. *Am J Psychiatry* 1983;140:734–739.
2. Fleming KC, Evans JM, Weber DC, Chutka DS. Practical functional assessment of elderly patients: a primary care approach. *Mayo Clin Proc* 1995;70;890–910.
3. Patterson CJ, Gauthier S, Bergman H, et al. The recognition, assessment and management of dementing disorders: conclusions from the Canadian Consensus Conference on Dementia. *CMAJ* 1999;160:S1–S15.
4. Sano M, Ernesto C, Thomas RG, et al. A controlled trial of selegiline, alpha-tocopherol, or both as treatment for Alzheimer's disease. The Alzheimer's Disease Cooperative Study. *N Engl J Med* 1997;336:1216–1222.
5. Miller ER, Pastor-Barriuso R, Dalal D, et al. Meta-analysis: high-dosage vitamin E supplementation may increase all-cause mortality. *Ann Intern Med* 2005;142:37–46.
6. Reisberg B, Doody R, Stöffler A, et al. Memantine in moderate to severe Alzheimer's disease. *N Engl J Med* 2003;348:1333–1341.
7. Tariot P, Farlow MR, Grossberg GT, et al. Memantine treatment in patients with moderate to severe Alzheimer's disease already receiving donepezil: a randomized controlled trial. *JAMA* 2004;291:317–324.
8. Schneider LS, Tariot PN, Dagerman KS, et al. For the CATIE-AD Study Group. Effectiveness of atypical antipsychotic drugs in patients with Alzheimer's disease. *N Eng J Med* 2006;355:1525–1538.
9. Rayner AV, O'Brien JG, Shoenbachler B. Behavior disorders of dementia: recognition and treatment. *Am Fam Physician* 2006;73:647–654.
10. Schneeweiss S, Setoguchi S, Brookhart A, et al. Comparative Safety of Conventional and Atypical Antipsychotics Medications: Risk of Death in British Columbia Seniors. Effective Health Care Research (HSA290200500161). Rockville, MD: Agency for HealthCare Research and Quality, 2007. http://effectivehealthcare.ahrq.gov/repFiles/DEcIDE_Atypical_Antipsychotics_Seniors.pdf. Accessed December 18, 2009.
11. Rochon PA, Normand SL, Gomes T, et al. Antipsychotic therapy and short-term serious events in older adults with dementia. *Arch Intern Med* 2008;168:1090–1096.
12. Public health advisory: deaths with antipsychotics in elderly patients with behavioral disturbances. Washington DC: U.S. Food and Drug Administration, 2009. http://www.fda.gov/Drugs/DrugSafety/PublicHealthAdvisories/ucm053171. htm. Accessed December 18, 2009.
13. Jest DV, Blazer D, Casey D, et al. ACNP White Paper: update on use of antipsychotic drugs in elderly persons with dementia. *Neuropsychopharmacology* 2008;33:957–970.
14. Wilkins CH, Moylan KC, Carr DB. Diagnosis and management of dementia in long-term care. *Ann Long Term Care* 2008;16(Suppl 1):30–38.
15. Snowdon DA, Greiner LH, Mortimer JA, et al. Brain infarction and the clinical expression of Alzheimer disease. The Nun Study. *JAMA* 1997;277:813–817.
16. Burns J, Church JA, Johnson DK, et al. White matter lesions are prevalent but differentially related with cognition in aging and early Alzheimer's disease. *Arch Neurol* 2005;62:1870–1876.
17. Rudolph JL, Salow MJ, Angelini MC, McGlinchey RE. The anticholinergic risk scale and anticholinergic adverse effects in older persons. *Arch Intern Med* 2008;168:508–513.
18. Tune L, Carr S, Hoag E, Cooper T. Anticholinergic effects of drugs commonly prescribed for the elderly: potential means of assessing risk of delirium. *Am J Psychiatry* 1992;149:1393–1394.

19. Podsiadlo D, Richardson S. The timed "Up & Go": a test of basic functional mobility for frail elderly persons. *J Am Geriatr Soc* 1991;39:142–148.
20. Guralnik JM, Ferrucci L, Simonsick EM, et al. Lower-extremity function in persons over the age of 70 years as a predictor of subsequent disability. *N Engl J Med* 1995;332:556–561.
21. Fuller GF. Falls in the elderly. *Am Fam Physician* 2000;61:2159–2168.
22. Guideline for the prevention of falls in older persons. American Geriatrics Society, British Geriatrics Society, and American Academy of Orthopaedic Surgeons Panel on Falls Prevention. *J Am Geriatr Soc* 2001;49:664–672.
23. American Medical Association, National Highway Traffic Safety Administrations. Physician's Guide to Assessing and Counseling Older Drivers. Chicago: American Medical Association, 2003.
24. Morley J. Anorexia of aging: physiologic and pathologic. *Am J Clin Nutr* 1997;66:760–773.
25. Finucane TE, Christmas C, Travis K. Tube feeding in patients with advanced dementia: a review of the evidence. *JAMA* 1999;282:1365–1370.
26. Miller SS, Marin DB. Assessing capacity. *Emerg Med Clin North Am* 2000;18:233–242.
27. Wong JG, Clare IC, Gunn MJ, Holland AJ. Capacity to make health care decisions: its importance in clinical practice. *Psychol Med* 1999;29:437–446.

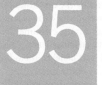

35 Allergy and Immunology

Jinny E. Chang and Shirley D. Joo

ALLERGY

General Principles

Epidemiology

- Allergy is highly prevalent in the United States, affecting about 50 million people suffering from some type of allergy.
- About 20 to 40 million people in the United States have seasonal and perennial allergies.[1] Food allergies have been reported in up to 21% of the adult population,[2] while Hymenoptera venom allergy has been reported in approximately 3% of adults[3] and 1% of children.[4]
- Medication allergies have been hard to study and vary greatly among populations.

Classification

The classic **Gel and Coombs classification** is as follows:

- Type I reaction (immediate hypersensitivity): Immunoglobulin E (IgE)-mediated release of histamine and other mediators from mast cells and basophils. Allergic reactions further characterized in this section involve the type I reaction.
- Type II reaction (cytotoxic hypersensitivity): Immunoglobulin G (IgG) or immunoglobulin M (IgM) antibodies bound to cell surface antigens, with subsequent complement fixation.
- Type III reaction (immune-complex hypersensitivity): Circulating antigen-antibody immune complexes that deposit in postcapillary venules, with subsequent complement fixation.
- Type IV reaction (cell-mediated delayed hypersensitivity): Mediated by T cells.

Pathophysiology

- For an **allergic reaction** to occur, **allergen-specific IgE** must be cross-linked on the surface of mast cells and basophils. This leads to release of initial mediators from mast cells and basophils within minutes of exposure to the allergen, a response that is known as the **early phase.** Lymphocytes and eosinophils arrive at the site 4 to 72 hours after the initial event, the so-called **late-phase** response. Often symptoms subside or disappear completely after the early phase only to reappear with the late phase.
  - **Early phase: Mast cells** release histamine, cytokines, leukotrienes, prostaglandins, and tryptase. Because mast cells are the only cells in the body that release **tryptase,** the serum level of this enzyme is increased after a systemic allergic reaction. **Basophils** also release **histamine and various cytokines.** Histamine mainly binds to the H_1 receptor, leading to increased vascular permeability and edema. In addition, perturbation of nerve endings leads to increased mucus production and the sensation of itch.

- **Late phase: Lymphocytes** are recruited to the site of the reaction by the cytokines that are released in the early-phase response. These cells further exacerbate the reaction through the **release of additional cytokines.** The presence of certain cytokines and leukotrienes then attracts **eosinophils,** and they release **additional leukotrienes,** which can lead to bronchoconstriction. They also release several **toxic proteins,** including major basic protein, which leads to disruption of the airway epithelium.
- **Allergen** is a protein or carbohydrate against which the body can produce IgE. Allergens may be inhaled, ingested, or injected into the body, where they encounter IgE bound to mast cells or basophils and an allergic reaction occurs. The first time that a person is exposed to a specific allergen, no allergic response can occur because this initial exposure is required for the immune system to make IgE against the allergen.
  - **Seasonal allergens** are certain airborne allergens that are more prevalent at specific times of the year. These seasonal allergens include tree, grass, and weed pollens (most often seen in the spring, early summer, and early fall, respectively).
  - **Perennial allergens** are present all year and include dust mites, cockroaches, and molds (although some molds have a seasonal increase in midsummer).
  - Other allergens are encountered only through specific exposures. These include medications, stinging insect venoms, animal danders, and foods.
- **Haptenation:** Most medications are too small to elicit an IgE response; however, the drug may bind to serum proteins, which then allow for sensitization. The IgE that is produced in this manner is directed against a medication, and subsequent exposure leads to binding of IgE to the drug alone, without any binding to serum proteins.

Diagnosis

Clinical Presentation

History

- **Symptoms:** Runny nose, sneezing, wheezing, conjunctivitis, rashes, or swelling, year round (perennial) or are they restricted to specific exposures.
- **Exacerbating/alleviating factors:** Pets, smoke, perfume, change in air temperature, and certain seasons.
- **Environmental history:** Where does the patient work, live, and play? What exposures are present in each of these environments? Does the patient have a pet?
- **Family history:** Are there other members of the family with allergic diseases (including asthma)? A child with one parent with allergic disorders has a 40% chance of having allergies (and/or allergic asthma). Two parents increase the risk to 60% to 80%.
- **Psychosocial issues:** It is important to determine if any psychosocial issues exist that may interfere with the patient's care. For example, one should determine if the patient has appropriate social support. It is also helpful to determine the patient's goal for the visit.

Physical Examination
Appearance

- **Mouth breathing** due to nasal congestion may be present.
- Because of edema in the nasal tissues, the draining veins under the eyes may be compressed, leading to pooling of blood and darkening of the region under the eyes. This is known as **allergic shiner.**
- Patients may also have infraorbital folds or **Dennie lines,** as well as a **nasal crease,** a transverse line across the lower portion of the nose.
- Patients with the hyper-IgE syndrome have a coarse facies and may have recurrent "cold" soft-tissue abscesses, which are abscesses that lack erythema.

Skin Examination

- **Urticaria,** or hives, is a maculopapular erythematous, often pruritic, eruption in the cutaneous tissues.
- **Angioedema** is edema in the SC tissues and is often painful but not pruritic.
- **Dermatographism** (or dermographism) is the tendency to form wheal-and-flare responses (urticate) to firm pressure applied to the skin. These patients may have physical urticarias as the etiology of their recurrent skin rashes.
- **Head, ears, eyes, nose, and throat:** The anatomy of the nose must be clearly evaluated, looking for the presence of swollen and edematous turbinates, pale- or blue-tinged nasal mucosa, polyps (whitish to clear sacs often hanging from the underside of the turbinates), and any septal deviation, ulceration, or perforation that may alter airflow.

Pulmonary

- A thorough lung examination is required, including auscultation of the lung fields, listening for any evidence of wheezing or an increased expiratory phase.
- In some patients, the use of a forced expiratory maneuver helps to expose underlying wheezing that cannot be heard at rest.

Diagnostic Testing

- All testing modalities may have false positives, and, therefore, correlation with the patient's symptoms and exposures is necessary.
- **Epicutaneous: This is the most specific test available and identifies most clinically significant allergens.** Although sensitivity to most allergens can be evaluated using epicutaneous and intradermal skin tests, food allergens should only be evaluated using epicutaneous methods.
- **Intradermal:** This type of skin test is more sensitive than epicutaneous testing but less specific. Irritant effects may cause many more false positives with this test. The risk of a systemic reaction is also increased with intradermal testing.
- **In vitro tests (radioallergosorbent test [RAST] or PRIST test):** These tests evaluate for the presence of IgE in the patient's serum against specific allergens, which are usually immobilized on a disk or plastic plate. They only determine whether specific IgE exists in the blood and have the potential to give positives to allergens to which the patient is not being exposed or to allergens to which the patient is not clinically allergic. In general, the sensitivity and specificity of in vitro tests are similar to those of intradermal skin testing alone.

Treatment

Environmental Control

Environmental control measures are the first and most important therapy for allergic disorders because these interventions limit or prevent exposure of patients to the allergens to which they are sensitive. Examples of appropriate control measures include the following

- **Pets** (in particular furred pets):
  - Keep pet out of home or at least out of the bedroom.
  - Remove carpeting.
  - Wash the pet regularly.
- **Dust mites:**
  - Wash bedding in hot water ($\geq 130°F$) weekly.
  - Use synthetic pillows, blankets, and mattresses.
  - Encase the pillows and mattress in dust mite–proof encasings.
  - Maintain home humidity level at approximately 45%.

Medications

Medications commonly used for allergic conditions are detailed in Table 1.

Corticosteroids

- **Mechanisms of action** of steroids include inhibiting the production of cytokines, which effectively prevents the late-phase response. Steroids do not block the immediate-phase response and are **not a contraindication to skin testing.**
- Long-term use of steroids is associated with **side effects.** The risk of side effects is much greater with systemic (oral) steroids than with topical (inhaled) steroids.
- **Posterior capsular cataracts** are associated with prolonged use, and annual ophthalmologic examinations are recommended for patients on any continual steroid dose (inhaled or oral).
- **Adrenal suppression** occurs with extended use of oral (any dose) or high-dose inhaled steroids. Short courses (less than a month) of oral steroids do not appear to have a significant effect on the hypothalamus-pituitary-adrenal axis.
- **Osteoporosis** is a risk of corticosteroid use; patients should be encouraged to take supplemental calcium and may require bone density scans to evaluate their risk.
- Newer studies suggest that **growth retardation** in the pediatric population **does not** occur with moderate-inhaled corticosteroid doses.[5]

Immunotherapy

- **Indications** are for **allergic rhinitis, asthma with or without an allergic rhinitis component,** and **venom hypersensitivity.** The mechanisms of action are still under investigation.
- **Treatment** consists of initial SC injections that contain increasing doses of the allergen extracts to which the patient is sensitive. Once the "buildup" phase is completed, the patient is kept at a maintenance dose for several years. The recommended length of therapy is variable (usually at least 3 to 5 years). Immunotherapy **should be prescribed by an allergist only** after the patient's response to skin tests or, under special circumstances, based on the results of in vitro testing.
- **Adverse reactions** are usually mild, with only localized pruritus, erythema, and edema. However, some reactions can be severe enough to include asthmatic flares, diffuse urticaria, and even anaphylactic shock.
  - The highest risk of a reaction is during the initial buildup phase; however, **a reaction may occur at any dose.**
  - A physician and staff who are experienced in treating anaphylactic shock and an emergency cart **must** be immediately available.
  - The risk for a reaction from an injection is greatest, up to 30 minutes following the shot, and patients should not be allowed to leave the office until this period has passed.
  - Any time that a patient has had a significant reaction, immunotherapy should be held, pending discussion with an allergist.
  - The only exception to this rule is venom immunotherapy, in which the risk of a reaction is greatest for up to 60 minutes after the shot, and, therefore, patients need to wait for an hour before leaving the office.

ANAPHYLAXIS

General Principles

- Anaphylaxis represents the rapid release of mast cell mediators, preformed as well as newly synthesized. The symptoms of anaphylaxis may be related to one or, more

TABLE 1	Commonly Used Outpatient Medications in Allergy and Immunology				
Medication	Class	Usual Adult Dosage	Indications	Major Side Effects	Other
Chlorpheniramine	CA	4 mg q12 hours	AR, UR, ANA	Fatigue/drowsiness/impaired mental performance	72 hours[a]
Diphenhydramine	CA	25–50 mg q6–8 hours	AR, UR, ANA	Fatigue/drowsiness/impaired mental performance	72 hours[a]
Cetirizine	NA	10 mg qd	AR, UR, ANA	Minimal sedation	7–10 days[a]
Levocetirizine	NA	5 mg qd	AR, UR, ANA		7–10 days
Fexofenadine	NA	60 mg bid 180 mg qd	AR, UR, ANA	None	5–7 days[a]
Loratadine	NA	10 mg qd	AR, UR, ANA	None	7–10 days[a]
Azelastine	IA	2 sprays bid	AR	Some sedation possible	7 days[a]
Olopatadine	IA/MS	2 sprays bid	AR		7 days
Budesonide	IS	200 µg/puff 2 puffs qd	AS	Steroid side effects and oral thrush	
	NS	32 µg/spray 2 sprays qd	AR	Steroid side effects	
Ciclesonide	IS	80, 160 µg/puff 1 puff bid	AS	Steroid side effects and oral thrush	
	NS	50 µg/spray 2 sprays qd	AR	Steroid side effects	
Flunisolide	IS	250 µg/puff 2 puffs bid	AS	Steroid side effects and oral thrush	
	NS	25 µg/spray 2 sprays bid	AR	Steroid side effects	

(continued)

TABLE 1 Commonly Used Outpatient Medications in Allergy and Immunology (*Continued*)

Medication	Class	Usual Adult Dosage	Indications	Major Side Effects	Other
Fluticasone	IS	44–220 µg/puff 2 puffs bid or qd	AS	Steroid side effects and oral thrush	
	NS	50 µg/spray 2 sprays qd	AR	Steroid side effects	
Mometasone	NS	50 µg/spray 2 sprays qd	AR	Steroid side effects	
Triamcinolone	IS	75 µg/puff 2 puffs tid-qid	AS	Steroid side effects and oral thrush	
	NS	55 µg/spray 1–2 sprays qd	AR	Steroid side effects	
Fluticasone/salmeterol diskus	IS/LBD	100, 250, 500 µg fluticasone/puff 50 µg salmeterol/puff	AS	Steroid side effects, oral thrush, and must be used no >1 inhalation bid	
Fluticasone/salmeterol HFA	IS/LBD	1 inhalation bid 45, 115, 230 µg fluticasone/puff 21 µg/puff Salmeterol	AS	Steroid side effects, oral thrush, and must be used no more than 2 puffs bid	
Salmeterol diskus	LBD	50 µg/inhalation 1 inhalation bid	AS	None Must not be used >1 inhalation bid and not recommended without use of inhaled steroid	

Salmeterol inhaler	LBD	21 μg/puff 2 puffs bid	AS	None Must not be used >2 puffs bid and not recommended without use of inhaled steroid
Albuterol	SBD	90 μg/puff 2 puffs q6 hours prn	AS	May make patient shaky, nervous, and anxious
Zafirlukast	LTA	20 mg bid (>12 y/o) For 7–11 y/o: 10 mg bid	AS, AR	None
Montelukast	LTA	10 mg qhs	AS, AR	None
Zileuton	LTA	600 mg qid (>12 y/o)	AS, AR	May cause liver damage (need to monitor LFTs before initiation of and during therapy)
Ipratropium bromide	NAC	21 or 42 μg/spray 2 sprays q8 hours prn	NAR	Dry mouth, nasal mucosa, epistaxis
	IAC	18 μg/spray 2 puffs q8 hours prn	AS	Dry mouth, cough

ANA, anaphylaxis; AR, allergic rhinitis; AS, asthma; CA, classic antihistamine; IA, intranasal antihistamine; IAC, inhaled anticholinergic; IS, inhaled steroid; LBD, long-acting bronchodilator; LFTs, liver function tests; LTA, leukotriene antagonist; MS, mast cell stabilizer; NA, newer antihistamine; NAC, intranasal anticholinergic; NAR, nonallergic rhinitis; NS, nasal steroid; SBD, short-acting bronchodilator; UR, urticaria; y/o, years old.
[a]Time before skin testing that antihistamine should be discontinued.

TABLE 2	Estimated Incidence or Prevalence of Acute Anaphylactic Reactions

Cause	Incidence or Prevalence
General cause	1/2,700 hospitalized patients
Chymopapain	2% of females; 0.2% of males
Insect sting	0.4%–0.8% of U.S. population
Radiographic contrast material	1/1,000–14,000 procedures
Penicillin (fatal outcome)	1.0–7.5/million treatments
General anesthesia	1/300 treatments
Hemodialysis	1/1,000–5,000 treatments
Immunotherapy (severe reaction)	0.1/million injections

Modified from Sim TC. Anaphylaxis. How to manage and prevent this medical emergency. *Postgrad Med* 1992;92:277.

commonly, multiple organ systems and are among the most rapid and profound of the allergic reactions; without rapid treatment, they may prove to be fatal.
- Anaphylactic reactions are not rare. Common causes of anaphylaxis and their incidence are shown in Table 2.
- Although the office management is essentially identical, anaphylaxis can be divided into two broad categories: IgE mediated and non-IgE mediated **(formerly known as anaphylactoid reactions).**

Classification
- Anaphylactic reactions can be classified according to the severity of the reaction. The most common classification is shown in Table 3.
- Anaphylaxis may be monophasic, biphasic, or, in rare cases, prolonged. As noted previously, classic allergic reactions may have an early and a delayed or late phase.
- It is not uncommon to see a patient who was successfully treated for anaphylaxis have a **second,** often as profound, reaction 4 to 12 hours following the initial anaphylactic reaction.

TABLE 3	Classification of Anaphylactic/Anaphylactoid Reactions According to Severity

Grade	Skin	GI	Respiratory	Cardiovascular
I	Pruritus, urticaria, flush, etc.	None	None	None
II	Pruritus, urticaria, flush, etc.	Nausea	Dyspnea Hypotension	Tachycardia
III	Pruritus, urticaria, flush, etc.	Vomiting Defecation	Bronchospasm Cyanosis	Shock
IV	Pruritus	Vomiting	Respiratory	Cardiac

Pathophysiology

- The rapid release of vasoactive mediators results in a loss of vascular tone, resultant pooling in the splanchnic bed, and functional hypovolemia. Because of increased capillary permeability, fluid and colloid are lost into the extravascular space.
- The net result of these two alterations is a profound decrease in blood pressure (BP). Other manifestations of anaphylaxis include bronchospasm, laryngeal edema, profuse nasal discharge, watery itchy eyes, marked postnasal drip, nausea, vomiting, diarrhea, abdominal cramping, uterine cramping, urticaria, angioedema, and rarely anaphylactic-induced pulmonary edema and acute heart failure.

Diagnosis

The **criteria** for the diagnosis include at least one of the following:

- **Laryngeal edema, bronchospasm or hypotension,** and the presence of other distinctive signs of allergy, such as urticaria or angioedema, or both; sneezing or rhinorrhea (often profuse); nausea; vomiting or diarrhea; and uterine cramping.
- A history of recent exposure to the agent is associated with anaphylaxis.
- A few conditions that might **mimic** anaphylaxis include vasovagal syncope, hyperventilation syndrome, globus hystericus, hereditary angioedema, carcinoid syndrome, systemic mastocytosis, and fictitious anaphylaxis.

Treatment

Recognition

Perhaps, the most important aspect of the treatment of anaphylaxis is the early recognition and treatment. **If anaphylaxis is suspected, treatment should be initiated without waiting to see if the reaction becomes worse.** True anaphylaxis rarely goes away without treatment.

Therapy

- The cornerstone of the treatment for anaphylaxis is placing the **patient in supine position** with rapid introduction of **epinephrine** and **fluid.** Other therapies may be added later. Most studies of fatal anaphylaxis have demonstrated failure to introduce these measures as a major contributor to the adverse outcome.
- Patients with acute anaphylaxis are often hypoxic. Thus, the rapid establishment of an **adequate airway** is critical.
- The outpatient treatment of anaphylaxis should be directed toward stabilizing the patient to assure a patent airway and maintain an adequate BP. Once this has been established, the patient should be **rapidly transported to an emergency care facility.**

Adrenergic or Sympathomimetic Agents

- The most important agent for the treatment of anaphylaxis is **epinephrine,** which should be used as soon as the reaction is recognized. The usual doses for epinephrine are shown in Table 4. It is important to remember that in most cases, SC or IM epinephrine is adequate, with recent data suggesting that IM administration is preferred.
- **Intravenous epinephrine should always be given using 0.1 mg/mL or 1:10,000 aqueous** rather than the 1:1,000 concentrations. Intermittent epinephrine can be repeated at 15- to 20-minute intervals, and after four doses, if necessary, can be followed by continuous intravenous therapy until the BP is stabilized.

TABLE 4	Doses for Epinephrine in the Treatment of Anaphylaxis

Minor-to-Moderate Manifestations	Dose and Route
Type I or II	0.3–0.5 mg (1:1,000) SC or IM adults 0.01 mg/kg (1:1,000) SC or IM children Repeat every 12–20 minutes × 4
Severe reaction—type III	0.5–1.0 mg (1:1,000) SC or IM adults 0.01–0.02 mg/kg SC or IM children Repeat every 3 minutes × 4
Severe reaction—type IV	0.1–1.0 mg (1:10,000) IV adults 0.01–0.02 mg (1:10,000) IV children
Continuous IV therapy, if intermittent therapy fails	0.1–1.0 µg/kg/min; titrate to maintain blood pressure
Upper-respiratory compromise	1.0–4.0 mg (racemic) by inhalation (meter-dose inhaler or nebulizer)

- Other sympathomimetic agents that may be useful include terbutaline (given SC or IM), dopamine, dobutamine, and norepinephrine. In general, these agents are sued in profound and prolonged anaphylactic reactions and are beyond the scope of this chapter.
- Aerosolized racemic epinephrine can be tried in patients who have laryngeal edema; however, if this is not available or is not rapidly effective, use of an endotracheal tube, cricothyroid puncture, or tracheotomy may be necessary to protect the airway. The establishment of an airway should be accompanied by the use of oxygen therapy.

Fluids
- Establishment of IV access and the institution of fluid replacement therapy should be accomplished as soon as epinephrine has been given.
- Two types of fluids are available for therapy: colloid (albumin, hydroxyethyl starch [hetastarch], pentastarch, dextrans, and blood and blood products) and crystalloid (dextrose, saline, and Ringer lactate).
- The choice between colloid and crystalloid has received significant attention. In general, colloid has the benefit of increasing oncotic pressure, which has been lost due to capillary leakage. Colloid solutions have been associated with increased oxygen saturation and less increase in lung water than crystalloid solutions.
- **Some colloid solutions are associated with adverse side effects,** such as anaphylactoid reactions (dextrans) and potential for infectious diseases (blood and blood products). Of the colloid solutions, hydroxyethyl starch is the preferred solution. An initial infusion of 500 mL is followed by crystalloid therapy. The choice of crystalloid solution is arbitrary, and any of the solutions mentioned above is adequate. The goal of therapy is to maintain adequate BP.

Antihistamines
- Antihistamines are a useful adjunct (IV, IM, PO), particularly for patients who experience urticaria or generalized skin pruritus.
- However, **antihistamines are not a substitute for epinephrine and fluids.** One should not give an antihistaminic and then wait to see if it is effective, even in mild anaphylaxis.

Other Agents
- **Glucagon:** May be effective in patients taking β-blockers.
- **β-Agonists:** Patients who experience significant bronchospasm should receive a short-acting β-agonist.

Basic Office Emergency Kit
This should include the following:
- Epinephrine: 1:1,000 aqueous for SC and IM use and 1:10,000 aqueous for IV use.
- Racemic epinephrine: Meter-dose inhaler or nebulizer use.
- IV fluids: Colloid and crystalloid.
- Large-bore IV catheter.
- Tourniquet.
- Oxygen with face mask or nasal prongs.
- Ambu-bag.
- Additional medications: H_1 antihistamines, H_2 antihistamines, and corticosteroids.

Prevention

- Prevention is one of the most important aspects of treatment for the practitioner.
- Emphasis should include instructing the patient that **most severe reactions** (including those to food, drugs, stinging insects, and radiocontrast media) **rarely go away.** If these reactions are identified, the patient should be advised to avoid that agent in the future. Individuals who are food sensitive should read all labels for prepared food and inquire for the presence of that food at restaurants. The "Food Allergy and Anaphylaxis Network" (http://www.foodallergy.org) can help individuals by identifying food that contains potent allergens and in designing meals that avoid those allergens.
- Every patient who has experienced anaphylaxis in the past should have a **self-injectable epinephrine prescribed and to be carried at all times.** A medical alert bracelet or necklace that identifies important allergens (especially drug allergy) is also an important preventive measure.

VENOM HYPERSENSITIVITY

General Principles

Definition
- Only insects with true stingers are included within the order Hymenoptera. Some examples are yellow and bald-faced hornet, yellow jacket, paper wasp, honeybee, and fire ants.
- A sting introduces roughly 20 to 50 mg venom protein.
- Included in this mix of proteins are many vasoactive amines, alkaloids, and species-specific proteins, such as hyaluronidase, acid phosphatase, and phospholipase A.

Epidemiology
- Estimates suggest that 6% to 17% of the population in the United States have specific IgE against Hymenoptera venoms[6] with a small predilection toward males.
- Clinically significant Hymenoptera venom–allergic reactions occurs in approximately 3% of adults[3] and 1% of children.[4]

Classification
- **Large local reactions** are characterized by induration, erythema, and pain at the sting site. The area involved can spread to regions of the body that are directly

adjacent to the sting site, but, **as long as these sites are contiguous, the reaction is still considered local.** These reactions are often quite dramatic and may last for up to a week, but they **rarely progress and need no further evaluation.**

- **Systemic reactions** include any reactions that occur **away from the initial sting site.** For example, facial urticaria immediately following a sting on the left hand is considered a systemic reaction, whereas edema of the entire left arm is not considered as such.
  - Systemic reactions can include urticaria, bronchospasm, laryngeal edema, hypotension, and other symptoms of anaphylaxis.
  - Most patients who have a severe reaction have no history of venom-induced anaphylaxis.
  - In patients with a history of a systemic reaction, 60% have a similar reaction with a re-sting, whereas only 11% have a worse reaction.

Pathophysiology

- A prior sting sensitizes the individual to the Hymenoptera venom, producing a specific IgE. Each subsequent sting can cause an increased likelihood of sensitization.
- Large local and systemic reactions to stinging insects are via the IgE-mediated pathway with mast cell and basophil degranulation as previously described in this chapter.

Diagnosis

Clinical Presentation

- **Type of insect:** It is important to try and identify the stinging insect, as this will guide skin testing and ultimate therapy. It is also helpful to determine if the patient was stung once or multiple times and by one or more insects.
- **Site of sting:** The location of the sting may be important in determining whether or not a systemic reaction occurred. It can also aid in identification of the insect involved. For example, honeybees usually sting when they are stepped on and are not normally known to attack people. Yellow jackets, however, attack people when their food source is threatened. This usually happens in the late fall, when they can be found scavenging for food in garbage containers.

Diagnostic Testing

- Various concentrations of the venoms are used to determine sensitivity to Hymenoptera venoms. False-positive skin test results are possible due to venom cross reactivity.
- **RAST inhibition** is an in vitro test that involves adding specific antigens to determine the level of cross reactivity. Usually, this test isolates the important insects.

Treatment

Local Reaction

- Local reactions require supportive care of ice, compression, and elevation. In severe local reactions, corticosteroids (usually 0.5 mg/kg prednisone) are sometimes prescribed to help decrease the edema and irritation.
- In addition, antihistamines can help alleviate the pruritus that is often associated with a sting.

Systemic Reaction

- Acute treatment of a systemic reaction includes the liberal use of IM (preferable) or SC **epinephrine** (Table 4) to treat anaphylaxis rapidly.
- **β-Agonists** are useful if bronchospasm develops from the sting (albuterol meter-dose inhaler or by nebulization).
- **Antihistamines** are also helpful in the acute treatment to block the effects of histamine release.
- **Corticosteroids** (0.5 to 1.0 mg/kg prednisone for 7 to 10 days) are helpful as well in the treatment of acute stings. These medications help abrogate the edema as well as help modify a late-phase response from occurring.
- **Long-term therapy** involves initiation of venom immunotherapy, which has been shown to reduce the patient's risk of a systemic reaction from a subsequent sting to that of the general population. In addition to immunotherapy, any patient who has had a systemic reaction to a sting should have self-injectable epinephrine (Epi-Pen) prescribed and be taught how to use it appropriately. Besides epinephrine, these patients should have antihistamines with them at all times. Patients are also encouraged to wear a medical alert bracelet that identifies them as venom allergic.

Immunotherapy

- Once patients begin venom immunotherapy, they are protected from subsequent stings—even if they are just in the buildup phase of the injections.
- The maintenance dose of the injections usually contains 100 mg venom proteins—roughly 1.5 to 2.0 times the amount in a single sting.
- The question of how long a patient should continue to receive immunotherapy is still under investigation. Some physicians treat for 5 years and then discontinue the shots, whereas others continue immunotherapy until the patient's skin test results become negative or at least a log-fold less reactive. The patient, primary care physician, and allergist should all be involved in the decision of when to discontinue immunotherapy.

URTICARIA AND ANGIODEDEMA

General Principles

Definition

Urticaria

- Urticaria is an erythematous maculopapular eruption in the superficial layers of the dermis and is associated with pruritus.
- It can further be divided into acute and chronic lesions based on the temporal nature of the rash.

Angioedema

- Angioedema, by contrast, consists of edema in the deep layers of the dermis and is usually characterized by pain rather than pruritus. Angioedema without urticaria usually presents as a painful, nonpruritic swelling of the deep dermis.
- The most often affected areas are the soles of the feet, palms of the hands (including the thenar eminence), buttocks, and face (including the larynx, lips, tongue, and periorbital regions).
- Attacks often occur after even minimal trauma and may progress around the body. The greatest danger with angioedema is that it may involve the larynx and can lead to complete obstruction of the airway.

- **Allergic angioedema** is an IgE-mediated hypersensitivity reaction to drugs, environmental contacts, insect stings, or other substances and can be idiopathic.
- **Nonallergic angioedema** occurs primarily as a result of increased bradykinin levels and can be further classified into hereditary, drug induced, acquired, and miscellaneous.

Classification

Urticaria
- **Acute** urticaria is any urticarial episode that lasts for <6 weeks.
- **Chronic urticaria** is when the episode lasts for >6 weeks. An urticarial episode consists of a period when hives are present daily or nearly daily. It should be noted that a given crop of hives will likely be present only for a short period, but the patient may have multiple crops of hives during the episode.

Angioedema
Acquired Angioedema
- **Acute:** Allergic, IgE mediated drugs (angiotensin-converting enzyme [ACE] inhibitors, nonsteroidal anti-inflammatory drugs [NSAIDs], fibrinolytic agents, estrogen, narcotics, some antibiotics), foods, insect bites, pollens and fungi, contrast dyes/drugs, serum sickness, and necrotizing vasculitis.
- **Chronic:** Idiopathic, acquired C1 inhibitor deficiency, angioedema-eosinophilia syndrome, and vibratory angioedema.
  - Type 1: Can be secondary to disease such as B-cell lymphomas, which produce excessive antibodies that lead to immune complexes and consumption of complement.
  - Type 2: Secondary to autoimmune diseases that generate autoantibodies against C1-esterase inhibitor.
  - Can be subcategorized into acquired C1-INH deficiency angioedema, idiopathic, allergic, drug induced, and miscellaneous.

Hereditary Angioedema
- The kallikrein-kinin system fails to be inhibited because of C1 inhibitor absence/dysfunction and leads to early-acting complement components C4 and C2 to be low.[7]
  - Type 1: C1 inhibitor deficient or absent due to mutation of *SERPING1* gene (80% to 85% of hereditary angioedema patients).
  - Type 2: C1 inhibitor dysfunctional (15% to 20% of hereditary angioedema patients from point mutation).
  - Type 3: C1 inhibitor level normal. Occurs in X-linked dominant fashion and therefore affects mainly women. Has been linked to mutations in the *Factor XII* gene.[8]

Epidemiology

- Approximately 15% to 24% of the U.S. population will experience at least one episode of urticaria (hives), angioedema, or both in their lifetime.[9]
- Among those experiencing either angioedema or urticaria, approximately 40% will present with both conditions simultaneously.[10]

Etiology

Acute Urticaria
- Most of the inciting agents that lead to acute urticaria can be easily identified because of the close temporal relationship between exposure and hive development.
- Often the patient has already identified the responsible agent before seeking medical attention.

- **Foods:** For example, peanuts and shellfish.
- **Medications:** For example, penicillin.
- **Infections:** Usually viral infections.
- **Physical causes:**
  - Cold, heat, pressure, sun, water, vibration, cholinergic stimulation, and exercise.
  - In some patients, exercise is a trigger only when closely preceded by eating.

Chronic Urticaria
- The inciting agents that lead to chronic urticaria are much more difficult to identify because the temporal relationship is not as clear as in acute urticaria.
- These patients tend to be more emotionally and physically affected by their disease and its chronicity.
- Chronic urticaria has been attributed to the following:
- **Medications:** For example, NSAIDs.
- **Collagen vascular disease:** For example, systemic lupus erythematosus.
- **Neoplasia.**
- **Autoimmune diseases.**
  - The autoimmune phenomenon that is most often associated with urticaria is **thyroid disease.**
  - Patients may be hypo-, hyper-, or even clinically euthyroid but usually have **antithyroid peroxidase autoantibodies** (also known as **antimicrosomal antibodies**).
  - In these patients (including the clinically euthyroid), treatment with physiologic doses of thyroid hormone often leads to resolution of the urticaria.
- **Diet:** Chronically eaten foods.
- Patients with chronic urticaria who have **autoantibodies** directed **against** either **IgE** or the **high-affinity IgE receptor (FcεRI)** do not respond well to antihistamines alone and often require corticosteroids for relief of their hives. Further treatment options for these patients are still being investigated.
- **Idiopathic urticaria,** the largest set of urticarias, is a catchall group that represents those cases in which no etiology for the urticaria can be discerned.

Angioedema
In most cases, angioedema is due to either a drug (such as an ACE inhibitor, an angiotensin receptor blocker [ARB], aspirin, an antibiotic, or an NSAID) or a deficiency in the complement component C1 esterase inhibitor (C1INH).
- Angioedema from an ACE inhibitor or ARB can occur at any point during a course of treatment and necessitates discontinuation of the drug, even if it is not the cause, because these drugs can enhance angioedema caused by other factors.
  - Clearly, all drugs of the same class need to be avoided; however, it is less clear whether sensitivity to one class necessitates avoidance of the other. However, several case histories have been reported in which angioedema has developed in patients with ACE inhibitor–induced angioedema when treating with an ARB therapy.[11]
  - Therefore, if possible, it is probably best to avoid both classes of medications if a patient develops sensitivity to one of them.
- A deficiency in C1INH can be either acquired or hereditary (known as hereditary angioedema). The acquired form of the disease is often associated with a hematologic malignancy and the subsequent production of an autoantibody that blocks the function of C1INH.
  - To evaluate for a possible deficiency in C1INH, a C4 level can be obtained. This is low even between attacks in hereditary angioedema.

- Further evaluation includes a quantitative C1INH level.
- If this is not significantly decreased, a functional C1INH level should be obtained. This is reduced in either acquired or hereditary forms.
- Finally, mixing studies and an anti-C1INH antibody enzyme-linked immunosorbent assay (ELISA) can be obtained to evaluate for the presence of an inhibiting autoantibody (often associated with an underlying hematologic malignancy).
- Patients with known or suspected angioedema due to a complement deficiency should be evaluated by an allergist/immunologist.

Pathophysiology

Urticaria

- Urticaria is dermal edema resulting from vascular dilatation and leakage of fluid into the skin in response to molecules (histamine, bradykinin, leukotriene C4, prostaglandin D_2, and other vasoactive substances) released from mast cells and basophils.[12]
- The prototypical lesion and pruritus are the result of H_1 histamine receptor activation on endothelial and smooth muscle cells leading to increased capillary permeability and H_2 histamine receptor activation leading to arteriolar and venule vasodilation.
- Urticaria are distinguished between immunologic and nonimmunologic mechanisms.

Immunological Urticaria

- Includes processes mediated by antibodies and/or T cells that result in mast cell activation.
- Urticaria may result from the binding of IgG autoantibodies to IgE and/or to the receptor for IgE molecules on mast cells, thus corresponding to a type II hypersensitive reaction. These autoimmune urticarias represent 30% to 50% of patients with chronic urticaria.
- Mast cell activation can also result from type I via IgE and type III through the binding of circulating immune complexes to mast cell–expressing Fc receptors for IgG and IgM.
- Finally, under certain circumstances, T cells can induce activation of mast cells, as well as histamine release (type IV HS).

Nonimmunological Urticarias

Result from mast cell activation through membrane receptors involved in innate immunity (e.g., complement, toll like, cytokine/chemokine, and opioid) or by direct toxicity of xenobiotics (haptens, drugs). Urticaria may result from different pathophysiological mechanisms that explain the great heterogeneity of clinical symptoms and the variable responses to treatment.[13]

Angioedema

- An **IgE-mediated hypersensitivity reaction** to drugs, foods, environmental exposures, insect stings, or other substances resulting in histamine release from mast cells results in allergic angioedema.[14] Most cases, however, are idiopathic.
- **Nonallergic angioedema** (see classifications above including hereditary, drug-induced, acquired, and miscellaneous angioedema) occurs mostly as a result of increased bradykinin levels.[15,16]

Diagnosis

Clinical Presentation

History
- Determine whether the urticaria is **acute or chronic.**
- It is also important to determine whether the lesions are **pruritic or painful.** Because vasculitis may present with urticarial lesions, it is critical to determine whether the individual crops of hives **last for >24 hours** and whether they **resolve with scarring.** Both of these conditions are associated with urticarial vasculitis, not urticaria.

Physical Examination
- Specifically, the physician should look for evidence of thyroid disease, collagen vascular disease, occult infection, or malignancy.
- Several types of urticaria can develop from physical causes. These **physical urticarias** can be diagnosed during the examination by using various maneuvers to reproduce each of them. For example, cold urticaria can be diagnosed by placing an ice cube on the forearm for 4 minutes. The cube is then removed and the arm observed for 10 minutes. A hive that develops at the same location where the ice cube was indicates a positive test result.

Diagnostic Testing

- Reasonable common laboratories to obtain include complete blood cell count sedimentation rate, liver function tests, anaphylaxis, antithyroid peroxidase antibodies, and urinalysis.
- Chronic urticaria index: Commercially available test to detect presence of anti-FcεRI autoantibodies.
- Skin and RAST testing:
  - Although the specific antigens that are responsible for urticaria are often hard to discern, it may be helpful in some patients to perform skin or RAST testing.
  - These tests tend to be more useful in patients with acute urticaria in whom a specific food or medication is believed to be the offending agent.
  - As mentioned previously, skin testing is the preferred modality to evaluate for allergy; however, some patients with urticaria have such severe skin disease that RAST testing may be more feasible.
- In addition to specific food allergens, urticaria can develop from sensitivity to food additives. **The only reliable test for sensitivity to food additives is a double-blind placebo-controlled challenge.** These are usually performed in an allergist's office and take several hours to complete.

Treatment

The most important therapeutic intervention is to **avoid the inciting agent(s)** and/or **treat the underlying condition.**

Urticaria

- Medications include use of antihistamines often in escalating doses, to control the pruritus and urticarial flares. In addition to the traditional H_1-receptor antagonist antihistamines (see Table 1 for medications and doses), patients may benefit from the addition of an H_2-receptor antagonist (cimetidine, ranitidine, famotidine, etc.).

- **Tricyclic antidepressants,** such as doxepin (starting dose, approximately 10 to 25 mg daily), are often used because of their strong antihistaminic activity. Because these medications are often sedating, they should be given shortly before or at bedtime.
- **Corticosteroids** can be used (often prednisone, 0.5 mg/kg daily) to alleviate urticarial flares, but the numerous side effects of chronic use limit their feasibility in chronic urticaria.
- In patients with **chronic idiopathic urticaria,** it is helpful to control their urticaria with appropriate doses of medications and then to withdraw the medications after a specified duration of time (6 weeks to 6 months) to evaluate for the continued presence of urticarial lesions. If the hives recur, restart the medications for another period of time.

Angioedema

- **Avoidance** of the causative agent is the primary treatment in drug-induced angioedema. As mentioned above, a reaction to an ACE inhibitor or ARB may be the reason to avoid all drugs of both classes. In cases in which angioedema is secondary to a malignancy, **treatment of the underlying disease** leads to resolution of the angioedema.
- **For chronic therapy** of hereditary angioedema, **androgens** (usually stanozolol) can be used. These increase the levels of C1INH and prevent attacks of angioedema. These patients should be referred to an allergist/immunologist for diagnosis and therapy. Because of their masculinizing effects, androgens should be particularly avoided in the treatment of female patients. Primary care physicians should not attempt to treat hereditary angioedema.
- **For acute therapy** of angioedema, **epinephrine** can be used. Unfortunately, patients with hereditary angioedema usually respond poorly to epinephrine alone. In these cases, **fresh frozen plasma (FFP)** (which contains C1INH) can be given; however, in some patients, this worsens the swelling. **Purified C1INH** is in clinical trials; when commercially available, it could be used to acutely treat patients with angioedema. As **preparation for surgery,** patients can be given FFP or C1INH before the operation to prevent peri- and postoperative angioedema.
- **Supportive therapy** is always important. Laryngeal angioedema may develop, and therefore it is always important to safeguard the airway. Some patients may even require intubation or tracheostomy during their attacks.

DRUG ALLERGIES

General Principles

Epidemiology

- Allergic reactions to drugs represent a major contributor to the spectrum of adverse drug reactions.
- Studies suggest that as many as 40% of all hospitalizations in the United States are in one way or another related to an adverse drug reaction.

Classification

- **Reactions related to the pharmacologic properties of the drug** such as side effects, toxic reactions, and drug interactions. Because these reactions are based on the chemical properties of the drug, they occur in all patients if a sufficient amount of drug is given. Therefore, in many cases, the reaction may be lessened by alteration in the dose of the drug.

- **Reactions due to toxic metabolites** may mimic immunologic reactions or side effects. In this case, the biotransformation product rather than the drug itself is the offending agent. The reaction to sulfa-containing drugs (mostly sulfamethoxazole in patients who are HIV positive) is an example of this reaction. These reactions are different from other side effects, and the method for abrogating the reaction differs from that of other types of adverse drug reactions.
- **Idiosyncratic reactions** are adverse effects with an unknown mechanism.
  - They are seen in susceptible individuals, but the basis for the susceptibility is not known.
  - These reactions may occur **at any point during therapy.**
  - The reactions may be mild, such as the facial dyskinesis that is seen with phenothiazines, or devastating, such as the aplastic anemia with chloramphenicol.
  - What is clear is that **idiosyncratic reactions almost invariably recur if the drug is reintroduced.**
- **Immunology-based reactions.**
  - Adverse reactions may be the result of production of antibodies or cytotoxic T cells directed against the drug or a biotransformation of the drug.
  - The types of reactions include contact sensitivity of fixed drug reactions (type IV or cell-mediated reaction); tissue-specific reactions due to T-cell immunity, such as drug-induced hepatitis; tissue-specific damage due to IgG antibodies (type II or III); and drug allergy due to IgE antibodies (type I).
  - Other reactions are believed to have an immunologic basis, but the exact mechanism has not been elucidated. Examples include drug fever and erythema multiforme minor and major (Stevens-Johnson syndrome) and toxic epidermal necrolysis.

Pathophysiology

- **Mechanism of drug allergy:**
  - The majority of the therapeutic agents are low-molecular-weight organic compounds and are not capable of inducing the production of either antidrug antibodies or T-cell proliferation on its own. It is only when the drug (or one or more of its biotransformation products) reacts covalently with a tissue protein (or carbohydrate) that acts as a hapten that is capable of inducing an immune response.
  - The actual immunogen may be the hapten itself, the hapten-protein conjugate, or a tissue protein that has been altered by interaction so that it is now recognized as a foreign body.
  - Because a chemical bond must occur between the drug and the tissue protein, the propensity of that drug to bind to protein either in its native state or following metabolism determines the allergenic potential of that drug. Thus, β-lactam antibiotics are very reactive with tissue protein and are major allergens, whereas cardiac glycosides are very nonreactive, and true allergy to this class of drugs is rarely seen.
- **Route of administration** is important in the induction phase of drug allergy.
  - Parenteral administration of a drug has the highest potential for inducing an immunologic reaction.
  - Oral administration is much less likely to result in an immunologic reaction to a drug.
  - Application of a drug to the skin may result in a contact sensitivity (type IV) rather than the production of antidrug IgE.
- **In all but the rarest cases, the actual immunogen is not known.**
  - This is important because the development of in vivo tests (skin tests) or in vitro tests (RAST or ELISA) is based on a thorough knowledge of the chemical structure of the allergen.

- For the first-generation β-lactam antibiotics (penicillins and first-generation cephalosporins), the immunogens are well described or are surmised from extensive skin testing. Thus, 75% of patients with a history of penicillin reaction have a positive skin test result to penicilloyl-polylysine (Pre-Pen), whereas 6% of patients react to penicillin G and 7% of patients react to penicilloic acid. The latter two reagents are used to conjugate rapidly with tissue proteins and provide the appropriate antigen. With a knowledge of the allergens, the results of this skin test has high sensitivity and specificity.
- Other drug classes have not been studied, and, thus, the allergen(s) are not known. It is possible to use the native drug as an allergen in the hope that the drug or its metabolite will provide an appropriate allergenic structure; however, the predictive value of these tests is questionable.

Diagnosis

The diagnosis of drug allergy is based on a thorough history, physical examination, in vivo or in vitro testing or both, and, when necessary, a provocative challenge.

Clinical Presentation

- **The drug or drugs that the patient had been taking at the time of the reaction.** If the reaction occurred in the past, a chart review may be necessary.
- **The type of reaction** and the potential for that reaction to be immunologic in nature. It is often helpful for the physician to make a list of the potential offending drugs and then to rank the drugs by allergenic potential. Although all drugs are potential allergens, as mentioned previously, **some are much more allergenic than others.**
- **The severity of the reaction** is also very important, as it determines the steps that may have to be taken to abrogate a similar reaction. An anaphylactic reaction is much more significant than a minor skin rash.
- **A history of reactions** to drugs is very helpful. Several groups have demonstrated that a patient who has had one reaction to a drug is more likely to have another than is a patient who has never reacted. For some patients, true reactions are seen to multiple drug classes and probably represent an increased ability to react to haptenated proteins. This has been referred to as the **multiple drug allergy syndrome.**
- **A family history of drug allergy** is also a predictive factor. The relative risk of a drug reaction is multifold higher if the patient's mother or father has also had a drug reaction.
- Finally, **the nature of concurrent illness** should be established to ensure that the reaction is due to a drug and not from the illness. For example, a facial rash in a patient with lupus erythematosus is most likely the result of the disease process and not a drug reaction.

Diagnostic Testing

In Vivo or In Vitro Testing
- Skin testing is the most important technique for the diagnosis of a true drug allergy.
- In the case of penicillin or the first-generation cephalosporins, skin testing is easily performed and highly predictive of an allergic reaction.
- Referral to an allergist/immunologist is necessary for skin testing to be performed.
- In vitro testing, such as RAST or ELISA tests, has the same drawback as skin testing, as it relies on knowledge of the actual allergen.

- These tests are further compromised by the amount of time that is necessary for the test to be performed (usually >24 hours), and, thus, they are not applicable to the acute situation.
- Evidence has demonstrated that skin testing may not be reliable within the first several weeks after a severe drug reaction, and this may be the one situation in which in vitro testing is necessary.

Provocative Dose Challenge

- A provocative dose challenge provides a method for determining a patient's sensitivity to a given drug or drug class and for initiating therapy to that drug. Indeed, in practice, this is performed only when a decision to start the patient on the drug has been made.
- The challenge begins with a small (1 mg) dose of the drug and proceeds rapidly to higher doses. In practice, we generally base the dose for challenge on the dose of drug that is necessary for therapy.
- If the patient tolerates a 1-mg to 10-mg dose, then one-tenth the therapeutic dose followed by one-fourth the therapeutic dose and then one-half the therapeutic dose at 15- to 30-minute intervals are given.
- The provocative dose challenge should be performed in a medical setting, where appropriate resuscitative measures are available.

Treatment

Alternate Drug Class

- The most effective therapy for drug allergy is the selection of an alternative drug class.
- The selection of an alternative drug should always be the first consideration in approaching a drug-allergic patient.
- In most cases, an effective therapeutic agent is available that does not cross react with the drug to which the patient is sensitive.
- In some cases, an alternative drug may be of the same drug class but lacks a reactive side chain.
  - An example is the substitution of lisinopril or enalapril, which does not have a sulfonamide side chain, and of captopril, which contains a sulfonamide.
  - Similarly, ethacrynic acid may substitute for furosemide.
  - The substitution of an alternative antibiotic, which may differ only in a reactive side chain, is often very effective and precludes the need for skin testing and desensitization.
- The selection of an **alternative modality** is also effective in anaphylactoid reactions. For example, the selection of a low–ionic strength radiocontrast medium rather than the high-strength material decreases the potential for a reaction greatly.

Provocative Dose Challenge

- This can often be effective when skin testing or in vitro testing is not available.
- The physician should choose the drug class that is least likely to give a positive reaction.
- For example, patients who have a history of a reaction to a local anesthetic (which almost never causes a true allergic reaction) can receive a provocative challenge with the least reactive group of agents.
  - The least reactive agents do not contain a para-aminobenzoic acid ester group.

TABLE 5	Protocol for Pretreatment of Patients with a History of Radiocontrast Media Reactions		

| Time Before the Procedure | Drug and Dose | | |
	Prednisone[a]	Cimetidine[b]	Diphenhydramine[c]
13 hours	50 mg PO or IV	300 mg PO or IV	
7 hours	50 mg PO or IV	300 mg PO or IV	
1 hours[d]	50 mg PO or IV	300 mg PO or IV	50 mg PO or IV

[a]Other agents include methylprednisolone, 40 mg IV.
[b]Other agents include ranitidine, 150 mg.
[c]Other agents include chlorpheniramine, 10–12 mg.
[d]Can also add ephedrine, 25 mg PO, 1 hour before procedure.

- Because preservatives such as parabens or additional agents such as β-adrenergic agonists can cause reactions, we recommend that the provocative challenge be carried out using **preservative-free solutions.**
- These are available as obstetric preparations of most local anesthetics. If a small (1 mL) dose of the local anesthetic does not provoke a reaction, this anesthetic can be used without hesitation.

Pretreatment Protocols

Pretreatment protocols are available for a number of drug classes that cause reaction by anaphylactic or anaphylactoid mechanisms, and the protocol may prevent or decrease any reaction that might occur. The protocol that is used in the reintroduction of radiocontrast media is presented in Table 5.

Drug Desensitization

- The purpose of desensitization is to prevent a potentially life-threatening reaction. The procedure does not prevent the appearance of mild skin reactions such as pruritus or urticaria.
- This should only be performed under the supervision of an allergist/immunologist and only in a location that is capable of treating significant and potentially prolonged anaphylaxis.
- The desensitization procedure involves the introduction of minute amounts of the drug and then slowly increasing the dose (usually by doubling) every 15 to 20 minutes until a full therapeutic dose is achieved.
- The potential for a reaction is much less when oral medication is used. Therefore, when possible, the initiation of the desensitization procedure is by the oral route followed by parenteral medication if indicated.
- Importantly, **the desensitized state lasts only as long as the drug is given.** Once the drug has been stopped, the patient becomes sensitive again in 8 to 48 hours. It is not possible to predict when the patient will become sensitive; thus, **if the patient misses taking the drug for >12 hours, the procedure has to be repeated.** If the physician foresees a need to retreat with the same medication in a short period of time, the drug should be continued (usually orally) to avoid having to undergo another desensitization.

FOOD ALLERGIES

General Principles

- General "sensitivity" to foods is common, but food allergy is a term reserved for an immunologic-mediated sensitivity (i.e., IgE mediated, cell mediated, and mixed).
- Patients may present with a number of varying symptoms: urticaria/angioedema, asthmatic flares, abdominal cramping, diarrhea, rhinoconjunctivitis flares, and anaphylaxis.
- Food allergy is thought to occur in up to 6% of children and in <3% to 4% of adults. The overall prevalence is growing, particularly in developed countries.

Classification

- **IgE mediated:** Acute onset including symptoms of urticaria/angioedema, oral allergy syndrome (pruritus and mild edema confined to oral cavity), rhinitis, asthma, anaphylaxis, and food-dependent/exercise-induced anaphylaxis (food triggers anaphylaxis only if ingestion followed by exercise).
- **Cell mediated:** Delayed onset with possible chronic clinical picture with symptoms of atopic dermatitis (associated with food in 35% of kids with moderate-to-severe rash) and/or eosinophilic gastroenteropathies (varying degrees of dysphagia or odynophagia).
- **Mixed IgE and cell mediated:** Delayed onset with dietary protein enterocolitis (seen in infants with chronic exposure leading to emesis, diarrhea, and growth retardation), as well as dietary protein proctitis giving mucus-laden bloody stools in infants.[17,18]
- **Nonimmunologically mediated** mechanisms fall into the categories of enzymatic or transport deficiencies (e.g., lactase deficiency or glucose/galactose malabsorption, respectively).

Pathophysiology

- The mechanisms of allergy and tolerance have been under investigation, with the breakdown of gastrointestinal barrier[19] and nonoral exposure (via respiratory sensitization[20] and skin sensitization[21]) as possible contributors to food allergies.
- Proteins easily degraded by heat and chemicals are less likely to cause severe reactions in contrast to stable proteins as found in nuts and seeds.[22]
- Genetic influences have also been identified, as peanut allergy is much more likely in a child with a sibling with known peanut allergy.[23]
- Hygiene theory postulates that decreased exposures to bacteria and infections may influence immune function with a more atopic clinical picture[24,25] and an immune deviation toward a Th2 response, where IL-4, IL-5, and IL-13 induce IgE and eosinophilic inflammation leading to disease.

Diagnosis

Determine what type of reaction occurred, and whether it was IgE mediated.

IgE-Mediated Food Allergy

- Determine the timing of the reaction after ingestion of the suspected food.
- Most allergic reactions occur within 15 to 30 minutes of ingestion.
- Reactions that occur hours after eating are much less likely to represent an allergic response.
- Determine the suspected foods that are involved.

- In food allergy in adults, the most often offending agents are peanuts, tree nuts, and shellfish. In children, the common offending foods also include milk, wheat, soy, and egg.

Non–IgE-Mediated Food Allergy

- Non–IgE-mediated food allergies can also present as food intolerance as described above.
- **Eosinophilic gastroenteritis** is a disorder that is characterized by eosinophilic infiltration of the gastrointestinal wall and peripheral eosinophilia. These patients often present with malabsorption and usually have allergic diseases as well. They should be evaluated and treated by a specialist.

Diagnostic Testing

- A positive test result must correlate with the patient's history for that allergen to be associated with the patient's symptoms.
- These tests should be performed in an allergist/immunologist's office.
- Skin testing for the various food allergens is often performed.
  - Because of the irritant nature of many food allergen preparations and the possibility of systemic reactions, only epicutaneous and not intradermal testing should be performed.
  - In some cases, testing is done with fresh fruits or vegetables, which are pricked with the testing device.
- CAP-RAST testing allows for the determination of specific IgE against various food allergens.
- **The gold standard for diagnosing food allergy is the double-blind placebo-controlled food challenge.** These challenges can be dangerous and should be performed by allergists either in their clinic or in the hospital. If this food challenge does not show sensitivity to the suspected food, an open-label challenge with the food is usually performed.

Treatment

- **Avoid the offending food.**
- Educate the patient and family members/friends about how allergic reactions to foods occur, how to avoid these reactions, and how to treat when a reaction occurs.
- In children, it is important that all potential caregivers (including, e.g., the parents of the child's friend) understand the disease and how to avoid and treat reactions.
- To treat episodes, the patient (and caregivers) should always have immediately available self-injectable epinephrine (Ana-Kit or Epi-Pen).
  - Any patients for whom self-injectable epinephrine is prescribed should have the proper use of the injector demonstrated to them in the physician's office.
  - Before leaving the office, patients should demonstrate to the physician that they understand the proper use of self-injectable epinephrine.
  - They should also be aware that whenever they have used their epinephrine, they should seek immediate medical attention.
- The risk of death from food allergies is increased (especially with children) when patients have asthma (see Chapter 12) and are unaware that they have ingested a food to which they are sensitive, patients are away from home or from a primary caregiver when the reaction occurs, and the time to epinephrine injection is >30 minutes.[26]

- **Allergen-specific immunotherapeutics** are designed to present the allergen in a context that stimulates a Th1 immune response (e.g., IFN-γ) or generates suppressive (regulatory) T cells that results in downregulation of Th2 responses.
- **Anti-IgE antibodies** (omalizumab) as well as cytokine/anticytokine medications are considered not allergen specific and designed to modulate or interrupt the allergic responses.

RHINITIS AND RHINOCONJUNCTIVITIS

General Principles

Definition

- Allergic rhinitis is inflammation of the nasal mucosa, and allergic rhinoconjunctivitis is the combination of inflammation of nasal mucosa and conjunctiva due to allergies.
- The disease tends to occur predominately in childhood, and the onset is usually before puberty.
- Untreated, rhinoconjunctivitis can lead to several other diseases, including sinusitis, otitis media, and asthma.
- Nearly one-fifth of the general population has a form of seasonal or perennial allergic rhinoconjunctivitis, or both.
- In the United States, approximately 20 to 40 million people are affected, 10% to 30% of adults and up to 40% of children.

Classification

Inflammatory

- **Allergic:** Rhinitis due to the presence of specific IgE against seasonal or perennial allergens, or both.
- **Infectious:** Often associated with viral upper-respiratory infections.
- **Nonallergic rhinitis with eosinophilia syndrome:** A not well-characterized syndrome consisting of nasal eosinophilia in a patient with rhinitis and no evidence of allergic sensitization.
- **Atrophic:** More common in elderly patients; occurs as a result of thinning of the nasal mucosa.

Noninflammatory

- **Vasomotor/gustatory:** Occurs within minutes of exposure to cold or foods, or both (or even with the thought of eating).
- **Rhinitis medicamentosa:** The result of overuse of an intranasal decongestant.
- **Hormonal:** For example, pregnant and thyroid disease; resolves with treatment of the thyroid disease or conclusion of the pregnancy.

Structural

- **Foreign body:** Usually a unilateral rhinitis.
- **Tumor/granuloma/hypertrophic sinuses:** Often unilateral rhinitis (except with hypertrophic sinuses).
- **Cerebrospinal fluid leak:** Unilateral rhinorrhea that contains glucose (nasal discharges have no glucose, but cerebrospinal fluid does).
- **Ciliary dysfunction:** Diagnosed by an abnormally increased sugar transit time (saccharin test) from the anterior nares to the pharynx or by abnormal ciliary anatomy identified by electron microscopy of nasal mucosa biopsies.

Pathophysiology

Inhaled allergens are noticed and processed by dendritic cells (APCs). The allergen is presented to CD4+ T cells, which produce cytokines that influence basophil proliferation (IL-13), B-cell class switching to IgE synthesis (IL-4), eosinophil proliferation (IL-5), and mast cell proliferation (IL-9).[27]

Diagnosis

Clinical Presentation

History
- Determine the patients' symptoms including nasal discharge, nasal pruritus, sneezing, headaches, and unilateral or bilateral nares involvement. It is important to determine whether other organ systems are involved (such as the lungs or eyes).
- Determine seasonality of the patient's symptoms. Allergic sensitivity to tree, grass, and weed pollens tends to occur in the spring, summer, and fall, respectively, whereas allergies to dust mites, molds, and pets generally do not have a seasonal distribution.
- Obtain a history of aggravating and alleviating factors. Often, patients know that their symptoms are worse when they visit a friend with a cat or, perhaps, when they dust or go outside. They might note that they are better in less humid environs, for example.

Physical Examination
Refer to the Allergy section above.

Diagnostic Testing

To identify the allergens to which a patient is sensitive, either skin testing (epicutaneous and intradermal) or RAST testing can be performed. However, it is important that any positive results be clinically correlated with the patient's symptoms.

Treatment

Environmental Control

- **Environmental control measures are the most important therapeutic intervention** that can be made.
- If patients are sensitive to dust mites, (ideally) they should remove all carpet in the home, use dust mite–proof encasings on their pillows and mattress, use synthetic pillows and comforters, wash all bedding in water with a temperature of ≥130°F weekly, and keep home humidity level at <45%.
- Pet-sensitive patients should keep their pets out of the house, if possible, or, if not, the animals should be excluded from the bedroom at all times. Cats and dogs that have access to the indoors should be washed on a regular basis.

Antihistamines

- Once environmental control measures have been undertaken, the next intervention is the use of a nonsedating antihistamine to block the symptoms associated with histamine release.
- The U.S. Food and Drug Administration considers loratadine and fexofenadine (both oral preparations) as the only nonsedating antihistamines, because their incidence of net sedation is <2%.

- Second-generation antihistamines with very low sedation are cetirizine (oral preparation; net sedation approximately 7%) and azelastine (nasal spray preparation only; net sedation approximately 6%).

Anti-inflammatory Agents

- Intranasal nonsteroidal anti-inflammatory medications, such as **cromolyn sodium,** are the safest agents to use and are now available over the counter. Unfortunately, for maximum effectiveness, cromolyn sodium (2 squirts/nostril) needs to be used four times per day.
- The most effective anti-inflammatory medications for rhinitis (not just allergic but any inflammatory etiology) are **intranasal corticosteroids** (refer to Table 1 for doses).
  - The same corticosteroids that are found in asthma inhalers are also available for intranasal inhalation.
  - Improvement may occur within 24 to 48 hours of starting the medication but often takes up to a week before a full therapeutic effect is reached.
  - The doses given are much lower than those used in asthma, and, therefore, risks of systemic side effects from intranasal steroids are much lower.
  - The major side effect of these medications is epistaxis. If this occurs, the patient should stop using the nasal spray for several days until the bleeding stops (they can use intranasal saline during this period), and then they can restart the steroid spray.

Decongestants

- **Oral decongestants** (such as pseudoephedrine) are useful in treating nonallergic rhinitis, especially in patients whose major symptom is nasal congestion.
- **Nasal decongestants** (β-adrenergic medications), although available over the counter, should be **avoided if possible.**
  - These medications provide immediate relief of nasal congestion; however, **tachyphylaxis** develops quickly.
  - Because the withdrawal of the drug leads to a **rebound** hyperemia with worsening nasal congestion, patients' nostrils are often addicted to these medications by the time they see a physician (a condition known as rhinitis medicamentosa).
  - If patients must use an intranasal decongestant, they should use it for **no >3 days** at a time.
  - Addicted patients often require a short course of systemic corticosteroid therapy to get them off the decongestant. Once the systemic corticosteroids have been started, patients should stop using their nasal decongestant and start an intranasal corticosteroid regimen.

Intranasal Anticholinergics

- Intranasal anticholinergics are useful in patients with noninflammatory rhinitis.
- For example, an intranasal anticholinergic (ipratropium bromide 0.03%, 1 to 2 sprays/nostril) can be used 10 to 15 minutes before each meal **to help alleviate gustatory rhinorrhea.**

Immunotherapy

Immunotherapy (discussed above) is quite helpful in allergic rhinitis and can be thought of as a corticosteroid-sparing anti-inflammatory agent.

Antibiotics

- Antibiotics are **not usually indicated** in rhinitis unless there is reason to believe that the patient may have an underlying sinusitis.

- In these cases, an antibiotic that has good sinus penetration and is active against *Streptococcus pneumoniae, Haemophilus influenzae,* and *Moraxella catarrhalis* is indicated (mainly β-lactam antibiotics [with or without a β-lactamase inhibitor] or a sulfa drug, or macrolide antibiotic in β-lactam–sensitive individuals).

Surgery

- Surgery is reserved for those patients who have chronic sinusitis and in whom no other therapy is able to control their rhinitis.
- In many cases, the surgery provides only temporary relief and is not curative.

Additional Resources

Physician

- National Institute of Allergy and Infectious Diseases (http://www.niaid.nih.gov).
- National Heart, Lung, and Blood Institute Information Center (http://www.nhlbi.nih.gov).
- American Academy of Allergy, Asthma, & Immunology (http://www.aaaai.org).
- American College of Allergy, Asthma & Immunology (http://www.acaai.org).

Patient

- Food Allergy and Anaphylaxis Network (http://www.foodallergy.org).
- Asthma and Allergy Foundation of America (http://www.aafa.org).
- American Lung Association (http://www.lungusa.org).
- Allergy and Asthma Network—Mothers of Asthmatics (http://www.aanma.org).

REFERENCES

1. Skoner DP. Allergic rhinitis: definition, epidemiology, pathophysiology, and diagnosis *J Allergy Clin Immunol* 2001;108(Suppl 1):S2–S8.
2. Saefer T. Epidemiology of food allergy/food intolerance in adults:associations with other manifestation of atopy. *Allergy* 2001;56:1172–1179.
3. Golden DB. Epidemiology of allergy to insect venoms and stings. *Allergy Proc* 1989;10:103–107.
4. Lockey RF, Turkeltaub PC, Baird-Warren IA, et al. The Hymenoptera venom study I, 1979–1982: demographics and history-sting data. *J Allergy Clin Immunol* 1988;82:370–381.
5. Szefler S, Weiss S, Tonascia J. Long-term effects of budesonide or nedocromil in children with asthma. *N Engl J Med* 2000;343:1054–1063.
6. Golden DB. Epidemiology of insect venom sensitivity. *JAMA* 1989;262:3269–3270.
7. Waytes AT, Rosen FS, Frank MM. Treatment of hereditary angioedema with a vapor-heated C1 inhibitor concentrate. *N Eng J Med* 1996;334:1630–1634.
8. Cichon S, Martin L, Hennies HC, et al. Increased activity of coagulation factor XII (Hageman factor) causes hereditary angioedema type III. *Am J Hum Genet* 2006;79:1098–1104. Epub 2006 Oct 18.
9. Yates C. Parameters for the treatment of urticaria and angioedema. *J Am Acad Nurse Pract* 2002;14:478–483.
10. Greaves M, Lawlor F. Angioedema: manifestations and management. *J Am Acad Dermatol* 1991;25:155–165.
11. Cha YJ, Pearson VE. Angiooedema due to losartan. *Ann Pharmacother* 1999;33:936–938.
12. Zuberbier T, Maurer M. Urticaria: current opinions about etiology, diagnosis and therapy. *Acta Derm Venereol* 2007;87:196–205.
13. Hennino A. Pathophysiology of urticaria. *Clin Rev Allergy Immunol* 2006;30:3–11.

14. Kulthanan K, Jiamton S, Boochangkool K, Jongjarearnprasert K. Angioedema: clinical and etiological aspects. *Clin Dev Immunol* 2007;2007:26438.

15. Bas M, Adams V, Suvorava T, Niehues T, Hoffmann TK, Kojda G Nonallergic angioedema: role of bradykinin. *Allergy* 2007;62:842–856.

16. Agostoni A, Aygören-Pürsün E, Binkley K, et al. Hereditary and acquired angioedema: problems and progress: proceedings of the third C1 esterase inhibitor deficiency workshop and beyond. *J Allergy Clin Immunol* 2004;114:S51–S131.

17. Sicherer SH, Sampson HA. Food allergy: recent advances in pathophysiology and treatment. *Annu Rev Med* 2009;60:261–277.

18. Sampson HA. Food allergy. Part 1: Immunopathogenesis and clinical disorders. *J Allergy Clin Immunol* 1999;103:717–728.

19. Chehade M, Mayer L. Oral tolerance and its relation to food hypersensitivities. *J Allergy Clin Immunol* 2005;115:3–12.

20. Fernandez-Rivas M, Bolhaar S, Gonzalez-Mancebo E, et al. Apple allergy across Europe: how allergen sensitization profiles determine the clinical expression of allergies to plant foods. *J Allergy Clin Immunol* 2006;118:481–488.

21. Strid J, Thomson M, Hourihane J, et al. A novel model of sensitization and oral tolerance to peanut protein. *Immunology* 2004;113:293–303.

22. Steckelbroeck S, Ballmer-Weber BK, Vieths S. Potential, pitfalls, and prospects of food allergy diagnostics using recombinant allergens or synthetic sequential epitopes. *J Allergy Clin Immunol* 2008;121:1323–1330.

23. Sicherer SH, Furlong TJ, Maes HH, et al. Genetics of peanut allergy: a twin study. *J Allergy Clin Immunol* 2000;106:53–56.

24. Voelker R. The hygiene hypothesis. *JAMA* 2000;283:1282.

25. Lynch NR, Goldblatt J, LeSouef PN. Parasitic infections and risk of asthma and atopy. *Thorax* 1999;54:659–660.

26. Sampson HA, Mendelson L, Rosen JP. Fatal and near-fatal anaphylactic reactions to food in children and adolescents. *N Engl J Med* 1992;327:380–384.

27. Broide D. The Pathophysiology of allergic rhinoconjunctivitis. *Allergy Asthma Proc* 2007;28:398–403.

36

Otolaryngology
Thomas M. De Fer

CERUMEN IMPACTION

General Principles

- Cerumen is composed of desquamated skin and adnexal gland lipid secretions (sebaceous and apocrine sweat glands) in the external auditory canal (EAC).
- The EAC is normally self-cleaning with epithelial migration from the tympanic membrane (TM) outward.
- Risk factors for cerumen accumulation/impaction include age >60 years, cognitive impairment, obstruction of EAC by hair proliferation or narrowing (e.g., scarring from chronic infection or in Down syndrome), foreign bodies (e.g., hearing aids or earplugs), the use of cotton-tipped swabs, skin conditions that affect the EAC, and impairment of self-migration of cerumen out of the EAC.
- There do appear to be genetic factors as well.
- Cerumen impaction may cause hearing loss, otalgia, fullness, itching, tinnitus, cough, and perhaps dizziness/vertigo.

Diagnosis

- Diagnosis is, of course, via otoscopy.
- Cerumen ranges widely in texture (soft and liquid to hard and dry) and color (nearly white to nearly black).
- Cerumen accumulation may partially or totally obscure visualization of the TM and is, therefore, often rather problematic when attempting to diagnose ear complaints that require adequate visualization of the TM.
- Cerumen impaction may abut the TM.
- Patients who use hearing aids should be occasionally examined for cerumen accumulation.[1]
- Patients should be asked about known TM perforation, tympanostomy tubes, and other prior ear surgeries.

Treatment

- **Removal of cerumen is recommended when accumulation/impaction causes symptoms or prevents adequate and necessary examination.**[1]
- "Asymptomatic" nonimpacted cerumen does not necessarily require any treatment.
- Cerumen impaction may be achieved via **irrigation, cerumenolytics,** or **manual removal other than irrigation.**[1]
- Disimpaction should be done with care.
- The bony portion of the EAC can be quite sensitive and is easily abraded or lacerated.
- The TM may be inadvertently punctured.

- Home use of cotton swabs, oral jet irrigators, and ear "candling" is strongly discouraged.[1]

Irrigation

- This consists of flushing cerumen from the ear canal with a large syringe with the patient sitting up.
- The water should be approximately body temperature and directed toward the superior wall of the EAC (rather than at the TM) until the impaction is extruded. An emesis basin placed beneath the ear catches the irrigant.
- Irrigation is **contraindicated** when a history of perforation exists, infection is present or recurrent, or the patient has had a prior ear surgery/mastoidectomy.[1]
- Excessive force induces pain and may result in EAC lacerations or TM perforation, but the latter is a rare complication.
- Irrigation with plain tap water may be associated with malignant otitis externa (OE) in diabetics. Otorrhea and/or otalgia should be reported promptly to the physician. Alternatively, irrigation may be done with hydrogen peroxide or a 50% solution of white vinegar.[1]

Cerumenolytics

- This entails instilling substances into the EAC, resulting in thinning of the cerumen and promoting its egress from the EAC.
- These topical agents are of three types[1,2]:
  - **Water based,** such as plain water/saline, 3% hydrogen peroxide, 2% acetic acid (Acetasol), docusate 1% liquid (Colace), 10% sodium bicarbonate, and 10% triethanolamine polypeptide oleate condensate (Cerumenex). Triethanolamine polypeptide should not be left in the ear for >15 to 30 minutes and afterwards it should be flushed out. It may also cause a local dermatitis, which may be mild to severe. Because of this concern, Cerumenex is no longer available in the United States.
  - **Oil based,** including olive oil, almond oil, mineral oil, and arachis (peanut) oil. Oil-based products are not actually cerumenolytics but lubricants/softeners.
  - The **non–water, non–oil-based** product available in the United States is 6.5% carbamide peroxide (urea hydrogen peroxide) (Debrox, Murine).
- All of these agents (including water or saline) may be superior to no treatment for clearing cerumen and avoiding irrigation.[1–3]
- It is unclear that any particular agent is more effective; however, non–water, non–oil-based products may be superior to oil-based products.[1–3]
- Longer use (1 day vs. 4 days) may be more effective.[2]
- All cerumenolytics may also be used prior to irrigation to potentially increase the chances of success.[1,2]
- Use of cerumenolytics is **contraindicated** in patients with OE, otitis media, and TM puncture.

Manual Removal other than Irrigation

- Manual removal requires care, clinician skill, adequate illumination, and the proper equipment.
- In the right hands, manual removal can be effective and quick.
- Typically a metal or plastic loop or spoon is used with direct visualization through a hand-held otoscope.

• Potential harms include pain, laceration of the EAC, perforation of the TM, and infection.

Referral

• Referral to an otolaryngologist is appropriate for use of a binocular microscope and otologic instruments when the cerumen is severely impacted or when other attempts have failed.
• Other factors that make referral appropriate include TM perforation, a history of TM or mastoid surgery, EAC stenosis, or pain with other attempts at removal.

OTITIS EXTERNA

General Principles

• OE is defined as inflammation of the EAC, with acute OE (AOE) being the most common infection.
• OE is classified into three stages: preinflammatory, acute inflammatory, and chronic inflammatory (>6 weeks).[4] Chronic OE is usually not bacterial in origin.
• **AOE is specifically defined as follows**[5]:
  • Rapid onset of symptoms (with 48 hours) in the past 3 weeks with symptoms and signs of EAC inflammation.
  • Symptoms of EAC inflammation: Otalgia, itching, or fullness, with or without herring loss or jaw pain.
  • Signs of EAC inflammation: Tenderness of the tragus/pinna or diffuse ear canal edema/erythema, with or without otorrhea, regional lymphadenitis, TM erythema, or cellulitis of the pinna and adjacent skin.
• AOE is particularly common after swimming (swimmer's ear) or after local trauma with a foreign body. Other risk factors are insufficient or excess cerumen, excess cleaning/scratching of the EAC, high humidity (tropical ear), warm temperatures, and hearing aid/ear plug use.
• Cultures of purulent secretions in AOE typically reveal *Pseudomonas aeruginosa* and *Staphylococcus aureus*.[5] Polymicrobial infections are not unusual and may include anaerobic organisms.
• Otomycosis is a superficial mycotic infection of the EAC caused by fungi such as *Aspergillus niger* and *Candida albicans*. These do not usually present as AOE.[5]
• **Necrotizing (malignant)** OE is a severe complication of AOE seen most commonly in elderly diabetics and the immunocompromised. Infection aggressively spreads to the surrounding tissue including cartilage, temporal bone, and skull base. It is most often caused by *P. aeruginosa*. It has also been reported to be due to *A. niger*.

Diagnosis

Clinical Presentation

History
• Symptoms include itching or pain, hearing loss, and/or fetid drainage.
• The complaints are almost always unilateral and usually follow a precursor event or recent travel in a tropical environment.
• Pain is the most common complaint and ranges from dull achiness to an intense incapacitating level. Fever may occur when the inflammation is severe.

- Patients with necrotizing OE may have a less severe initial presentation but classically develop severe protracted pain, which seems to be out of proportion to examination findings.

Physical Examination
- Physical examination of an ear with AOE reveals a normal auricle but tenderness with tragal manipulation.
- The EAC skin is erythematous, and induration ranges from mild to severe, in which the canal lumen obstructs secondary to edema.
- The lumen contains moist desquamated debris, serum, or seropurulent secretions.
- The TM appears lusterless or erythematous or may not be visible secondary to narrowing of the lumen.
- In severe cases, fever, temporomandibular joint (TMJ) tenderness, periauricular erythema, and cervical lymphadenopathy may be found.
- EAC skin necrosis or granulation tissue at the cartilage-bone junction, high fever, significant otorrhea, and facial nerve palsy are all consistent with necrotizing OE.

Differential Diagnosis

The differential diagnosis of OE is presented in Table 1.

Treatment

Otic Toilet
- The EAC should be carefully cleansed by flushing out excess cerumen, desquamated skin, purulent material, and any foreign body thereby allowing topical treatments to reach the affected skin.
- This may be done with an ear syringe and 50:50 hydrogen peroxide and water.
- If the TM is ruptured, then irrigation should not be done.
- In more severe cases, proper cleansing may require referral to an otolaryngologist and the use of a binocular microscope and otologic instruments.

Topical Agents
- There are a large number of topical otic preparations for this purpose: acidifying agents, antiseptics, antibiotics, and corticosteroids, individually or in combination of some or all. All appear to have efficacy.[6]

TABLE 1	Differential Diagnosis of Otitis Externa

Cerumen accumulation/impaction
Dermatitides of the EAC (e.g., allergic, atopic, and seborrheic) of the EAC
Furuncles of the EAC
Perichondritis (painful inflammation of the auricle)
Herpes zoster oticus (pain usually precedes the development of vesicles; facial nerve paresis confirms the Ramsay Hunt syndrome)
Suppurative OM with TM rupture
Cholesteatoma
Carcinoma of the EAC

EAC, external auditory canal; OM, otitis media; TM, tympanic membrane.

- **Acidifying agents** include 2% acetic acid (VoSoL, Domeboro) and boric acid. Acidification may be particularly useful for otomycosis.
- The most common **antiseptic** is alcohol, which also evaporates quickly drying the EAC. Alcohol is a common additive to many otic solutions. Otic antiseptics appear to have similar efficacy as do topical antibiotics.[6]
- The most common **topical otic antibiotics** are as follows:
  - **Polymyxin B and neomycin** (with 1% hydrocortisone, previously sold under the brand name Cortisporin Otic, now generic, 4 drops tid-qid for up to 10 days). The former is active against *P. aeruginosa* and the latter against *S. aureus.* With prolonged use, neomycin may actually cause chronic OE secondary to allergic dermatitis.
  - **Ciprofloxacin** 0.2% (with 1% hydrocortisone, Cipro HC Otic, 3 drops bid for 7 days) and 0.3% (with 0.1% dexamethasone, Ciprodex Otic, 4 drops bid for 7 days). Ciprofloxacin is active against both *P. aeruginosa* and *S. aureus.*
  - **Ofloxacin** 0.3% (Floxin Otic, 10 drops/0.5 mL qd for 7 days), active against both *P. aeruginosa* and *S. aureus.*
  - Gentamicin and tobramycin ophthalmic solutions have also been used to treat OE.
  - **Antibiotics are clearly better than placebo** and no single antibiotic has been clearly shown to be superior to any other. However, those treated with a quinolone may improve somewhat faster than those treated with a nonquinolone.[6]
  - **Oral antibiotics** are usually unnecessary (except, e.g., those with diabetes, immunodeficiency, or infection beyond the EAC and when topical therapy cannot be effectively delivered).[5]
- Typical topical **corticosteroids** include 1% hydrocortisone and 0.1% dexamethasone. The addition of topical steroids to topical antibiotics does not seem to substantially improve clinical cure rates though they may speed pain relief.[5,6]
- When there is a suspected or known TM rupture, ototoxic agents (alcohol, acidifiers, Cortisporin, and aminoglycosides) should not be used. Ofloxacin and ciprofloxacin/dexamethasone are approved for middle-ear use.[5]
- If the EAC is significantly narrowed because of edema, topical therapy may be difficult to deliver and a wick (Oto-Wick, Merocel, or ribbon gauze) should be placed.[5] The wick should be gently inserted with fingers into the EAC to provide a conduit for the antibiotic drops. As the edema recedes, the wick can be removed, usually 24 to 72 hours.

Pain Control

- While usually modest, the pain from AOE can be severe and analgesic therapy should be recommended.[5]
- Analgesics such as acetaminophen, nonsteroidal anti-inflammatory drugs (NSAIDs), and opiates are all appropriate depending on the degree of pain.[5]
- Topical otic analgesics such as 1.4% benzocaine (with 5.4% antipyrine, previously sold under the brand name Auralgan, now generic) are generally not recommended.[5]
- As noted above, topical steroids may hasten pain relief.[5]

Necrotizing Otitis Externa

- Prompt referral to an otolaryngologist is crucial.
- Computed tomography (CT), magnetic resonance imaging (MRI), and bone scanning can confirm this diagnosis.
- Cultures should be taken.
- Hospital admission for topical and intravenous high-dose antipseudomonal antibiotic therapy, cleaning, and debridement is required.

OTITIS MEDIA

General Principles

- Otitis media simply signifies inflammation of the middle ear.
- **Acute otitis media** (AOM) is defined by the presence of **middle effusion ear with acute symptoms and signs of illness and middle-ear inflammation.**[7] **It is an infectious process** caused by viruses or bacteria and is far more common in young children than adults, but it does occur in adults. Most of the studies regarding AOM have, therefore, been done in children.
  - The most common viruses are rhinoviruses, influenza viruses, adenoviruses, and respiratory syncytial virus.
  - The most common bacteria are *Streptococcus pneumoniae*, *Haemophilus influenzae*, and *Moraxella catarrhalis*. *Mycoplasma pneumoniae* is an uncommon cause. The bacterial causes in adults are likely similar to those in children.[8]
  - Combine viral and bacterial infections appear to be common, at least in children.
  - AOM is generally thought to be preceded by inflammation of the upper respiratory tract (e.g., a viral infection of allergic) resulting in obstruction of the isthmus of the Eustachian tube (ET). Fluid accumulates in the middle ear, and there is subsequent growth of microorganisms.
- **Otitis media with effusion** (OME, otherwise known as serous otitis) is a chronic form of middle-ear inflammation.
  - OME is typified by a **middle-ear effusion without acute signs of infection.**[9]
  - Although OME usually follows an upper respiratory tract infection (URI), it is itself **not an infectious process** and it may result from noninfectious causes such Eustachian tube dysfunction (ETD).
  - As with AOM, it is most commonly seen in children.
  - OME may persist for week to months.

Diagnosis

Clinical Presentation
History
- The most common symptoms of AOM are abrupt onset of otalgia, hearing loss, vertigo, and fever, but these are relatively nonspecific.
- Adults with AOM complain more of otalgia, hearing difficulty, sore throat, and otorrhea than children.[10]
- OME typically presents with ear fullness and hearing loss. Symptoms of acute infection are absent.

Physical Examination
- Physical examination is key to differentiating AOM and OME. This differentiation can, however, be challenging.
- Cerumen obstructing good visualization of the TM should be removed (see the "Cerumen Impaction" section above).
- Middle-ear effusions are suggested by the following[7,9]:
  - Absent or decreased TM motility on pneumatic otoscopy. Requires careful technique and a tight seal.
  - Bulging of the TM.

- Air-fluid level behind the TM.
- Otorrhea.
- Acute middle-ear inflammation is signified by the following[7]:
  - Distinct erythema of the TM. Erythema can also be caused by manipulation of the EAC, crying, fever, and URI.
  - Distinct otalgia.
- Those with AOM will have evidence of an effusion and acute inflammation, while those with OME will only have evidence of an effusion.
- **Tympanocentesis,** performed by an otolaryngologist, for culture is rarely necessary but may be helpful in immunocompromised patients, patients whose symptoms fail to respond, or patients in whom complications of AOM, such as intracranial infection, develop.

Treatment

Acute Otitis Media

- There are no evidence-based treatment recommendations specifically for adults with AOM. The recommendations here are based on those for pediatric patients.[7]
- **Observation** of otherwise healthy adults with mild-to-moderate uncomplicated AOM for 2 to 3 days is appropriate.
- **Antibiotic therapy** may be helpful for those who are initially severely symptomatic or for those with persistent symptoms after 2 to 3 days.
- **Amoxicillin** 500 mg tid for 5 to 10 days is a reasonable first-line choice for the majority of patients.
- Alternative first-line antibiotics include trimethoprim-sulfamethoxazole DS, 1 bid; azithromycin, 500 mg qd; or clarithromycin, 500 mg bid.
- When patients fail to respond to first-line treatment or when there are significant concerns regarding resistance, amoxicillin-clavulanate, 875 mg bid, or cefuroxime axetil, 500 mg bid, may be used.

Otitis Media with Effusion

- Because OME is not itself an infectious process, antibiotic therapy is usually not indicated.
- Watchful waiting is a reasonable approach in the large majority of adults.
- Tympanostomy tubes are sometimes indicated in children.[9]
- Antihistamines, decongestants, and corticosteroids are of uncertain efficacy specifically with regard to OME.

EUSTACHIAN TUBE DYSFUNCTION

General Principles

- The ET provides ventilation of the middle ear, protection from reflux of nasopharyngeal secretions, and drainage of the middle-ear space. Normally the ET is closed but opens easily to equalize pressure in the middle ear.[11]
- ETD resulting from obstruction and abnormal patulous Eustachian tube (PET) can subsequently affect the middle ear.
- Obstruction interferes with the ventilation and drainage functions of the ET. It also leads to the development of negative pressure in the middle ear.

TABLE 2	Causes and Risk Factors for Eustachian Tube Dysfunction

Intrinsic mechanical obstruction	**Extrinsic mechanical obstruction**
Viral URIs	Recurrent adenotonsillitis
Allergic rhinosinusitis	Adenoid hypertrophy
Chronic sinusitis	Congenital cholesteatoma
Gastropharyngeal reflux	Nasopharyngeal polyps
Ciliary dyskinesis	Nasopharyngeal neoplasms
Tobacco smoke	**Congenital**
XRT to the head and neck	Cleft palate
Reduced mastoid air cell system	Craniofacial syndromes (e.g., Down
"Buffer zone" for middle-ear pressure equalization	and Turner syndromes)

URI, upper respiratory tract infection; XRT, radiation therapy.

- ET obstruction, and therefore ETD, can be temporary, fluctuating/recurrent, or chronic.
- Chronic ET obstruction and negative pressure can lead to weakening of the TM with retraction into the middle-ear space (this is referred to as atelectasis).
- PET diminishes the protective function of the ET by more easily allowing reflux of nasopharyngeal secretions to the middle ear.
- Causes and risk factors for ETD are presented in Table 2.[11–13]
- PET has been associated with weight loss, pregnancy, oral contraceptives/estrogen treatments, and muscular disorders, but it is often idiopathic.[14]
- ETD can lead to chronic annoying symptoms, hearing loss, otic barotrauma (e.g., during air travel, scuba diving), OME, AOM, atelectasis, and acquired cholesteatoma.[13]

Diagnosis

Clinical Presentation

History
- The symptoms of ETD depend on the degree, constancy, and chronicity of obstruction.
- Symptoms of ETD can include ear fullness/blockage/pressure, otalgia, abnormal hearing, muffled sound of one's own voice, popping/crackling/squeaking sounds, tinnitus, vertigo, and problems with flying.[11–13]
- Patients with a PET may complain of hearing their own breathing and an unusually loud volume of their own voice (autophony). This symptom may disappear when the patient lies down. Oddly these patients also complain that the ear feels blocked.[14]

Physical Examination
- Otoscopy with ETD is not uncommonly normal. There may be evidence of a middle-ear effusion (see OME above).
  - Atelectasis is revealed by a thinned sunken-in TM and readily visible incudostapedial joint of the ossicles.
- With PET, otoscopy may reveal motion of the TM, medially with inspiration and laterally with expiration, which is exacerbated by forced respiration. Because venous

engorgement may relieve the patency when patients are supine, the ear should be examined with the patient in the sitting position.

Diagnostic Testing

- Tympanometry can detect even subtle negative middle-ear pressure with ETD and excessive TM movement with PET.
- Audiometry may reveal mild conductive hearing loss (CHL).
- Flexible endoscopy may be necessary to visualize the nasopharynx and the ET ostia.

Treatment

- Treatment of ETD requires interruption of the persistent ET obstruction and negative pressure.
- **Medical therapy** should be directed toward resolving the underlying inflammatory disorder, as well as ET inflammation. There is no clear consensus, but treatments typically used include the following:
  - Topical oxymetazoline, 2 puffs in both nostrils bid for 5 days only.
  - Oral decongestants such as pseudoephedrine, 60 to 120 mg/day bid prn.
  - Oral antihistamines, both nonselective and selective; diphenhydramine 25 to 50 mg qid prn; fexofenadine 60 mg bid or 180 mg daily; and cetirizine 5 to 10 mg daily.
  - Topical nasal steroids such as beclomethasone 1 to 2 sprays (42 μg/spray) bid.[15]
  - Whether or not more aggressive treatment for allergic rhinitis, such as immunotherapy, is unclear.
- Frequent **autoinflation** of the middle ear may also be useful (accomplished by Valsalva with the nose pinched and mouth closed).[16]
- **Surgical therapy** generally consists of myringotomy and placement of a tympanostomy tube. The TM often reverts to normal while the tube remains in place. Other possible surgical options are laser Eustachian tuboplasty and laser myringotomy.
- Treatment of PET depends on the severity of the disturbance. Most often reassurance alone satisfies a patient's concern. When symptoms are chronic and annoying, referral to an otolaryngologist is indicated.[14]

TINNITUS

General Principles

- Tinnitus is a very common complaint and is defined as the perception of sound that is not related to any external source. It can affect one or both ears and be intermittent or continuous.
- **Objective tinnitus** is the perception of sound arising from sounds within the body that an examiner can also perceive. It is usually secondary to acoustic energy that is created by turbulent blood flow through vessels near the ear.
- **Subjective tinnitus,** on the other hand, is the perception of sound in the absence of an actual acoustic stimulus (internal or external). Subjective tinnitus is much more common than objective tinnitus.
- Chronic tinnitus can have a very significant effect on quality of life.
- The prevalence of tinnitus increases with age, and it is **often associated with hearing loss.**
- There are many potential etiologies, some of them quite serious, but the cause is usually benign in the majority of patients (Table 3).[17]

TABLE 3	Causes of Tinnitus

Objective	Subjective
Pulsatile/vascular[a]	**Otologic**
Arterial bruits (e.g., carotid stenosis)	Sensorineural hearing loss (e.g., presbycusis, noise induced, and other causes of sudden sensorineural hearing loss)
Valvular disease (e.g., aortic stenosis and other causes of a heart murmur)	
High cardiac output (e.g., systemic AVFs, hyperthyroidisms, anemia, drug toxicity)	Conductive hearing loss (e.g., otosclerosis, cerumen, OE, AOM, OME, ETD, TM perforation, and cholesteatoma)
Cranial/cervical AVMs/AVFs (e.g., dural AVFs)	Autoimmune hearing loss (e.g., rheumatoid arthritis, lupus, Cogan syndrome, and others)
Venous hum (thought to be caused by turbulent blood flow in the internal jugular veins)	Multiple other causes of hearing loss (e.g., ischemia/infarct, endocrine, and metabolic)
Vascular tumors (e.g., paraganglioma/ glomus tumor of the jugular bulb or middle ear)	Ménière disease
Neuromuscular/anatomic	Barotrauma (middle and/or inner ear)
Palatal myoclonus (essential or acquired due to lesions in the triangle of Guillain-Mollaret, "myoclonic triangle")	Ototoxic medications (e.g., aminoglycosides, vancomycin, and loop diuretics, salicylates/NSAIDs, cisplatin, antimalarials, and many others)
Stapedial muscle spasm	**Neurologic**
Tensor tympani spasm	Acoustic neuroma (vestibular schwannoma)
Patulous Eustachian tube	
Spontaneous	Other tumors in the cerebellar-pontine angle
Spontaneous otoacoustic emissions	Chiari malformations
Possible/uncertain cause/origin	Multiple sclerosis
Temporomandibular joint dysfunction	Head injury
	Infectious
Cervical spine disorders (e.g., whiplash)	OE/AOM
Other dental disorders	Meningitis
	Viral cochleitis (e.g., herpesviruses, influenza, mumps, measles, rubella, HIV, and others)
	Lyme disease
	Syphilis

AOM, acute otitis media; AVF, arteriovenous fistula; AVM, arteriovenous malformation; ETD, Eustachian tube dysfunction; HIV, human immunodeficiency virus; NSAID, nonsteroidal anti-inflammatory drug; OE, otitis externa; OME, otitis media with effusion; TM, tympanic membrane.
[a]Vascular causes do not always produce pulsatile tinnitus.
Modified from Lockwood AH, Salvi RJ, Burkard RF. Tinnitus. *N Engl J Med* 2002;347: 904–910.

Diagnosis

Clinical Presentation

History
- Tinnitus may be described by patients in many ways including pulsing, humming, rushing, whooshing, clicking, cricket-like ringing, buzzing, hissing, whining, whistling, and high or low pitched.
- Pulsatile tinnitus is usually objective/vascular in origin (see Table 3).
- Particular attention should obviously be paid to the otoneurologic history including indications of hearing loss, noise exposure, otalgia, cerumen impaction, OE, AOM, OME, ETD, PET, vertigo, focal neurologic deficits, exposure to ototoxins, etc.
- Some patients complain of sleep disturbance or impaired concentration.

Physical Examination
- A careful otoscopic examination should be performed as well as the rest of the head and neck.
- A neurological examination is also generally useful (particularly if there are other focal neurologic complaints).
- Auscultation can reveal the sound of pulsatile tinnitus when listening over the mastoid, the infra-auricular region, or the carotid artery.
- Cardiac auscultation may disclose a murmur or evidence of high cardiac output.

Diagnostic Testing
- **Audiometry will be indicated for most patients.**
- Depending on the specific clinical situation, those with pulsatile tinnitus may require carotid artery Dopplers, echocardiography, and other vascular studies as indicated. Referral to an otolaryngologist is also warranted for such patients.
- Those with focal neurologic signs may benefit from imaging of the brain.

Treatment

- Objective tinnitus, while much less common, may be amenable to specific therapies, such as, surgery for vascular disorders.
- When warranted, patients should be reassured of the low likelihood of life-threatening conditions.
- A brief explanation of how competing environmental sounds can mask the tinnitus is useful. Common choices for masking include soft music on the radio, television, or a room fan.
- **Masking devices** are sometimes necessary to provide relief from intractable tinnitus. These are essentially sound generators worn like a hearing aid that produce low-level broadband noise and are available from audiologists.
- All drugs that are known to cause tinnitus should be discontinued if possible.
- There are currently no drugs specifically approved by the FDA for the treatment of tinnitus.
- Tinnitus is known to be associated with depression and anxiety, and there is some data to suggest that antidepressant treatment may be effective but the data are mixed.[17,18]
- More recent research does not support the use of gabapentin for tinnitus.[19]
- Tinnitus retraining therapy entails counseling to enhance the patient's understanding of the problem, as well as sound therapy several hours a day may be helpful.[20] The goal is to habituate the patient to the sound and to decrease its negative associations.

VERTIGO AND DIZZINESS

General Principles

- The neurological perspective on dizziness and vertigo can be found in Chapter 41.
- Dizziness is a common symptom that can be quite challenging to correctly diagnose and treat. Many patients have difficulty spontaneously expressing what exactly they mean by "dizziness" and the potential causes are many and varied.
- The goal of the initial evaluation is to categorize the patient's dizziness into one of the following categories:
  - Vertigo (the illusion of movement, either of self or the environment).
  - Disequilibrium (the sensation of imbalance/unsteadiness, particularly when walking).
  - Presyncope (the sensation of nearly passing out, blacking out, and fainting).
  - Nonspecific dizziness/lightheadedness (the patient cannot specifically endorse any of the above and may only be able to state something along the lines of "I don't know doctor, I'm just dizzy/lightheaded").
- **Vertigo is the most common specific complaint and will be discussed in detail here.** The evaluation of presyncope/syncope is discussed in Chapter 7.
- Dizziness is more common in the elderly and often multifactorial in origin.
- Most of the many causes of dizziness and vertigo are presented in Table 4.

Diagnosis

Clinical Presentation

History

- As indicated above, the history is critical to categorizing the symptom of dizziness. Patients should first be given the opportunity to describe their symptoms with open-ended questioning but specific questions are often necessary.
- **Asking specific questions to rule in or to rule out vertigo is a reasonable first step.** It is important to remember that vertigo, while often described as spinning, can be **any sense of motion** (of self or the environment), such as tilting, swaying, rocking, side to side, and up and down.
- Although vertigo specifically points to the vestibular system, it does not exclude other contributing factors. In addition, some instances of disequilibrium and nonspecific dizziness/lightheadedness may ultimately prove to be vestibular in origin.
- **Disequilibrium** is indicated by the sensation of imbalance/unsteadiness, particularly when walking. Follow-up questions regarding symptoms of neuropathy, musculoskeletal limitations, Parkinsonism, vision, and falls are appropriate.
- **Presyncope** is characterized by the sensation of wooziness and nearly passing out, blacking out, and fainting. If this is most likely to match with the patients' symptoms, then further questioning in this vein is indicated (e.g., orthostasis, palpitations, chest pain, vasovagal symptoms).
- **Nonspecific dizziness/lightheadedness** is typified by a patient who cannot specifically endorse any of the above descriptions.
- **The remainder of this discussion will focus specifically on vertigo.**
- Specifics of duration, recurrence, frequency of episodes, and exacerbating factors of vertigo should be detailed.
- In general, head motion can make all forms of vertigo worse.

TABLE 4	Causes of Dizziness and Vertigo

Vertigo	Disequilibrium
Peripheral	Peripheral neuropathy
Benign positional vertigo	Musculoskeletal problems affecting
Vestibular neuronitis	gait (e.g., arthritis and muscular
Labyrinthitis	weakness)
Ménière disease (endolymphatic	Poor vision
hydrops)	Parkinson disease
Herpes zoster oticus (Ramsay	Cerebellar atrophy
Hunt syndrome)	Medications (e.g., antiepileptics,
Perilymphatic fistula	sedative hypnotics)
Otitis media	Vestibular disorders
Cholesteatoma	**Presyncope**
Labyrinthine concussion	Orthostatic hypotension
Ototoxic medications	Vasovagal
Cogan syndrome	Arrhythmia
Recurrent vestibulopathy	Carotid sinus hypersensitivity
Acoustic neuroma (vestibular	Other causes of reduced cardiac output
schwannoma)	(e.g., aortic stenosis, hypertrophic
Central	obstructive cardiomyopathy)
Brainstem ischemia/infarction	Vertebrobasilar insufficiency
(e.g., Wallenberg syndrome)	**Nonspecific dizziness/**
Cerebellar ischemia/infarction/	**lightheadedness**
hemorrhage	Hyperventilation
Migraine associate vertigo	Hypoglycemia
Basilar migraine	Medications
Multiple sclerosis	Depression
Chiari malformation	Anxiety
	Panic disorder
	Somatization disorder
	Vestibular disorders

- Nausea and vomiting are common accompaniments of acute vertigo except when the individual episodes are very short.
- Patients should be asked about headache and other migrainous features, otalgia, hearing loss, postural instability, other focal neurologic symptoms, head trauma, past medical history, and medication use.
- Table 5 presents a summary of the symptomatic characteristics of the more common causes of vertigo.

Physical Examination
- The distinction between central and peripheral vertigo is important in terms of narrowing the differential diagnosis and identifying those who may require prompt and more aggressive evaluation and treatment (i.e., those with central vertigo). Table 6 summarizes some of the distinguishing features.[21]
- Otoscopy should be done on all patients.
- The **head thrust test** (also known as the head impulse test) consists of first asking the patient to visually fixate on a distant object with the eyes about 10° away from the

TABLE 5 Clinical Features of Common Causes of Vertigo

Condition	Onset and Time Course of Vertigo	Typical Scenario	Auditory Symptoms	Associated CNS Symptoms and Signs	Nystagmus	Vestibular Exam Findings
Benign paroxysmal positional vertigo (BPPV)	Recurrent episodes ≤1 minute over weeks to months Recurrences wax and wane over time with spontaneous remissions	Most common cause of vertigo Distinctly caused by change in position often while in bed, looking up, and bending forward Sometimes associated with nausea and vomiting	No	No	Positionally provoked with rotatory and upward components (prototypical posterior canal involvement) Latency 3–5 seconds, duration 5–15 seconds Fatigable May be suppressed by visual fixation	Typical nystagmus provoked by the Dix-Hallpike maneuver
Vestibular neuronitis	Abrupt onset over a few hours Resolves after a few days to weeks May be followed by months of vague dizziness	May have viral prodrome Severe vertigo worsened by head movement Often with severe nausea and vomiting Gait instability but able to walk, sway toward the side of the lesion	No	No	Spontaneous, unidirectional, usually horizontal/torsional May be suppressed by visual fixation	Positive head thrust test

(continued)

TABLE 5 Clinical Features of Common Causes of Vertigo (*Continued*)

Condition	Onset and Time Course of Vertigo	Typical Scenario	Auditory Symptoms	Associated CNS Symptoms and Signs	Nystagmus	Vestibular Exam Findings
Labyrinthitis	Same as vestibular neuronitis	Same as vestibular neuronitis	Unilateral sensorineural hearing loss	No	Same as vestibular neuronitis	Same as vestibular neuronitis
Ménière disease	Episodic over years with prolonged remissions. Episodes may occur in clusters. Episodes minutes to hours duration	Triad of episodic vertigo, tinnitus, and hearing loss. May be secondary to other inner-ear disorders. Some patients have relatively less vertigo and more hearing problems	Low-pitched tinnitus. Sensorineural hearing loss, fluctuating but progressive and permanent over years duration. Ear fullness. Otalgia	No	During episodes unidirectional, usually horizontal/torsional	Dix-Hallpike maneuver unnecessary given characteristic history
Migraine-associated vertigo	Recurrent spontaneous or positional episodes that last minutes to hours to days. Severity is variable. Some may report episodes of disequilibrium,	History of migraines. Vertigo with migraine headache. May be precipitated by typical migraine triggers. Some feel this	Usually no but mild sensorineural hearing loss (not progressive) and tinnitus have been reported	Headache with or following vertigo. Headache may not always occur with episodes of vertigo and vice versa	Nystagmus during episodes may have central or peripheral features	Dix-Hallpike maneuver may elicit symptoms of vertigo

	imbalance, unsteadiness, or lightheadedness rather than true vertigo Some may have more chronic dizziness and/or motion sensitivity	is an under-appreciated very common cause of episodic vertigo		Typical migrainous features often present (e.g., aura, unilateral, pulsating, photophobia, other visual symptoms, phonophobia, nausea, vomiting)	
Brainstem infraction	Abrupt onset, sometimes very severe Duration of minuets to weeks but may be chronic	Older patients with vascular risk factors Nausea and vomiting may be prominent Severe gait instability, may fall when attempting to walk	No	Other findings of brainstem infarction including dysphagia, dysarthria, diplopia, Horner syndrome, deficits in pain and temperature sensation, etc.	Spontaneous nystagmus, may have any trajectory but usually horizontal/rotatory Slow nystagmus gazing to ipsilateral side Fast nystagmus gazing to contralateral side Not fatigable Not affected by visual fixation Dix-Hallpike maneuver generally unnecessary No latency, >1 minute, not fatigable, may change direction with head position change

(continued)

767

TABLE 5	Clinical Features of Common Causes of Vertigo (*Continued*)						
Condition	Onset and Time Course of Vertigo	Typical Scenario	Auditory Symptoms	Associated CNS Symptoms and Signs	Nystagmus	Vestibular Exam Findings
Cerebellar infarction or hemorrhage	Same as brainstem infarction Vertigo is not always present	Same as brainstem infarction Headache may occur	No	Findings depend on area and degree of cerebellar involvement Gait ataxia, truncal lateropulsion, limb incoordination May be accompanied by medullary infarction with the findings as above	Same as brainstem infarction	Same as brainstem infarction

TABLE 6	Distinguishing Peripheral and Central Vertigo	
	Peripheral	**Central**
Vertigo	Often severe	Often less severe
Nystagmus		
Type/direction	Positional[a] or spontaneous[b]	Spontaneous
	Horizontal with rotatory component or vertical with a torsional component (never exclusively vertical or rotatory)	Horizontal, vertical, or rotatory, including exclusively vertical or rotatory (which does not occur with peripheral causes)
		May change direction with gaze
	Unidirectional	Not inhibited
	Inhibited	Finite (weeks to months[c])
Effect of visual fixation	Finite[b] (days to weeks) or chronically[c] episodic/	More persistent than episodic
Duration	recurrent[a] (individual episodes lasting ≤1 minute to hours)	
Nausea and vomiting	May be severe but can be minimal	Variable
Postural/gait instability	Mild to moderate, usually able to walk, sway toward side of lesion	Often severe, may not be able to walk without falling
Hearing loss/ tinnitus	Sometimes[d]	Usually not
Other neurologic findings	No	Often
Head thrust test	Often abnormal[b], eyes pulled off target and saccade back to target	Usually normal, eyes remain on target
Dix-Hallpike maneuver[e] for positional nystagmus		
Latency	2–15 seconds	None
Duration	5–30 seconds	30–120 seconds
Fatigability	Yes	Sometimes yes, sometimes no
Provoked vertigo	Often severe	Absent or less severe
Fixation	Suppression	No suppression
Type/direction	Horizontal/rotary	Vertical/horizontal
Characteristic	Direction fixed	Direction changing

[a]Benign paroxysmal positional vertigo (BPPV), Ménière disease, and migraine-associated vertigo.
[b]Vestibular neuronitis, labyrinthitis.
[c]Vertigo is never truly chronic (i.e., continuous symptom with absolutely no remissions).
[d]Labyrinthitis, Ménière disease.
[e]The Dix-Hallpike maneuver is a provocative test most useful for those with positional (rather than spontaneous) vertigo and in particular, BPPV involving the posterior canal (>90% of cases).
Modified from Goebel JA. Practical Management of the Dizzy Patient. 2nd Ed. Philadelphia, PA: Lippincott Williams & Wilkins, 2008.

primary position. Then the examiner quickly turns the head horizontally about 10° to 15°, first to one side and then the other. The normal response is for the eyes to remain on target. Abnormal responses occur in peripheral conditions—the eyes are pulled off target and saccade back on target.

- **Dix-Hallpike maneuver** is presented in Figure 1.[22] The classical findings of this test are strongly suggestive of posterior canal benign paroxysmal positional vertigo (BPPV),

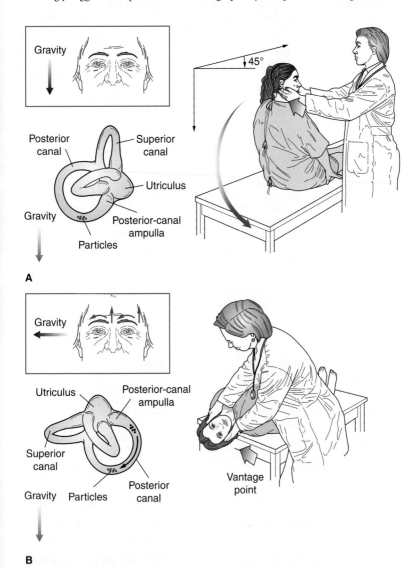

Figure 1. Dix-Hallpike Maneuver. (From Furman JM, Cass SP. Benign paroxysmal positional vertigo. *N Engl J Med* 1999;341:1590–1596, with permission.)

that is, vertigo and mixed rotatory and vertical nystagmus, with the upper poles of the eyes beating toward the floor.

- Table 5 also presents a summary of the physical examination findings in the more common causes of vertigo.

Diagnostic Testing

- When the history and physical examination are clearly suggestive of a peripheral lesion, diagnostic testing per se is generally unnecessary.
- **Brain CT scan or MRI** is indicated when the history and physical examination suggest a central cause or an acoustic neuroma.
- **Audiometry** is sometimes indicated (e.g., for Ménière disease).
- Otolaryngologists may sometimes order more sophisticated diagnostic testing such as electronystagmography (ENG). ENG records eye motion during vestibular and oculomotor manipulation. It can measure unilateral or bilateral labyrinthine or hyper- or hypofunction or disorders of oculomotor control.
- **Rotary chair testing** measures vestibular response to angular acceleration and is useful to assess patients who are suspected of having bilateral hypofunction or cerebellar abnormalities.

Treatment

Nonspecific Symptomatic Treatment

- Several classes of medication are frequently given for the symptomatic treatment of vertigo and associated nausea and vomiting.
- These medications seem to be most effective for acute vertigo with nausea and vomiting. They may not be very helpful for brief spells of vertigo.
  - **Antihistamines:** The efficacy of antihistamines is due to their **anticholinergic** properties, such as **diphenhydramine,** 25 to 50 mg PO/IM/IV every 4 to 6 hours prn; **meclizine,** 25 to 50 mg PO every 6 hours prn; **dimenhydrinate,** 50 to 100 mg every 4 to 6 hours prn; and **scopolamine,** 0.4 to 0.8 mg PO every 6 hours prn or 0.3 to 0.6 mg IM/IV every 6 hours prn or 1.5 mg patch every 3 days prn.
  - **Phenothiazines:** Most have anticholinergic and dopamine antagonist properties. **Promethazine** (12.5 to 25 mg PO/IM every 4 to 6 hours) is a phenothiazine derivative, but its antiemetic properties are due largely to its anticholinergic effects. The much more antidopaminergic drugs include **prochlorperazine** 5 to 10 mg PO/IM/IV every 6 hours.
  - **Benzodiazepines:** Drugs such as diazepam and lorazepam are sometimes used for their mild antiemetic and sedative properties.

Benign Paroxysmal Positional Vertigo

- BPPV episodes, if left untreated, will frequently resolve themselves in days to weeks.
- The most specific treatment for BPPV is otolith repositioning with the **Epley maneuver** (Fig. 2).[22]
- Recurrences are common.
- Nonspecific vestibular suppressants are also sometimes used to lessen symptoms.

Vestibular Neuronitis

- Treatment of vestibular neuronitis is typically supportive.[23]
- Vestibular suppressants can be effective.
- Spontaneous recovery occurs in days to weeks.

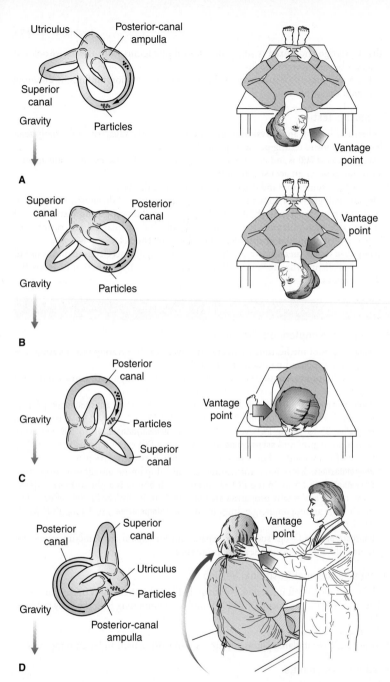

Figure 2. Epley Maneuver. (From Furman JM, Cass SP. Benign paroxysmal positional vertigo. *N Engl J Med* 1999;341:1590–1596, with permission.)

- Early ambulation and vestibular exercises are often recommended to facilitate recovery of balance.

Ménière Disease

- Vestibular suppressants/antiemetics are used to treat acute vertigo and nausea and vomiting.[24]
- Attacks may be lessened by avoiding high salt intake, monosodium glutamate, alcohol, caffeine, nicotine, and stress.
- Diuretics (e.g., hydrochlorothiazide, triamterene, and acetazolamide), but there is limited quality data in support of this form of treatment.
- Invasive/surgical treatments may be necessary for intractable symptoms.

HEARING LOSS

General Principles

- Ten percent of Americans have some degree of hearing loss.[25]
- Causes of hearing loss are numerous and may be congenital, infectious, traumatic, toxic, neoplastic, vascular, immunologic, neurologic, metabolic, or hereditary (Table 7).
- Hearing loss is subtyped into conductive, sensorineural, or mixed based on audiometric measures.
  - **Conductive hearing loss** is caused by a disturbance of the mechanism that transmits sound waves from the environment to the cochlea.

TABLE 7	Causes of Hearing Loss
Conductive	**Sensorineural**
Congenital malformations	Congenital/hereditary
Cerumen impaction	Presbycusis
Foreign body in the EAC	Ménière disease
Otitis externa	Acoustic neuroma
Trauma to the EAC	Meningioma
Tumors of the EAC (e.g., squamous cell carcinoma and basal cell carcinoma)	Ototoxins (e.g., aminoglycosides, loop diuretics, antimetabolites, salicylates)
Bony tumors impinging on the EAC (e.g., osteoma and exostosis)	Autoimmune inner-ear disease
Barotrauma	Perilymphatic fistula
Tympanic membrane perforation	Barotrauma
Eustachian tube dysfunction	Infections
Otitis media	Meningitis
Cholesteotoma	Syphilis
Otosclerosis	Viral cochleitis
Glomus tumor	Multiple sclerosis
	Stroke
	Trauma
	Idiopathic

EAC, external auditory canal.

- **Sensorineural hearing loss** (SNHL) represents a dysfunction of the cochlea, auditory nerve, or auditory pathway of the CNS. Most SNHLs are not reversible, but several exceptions are known. Therefore, accurate diagnosis is essential.
- **Mixed hearing** loss involves dysfunction in both pathways.

Etiology/Pathophysiology

- **Otosclerosis** is a common cause of CHL that may also cause progressive SNHL.
  - It occurs as uncontrolled new bone formation in the otic capsule, resulting in fixation of the stapes.
  - Otosclerosis can be passed on by autosomal dominant transmission with incomplete penetrance (approximately 40%) and is most prevalent in Caucasians and women and young adults.[26]
  - The disease process is accelerated by pregnancy.
- **Cholesteatoma** is defined as a squamous epithelium pocket or sac filled with keratin debris within the middle ear or mastoid.
  - It manifests with bone destruction secondary to enzymatic activity at a bone interface and often becomes chronically infected, causing fetid drainage.
  - Types of cholesteatomas include **congenital** (an epithelial cyst in the mastoid air cells or middle ear without communication with the external ear); **primary acquired** (develops from perforation of the flaccid portion of the TM); and **secondary acquired** (develops from a progressive retraction pocket of an atrophic TM).
- **Slowly progressive SNHL (presbycusis)** is a nontreatable hearing loss that is secondary to aging and persistent noise exposure.
- **Fluctuating or rapidly progressive SNHL** is sometimes reversible and may occur with a handful of conditions:
  - Ménière disease (believed to be due to an increase in fluid pressure of the endolymph in the inner ear).
  - Acoustic neuroma (schwannoma of the eighth cranial nerve).
  - Autoimmune inner-ear disease.
  - Perilymphatic fistula (PLF) occurs when perilymph of the inner ear is exposed to the middle ear and thus results in dysfunction of the inner ear.
  - Idiopathic.
- **Sudden SNHL** is defined as ≥ 30 dB of SNHL over at least three contiguous audiometric frequencies occurring in ≤ 3 **days.** It is usually unilateral and thought to be most often secondary to a viral etiology, although a vascular interruption etiology is known to exist.

Risk Factors

- Risk factors for hearing loss vary with age.
- In children, low-birth-weight intrauterine infections, meningitis, and a family history are risk factors.
- In adults, unprotected noise exposure, head trauma, exposure to ototoxins (such as aminoglycosides), or radiation to the head is associated with a greater risk of hearing loss.

Diagnosis

Clinical Presentation

History

- History that is important to elicit is whether hearing loss is unilateral or bilateral, age at onset, and course of hearing loss (i.e., sudden, progressive, or fluctuating).

- Associated symptoms may include tinnitus, dizziness, aural fullness, otalgia, or otorrhea.
- History should include past ear infections or surgery, head trauma, the presence of other illnesses, and ototoxic exposures such as noise or medications.
- Commonly implicated **medications** include aminoglycosides, vancomycin, cisplatinum, nitrogen mustard, furosemide, ethacrynic acid, salicylates, and quinine.
- Symptoms of **Ménière disease** include unilateral fluctuating SNHL, tinnitus, recurrent attacks of vertigo (see the "Vertigo and Dizziness" section above), and a sense of aural fullness. Alternating remissions and exacerbations of symptoms are common, but after several years, the vertigo has a tendency to subside and hearing loss stabilizes at the moderate-to-severe level.
- Progressive growth of an **acoustic neuroma** results in unilateral progressive SNHL and in some cases tinnitus, vertigo, and ataxia.
- **Autoimmune inner-ear disease** presents with bilateral SNHL and progressive loss in at least one ear over days to months. Some patients also complain of dizziness/vertigo and some have other autoimmune disorders (e.g., Cogan syndrome and Wegener granulomatosis).[27]
- Patients with **PLF** note sudden or fluctuating hearing loss, with tinnitus and vertigo, and may reveal antecedent trauma to the head.

Physical Examination

- Physical examination includes the assessment of normality of anatomy as well as abnormal findings.
- Inspection of the EAC and TM can be performed with otoscope or microscope.
- In the EAC, identification of cerumen, blood, pus, fungus, granulation tissue, keratinaceous debris, or foreign body may be noted and removed.
- Polyps, osteomas, exostoses, or tumors may be found and prevent visualization of the TM.
- TM mobility can be assessed by pneumatic otoscopy (gentle insufflation of the EAC with a rubber bulb attached to the otoscope).
- Inspection of the TM may reveal TM scarring, perforation, atrophic segments, or retraction pockets.
- Middle-ear serous fluid appears amber, pus looks white, and hemotympanum is reddish blue.
- Masses may be seen and appear white (cholesteatoma) or red (glomus tumor).
- **Tuning fork testing** suggests CHL or SNHL. The Weber and Rinne tests are used together.
  - The **Weber** test places the vibrating fork in the midline of the head. The sound is perceived louder in the ear with conductive loss or in the better-hearing ear with SNHL.
  - The **Rinne** test places a vibrating fork on the mastoid and then over the EAC. The sound is louder with the fork on the mastoid with CHL and louder over the EAC when conductive loss is not present.

Diagnostic Testing

Audiologic Testing

- Audiologic testing is the measure of choice with suspected hearing loss. This examination includes testing of pure tone thresholds for air and bone conduction in a soundproof booth.
- SNHL is identified when the two thresholds match.
- Conductive hearing is present if air thresholds are below bone thresholds.

- Speech discrimination measures a patient's ability to perceive and repeat words.
- Tympanometry measures TM mobility and is reduced with middle-ear fluid, infection, or mass.
- Acoustic reflex testing determines the intactness of a reflex arc passing through the cochlear nerve brainstem, facial nerve, and stapedial muscle. Abnormal reflex tests suggest cochlear nerve or brainstem pathology such as an acoustic neuroma or meningioma.

Laboratories
- Laboratory testing is directed at uncovering systemic disease that results in hearing loss.
- When the erythrocyte sedimentation rate is elevated, inner-ear antigen-specific tests can reveal autoimmune SNHL, a condition that is potentially reversible with high-dose steroid therapy.[27]
- Other tests include thyroid function tests, fasting glucose, cholesterol and triglycerides, and the fluorescent treponemal antibody absorption test (FTA-Abs).
- Congenital or acquired syphilis can result in hearing loss, and therefore a positive FTA-Abs should be followed by a Venereal Disease Research Laboratory (VDRL) test to determine active infection. When hearing loss is associated with positive syphilis serology, neurosyphilis should be suspected and a lumbar puncture performed for cerebrospinal fluid testing.

Imaging
- Radiologic evaluation uses high-resolution CT when temporal bone pathology or trauma is suspected.
- MRI with gadolinium as contrast is used for suspected pathology of the cochlear nerve, brainstem, or brain.
- Acoustic neuromas are enhancing lesions on CT and MRI near the internal auditory canal, with variable extension into the cerebellopontine angle.

Treatment

- **CHL** etiologies are treated by the removal of obstructive wax, debris, or lesions; evacuation of the fluid in otitis media; or microsurgical repair of anatomic defects, such as TM perforation, ossicular chain disruption, or cholesteatoma.
- **Otosclerosis** treatment is surgical, with replacement of the stapes by prosthesis or aural amplification by hearing aid to compensate for the loss.
- **Slowly progressive SNHL (presbycusis):**
  - Patients who are most likely to benefit from a **hearing aid** have moderate-to-severe loss that impairs their understanding of conversational speech. In general, bilateral amplification is recommended, as patients are more likely to understand speech, justifying the extra cost. Unfortunately, many people do not take advantage of hearing aids.
  - **Use noise protection strategies** (earplugs) when exposure to loud noises is anticipated (i.e., weapons firing, power tools, lawnmowers, or vacuuming).
  - Profound loss is best treated by implantable hearing aids or cochlear implantation, but assistive listening devices are also helpful for enhancing face-to-face communication, telecommunications, and alerting devices.
- **Ménière disease** is treated as discussed above in the "Vertigo and Dizziness" section.

- **Acoustic neuroma** treatment consists of surgical removal by skull base otolaryngologists and neurosurgeons or, more recently, by gamma knife obliteration in controlled studies.
- **Autoimmune inner-ear disease** is the most responsive etiology of rapidly progressive SNHL.
  - Treatment consists of prednisone (1 mg/kg/day to a maximum of 60 mg/day) for 4 weeks, at the end of which time an audiogram is repeated.[27,28]
  - Responders are continued until recovery plateaus and then are decreased to 10 mg/day for 6 months. Nonresponders are tapered off prednisone over 14 days.
- Idiopathic causes fluctuating or rapidly progressive SNHL should be treated with a 10-day course of prednisone, 1 mg/kg/day up to 60 mg/day, and then tapered over 14 days, with repeat audiometry at 2 weeks into treatment.
- **PLF** treatment is initially conservative, with bed rest, head elevation, and avoidance of straining. If symptoms persist or progress, surgical exploration of the middle ear is performed to search for a perilymph leak. If a leak is found, it is patched with fascia.
- The most commonly used treatment **for sudden SNHL** is the administration of corticosteroids as quickly as possible; however, data are conflicting.[29,30] Some cases resolve spontaneously.
  - Prednisone, 60 mg/day, should be initiated for 1 week and then tapered anytime within 4 weeks of the sudden loss.
  - Vasodilators and anticoagulants have not proved to be effective.
  - The use of antiviral agents is of uncertain benefit.

TRIGEMINAL NEURALGIA

General Principles

- Trigeminal neuralgia (TN) is one of the most common facial pain syndromes.
- The incidence increases with age.
- Classically there is no demonstrable neurologic deficit.
- Classical TN is usually caused by vascular compression of the trigeminal nerve root causing focal demyelination but may also be idiopathic. Secondary TN can result from conditions such as multiple sclerosis and tumors.

Diagnosis

- It is characterized by sudden episodic attacks of unilateral severe sharp pain in the distribution of a branch of the trigeminal nerve (most often V2 and/or V3).
- The attacks last seconds to minutes and are triggered by light touch of the face or oral cavity.
- Episodes of pain typically come and go with intermittent exacerbations.
- As noted, the physical examinations should not reveal deficits of the trigeminal nerve. If it does, consideration of a secondary cause or alternative diagnosis must be entertained.
- MRI has variable sensitivity and specificity for identifying patients with neurovascular compression.[31]
- If a secondary cause is suspected, an MRI should probably be done.
- Abnormal trigeminal evoked potentials may be helpful in identifying patients with secondary TN.[31]

Treatment

- Many patients can be managed medically.
- The best supported treatment is **carbamazepine,** 200 to 1,200 mg/day, divided bid. **Oxcarbazepine,** 300 to 1,200 mg bid, is also probably effective.[31,32]
- Possibly effective medications are baclofen (5 to 20 mg tid), lamotrigine, and pimozide.[31]
- Many other medications have been tried but conclusive data are lacking.[31]
- Patient with refractory pain can be referred for possible surgical therapy.

EPISTAXIS

General Principles

- Epistaxis (nasal bleeding) can be a single prolonged episode or multiple minor episodes.
- The incidence of epistaxis is greatest in older patients.
- Nasal bleeding is more common during winter months due to decreased humidity and frequent URI.
- The vascular anatomy of the nose and clinical experience have led to the **division of epistaxis into anterior and posterior locations.**
- >80% of the time, the location of epistaxis is easily visible in the front of the nose and is designated as anterior. This usually involves an area of anterior septum known as **Kiesselbach plexus,** where multiple vessels anastomose.

Etiology/Pathogenesis

- The causes of epistaxis are presented in Table 8.
- **Mechanical or traumatic causes** may result in mucosal lacerations and epistaxis.
  - Chronic trauma from recurrent nasal picking may result in anterior ulceration and bleeding.
  - Other sources of chronic mucosal trauma include administration of steroid nasal sprays and recurrent use of intranasal cocaine.
  - Occasionally, epistaxis may occur weeks after head trauma with the formation of a traumatic aneurysm. Bleeding is recurrent and heavy and may be fatal.
- **Septal deformities** may cause turbulent airflow, resulting in excessive drying and subsequent epistaxis. These deformities include deviations, spurs, and perforations.
- **Inflammation** may result from URIs, sinusitis, nasal allergy, or exposure to toxic inhalants.
- **Neoplasms,** benign or malignant, of the nose, sinuses, or nasopharynx may result in recurrent bouts of epistaxis.
- **Coagulation abnormalities** (particularly von Willebrand disease and hemophilia) should be suspected when easy bruisability, prolonged bleeding after surgery or laceration, and a positive family history are present.
- **Hereditary hemorrhagic telangiectasia** (Osler-Weber-Rendu disease) is an autosomal dominant disease characterized by diffuse mucocutaneous telangiectasias. A positive family history is found in 80% of patients.
- The contribution of **hypertension** is debated. Several studies have failed to show a clear association. Patients presenting with epistaxis are often very anxious and this may contribute considerably to elevations of blood pressure. Treatments for epistaxis can be rather uncomfortable and frightening, only exacerbating the problem.

TABLE 8 Causes of Epistaxis

Environmental factors
Low humidity
Low air temperature
Airborne irritants (including smoking)
Toxic chemicals

Local causes
Trauma
Excessive picking
Forceful/excessive nose blowing
Accidents with facial trauma
Foreign bodies
Nasal septal deviation
Acute URIs
Allergic rhinitis
Nasal polyps
Aneurysms
Neoplasms of the nose, sinuses,
   or nasopharynx (e.g., squamous
   cell carcinoma, adenoid cystic
   carcinoma, inverted papilloma,
   melanoma)
Cocaine snorting

Systemic/secondary causes
Hypertension (uncertain association)
Atherosclerosis
Coagulopathies (e.g., von Willebrand
   disease, hemophilia)
Thrombocytopenia or reduced
   platelet function
Vascular disorders (e.g., HHT,
   scurvy, vasculitides)
Endocrine disorders (e.g.,
   pheochromocytoma,
   glucocorticoid excess, pregnancy)
Endometriosis

Medications
NSAIDs
Warfarin
Aspirin
Nasal/oral steroids

Pseudoepistaxis
Hemoptysis
Hematemesis
Injury to the internal carotid artery

HHT, hereditary hemorrhagic telangiectasia; NSAID, nonsteroidal antiinflammatory drug; URI, upper respiratory infection.

Diagnosis

- Evaluation begins with a history to discern severity, location, duration, and frequency of bleeding as well as the presence of other nasal symptoms including obstruction or rhinorrhea.
- The general history should investigate traumatic injuries, underlying medical conditions, medications, use of tobacco or alcohol, and family history.
- Anterior rhinoscopy is facilitated by applying topical nasal decongestant spray (phenylephrine 0.25%, 2 puffs each nostril).
- Endoscopes are used to visualize the remaining mucosal surfaces to identify posterior epistaxis and to search for tumors.
- Laboratory testing is appropriate to assess severity of blood loss or coagulopathy.
- CT or MRI is indicated to evaluate neoplasms.

Treatment

Anterior Epistaxis

- Systemic coagulopathies should be corrected.
- Treatment of anterior epistaxis should occur with the patient seated, adequate light, suction, cautery, and packing materials available.

- On removal of clots, **topical 4% lidocaine and phenylephrine** are sprayed into the nose. If bleeding is not active, a suction or cotton-tipped applicator can gently abrade likely source vessels on the anterior septum to identify the bleeding site.
- **Simple tamponade** will stop the majority of anterior nosebleeds.
  - The nostrils should be pinched shut against the nasal septum using the thumb and forefinger for at least 5 uninterrupted minutes.
  - An ice pack may be applied to the dorsum of the nose.
  - Patients should be encouraged to spit blood out of the mouth rather than swallowing it.
  - Once bleeding has stopped, the patient should be instructed to gently apply petroleum jelly to the area several times a day for about a week. The use of a humidifier or saline nasal spray may be helpful. **Epistaxis precautions** include avoidance of nose blowing, nasal picking, heavy lifting or straining, and aspirin or NSAIDs.
  - If the above is not successful, it may be attempted again for a longer period of gentle but firm pressure. A vasoconstricting agent may be applied prior to holding pressure.
- **Cautery** comes in two forms, chemical and electrical.
  - **Silver nitrate** on applicator sticks provides an effective chemical cauterization with only a mild burning sensation when applied to bleeding vessels. Care should be taken not to cauterize large areas or on both sides of the septum as this can lead to septal perforation.
  - **Electrocautery** is available from a hand-held cautery device and is also very effective; however, because it is associated with greater pain, it may require the injection of a local anesthetic.
  - After cautery, a piece of absorbable oxidized cellulose (Surgicel) is placed over the newly created eschar to provide additional protection, and the patient is advised to apply saline spray every 2 hours while awake and to practice epistaxis precautions for 5 days.
- **Packing** is indicated when cauterization fails but is generally achieved by referral to an otolaryngologist.
  - First, expandable compressed sponges ("nasal tampons," Merocel) are easily inserted with minimal discomfort to tamponade anterior bleeding rapidly, but they sometimes fail to apply adequate pressure.
  - If they fail, an inflatable balloon or petrolatum ribbon gauze should be inserted instead. This technique can be quite difficult for the inexperienced and seldom results in a neat, textbook appearance. It is moderately painful to undergo but can be tolerated after topical anesthesia.
- Once epistaxis is controlled by packing, the **packing should be removed 2 or 3 days later** and the nose inspected. Mild pain medications should be given for comfort, and oral cephalexin, 500 mg tid, may be administered until the packs are removed. Antibiotics are presumably given to prevent toxic shock syndrome secondary to *S. aureus* colonization, but data in support of this are lacking.

Posterior Epistaxis

- Posterior nosebleeds are much more difficult to treat and are associated with more discomfort, severe bleeding, morbidity, and mortality.
- Systemic coagulopathies should be corrected.
- Treatment of posterior epistaxis should then follow a stepwise approach in the hands of an otolaryngologist.

- **Packing** traditionally uses a gauze sponge pulled into the nasopharynx via strings through the nostrils. This is combined with an anterior pack and left in place for 3 days. However, this is cumbersome and painful. Now, inflatable balloons are available that insert easily and can be gradually filled with water by a syringe until bleeding stops.
- Patients who require posterior packing should be admitted for careful observation.
- Pain control usually requires oral or intramuscular opioids and occasional benzodiazepines to sleep.
- Cephalexin, 500 mg tid, may be given until the packs are removed to prevent toxic shock syndrome secondary to *S. aureus* colonization.
- **Endoscopic cautery** has become an effective means of controlling posterior epistaxis because the fiberoptic nasal endoscopes provide excellent visualization of the mucosal surface of the nose, allowing for accurate localization of the bleeding source. The procedure is best tolerated in the operating room with anesthesia. This method is 90% effective.[33]
- **Arterial embolization** is particularly useful when bleeding is too heavy for visualization with endoscopes, the patient is too ill for anesthesia, or surgical intervention fails. The major risks from embolization are rare but include cerebrovascular accident.
- **Arterial ligation** is a 75% to 100% effective technique of obtaining epistaxis control.[34] The specific vessels to ligate depend on the location of the likely bleeding site. Occasionally, bilateral ligation is necessary.

HOARSENESS

General Principles

- Hoarseness (dysphonia) is a nondescript term that is intended to mean an impairment in the sound of one's voice.
- Risk factors for voice disruption include smoking, voice abuse, gastroesophageal reflux disease (GERD), and cervical or mediastinal surgery.
- Disruption of muscular or epithelial layers, or both, of the vocal cords results in dysphonia. Both layers may be destroyed with invasion by malignancy or fibrosis from radiation therapy.

Etiology/Pathogenesis

- The causes of hoarseness are listed in Table 9.
- **Acute laryngitis, the most common malady that results in hoarseness,** is most often secondary to mucosal edema from a URI or may follow an episode of vocal abuse.
- **Chronic laryngitis** is created by long-term inflammatory conditions such as smoking, **laryngopharyngeal reflux** (LPR), and postnasal drip (caused by allergic rhinitis or chronic sinusitis).
  - Many patients with LPR do not report heartburn (i.e., GERD) and the diagnostic criteria for LPR are not well defined.[35]
  - The mechanisms of symptoms (i.e., hoarseness in this context) are presumed to be direct irritation from gastric secretions and/or indirect laryngeal irritation due to chronic vagally mediated reflexes (e.g., cough, throat clearing) secondary to the presence of gastric secretion in the esophagus.
- **Vocal fold nodules** are bilateral calluses that form in response to repeated forceful closure, as occurs with screaming, speaking too loudly, throat clearing, and chronic coughing and prevent full closure of the vocal cords.

TABLE 9	Causes of Hoarseness

Infectious
Upper respiratory infections
Acute bronchitis
Acute/chronic sinusitis
Acute viral laryngitis
Common cold

Inflammatory/irritant
Acute/chronic vocal abuse
Alcohol
Allergic rhinitis
Chemical fumes
Chronic cough
Chronic sinusitis
Habitual throat clearing
Inhaled corticosteroids
Laryngopharyngeal reflux
Smoking

Vocal fold lesions
Direct trauma (e.g., intubation)
Laryngeal papillomatosis
Vocal fold bowing (presbylarynges)
Vocal fold/laryngeal malignancy
Vocal fold nodules
Vocal fold polyps

Neurologic
Neuromuscular disorders (e.g., multiple sclerosis, myasthenia gravis, Parkinson disease)
Spasmodic dysphonia
Stroke
Vocal cord paralysis (e.g., postsurgical, mass/tumor related)

Systemic diseases
Acromegaly
Amyloidosis
Hypothyroidism
Lupus
Relapsing polychondritis
Rheumatoid arthritis
Sarcoidosis

Psychogenic
Functional/conversion aphonia

Other
Muscle tension dysphonia

- **Vocal fold polyps** generally result from vocal abuse or smoking. When smoking is the etiologic agent, the polyps are more often bilateral.
- **Laryngeal papillomatosis** can occur in adults when human papilloma virus, types 6 or 11, infests epithelium in the border between ciliated and squamous cells.
- **Vocal fold/laryngeal malignancy** usually occurs in smokers and alcohol abusers.
- **Vocal fold paralysis** results from temporary or permanent interruption of the vagus nerve or its branch, the recurrent laryngeal nerve.
  - This can occur after cervical or thoracic surgery (the most common etiology), trauma, forceps delivery, aortic aneurysm, congestive heart failure, or cerebrovascular accident or secondary to neoplasm along the course of the vagus or recurrent laryngeal nerve.
  - Loss of neural innervation prevents adduction (closure) of the vocal fold and arytenoid cartilage; thus, contact between the cords for phonation is lost.
- **Vocal fold bowing,** presbylarynges, results when vocalis muscle atrophy occurs as a result of decreased usage and aging. The patient is chronically soft spoken. The voice is breathy and weak and often trails off to inaudible levels. Projection is lost, but cough is mildly weakened or intact.
- **Spasmodic dysphonia,** a focal dystonia of adductor or abductor muscles in the larynx, results in spasms that interrupt phonation. Patients complain of a choked-off sound to the voice. Spoken words beginning with "h" are common triggers. Because stress frequently exacerbates the severity, and patients sound as if they are on the verge of crying, they are often misdiagnosed with psychiatric disorders.

Diagnosis

Clinical Presentation

History

- The history should solicit information about the character of the hoarseness, the onset and duration, and the course, as well as associated symptoms, the patient's voice-use patterns, and social habits (smoking and alcohol use).[36]
- Ask questions relevant to GERD and neurologic disorders (e.g., Parkinson disease, myasthenia gravis, and stroke).
- Any history of neck trauma, surgery, or radiation therapy should be ascertained.
- Worrisome co-occurring symptoms such as dyspnea, cough, hemoptysis, odynophagia, dysphagia, aspiration, fever, and weight loss should be sought.

Physical Examination

- The examination must include the ear, nose, and throat in addition to the larynx.
- Assessment of hearing, sinus function, and oral cavity disease may reveal clues to the etiology of hoarseness.
- Palpate the neck for masses or any other abnormalities.
- Consideration of general health is appropriate to realize the impact of respiratory conditions or neuromuscular disorders on phonation.

Diagnostic Testing

- Visualization of the larynx can be readily achieved by indirect mirror inspection or flexible fiberoptic laryngoscopy. Laryngoscopy should be done in most patients with unexplained, persistent hoarseness.
  - The mirror examination gives a true-color reflection of the larynx by positioning the mirror against the soft palate, avoiding contact with the base of the tongue to prevent gagging and retracting the tongue forward while a light is reflected against the downward-angled mirror.
  - The fiberscope, passed through the nose to the pharynx, is well tolerated and allows thorough examination of the larynx structure and function (phonation).
- Upper esophageal sphincter pH monitoring might be useful in the diagnosis of LPR.
- CT scanning of the neck and chest will often be indicated when there is a clinical suspicion of malignancy or other mass lesion.

Treatment

- Hoarseness due to **acute laryngitis** is short lived (<2 weeks) but may be severe for several days.
  - If a URI initiates the dysphonia, treatment with humidity, hydration, and voice rest is indicated.
  - **Voice rest** usually corrects edema secondary to vocal abuse.
- **The mainstay of treatment for chronic hoarseness is eliminating the inciting problem** and maintaining proper hydration.
- Proton pump inhibitors are very often given for LPR. Data are conflicting regarding efficacy. Patients with coexistent GERD may respond better. LPR symptoms may take longer to respond than do GERD symptoms. Typical GERD lifestyle/dietary modification may be of benefit.[35]
- The treatment for vocal fold nodules is to eliminate the abusive patterns of voice use and is directed under the care of a speech therapist. Rarely, nodules persist after therapy and require microscopic removal.

- Microscopic excision of vocal fold polyps is the treatment of choice.
- The lesions of papillomatosis can be removed by laser ablation to palliate symptoms, but they usually recur over several months to a year.
- Treatment for vocal fold malignancy involves surgical resection or radiotherapy, either is highly effective for early disease.
- Treatment for vocal fold paralysis consists of repositioning the immobile vocal fold to the midline by placing an implant or injecting the vocal cord with fat or collagen. Speech therapy is helpful to control potentially damaging compensatory mechanisms.
- Speech therapy can often restore some muscle bulk and improve vocal performance with vocal fold bowing/presbylarynges. Rarely, bilateral vocal cord medialization laryngoplasty is required for restoration of adequate voice.
- For spasmodic dysphonia, injection of the affected muscles with botulinum toxin (Botox) can prevent the spasms and restore adequate phonation temporarily. Repeat injections are required every 4 to 5 months.

SIALOLITHIASIS

General Principles

- Salivary gland duct stones may result in blockage of gland secretions and subsequent inflammation of the gland and sometimes sialadenitis (also called sialoadenitis).
- The process may occur in any of the salivary glands: parotid, submandibular, bilingual, and minor. Most often it is the submandibular glands.
- The pathophysiology of stone formation is not well understood. Slow ductal flow and prior inflammation may probably are involved.

Diagnosis

- Some salivary gland stones are asymptomatic.
- Patients present with a painful and swollen mass at the site of the involved gland.
- Symptoms may be intermittent due to episodic duct obstruction.
- Those with sialadenitis have more significant local signs of inflammation, possibly purulent discharge from the involved gland duct, and fever.
- Long-term complete obstruction can result in a firm chronically inflamed gland.
- Palpation of the floor of the mouth or the buccal mucosa may reveal the presence of a stone.
- The differential diagnosis of symptomatic sialolithiasis includes viral sialadenitis (e.g., mumps, HIV, coxsackievirus, influenza, parainfluenza, herpes), bacterial sialadenitis (e.g., *S. aureus* and others), salivary gland tumors (benign or malignant and primary or secondary), Sjögren syndrome, sarcoidosis, malnutrition/alcoholism, and radiation.
- CT scanning can not only readily identify stones but also demonstrate abscess formation or invasive processes.
- At present, sialography is rarely necessary.
- Clinical presentations suggestive of more serious differential items should most likely be imaged and possibly biopsied.

Treatment

- In general, the treatment of sialolithiasis is conservative and includes good hydration, sialogogues (most commonly sour candy), messaging the gland/duct, warm compresses, eliminating if possible drugs with anticholinergic properties, and analgesics.

- Those with possible bacterial sialadenitis are treated with dicloxacillin or cephalexin.
- Persistent, severe, and recurrent symptoms should be referred to an otolaryngologist.
- Multiple or more or less invasive procedures are available for stone removal/destruction.

REFERENCES

1. Roland PS, Smith TL, Schwartz SR. Clinical practice guideline: cerumen impaction. *Otolaryngol Head Neck Surg* 2008;139(3 Suppl 2):S1–S21.
2. Hand C, Harvey I. The effectiveness of topical preparation for the treatment of earwax: a systematic review. *Br J Gen Pract* 2004;54:862–867.
3. Burton MJ, Dorée CJ. Ear drops for the removal of ear wax. *Cochrane Database Syst Rev* 2009;(1):CD004326.
4. Senturia BH, Marcus MD. Diseases of the External Ear: An Otologic-Dermatologic Manual. New York: Grune & Stratton, 1980.
5. Rosenfeld RM, Brown L, Cannon CR, et al.; American Academy of Otolaryngology—Head and Neck Surgery Foundation. Clinical practice guideline: acute otitis externa. *Otolaryngol Head Neck Surg* 2006;134(4 Suppl):S4–S23.
6. Rosenfeld RM, Singer M, Wasserman JM, Stinnett SS. Systematic review of topical antimicrobial therapy for acute otitis externa. *Otolaryngol Head Neck Surg* 2006;134(4 Suppl): S24–S48.
7. American Academy of Pediatrics Subcommittee on Management of Acute Otitis Media. Diagnosis and management of acute otitis media. *Pediatrics* 2004;113:1451–1465.
8. Celin SE, Bluestone CD, Stephenson J, et al. Bacteriology of acute otitis media in adults. *JAMA* 1991;266:2249–2252.
9. American Academy of Family Physicians; American Academy of Otolaryngology—Head and Neck Surgery; American Academy of Pediatrics Subcommittee on Otitis Media With Effusion. Otitis media with effusion. *Pediatrics* 2004;113:1412–1429.
10. Culpepper L, Froom J, Bartelds AI, et al. Acute otitis media in adults: a report from the International Primary Care Network. *J Am Board Fam Pract* 1993;6:333–339.
11. Seibert JW, Danner CJ. Eustachian tube function and the middle ear. *Otolaryngol Clin North Am* 2006;39:1221–1235.
12. Derebery MJ, Berliner KI. Allergic eustachian tube dysfunction: diagnosis and treatment. *Am J Otol* 1997;18:160–165.
13. Grimmer JF, Poe DS. Update on eustachian tube dysfunction and the patulous eustachian tube. *Curr Opin Otolaryngol Head Neck Surg* 2005;13:277–282.
14. Poe DS. Diagnosis and management of the patulous eustachian tube. *Otol Neurotol* 2007;28:668–677.
15. Tracy JM, Demain JG, Hoffman KM, Goetz DW. Intranasal beclomethasone as an adjunct to treatment of chronic middle ear effusion. *Ann Allergy Asthma Immunol* 1998;80: 198–206.
16. Perera R, Haynes J, Glasziou P, Heneghan CJ. Autoinflation for hearing loss associated with otitis media with effusion. *Cochrane Database Syst Rev* 2006;(4):CD006285.
17. Lockwood AH, Salvi RJ, Burkard RF. Tinnitus. *N Engl J Med* 2002;347:904–910.
18. Robinson SK, Viirre ES, Stein MD. Antidepressant therapy in tinnitus. *Hear Res* 2007;226:221–231.
19. Piccirillo JF, Finnell J, Vlahiotis A, et al. Relief of idiopathic subjective tinnitus: is gabapentin effective? *Arch Otolaryngol Head Neck Surg* 2007;133:390–397.
20. Herraiz C, Hernandez FJ, Plaza G, de los Santos G. Long-term clinical trial of tinnitus retraining therapy. *Otolaryngol Head Neck Surg* 2005;133:774–779.
21. Goebel JA. Practical Management of the Dizzy Patient. 2nd Ed. Philadelphia, PA: Lippincott Williams & Wilkins, 2008.

22. Furman JM, Cass SP. Benign paroxysmal positional vertigo. *N Engl J Med* 1999;341: 1590–1596.

23. Baloh RW. Clinical practice. Vestibular neuritis. *N Engl J Med* 2003;348:1027–1032.

24. Coelho DH, Lalwani AK. Medical management of Meniere's disease. *Laryngoscope* 2008; 118:1099–1108.

25. Nadol JB Jr. Hearing loss. *N Engl J Med* 1993;329:1092–1102.

26. Moumoulidis I, Axon P, Baguley D, Reid E. A review on the genetics of otosclerosis. *Clin Otolaryngol* 2007;32:239–247.

27. Ruckenstein MJ. Autoimmune inner ear disease. *Curr Opin Otolaryngol Head Neck Surg* 2004;12:426–430.

28. Harris JP, Weisman MH, Derebery JM, et al. Treatment of corticosteroid-responsive autoimmune inner ear disease with methotrexate: a randomized controlled trial. *JAMA* 2003 Oct 8;290(14):1875–1883.

29. Conlin AE, Parnes LS. Treatment of sudden sensorineural hearing loss: I. A systematic review. *Arch Otolaryngol Head Neck Surg* 2007;133(6):573–581.

30. Conlin AE, Parnes LS. Treatment of sudden sensorineural hearing loss: II. A Meta-analysis. *Arch Otolaryngol Head Neck Surg* 2007;133:582–586.

31. Gronseth G, Cruccu G, Alksne J, et al. Practice parameter: the diagnostic evaluation and treatment of trigeminal neuralgia (an evidence-based review): report of the Quality Standards Subcommittee of the American Academy of Neurology and the European Federation of Neurological Societies. *Neurology* 2008;71:1183–1190.

32. Sindrup SH, Jensen TS. Pharmacotherapy of trigeminal neuralgia. *Clin J Pain* 2002;18: 22–27.

33. O'Leary-Stickney K, Makielski K, Weymuller EA Jr. Rigid endoscopy for the control of epistaxis. *Arch Otolaryngol Head Neck Surg* 1992;118:966–967.

34. Metson R, Lane R. Internal maxillary artery ligation for epistaxis: an analysis of failures. *Laryngoscope* 1988;98:760–764.

35. Gupta R. Sataloff RT. Laryngopharyngeal reflux: current concepts and questions. *Curr Opin Otolaryngol Head Neck Surg* 2009;17:143–148.

36. Syed I, Daniels E, Bleach NR. Hoarse voice in adults: an evidence-based approach to the 12 minute consultation. *Clin Otolaryngol* 2009;34:54–58.

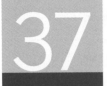

Women's Health

Karen S. Winters and Kathryn M. Diemer

OSTEOPOROSIS

General Principles

- Peak bone mineral density (BMD) is attained by 18 to 25 years of age and is determined mostly by genetic factors.
- Osteoporosis is defined as a disease of low bone mass and microarchitectural deterioration of bone tissue that leads to enhanced bone fragility and a consequent increase in fracture risk.[1]
- It can have serious consequences on quality of life:
  - Pain, possible permanent disfigurement, loss of height, loss of self-esteem, and increased risk of hip fracture.
  - Only one-third of patients who experience a hip fracture are able to return to their prefracture level of function.
  - Half of all women who have a hip fracture spend time in a nursing home.
  - The 1-year mortality after a hip fracture has been reported as high as 27%.[2]
- Osteoporosis is clinically silent until the first fracture occurs; therefore, it is imperative that those at risk for this disease are recognized early and that steps are taken to prevent bone loss and fracture.

Risk Factors

- Risk factors for low bone density have limited value in estimating a woman's actual bone density.[3]
- Risk factors for fracture that are independent of BMD are presented in Table 1.
- **Low bone mass is the single most accurate predictor of fracture.**
- Ten-year fracture risk may also be estimated using the **World Health Organization (WHO) Fracture Risk Assessment Tool (FRAX)** available at http://www.shef.ac.uk/FRAX.[4]

Diagnosis

Clinical Presentation

History
- Risk factor screening is a useful tool in the evaluation of patients with osteoporosis, as it allows the physician to recognize factors that can influence bone density and fracture risk (Table 1).
- Essential historical information includes the following:
  - Height at age 30 years and any loss of height.
  - Medications, including heparin, thyroid medications, diuretics, hormone replacement/oral contraceptive pills (OCPs), phenytoin/phenobarbital, prednisone, calcium, calcitonin, vitamins, raloxifene, or bisphosphonates.

TABLE 1	Risk Factors for an Osteoporotic Fracture or Low Bone Density

Associated with increased risk of fracture independent of BMD:	**Associated with low BMD:**
Advanced age	Female sex
History of fracture during adulthood	Caucasian or Asian ethnicity
Family history of an osteoporotic fracture	Prolonged calcium deficit
Prolonged use of corticosteroids	Vitamin D deficiency
Low body weight (<127 lb/58 kg)	Sedentary lifestyle
Smoking	Early menopause (before 45 years of age)
Excessive alcohol intake	Prolonged amenorrhea
	Bilateral oophorectomy
	History of gastric surgery
	Many medical conditions (including endocrine, gastrointestinal, rheumatologic, bone/marrow-related, and genetic disorders; organ transplantation)
	Drugs (e.g., corticosteroids, immunosuppressants, anticonvulsants, heparin, chemotherapy, thyroid hormone)

- Dietary history, specifically dairy products, lactose intolerance, vegetarian or other restrictive diets, or caffeine intake.
- Fractures as an adult.
- Family history of fractures, dowager's hump, or osteoporosis.
- Physical activity.
- Menstrual history.
- Pain and functional limitations of activities of daily living.
- Falls.

Physical Examination
- A complete physical examination should be performed on each patient, with emphasis on the accurate measurement of height and weight.
- A spinal examination should be included, noting evidence of kyphosis, pain, and muscle spasm.
- A breast examination should be performed on any woman in whom estrogen replacement is being considered.
- Gait stability and fall risk should be assessed including balance, proprioception, and muscle strength.

Diagnostic Testing

Laboratories
- Laboratory studies should be limited and directed by the history and physical examination.
- **Comprehensive biochemical profile** allows simple screening for secondary causes, that is, calcium-phosphorus ratio for hyperparathyroidism, total protein-albumin ratio for myeloma, and screening for liver and kidney disease.

TABLE 2	Indications for Bone Mineral Densitometry, Bone Mass Measurement Act of 1998

- An estrogen deficient women at clinical risk of osteoporosis as determined by a physician or qualified nonphysician practitioner based on her medical history and other findings
- Postmenopausal women deciding whether to begin estrogen replacement therapy (ERT) or other osteoporosis therapy
- Radiologically suspected osteopenia
- Receiving or expecting to receive glucocorticoids ($\geq$7.5 mg/day for $\geq$3 months)
- Primary hyperparathyroidism
- Serial monitoring to follow therapy

- **Thyroid-stimulating hormone (TSH)** should be measured in patients with symptoms of hyperthyroidism or those who are receiving thyroid replacement.
- **25-Hydroxyvitamin D** screens for body stores of vitamin D (desirable $\geq$30 ng/mL).
- Additional studies can be considered for those with very low bone mass or those who continue to lose bone despite antiresorptive therapy, including parathyroid hormone (PTH) battery, 24-hour urine for calcium excretion, serum protein electrophoresis (SPEP), cortisol levels, estradiol levels in women, testosterone levels in men, and bone biopsy (rarely required).

Bone Density Testing
- Bone densitometry has improved the diagnosis and treatment of osteoporosis. It allows the clinician to diagnose low bone mass before fracture occurs. Bone mass measurement is an accurate predictor of fractures.[5]
- The indications for bone mineral densitometry according to the **Bone Mass Measurement Act of 1998** are presented in Table 2 and those of the **National Osteoporosis Foundation** (NOF) in Table 3.[6]

TABLE 3	National Osteoporosis Foundation Indications for Bone Mineral Density Testing

- All women 65 years of age and older
- All men 70 years of age and older
- Postmenopausal women <65 years old in whom there is a concern for osteoporosis based on clinical risk profile
- Men 50–69 years old in whom there is a concern for osteoporosis based on clinical risk profile
- Perimenopausal women with a specific risk factor associated with increased fracture risk (Table 1)
- Adults who have a fracture after the age of 50
- Adults with a medical condition or taking a medication associated with low BMD
- Anyone being considered for pharmacologic therapy for osteoporosis
- Anyone being treated for osteoporosis, to monitor treatment effect
- Anyone not receiving therapy in whom evidence of bone loss would lead to treatment

TABLE 4	World Health Organization Criteria for the Diagnosis of Osteoporosis[a]

Category	T Score
Normal	<-1 SD from peak bone mass
Low bone mass/osteopenia	-1 SD to -2.5 SD from peak bone mass
Osteoporosis	≤-2.5 SD from peak bone mass
Severe osteoporosis	≤-2.5 SD with fragility fracture

SD, standard deviation.
[a]Diagnostic guidelines developed for postmenopausal women.

- All bone mass measurement techniques are valuable for making the diagnosis of osteoporosis and predicting fracture risk.
  - The most widely available methods are single x-ray absorptiometry, dual x-ray absorptiometry, quantitative computed tomography, and ultrasound densitometry.
  - The techniques vary in terms of precision, cost, radiation exposure, and ability to follow serial changes.
  - The most common method of measuring bone mass and currently the "gold standard" is dual x-ray absorptiometry.
- For the diagnosis of osteoporosis, the bone density of a patient is compared with the mean young adult normal reference range (the T score).
- The WHO has developed **diagnostic criteria** for osteoporosis using **T scores** (compared with young normal adults of the same sex) (Table 4)[7]:
  - The -2.5 T score or less standard deviation was chosen because more than half of osteoporotic fractures occur below that level.
  - Z scores, which compare a patient's BMD with that of age-matched controls, are also reported on bone mass measurement.
  - If the Z score is more than two standard deviations below age-matched subjects, a cause other than age-related bone loss should be considered, and a secondary cause of osteoporosis should be sought.
- Serial BMD measurements can be used to **monitor the effect of treatment or the clinical course of a specific medical condition.**
- The usefulness of serial measurements is dependent on the precision error of the measuring device used.
  - Change in any biologic test should be at least 2.8 times the precision of the technique to be 95%, confident that the change is real and not due to a measurement error in the machine.
  - For example, if a densitometer has a 1% precision error, there should be at least a 2.8% change to be confident that this change is real.

Treatment

Universal Recommendations
Diet Therapy
- Diet therapy is essential in the prevention and treatment of osteoporosis.
- Calcium supplementation alone has a small positive effect on BMD.[8]
- **The calcium intake for postmenopausal women should be 1,200 to 1,500 mg/ day.**

- Examples of the elemental calcium content of various foods include the following: 8-oz glass of milk contains 300 mg, 1 oz of Swiss cheese contains 270 mg, and 1 cup of cooked broccoli contains 100 mg.[9]
- Eating calcium-fortified foods should be encouraged.
- **Calcium supplements:** Calcium carbonate is acceptable for most patients for supplementation. It is cheap and has relatively few side effects. Guidelines for calcium supplement use include the following:
  - Calcium is best absorbed in small amounts; consider dividing the daily dose if >500 mg.
  - Synthetic calcium supplements are optimal. Oyster shell calcium, dolomite, and bone meal can contain heavy metal contaminants.[10]
- **Vitamin D (800 to 1,000 IU PO daily)** is beneficial for patients with osteoporosis. Ambulatory men and women older than the age of 65 years who were given calcium carbonate and vitamin D had a significant reduction in nonvertebral fractures.[11] Patients with significant hypovitaminosis D require more aggressive repletion.

Fall Prevention
- Patient education is essential for the prevention and treatment of osteoporosis particularly with regard to fall prevention.
- Look for and remove throw rugs, loose carpets, slippery floors, cords and wires, or anything that can cause a patient to slip.
- Inspect for unstable furniture and clutter that can obstruct mobility.
- Ensure adequate lighting, especially at night.
- Install grab bars for the toilet, place a nonslip surface in the shower.
- Wear properly fitting shoes.
- Repair or remove irregular sidewalks, ice or snow, and uneven surfaces.
- Correct vision and hearing problems.
- Eliminate causes of postural hypotension if possible. Otherwise advise patients to get up slowly.
- **Hip protectors** may reduce hip fractures in nursing home patients.[12,13] Acceptance to and adherence with hip protectors is relatively low.

Exercise
- Exercise should be encouraged in patients with osteoporosis as allowed by their functional status.
- Weight-bearing exercise, such as walking, jogging, basketball, dancing, and cycling, should be initiated at least three times per week.[14]
- Avoid unsafe forces, including flexion and forward bending of the vertebral column, as they can increase the risk of a compression fracture. Rotation of the spinal column also increases compressive forces on the spine.

Medications
Regardless of the specific treatment for the prevention or treatment of osteoporosis, all patients should receive adequate calcium and vitamin D, partake in regular weight-bearing exercise, and stop smoking.

Who Should Be Treated
According to the NOF, treatment should be considered in postmenopausal women and men aged 50 years or older with the following[5]:
- Hip or vertebral fracture.
- T score of ≤−2.5 at the femoral neck or spine (after appropriate evaluation to exclude secondary causes).

- Low BMD (T score of -1.0 to -2.5 at the femoral neck or spine) and a 10-year risk of hip fracture of $\geq 3\%$ or a 10-year risk of any major osteoporotic fracture of $\geq 20\%$ (based on the WHO FRAX algorithm, http://www.shef.ac.uk/FRAX).

Bisphosphonates
- Bisphosphonates inhibit the action of osteoclasts.
- The bisphosphonates alendronate, risedronate, and ibandronate are approved for the prevention and treatment of osteoporosis, while zoledronic acid is approved for treatment.
- For most patients, bisphosphonates are first-line therapy.
- All increase the BMD and reduce the risk of fractures.
- Orally administered bisphosphonates are poorly absorbed and, therefore, should be taken first thing in the morning, on an empty stomach, and no liquid, food, or other medications taken for at least 30 minutes. Calcium supplements should not be taken for at least 1 hour afterwards.
- When taken orally, bisphosphonates may cause esophagitis. Therefore, patients should sit or stand for at least 30 minutes after taking the drug with at least 8 oz of water. If taken properly, tolerance is excellent.[15] Less frequent administration may also improve gastrointestinal tolerability.[16]
- There may also be a link between the administration of bisphosphonates and osteonecrosis (avascular necrosis) of the jaw. The level of risk is not precisely known but is most likely very small. Risk factors appear to be high-dose IV administration, cancer, and dental procedures.[17–21]
- IV administration can result in flu-like symptoms (fever, arthralgias, myalgias, and headache) and transient hypocalcemia. The latter underscores the importance of calcium and vitamin D supplementation.
- The maximal duration of bisphosphonates therapy is uncertain.
- An increasing or stable BMD (generally measured every 2 years) is indicative of a treatment effect.

Alendronate
- Alendronate has been shown to improve BMD in the spine by 8.8% and in the hip by 5.9% after 3 years of therapy.[22] A meta-analysis of 11 randomized trials found that after 3 years of ≥ 10 mg of alendronate a 7.48% increase in BMD of the lumbar spine and 5.60% of the hip.[23]
- Women with osteoporosis treated with alendronate therapy for 3 years (2 years of 5 mg and 1 year of 10 mg) had a reduction in vertebral fractures by 47% and hip fractures by 51%.[24] The above meta-analysis found a pooled relative risk (RR) of fracture of 0.52 for vertebral fractures and 0.51 for nonvertebral fractures.[23]
- The recommended dosage for the treatment of osteoporosis in men and women is alendronate, 10 mg PO daily or 70 mg PO once weekly.[25]
- The dosage for the prevention of osteoporosis in postmenopausal women is 5 mg/day or 35 mg once weekly.
- The dose for the treatment of corticosteroid-induced osteoporosis is 5 mg/day, except in postmenopausal women not receiving estrogen, for whom the recommended dosage is 10 mg/day.

Risedronate
- Risedronate has been shown to improve BMD in the spine by 4% to 6% and in the hip by 1% to 3%.[26]
- The Vertebral Efficacy with Risedronate Trial (VERT) showed a 41% to 49% reduction in spinal fractures and a 39% reduction in nonvertebral fractures.[26,27]

Women aged 70 to 79 years with confirmed osteoporosis had a 40% reduction in hip fractures with 5 mg/day.[28]

- A meta-analysis of eight randomized trials found that after at least 1 year of 5 mg risedronate an increase in BMD of 4.54% for the lumbar spine and 2.75% for the femoral neck. The RR of fracture after at least 1 year of $\geq$2.5 mg of risedronate was 0.64 for vertebral fractures and 0.73 for nonvertebral fractures.[29]
- Recommended dosage for treatment and prevention of postmenopausal osteoporosis is risedronate, 5 mg PO daily. The dose for the prevention and treatment of corticosteroid-induced osteoporosis is 5 mg/day, or 35 mg once weekly,[30] or 75 mg on 2 consecutive days a month,[31] or 150 mg once monthly.[32]

Ibandronate

- Ibandronate daily or intermittently has also been shown to significantly increase BMD and decrease fractures.[33-36]
- The recommended dosage of ibandronate is 150 mg monthly.[37,38]
- Ibandronate can also be administered IV, 3 mg every 3 months.[39,40] This regimen may be effective for those who cannot tolerate oral administration or who cannot follow oral dosing precautions.

Zoledronic Acid

- IV zoledronic acid is approved for the treatment of osteoporosis.
- Once yearly administration **increases BMD** as well as intermittent administration[41] and **reduces the risk of vertebral** (70%) **and hip fractures** (41%).[42]
- If given within 90 days after repair of a hip fracture, zoledronic acid reduces the risk of new fractures (35%) and improves survival (28%).[43]
- The recommended dosage is 5 mg IV over at least 15 minutes.
- Zoledronic acid also has indications for hypercalcemia of malignancy, multiple myeloma, and bone metastases from solid tumors.

Raloxifene

- Raloxifene is a selective estrogen receptor modulator. It inhibits the loss of BMD but does not cause endometrial hyperplasia.
- In the Multiple Outcomes of Raloxifene Evaluation (MORE) trial, 7,705 women were assigned to receive placebo or raloxifene at 60 or 120 mg. Treatment with raloxifene **increased the BMD** of the femoral neck and spine by 2.1% to 2.3% and 2.5% to 2.6%, respectively, compared with placebo.[44,45] During the 4-year continuation of a subset of MORE subjects (Continuing Outcome Relevant to Evista, CORE), differences in BMD between raloxifene and placebo were maintained.[46]
- **Vertebral fractures were reduced by 30% to 50%.**[44,45,47]
- **No data support reduction in nonvertebral fractures** at this time.[44-47]
- The MORE trial revealed a **70% reduction in the development of invasive breast cancer** in patients who were treated with raloxifene and had no effect on the endometrium.[48] The Raloxifene Use for The Heart (RUTH) trial demonstrated a 43% reduction in invasive breast cancer.[49] During the combined MORE/CORE 8 years, there was a 66% reduction in invasive breast cancer and a 76% reduction in estrogen receptor (ER)-positive invasive breast cancer by 76%.[50] There was no change in the incidence of ER-negative invasive breast cancer.
- Total serum cholesterol and low-density lipoprotein cholesterol levels decreased significantly without change in high-density lipoprotein or triglyceride levels. Raloxifene 60 mg daily reduced the total cholesterol level by 6.4% and the low-density lipoprotein level by 10.1%.[51]

- Raloxifene **does not appear to have a significant effect on the risk of coronary events.**[49,52]
- **The risk of venous thromboembolism with raloxifene may be elevated:** MORE trial RR 2.1 to 3.1, CORE study RR 2.17, and RUTH trial hazard ratio (HR) 1.44.[44,49,50,52,53] The risk is probably not as much as with tamoxifen.[54]
- In the RUTH trial, raloxifene was associated with an **increased risk of fatal stroke** (HR 1.49) but not with total stroke or all cause mortality.[49]
- Other side effects include hot flashes and leg cramps.
- The recommended dosage for prevention and treatment is raloxifene 60 mg daily.

Calcitonin
- Salmon or human calcitonin can be given as an SC injection or as a nasal spray.
- Calcitonin improves BMD by 1% to 2% in patients who are treated with calcitonin, 200 IU nasal spray daily.
- The Prevent Recurrence of Osteoporotic Fracture (PROOF) trial showed a reduction in vertebral fractures by 36% with the nasal spray in women who were 5 years postmenopausal with vertebral fractures. However, 59% of participants withdrew prematurely; therefore, results of this study should be interpreted cautiously. No significant reduction in hip fractures occurred.[55]
- A meta-analysis showed a reduction in vertebral fractures (RR 0.46) and nonvertebral fractures (RR 0.52).[56]
- Most consider calcitonin less effective than bisphosphonates.
- Calcitonin has an analgesic effect when given in the treatment of compression fractures.[57]
- Recommended dosage for the treatment of women >5 years postmenopausal with low bone mass is one spray (200 IU) in one nostril daily. The patient should alternate nostrils each day. The SC dose is 100 IU/day.

Parathyroid Hormone
- PTH is considered to be an "anabolic" treatment, in that it stimulates bone formation rather than acting as an antiresorptive.
- Intermittent PTH administration, as opposed to chronic elevations (as in chronic kidney disease or primary hyperparathyroidism), stimulates the maturation of osteoblasts and, therefore, bone formation. The explanation for this incongruity is not fully understood.
- PTH affects trabecular bone more than cortical bone and qualitatively improves trabecular architecture.
- PTH is usually given as recombinant human PTH amino acids 1 to 34, known as **teriparatide.** Intact PTH is also effective.[58]
- In the Fracture Prevention Trial (FPT) of 1,637 postmenopausal women with a prior vertebral fracture randomized to placebo or 20 or 40 μg teriparatide daily, BMD increased in the spine and hip but not in the radial shaft.[59]
- After a median treatment period of 21 months in FPT, there was significant reduction in vertebral fractures (RR 0.31 to 0.35) and nonvertebral fractures (RR 0.46 to 0.47).[59] BMD increases before fracture reduction occurs.
- Side effects include hypercalcemia, nausea, headache, leg cramps, and dizziness.
- Animal studies suggest an increased risk of osteosarcoma. Teriparatide should not be given to those with increased risk such as Paget disease, skeletal radiation therapy, or a history of bone malignancy.
- The recommended dosage of teriparatide is 20 μg subcutaneously daily for a maximum of 2 years. A bisphosphonates is typically given after this.[60]

- Concurrent administration of alendronate does not produce an additive effect and may actually reduce the effects of PTH.[61]

Estrogen Replacement Therapy

- Estrogen therapy (ET) has been shown to slow down bone loss following menopause or to increase it by as much as 6%.[62]
- Numerous observational studies support ET as effective in the reduction of vertebral fractures by as much as 50% to 80%. A study of osteoporotic fractures suggested that women who started ET within 5 years of menopause and used ET for >10 years had a relative risk for wrist fractures of 0.25 and a relative risk for hip fractures of 0.27.[63] A meta-analysis of seven trial found the RR of vertebral fracture of 0.66 and nonvertebral fractures of 0.87; however, the 95% confidence intervals (CI) for both crossed 1.0.[64]
- Since the results of the Women's Health Initiative (WHI) (excess coronary events, strokes, pulmonary emboli, and invasive breast cancer) and the availability of other effective drugs, ET is no longer considered appropriate for first-line therapy for the prevention and treatment of osteoporosis.[65]
- Dosing is discussed in the "Menopause" section below.

Management of Corticosteroid-Induced Osteoporosis

- Skeletal effects of corticosteroids include decreased BMD and increased fracture risk and are related to dose and duration of therapy.
- Daily prednisone doses of ≥7.5 mg/day can result in significant bone loss. Lower doses can also have an effect on bone metabolism.
- Alternate-day regimens have not been shown to be protective on bone loss.
- Bone densitometry should be considered on any patient who is presently receiving corticosteroids or if long-term therapy is initiated.
- Patients who are on corticosteroids should receive adequate calcium intake (1,500 mg/day) and vitamin D (800 IU).
- Weight-bearing exercise should be encouraged.
- **Alendronate** has been shown to prevent bone loss in patients receiving corticosteroid therapy and to reduce the risk of fractures in postmenopausal women who are taking steroids.[66,67]
- **Risedronate and zoledronic acid** are similarly effective.[68–71]
- **Calcitonin** may preserve bone loss, but it has not been shown to prevent fractures in the setting of corticosteroid treatment.[72,73]
- Teriparatide may be more effective than alendronate in patients who have osteoporosis and have received corticosteroids for at least 3 months.[74]

Management of Osteoporosis in Men

- If a male patient presents with a fracture that is associated with mild-to-moderate trauma, BMD testing should be performed, and a search for secondary causes of bone loss should be considered.
- Evaluation should evaluate for risk factors for osteoporosis including possible drugs that could affect BMD, such as corticosteroids, anticonvulsants, history of alcohol ingestion (>100 g/day), or nicotine use.
- Appropriate laboratory studies should be done such as SPEP, complete blood cell count, calcium, phosphate, albumin, creatinine, alkaline phosphatase, PTH battery, TSH, free testosterone, 25-hydroxyvitamin D, 24-hour urine collection for calcium and creatinine excretion, and cortisol levels.

- Causes of hypogonadism, such as Klinefelter syndrome, hyperprolactinemia, anorexia nervosa, and hemochromatosis, should also be considered. Bone biopsy may be needed if no etiology is found.
- As with female patients, sufficient calcium and vitamin D is important. Patients should be encouraged to stop smoking and drinking alcohol.
- If a secondary cause is found, it should be treated.
- Hypogonadism is a relatively common cause, and testosterone replacement increases BMD.[75–77] **Alendronate** has been shown to maintain BMD and prevent fractures in men with osteoporosis, vertebral fracture odds ratio (OR) 0.44 and nonvertebral fracture OR 0.60.[78]
- **Risedronate** has been shown to reduce vertebral fractures and increase the bone mass in men treated with corticosteroids.[79–82]
- **Teriparatide** has also been shown to be effective in men.[83–85]

MENOPAUSE

General Principles

- The menopausal transition period is typified by variation in menstrual cycle length and eventual skipped periods.
- Menopause is technically defined as the first 12 months after the last period. The postmenopausal phase begins after that.
- The average age of menopause is 50 to 51 years.[86]
- With ovarian failure, follicle-stimulating hormone and luteinizing hormone levels rise and estradiol levels fall.
- Other causes of amenorrhea and menopausal symptoms should be considered: excessive weight loss, concurrent medical illnesses, pregnancy, thyroid disease, pituitary disease, and medications.

Diagnosis

Clinical Presentation

- Symptoms associated with menopause include the following:
  - Irregular bleeding.
  - Hot flashes/night sweats.
  - Sleep disturbance.
  - Vaginal dryness/itching/dyspareunia.
  - Sexual dysfunction.
  - Urinary incontinence.
  - Mood changes (inconsistent degree of association).
- Menopausal symptoms typically last for a few months but can persist for several years.[86]
- **Hot flashes** affect approximately 75% of menopausal women. They occur most frequently at night and are due to estrogen deficiency. It is believed that estrogen withdrawal lowers the temperature set point in the hypothalamus to reduce the body thermostat. As a result, vasodilatation of the vessels in the hands and upper body occurs so that the heat in the central organs is lost at the periphery.[87]
  - Hot flashes are not synonymous with estrogen deficiency.
  - Other causes of hot flashes should be considered, such as pheochromocytoma, carcinoid, pregnancy, and panic disorder.

- Long-term effects in the postmenopausal period include the following:
  - Osteoporosis.
  - Increased cardiovascular disease risk.

Diagnostic Testing

- Diagnostic testing is generally unnecessary.
- As noted, follicle-stimulating hormone and luteinizing hormone levels are high and estradiol levels are low.
- Other tests may be indicated to rule out other possible causes of amenorrhea.

Treatment

Hot Flashes

Estrogen Therapy
- **ET is the most effective treatment.**[86,88,89]
- However, the results of the Women's Health Initiative and the Heart and Estrogen/progestin Replacement Study (HERS) have greatly called into question the advisability of long-term (i.e., >approximately 5 years) or chronic indefinite ET, most specifically with regard to combined estrogen and progestin treatment.[65,90] It is important to recognize that the direct applicability of these studies to all menopausal women is somewhat tenuous.[91]
- As well, quality of life is also a very important consideration.[92]
- The balance of risks and benefit appears to be more favorable for women who have had a hysterectomy receiving estrogen-only treatment in comparison with women with a uterus receiving combined estrogen-progestin treatment.
- On balance, short-term (i.e., <approximately 2 to 3 years) administration of the lowest effective dose of estrogen is a viable option for women with moderate-to-severe vasomotor symptoms who have no history of cardiovascular disease, breast cancer, endometrial cancer, or venous thromboembolism.[89,91,92]
  - Low-dose estrogen therapies include 0.3 mg oral conjugated estrogen, 0.25 to 0.5 mg micronized 17β-estradiol, or 0.025 mg transdermal 17β-estradiol patch.[91] Higher doses may be necessary in some patients for symptom control.
  - **A progestin must be added in women with an intact uterus.**[93]
  - Low-dose (i.e., containing 20 μg of ethinyl estradiol) OCPs are also a reasonable option for women less than approximately 50 years old.
- ET can generally be tapered off gradually after a year or two. Some women may have return of hot flashes.
- **Other side effects of estrogen** include abdominal bloating, cramps, breast tenderness, hypertriglyceridemia (oral estrogen only), breakthrough bleeding, weight changes, enlargement of benign tumors of the uterus, dry eyes, and skin changes.
- **Side effects of progestins** include breakthrough bleeding, edema, weight changes, rash, insomnia, and somnolence.

Other Treatments
- Simple **environmental changes,** including keeping the room cool and dressing in layers, may make hot flashes more tolerable.
- **Serotonin-reuptake inhibitors** (SSRIs, e.g., paroxetine and fluoxetine) and **serotonin-norepinephrine reuptake inhibitors** (SNRIs, e.g., venlafaxine) are effective for vasomotor symptoms but not as much as ET.[86,89,94]

- **Gabapentin** appears to be effective at reducing the frequency of hot flashes.[86,89,95] Doses up to 900 mg/day may be required. Common side effects of gabapentin include dizziness/unsteadiness and fatigue/somnolence.
- Studies regarding clonidine are mostly of fairly low quality and conflicting.[86,94]
- The effectiveness of soy foods, soy extracts, red clover extracts, and black cohosh is questionable[86,89,94,96,97]

Genitourinary Symptoms

- Vaginal atrophy presents with dyspareunia, vaginal dryness, itching, and irritation. Oral and topic estrogen is useful for symptoms associated with vaginal atrophy. Systemic effects of vaginal estrogen are probably quite low. Concomitant progestin therapy is not necessary for women with a uterus receiving topical vaginal estrogen.
- The terminal urethra is embryonically related to the vagina. As it becomes thinner, there is more risk of infection and incontinence. Dysuria without evidence of infection is due to the thinning of the epithelium, allowing urine in close contact with the sensory nerves. Also, the normal urethral pressures created by the urethra and surrounding tissues are decreased. Topical estrogen in some studies has been shown to reduce the incidence of urinary tract infections.[86,98]

CERVICAL CANCER SCREENING

- Cervical cancer screening has reduced the incidence of invasive cervical cancer by 95%. Half of the women in the United States with invasive cervical carcinoma have never had a Pap smear, and another 10% have not had a Pap smear in 5 years.[99]
- Risk factors for cervical cancer include smoking, multiple sex partners, sexual activity at an early age, and sex with a "high-risk" partner, characterized by multiple sex partners or a partner who has developed genital neoplasia, history of a sexually transmitted infection, HIV, and prolonged OCP use.[100–102]
- Human papilloma virus (HPV) appears to be the link between sexual activity and cervical neoplasia. Evidence of HPV infection is consistently found in 90% of cervical cancers.
- Cervical cancer screening with the Pap smear is recommended for all women who have ever been sexually active and who have a cervix. The American Cancer Society (ACS), United States Preventative Services Task Force (USPSTF), and American College of Obstetrics and Gynecology (ACOG) have similar but not identical recommendations.
- Begin screening by approximately 3 years after first sexual intercourse or by age 21, whichever comes first (ACS, USPSTF).
- In November, 2009 ACOG amended their guidelines recommending that screening should begin at 21 years regardless of sexual history.
- Testing interval recommendations vary:
  - **USPSTF** recommends the following:
    - Screening at least every 3 years.
    - The evidence is insufficient to recommend for or against the routine use of liquid-based cytology or the routine use of HPV testing as a primary screening test for cervical cancer.
  - **ACS** recommends the following:
    - Screening should be done every year with the regular Pap test or every 2 years using the newer liquid-based Pap test.

- o Beginning at age 30, women who have had 3 normal Pap test results in a row may get screened every 2 to 3 years.
  - o Another reasonable option for women over 30 is to get screened every 3 years (but not more frequently) with either the conventional or liquid-based Pap test, plus the DNA test for HPV.
- **ACOG** recommends the following:
  - o For women age 21 to 29 cervical cytology screening is recommended every 2 years.
  - o If a woman age 30 and older has had negative results on three consecutive cervical cytology tests, then she may be rescreened with cervical cytology alone every 3 years.
  - o Combined cytology and HPV DNA testing is an appropriate screening test for women >30 years. The combined testing is not appropriate for women under age 30, since they frequently test positive for HPV that will clear up on its own.
- **Cervical intraepithelial neoplasias** are usually divided into categories based on cytologic grades. The **Bethesda system** is the currently recognized reporting system. Included in this system is the pathologist's interpretation of the smear, including the presence of benign cellular changes or evidence of cellular atypia, or both. Infectious processes such as *Trichomonas*, *Candida*, *Actinomyces*, or cellular changes associated with herpes simplex virus are reported. Reactive (but benign) changes associated with inflammation, atrophy, radiation, or intrauterine contraceptive device are also reported. The four categories of squamous cell abnormalities are as follows:
- Atypical squamous cells (ASC).
- Low-grade squamous intraepithelial lesions (LSIL).
- High-grade squamous intraepithelial lesions (HSIL).
- Squamous carcinoma.
- **ASC of undetermined significance (ASC-US)** are no uncommonly associated with lesions that regress spontaneously, and the risk of invasive cervical cancer is low.
  - The preferred management for nonadolescent women is reflex HPV testing. That is, the specimen is collected at the time of the cervical smear and HPV testing ordered if the cytologic results are ASC-US.[103]
  - Those with positive testing for high-risk HPV types should be referred for colposcopy.
  - Those with negative testing, cytology should be repeated in 12 months.
  - In adolescents (<20 years old), repeat cytology in 12 months is recommended due to the very high prevalence of HPV infection and the extremely low prevalence of invasive cancer.
- **ASC but HSIL cannot be ruled out (ASC-H)** should be evaluated with colposcopy.[103]
- **LSIL** should be further evaluated with colposcopy in most women. In adolescents, however, repeat cytology at 12 months is recommended.[103] HPV testing is an option for postmenopausal women.
- **HSIL** must be further evaluated with colposcopy.[103]

NIPPLE DISCHARGE

General Principles

- Nipple discharge is common and mostly benign.
- Nipple discharge can be classified as galactorrhea, physiologic, or pathologic.

- **Galactorrhea** is bilateral, milky, involves multiple ducts, and is not associated with pregnancy or lactation.
  - It is very unusual for nulligravid women to secrete breast milk spontaneously, although this may occur in girls as they enter puberty.
  - Breast secretions can be demonstrated in 25% of normal women who have been pregnant; this percentage is even higher when breast massage is performed.
  - Galactorrhea suggests an effect of **prolactin** either through drugs, pituitary tumors, or an endocrine effect.
  - **Drugs** that are associated with galactorrhea include oral contraceptives, tricyclic antidepressants, antipsychotics, methyldopa, reserpine, cimetidine, and antiemetics.[104]
- **Physiologic nipple discharge** is usually bilateral and serous. It is believed to be a consequence of local breast stimulation or irritation in women with hormonally primed breast tissue (either by pregnancy or oral contraceptives). Gonadal function is preserved. Avoiding breast stimulation should resolve this condition.
- **Pathologic nipple discharge** is usually unilateral and localized to a single duct. It is spontaneous, intermittent, and persistent.
  - The fluid can be serosanguineous, bloody, greenish, or clear.
  - The most common cause of unilateral discharge is intraductal papilloma, followed by mammary duct ectasia.[104]
  - About 10% to 15% of cases are due to breast carcinoma.[104]
  - Purulent discharge can be caused by mastitis.

Diagnosis

Clinical Presentation

- The history should include questioning in regard to menstrual pattern, recent pregnancy, infertility, medications, symptoms of hypothyroidism, breast stimulation, and presence of headaches or visual complaints.
- Any medications associated with galactorrhea should be stopped, and pregnancy should be ruled out.
- Physical examination should include a complete breast examination and evaluation for signs of hypothyroidism or pituitary tumor.
- Try to determine if the discharge is from one (more concerning) or multiple ducts.

Diagnostic Testing

- If fluid is expressed and not grossly, it should be evaluated for occult blood.
- Cytology of the discharge has low sensitivity and specificity.
- Measurement of TSH, prolactin, and a pregnancy test are indicated with discharge from multiple ducts. Excluding pregnancy, a prolactin level of >300 ng/mL is almost always the result of a prolactinoma.
- Mammography should be obtained in patients >35 years with a pathologic discharge or if a mass is palpated. A negative mammogram does not exclude malignancy.[104]
- Ultrasound is reasonable in those >35 years, but if it is negative, a mammogram should subsequently be obtained.[104] Ultrasound is also frequently preformed in women >35 years.
- Galactography (also called ductography, cannulation of the secreting duct followed by injection of contrast material) can be considered to identify intraductal

lesions but the technique is difficult. A negative test does not completely exclude cancer.

- Magnetic resonance imaging and ductoscopy are also available diagnostic tests.

Treatment

- Galactorrhea:
  - Patients with normal periods and normal prolactin levels do not require treatment.
  - Breast stimulation is discouraged.
  - If the patient is receiving a medication that is associated with galactorrhea, the dose can be decreased or the drug stopped and the patient followed.
  - The management of prolactinoma is discussed in Chapter 17.
- Patients with pathologic discharge should be referred for evaluation by a surgeon who is experienced with diseases of the breast.

BREAST MASSES

- Risk factors for breast cancer include female gender, increasing age, first-degree relative (mother or sister) with breast cancer (highest risk is if the relative was premenopausal and the cancer was bilateral), previous breast cancer, late age of first pregnancy, and nulliparity.
- The patient should be questioned for any associated symptoms, such as pain and nipple discharge. Menstrual history should be obtained, and she should be questioned to determine the possibility of pregnancy. Medications should be reviewed, and any history of trauma should be obtained. An accurate family history should be elicited. If a history of breast, ovarian, colon, or prostate cancer is found in numerous family members, genetic counseling should be considered.
- Physical examination should include inspection and palpation of the breast with the patient seated and then lying flat. The breasts should be observed for skin dimpling or changes in contour. The nipple should be inspected for spontaneous discharge. The axillary and supraclavicular area should be palpated for any evidence of a mass or enlarged lymph nodes. The breast should be palpated gently, including the nipple, areola, and breast tissue. The breast should be palpated circumferentially to the axilla. The nipple should be closely evaluated for discharge, and the character of the discharge should be noted. A ductal carcinoma may present with an isolated spontaneous serosanguineous discharge.
- **Differential diagnosis** for a discrete nodule includes fibroadenoma, cysts, fibrocystic changes, malignancy, and trauma. A dominant nodule remains unchanged throughout the menstrual cycle. In fibrocystic disease, the palpable nodules frequently feel cystic and are subject to change during the menstrual cycle. Benign nodules have characteristics such as easy mobility, regular borders, and a soft or cystic feel. However, **physical examination alone cannot exclude malignancy;** therefore, other diagnostic tests are indicated.
- **Women <30 years** with a breast mass and no other symptoms can be observed through one menstrual cycle, and if it resolves, no further treatment is indicated. If the mass persists, ultrasound is a reasonable next step.
- **Women >30 years** should have a mammogram. Ultrasound may also be indicated.
- **Routine screening mammography** recommendations are discussed in Chapter 43.

VAGINITIS

- The presence of vaginal discharge is not always abnormal.
- Symptoms are usually nonspecific.
- The vagina has 25 bacterial species, and pH is usually 4.0 due to lactobacilli.
- Semen, menses, and ectropion may alter the pH.
- Fifty percent of vaginitis is from bacterial vaginosis (BV), 25% from *Trichomonas vaginitis*, and 25% from *Candida vaginitis*.
- Management of sexually transmitted infections is discussed in Chapter 23.

BACTERIAL VAGINOSIS

General Principles

- BV is thought to result from a polymicrobial alteration in the normal vaginal flora, a dramatic reduction in lactobacilli with marked increase in anaerobes, an overgrowth of *Gardnerella* spp., or genital mycoplasmas.
- *G. vaginalis* may be cultured from 30% to 70% of healthy asymptomatic women.

Diagnosis

- BV is characterized by malodorous vaginal discharge, with or without vaginal pruritus.
- Usually, there is no external genital irritation or dysuria.
- The discharge is a homogeneous, nonviscous, milky-white fluid that coats the vagina and cervix.
- The presence of **"clue cells"** (epithelial cells that have lost their sharp margins and have a granular appearance because of the adherence of bacteria over the surface) is an accepted criterion for diagnosis.
- **The pH should be >4.5.**
- Another common test **(whiff test)** involves the amine (fishy) odor released when the vaginal discharge is alkalinized by mixing with 10% KOH.
- No cultures are needed in clinical diagnosis of BV.

Treatment

- **Metronidazole** is the most effective antimicrobial for BV, with cure rates >90%.
  - Standard treatment is metronidazole, 500 mg PO bid for 7 days.[105]
  - Alternative treatments are metronidazole ER, 750 mg PO qd for 7 days; and metronidazole gel, one application intravaginally every night for 5 nights.
  - Patients should be advised to avoid alcohol consumption during treatment with metronidazole due to a possible disulfiram-type reaction.
  - Nausea and metallic taste are common side effects.[106]
- Alternatives are **clindamycin** cream 2% intravaginally for 7 nights or clindamycin 300 mg PO bid for 7 days.
- The effectiveness of probiotics is uncertain.[107]
- Relapses are relatively common after treatment.
- The treatment of sexual partners remains controversial. *Gardnerella vaginalis* has been found in the urethra of >9% of male partners of affected women. No data

about the effect of treatment of the partner are available. Some physicians prefer to treat partners only if bacterial vaginosis fails to respond or recurs. It is unknown if abstinence or condom use affects recurrences.

TRICHOMONAS VAGINITIS

General Principles

- *Trichomonas vaginalis* is a contagious parasite that is acquired through sexual contact.
- It is often found in the presence of other sexually transmitted infections.
- Many women are asymptomatic.
- *T. vaginalis* may also cause urethritis in men but is usually asymptomatic.

Diagnosis

- *T. vaginalis* causes profuse, purulent, malodorous, sometimes foamy vaginal discharge. Pruritus may be present.
- **pH of >4.5 and whiff test may be positive.**
- The "strawberry cervix" caused by cervical petechiae is a characteristic manifestation.
- Diagnosis can be made by microscopic detection of motile trichomonads on examination of a saline wet prep or vaginal or urethral secretions. The slide should be examined soon after preparation to detect motility. Organisms are detected in 60% to 70% of infected women.
- The reliability of the Pap smear is quite variable.
- Culture is available but generally not necessary.

Treatment

- **Standard treatment is single-dose metronidazole** (2 g PO) or 500 mg PO bid for 7 days.[105,108] Patients should be warned not to drink alcohol during the course of treatment.
- The cure rate is approximately 90%.
- Most physicians advocate treating all patients who have detectable organisms to reduce the sexual transmission of the organism.
- Treatment of male sexual partners is usually recommended.[105]

VULVOVAGINAL CANDIDIASIS

General Principles

- This "yeast infection" is suggested by the presence of vulvovaginal soreness, dyspareunia, vulvar pruritus, external dysuria, and thick or "cheesy" vaginal secretions.
- It is typically caused by *Candida albicans* but can sometimes be caused by other *Candida* spp.
- Factors that predispose to colonization and infection include diabetes, steroid therapy, pregnancy, antibiotics, obesity, OCPs, immunosuppressant drugs, and HIV infection.
- Candidiasis is usually not transmitted sexually.

- Ten to twenty percent of women normally have yeast colonized in the vagina; 75% of women have at least one episode of *Candida vaginitis*, and 45% have two or more episodes during their lifetime.

Diagnosis

- Speculum examination may reveal candidal plaques adherent to the vaginal mucosa with erythema or edema of the introitus.
- **The vaginal pH is usually <4.5.**
- Diagnosis can be made by inspection of the typical vaginal lesions or by observation of fungal elements (budding yeast and pseudohyphae) in a KOH preparation.
- Cultures are not recommended.
- It is justifiable to treat an apparent or suspected candidal vulvovaginitis even with a negative KOH preparation (only 40% to 80% sensitive).

Treatment

- Treatment is with one of the **imidazole antifungal drugs,** such as butoconazole, clotrimazole, miconazole, terconazole, or tioconazole. All are more effective than nystatin.[105]
  - Courses of treatment range from single dose to 3 to 7 days depending on the agent and dosage.
  - Most come in cream or suppository for intravaginal use.
- If the woman is menstruating, she should not use tampons, which may absorb the drug.
- **Single-dose oral fluconazole,** 150 mg, is an expensive but very effective alternative.
- Treatment of asymptomatic male partners is not indicated except in some cases of recurrent candidiasis.
- **Recurrent candidal infections** are common and can be distressing. All predisposing factors should be addressed. Each recurrent episode generally responds to topical treatment, longer treatment may be indicated. Oral fluconazole 100 to 200 mg every third day for 3 doses is an option followed by maintenance suppression with fluconazole 100 to 200 mg weekly for 6 months may be effective.[105,109]

REFERENCES

1. Consensus development conference: diagnosis, prophylaxis, and treatment of osteoporosis. *Am J Med* 1993;94:646–650.
2. Miller CW. Survival and ambulation following hip fracture. *J Bone Joint Surg* 1978;60: 930–934.
3. Slemenda CW, Hui SL, Longcope C, et al. Predictors of bone mass in perimenopausal women. A prospective study of clinical data using photon absorptiometry. *Ann Intern Med* 1990;112:96–101.
4. WHO Scientific Group on the Assessment of Osteoporosis at Primary Health Care Level. Geneva: World Health Organization, 2007.
5. Cummings SR, Nevitt MC, Browner WS, et al. Risk factors for hip fracture in white women. Study of Osteoporotic Fractures Research Group. *N Engl J Med* 1995;332:767–773.
6. Clinician's Guide to Prevention and Treatment of Osteoporosis. Washington, DC: National Osteoporosis Foundation, 2008.
7. Kanis JA, Melton LJ III, Christiansen C, et al. The diagnosis of osteoporosis. *J Bone Miner Res* 1994;9:1137–1141.
8. Shea B, Wells G, Cranney A, et al.; Osteoporosis Methodology Group and The Osteoporosis Research Advisory Group. Meta-analyses of therapies for postmenopausal osteoporosis. VII.

Meta-analysis of calcium supplementation for the prevention of postmenopausal osteoporosis. *Endocr Rev* 2002;23:552–559.

9. NIH Consensus conference. Optimal calcium intake. NIH Consensus Development Panel on Optimal Calcium Intake. *JAMA* 1994;272:1942–1948.

10. Whiting SJ. Safety of some calcium supplements questioned. *Nutr Rev* 1994;52:95–97.

11. Dawson-Hughes B, Harris SS, Krall EA, Dallal GE. Effect of calcium and vitamin D supplementation on bone density in men and women 65 years of age or older. *N Engl J Med* 1997;337:670–676.

12. Parker MJ, Gillespie WJ, Gillespie LD. Hip protectors for preventing hip fractures in older people. *Cochrane Database Syst Rev* 2005;(3):CD001255.

13. Sawka AM, Boulos P, Beattie K, et al. Do hip protectors decrease the risk of hip fracture in institutional and community-dwelling elderly? A systematic review and meta-analysis of randomized controlled trials. *Osteoporos Int* 2005;16:1461–1474.

14. Bonaiuti D, Shea B, Iovine R, et al. Exercise for preventing and treating osteoporosis in postmenopausal women. *Cochrane Database Syst Rev* 2002;(3):CD000333.

15. Cryer B, Bauer DC. Oral bisphosphonates and upper gastrointestinal tract problems: what is the evidence? *Mayo Clin Proc* 2002;77:1031–1043.

16. Strampel W, Emkey R, Civitelli R. Safety considerations with bisphosphonates for the treatment of osteoporosis. *Drug Saf* 2007;30:755–763.

17. King AE, Umland EM. Osteonecrosis of the jaw in patients receiving intravenous or oral bisphosphonates. *Pharmacotherapy* 2008;28:667–677.

18. Pazianas M, Miller P, Blumentals WA, et al. A review of the literature on osteonecrosis of the jaw in patients with osteoporosis treated with oral bisphosphonates: prevalence, risk factors, and clinical characteristics. *Clin Ther* 2007;29:1548–1558.

19. Khan AA, Sándor GK, Dore E, et al; Canadian Taskforce on Osteonecrosis of the Jaw. Bisphosphonate associated osteonecrosis of the jaw. *J Rheumatol* 2009;36:478–490.

20. Rizzoli R, Burlet N, Cahall D, et al. Osteonecrosis of the jaw and bisphosphonate treatment for osteoporosis. *Bone* 2008;42:841–847.

21. Woo SB, Hellstein JW, Kalmar JR. Narrative [corrected] review: bisphosphonates and osteonecrosis of the jaws. *Ann Intern Med* 2006;144:753–761.

22. Liberman UA, Weiss SR, Bröll J, et al. Effect of oral alendronate on bone mineral density and the incidence of fractures in postmenopausal osteoporosis. The Alendronate Phase III Osteoporosis Treatment Study Group. *N Engl J Med* 1995;333:1437–1443.

23. Cranney A, Wells G, Willan A, et al.; Osteoporosis Methodology Group and The Osteoporosis Research Advisory Group. Meta-analyses of therapies for postmenopausal osteoporosis. II. Meta-analysis of alendronate for the treatment of postmenopausal women. *Endocr Rev* 2002;23:508–516.

24. Black DM, Cummings SR, Karpf DB, et al. Randomised trial of effect of alendronate on risk of fracture in women with existing vertebral fractures. Fracture Intervention Trial Research Group. *Lancet* 1996;348:1535–1541.

25. Rizzoli R, Greenspan SL, Bone G III, et al.; Alendronate Once-Weekly Study Group. Two-year results of once-weekly administration of alendronate 70 mg for the treatment of postmenopausal osteoporosis. *J Bone Miner Res* 2002;17:1988–1996.

26. Harris ST, Watts NB, Genant HK, et al. Effects of risedronate treatment on vertebral and nonvertebral fractures in women with postmenopausal osteoporosis: a randomized controlled trial. Vertebral Efficacy With Risedronate Therapy (VERT) Study Group. *JAMA* 1999;282:1344–1352.

27. Reginster J, Minne HW, Sorensen OH, et al. Randomized trial of the effects of risedronate on vertebral fractures in women with established postmenopausal osteoporosis. Vertebral Efficacy with Risedronate Therapy (VERT) Study Group. *Osteoporos Int* 2000;11:83–91.

28. McClung MR, Geusens P, Miller PD, et al.; Hip Intervention Program Study Group. Effect of risedronate on the risk of hip fracture in elderly women. Hip Intervention Program Study Group. *N Engl J Med* 2001;344:333–340.

29. Cranney A, Tugwell P, Adachi J, et al.; Osteoporosis Methodology Group and The Osteoporosis Research Advisory Group. Meta-analyses of therapies for postmenopausal

osteoporosis. III. Meta-analysis of risedronate for the treatment of postmenopausal osteoporosis. *Endocr Rev* 2002;23:517–523.

30. Harris ST, Watts NB, Li Z, et al. Two-year efficacy and tolerability of risedronate once a week for the treatment of women with postmenopausal osteoporosis. *Curr Med Res Opin* 2004;20:757–764.

31. Delmas PD, Benhamou CL, Man Z, et al. Monthly dosing of 75 mg risedronate on 2 consecutive days a month: efficacy and safety results. *Osteoporos Int* 2008;19: 1039–1045.

32. Delmas PD, McClung MR, Zanchetta JR, et al. Efficacy and safety of risedronate 150 mg once a month in the treatment of postmenopausal osteoporosis. *Bone* 2008;42:36–42.

33. Delmas PD, Recker RR, Chesnut CH III, et al. Daily and intermittent oral ibandronate normalize bone turnover and provide significant reduction in vertebral fracture risk: results from the BONE study. *Osteoporos Int* 2004;15:792–798.

34. Chesnut CH III, Skag A, Christiansen C, et al.; Oral Ibandronate Osteoporosis Vertebral Fracture Trial in North America and Europe (BONE). Effects of oral ibandronate administered daily or intermittently on fracture risk in postmenopausal osteoporosis. *J Bone Miner Res* 2004;19:1241–1249.

35. Harris ST, Blumentals WA, Miller PD. Ibandronate and the risk of non-vertebral and clinical fractures in women with postmenopausal osteoporosis: results of a meta-analysis of phase III studies. *Curr Med Res Opin* 2008;24:237–245.

36. Cranney A, Wells GA, Yetisir E, et al. Ibandronate for the prevention of nonvertebral fractures: a pooled analysis of individual patient data. *Osteoporos Int* 2009;20:291–297.

37. Miller PD, McClung MR, Macovei L, et al. Monthly oral ibandronate therapy in postmenopausal osteoporosis: 1-year results from the MOBILE study. *J Bone Miner Res* 2005; 20:1315–1322.

38. Reginster JY, Adami S, Lakatos P, et al. Efficacy and tolerability of once-monthly oral ibandronate in postmenopausal osteoporosis: 2 year results from the MOBILE study. *Ann Rheum Dis* 2006;65:654–661.

39. Delmas PD, Adami S, Strugala C, et al. Intravenous ibandronate injections in postmenopausal women with osteoporosis: one-year results from the dosing intravenous administration study. *Arthritis Rheum* 2006;54:1838–1846.

40. Eisman JA, Civitelli R, Adami S, et al. Efficacy and tolerability of intravenous ibandronate injections in postmenopausal osteoporosis: 2-year results from the DIVA study. *J Rheumatol* 2008;35:488–497.

41. Reid IR, Brown JP, Burckhardt P, et al. Intravenous zoledronic acid in postmenopausal women with low bone mineral density. *N Engl J Med* 2002;346:653–661.

42. Black DM, Delmas PD, Eastell R, et al.; HORIZON Pivotal Fracture Trial. Once-yearly zoledronic acid for treatment of postmenopausal osteoporosis. *N Engl J Med* 2007 May 3;356(18):1809–1822.

43. Lyles KW, Colón-Emeric CS, Magaziner JS, et al.; HORIZON Recurrent Fracture Trial. Zoledronic acid and clinical fractures and mortality after hip fracture. *N Engl J Med* 2007;357:1799–1809.

44. Ettinger B, Black DM, Mitlak BH, et al. Reduction of vertebral fracture risk in postmenopausal women with osteoporosis treated with raloxifene: results from a 3-year randomized clinical trial. Multiple Outcomes of Raloxifene Evaluation (MORE) Investigators. *JAMA* 1999;282:637–645.

45. Delmas PD, Ensrud KE, Adachi JD, et al.; Multiple Outcomes of Raloxifene Evaluation Investigators. Efficacy of raloxifene on vertebral fracture risk reduction in postmenopausal women with osteoporosis: four-year results from a randomized clinical trial. *J Clin Endocrinol Metab* 2002;87:3609–3617.

46. Siris ES, Harris ST, Eastell R, et al.; Continuing Outcomes Relevant to Evista (CORE) Investigators. Skeletal effects of raloxifene after 8 years: results from the continuing outcomes relevant to Evista (CORE) study. *J Bone Miner Res* 2005;20:1514–1524.

47. Cranney A, Tugwell P, Zytaruk N, et al.; Osteoporosis Methodology Group and The Osteoporosis Research Advisory Group. Meta-analyses of therapies for postmenopausal

osteoporosis. IV. Meta-analysis of raloxifene for the prevention and treatment of post-menopausal osteoporosis. *Endocr Rev* 2002;23:524–528.

48. Cummings SR, Eckert S, Krueger KA, et al. The effect of raloxifene on risk of breast cancer in postmenopausal women: results from the MORE randomized trial. Multiple Outcomes of Raloxifene Evaluation. *JAMA* 1999;281:2189–2197.

49. Barrett-Connor E, Mosca L, Collins P, et al.; Raloxifene Use for The Heart (RUTH) Trial Investigators. Effects of raloxifene on cardiovascular events and breast cancer in postmenopausal women. *N Engl J Med* 2006;355:125–137.

50. Martino S, Cauley JA, Barrett-Connor E, et al.; CORE Investigators. Continuing outcomes relevant to Evista: breast cancer incidence in postmenopausal osteoporotic women in a randomized trial of raloxifene. *J Natl Cancer Inst* 2004;96:1751–1761.

51. Delmas PD, Bjarnason NH, Mitlak BH, et al. Effects of raloxifene on bone mineral density, serum cholesterol concentrations, and uterine endometrium in postmenopausal women. *N Engl J Med* 1997;337:1641–1647.

52. Collins P, Mosca L, Geiger MJ, et al. Effects of the selective estrogen receptor modulator raloxifene on coronary outcomes in the Raloxifene Use for The Heart trial: results of subgroup analyses by age and other factors. *Circulation* 2009;119:922–930.

53. Grady D, Ettinger B, Moscarelli E, et al.; Multiple Outcomes of Raloxifene Evaluation Investigators. Safety and adverse effects associated with raloxifene: multiple outcomes of raloxifene evaluation. *Obstet Gynecol* 2004;104:837–844.

54. Vogel VG, Costantino JP, Wickerham DL, et al.; National Surgical Adjuvant Breast and Bowel Project (NSABP). Effects of tamoxifen vs raloxifene on the risk of developing invasive breast cancer and other disease outcomes: the NSABP Study of Tamoxifen and Raloxifene (STAR) P-2 trial. *JAMA* 2006;295:2727–2741.

55. Chesnut CH III, Silverman S, Andriano K, et al. A randomized trial of nasal spray salmon calcitonin in postmenopausal women with established osteoporosis: the prevent recurrence of osteoporotic fractures study. PROOF Study Group. *Am J Med* 2000;109:267–276.

56. Cranney A, Tugwell P, Zytaruk N, et al.; Osteoporosis Methodology Group and The Osteoporosis Research Advisory Group. Meta-analyses of therapies for postmenopausal osteoporosis. VI. Meta-analysis of calcitonin for the treatment of postmenopausal osteoporosis. *Endocr Rev* 2002;23:540–551.

57. Knopp JA, Diner BM, Blitz M, et al. Calcitonin for treating acute pain of osteoporotic vertebral compression fractures: a systematic review of randomized, controlled trials. *Osteoporos Int* 2005;16:1281–1290.

58. Greenspan SL, Bone HG, Ettinger MP, et al.; Treatment of Osteoporosis with Parathyroid Hormone Study Group. Effect of recombinant human parathyroid hormone (1–84) on vertebral fracture and bone mineral density in postmenopausal women with osteoporosis: a randomized trial. *Ann Intern Med* 2007;146:326–339.

59. Neer RM, Arnaud CD, Zanchetta JR, et al. Effect of parathyroid hormone (1–34) on fractures and bone mineral density in postmenopausal women with osteoporosis. *N Engl J Med* 2001;344:1434–1441.

60. Black DM, Bilezikian JP, Ensrud KE, et al.; PaTH Study Investigators. One year of alendronate after one year of parathyroid hormone (1–84) for osteoporosis. *N Engl J Med* 2005;353:555–565.

61. Black DM, Greenspan SL, Ensrud KE, et al.; PaTH Study Investigators. The effects of parathyroid hormone and alendronate alone or in combination in postmenopausal osteoporosis. *N Engl J Med* 2003;349:1207–1215.

62. Effects of hormone therapy on bone mineral density: results from the postmenopausal estrogen/progestin interventions (PEPI) trial. The Writing Group for the PEPI. *JAMA* 1996;276:1389–1396.

63. Cauley JA, Seeley DG, Ensrud K, et al. Estrogen replacement therapy and fractures in older women. Study of Osteoporotic Fractures Research Group. *Ann Intern Med* 1995; 122:9–16.

64. Wells G, Tugwell P, Shea B, et al.; Osteoporosis Methodology Group and The Osteoporosis Research Advisory Group. Meta-analyses of therapies for postmenopausal osteoporosis.

V. Meta-analysis of the efficacy of hormone replacement therapy in treating and preventing osteoporosis in postmenopausal women. *Endocr Rev* 2002;23:529–539.

65. Rossouw JE, Anderson GL, Prentice RL, et al.; Writing Group for the Women's Health Initiative Investigators. Risks and benefits of estrogen plus progestin in healthy postmenopausal women: principal results From the Women's Health Initiative randomized controlled trial. *JAMA* 2002;288:321–333.

66. Saag KG, Emkey R, Schnitzer TJ, et al. Alendronate for the prevention and treatment of glucocorticoid-induced osteoporosis. Glucocorticoid-Induced Osteoporosis Intervention Study Group. *N Engl J Med* 1998;339:292–299.

67. Adachi JD, Saag KG, Delmas PD, et al. Two-year effects of alendronate on bone mineral density and vertebral fracture in patients receiving glucocorticoids: a randomized, double-blind, placebo-controlled extension trial. *Arthritis Rheum* 2001;44:202–211.

68. Cohen S, Levy RM, Keller M, et al. Risedronate therapy prevents corticosteroid-induced bone loss: a twelve-month, multicenter, randomized, double-blind, placebo-controlled, parallel-group study. *Arthritis Rheum* 1999;42:2309–2318.

69. Reid DM, Hughes RA, Laan RF, et al. Efficacy and safety of daily risedronate in the treatment of corticosteroid-induced osteoporosis in men and women: a randomized trial. European Corticosteroid-Induced Osteoporosis Treatment Study. *J Bone Miner Res* 2000;15:1006–1013.

70. Mok CC, Tong KH, To CH, et al. Risedronate for prevention of bone mineral density loss in patients receiving high-dose glucocorticoids: a randomized double-blind placebo-controlled trial. *Osteoporos Int* 2008;19:357–364.

71. Reid DM, Devogelaer JP, Saag K, et al.; HORIZON investigators. Zoledronic acid and risedronate in the prevention and treatment of glucocorticoid-induced osteoporosis (HORIZON): a multicentre, double-blind, double-dummy, randomised controlled trial. *Lancet* 2009;373:1253–1263.

72. Montemurro L, Schiraldi G, Fraioli P, et al. Prevention of corticosteroid-induced osteoporosis with salmon calcitonin in sarcoid patients. *Calcif Tissue Int* 1991;49:71–76.

73. Luengo M, Pons F, Martinez de Osaba MJ, Picado C. Prevention of further bone mass loss by nasal calcitonin in patients on long term glucocorticoid therapy for asthma: a two year follow up study. *Thorax* 1994;49:1099–1102.

74. Saag KG, Shane E, Boonen S, et al. Teriparatide or alendronate in glucocorticoid-induced osteoporosis. *N Engl J Med* 2007;357:2028–2039.

75. Anderson FH, Francis RM, Faulkner K. Androgen supplementation in eugonadal men with osteoporosis-effects of 6 months of treatment on bone mineral density and cardiovascular risk factors. *Bone* 1996;18:171–177.

76. Katznelson L, Finkelstein JS, Schoenfeld DA, et al. Increase in bone density and lean body mass during testosterone administration in men with acquired hypogonadism. *J Clin Endocrinol Metab* 1996;81:4358–4365.

77. Behre HM, Kliesch S, Leifke E, et al. Long-term effect of testosterone therapy on bone mineral density in hypogonadal men. *J Clin Endocrinol Metab* 1997;82:2386–2390.

78. Sawka AM, Papaioannou A, Adachi JD, et al. Does alendronate reduce the risk of fracture in men? A meta-analysis incorporating prior knowledge of anti-fracture efficacy in women. *BMC Musculoskelet Disord* 2005;6:39.

79. Ringe JD, Faber H, Farahmand P, Dorst A. Efficacy of risedronate in men with primary and secondary osteoporosis: results of a 1-year study. *Rheumatol Int* 2006;26:427–431.

80. Ringe JD, Farahmand P, Faber H, Dorst A. Sustained efficacy of risedronate in men with primary and secondary osteoporosis: results of a 2-year study. *Rheumatol Int* 2009;29:311–315.

81. Boonen S, Orwoll ES, Wenderoth D, et al. Once-weekly risedronate in men with osteoporosis: results of a 2-year, placebo-controlled, double-blind, multicenter study. *J Bone Miner Res* 2009;24:719–725.

82. Majima T, Shimatsu A, Komatsu Y, et al. Effects of risedronate or alfacalcidol on bone mineral density, bone turnover, back pain, and fractures in Japanese men with primary osteoporosis: results of a two-year strict observational study. *J Bone Miner Metab* 2009;27:168–174.

83. Kurland ES, Cosman F, McMahon DJ, et al. Parathyroid hormone as a therapy for idiopathic osteoporosis in men: effects on bone mineral density and bone markers. *J Clin Endocrinol Metab* 2000;85:3069–3076.

84. Orwoll ES, Scheele WH, Paul S, et al. The effect of teriparatide [human parathyroid hormone (1–34)] therapy on bone density in men with osteoporosis. *J Bone Miner Res* 2003;18:9–17.

85. Finkelstein JS, Hayes A, Hunzelman JL, et al. The effects of parathyroid hormone, alendronate, or both in men with osteoporosis. *N Engl J Med* 2003;349:1216–1226.

86. Nelson HD. Menopause. *Lancet* 2008;371:760–770.

87. Bäckström T. Symptoms related to the menopause and sex steroid treatments. *Ciba Found Symp* 1995;191:171–186.

88. Maclennan AH, Broadbent JL, Lester S, Moore V. Oral oestrogen and combined oestrogen/progestogen therapy versus placebo for hot flushes. *Cochrane Database Syst Rev* 2004;(4): CD002978.

89. American College of Obstetricians and Gynecologists Women's Health Care Physicians. Vasomotor symptoms. *Obstet Gynecol* 2004;104(4 Suppl):106S–117S.

90. Hulley S, Grady D, Bush T, et al. Randomized trial of estrogen plus progestin for secondary prevention of coronary heart disease in postmenopausal women. Heart and Estrogen/progestin Replacement Study (HERS) Research Group. *JAMA* 1998;280:605–613.

91. North American Menopause Society. Estrogen and progestogen use in peri- and postmenopausal women: March 2007 position statement of The North American Menopause Society. *Menopause* 2007;14:168–182.

92. ACOG Task Force for Hormone Therapy American College of Obstetricians and Gynecologists Women's Health Care Physicians. Summary of balancing risks and benefits. *Obstet Gynecol* 2004 Oct;104(4 Suppl):128S–129S.

93. American College of Obstetricians and Gynecologists Women's Health Care Physicians. Ovarian, endometrial, and colorectal cancers. *Obstet Gynecol* 2004;104(4 Suppl):77S–84S.

94. Nelson HD, Vesco KK, Haney E, et al. Nonhormonal therapies for menopausal hot flashes: systematic review and meta-analysis. *JAMA* 2006;295:2057–2071.

95. Toulis KA, Tzellos T, Kouvelas D, Goulis DG. Gabapentin for the treatment of hot flashes in women with natural or tamoxifen-induced menopause: a systematic review and meta-analysis. *Clin Ther* 2009;31:221–235.

96. Lethaby AE, Brown J, Marjoribanks J, et al. Phytoestrogens for vasomotor menopausal symptoms. *Cochrane Database Syst Rev* 2007;(4):CD001395.

97. Krebs EE, Ensrud KE, MacDonald R, Wilt TJ. Phytoestrogens for treatment of menopausal symptoms: a systematic review. *Obstet Gynecol* 2004;104:824–836.

98. American College of Obstetricians and Gynecologists Women's Health Care Physicians. Genitourinary tract changes. *Obstet Gynecol* 2004;104(4 Suppl):56S–61S.

99. Spitzer M. Cervical screening adjuncts: recent advances. *Am J Obstet Gynecol* 1998;179: 544–556.

100. International Collaboration of Epidemiological Studies of Cervical Cancer. Cervical carcinoma and reproductive factors: collaborative reanalysis of individual data on 16,563 women with cervical carcinoma and 33,542 women without cervical carcinoma from 25 epidemiological studies. *Int J Cancer* 2006;119:1108–1124.

101. International Collaboration of Epidemiological Studies of Cervical Cancer. Cervical carcinoma and sexual behavior: collaborative reanalysis of individual data on 15,461 women with cervical carcinoma and 29,164 women without cervical carcinoma from 21 epidemiological studies. *Cancer Epidemiol Biomarkers Prev* 2009;18:1060–1069.

102. International Collaboration of Epidemiological Studies of Cervical Cancer, Appleby P, Beral V, Berrington de González A, et al. Cervical cancer and hormonal contraceptives: collaborative reanalysis of individual data for 16,573 women with cervical cancer and 35,509 women without cervical cancer from 24 epidemiological studies. *Lancet* 2007;370:1609–1621.

103. Wright TC Jr, Massad LS, Dunton CJ, et al.; 2006 American Society for Colposcopy and Cervical Pathology-sponsored Consensus Conference. 2006 consensus guidelines for the management of women with abnormal cervical cancer screening tests. *Am J Obstet Gynecol* 2007;197:346–355.

104. Hussain AN, Policarpio C, Vincent MT. Evaluating nipple discharge. *Obstet Gynecol Surv* 2006;61:278–283.

105. Centers for Disease Control and Prevention, Workowski KA, Berman SM. Sexually transmitted diseases treatment guidelines, 2006. *MMWR Recomm Rep* 2006;55:1–94.

106. Oduyebo OO, Anorlu RI, Ogunsola FT. The effects of antimicrobial therapy on bacterial vaginosis in non-pregnant women. *Cochrane Database Syst Rev* 2009;(3):CD006055.

107. Senok AC, Verstraelen H, Temmerman M, Botta GA. Probiotics for the treatment of bacterial vaginosis. *Cochrane Database Syst Rev* 2009;(4):CD006289.

108. Forna F, Gülmezoglu AM. Interventions for treating trichomoniasis in women. *Cochrane Database Syst Rev* 2003;(2):CD000218.

109. Sobel JD, Wiesenfeld HC, Martens M, et al. Maintenance fluconazole therapy for recurrent vulvovaginal candidiasis. *N Engl J Med* 2004;351:876–883.

Men's Health
Melvin Blanchard

Disorders in men's health range from benign conditions that primarily affect quality of life to life-threatening malignancies and organ-threatening emergencies. Traditionally, many of these conditions have received little attention from primary care physicians because of limited understanding and therapeutic options and a reluctance to initiate discussion on the part of both patients and physicians. Advances in pharmacologic and nonpharmacologic therapies now allow primary care physicians to provide initial treatment and urology referrals for men who fail initial therapy or have urgent indications.

PROSTATE CANCER SCREENING

General Principles

- Prostate cancer is the most common noncutaneous malignancy in older men and is the second most common cause of cancer mortality after lung cancer.
- Approximately 190,000 men will be diagnosed in 2009 and 27,000 will die from this malignancy.[1]
- The introduction of available screening tests has led to intense debate and varying societal recommendations.
  - The variable course of prostate cancer makes screening for the presence of disease a complicated decision. Some men have subclinical prostate cancer that progresses slowly and never contributes to mortality, whereas others have disease aggressive enough to cause premature death.
  - The American Cancer Society and the American Urological Society recommend screening and early detection programs for men at high risk for prostate cancer (positive family history and African American) starting as early as 40 to 45 years of age.
- Unfortunately, neither highly sensitive screening tests that detect cancers likely to be clinically significant nor highly specific tests, which identify low-grade disease not likely to cause death, are available.
- Early detection and treatment are the only ways to decrease mortality from prostate cancer since it is incurable once spread beyond the capsule.
- Screening has effectively increased the identification of organ confined and potentially curable cancer, from 30% to 70%.
  - Consequently, the 5-year survival rate for men (from the time of diagnosis) has increased from 61% to almost 100% over approximately the last 30 years.[1]
  - However, the apparent gain in survival resulting from early detection may be due to **lead-time bias,** as men who would otherwise never be diagnosed or have any sequelae of prostate cancer are having it detected earlier.
- The benefit of treatment in clinically localized prostate cancer has not been definitively proven.
  - In men with well and moderately differentiated cancers, observation alone is associated with high prostate cancer-specific survival rates.[2,3]

- The primary treatment modalities, radical prostatectomy and radiation therapy, are associated with significant rates of complications, including erectile dysfunction (ED), urinary incontinence, and urethral or rectal injury.
- Controversy persists as to whether screening for prostate cancer decreases its morbidity or mortality.
  - Two large multicenter randomized prospective clinical trials, one conducted in Europe and another in the United States reported conflicting results on this question.[4,5]
  - The European study reported a 20% decline in mortality, whereas the U.S. study found no significant difference in death rate.
  - Although these results are interim, the 9-year follow-up is significant. Future results may not settle this important question.

Screening Tests

Digital Rectal Examination

- The digital rectal examination (DRE) is a nonstandardized examination of the prostate which produces abnormalities in 3% to 12% of patients.[6]
- An **abnormal DRE** has a positive predictive value for cancer of 18% to 28%.[7]
  - However, when abnormal, it necessitates a transrectal ultrasound-guided prostate biopsy.
  - Therefore, 72% to 82% of patients with an abnormal DRE will have a prostate biopsy that is negative for malignancy.

Prostate-Specific Antigen

- Prostate-specific antigen (PSA) is a 240-amino acid serine protease secreted by prostatic epithelial cells that lyses the clotted ejaculate to enhance sperm motility.
- Some of this naturally leaks into blood and to a greater extent in prostate cancer.
- In addition, ejaculation and prostate manipulation raise PSA levels. **A routine DRE does not clinically change the results of PSA testing.**[8]
- The 5-α-reductase inhibitor, finasteride, reduces total PSA (tPSA) by about 50% in 6 to 12 months.[9]
- The positive predictive value of a total PSA (tPSA) >4.0 ng/mL is about 30% but it is a continuum, as the risk of prostate cancer increases significantly even within the normal range.[10] **The sensitivity of this cutoff is 70% to 80%, but the specificity is low,** as multiple conditions besides cancer can elevate tPSA (Table 1).

TABLE 1	Processes That Affect Prostate-Specific Antigen (PSA) Besides Prostate Cancer	
Increase PSA	**No Effect on PSA**	**Decrease PSA**
Age	α-Blocker therapy	Finasteride therapy
Benign prostatic hyperplasia	Cystoscopy	Prostate resection
Prostate biopsy	Routine digital rectal examination	
Prostatitis	Testosterone replacement	
Recent ejaculation	Urethral catheterization	
Urinary tract infection		
Vigorous prostate massage		

Prostate-Specific Antigen Velocity
- PSA velocity (PSAV), the rate of change in PSA over time, is **abnormal when it is >0.75 ng/mL/year.**
- **It increases the specificity of PSA** for identifying prostate cancer and is most reliable when three values are obtained at the same laboratory over at least 18 months.
- High PSAV, however, may be indicative of prostatitis.
- One study suggests that PSAV may be prognostic when obtained in the year before the diagnosis of prostate cancer.[11]

Free Prostate-Specific Antigen
- Percent free PSA (fPSA), the ratio of free circulating to bound PSA in serum, is **lower in men with prostate cancer than in those with benign prostatic diseases.**
- It is most useful in deciding which patients with a mildly elevated PSA (4 to 10 ng/mL) should undergo biopsy.
- An **upper cutoff of 25%** significantly decreases the number of false-positive biopsies while maintaining a high level of sensitivity.[12]
- The complexed PSA (cPSA) is also measurable but, practically, has no significant advantage over fPSA.

Prostate-Specific Antigen Density
PSA density, the PSA divided by prostate volume (measured by transrectal ultra-sound), and **age/race-specific reference ranges** either require additional cost or have less clear benefit on cancer detection rates and are **not a part of routine guidelines.**

Screening Recommendations

- **The decision as to whether to screen for prostate cancer must be individualized,** as the lack of evidence from clinical trials has led the different major societies to have very different recommendations on screening.
- See Figure 1 for a rational approach to prostate cancer screening.
- The **United States Preventive Services Task Force** (USPSTF) concludes that current evidence is insufficient to assess the balance of benefits and harms of prostate cancer screening in men <75 years of age and recommends against screening in men aged ≥75 years.
- The **American Cancer Society** recommends offering annual PSA to all men 50 years and older with a life expectancy of at least 10 years; men at high risk (African American, men with one or more first-degree relatives with prostate cancer prior to age 65) should be screened starting at age 45.
- The **American urological Association** recommends offering DRE and PSA screening to all men 50 years and older who have a life expectancy of at least 10 years.

BENIGN PROSTATIC HYPERPLASIA

General Principles

- Benign prostatic hyperplasia (BPH) is defined histologically as hypertrophy of epithelia glandular and stromal tissue.
- It is present primarily in older men with functioning testicles.
- The prevalence of BPH increases with age from 8% among men in their fourth decade of life to 80% among those >80 years of age, with lower urinary tract symptoms (LUTS) in about 25% to 45% of men >70 years of age.[13]

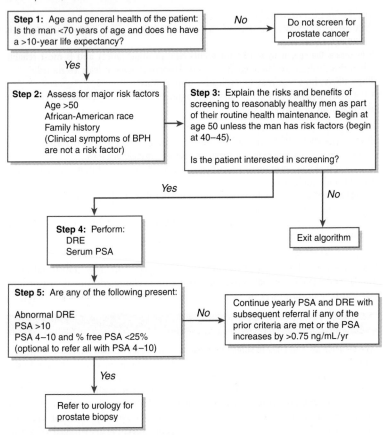

Figure 1. Prostate cancer screening algorithm. BPH, benign prostatic hyperplasia; DRE, digital rectal examination; PSA, prostate-specific antigen.

- BPH may be complicated by recurrent urinary tract infections (UTIs), urinary bladder stones, and acute urinary retention.

Diagnosis

Clinical Presentation

History

- Patients with LUTS complain of urgency, frequency, nocturia, weak stream, hesitancy, and incomplete emptying.
- The **American Urological Association Symptom Index** (AUA-SI) (Table 2), a standardized questionnaire that quantifies these symptoms, should be administered to all men with BPH.[14]
  - The AUA-SI score is used to classify symptom severity, guide treatment recommendations, and follow response to therapy.

TABLE 2	American Urological Association Symptom Index					
During the Past Month, How Often Have You . . .	Not At All	Less Than 1 Time in 5	Less Than Half the Time	Half the Time	More Than Half the Time	Almost Always
1. Had the sensation of not emptying your bladder completely after you finished urinating?	0	1	2	3	4	5
2. Had to urinate <2 hours after you finished urinating?	0	1	2	3	4	5
3. Found you stopped and started several times when you urinated?	0	1	2	3	4	5
4. Found it difficult to postpone urination?	0	1	2	3	4	5
5. Had a weak urinary stream?	0	1	2	3	4	5
6. Had to push or strain to begin urination?	0	1	2	3	4	5
7. Typically needed to get up to urinate from the time you went to bed at night until the time you got up in the morning?	None	1 (time)	2 (times)	3 (times)	4 (times)	5 (times)

0–7 points = mild symptoms.
8–19 points = moderate symptoms.
20–35 points = severe symptoms.
Modified from Barry MJ, Fowler FJ Jr, O'Leary MP, et al. The American Urological Association Symptom Index for benign prostatic hyperplasia. The Measurement Committee of the American Urological Association. *J Urol* 1992;148:1549.

- The history should also assess for sexual dysfunction; neurogenic bladder; prior urethral trauma or urethritis; diabetes; and drugs that decrease bladder function or increase tone at bladder neck (anticholinergics, sympathomimetic amines).

Physical Examination
- The prostate should be palpated for nodules and an estimation of its size.
- Men with oversized prostates are at increased risk of experiencing complications and undergoing prostate surgery.

Diagnostic Testing

Laboratories

- **Urinalysis** should be obtained to rule out infection and assess for complications (hematuria, UTI) and glycosuria.
- **Serum creatinine** should be obtained as it may indicate underlying kidney disease which could contribute to LUTS.
- **PSA testing** serves two potential purposes:
  - **Screening for prostate cancer is optional,** as its prevalence is not increased despite the fact that PSA is elevated in 25% to 30% of men with BPH.
  - **Percent free PSA** testing should be considered in men with a PSA of 4 to 10 ng/mL (see the "Prostate Cancer Screening" section).
  - **PSA is predictive of prostate size,** as PSA values of >1.6, 2.0, and 2.3 correlate with 70% sensitivity and specificity to prostates >40 mL in size in men in their 50s, 60s, and 70s, respectively.[15]

Imaging

Renal imaging (ultrasound or intravenous pyelography) should be performed in patients with complications such as hematuria, recurrent UTIs, or unexplained chronic kidney disease.

Diagnostic Procedures

Urodynamic testing (peak flow rate and pressure volume studies) should be reserved for patients with an unclear diagnosis, suspected neurogenic bladder dysfunction, or moderate to severe disease that fails to respond to initial therapy.

Treatment

- The major factors to consider in determining the choice of therapy are the man's AUA-SI score and prostate size.
- Other factors to consider are his age, concomitant hypertension, current medications, sexual history, and the degree to which his symptoms affect his quality of life.

Watchful Waiting

- Watchful waiting without treatment is **recommended for patients with mild symptoms (AUA-SI ≤7) and is an option for those with moderate symptoms who do not want to initiate lifelong medical therapy and do not have BPH complications** (urinary retention, renal insufficiency, UTI).
- Patients should minimize fluids before bedtime and avoid medications with anticholinergic or sympathomimetic properties (including antihistamines, tricyclic antidepressants, and decongestants), caffeinated beverages, and alcohol.
- Many patients with mild symptoms have no change or improve without treatment; however, there is some concern that delay in treatment may result in bladder decompensation.[16]

Medications

Pharmacologic therapy is recommended for patients with moderate symptoms who request treatment and for those with severe symptoms.

First Generation α-Blockers

- **Terazosin and doxazosin are α-1-adrenergic blockers** that relax smooth-muscle cells in the prostate and lead to an improvement of symptoms (decrease of 4 to 6 points on AUA-SI) within weeks of initiating therapy.[17]

- Symptomatic improvement is maintained with long-term therapy, but α-1-blockers do not decrease prostate size, the rate of urinary retention, the need for surgery, or PSA.
- α-1-blockers are effective in men with small and large prostates.
- These agents are possible choices for men with concomitant hypertension that requires treatment. Terazosin and doxazosin decrease blood pressure (BP) by approximately 10 to 15/10 to 15 mm Hg in men with elevated BP but have no clinically significant effect on BP in normotensive patients.[18] However, they should not be used at the expense of other drugs for overriding indications (see Chapter 3).
- Treatment is initiated at night with dose titration over 2 to 3 weeks to minimize side effects.
  - Terazosin is titrated weekly from 1 to 2 to 5 mg PO qh and can subsequently be increased to 10 to 20 mg PO qh.
  - Doxazosin is titrated from 1 to 2 to 4 mg PO qh and can be subsequently increased to 8 to 16 mg PO qh.
- Common side effects are dizziness, orthostatic hypotension, and fatigue.
- **Hypotension and orthostasis are exacerbated with concomitant use of phosphodiesterase inhibitors for ED** (e.g., sildenafil, vardenafil, tadalafil).
- The Food and Drug Administration (FDA) has posted a drug safety alert indicating that α-1-blockers increase the risk of floppy iris syndrome in patients with cataract surgery.

Second Generation α-Blockers
- **Alfuzosin, silodosin, and tamsulosin, are uroselective α-1$_a$-blockers** with pharmacologic activity that is limited to the prostate with minimal systemic effects on BP.
- They are good choices for men who want rapid symptom relief who are prone to orthostasis.
- The dose for alfuzosin is 10 mg PO daily, silodocin is 8 mg PO daily, and tamsulosin is 0.4 to 0.8 mg PO daily.
  - Dose titration and nocturnal dosing are unnecessary for these three agents.
  - The dose of silodosin should be halved for patients with a creatinine clearance of 30 to 49 mL/minute.
  - Both silodosin and alfuzosin should be avoided in patients with a creatinine clearance of <30 mL/minute.
- Common side effects of these agents are ejaculatory problems and dizziness.
- The FDA has posted a drug safety alert indicating that tamsulosin and other α_1-blockers increase the risk of floppy iris syndrome in patients with cataract surgery.

5-α-Reductase Inhibitors
- **Finasteride and dutasteride are 5-α-reductase inhibitors** (inhibit conversion of testosterone to dihydrotestosterone, reverse epithelial glandular hyperplasia, and shrink the prostate by approximately 15% to 30% within several months).
- Symptomatic improvement is sustained for long term and they are the only drug class that have been shown to decrease the rate of urinary retention and need for prostate surgery.[19–21]
- However, these agents are **effective only in men with enlarged prostates >40 mL in size.**[22]
- PSA can predict which patients are candidates for treatment with finasteride (see the "Prostate-Specific Antigen" section above).
- The **symptomatic response to these agents is delayed** for 6 to 12 months.
- The dose **for finasteride** is 5 mg PO daily and for dutasteride, it is 0.5 mg PO daily.
- The only common side effects are sexual, including ED, decreased libido, and ejaculatory dysfunction.
- After 6 months of therapy, finasteride decreases PSA by approximately 50%.

- **tPSA retains its ability to be used as a screening test for prostate cancer provided that the tPSA value is doubled.**[23]
- fPSA is unchanged by treatment.
- Questions have been raised about the safety of these agents in the Prostate Cancer Prevention trial. This 7-year study showed that, compared with placebo, finasteride reduced the risk of prostate cancer. However, participants who developed prostate cancer while on study drug were more likely to develop higher-grade cancers.

Combination Therapy
- Combination therapy with an α-1-blocker and finasteride makes theoretical sense for men with large prostates and is frequently attempted but research study results are mixed.
- It is a general practice among many to use combination therapy in symptomatic men with large prostate and monotherapy (α-1-blockers) in patients with small gland size.[24,25]

Herbal Treatment
- Several different forms of herbal therapy, including saw palmetto (*Serenoa repens*), *Pygeum africanum*, cernilton, and β-sitosterols, are available and self-prescribed by patients to treat BPH.
- These agents have been shown to be effective in the short term but their mechanism of action and long-term efficacy are unknown.[26]
- **Saw palmetto** (160 mg PO bid) is the most commonly used herb in the United States.

Surgical Management
- **Indications for referral to urology** include refractory LUTS, complications such as recurrent hematuria or recurrent UTIs, bladder stones, acute urinary retention and renal insufficiency with hydronephrosis, a rectal examination or PSA suspicious for prostate cancer, and an unclear diagnosis when urodynamic testing may be helpful.
- **Transurethral resection of the prostate (TURP),** the "gold standard" for BPH treatment, has a much greater benefit in reducing symptoms than medical therapy.
  - TURP results in retrograde ejaculation and ED in a significant percentage of patients, and approximately 20% have unsatisfactory results and require further therapy.
  - As TURP removes only central prostatic tissue, it does not eliminate the chance of developing prostate cancer.
  - Several new **minimally invasive surgical procedures** have been introduced as alternatives to TURP.

PROSTATITIS

General Principles

- Prostatitis is the most common urologic complaint among men <50 years of age.
- The prostatitis syndromes are classified by their acuity of presentation and findings on urinalysis and culture before and after prostatic massage.
  - Acute prostatitis
  - Chronic bacterial prostatitis
  - Chronic prostatitis/chronic pelvic pain syndrome
    - Inflammatory
    - Noninflammatory
  - Asymptomatic inflammation of the prostate
- **Only 5% to 10% of cases are due to bacterial causes.**[27]

Diagnosis

Acute Bacterial Prostatitis

- Patients present with symptoms of a UTI (e.g., dysuria, frequency, urgency) and systemic symptoms such as fever, malaise, and lower-abdominal or back pain.
- A gentle prostate examination might reveal an enlarged, warm, and tender prostate.
- **Vigorous massage is contraindicated** as this could cause bacteremia and sepsis.
- Urinalysis and culture are positive, most often for *Escherichia coli* or other gram-negative organisms.
- An abdominal ultrasound or CT scan to rule out a prostatic abscess should be considered if initial treatment fails.

Chronic Prostatitis Syndromes

- Patients with the three chronic prostatitis syndromes present with similar symptoms, classically a triad of recurrent voiding symptoms, pain (pelvic, perineal, inguinal, back, penile, or scrotal), and ejaculatory symptoms (pain, hematospermia).
- Patients with **chronic bacterial prostatitis** are usually older, frequently have recurrent UTIs with the same organism, and may have a history of acute prostatitis.
- Patients with the two **chronic nonbacterial prostatitis syndromes** are often younger and do not have a history of recurrent UTIs.
  - The predominant pain and predilection to occur in younger men distinguish it from BPH.
  - Chronic nonbacterial prostatitis is the most common urologic diagnosis in men <50 years of age.
- The prostate examination is often normal in men with each of the chronic prostatitis syndromes. A **diagnostic prostate massage** comparing a midstream urine specimen (the second 10 mL of urine voided) with one after a vigorous prostate massage is the test of choice to correctly diagnose the three syndromes (Table 3).

Treatment

Acute Prostatitis

- Patients should be initially treated with broad-spectrum parenteral antibiotics followed by oral agents if they respond.
  - Potential oral regimens include trimethoprim-sulfamethoxazole, 1 DS tablet PO bid; doxycycline, 100 mg PO bid; ciprofloxacin, 500 mg PO bid; or levofloxacin, 500 mg PO daily for 4 to 6 weeks.
  - Severely ill patients with suspected bacteremia require admission for IV antibiotics.
- Supportive care with analgesics, stool softeners, and vigorous oral hydration may be beneficial.
- Because of the relatively high risk for urinary retention, bladder scanning should be done to assess the postvoid residual. For patients who require short-term drainage, a small urethral catheter may be sufficient; those who require long-term drainage will need a suprapubic catheter.

Chronic Prostatitis Syndromes

- **Prolonged courses of antibiotics** (4 to 6 weeks), preferably with a fluoroquinolone (has excellent prostate penetration), are recommended.

TABLE 3	Diagnostic Prostate Massage Results		
Type of Prostatitis	Prostate Examination	Postmassage Urinalysis	Postmassage Culture
Acute bacterial (5%)	Warm, boggy, enlarged, tender	Vigorous massage contraindicated	Vigorous massage contraindicated
Chronic bacterial (5%–10%)	Can be mildly tender and boggy or can be normal	Positive[a]	Positive[b]
Inflammatory chronic nonbacterial (50%–60%)	Usually normal	Positive[a]	Negative
Noninflammatory chronic nonbacterial (prostatodynia) (30%–40%)	Usually normal	Negative	Negative

[a]A positive urinalysis is >10 to 15 WBCs/high-power field.
[b]A positive culture has a colony count that is at least 10-fold greater than the premassage culture.

- **α-1-adrenergic blockers** (see the "Benign Prostatic Hyperplasia" section above) may provide additional symptomatic relief.
- Patients' recurrences require retreatment.
- **Treatment of both types of chronic nonbacterial prostatitis is difficult** and often prolonged. Recommendations are based primarily on clinical experience, as controlled trial data are limited.[28]
  - Patients with **inflammatory chronic nonbacterial prostatitis** should receive a trial of 4 to 6 weeks of antibiotics (doxycycline, erythromycin, or a fluoroquinolone), with continuation for 12 weeks if improvement occurs because of anecdotal evidence that links the syndrome to atypical pathogens. Repetitive prostate massage two to three times per week, α-1-adrenergic blockers, nonsteroidal anti-inflammatory drugs, and lifestyle changes (e.g., minimizing spicy foods, alcohol, and caffeine) may all be helpful.
  - Treatment options for **noninflammatory chronic nonbacterial prostatitis** (prostatodynia) include α-1-adrenergic blockers, nonsteroidal anti-inflammatory drugs, "muscle relaxants" such as diazepam, and anticholinergic agents.[29]

ERECTILE DYSFUNCTION

General Principles

- ED is the **consistent** inability to attain or maintain an erection that is satisfactory for successful intercourse.[30]
- The prevalence increases with advancing age and the impact on quality of life is substantial.[31]

TABLE 4	Common Risk Factors for Erectile Dysfunction
Category	**Examples**
Vascular disease	Coronary artery disease, diabetes, hyperlipidemia, hypertension, peripheral vascular disease
Neurologic disorders	Multiple sclerosis, Parkinson disease, spinal cord injury, stroke
Endocrine disorders	Hyperprolactinemia, hyperthyroidism, hypothyroidism, primary hypogonadism (testicular), secondary hypogonadism (CNS)
Chronic medical disorders	Chronic renal insufficiency, cirrhosis, COPD
Psychogenic	Anxiety disorder, depression, marital/relationship discord
Urologic disorders	Advanced prostate cancer, colorectal, bladder, or prostate surgery, pelvic trauma/fracture, Peyronie disease, radiation therapy
Medications	Antihypertensives (especially thiazide diuretics, beta-blockers, clonidine), psychiatric medications (anticholinergics, MAO inhibitors, phenothiazines, SSRIs, TCAs), antiandrogens (cimetidine, digoxin, estrogens, finasteride, ketoconazole, LHRH agonists, spironolactone)
Illicit substances	Alcohol, amphetamines, cocaine, marijuana, opiates, tobacco

CNS, central nervous system; COPD, chronic obstructive pulmonary disease; LHRH, luteinizing hormone-releasing hormone; MAO, monoamine oxidase; SSRIs, selective serotonin reuptake inhibitors; TCAs, tricyclic antidepressants.

- Many men are embarrassed to raise the subject, so it is important that primary care physicians initiate the subject with their patients.
- The risk factors for ED are presented in Table 4.

Diagnosis

Clinical Presentation

History
- A detailed **sexual history** should assess the severity, onset, duration, progression, and situational nature of the problem to confirm that the patient has erectile failure and not a problem with libido or ejaculation.
  - A gradual progressive onset of ED with absence of nocturnal or morning erections suggests an **underlying medical cause.**
- ED that develops suddenly is likely either **psychogenic** or due to a **medication.**
- **Risk factors** for ED should be reviewed (Table 4).
- The **potential cardiovascular risk of intercourse** to the patient should be assessed, given the strong association between ED and coronary artery disease.
  - Patients who can safely exercise to a level of five metabolic equivalents (see Chapter 2, Table 3) are at low risk for coronary ischemia during intercourse.

- Stress testing should be considered, before the initiation of therapy or resumption of intercourse, in sedentary men with multiple cardiac risk factors who cannot safely exercise to this level.[32]

Physical Examination

The physical examination should assess for evidence of vascular or neurologic disease, stigmata of hypogonadism (small testicles, gynecomastia), prostate abnormality (with DRE), and penile anatomic abnormalities (Peyronie disease).

Diagnostic Testing

- **Routine laboratory evaluation** should include serum glucose, renal function, complete blood count, and lipid analysis.
- A **PSA** should be considered if testosterone therapy needs to be initiated.
- Thyroid-stimulating hormone and liver function tests should be performed if the initial history or physical examination is suggestive of thyroid or liver disease.
- **Routine testosterone assessment in patients with ED is controversial.**
  - Hypogonadism is the cause of ED in 5% to 10% of patients but only approximately one third of these patients improve with testosterone replacement.[33]
  - Testing with morning total and free serum testosterone is initially recommended only for patients with low libido or evidence of hypogonadism.
  - Testing should otherwise be deferred until patients have failed oral pharmacologic therapy.
  - Abnormal initial testosterone levels should be repeated for confirmation along with serum luteinizing hormone (LH), follicle-stimulating hormone (FSH), and prolactin to determine the source of hypogonadism.
- **Urologic testing** with nocturnal penile tumescence or vascular studies is unnecessary in the primary care setting.

Treatment

- In 80% to 90% of men, erectile function should be able to be restored with some form of therapy.
- Attempts should be made to **improve uncontrolled risk factors,** such as diabetes and hypertension, and to decrease the use of tobacco, alcohol, and other illicit substances.
- If possible, **potentially contributing medications** should be stopped or have their doses decreased.
- **Reassurance** may be curative in young men with psychogenic ED. Referral to a psychologist for **marital or couples counseling** may be helpful as an adjunctive form of therapy for psychogenic ED that has failed to respond to oral pharmacologic therapy.

Medicines

Phosphodiesterase Inhibitors
- Phosphodiesterase inhibitors include sildenafil, tadalafil, and vardenafil (see Table 5).
- These agents selectively inhibit PDE5, which is found in high concentrations within the corpus cavernosum, and are the treatment of choice for ED.
- They require sexual stimulation to precipitate an erection and are **effective in all forms of organic and psychogenic ED** but response rates are lower in patients with complete ED, diabetes, and after radical prostatectomy.[34]
- They do not increase libido.

TABLE 5	Phosphodiesterase Inhibitors for Erectile Dysfunction

Drug	Onset (Duration) of Action	Dose Range	Food Interaction	Comments
Vardenafil	1 hour (4 hours)	5 mg, 10 mg, 20 mg Dose adjustment not required for renal impairment. Not studied in dialysis patients.	May take with or without food.	Prolongs QT interval. Should not be prescribed to patients with congenital long QT syndrome or those taking antiarrhythmics (amiodarone, sotalol, procainamide, or quinidine)
Sildenafil	1 hour (4 hours)	25 mg, 50 mg, 100 mg Start with 25 mg if CrCl <30 mL/min or liver dysfunction	High fat Grapefruit juice may increase drug levels and toxicity	
Tadalafil	1 hour (36 hours)	2.5 mg, 10 mg, 20 mg 2.5 mg used in once daily dosing Dosing adjustment required when creatinine clearance ≤50 mL/min or hepatic dysfunction.	Grapefruit juice may increase drug levels and toxicity	

- **The three agents available are thought to have similar efficacy** (no head-to-head trials yet done).
- Side effects include headaches, flushing, dyspepsia, visual disturbance, rhinitis, priapism, and dizziness.
- Patients with symptoms of cardiac disease should be referred for cardiac evaluation before initiation of these agents.
- The PDE5 inhibitors **potentiate the effect of nitrates** causing severe and refractory hypotension, so the combination of these agents with nitrates in any form (oral, transdermal, IV) is **absolutely contraindicated.**[35]
- The combination **with α-1-adrenergic blockers can also cause orthostatic hypotension** and even severe hypotension. Alcohol potentiates the hypotensive effects of these agents.
- They are metabolized in the liver by cytochrome P450 CYP3A4 and thus, caution must be exercised when prescribing with inhibitors such as ketoconazole, itraconazole, protease inhibitors, and cimetidine.

Testosterone Replacement

- **Testosterone replacement is only indicated for patients with documented hypogonadism.**
- Currently, there are no oral preparations of testosterone sold in the United States.
- Since prostate cancer is hormone sensitive, before initiating testosterone, it is necessary to ensure that the patient does not have prostate cancer. After starting testosterone replacement, PSA, prostate examination, testosterone levels, liver function tests, and cholesterol should be monitored.
- **Intramuscular injections of testosterone enanthate** or **testosterone cypionate** are initiated at dosages of 150 to 200 mg IM every 2 to 3 weeks.
- **Testosterone patches** provide physiologic doses of hormone replacement. **Androderm,** 2.5 to 7.5 mg, is applied daily to clean, dry, non–hair-bearing areas.
- **Two testosterone gels are available (AndroGel and Testim).** They are applied to clean, dry skin via metered-dose device in a dosage range of 5 to 10 g/day.
- **One buccal form of testosterone is available (Striant).** It is dosed as 30 mg every 12 hours, applied to the gum area above the upper incisors.

Other Treatment

- More invasive nonsurgical treatment options include **intracorporeal and intraurethral injections of alprostadil and external vacuum constriction devices.**
- Intracorporeal injections and vacuum devices are very effective but suffer from high dropout rates.
- These forms of therapy should be deferred to a urologist unless the primary care physician has undergone appropriate training in the administration of these modalities, which require significant office-based patient education and training.

Referral

- Indications for referral to urology include a history of pelvic trauma, abnormal genital examination, contraindications to or intolerable side effects from oral pharmacologic therapy, and failure of oral therapy in patients who wish to try a more invasive modality.
- Priapism is an indication for an emergent urology consult.

TESTICULAR MASSES

General Principles

- Patients with testicular masses may present with a painless lump or scrotal discomfort, ranging from a dull ache that worsens with exercise to severe testicular pain.
- **Benign causes** include fluid collections, infection (e.g., acute orchitis, focal or subacute orchitis, or postinflammatory scarring), infarction (idiopathic or secondary to torsion), and cysts.
  - A **hydrocele** is a collection of peritoneal fluid between the parietal and visceral layers of the tunica vaginalis, a potential space surrounding the testicle. A communicating hydrocele allows peritoneal fluid to pass between the peritoneal cavity and the layers of the tunica vaginalis. A noncommunicating hydrocele represents an imbalance in the secretory and absorptive capacities of the layers of the tunica vaginalis. This is most often due to injury or infection with resultant inflammatory reaction. A hydrocele may also accompany a testicular neoplasm or torsion.

- A **varicocele** is an abnormal tortuosity and dilation of the pampiniform venous plexus and internal spermatic vein. Varicoceles are found in 20% of men and are usually asymptomatic. It constitutes the most common surgically correctable cause of male factor infertility (30% of infertile men).
- A **spermatocele** is a painless cystic mass separate from the testis (<2 cm, this is called an epididymal cyst).
- **Malignant causes** include primary testicular cancer and extratesticular malignancies such as leukemia or lymphoma.
  - **Testicular cancer** accounts for only 1% of all cancers in men but is the most common cancer in men 15 to 34 years of age.
  - A significantly increased number of testicular cancers are found in patients with cryptorchidism, with neoplasms developing in the undescended and the contralateral descended testis.[36–38]
  - **Lymphomas and leukemia are the most common extratesticular malignancies to involve the testicles.** Lymphoma accounts for 1% to 7% of all testicular tumors and is a frequent cause of testicular enlargement in men >50 years of age. Involvement is bilateral in 50% of cases either simultaneously or successively. Leukemic infiltration (50% have bilateral involvement) is usually seen in children, and the testis is the most common site of relapse of acute leukemia.

Diagnosis

Clinical Presentation

History

- Men with **hydrocele** present with a painless scrotal swelling that can be transilluminated. The swelling may be small and soft on awakening but worsens during the day, becoming large and tense.
- Most **varicoceles** occur on the left side as the left testicular vein drains into the left renal vein, whereas the right testicular vein drains directly into the large inferior vena cava. Patients generally report a mass that lies posterior to and above the testis. The sudden onset of a left-sided varicocele in an elderly man may be indicative of a renal cell carcinoma and should be evaluated with a renal ultrasound. Sudden development of a right-sided varicocele may occur with inferior vena cava obstruction. The venous dilation is commonly decreased when the patient is supine and increases when he is upright.
- A painless testicular mass is suggestive of a **primary testicular tumor** but occurs only in a minority of patients. Most present with diffuse testicular pain, swelling, hardness, or some combination of these findings.

Physical Examination

- **The testes** should be palpated for masses, volume, tenderness, and cryptorchidism.
- A testicle that is <4 cm long is considered small.
- All masses and swellings should be **transilluminated.**
  - Solid tumors do not transmit light, whereas a **hydrocele** glows a soft red color.
- If a testicle cannot be palpated within the scrotum, the inguinal canals and lower abdomen should be examined.
- **The epididymis, spermatic cord, and vas deferens** are examined next.
  - The epididymis is located posterior to the testicle.
  - Have the patient perform the Valsalva maneuver while standing.
  - Palpate for a mass of dilated testicular veins in the spermatic cord, forming a varicocele above and behind the testis.

- The **inguinal canals** should be explored for hernias or cord tenderness. Inflammation of the cord structures can cause inguinal or scrotal pain, with a normal testis.
- Classically, a **varicocele** feels like a "bag of worms" above the testicle. Examine the patient in both positions. Have him perform the Valsalva maneuver when standing, which accentuates the dilation.
- **Spermatoceles** are typically located superior and posterior to the testis, freely movable, and **transilluminate** easily. Aspiration of the contents usually reveals dead sperm.
- Evaluate men for the presence of **gynecomastia**, as 30% of Leydig cell tumors produce testosterone, which is converted to estrogen.
- Rarely, testicular tumors present with disseminated disease, such as supraclavicular lymphadenopathy or abdominal masses from retroperitoneal lymph node spread or as a result of a tumor that arises within an undescended intra-abdominal testis.

Diagnostic Testing

Laboratories

The following **tumor markers** may be useful in supporting a diagnosis of primary testicular cancer.

- **α-Fetoprotein** is produced by nonseminomatous germ cell tumors (embryonal carcinomas and yolk sac tumors). An elevated α-fetoprotein may be seen at any stage, although 40% to 60% of patients with metastases have increased serum concentrations.
- **β-Human chorionic gonadotropin** is increased in seminomatous and nonseminomatous tumors. Elevations occur in 40% to 60% of patients with metastatic nonseminomatous germ cell tumors and 15% to 20% of patients with metastatic seminomas.
- **Lactic dehydrogenase** elevation is nonspecific but has prognostic value in patients with advanced germ cell tumors. It is increased in 60% of patients with nonseminomatous germ cell tumors and 80% of those with seminomatous germ cell tumors.

Imaging

- Testicular **ultrasound** is a highly reliable way of differentiating intratesticular from extratesticular lesions and should be the initial imaging study of choice.
- Gray-scale sonography of lymphomatous and leukemic testicular involvement reveals diffuse or multifocal decreased echogenicity, which can be more subtle and ill defined than the typical well-circumscribed hypoechoic mass of primary testicular cancer.
- Germ cell tumors are typically intratesticular and may produce one or more hypoechoic masses or show diffuse abnormalities with microcalcifications.
- **CT scans and MRI** of malignancy demonstrate a mass that is relatively isointense to the surrounding normal testicular parenchyma on T1-weighted images and exhibits brisk and early enhancement after IV gadolinium.

Treatment

Benign Masses

Hydrocele

- Management of hydrocele may require aspiration of the fluid (by a urologist) to be able to palpate the testis carefully.
- A scrotal ultrasound should always be considered if the diagnosis is in question, as a reactive hydrocele may occur with a testicular neoplasm.

- Generally, no therapy is needed except in the setting of either discomfort from a bulky mass or a tense hydrocele, which decreases circulation to the testis.
- Tense or uncomfortable hydroceles should always be aspirated.

Varicocele
- Not all varicoceles are associated with infertility, and not all need to be corrected.
- If the patient has an abnormal semen analysis and is infertile or if the patient is symptomatic with a dull ache or feeling of heaviness in the testicle, the varicocele should be treated.
- Therapy consists of surgical ligation or sclerotherapy of the pampiniform plexus.

Malignant Masses
- Management of suspicious masses should be with urologic consultation.
- For lesions that are likely malignant, a radical orchiectomy with ligation of the spermatic cord at the internal ring is required.
- The primary lymphatic and vascular drainage of the testis is to the retroperitoneal lymph nodes and the renal or great vessels, respectively. Therefore, direct testicular biopsy through the scrotum is contraindicated.
- The staging workup includes CT scans of the abdomen and pelvis and a chest x-ray.

PRIAPISM

- Priapism is a prolonged (>6 hours), usually painful, erection that is not initiated by sexual stimuli. It results from a disturbance in the normal regulatory mechanisms that initiate and maintain penile flaccidity.
- **Low-flow, or ischemic, priapism** is due to decreased penile venous outflow.
  - The etiology includes sickle cell disorders, tumor infiltrates, and oral or injected medications.
  - It can also be idiopathic.
- **High-flow, or arterial, priapism** produces painless, persistent semirigid to rigid erections that may still increase in tumescence in response to sexual stimuli.
  - It results from increased arterial inflow into the cavernous sinusoids, which overwhelms venous outflow.
  - The etiology is usually groin or straddle trauma that causes injury to the internal pudendal artery or its branches. This establishes a direct arterial-to-cavernous shunt that bypasses the normally regulatory helicine arteries.
- Patients with priapism should be **emergently managed in consultation with a urologist.** Evaluation may include blood gas assessment of cavernosal aspitate.
- Therapeutic options range from aspiration to embolization and surgical intervention.[39]

ANDROGENETIC ALOPECIA

General Principles

- Androgenetic alopecia is a hereditary thinning of the hair that is induced by androgens in genetically susceptible men.
- It is also known as **male pattern hair loss** or **common baldness.**
- Thinning of the hair usually begins between 12 and 40 years of age, and approximately half the population expresses this trait to some degree before the age of 50 years.

- The pattern of inheritance is polygenic.
- The onset is gradual, and the condition slowly develops over years.
- It is important to rule out other causes of alopecia, such as has hypo- or hyperthyroidism, iron deficiency, acute illness, and effects of drugs such as anticonvulsants.

Treatment

Topical Minoxidil

- Topical minoxidil, a potassium channel agonist and vasodilator, is able to increase survival time and delay senescence of cultured keratinocytes in vitro.
- After topical application, minoxidil increases the duration of the anagen phase, leading to production of hairs that are progressively thicker and longer.
- Minoxidil lotion 2% or 5%, 1 mL should be applied twice per day to the affected scalp. Twice-daily application has no significant systemic side effects.
- The percentage of patients who show cosmetically acceptable hair regrowth after 1 year ranges from 40 to 60, depending on patient selection.
- Adverse effects include allergic contact dermatitis and reversible hypertrichosis.

Finasteride

- Oral finasteride, 1 mg/day, is also FDA approved for androgenic alopecia.
- It decreases dihydrotestosterone levels in scalp and blood by 60%.
- This drug is also used to treat BPH, but at a dose of 5 mg/day.
- Effects on testosterone, PSA, and libido are minimal at the dose for alopecia compared with those seen at the higher dose.[40-43]

Other Treatments

- **Surgical options** including hair transplantation, scalp flaps, and excision of bald scalp with or without tissue expansion are options to treat advanced androgenetic alopecia.

REFERENCES

1. Jemal A, Siegel R, Ward E, et al. Cancer statistics, 2009. *CA Cancer J Clin* 2009; 59:225–249.
2. Chodak GW, Thisted RA, Gerber GS, et al. Results of conservative management of clinically localized prostate cancer. *N Engl J Med* 1994;330:242–248.
3. Thompson I, Thrasher JB, Aus G, et al. Guideline for the management of clinically localized prostate cancer: 2007 update. *J Urol* 2007;177:2106–2131.
4. Schröder FH, Hugosson J, Roobol MJ, et al. Screening and prostate-cancer mortality in a randomized European study. *N Engl J Med* 2009;360:1320–1328.
5. Andriole GL, Crawford ED, Grubb RL III, et al. Mortality results from a randomized prostate-cancer screening trial. *N Engl J Med* 2009;360:1310–1319.
6. Thompson IM, Ankerst DP. Prostate-specific antigen in the early detection of prostate cancer. *CMAJ* 2007;176:1853–1858.
7. Wilbur J. Prostate cancer screening: the continuing controversy. *Am Fam Physician* 2008;78:1338.
8. Crawford ED, Schutz MJ, Clejan S, et al. The effect of digital rectal examination on prostate-specific antigen levels. *JAMA* 1992;267:2227–2228.
9. Roehrborn CG, Marks LS, Fenter T, et al. Efficacy and safety of dutasteride in the four-year treatment of men with benign prostatic hyperplasia. *Urology* 2004;63:709–715.
10. Gann PH, Hennekens CH, Stampfer MJ. A prospective evaluation of plasma prostate-specific antigen for detection of prostatic cancer. *JAMA* 1995;273:289–294.

11. D'Amico AV, Chen MH, Roehl KA, Catalona WJ. Preoperative PSA velocity and the risk of death from prostate cancer after radical prostatectomy. *N Engl J Med* 2004;351:125–135.

12. Lee R, Localio AR, Armstrong K, et al. A meta-analysis of the performance characteristics of the free prostate-specific antigen test. *Urology* 2006;67:762–768.

13. Guess HA, Arrighi HM, Metter EJ, Fozard JL. Cumulative prevalence of prostatism matches the autopsy prevalence of benign prostatic hyperplasia. *Prostate* 1990;17:241–246.

14. Barry MJ, Fowler FJ Jr, O'Leary MP, et al. The American Urological Association Symptom Index for benign prostatic hyperplasia. The Measurement Committee of the American Urological Association. *J Urol* 1992;148:1549.

15. Roehrborn CG, Boyle P, Gould AL, Waldstreicher J. Serum prostate-specific antigen as a predictor of prostate volume in men with benign prostatic hyperplasia. *Urology* 1999;53:581–589.

16. Flanigan RC, Reda DJ, Wasson JH, et al. 5-year outcome of surgical resection and watchful waiting for men with moderately symptomatic benign prostatic hyperplasia: a Department of Veterans Affairs cooperative study. *J Urol* 1998;160:12–16.

17. AUA Practice Guidelines Committee. AUA guideline on management of benign prostatic hyperplasia (2003). Chapter 1: diagnosis and treatment recommendations. *J Urol* 2003; 170(2 Pt 1):530–547.

18. Lepor H, Kaplan SA, Klimberg I, et al. Doxazosin for benign prostatic hyperplasia: long-term efficacy and safety in hypertensive and normotensive patients. The Multicenter Study Group. *J Urol* 1997;157:525–530.

19. Thorpe A, Neal D. Benign prostatic hyperplasia. *Lancet* 2003;361:1359–1367.

20. McConnell JD, Bruskewitz R, Walsh P, et al. The effect of finasteride on the risk of acute urinary retention and the need for surgical treatment among men with benign prostatic hyperplasia. Finasteride Long-Term Efficacy and Safety Study Group. *N Engl J Med* 1998;338:557–563.

21. Roehrborn CG, Boyle P, Nickel JC, et al. Efficacy and safety of a dual inhibitor of 5-alpha-reductase types 1 and 2 (dutasteride) in men with benign prostatic hyperplasia. *Urology* 2002;60:434–441.

22. Lepor H, Williford WO, Barry MJ, et al. The impact of medical therapy on bother due to symptoms, quality of life and global outcome, and factors predicting response. Veterans Affairs Cooperative Studies Benign Prostatic Hyperplasia Study Group. *J Urol* 1998;160:1358–1367.

23. Andriole GL, Guess HA, Epstein JI, et al. Treatment with finasteride preserves usefulness of prostate-specific antigen in the detection of prostate cancer: results of a randomized, double-blind, placebo-controlled clinical trial. PLESS Study Group. Proscar Long-term Efficacy and Safety Study. *Urology* 1998;52:195–201.

24. Lepor H, Williford WO, Barry MJ, et al. The efficacy of terazosin, finasteride, or both in benign prostatic hyperplasia. Veterans Affairs Cooperative Studies Benign Prostatic Hyperplasia Study Group. *N Engl J Med* 1996;335:533–539.

25. McConnell JD, Roehrborn CG, Bautista OM, et al. The long-term effect of doxazosin, finasteride, and combination therapy on the clinical progression of benign prostatic hyperplasia. *N Engl J Med* 2003;349:2387–2398.

26. Wilt TJ, Ishani A, Stark G, et al. Saw palmetto extracts for treatment of benign prostatic hyperplasia: a systematic review. *JAMA* 1998;280:1604–1609.

27. Benway BM, Moon TD. Bacterial prostatitis. *Urol Clin North Am* 2008;35:23–32.

28. McNaughton Collins M, MacDonald R, Wilt TJ. Diagnosis and treatment of chronic abacterial prostatitis: a systematic review. *Ann Intern Med* 2000;133:367–381.

29. Pontari MA. Chronic prostatitis/chronic pelvic pain syndrome. *Urol Clin North Am* 2008; 35:81–89.

30. NIH Consensus Conference. Impotence. NIH Consensus Development Panel on Impotence. *JAMA* 1993;270:83–90.

31. Feldman HA, Goldstein I, Hatzichristou DG, et al. Impotence and its medical and psychosocial correlates: results of the Massachusetts Male Aging Study. *J Urol* 1994;151:54–61.

32. Cheitlin MD, Hutter AM Jr, Brindis RG, et al. Use of sildenafil (Viagra) in patients with cardiovascular disease. Technology and Practice Executive Committee. *Circulation* 1999;99: 168–177.

33. Buvat J, Lemaire A. Endocrine screening in 1,022 men with erectile dysfunction: clinical significance and cost-effective strategy. *J Urol* 1997;158:1764–1767.

34. Cohan P, Korenman SG. Erectile dysfunction. *J Clin Endocrinol Metab* 2001;86:2391–2394.

35. Webb DJ, Freestone S, Allen MJ, Muirhead GJ. Sildenafil citrate and blood-pressure-lowering drugs: results of drug interaction studies with an organic nitrate and a calcium antagonist. *Am J Cardiol* 1999;83:21C–28C.

36. Bosl GJ, Motzer RJ. Testicular germ-cell cancer. *N Engl J Med* 1997;337:242–253.

37. Shaw J. Diagnosis and treatment of testicular cancer. *Am Fam Physician* 2008;77:469–474.

38. Tiemstra JD, Kapoor S. Evaluation of scrotal masses. *Am Fam Physician* 2008;78:1165–1170.

39. Burnett AL, Bivalacqua TJ. Priapism: current principles and practice. *Urol Clin North Am* 2007;34:631–642, viii.

40. Sinclair R. Male pattern androgenetic alopecia. *BMJ* 1998;317:865–869.

41. Price VH. Treatment of hair loss. *N Engl J Med* 1999;341:964–973.

42. Kaufman KD, Olsen EA, Whiting D, et al. Finasteride in the treatment of men with androgenetic alopecia. Finasteride Male Pattern Hair Loss Study Group. *J Am Acad Dermatol* 1998;39:578–589.

43. Otberg N, Finner AM, Shapiro J. Androgenetic alopecia. *Endocrinol Metab Clin North Am* 2007;36:379–398.

Dermatology
Ilana Rosman, Brendan Lloyd, and Omar Jassim

GENERAL OVERVIEW

- Compromise to the skin and its functions can lead to disfigurement, discomfort, and disability. In the United States, one in three people develops a skin problem each year. Of outpatient visits to physicians, 10% are for a skin disorder, and two thirds of these visits are to nondermatologists. Skin disease accounts for 5% of inpatient admissions. Skin findings are valuable diagnostic and prognostic markers of internal disease that may precede other signs.
- Skin disorders can cause significant psychological and emotional distress. Support foundations for patients with skin disorders can be accessed through the American Academy of Dermatology (866-503-7546 or http://www.aad.org).
- Skin cancer is the most common type of cancer. The American Cancer Society recommends that everyone practice monthly skin checks and have regular total body skin examinations performed by a physician every 3 years from age 20 to 40 and yearly after age 40 (http://cancer.org).

Dermatologic History and Physical Examination

Elements of the Clinical Dermatologic History
The elements of the dermatologic history are presented in Table 1.

Medical History
- Certain conditions may predispose to or may be associated with skin disease. These include the following:
  - Autoimmune disease (lupus, dermatomyositis, etc.).
  - Endocrinopathy (e.g., diabetes mellitus, thyroid disease).
  - Hepatic dysfunction.
  - Genetic disorders (neurofibromatosis, Down syndrome, etc.).
  - Immunosuppression (HIV/AIDS, transplant recipients, etc.).
  - Malignancy.
  - Renal dysfunction.

Medications
Systemic medications (especially new medication and antibiotics, antihypertensives, and antiepileptics), herbal supplements, and topical medication should be noted.

Family History
Primary skin diseases such as psoriasis, eczema, and skin cancer should be noted. Family history of autoimmune disorders or allergies may also be important.

TABLE 1	Elements of the Dermatologic History

Subjective skin complaints
Pruritus
Pain
Crusting
Discharge
Redness
Scaling

Timing
Acute (hours)
Subacute (days)
Chronic (weeks to months)

Severity
Transient vs. constant
Subjective rating of discomfort

Constitutional symptoms
Fevers
Abdominal pain
Weakness

Prior skin history
Trauma
Previous surgery
Allergic reactions
Skin cancer

Prior treatment
Topical preparations
Antihistamines
Steroids
UV light treatment

Social History
Occupational exposures, living conditions, and sexual history can be contributory.

Physical Examination

Skin Examination
- Ask your patient to disrobe and put on a gown. Very few patients are embarrassed or bothered by this, and most people expect to put on a gown when they go to the physician.
- Examine the entire skin surface as well as the palms and soles, genitals, oropharynx, and eyes. If there is a concern for or history of melanoma, examine the neck, axillae, and groin for lymphadenopathy.
- If a lesion is identified, classify it (Table 2).

TABLE 2	Classification of Lesions

Primary lesions are induced by disease

Macule	<1-cm area of circumscribed color change, not palpable
Patch	>1-cm macule
Papule	<1-cm palpable mass
Plaque	>1-cm papule
Nodule	>1-cm spherical papule
Vesicle	<1-cm fluid-filled papule
Bulla	>1-cm fluid-filled papule
Pustule	Pus-filled papule
Wheal	Edematous papule or plaque

Secondary lesions are induced by the patient

Excoriation	Linear erosions
Lichenification	Skin thickening, hyperpigmentation, and accentuated skin markings

Dermatologic Therapies

Skin disorders are characterized by pruritus, inflammation, alterations in hydration, and susceptibility to irritation. Identification and treatment of specific underlying conditions should always be attempted.

Dry Skin Care

Almost all itchy skin conditions are improved by the following regimen:
- Take short, cool baths or showers (<5 minutes).
- Use mild, nondrying soaps, including Dove, Oil of Olay, and Cetaphil. Use of washcloths and loofahs should be discouraged. Limiting the use of soap to the axilla and groin may be necessary.
- After bathing, pat dry and apply thick moisturizers such as Vaseline or Aquaphor ointments, Eucerin or Cetaphil creams, or Aveeno or Lubriderm lotions. These should be applied while the skin is still damp. Apply moisturizers as often as needed.
- Apply any prescribed medications as directed.

Wet Skin Care

Excessive moisture in intertriginous areas can lead to infection. Prevent as follows:
- Dry the area and apply powder or dry dressing of absorptive material.
- In severe cases with maceration, exudation, and erosion, apply drying dressings.
- Separate skin surfaces with absorptive materials.

Antipruritics

- Pruritus and burning can lead to uncontrolled scratching and can perpetuate an underlying condition.
- Topical agents can be used to control symptoms.
  - Camphor 1% to 3% and menthol provide a cooling sensation and should be stored in the refrigerator.
  - Phenol 0.25% to 2.00% causes local hypoesthesia but should not be used on raw or ulcerated skin.
  - Topical anesthetics (benzocaine), antihistamines (diphenhydramine), and neomycin are best avoided because of a high rate of contact dermatitis.
- Systemic antihistamines (H_1-receptor antagonists) are most useful in the treatment of urticaria, but are also helpful in pruritic skin disorders due to their sedative effect.

Protection

- Cotton and rubber gloves can be used to avoid excessive contact with water or chemical irritants. Cotton absorbs palmar sweat and should be cleaned or changed frequently.
- Barrier creams and ointments may prevent contact of irritating chemicals with sensitive skin, but are not substitutes for mechanical barriers.

Topical Steroids

- Topical steroids are first-line therapy for many dermatologic conditions (Table 3). However, they can have significant side effects. Topical steroids can cause skin atrophy, striae, acne, infection, and suppression of the pituitary-adrenal axis. Side effects tend to occur with repeated application or application to the face, thin-skinned areas (neck, antecubital/popliteal fossae), or occluded areas (axillae, groin, inframammary

TABLE 3	Topical Steroids

Low strength
Hydrocortisone 1%, 2.5% (Class 7)
Desonide 0.05% (Class 6)

Medium strength
Fluocinolone acetonide 0.025% (Class 5)
Triamcinolone acetonide 0.1% (Class 4)

High strength
Fluocinonide 0.05% (Class 2)

Highest strength
Betamethasone dipropionate 0.05% (Class 1)
Clobetasol propionate 0.05% (Class 1)

Note: Classes 6 and 7 are indicated for facial use. Classes 1 and 2 are indicated for palmar/plantar areas or severe/resistant lesions.

folds). Patients should be cautioned to use a small amount of topical steroid only on the affected areas of skin and never on normal skin.
- Several factors are important in determining the optimal steroid for a particular condition. Accurate diagnosis obviates the need for combination agents such as a weak azole antifungal and a high-strength topical steroid.
- **Base or vehicle:**
  - Ointments are more lubricating as well as more occlusive, making them more potent. A lubricating ointment is best for dry dermatitis.
  - Creams are less lubricating than ointments, but more so than gels, lotions, and solutions. A cream would be more appropriate for a weeping dermatitis. Creams are more likely to have additives that may irritate skin. If a patient complains of burning or stinging with a cream, it may be appropriate to switch to a comparable ointment.
  - Lotions, gels, foams, and solutions are easier to use in hair-bearing areas, and are most often used in dermatitis of the scalp. Gels may also be appropriate for the oropharynx.
- **Strength:**
  - Higher-strength (Classes 1 to 2) topical steroids are used for palmar/plantar areas or for severe or resistant lesions.
  - Lower-strength (Classes 6 to 7) topical steroids are indicated for intermittent facial use.
- **Dosage:**
  - Applications should be performed twice daily.
  - When a cream or ointment is used, 1 g covers the face and 30 g covers the body of an adult.
- **Occlusion:**
  - Occlusion with plastic wrap or gloves increases the potency of the products but should be reserved for severe, resistant lesions. A limited time course for occlusion should be specified.
  - Occlusion increases both the potency and the risk of side effects.

SKIN NEOPLASMS

Half of all primary cancers in the United States are basal cell carcinoma (BCC) and squamous cell carcinoma (SCC) of the skin. Melanoma has the fastest rising incidence among solid tumors. However, many benign skin growths may be mistaken for skin cancer. It is important to distinguish between benign and malignant lesions and to determine which lesions should be biopsied.

Skin Cancer Prevention

- Patients should be advised to avoid sun exposure between 10 AM and 3 PM.
- Clothing (including hats and swimwear) with SPF (sun protection factor) can be purchased online and in many active-wear stores.
- Sunscreens are useful adjuncts to long sleeves and wide-brimmed hats for fair-skinned people or patients with dermatoses induced by ultraviolet light. A daily moisturizer with UVB protection (SPF 15 to 30) is appropriate for most fair-skinned individuals.
  - For certain light-sensitive disorders (e.g., systemic lupus erythematosus) and photosensitizing drugs (e.g., tetracycline, sulfonamides, thiazides, quinolones), combination sunscreens (UVA [ultraviolet A] and UVB [ultraviolet B]) are necessary.
  - All sunscreens should be applied 30 to 60 minutes before exposure and should be reapplied at least every 90 minutes and after bathing, swimming, or excessive sweating.
  - Allergic and photosensitivity reactions occur to para-aminobenzoic acid, especially in patients who are sensitive to benzocaine, procaine, thiazides, and sulfonamides. Very few sunscreen products contain para-aminobenzoic acid anymore.
  - Titanium dioxide and zinc oxide are opaque sunscreens that shield against UVA and UVB by providing a physical block. They are particularly useful on the nose and lips.
- Patients should perform skin examinations monthly. Encourage patients to use the ABCDEs when examining their own skin. Lesions with the following traits are more likely to be malignant and should be evaluated by a physician for consideration of biopsy.
  - **Asymmetry:** If you draw a line through the lesion, the two sides do not match.
  - **Border:** Irregular, notched, or scalloped borders are worrisome for melanoma.
  - **Colors:** Melanoma may have different shades of brown, tan, or black within one lesion. Red, blue, and white areas may also be present.
  - **Diameter:** A diameter of >6 mm is concerning for melanoma.
  - **Evolution:** Any change in size, shape, color, or other characteristic is more likely to be present in a malignant lesion. Development of pain, pruritus, or bleeding of the lesion is concerning for skin cancer.

Seborrheic Keratosis

- Seborrheic keratoses are hyperkeratotic epidermal papules commonly found in middle-aged and elderly patients.
- They are benign skin neoplasms that can be confused with skin cancer. They essentially have the same malignant potential of normal skin.
- On exam, they have a waxy, "stuck-on" appearance and may be tan, yellow, dark brown, or black in color. White horn cysts may be visible on close inspection. There is always a well-defined border. They usually appear on the face, chest, and back.

- **Stucco keratoses** are a variant consisting of small white papules on the lower legs.
- **Dermatosis papulosa nigra** is a form of seborrheic keratosis that appears as multiple, small, darkly pigmented, possibly pedunculated papules on the cheeks and periorbital areas of black, Hispanic, and Asian patients.
- If symptomatic, irritated seborrheic keratoses may be removed using cryosurgery (liquid nitrogen), curettage, or scissors excision. Most seborrheic keratoses, however, do not require treatment or are treated for cosmetic reasons. If a clinician is not certain of the diagnosis, these destructive measures must be avoided as the differential of pigmented lesions includes melanoma.

Skin Tag

- Also called acrochordons, skin tags are pedunculated skin-colored to brown papules commonly occurring on skin experiencing friction, specifically the neck, axillae, and groin.
- Obesity predisposes to the formation on skin tags.
- Treatment options for irritated or cosmetically troubling lesions include snipping with scissors and, less commonly, electrodesiccation or cryosurgery.

Keratinous Cyst

- Cysts on the skin present as firm subcutaneous nodules often with a central black punctum. They are freely mobile.
- **Pilar cysts** frequently occur on the scalp.
- Inflamed cysts may be treated with corticosteroid injection or, if necessary, incision and drainage. Once inflammation has subsided, definitive treatment consists of excision. The entire epithelial lining surrounding the cyst must be removed to prevent recurrence.

Lipoma

- Lipomas present as rubbery, well-defined subcutaneous tumors. They are freely mobile.
- Lipomas are benign lesions.
- Angiolipomas are often painful.
- Treatment consists of excision, but is generally reserved for changing, symptomatic, or cosmetically undesirable lesions.

Melanocytic Nevus

- By definition, a melanocytic nevus is a **benign skin neoplasm.** They are common growths and usually appear from childhood through ages 35 to 40.
- **Melanocytic nevi** are flesh-colored, light brown or dark brown smooth, circumscribed papules or macules. They present on any area of the skin but often are concentrated in sun-exposed areas.
- Unlike melanomas, nevi are symmetric with well-defined borders and uniform color. They are usually <6 mm in diameter.
- **Dysplastic nevi** may have many of the characteristics of melanoma. Patients with a large number of nevi or with dysplastic nevi are at higher risk for melanoma and should be examined more frequently.

- **Recurrent nevi** returning after incomplete excision may be very difficult to distinguish from malignant melanoma. Obtaining an accurate history of a pigmented lesion is critical in avoiding this pitfall and must be included in submitting a specimen for pathologic examination.

Solar Lentigo

- Solar lentigines are **benign** pigmented lesions caused by chronic sun exposure.
- On examination, they appear as tan to dark brown macules often on the face and dorsal hands.
- Special attention should be paid to lesions that violate the ABCDEs as the differential includes lentiginous-type melanoma (lentigo maligna). Biopsy of the entire clinical lesion is preferred to avoid sampling bias.

Cherry Angioma

- Cherry angiomas are **benign** collections of blood vessels appearing as round, red papules.
- No treatment is necessary unless lesions become irritated or bleed.

Actinic Keratosis

- Actinic keratoses (AK) are **premalignant lesions** caused by chronic sun exposure. If left untreated, they may develop into SCC.
- On examination, they appear as erythematous, raised papules with a firm scaly texture. On palpation, they have a "sandpaper" feel.
- Typically, actinic keratoses are treated with cryosurgery. Other therapeutic options for patients with persistent or widespread lesions include curettage, topical 5-fluorouracil, and photodynamic therapy.

Basal Cell Carcinoma

General Principles
- BCC is the **most common type of skin cancer.** It is caused by chronic sun exposure. Fair-skinned individuals are at the highest risk.
- Patients have a 50% risk of developing a second primary within 5 years. There is a very low metastatic potential, but BCCs can cause significant local tissue destruction.
- Patients with BCC should be examined every 6 to 12 months.

Diagnosis
- BCC presents most commonly as a pearly, telangiectatic papule on the face or trunk.
- Superficial BCC may occur on the trunk and extremities and appear as a scaly plaque with raised borders.
- Ulceration is common.
- Diagnosis is made by shave or punch biopsy.

Treatment
- Surgical options include excision, Mohs micrographic surgery, and electrodesiccation and curettage.

- Medical therapies include imiquimod and 5-fluorouracil for superficial BCCs.
- Radiation may be used to treat BCC in some instances.
- Location, size, histologic features, and patient preference guide the choice of definitive therapy.

Squamous Cell Carcinoma

General Principles
- SCC is caused by chronic sun exposure. SCC may also arise in chronic ulcers **(Marjolin ulcer)** or other chronic skin lesions.
- People with fair skin and history of actinic keratoses are at higher risk of developing SCC. The risk of SCC is significantly increased in patients with a history of solid organ transplantation.
- Patients are at high risk of developing a second primary lesion. Metastasis is uncommon, occurring in <5% of cases. Risk factors for metastasis include location (e.g., lips, ears, and genitalia), immunosuppression, and carcinomas arising from non-UV causes (e.g., longstanding discoid lupus or burns).
- Patients with SCC should be followed closely in the near-term and at least every 12 months in the longer-term. Examination of lymph nodes is recommended.

Diagnosis
- SCC is characterized by a red scaly papule, plaque, or nodule on the face, scalp, trunk, or extremities. Lesions may have a verrucous appearance.
- Diagnosis is made by shave or punch biopsy.

Treatment
Surgical options include excision with 4 mm margins, Mohs micrographic surgery, and electrodesiccation and curettage.

Melanoma

General Principles
- Melanoma can develop anywhere. In Caucasian men, the back is the most common location, whereas in Caucasian women, the legs and back are most common. The palms, soles, and nail beds are most common in Asians, Hispanics, and African-Americans.
- People with a family history of melanoma are at higher risk for developing melanoma; however, most melanomas are diagnosed in patients with no family history of melanoma.
- Unlike BCC and SCC, melanoma has a high potential for metastasis.
- Patients with melanoma should be examined for lymphadenopathy. Sentinel node biopsy may also be performed for cancer staging.

Diagnosis
- On examination, asymmetry, irregular borders, multiple colors, and a diameter >6 mm are worrisome signs for a malignant lesion.
- Excisional biopsy should be performed on any concerning or changing lesion. It is preferable not to sample a lesion but to provide the entire clinical lesion for pathologic examination, as the malignancy may be present only in a portion of the clinical lesion.

- The estimate of tumor volume (Breslow thickness) provides prognostic information. Transecting a lesion during biopsy may destroy this information.

Treatment

- Wide local excision is the definitive treatment for melanoma. Excisional margins and the need for sentinel lymph node biopsy are based on the Breslow thickness of the lesion.
- The role of complete lymphadenectomy in the surgical treatment of patients with positive sentinel nodes remains controversial.
- Metastatic melanoma may be treated with chemotherapy but prognosis is extremely poor.

DERMATITIDES

Contact Dermatitis

General Principles

- **Irritant contact dermatitis** is a nonallergic reaction of the skin due to chemical or physical agents. Mild irritants require repeated or prolonged contact to cause dermatitis (e.g., soaps, detergents, and solvents). Strong irritants can cause dermatitis following a single exposure (e.g., strong acids or alkali).
- **Allergic contact dermatitis** is a form of delayed hypersensitivity (type IV reaction) that develops only in sensitized individuals. The distribution and pattern of the dermatitis may suggest a specific allergen. Patch testing may be necessary to identify the offending allergen. Common allergens include the following:
  - **Plants** (e.g., Rhus dermatitis otherwise known as urushiol-induced dermatitis, or **poison ivy, oak, and sumac**): characterized by linear, vesicular lesions.
  - **Metals** (e.g., nickel, chrome): affect skin that touches jewelry and fasteners, especially on the earlobes and in the periumbilical area.
  - **Rubber/latex:** affects skin in contact with gloves, condoms, and elastic.
  - **Topical medications:** specifically neomycin, benzocaine, additives in creams, and other vehicles.
  - **Cosmetics:** preservatives in makeup, perfume, and hair dye.
  - **Other:** adhesives, inks, and antibacterials in cutting oils.

Diagnosis

- Acute dermatitis is characterized by erythema, weeping/oozing, crusting, and vesiculation. Poison ivy often produces linear vesicles. Severe lesions may demonstrate edema, ulceration, and large bullae.
- Chronic dermatitis is characterized by scale, dry skin, and eventually lichenification of (thick, hyperkeratotic) skin.
- The diagnosis is made largely by history of exposure to irritants or allergens.
- Skin examination may reveal a particular pattern associated with a type of dermatitis.

Treatment

- **Mild dermatitis** is treated with topical steroids, topical or systemic antipruritics, and avoidance of the offending agent.
- **Severe blistering reactions** are treated with oral prednisone, 0.5 to 1.0 mg/kg tapered over 10 to 21 days, antipruritics, and drying agents.

Atopic Dermatitis (Eczema)

- Atopic dermatitis presents as erythematous, scaly plaques that may demonstrate lichenification and pigment alteration (hyper or hypopigmentation).
- **Dyshidrotic eczema** is characterized by vesiculation. Scratching or rubbing worsens the condition.
- Commonly affected areas include skin flexures, hands, and feet.
- Effective therapy includes emollients, dry skin care, topical steroids, and antihistamines for reduction of pruritus. Choice of topical steroid depends on the location and severity of the lesion as well as the age of the patient.
- Recalcitrant cases may be treated with UV light therapy or immunosuppressants.
- Superinfection is common and should be treated with antibiotics targeting staph and strep.

Stasis Dermatitis

- Stasis dermatitis is characterized by bilateral erythema, hyperpigmentation, and scaling most prominent on the lower legs. It is often confused for cellulitis, an infection that is almost always unilateral.
- Successful treatment of stasis dermatitis requires reduction of lower-extremity edema with compression stockings. Triamcinolone, 0.1% ointment applied bid, is an appropriate topical steroid.
- Stasis dermatitis may progress to lipodermatosclerosis and ulceration.

Keratosis Pilaris

- Keratosis pilaris is a chronic papular eruption that occurs on the proximal extensor surfaces of the extremities and cheeks throughout life.
- The rash is characterized by scaly follicular papules and is usually asymptomatic.
- Treatment is limited to emollients and keratolytics.

Seborrheic Dermatitis

- Seborrheic dermatitis is a very common, mild dermatitis in adults. However, it can be quite severe in patients with HIV or Parkinson disease.
- In adults, erythema with fine white or greasy scale is seen on the scalp (dandruff), eyebrows, eyelids, nasolabial folds, ears, sternal area, axillae, inframammary folds, and perineum.
- Antiseborrheic shampoos, such as selenium sulfide, zinc pyrithione, tar, or 2% ketoconazole, are used at least every other day for 10 to 15 minutes. For the face or trunk, ketoconazole cream or 1.0% to 2.5% hydrocortisone cream bid is used.

Psoriasis

General Principles

- Psoriasis is a chronic recurring condition with varying degrees of severity. While some patients suffer from widespread disease, others may have only a few small patches of involvement. Psoriatic arthritis involves the joints and may cause significant disfigurement and disability.

- Psoriasis has been associated with higher rates of cardiac disease and depression.
- Although the etiology is unknown, there is likely a genetic component.
- Stress, smoking, alcohol consumption, and certain medications (e.g., lithium, beta-blockers) can aggravate the disease. There may also be worsening of psoriasis after systemic steroids.

Diagnosis

- Examination reveals erythematous plaques with silvery scale on the elbows, knees, scalp, and trunk. Nail changes including pitting and "oil spots" may also be present. Psoriasis can progress to generalized erythroderma.
- Joint pain and stiffness should be characterized if present.
- **Guttate ("droplike") psoriasis** is characterized by small, erythematous papules on the trunk and may be associated with streptococcal pharyngitis.

Treatment

- **Mild to moderate psoriasis** is treated topically with topical steroids, vitamin D_3 analogues (calcipotriene), retinoids (tazarotene), tar derivatives, natural sunlight, or narrow-band ultraviolet B radiation. Calcipotriene and tazarotene are more expensive than topical steroids but less likely to cause skin atrophy and tachyphylaxis. Calcipotriene can cause hypercalcemia if it is used on >10% of the body. Tazarotene can cause burning, erythema, and desquamation. Sunlight and UVB radiation can cause burning and increase the risk of skin cancer.
- **Severe psoriasis** may require phototherapy or systemic agents (methotrexate, acitretin, cyclosporine, etanercept, adalimumab, infliximab). These therapies must be closely monitored. The biologic agents increase the risk of infection, especially reactivation of tuberculosis. Tuberculosis skin tests (PPDs) must be placed yearly. Systemic therapies are for patients who are incapacitated by their disease and resistant to less toxic forms of treatment. They are the only therapies appropriate for psoriatic arthritis.
- **Scalp psoriasis** is treated topically with tar shampoo and steroid solutions. Prominent scale needs to be removed before other treatments will work.
- **Guttate psoriasis** may respond to penicillin or amoxicillin, presuming that there is an underlying streptococcal infection. Phototherapy is also particularly effective for guttate psoriasis.
- **Inverse psoriasis** affects the axillae, inframammary folds, and groin. Topical agents appropriate for these locations should be prescribed.

Pityriasis Rosea

- Pityriasis rosea is characterized by pink, oval papules with minimal peripheral scale. The rash commonly appears in a "Christmas tree" distribution on the trunk. The herald patch is a larger pink plaque.
- Pityriasis rosea is mildly pruritic and resolves in 6 to 12 weeks.
- Treatment includes sunlight, phototherapy, topical steroids, erythromycin, and antipruritics.
- The rash of secondary syphilis can closely mimic pityriasis rosea. If there is clinical suspicion, an RPR may be indicated.

Lichen Planus

- Lichen planus is characterized by pruritic, purple, polygonal papules that favor the volar wrists, ankles, and genitals. Lesions have lacy white scale (Wickham striae). Oral lesions are common and appear as lacy white plaques or erosions often on the buccal mucosa.
- Occasionally, lichen planus is associated with hepatitis and angiotensin-converting inhibitors.
- Treatment is with topical steroids with occlusion when possible, emollition, and antipruritics. Severe, generalized cases may require oral prednisone or phototherapy. There are case reports of effectiveness of oral metronidazole.

Thermal Burns

- Dermatitis of varying intensity may be caused by the action of excessive heat on the skin. If the heat is extreme, the skin and underlying tissue may be destroyed.
- **First-degree burns** congest superficial blood vessels, causing erythema that may be followed by desquamation (e.g., sunburn). Treatment includes prompt cold application and emolliation.
- **Second-degree burns** cause edema and vesicles. Treatment includes prompt cold application and emolliation. Vesicles should not be opened unless they are tense and painful. When required, drainage under aseptic technique is recommended.
- **Third-degree burns** cause full-thickness necrosis of the skin and anesthesia. Severe second- and third-degree burns benefit from specialized teams of physicians. Third-degree burns require skin grafting and heal with scarring.

ACNE

Acne Vulgaris

General Principles
- Acne vulgaris tends to develop around puberty and may resolve later.
- Acne is an inflammatory condition with an infectious component. Scarring may be significant and should prompt consideration of more aggressive initial therapy.
- Treatments require at least 2 months to show significant improvement. Therapies should be continued for at least this long before changing.
- It may be improved by oral contraceptives (OCPs) but is worsened by medroxyprogesterone (Depo-Provera).
- **Papular acne** is characterized by open comedones (blackheads) and closed comedones (whiteheads).
- **Inflammatory acne** is characterized by erythematous papules and pustules.
- **Nodulocystic acne** is characterized by deep-seated nodules and results in scarring.

Treatment
- **Comedolytics** are the first-line therapy for papular acne.
  - Benzoyl peroxide, 2.5%, 5%, or 10%, is available as a wash or gel. Use higher concentrations and gels in patients with oily skin. Unlike topical antibiotics, benzoyl peroxide does not promote antibiotic resistance.

- Topical retinoids (tretinoin, adapalene, tazarotene) are available in creams and gels. They should be used in small quantities (a pea-sized amount covers the entire face) on clean, dry skin. Higher concentration creams and gels can be drying and can predispose to photosensitivity. Less frequent application may be necessary if irritation is significant.
- **Topical antibiotics** can be used in inflammatory acne.
- Clindamycin (Cleocin T) solution, lotion, or pledget one to two times daily.
- Erythromycin solution or pledget one to two times daily.
- **Systemic antibiotics** are often used in moderate to severe inflammatory acne and in nodulocystic acne. They should be tapered after several months of therapy, and an inability to discontinue may be an indication for referral to a dermatologist for oral isotretinoin (Accutane) therapy.
  - Doxycycline, tetracycline, and minocycline are most commonly used. Side effects include stomach upset and photosensitization. Blue discoloration has been described with chronic use of minocycline.
  - Erythromycin may also be used. Allergies and side effects may limit antibiotic choices in a given patient.
- **Systemic retinoic acid** is used in severe nodulocystic acne or acne vulgaris unresponsive to the therapies listed above. Isotretinoin (Accutane), 1 mg/kg/day, is prescribed for 5 to 6 months. All other acne therapies should be discontinued before starting isotretinoin.
  - Because of side effects and teratogenicity of the drug, isotretinoin is regulated by the government. Patients must register through an online monitoring system (iPLEDGE) and must present monthly for liver function tests and a lipid panel before obtaining a refill. Furthermore, sexually active women on isotretinoin are required to use two forms of birth control and have monthly pregnancy tests.
  - Side effects include liver function abnormalities, elevated triglycerides, photosensitivity, severe dryness of the lips and skin, and depression. There is also an increased risk for Staphylococcus infections and pyogenic granulomas.
  - Isotretinoin should only be prescribed by a physician familiar with its use.

Hidradenitis Suppurativa

- Hidradenitis suppurativa presents as multiple, recurrent painful cysts and nodules of the axillae, groin, and buttocks. Sinus tract formation is common.
- There is an association with obesity.
- Treatment ranges from topical and systemic antibiotics to intralesional corticosteroid injection to systemic retinoids and biologics. Excision is the definitive therapy.

Acne Rosacea

General Principles

- Acne rosacea usually affects patients between 30 and 60 years of age. It is more common among fair-skinned individuals.
- It is a chronic condition with intermittent exacerbations and remissions.
- There are several subtypes: erythematotelangiectatic, papulopustular, phymatous, glandular, and ocular.

Diagnosis

- On examination, erythema and telangiectasias on the cheeks and nose are the most common findings. Inflammatory papules and pustules may be present on the face, particularly in a perioral distribution.
- Rhinophyma may be present in long-standing rosacea and is more common in men.
- Ocular changes, including dryness, irritation, conjunctivitis, blepharitis, and rarely keratitis may occur.
- Flushing of the cheeks is common and may be brought on by alcohol, heat, sun exposure, strenuous exercise, stress, medications, and certain foods (e.g., spicy, hot beverages, citrus fruits).

Treatment

- Rosacea does not respond to comedolytics.
- Sunscreen is the first-line therapy for all patients. Sunlight, spicy foods, and hot beverages should be avoided.
- **Topical antibiotics** such as metronidazole gel or lotion (MetroGel or MetroLotion) and clindamycin (Cleocin T) are commonly used for papules and pustules. They are unlikely to have a significant effect on erythema and telangiectasias, which require cosmetic laser treatments.
- Sodium sulfacetamide wash or lotion (Plexion, Klaron) may also be effective.
- Systemic antibiotics (doxycycline, 50 to 100 mg bid) may effective for moderate to severe rosacea.

ULCERS

- Of leg ulcers, 90% result from of venous insufficiency, 5% result from arterial disease, and 5% are due to miscellaneous causes, including diabetic microangiopathy, pyoderma gangrenosum, malignancies, vasculitis, and infections.
- Diagnosis of the miscellaneous causes is often aided by skin biopsy, but consideration must be given to the long-healing time of biopsy sites in the lower leg, where ulcers are most common.

Venous Ulcers

- Venous ulcers tend to occur on the lower medial aspect of the legs in areas of preceding stasis dermatitis.
- Treatment aims to improve venous return with leg elevation and compression hose. Wet-to-dry dressings provide excellent debridement for 2 to 3 days, but longer use can interfere with wound healing. Most wounds improve with being kept clean, covered, and moist. This is often best achieved with occlusive dressings. Unna wraps may be particularly effective in severe cases.
- In cases recalcitrant to medical therapy, ablation of the superficial venous system (e.g., VNUS procedure) can be beneficial.

Arterial Ulcers

- Arterial ulcers tend to occur over the lateral malleolus and are often painful.
- Treatment includes local wound care and improving arterial blood flow.

BLISTERING DISORDERS

Pemphigus Vulgaris

General Principles
- Pemphigus vulgaris is characterized by flaccid bullae that break easily, leaving denuded areas that increase in size by progressive peripheral detachment. Oral lesions are common.
- Before corticosteroids became available, the mortality of this disease was 80%.
- **Pemphigus foliaceus** is characterized by flaccid bullae that usually arise on an erythematous base and superficial erosions that may accumulate thick scales. Oral lesions tend not to occur. Pemphigus foliaceus has a better prognosis than pemphigus vulgaris.

Diagnosis
- Physical examination reveals flaccid bullae and erosions.
- Nikolsky sign (spread of blister with application of horizontal, tangential pressure to the skin) is present.
- Diagnosis is confirmed by skin biopsy for routine histologic examination and direct immunofluorescence. Patient serum can also be submitted for indirect immunofluorescence to determine the titer of autoantibodies.

Treatment
- **High-dose prednisone,** 1 to 2 mg/kg/day, with transition to or concomitant use of a steroid sparing agent such as gold, cyclophosphamide, azathioprine, mycophenolate mofetil, or rituximab.
- Supportive care in a hospital setting may be required if large areas of skin are denuded.

Bullous Pemphigoid

General Principles
- Bullous pemphigoid (BP) is characterized by large tense bullae on an erythematous base that leave denuded areas. It often occurs in elderly patients.
- BP has a better prognosis than pemphigus.
- **Pemphigoid gestationis** characteristically occurs during pregnancy and presents on distended abdominal skin.

Diagnosis
- Physical examination reveals tense bullae. Occasionally, BP presents as urticarial or dermatitic plaques. It is less commonly seen on mucosal surfaces than pemphigus.
- Diagnosis is confirmed by biopsy for routine histologic examination and direct immunofluorescence.

Treatment
- Localized disease may be treated with high-potency topical steroids.
- Generalized or persistent BP is treated with **high-dose prednisone,** 1 to 2 mg/kg/day, or steroid-sparing immunosuppressants such as gold, cyclophosphamide, azathioprine, and mycophenolate mofetil.
- Tetracycline and niacinamide may also be used to treat BP.

Dermatitis Herpetiformis

General Principles
- Dermatitis herpetiformis presents in the second or third decade of life.
- It may be associated with gluten-sensitive enteropathy (celiac disease), which is sometimes asymptomatic.

Diagnosis
- Physical examination reveals eroded and crusted papules and vesicles that are symmetrically distributed on the extensor elbows, knees, and buttocks.
- Patients usually complain of intense pruritus.
- Diagnosis is confirmed by skin biopsy of lesional skin for routine histologic examination and perilesional skin for direct immunofluorescence. Laboratory tests for markers of celiac disease may also be useful in the diagnosis.

Treatment
- A gluten-free diet may be effective, but strict adherence is required.
- Dapsone, 50 to 150 mg/day is useful given that the inflammation consists largely of neutrophils.
- Antipruritics can be prescribed for symptomatic relief of the intense pruritus.

Erythema Multiforme

- Erythema multiforme is an acute, self-limited, often recurrent eruption characterized by "targetoid" lesions. The degree of severity varies widely.
- Lesions on the palms and soles are characteristic.
- Typical **erythema multiforme minor** is localized to the skin, does not involve the mucosa, and has minimal to no prodromal symptoms.
- **Erythema multiforme major** is often preceded by a prodromal phase and mucosal involvement is notable.
- The distinction between erythema multiforme major and Stevens-Johnson syndrome (SJS) (see below) may be challenging.
- Erythema multiforme is strongly associated with herpes simplex virus, Streptococcus, Mycoplasma, or other infections.

Stevens-Johnson Syndrome and Toxic Epidermolysis Necrosis

General Principles
- SJS and toxic epidermolysis necrosis (TEN) both present with a flu-like prodrome (particularly fever) rapidly progressing to skin pain, exanthem or targetoid lesions, and skin sloughing.
- Mucous membranes are always involved and consist of erosions of the mouth, eyes, genitalia, and lips with hemorrhagic crusts.
- The two conditions lie on a spectrum; categorization depends on how much of the body surface area (BSA) is involved. SJS involves <10% BSA, TEN involves >30% BSA, and SJS/TEN overlap involves 10% to 30% BSA.
- There is a strong association with medications including penicillins, sulfonamides (e.g., trimethoprim-sulfamethoxazole), anticonvulsants (e.g., phenytoin, carbamazepine,

lamotrigine), allopurinol, and nonsteroidal anti-inflammatory drugs (NSAIDs, e.g., piroxicam). However, many cases (up to 50%) are idiopathic.
* Mortality of SJS is 1% to 5%, whereas mortality of TEN can be as high as 35%.

Diagnosis

* Generalized skin sloughing is often seen on examination. The oral and genital mucosa should be examined; mucosal involvement presents with erosions and hemorrhagic crusts.
* Painful skin should be considered a strong warning sign.
* Sloughing may be confirmed by applying firm tangential pressure to affected skin and observing shearing.
* Diagnosis is confirmed by skin biopsy for routine histologic examination.

Treatment

* Treatment largely consists of **symptomatic and supportive care.** Admission to an intensive care unit is necessary if a significant portion of skin area is involved, and intubation is common. Any suspected offending agents should be eliminated.
* Systemic steroids in SJS/TEN are controversial and may contribute to secondary infections. There have been case reports of cyclosporine or intravenous immunoglobulin (IVIG) being helpful.
* Antimicrobial silver impregnated dressings (e.g., Acticoat) can be used to prevent secondary infection and can help limit painful dressing changes.

INSECT BITE

General Principles

Reactions to insect bites are usually triggered by a toxin or an allergen injected into skin by the offending arthropod.

Diagnosis

* Elements of the history that may be helpful include history of working in or cleaning a basement, activity in densely wooded areas, and recent travel.
* Diagnosis is largely based on examination of the bite. If a tick bite is suspected, inspect the skin for presence of the tick.
  * **Bee, wasp, and yellow jacket** bites consist of a painful red wheal with central punctum; the wheal fades in hours. A persistent local reaction with intense swelling around the bite area may arise and **does not indicate a systemic allergy.** In individuals with immediate systemic allergy, anaphylaxis may develop. Rarely, affected persons may manifest a delayed systemic allergic reaction that shows up as urticaria, polyarthritis, and lymphadenopathy.
  * **Fire ant** stings produce wheals with two hemorrhagic puncta. These usually evolve into pustules within hours.
  * **Mosquito** bites appear as pruritic wheals developing within hours. Patients with blood dyscrasias or malignancies may display exuberant, bullous reactions to bites.
  * **Flea** bites produce grouped urticarial papules, some with puncta, frequently on the legs.
  * **Tick** bites may not appear as typical insect bites on the skin but may result in fevers, spreading rashes, joint pain, and other systemic symptoms.

- **Spider** bites are usually mild. However, bites from brown recluse and black widow spiders can result in painful necrotic ulcers as well as systemic sequelae.

Treatment

- If insects are attached to the skin, they should be flicked (not squeezed) off the skin. Alternatively, they can be removed with fine forceps.
- Ticks are best removed by grasping them as close to the skin as possible with forceps and with a steady upward pull. It is important to confirm that the head has been removed. Clean the wound with soap, water, or mild disinfectant solution. The patient should report fever or unusual rashes to a physician.
- Ice, cold compresses, and phenolated calamine lotion are soothing agents. Topical steroids and oral antihistamines may be useful for itching and inflammation.
- Necrotic spider bites from a brown recluse or black widow may become superinfected and require antibiotics. Surgical debridement is rarely necessary.
- Anaphylactic reactions require emergency treatment (see Chapter 35).

DRUG REACTIONS

See Chapter 35.

URTICARIA

See Chapter 35.

ALOPECIA

Alopecias are divided into two major categories: nonscarring and scarring. Careful examination of the scalp for areas of regrowth and presence of follicular openings is important in distinguishing nonscarring from scarring. Nonscarring alopecias have the potential for regrowth, whereas scarring alopecias do not.

Nonscarring Alopecia

- **Androgenetic alopecia** has a genetic predisposition, with an interaction between circulating androgens and androgen receptors in hair follicles. Vellus hairs gradually replace terminal hairs. Androgenic alopecia affects 25% of patients >25 years of age and 50% of patients >50 years of age. Male pattern usually begins with bitemporal recession. Female pattern is usually more diffuse, with sparing of the frontal hairline. Men can be treated with 1 mL 5% minoxidil (Rogaine) bid or 1 mg finasteride (Propecia) daily. These agents cause some hair regrowth but are more effective at preventing further hair loss. Hair loss rapidly returns to normal on discontinuation. In women, there is no benefit to finasteride, and 2% minoxidil bid appears to be as effective as the 5% solution. Facial hypertrichosis is a more common side effect in women.
- **Alopecia areata** is characterized by rapid, complete hair loss in one or more oval patches. The scalp is most often affected, but any hair-bearing area may be involved. Alopecia areata totalis and alopecia areata universalis involve all the hair of the head or entire body, respectively. Hairs taper proximally to an attenuated bulb, producing "exclamation point hairs." Alopecia areata is considered to be an autoimmune disorder and can, although not usually, be associated with other autoimmune disorders; spontaneous regrowth often occurs within 6 months. Intralesional triamcinolone,

3 to 10 mg/mL every 4 to 6 weeks, is used for persistent or rapidly enlarging patches. Recurrence is common.

- **Telogen effluvium** is characterized by abrupt, diffuse hair loss over the entire scalp that results in decreased hair density. Anagen hairs (growing phase) are prematurely pushed into the telogen phase (resting) of the hair cycle (usually 2 to 4 months after the initiating event). Hair loss can continue for a subsequent 120 to 400 days, but then regrowth occurs. Causes include pregnancy, febrile illness, surgery, crash diets, systemic anticoagulant therapy, and stressful life episodes. Treatment consists of reassurance and should be directed at eliminating the underlying cause.
- **Anagen effluvium** is a widespread loss of anagen hairs from actively growing follicles due to arrest of cell division. It often manifests as acute, severe hair loss. Causes include cytotoxic agents for cancer chemotherapy, thallium, boron, and radiation therapy. Treatment consists of reassurance.
- **Trichotillomania** is excessive and repeated manipulation of hair by the patient that results in hair breakage. It typically produces a well-circumscribed area of broken hairs and alopecia. Treatment should be directed at discussing the nature of the problem with the patient, who may unknowingly persist in manipulating the hair. Extreme cases may require psychiatric evaluation and medication. Excess traction on hairs through certain hairstyles can cause hair loss through a similar mechanism. Although both trichotillomania and traction alopecia are considered nonscarring, prolonged trauma to the hair can cause permanent hair loss.
- Other causes of nonscarring alopecia include the following:
  - Endocrinologic abnormalities.
  - OCPs may initiate androgenic alopecia in predisposed women and telogen effluvium may develop 2 to 4 months after anovulatory agents are discontinued.
  - Nutritional causes include kwashiorkor, marasmus, zinc deficiency, essential fatty acid deficiency, and malabsorption.

Scarring Alopecia

- Hair follicles are scarred and thus **hair loss is permanent.** On physical examination the follicular openings are no longer seen.
- Causes include the following:
  - Infections including bacterial and fungal (e.g., tinea capitis).
  - Neoplasms, either primary or metastatic.
  - Physical and chemical agents.
  - Autoimmune disorders, including discoid lupus erythematosus (LE) and lichen planopilaris.
  - Neutrophilic scalp dermatoses (dissecting scalp cellulitis and folliculitis decalvans).
  - Idiopathic (e.g., sarcoid and central centrifugal scarring alopecia).

NAIL DISORDERS

Nail disorders are associated with systemic disease or congenital conditions, or can be the result of infection, injury, repeated trauma, or improper trimming.

Koilonychia

Koilonychia, or spoon-shaped nails, is associated with hematologic disorders (Plummer-Vinson syndrome, polycythemia vera); metabolic disorders (acromegaly, hyperthyroidism, hypothyroidism, malnutrition, porphyria); and traumatic/occupational disorders (acid/alkali, thermal burns, frostbite, petroleum, thioglycolate depilatory and permanent solution).

Leukonychia Striata

- Leukonychia striata are transverse white bands in the nail. Traumatic leukonychia striata are due to occupational trauma and manicuring.
- Discontinuous parallel, horizontal white bands are present in the nail plate but usually do not span the entire plate. Leukonychia striata are likely to be asymmetric and do not involve all nails.
- **Mees lines** are homogeneous white bands that span the nail plate. All nails are involved. Common causes include arsenic, carbon monoxide, cardiac failure, chemotherapy, Hodgkin disease, leprosy, renal failure, and sickle cell anemia.
- **Muehrcke lines** are paired white transverse lines spanning the nail plate that temporarily disappear with pressure and associated with chronic hypoalbuminemia.

Beau Lines

- Beau lines are characterized by a universal transverse depression spanning the nail plate that is associated with any systemic disease (e.g., chemotherapy, sepsis) that causes a temporary cessation of nail growth.
- The insult can be dated by measuring the distance between the proximal nail fold and the leading edge of the depression (fingernails grow 0.1 to 0.15 mm/day).

Onycholysis

- Onycholysis is distal separation of the nail plate from the nail bed.
- Common causes include trauma, drug reactions, contact dermatitis, and psoriasis.

Onychomycosis

See "Fungal Skin Infections" below.

Terry Nails

- Terry nails are a prominent erythematous band at the distal portion of the nail bed (<20% of the nail bed is involved) with a white proximal nail.
- They are associated with cirrhosis and renal failure but can be seen in healthy patients (especially children).
- **Half and half nails** are red, pink, or brown transverse distal bands with a white proximal nail. They are found in 15% of patients with chronic renal failure.

Paronychia

- Paronychias are pockets of localized infection at nail margins. They may be acute (usually trauma) or chronic (through occupational exposure).
- Cultures are positive for Staphylococcus (acute) or *Candida albicans* (chronic).

- Treatment is based on the underlying causative organism. In acute paronychia, saline soaks and topical antibiotics can be prescribed. If an abscess is detected, drainage and antibiotic treatment (often with a semisynthetic penicillin) is indicated. In the case of chronic paronychia, combination of antifungal and steroid ointment is required.

PIGMENT DISORDERS

Postinflammatory Pigment Alteration

- Any inflammation of the skin may result in pigment alteration. Postinflammatory hyperpigmentation is especially common in darker skin types. Treatment is not necessary and pigment will revert to normal over weeks to months.
- Areas of pigment alteration should not be treated as primary lesions. For example, patients treating eczematous rashes should be advised to taper topical steroids when redness, scale, and itching have resolved, not when pigment has normalized.

Vitiligo

- Vitiligo is characterized by depigmented patches, often symmetric, around the eyes, nose, mouth, ears, genitals, and dorsal hands. It can be segmental or become generalized.
- In severely affected individuals it can have significant psychosocial effects.
- It is rarely associated with other autoimmune diseases.
- Recommendations include broad-spectrum sunscreens and observation for cutaneous malignancies.
- Treatment includes topical steroids, psoralen ultraviolet A photochemotherapy, controlled exposure to sunlight, and punch grafts and is best performed under the care of a dermatologist.

Melasma

- Melasma is characterized by pigmented patches on the forehead, cheeks, lips, and extensor forearms.
- It is commonly seen with OCP use and pregnancy. Changing OCP pills has little effect.
- Treatment includes broad-spectrum sunscreens, topical hydroquinones, and tretinoin.

FUNGAL SKIN INFECTIONS

Candidiasis

See Chapter 22.

Tinea Versicolor

General Principles

- Tinea versicolor is a superficial cutaneous infection caused by the dimorphic organism Malassezia (particularly *M. globosa* and *M. furfur*).

- In yeast form, these are normal skin flora but conversion to the hyphal form is associated with the clinical condition. High heat and humidity seem to facilitate this transformation. Other associations include immunosuppression, malnutrition, Cushing disease, and perhaps genetic factors.
- In immunocompromised patients, Malassezia may cause more serious infections including folliculitis, catheter-related fungemia, and focal infections.

Diagnosis

- On physical examination, there are thin scaly papules and plaques on the trunk, extremities, and face. Papules and plaques may be, as the name implies, hypopigmented or hyperpigmented. Lesions often are more pronounced after sun exposure.
- KOH examination reveals spores and pseudohyphae ("macaroni and meatballs"). Tinea versicolor is difficult to culture.

Treatment

- Tinea versicolor is not responsive to **griseofulvin or systemic allylamines** such as terbinafine (Lamisil).
- **Selenium sulfide** 2.5% shampoo is used every day for 15 minutes for 7 days, weekly thereafter, and more often if needed. Medicated Head & Shoulders and Selsun Blue contain less selenium sulfide and need to be used more frequently.
- Any **topical azole antifungal cream** can be used twice daily for 2 weeks after the rash resolves.
- **Systemic ketoconazole,** 400 mg, once and then repeated 1 week later, may be prescribed. As the medication is excreted in sweat, patients should be instructed to exercise 90 minutes after ingestion and leave sweat on skin for as long as possible before bathing.

Tinea Capitis

General Principles

- Tinea capitis (scalp "ringworm") is rarely seen in patients >15 years of age.
- It may be confused with other more common scalp problems in adults.
- It is most often caused by *Trichophyton tonsurans.*

Diagnosis

- Physical examination reveals scaling alopecia with broken hairs. Posterior cervical lymphadenopathy often develops.
- Differential diagnosis includes alopecia areata and seborrheic dermatitis. However, alopecia areata has no scaling and seborrheic dermatitis has no alopecia.
- **Kerions** are boggy nodules that can drain pus and may develop in patients with untreated tinea capitis.
- KOH examination of scale reveals hyphae; microscopic examination of broken hairs reveals endospores or ectospores. Fungal culture should be performed.

Treatment

- **Griseofulvin,** 5 to 20 mg/kg/day for 4 to 8 weeks. The medicine should be taken with a fatty meal. It may cause photosensitivity.
- **Terbinafine, itraconazole,** and **fluconazole** have also been used successfully.

- Systemic therapy is required but can be supplemented with topical therapy to decrease the chance of spreading the disease. 2.5% selenium sulfide or 2% ketoconazole shampoo every other day is recommended.
- Children are no longer infectious once on treatment and can return to school.
- If **kerions** develop, treatment should consist of griseofulvin (5 to 20 mg/kg/day) for 6 to 8 weeks with prednisone (1 mg/kg/day) for the first 2 weeks.

Tinea Pedis and Tinea Manuum

General Principles

- These two dermatophyte infections are relatively uncommon in children.
- Acute tinea pedis is usually caused by *T. mentagrophytes*; the chronic form by *T. rubrum*. Both are contagious.

Diagnosis

- Physical examination reveals interdigital scaling and maceration. If soles are involved, the scaling is often in a "moccasin" distribution. Localized blisters can develop on the arch of the foot.
- On the hands, the infection resembles dyshidrotic eczema with localized blisters. However, tinea rarely involves both hands and both feet.
- Skin scraping with KOH preparation shows branched dermatophyte hyphae under magnification.

Treatment

- The areas involved should be kept clean and dry, with use of drying powders as needed.
- **Topical antifungal agents** are effective including terbinafine (Lamisil), naftifine (Naftin), clotrimazole (Lotrimin), ketoconazole (Nizoral), miconazole (Micatin/Monistat), and tolnaftate (Tinactin).
- Severe and/or chronic tinea may require oral antifungal treatment (e.g., griseofulvin, terbinafine, or itraconazole).

Onychomycosis

General Principles

- Generally, onychomycosis is any fungal infection of the finger and/or toenails. Involvement of the latter is much more common.
- **Tinea unguium** specifically refers to dermatophytic nail infections caused by *T. mentagrophytes* and *T. rubrum*.
- Fingernail onychomycosis is more often due to the yeast *C. albicans*.
- Onychomycosis can become a rather significant cosmetic concern for patients.

Diagnosis

- Onychomycosis is typified by thickened, yellow finger or toenails.
- Several patterns have been described: distal/lateral subungual (the most common type), proximal subungual (uncommon and characteristically occurring in immunocompromised patients), white superficial, and yeast. Total dystrophic onychomycosis signifies involvement of the entire nail unit.
- Examination of subungual debris or fragments of the thickened nail plate with KOH should reveal hyphae.
- Culture and biopsy may also be used to confirm the diagnosis if necessary.

Treatment

- Topical treatment (ciclopirox 8% solution, Penlac) is most often ineffective but is available for treating mild onychomycosis that does not involve the lunula.
- **Terbinafine,** 250 mg PO daily, may be more effective than other treatments. Fingernail infections should be treated for 6 weeks; toenails for 12 weeks. Liver function tests should be monitored during therapy.
- Alternatively, itraconazole, 200 mg PO twice daily, may be prescribed for 7 days, followed by a 3-week hiatus with two treatment cycles for fingernails and three for toenails.
- Removal of the nail and destruction of the nail matrix will also treat onychomycosis.
- The optimal clinical effect is related to the rate of outgrowth of healthy nail. It may take months after cessation of treatment before the healthy nail is seen.

Tinea Corporis

General Principles

- Tinea corporis ("ringworm") is a dermatophytic infection of the skin, excluding the scalp, hands, feet, nails, and groin.
- It is most often caused by *T. rubrum.*

Diagnosis

- Physical examination reveals advancing scaly, annular, slightly raised erythematous lesions. It may be pustular at the margins or hypopigmented centrally.
- Trunk and extremities are the most common areas.
- Diagnosis is usually clinical but can be confirmed with a KOH preparation demonstrating hyphae.
- **Majocchi granuloma,** or fungal folliculitis, has multiple pustules within a patch of tinea corporis. Diagnosis is often confirmed by biopsy when the folliculitis fails to respond to antibiotics.

Treatment

- The areas involved should be kept clean and dry, with use of drying powders as needed.
- Initial topical therapy includes **antifungal creams** such as clotrimazole 1% bid for up to 1 month.
- In severe cases, treatment with an oral antifungal agent (clotrimazole, terbinafine) may be required.
- **Majocchi granuloma** should be treated with oral antifungal therapy.
- For patients with recurrent, severe, or unresolving infection, referral to a dermatologist may be necessary. Consider diabetes mellitus or HIV in an adult with this diagnosis.

Tinea Cruris

General Principles

- Tinea cruris ("jock itch") is most often caused by *T. rubrum.*
- It is much more common in men than in women.
- Obesity, sweating, humidity, and autoinoculation for other sites of dermatophytic infection (e.g., tinea pedis, manuum, unguium) are contributing factors.

Diagnosis

- Tinea cruris is characterized by advancing scaly annular erythematous plaques. Central clearing, hyperpigmentation, or lichenification may be present. Pustules can occasionally be seen at the leading age.
- It is often present in the groin folds and bilateral buttocks but never involves the penis or scrotum.
- Differential diagnosis includes intertrigo or candidiasis and erythrasma. However, candidiasis often involves the scrotum and presents with satellite pustules and bright red plaques. Erythrasma is characterized by a hyperpigmented patch with fine scale and appears as coral red fluorescence on Wood lamp examination.
- Skin scraping from the active edge with KOH examination should show segmented hyphae.

Treatment

- The areas involved should be kept clean and dry, with use of drying powders as needed.
- **Topical antifungal agents** are the first line of therapy; these include terbinafine (Lamisil), naftifine (Naftin), clotrimazole (Lotrimin), ketoconazole (Nizoral), miconazole (Micatin/Monistat), and tolnaftate (Tinactin).

BACTERIAL SKIN INFECTIONS

See Chapter 22.

VIRAL SKIN INFECTIONS

Warts

General Principles

- Warts are intraepidermal tumors caused by infection with the human papilloma virus.
- **Verruca vulgaris,** or common warts, are flesh- to brown-colored hyperkeratotic papules. Acral areas, especially the hands, are most frequently involved, but any skin or mucous membrane may be involved.
- **Filiform warts** are fingerlike slender projections that arise particularly on the face or neck.
- Flat warts **(verruca plana)** are small, 1- to 3-mm flesh- to tan-colored papules on the face, neck, extensor upper extremities, and extensor lower extremities in females. They may be distributed in a linear pattern (koebnerization).
- **Plantar warts** are common warts that involve the thick skin of the sole.
- **Condyloma acuminata** are warts that grow on moist areas, especially the genital or perianal skin. These genital warts are the most common type of sexually transmitted disease.

Treatment

- Warts may resolve spontaneously or recur after apparent cure. Multiple treatments are usually necessary.
- Topical agents include keratolytic preparations, such as salicylic acid (Duofilm, Occlusal) as well as tretinoin (Retin A), fluorouracil, or podophyllum.
- Surgical destruction involves cryosurgery using liquid nitrogen, carbon dioxide laser, or electrodesiccation and curettage.

Molluscum Contagiosum

General Principles
- Mollusca are intraepidermal tumors caused by the molluscum contagiosum virus.
- They are very common in children and spread easily through physical contact.
- If widespread mollusca are seen in adults, HIV should be suspected.
- Mollusca can be transmitted through sexual contact and is most often seen as an STD in adults.

Diagnosis
- Mollusca appear as small (1 to 5 mm), discrete flesh-colored or pearly white waxy papules with central umbilication.
- They are commonly found on the face and flexures in children and on the genital area, lower abdomen, and thighs in adults.
- Lesions may become infected or inflamed in children who pick or scratch them.

Treatment
- Spontaneous resolution usually occurs in immunocompetent individuals.
- If treatment is desired, cryotherapy or topical cantharidin can be used.
- HIV patients often require more aggressive therapy and referral to a dermatologist is appropriate.

Herpes Simplex Virus

See Chapter 23.

Varicella Zoster Virus

See Chapter 22.

SKIN INFESTATIONS

Scabies

General Principles
- The causative agent is the mite, *Sarcoptes scabiei.*
- Patients give a history of intense pruritus often on the hands, feet, and genitalia.
- Multiple family members are often afflicted.
- In immunosuppressed or debilitated patients, the mites may be so numerous that the skin takes on a crusted appearance; hence the term crusted scabies **(Norwegian scabies).**

Diagnosis
Careful examination of the web spaces of the hands will often reveal the characteristic burrow made by a female mite. Scraping these burrows will produce the highest yield on scabies preps.

Treatment
Permethrin 5% cream is applied over the entire body from the neck down and left on overnight. Bedding must be washed and close contacts with symptoms should also be treated. The treatment can be repeated in 1 week.

Pediculosis

General Principles
- The causative agent is the louse. Different varieties infest different areas of the body.
- Commonly affected areas include the scalp (including eyelashes in children), body hair, and pubic hair.
- Lice lay eggs on hair shafts that can be seen as round white ovals (nits).
- Some diseases are transmitted between humans via louse vectors.
- Infestations may be asymptomatic or cause pruritus.

Treatment
Permethrin 1% rinse is the first-line therapy. Resistant cases may require permethrin 5% cream or lindane shampoo. Removal of all nits with a fine comb is essential to treatment success. Family members are often treated as well.

SKIN SIGNS OF AUTOIMMUNE DISEASE

Lupus Erythematosus

General Principles
- Lupus is a multisystem disorder. It can range from a relatively benign but disfiguring cutaneous eruption with no internal involvement to a severe systemic disease that is potentially fatal (see Chapter 28).
- **Chronic cutaneous lupus erythematosus** is also known as discoid lupus erythematosus (DLE). It is characterized by erythema, scaling, hypopigmentation, follicular plugging, scarring, and telangiectasias. The two forms are localized and widespread. Widespread discoid lesions occur above and below the neck. Systemic LE will develop in 5% of DLE patients.
- **Subacute cutaneous lupus erythematosus** is nonscarring with prominent photosensitivity. Most patients are antinuclear antibody positive and anti-Ro/SS-A positive. Of patients with subacute cutaneous lupus erythematosus, 50% meet clinical criteria for SLE.
- **Acute cutaneous** LE is characterized by malar rash, DLE lesions, photosensitivity, and oral ulcers.

Diagnosis
- Diagnosis is largely based on skin examination. Distribution of lesions and presence of scars should be noted.
- History of worsening of symptoms with sun exposure is important.
- Biopsy of active lesions may be helpful if there is uncertainty of the diagnosis. Biopsy for direct immunofluorescence (lupus band) has largely been supplanted by serologic testing in SLE. Direct immunofluorescence may be beneficial in cases of suspected DLE. In such cases, biopsy of longstanding lesions provides the highest yield.
- Serum tests for common markers of autoimmune disease, such as antinuclear antibody and anti-Ro/SS-a antibodies may be useful.

Treatment
- Cutaneous lupus often responds to the therapy for the systemic disease, such as broad-spectrum sunscreens, antimalarials (e.g., hydroxychloroquine), and topical steroids.
- Systemic prednisone has shown little benefit.

Dermatomyositis

General Principles

- Dermatomyositis combines an inflammatory myopathy with characteristic cutaneous findings (see Chapter 28).
- Dermatomyositis *sine* myositis has characteristic skin findings without evidence of myopathy.

Diagnosis

- Pathognomonic signs on examination include a heliotrope rash, a violaceous hue over the eyelids, and Gottron's papules, erythematous papules over the bony prominence/knuckles.
- Other cutaneous findings include periungual telangiectasias, photosensitivity, rash in the shawl distribution, calcinosis cutis (more common in children), cuticular hypertrophy, and splinter hemorrhages.
- Laboratory findings include elevated muscle enzymes, the presence of myositis antibodies, and a pauci-inflammatory interface dermatitis on biopsy.

Treatment

The cutaneous disease often responds to the therapy for the systemic disease, such as broad-spectrum sunscreens, antimalarials, topical steroids, and methotrexate.

Scleroderma

General Principles

- Scleroderma is characterized by thickening or hardening of the skin associated with increased dermal or subcutaneous sclerosis, or both.
- Localized cutaneous disease can occur, which includes morphea, linear scleroderma, and facial hemiatrophy.
- Systemic disease is further classified into two conditions:
  - **Limited scleroderma (CREST):** calcinosis, Raynaud phenomenon, esophageal dysmotility, sclerodactyly, telangiectasia.
  - **Diffuse scleroderma,** or progressive systemic sclerosis.
- **Nephrogenic systemic fibrosis** represents a sclerodermalike illness that presents in patients with renal failure and has been strongly linked to use of specific gadolinium MRI contrast media. Typically, nephrogenic systemic fibrosis starts distally on the extremities and progresses proximally.

Diagnosis

- Cutaneous manifestations include generalized sclerosis, acrosclerosis/sclerodactyly, calcinosis cutis, pruritus, nail fold capillary changes, matlike telangiectasias, Raynaud phenomenon, taut facies, and salt and pepper dyspigmentation.
- Skin biopsy for routine histologic examination confirms the diagnosis.

Treatment

Cutaneous sclerosis and pruritus respond somewhat to psoralen (a light sensitizer) combined with ultraviolet A therapy.

Vasculitis

General Principles
- Most cases of palpable purpura are caused by skin-limited small vessel leukocytoclastic vasculitis but can be associated with the systemic vasculitides.
- Fifty percent are idiopathic but potential causes include the following:
  - Infections: hepatitis, Streptococcus, respiratory viruses.
  - Drugs: acetylsalicylic acid, sulfonamides, penicillin, barbiturates, amphetamines, and propylthiouracil.
  - Autoimmune disease/idiopathic: SLE, rheumatoid arthritis, cryoglobulinemia, Henoch-Schönlein purpura, antineutrophil cytoplasmic antibody (ANCA)-associated vasculitides, and Churg-Strauss syndrome.

Diagnosis
- History of autoimmune disorder, infection, or new medication is important.
- On examination, palpable purpura is the hallmark of vasculitis.
- Skin biopsy for routine histologic examination confirms the diagnosis. Biopsy for direct immunofluorescence is useful in cases of suspected IgA-related vasculitis.
- Laboratory work to be considered in the appropriate clinical setting includes urinalysis, stool guaiac, CBC, erythrocyte sedimentation rate (ESR), chest radiography, hepatitis panel, antinuclear antibodies (ANA), ANCA, and cryoglobulins.

Treatment
- Most cases of cutaneous only small vessel leukocytoclastic vasculitis are self-limited. Treatment is aimed at removing the offending agent.
- Prednisone improves the cutaneous disease but does not change the course.
- Most patients are treated with rest, NSAIDs, or colchicine.

Erythema Nodosum

General Principles
- Erythema nodosum commonly presents in young women.
- Fifty percent of cases are idiopathic but potential causes include the following:
  - **Streptococcal pharyngitis** and other upper respiratory tract infections.
  - **Drugs:** OCPs, sulfonamides, trimethoprim-sulfamethoxazole, salicylates, phenacetin, iodides, and bromides.
  - **Bowel disease:** ulcerative colitis, Crohn disease, and infectious colitis.
  - **Pulmonary disease** (erythema nodosum with hilar lymphadenopathy): tuberculosis, sarcoid (Löfgren syndrome), coccidioidomycosis, histoplasmosis, blastomycosis, and lymphoma.
  - **Other infections:** leprosy, yersiniosis.
  - **Behçet disease.**
- It is most often presumed to represent some form of delayed hypersensitivity.

Diagnosis
- History of chronic pulmonary or bowel disease, infection, or new medication is important.

- Physical examination reveals tender, symmetric subcutaneous nodules, commonly on the shins.
- Skin biopsy confirms the diagnosis.
- Appropriate evaluation includes CBC, purified protein derivative, and chest x-ray. Effort should be made at identifying the underlying cause.

Treatment

- Most cases are self-limited, lasting 3 to 6 weeks. Treatment is aimed at removing the offending agent or treating the underlying disease.
- Initial therapy is NSAIDs.
- Alternate therapies include oral potassium iodide, indomethacin, or colchicine. Steroids, intralesional or systemic, should only be considered once infections have been excluded or for recalcitrant cases.

SKIN SIGNS OF INTERNAL MALIGNANCY

Cutaneous Metastases

- The overall incidence of metastasis to skin is low (2% to 8%).
- Metastatic carcinoma appears as firm, flesh-colored, red or blue nodules. The trunk and scalp are the most frequent sites.
- The most likely source of occult skin metastasis is the lung, breast, gastrointestinal tract, melanoma, ovary, and kidney.

Lymphoreticular and Hematologic Malignancies

- Metastasis or paraneoplastic phenomena may affect the skin.
- Leukemia cutis or lymphoma cutis can resemble carcinomatous skin metastasis and appear as firm papules, nodules, or plaques. It is more likely to be hemorrhagic or plum-colored.
- Gingival hypertrophy and bleeding are common with leukemia.
- **Sweet syndrome** (acute febrile neutrophilic dermatosis) is associated with hematologic malignancies in 10% of cases. Sweets presents as a febrile illness with characteristic "juicy" red nodules and plaques. Biopsy for routine histologic examination and for culture confirms the diagnosis.

Cutaneous T-Cell Lymphoma

- Also known as mycosis fungoides, cutaneous T-cell lymphoma may present with erythematous patches, plaques, nodules, tumors, generalized erythroderma, or its leukemic variant.
- **Sézary syndrome** should be considered in patients with persistent patches or plaques or generalized exfoliative erythroderma. It is a form of cutaneous T-cell lymphoma.
- Diagnosis is confirmed with biopsy.
- Treatments include psoralen ultraviolet A, topical mechlorethamine, methotrexate, interferon-alpha, and histone deacetylase inhibitors.

SKIN SIGNS OF ENDOCRINOLOGIC DISORDERS

Thyroid Disorders

- **Hyperthyroidism** is associated with fine thin hair that may progress to diffuse alopecia, fine velvety skin with increased warmth and sweating, palmar erythema, and diffuse hyperpigmentation.
- **Graves disease** is associated with ophthalmopathy (exophthalmos, lid puffiness, and proptosis), pretibial myxedema, thyroid acropachy (characterized by clubbing), soft-tissue swelling of the hands and feet, and periosteal new bone formation.
- **Hypothyroidism** is associated with cretinism or congenital hypothyroidism, generalized myxedema, xerosis, keratoderma, cold pale skin, carotenemia, brittle hair that may progress to alopecia, loss of lateral third of eyebrows, and brittle, slow-growing nails.

Diabetes Mellitus

- **Diabetic dermopathy** appears as atrophic hyperpigmented patches on the shins.
- **Necrobiosis lipoidica diabeticorum** is characterized by well-circumscribed, yellow-brown, shiny plaques with pronounced epidermal atrophy and telangiectasia, commonly seen on the shins.

Lipoprotein Disorders

- **Eruptive xanthomas** arise in crops and exhibit an inflammatory acneiform appearance. They may be mistaken for pustules. Patients are at risk for acute pancreatitis. Plasma triglycerides are markedly increased, but cholesterol is normal. Etiologic factors include genetic lipoprotein lipase deficiency, ethanol abuse, estrogens, or retinoids.
- **Tendon xanthomas** are subcutaneous nodules that affect the tendons with normal-looking overlying skin. They may be mistaken for rheumatoid nodules. If plasma cholesterol is increased, the most likely cause is familial hypercholesterolemia. Patients are at risk for atherosclerosis and coronary disease.
- **Xanthelasma** is the most common but least specific type of xanthoma. It arises in the periocular area, especially on the eyelids. Fifty percent of patients have increased cholesterol.

40 Psychiatry
Prateek C. Gandiga

OVERVIEW

- Mental health disorders include a heterogeneous collection of conditions related to behavior, mood, interpersonal interactions, cognition, and personal identity. All cause **impairment in personal well-being and meaningful function.**
- Internists are integral in the care of patients with mental illness. Primary care physicians provide the sole mental healthcare for 60% to 70% of patients in the United States with psychiatric disorders.[1]
- Denial or the fear of social stigma induces many patients with psychiatric symptoms to seek help from a primary care physician rather than a mental health professional. Alternatively, such patients may present with somatic or nonspecific complaints.[2]

Epidemiology

- **Approximately one in four American adults suffers from a diagnosable mental disorder annually.** Mental illness is widespread across the population, and approximately 6% suffer from "serious mental illness." Mental health disorders are the leading cause of disability for ages 15 to 44 in the United States and Canada.[3]
- Nearly half of patient with mental illness suffer from two or more psychiatric disorders at a single time. Symptoms may also overlap between several conditions. Disease severity sharply increases for coexisting mental illnesses.[1,3]

Associated Conditions

- Several neurogenetic syndromes (i.e., Turner syndrome, Down syndrome, fragile X syndrome, Prader-Willi syndrome) and medical diseases have associated psychiatric manifestations.
- Socioeconomic, environmental, and cultural stressors contribute to the pathogenesis and definition of psychiatric diseases.[4,5] The effective treatment and management of mental disorders requires a flexible, highly patient-specific approach.

Relationships between Psychiatric and Medical Illnesses

- **Psychiatric illnesses are intimately intertwined with medical illnesses.** Underlying medical ailments (including endocrine disorders, cardiovascular disease, and respiratory conditions) are associated with increased rates of mental health disorders. Conversely, patients with significant psychiatric conditions have an increased risk for virtually all medical disease categories.
- The severity of psychiatry illness is directly correlated to worsened disease control and morbidity in conditions such as diabetes and heart failure. For example, depression is predictive for the increased incident of stroke in hypertensive patients.

- Studies suggest that successful treatment of psychiatric symptoms is associated with significant improvement in physical health and medical outcomes.
- Medical illness is a risk factor for the development or exacerbation of depression, and depression is itself a risk factor for medical illness.[6]

Evaluation

- Patients with one mental health disorder should be screened for other coexisting mental health diseases.
- Patients should also undergo a thorough mental status examination, with evaluation of the following[7]:
  - **Appearance and general behavior** (i.e., dress, grooming, hygiene, level of distress, degree of eye contact, attitude toward the interviewer).
  - **Motor activity** (i.e., psychomotor agitation, tremors, dyskinesias, akathisia, mannerisms, tics, stereotypies, catatonic posturing, echopraxia, apparent responses to hallucinations, gait/neurological defects).
  - **Speech characteristics** including rate, rhythm, volume, inflection, and articulation.
  - **Mood** (internal/subjective emotional state) and **affect** (the range, stability, and appropriateness of emotional expression).
  - **Thought processes** (i.e., vagueness, incoherence, circumstantiality, tangentiality, neologisms, perseveration, flight of ideas, loose or idiosyncratic associations, self-contradictory statements).
  - **Thought content** including ideas of reference, overvalued ideas, ruminations, obsessions, compulsions, phobias, and delusions (i.e., erotomania, delusions of persecution, infidelity, infestation, somatic illness, guilt, worthlessness, thought insertion, thought withdrawal, thought broadcasting).
  - **Thoughts or impulses of harm to self or others** (i.e., intensity, specificity of plans, when they occur, what prevents the patient from acting on them).
  - **Perceptual disturbances** including hallucinations (a perception in the absence of a stimulus), illusions (an erroneous perception in the presence of a stimulus), and depersonalization (feeling detached from oneself).
  - **Sensorium/cognition** (i.e., level of consciousness, orientation, attention, concentration, memory).
  - **Insight** (i.e., understanding of current problems, motivation to change health risk behaviors).
  - **Judgment** (i.e., appropriate decision-making abilities).

DEPRESSION

General Principles

Classification

- Mood disorders form a phenotypic spectrum of abnormally altered emotional state.
- Mood disorders are subdivided into those with[8]:
  - Only abnormally low mood (unipolar depression syndromes).
  - Cycling between abnormally elevated and abnormally depressed moods (bipolar syndromes).
  - Simultaneous depression and mania (mixed mood syndromes).

- Mood disorders present with a **heterogeneous range of symptom severity and functional impairment.**

Epidemiology

- Depression is **extremely common** worldwide. Nearly 10% of American adults suffer from a medical mood disorder annually, and the lifetime prevalence of depressive illness is 15% to 20%.
- The median age of onset for mood disorders is 25 to 35 years of age.
- Depressive disorders are more common in women than in men.[3]

Etiology/Pathophysiology

- Mood disorders stem from incompletely understood interactions between psychophysiological stressors and alterations in neurohormonal pathways. Multiple different pathophysiological changes can cause similar phenotypes.
- Serotonin- and norepinephrine-dependent pathways in the limbic system play a key role in depression. Additional changes in the hypothalamus-pituitary-adrenal axis are also likely involved.[9,10] The contributions of other neurotransmitter pathways are less clear.
- Major depression exhibits complex inheritance patterns, likely involving multiple genes. Genetic predisposition is stronger in bipolar disorders and severe in recurrent depression.[9]

Risk Factors

- Depression syndromes are more likely in those with[4] history of depression, anxiety, and/or substance abuse; chronic medical illness; family history of major depression; domestic abuse/violence; stressful life events (i.e., death of a loved one, divorce, job changes, motor vehicle accident); recent myocardial infarction or stroke; and current or recent pregnancy.
- Patients should be evaluated for depression if they exhibit[4,11] work or relationship dysfunction, changes in interpersonal relationships, worsening performance in activities of daily living, poor follow-through with prior treatment recommendations, multiple unexplained symptoms or frequent medical visits, dampened affect, weight gain or loss, sleep disturbances or chronic fatigue, dementia or memory impairment, irritable bowel syndrome, fibromyalgia syndrome, and volunteered complaints of stress or mood disturbances.

Associated Conditions

- Anxiety disorders and substance abuse frequently co-occur with depressive disorders.[3]
- Significant medical, psychological, or environmental stressors precipitate the first episode of major depression in 40% to 60% of patients.[4]

Depression and Medical Illnesses

- Depression has a complex interdependent relationship with medical illness. Medical illnesses may[12,13]
  - be a direct biological cause of depression (i.e., thyroid disorder, stroke),
  - contribute to psychological stressors,
  - predispose to depression though changes in neurohormonal signaling, and
  - mimic signs and symptoms of depression (i.e., anemia).
- **Overwhelming evidence supports that depression is associated with worse outcomes, impaired control, and increased risk of complications in diseases such as diabetes mellitus, stroke, myocardial infarction, and congestive heart failure.**[12]

- Poor control of medical illnesses may also contribute to worsened outcomes in depression.
- Treatment of associated medical illnesses may improve depression and vice versa, though data are limited.

Diagnosis

Clinical Presentation

- Compared with nonpathological "normal" sadness, depression exhibits a greater intensity, a longer duration, associated physical symptoms, and a significant impact on patients' function.
- **Major depression is characterized by at least 2 weeks of persistently decreased mood and/or anhedonia** (a significant loss of interest in previously interesting activities). Patients also exhibit associated psychophysiological changes in sleep, thought patterns, motivation, and overall function (Table 1).[8]
- **"Minor" depression** patients meet two to three symptom criteria, rather than the three or more necessary to diagnose major depression.
- In **bipolar depression,** patients present with episodes identical to major depression but also have a history of manic or hypomanic episodes (abnormally and persistently elevated/expansive/irritable mood with distractibility, insomnia, grandiosity,

---

TABLE 1 Abridged DSM-IV-TR Criteria for Major Depression

A. Abnormally Depressed Mood
A 2-week period marked by either:
1. depressed mood most of the day, nearly every day, as indicated by either self-report or observation made by others, or
2. markedly diminished pleasure in almost all activities most of the day, nearly every day

B. Associated "SIGECAPS" Symptoms
During the period of mood disturbance, at least four of the following exist nearly every day and represent a change from previous function:
1. **S**leep disturbances, with insomnia or hypersomnia
2. **I**nterest lost in previously pleasurable or enjoyable activities
3. **G**uilt, with inappropriate or excessive feelings of worthlessness or responsibility
4. **E**nergy "loss," with feelings of fatigue
5. **C**oncentration difficulties or indecisiveness
6. **A**ppetite changes with significant weight gain or loss when not dieting (i.e., >5% of body weight in 1 month)
7. **P**sychomotor agitation or retardation, observable by others
8. **S**uicidal ideation with recurrent thoughts of death or a specific plan for committing suicide

To meet criteria for depression, the symptoms should cause clinically significant distress or impairment in function.
The symptoms should not be better accounted for due to the direct physiological effects of a substance, medication, or a general medical condition.

Modified from American Psychiatric Association. Diagnostic and Statistical Manual of Mental Disorders (DSM-IV-TR). Text Revision. 4th Ed. Arlington, VA: American Psychiatric Publishing, Inc., 2000.

flight of ideas/feelings, racing thoughts, agitation/increased goal-directed activity, increased/pressured speech, and/or risk taking/hedonism).

- **Mixed mood syndromes** manifest symptoms of both mania and depression during the same episode.[8]
- The "Two-Question Screen" is sensitive but not specific for depression[11,14]:
  - Over the past month, have you been bothered by little interest or pleasure in doing things?
  - Over the past month, have you been bothered by feeling down, depressed, or hopeless?
  - **If the patient answers "yes" to either screening question, evaluation should be performed using a quantitative standardized instrument** (i.e., the PHQ-9, Beck Depression Inventory, or Hamilton Depression Rating Scale).[4]
- Initial evaluation should also include the following:
  - Screening for suicidality or self-harm (see "Deliberate Self-Harm and Suicidality" section).
  - Assessment of depression severity.
  - Evaluation for bipolar and mixed mood disorders.
  - Screening for concurrent psychiatric issues including substance abuse.

Differential Diagnosis

- A great many medical conditions are strongly associated with or contribute to mood disorders including cardiac, endocrine infectious, metabolic neoplastic, neurological disorders, as well as effects due to medications, toxins, and elicit substances.
- Depression must be distinguished from other psychiatric conditions (Table 2).[5,8]

Diagnostic Testing

- Appropriate laboratory and radiographic testing should be performed to evaluate for medical conditions contributing to the patient's depression.
- EEG may assist in diagnosing behavioral changes due to frontal lobe status epilepticus, partial complex seizures, or encephalopathy from metabolic, autoimmune, or infectious causes.[15] However, EEG should **not** be performed unless there is an elevated index of suspicion based on history or physical examination.

Treatment

- Depression treatment consists of three phases[15]:
  - **Acute therapy** (usually 6 to 12 weeks).
  - **Continuation** (4 to 9 months), which targets prevention of relapse.
  - **Maintenance** (6 months to years), which targets prevention of a new distinct episode of major depression.
- **Bipolar and mixed mood syndromes require mood stabilizers (i.e., atypical antipsychotics, antiepileptics, lithium) before antidepressant treatment to prevent triggering mania.**
- Bipolar disorder eventually manifests in up to 10% of patients initially thought to have unipolar depression.
- Strongly consider treatment of patients with low mood who do not strictly meet criteria for depression (i.e., "minor" depression) but exhibit significant functional impairment.

TABLE 2	Psychiatric Differential Diagnosis for Major Depression[5,8]	
	Similarities to Major Depression	Differences from Major Depression
Bipolar disorders	• Depressive episodes identical to unipolar depression	• History of at least one manic or hypomanic episode • Antidepressant treatment of depression in bipolar disorder can precipitate a manic episode
Seasonal affective disorder (SAD)	• Symptoms identical to depression during episodes	• Depressive episodes show a seasonal pattern (typically a fall or winter predominance) • Episodes regress completely as the season changes
Dysthymia	• Low mood and affect • Chronic, recurrent course • Associated changes in sleep, energy, concentration, and appetite • May predispose to major depression	• Lesser symptom severity, without anhedonia • Depressed mood, more days than not, for at least 2 years • Lesser risk of self-harm or suicide
Adjustment disorder	• Low mood and affect • Precipitated by life stressors • High rates of coexistent anxiety	• Lesser symptom severity, without anhedonia • Symptoms resolve with resolution of the stressor • Lesser feelings of guilt/ worthlessness • Lesser changes in appetite, sleep, or energy • Lesser risk of self-harm or suicide
Bereavement	• Low mood and affect • Impaired function • Precipitated by loss of loved one • Potential hallucinations and illusions • May progress to major depression	• Symptoms last <2 months • Less severe impairment • Lesser feelings of guilt or suicidal ideation
Psychotic disorders (i.e., schizophrenia, schizoaffective disorder)	• May include symptoms of depression or mania • Hallucinations or delusions may resemble psychosis in mania or depression • May occur in concurrence with depression or mania	• Mood symptoms brief relative to the total duration of the psychotic disturbance • Significant "negative symptoms" (i.e., flattened affect, disorganized speech/ behavior)

(continued)

TABLE 2	Psychiatric Differential Diagnosis for Major Depression[5,8] (*Continued*)	
	Similarities to Major Depression	Differences from Major Depression
Dementia	• Cognitive symptoms similar to depression in elderly patients • Decreased motivation and function. Associated with physical symptoms including sleep dysfunction • May predispose to concurrent major depression	• Premorbid history of declining cognitive function • Variable rate of decline (i.e., rapid to subacute to chronic) depending on underlying etiology
Medical disorders (i.e., endocrine, neurological)	• Overlap in signs and symptoms with depression • May predispose to depression	• Symptoms improve with treatment of the underlying condition alone
Substance related (i.e., withdrawal, intoxication, pharmaceutical)	• Overlap in signs and symptoms with depression • Substance abuse may predispose to depression	• Symptoms improve with treatment of the underlying condition alone

Acute Therapy

- Patients and family members should be educated that[4]:
  - Depression is a medical illness not a sign of weak character,
  - Depression can be effectively treated,
  - Patients improve with treatment, and
  - Depression can recur, and patients should seek treatment early if symptoms return.
- Acute therapy should target symptom remission and not merely improvement.[4,13,17] Response to treatment is defined as a ≥50% reduction in symptomatology.[4]
- **Depression-specific psychotherapies and antidepressant medications** have similar response rates for **mild** depression. Both are acceptable initial approaches.
- **Antidepressants** should be started in patients with **moderate or severe** depression. Adjuvant psychotherapy may improve response, especially in severe, recurrent, or chronic depression.[4,13,16–20]
- **Depression with psychotic features** should be treated with a combination of selective serotonin reuptake inhibitors (SSRIs) or venlafaxine (a serotonin-norepinephrine reuptake inhibitor) and antipsychotics and/or electroconvulsive therapy (ECT).[6]
- Patients may require ≥6 weeks to achieve full symptom remission after treatment begins.[4,21]

- If a patient experiences a symptom reduction of ≥25% 4 to 6 weeks after treatment initiation but is not yet in remission, continue current therapy with medication up-titration if tolerated.[4]
- If there is <25% reduction of symptoms after 6 weeks of appropriate therapy, either adding or switching to another treatment both appear effective.[4]
- Patients who do not respond to an initial SSRI have a modestly better chance of response if changed to a non-SSRI rather than a different SSRI.[4,13,21]
- Augmentation may include the addition of serotonin-norepinephrine reuptake inhibitors (SNRIs), tricyclic antidepressants (TCAs), bupropion, mirtazapine, and/or adjuvant nonpharmacological interventions. Psychostimulants, atypical antipsychotics, monoamine oxidase inhibitors (MAOIs), thyroid hormone, and lithium have also been used.
- Figure 1 provides a recommended schema for acute treatment with antidepressant medications.
- Medications should be tapered when discontinued or added, with vigilance for drug-drug interactions and overlapping side effect profiles.
- Patients should be routinely **monitored for suicide risk** throughout therapy.

Duration of Treatment

- Treatment should be continued for **at least 4 to 9 months after remission of symptoms** (the continuation phase).[22] Recurrent episodes imply the need for longer medication maintenance.
  - First episode: continue medication for 6 to 12 months, withdraw gradually.
  - Second episode: continue medication for 3 years, withdraw gradually.
  - Three episodes or more: continue medication indefinitely.
- When antidepressants are discontinued, it is commonly recommended that the medications be tapered over 2 to 4 weeks to minimize side effects associated with abrupt cessation.[4]

Medications

- Data suggest **minimal difference in efficacy among antidepressants for the acute treatment** of depression.[23,24]
- While data are limited, **it appears that most medications are also equally effective in preventing relapse.** Side effect profiles and cost-considerations should guide treatment choices (Table 3).
- Adherence to medication therapy, even after symptom improvement, is key. Premature discontinuation of antidepressant treatment is associated with a 77% increase in the risk of relapse or symptom recurrence.[4]
- Risks for premature self-discontinuation include younger age, lower educational status, and higher self-perceived mental health.[21]
- **SSRIs and SNRIs are considered first-line agents given their side effect profiles.** There appears to be minimal within-class differences in efficacy.
- Mirtazapine may have a better tempo for symptom improvement compared with SSRIs but this effect is transient, idiosyncratic, and minimal.
- **TCAs** are effective but should be used cautiously given **cardiac side effects and risk for lethal overdose.** Higher doses of TCAs may be more effective in those who partially respond to lower doses.
- **MAOIs** should be restricted to patients unresponsive to other medications because of their potential for **drug interactions, serious side effects, and the necessity of dietary restrictions.**

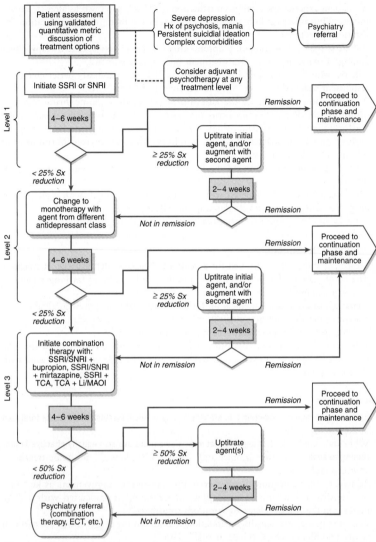

Figure 1. Suggested schema for acute therapy with antidepressant medications. LI, lithium; MAOI, monoamine oxidase inhibitor; SNRI, serotonin-norepinephrine reuptake inhibitor; SSRI, selective serotonin reuptake inhibitor; TCA, tricyclic antidepressant.

- Psychostimulants (i.e., dextroamphetamine, methylphenidate, methylamphetamine) are useful adjuvant treatments for depression but have not been adequately studied for use as monotherapy.
- Lithium augmentation has been used for unipolar depression but may cause serotonin syndrome when given with SSRIs.

TABLE 3   Antidepressant Medications

	Usual Starting Dose (mg/day)	Usual Total Therapeutic Dose (mg/day)	Side Effects and Clinical Notes	Qualitative Frequency of Common Side Effects								
				Headache	Insomnia or Agitation	Sedation	Nausea	Diarrhea	Dry Mouth	Weight Loss	Weight Gain	Anti-Cholinergic Effects
Tricyclics and tetra-cyclics (TCAs)			Affect multiple neurotransmitter systems. Risk of QTc prolongation, arrhythmia, MI. Anticholinergic effects include orthostasis and sexual dysfunction. Rare bone marrow and hepatic toxicity. Lower seizure threshold. Levels increased by concomitant SSRI. Potentially fatal at overdose.									
Amitriptyline (Elavil)	25–50	100–300	Metabol. to nor-triptyline by liver.	++	+	+++	+	+	+++	–	+++	+++
Amoxapine (Asendin)	50	100–400		+	+	++	+	–	++	–	+	+
Clomipramine (Anafranil)	25	100–250		+++	+++	+++	+++	+	+++	–	++	+
Desipramine (Norpramin)	25–50	150–200		+	+	+	+	+	+	+	+	+

(continued)

TABLE 3 Antidepressant Medications (Continued)

	Usual Starting Dose (mg/day)	Usual Total Therapeutic Dose (mg/day)	Side Effects and Clinical Notes	Qualitative Frequency of Common Side Effects								
				Headache	Insomnia or Agitation	Sedation	Nausea	Diarrhea	Dry Mouth	Weight Loss	Weight Gain	Anti-Cholinergic Effects
Doxepin (Adapin, Sinequan)	25–50	100–300		+	+	+++	+	+	++	−	++	++
Imipramine (Tofranil)	25–50	150–300	Metabol. to desipramine by liver. Increased orthostasis and arrhythmia vs. other TCAs.	+	+	++	+	+	+++	+	++	++
Maprotiline (Ludiomil)	50	100–225		+	+	+++	+	+	++	−	++	+
Nortriptyline (Pamelor)	25	75–100	Lower rates of orthostasis and arrhythmias vs. other TCAs.	+	−	+	+	+	+	+	+	++
Protriptyline (Vivactil)	10	15–60		+	+	+	+	+	++	−	−	+
Trimipramine (Surmontil)	25–50	100–300		+	−	+++	+	+	+	−	++	+
Selective serotonin reuptake inhibitors (SSRIs)			Sexual side effects. Headache and jitteriness often subside after first 4–7 days. Risk of birth malformations. Risk of seizures at very high doses. Risk of serotonin syndrome if given with MAOIs.									

Drug	Starting dose	Dose range	Notes									
Citalopram (Celexa)	10–20	20–60	Less Rx-Rx interactions than other SSRIs.	+	++	++	++	+++	+	+	+	−
Escitalopram (Lexapro)	10	10–20	Single isomer formulation of citalopram, similar SFx profile.	+++	++	++	++	++	+	−	+	−
Fluoxetine (Prozac)	5–10	20–60	CYP2D6 inhib. Take in morning to reduce insomnia. Active metabolites (long half-life, available in once-weekly formulation). Transiently decreases appetite.	++	+++	+++	+++	+++	+	++	+	−
Fluvoxamine (Luvox)	25	50–300	Affects multiple CYP isoforms. Increased risk of Rx-Rx interact vs. other SSRIs.	+++	+++	+++	+++	+++	++	++	+	−
Paroxetine (Paxil)	5–10	20–60	CYP2D6 inhib. Higher rates of extrapyramidal SFx and withdrawal SFx vs. other SSRIs. Less GI SFx if taken with food.	++	+++	+++	+++	+++	++	++	−	+
Paroxetine CR (Paxil CR)	12.5–25	25–75	CYP2D6 inhib. Same SFx as immediate release but possibly less GI SFx. Cannot crush or chew.	++	+++	+++	+++	+++	++	++	−	−

(continued)

TABLE 3 Antidepressant Medications (*Continued*)

	Usual Starting Dose (mg/day)	Usual Total Therapeutic Dose (mg/day)	Side Effects and Clinical Notes	Qualitative Frequency of Common Side Effects								
				Headache	Insomnia or Agitation	Sedation	Nausea	Diarrhea	Dry Mouth	Weight Loss	Weight Gain	Anti-Cholinergic Effects
Sertraline (Zoloft)	25–50	50–200	CYP2D6 inhib. but less potent inhib. than fluoxetine. Very sedating, best taken at night.	+++	++	++	+++	++	++	–	+	–
Dopamine-norepinephrine reuptake inhibitors												
Bupropion (Wellbutrin)	75–150	300–450	Risk of seizure. Mild stimulating properties. May be beneficial in treating SSRI-related sexual SFx. Caution in hepatic impairment.	+++	++	+	++	+	+++	++	–	–
Bupropion SR (Wellbutrin SR)	150	300–400		+++	++	+	++	+	+++	++	–	–
Bupropion XL (Wellbutrin XL)	150	300–450		+++	++	+	++	+	+++	++	–	–

	Starting dose	Dose range (mg)	Comments								
Serotonin-norepinephrine reuptake inhibitors (SNRIs)											
Venlafaxine (Effexor)	37.5	75–300	CYP2D6 inhib.: incr. SFx if switching from CYP2D6-metabol. agents. High risk of withdrawal SFx. HTN, MI at high doses.	+++	+++	++	+	+++	++	+	−
Venlafaxine XR (Effexor XR)	37.5	75–300		+++	+++	++	+	+++	++	+	−
Desvenlafaxine (Pristiq)	50	50	Active metabolite of venlafaxine: similar SFx but does not interact with CYP2D6. May increase LDL.	−	++	++	++	+++	++	−	−
Duloxetine (Cymbalta)	30	60–120	Contraind. if signif. renal/hepatic disease. May impair glycemic control in DM. Possible addition benefits in chronic pain control.	++	++	+++	++	+++	+++	+	−
Serotonin modulators											
Nefazodone (Serzone)	50	300–600	Potent CYP3A4 inhib. Increases REM sleep. Less sexual SFx than other antidepressants. Risk of QTc prolongs if given with cisapride. Risk of hepatotoxicity, Steven-Johnson syn.	+++	++	+++	+	+++	++	−	+

(continued)

875

TABLE 3 Antidepressant Medications (Continued)

	Usual Starting Dose (mg/day)	Usual Total Therapeutic Dose (mg/day)	Side Effects and Clinical Notes	Qualitative Frequency of Common Side Effects								
				Headache	Insomnia or Agitation	Sedation	Nausea	Diarrhea	Dry Mouth	Weight Loss	Weight Gain	Anti-Cholinergic Effects
Trazodone (Desyrel)	50	75–300	Postural hypotension and nausea. Risk of priapism, arrhythmias.	+++	+	+++	++	+	++	++	++	–
Noradrenergic agonist-specific serotonergic antagonist												
Mirtazapine (Remeron)	15	15–45	Neurotransmitters affected are dose-related. SFx may be greater at lower doses. Lower risk of sexual SFx than SSRI. Risk of bone marrow toxicity.	++	+	+++	+	+	+++	–	++	+

Monoamine oxidase inhibitors (MAOIs)			Risk of serotonin syndrome if given with or close to discontinuation of SSRIs.							
Phenelzine (Nardil)	15	15–90	Dose-related hypotension, sexual SFx, sleep disturbance. Rare hepatotoxicity.	++	++	+	+	+	–	++	–
Selegiline (Ensam)	6 (patch)	6–12		++	++	++	++	++	–	–	–
Tranylcypromine (Parnate)	10	30–60	Dose-related hypotension, sexual SFx, sleep disturbance. May cause transient hypertension for 3–4 hours after doses.	++	++	+	+	+	–	++	–

Contraind., contraindicated; CYP, cytochrome-P450; DM, diabetes mellitus; GI, gastrointestinal; HTN, hypertension; immed., immediate; inhib, inhibition; metabol., metabolized; LDL, low-density lipoprotein; MI, myocardial infarction; QTc, corrected QT interval; REM, rapid eye movement; Rx-Rx interact., drug-drug interaction; signif., significant; SFx, side effects; SR, sustained release; SSRIs, selective serotonin reuptake inhibitors; –, rare; TCAs; tricyclic antidepressants; XL, extended release; XR, extended release; +, seldom; ++, common; +++, frequent.

Modified from Depression Guideline Panel. U.S. Department of Health and Human Services. Agency for Health Care Policy and Research. Depression in Primary Care: Treatment of Major Depression. AHCPR Publication No. 93-0551. Rockville, MD: 1993; Gartlehner G, Hansen RA, Thieda P, et al. U.S. Department of Health and Human Services. Agency for Healthcare Research and Quality. Comparative Effectiveness of Second-Generation Antidepressants in the Pharmacologic Treatment of Adult Depression. AHRQ Publication No. 07-EHC007-EF. Bethesda, MD: 2007.

- St. John's wort and SAM-e (S-adenosyl methionine) are sometimes self-prescribed as "natural" antidepressants. Although potentially beneficial, serious drug-drug interactions and the heterogeneity of commercially available preparations argue against use.[4,18,25]
- Other herbals and dietary supplements, such as kava-kava, omega-3 fatty acid (docosahexaenoic acid), and valerian root, have not been proven effective for the treatment of depression.[4,25]

Nonpharmacologic Treatment

- **Several psychotherapy modalities are effective in the treatment of depression.**[19] Such interventions should be performed by counselors specifically trained in these techniques.
- **Combined therapy using both pharmacological and psychological therapy may be more effective than either intervention alone.**[4,19]
- **ECT** may benefit patients with refractory depression, depression with psychotic features, and geriatric patients.
- Repetitive transcranial magnetic stimulation, deep brain stimulation, vagus nerve stimulation, and acupuncture have not been adequately studied to recommend routine use against depression.[4]
- Seasonal affective disorder often improves with phototherapy using broad-spectrum bright light (typically 5,000 to 10,000 lux).[4] Such therapy should be initiated only by clinicians trained in prescribing phototherapy.
- Aerobic exercise may be of adjuvant benefit in reducing depressive symptoms.[4,18,26] Patients should aim for 30 minutes of moderate-intensity exercise, 3 to 5 days per week.

Referral

- Multiple trials demonstrate the added utility of a collaborative-care model with the close integration of physicians, mental health professionals, and case managers.[4] While both general medicine and psychiatric specialty settings yield good initial outcomes, therapeutic alliance with mental health specialists should be strongly considered.[21]
- Psychotherapy should be administered by a skilled therapist. Data suggest that the success of psychotherapy may be linked to the experience level of practitioners.
- Strongly consider **psychiatrist or mental health specialist referral** if there are intolerance or minimal benefit with first-line agents, signs of psychosis or suicidal ideation, severe symptoms or functional impairment, comorbid medical, psychiatric, or substance abuse disorders, symptoms or history suggestive of mania/bipolar disease or seasonal affective disorder, plans for psychotherapy, need for frequent or close follow-up, and patient requests for specialist treatment.
- Consider **hospitalization** if the patient[17] poses a serious risk for harm to self or others (involuntary hospitalization may be necessary), is severely ill and lacks adequate social supports, has not responded adequately to outpatient treatment, or has significant comorbid psychiatric or medical conditions.

Monitoring/Follow-Up

Expert opinion recommends patients should be[22]:
- Seen within 2 weeks after starting any medications to evaluate for tolerability, effectiveness, and appropriate dosage,

- Followed at least every 2 weeks until significant symptom improvement, and
- Followed at least every 3 months after symptom remission.

Outcome/Prognosis

- Depression is a heterogeneous disorder with a highly variable course.[9]
- In most patients, major depression is a relapsing-remitting illness with a >40% risk of recurrence within 2 years after the first depressive episode.[5]
- Repetitive episodes increase the risk of future recurrence.
- Relapse prevention with pharmacological and nonpharmacological modalities diminishes but does not completely prevent relapse.[19] Clinicians should be mindful to monitor for depression recurrence.

DELIBERATE SELF-HARM AND SUICIDALITY

General Principles

- Deliberate self-harm commonly involves self-cutting, self-poisoning, or intentional medication overdose.[27]
- Suicide is an act of self-harm with a fatal outcome, coconsciously initiated and performed with the expectation of death.[27]
- Individual self-harm acts vary in their associated
  - suicidal intent,
  - degree of planning (i.e., meticulous vs. impulsive, precautions against rescue), and
  - lethality of method (i.e., violent versus passive).

Epidemiology

- About 3% to 5% of the population have made an attempt at deliberate self-harm at some time during their lives.[27]
- Approximately one quarter of those with one self-harm attempt will reattempt self-harm within 4 years, with a long-term suicide risk of 3% to 7%.[3]
- The median mortality from suicide after an act of deliberate self-harm is 1.8% within the first year, 3.0% within 1 to 4 years, 3.4% within 5 to 10 years, and 6.7% within 9 years or longer.[27]
- Younger adults are more likely to attempt nonfatal self-harm, whereas older adults are more likely to complete suicide.
- Women attempt suicide two to three times as often as men, but men are four times as likely to die by suicide.[3]
- The highest suicide rates in the United States are found in white men >85 years of age.[3]
- >90% of those who commit suicide suffered from a mental illness, most commonly a mood or a substance abuse disorder.[3]

Etiology/Pathophysiology

- Evidence suggests that genetic predisposition, biological changes, and psychosocial factors all contribute to deliberate self-harm.[27]
- Reduced serotonin function and lowered cerebrospinal 5-hydroxyindoleacetic acid levels in the central nervous system may underpin the pathophysiologic changes of self-harm.
- Patients who deliberately self-harm also show personality traits of impulsiveness, aggression, inflexibility, and impaired judgment.

Risk Factors

- A large number of risk factors have been associated with the suicide attempts including the following[4,27,28]:
  - Suicidal thoughts, past attempts, specific/lethal plans, access to firearms.
  - Psychiatric illness (depression, bipolar disorder, schizophrenia, substance abuse).
  - Psychological features (shame, poor self-esteem, impulsiveness, aggression, hopelessness, severe anxiety).
  - Significant burden of medical illness.
  - Socioeconomic factors (lack of support, unemployment, recent stressful events).
  - Demographics (women/younger more likely to attempt, men/older more likely to succeed; widowed/divorced/single).
- Studies have not found racial predispositions for attempting suicide.[4,5]
- Factors with a protective effect include positive social support, children at home, responsibility to family, pregnancy (in the abscess of peripartum depression), religious beliefs, life satisfaction, and good judgment/problem-solving skills/coping skills.[28]
- **Antidepressants, including SSRIs and TCAs, may increase risk of self-harm during the initial treatment of psychiatric illness when compared with placebo.** The U.S. Food and Drug Administration issued a warning about the risks of suicidal thinking and behavior in adults aged 18 to 24 years during the first 1 to 2 months of treatment for major depression.[29]

Diagnosis

Clinical Presentation

At risk patients should be assessed for thoughts of causing deliberate harm to themselves or others.[4,28] Useful questions include the following:

- Do you feel that life is worth living?
- Do you wish you were dead?
- Have you thought about hurting yourself or ending your life?
- If so, how often have those thoughts occurred?
- If so, have you gone so far as to think about how you would do so?
- Do you have access to a way to carry out your plan?
- What keeps you from harming yourself?
- Do you feel that others are responsible for your problems?
- If so, have you thought about harming or punishing them?

Treatment

- Immediate **hospitalization** with close observation should strongly be considered for patients who[28] are deemed high risk for harm to self or others; evidence psychosis or command hallucinations; have current impulsive behavior, severe agitation, or poor judgment; have a specific suicide plan with persistent intent/ideation; have made precautions against discovery or rescue; have previously attempted suicide using means with high lethality; have significant comorbid psychiatric illness (including depression or substance abuse); and are male and >45 years of age.
- Reversible causes of suicidality or homicidality (i.e., substance withdrawal or intoxication, psychiatric illness, depression) should be identified and treated appropriately.
- Pharmacological and psychotherapeutic interventions may be beneficial for the treatment of those without underlying reversible causes, though data are limited and inconsistent.

Medications

- **Antidepressant medications** (i.e., SSRIs, SNRIs, TCAs) should be used to treat depressed patients with suicidal ideation (Table 3).[28]
- Lithium medications reduce the risk of both suicide and suicide attempts when used as long-term maintenance for recurring bipolar disorder and major depressive disorder.
- Anticonvulsant agents used as mood stabilizers (i.e., valproate, carbamazepine, lamotrigine) have **not** been shown to reduce risk of suicidal behavior.
- Clozapine reportedly decreases the rate of suicide and self-harm attempts in schizophrenia. Other antipsychotics may also reduce suicide risk in schizophrenic patients.
- Benzodiazepines may ameliorate the suicide risk in agitated patient because of anxiolytic effects but should be used cautiously as they also disinhibit behavior and enhance impulsivity, particularly in patients with borderline personality disorder.
- **No pharmaceutical treatments have clearly shown usefulness for reducing recurrent self-harm not associated with underlying psychiatric illness.**[27]
- Depot injections of flupentixol (an antipsychotic) may reduce the 6-month repeat self-harm risk in nonschizophrenic patients though data are limited.[31] The use of oral antipsychotics to prevent suicide in patients without schizophrenia has not been adequately studied.[27,30]
- Paroxetine has also not been shown to reduce recurrent deliberate self-harm in nondepressed patients.[27,30] Paroxetine and other SSRIs have been linked to suicidal ideation in children, adolescents, and young adults with depression but the implications of this association are unclear.[27,29,30]

Nonpharmacologic Treatment

- Clinical consensus suggests skilled psychosocial interventions and specific psychotherapeutic techniques (i.e., cognitive behavioral therapy, problem-solving therapy) be used in preventing recurrent self-harm.[27,28] Data evaluating these approaches are, however, limited.[27]
- ECT may provide short-term reduction in suicidal ideation, especially in cases of severe depression.[28,30]
- While recommended, intensive follow-up plus outreach, nurse-led management, emergency contact cards, and hospital admission have not consistently been shown to reduce recurrent self-harm compared with usual care.[27,30]

Referral

Patients with recurrent or persistent suicidal ideation or self-harm attempts should be cared for in collaboration with psychiatrists and other mental health professionals.

Follow-Up

- Patients who have attempted deliberate self-harm are at risk for future attempts. Repetition is more likely in patients[27] aged 25 to 49 years, unemployed or socioeconomic disadvantaged, divorced, living alone, or with unstable living situations, who have a criminal record, who have a history of stressful traumatic life events or come from a "broken home," and who have a history of substance abuse, depression, or personality disorder, and with recurrent feelings of hopelessness or powerlessness.
- Patients should be routinely monitored by clinicians and family members for evidence of suicidal ideation or recurrent self-harm behaviors. Repeat or long-term

hospitalization may be necessary if the patients are persistently a threat to themselves or others.

ANXIETY DISORDERS

- Anxiety disorders are the most common mental health illnesses, affecting nearly one in five American adults.[3] The disorders are **typified by increased agitation, nervousness, and autonomic tone which disrupt general well-being and function.**
- Anxiety disorders include panic disorder, obsessive-compulsive disorder, posttraumatic stress disorder, generalized anxiety disorder (GAD), and phobias (Table 4).[5,8]
- Anxiety disorders frequently co-occur with depressive disorders or substance abuse. In addition, most people with one anxiety disorder also have another anxiety disorder.[3]
- Medical issues such as hypoglycemia, hyperthyroidism, respiratory disease, gastrointestinal disease, and medication side effects all predispose to anxiety disorders. Improvement of these conditions may improve the patients' psychiatric issues.

GENERALIZED ANXIETY DISORDER

General Principles

GAD is characterized by **unreasonably excessive concern** about common issues such as finances, family, or work. In GAD, worries become so exaggerated that there is difficulty in performing day-to-day tasks (Table 5).[8]

Epidemiology

- About 3% of American adults suffer from GAD.[3] However, studies suggest that GAD may be more prevalent in primary care settings, and suggest that GAD is the anxiety disorder most often seen by general internists.[31]
- GAD develops gradually and may present at any age, though the median age of onset is about 30 years.
- Similar to other anxiety disorders, GAD is more common in women than in men.[3]

Etiology/Pathophysiology

- GAD develops from a combination of biological and psychosocial factors.
- Multiple neurotransmitter and endocrine pathways, including the hypothalamic-pituitary-adrenal axis, have been implicated.[32] Medical disorders such as chronic pain, endocrine diseases, and pulmonary conditions may predispose to generalized anxiety.
- Social and environmental stressors, including recent unfavorable events, also likely contribute to GAD.[33]
- Maladaptive cognitive strategies play a prominent role in GAD. "Worry" subjectively increases preparedness for feared events but also causes distress over them. GAD patients subconsciously overvalue the "worry process" and, over time, develop a cycle of worry-proneness.[31]
- Predisposition to GAD appears modestly inheritable but incompletely understood.[32,33]

Associated Conditions

- Patients with GAD may exhibit worsening job performance, changes in interpersonal relationships, multiple unexplained symptoms or frequent medical visits,

TABLE 4	Characteristics of Common Anxiety Disorders[5,8]	
	Defining Characteristics	**Additional Features**
Panic disorder	• Recurrent unexpected short-lived episodes of marked autonomic arousal (i.e., tachycardia, palpitations, sweating, shortness of breath) and catastrophic thinking (i.e., fear of fainting, dying, "depersonalization"). • Attacks are abrupt in onset, unprovoked and, unexplained.	• Impairment stems from worry about potential future panic episodes. • Possible evolution into avoidance of places or situations associated with past panic episodes (a.k.a., agoraphobia). • Panic episodes may awaken patient from sleep during non-REM states. • Symptoms may fluctuate in intensity.
Generalized anxiety disorder	• Excessive worry about multiple foci of concern for more days than not with significant disruption of daily life.	• Association with nonspecific somatic complaints including fatigue, insomnia, muscle tension. • Related concentration difficulties, irritability, or restlessness. • Symptoms may fluctuate in intensity.
Posttraumatic stress disorder	• Intense fear, helplessness, and "flashbacks" following an extreme traumatic stressor with perceived risk of death or serious injury. • Patients avoid reminders of the trauma and experience hyperarousal (i.e., easy startle, irritability, difficulty concentrating, insomnia).	• Possible traumas may include violent or sexual assault, kidnapping, incarceration, natural disasters, or severe accidents. • Patients may also experience posttraumatic stress disorder from witnessed events or events experienced by a family member or loved one.
Phobias	• Unreasonably excessive and persistent fear triggered by the presence or anticipation of a specific stimulus. • Phobias cause significant impairments in function due to avoidance behaviors.	• Common phobias include animals (i.e., dogs, insects, spiders); environmental features (i.e., closed spaces, heights, darkness); and social situations (i.e., public speaking, eating in public).
Obsessive-compulsive disorder	• Presence of either obsessions (repetitive intrusive anxiety-provoking thoughts) or compulsions (repetitive anxiety-relieving behaviors or mental acts designed to neutralize obsessions)	• Patients often recognize the irrationality of their obsessions. • The nature of the patients' obsessions and compulsions may change over time.

TABLE 5	Abridged DSM-IV-TR Criteria for Generalized Anxiety Disorder

A. Excessive Anxiety and/or Worry

Excessive, difficult-to-control anxiety and "worry" (apprehensive expectation) about a number of events or activities of daily life (i.e., work, school) occurring most days for at least 6 months.

B. Associated Psychiatric and/or Somatic Symptoms

The anxiety and worry are associated with three or more of the following:

1. Restlessness or feeling keyed up or on edge
2. Fatigue, or easy fatigability
3. Difficulty concentrating, or mind going blank
4. Irritability
5. Muscle tension
6. Sleep disturbances (i.e., insomnia, difficulty staying asleep, restless/ unsatisfying sleep)

C. Exclusion of Other Anxiety Disorders

The focus of the anxiety is *not confined* to worry about:

1. Having a panic attack (i.e., panic disorder)
2. Being embarrassed in public (i.e., social phobia)
3. Being contaminated (i.e., obsessive-compulsive disorder)
4. Being away from home or close relatives (i.e., separation anxiety disorder)
5. Gaining weight (i.e., anorexia nervosa)
6. Having multiple physical complaints (i.e., somatization disorder)
7. Having a serious illness (i.e., hypochondriasis)

The anxiety and worry *should not* occur exclusively during posttraumatic stress disorder.

D. Exclusion of Other Psychiatric Disorders

The disturbance does not occur exclusively during a mood disorder, a psychotic disorder, or a pervasive developmental disorder.

To meet criteria for generalized anxiety disorder, the symptoms should cause clinically significant distress or impairment in function.

The symptoms should not be better accounted for due to the direct physiological effects of a substance, medication, or a general medical condition.

Modified from American Psychiatric Association. Diagnostic and Statistical Manual of Mental Disorders (DSM-IV-TR). Text Revision. 4th Ed. Arlington, VA: American Psychiatric Publishing, Inc., 2000.

concentration difficulties, sleep disturbances or chronic fatigue, and increasing alcohol/tobacco use.

- Patients with GAD are at high risk for developing another anxiety disorder or major depression.[33,34]
- More than one third of GAD patients "self-medicate" with the abuse of alcohol or illicit drugs.[31]
- **GAD is a chronic condition but can be improved or controlled with treatment.** Twenty-five percent of adults with GAD will be in full remission after 2 years and thirty-eight percent will have a remission after 5 years.[33]

- However, nearly one third of patients in full remission will have a clinically significant relapse within 5 years; the rate is even higher for those with only partial remission.[33]

Diagnosis

Clinical Presentation

- The hallmark of GAD is **excessive and difficult-to-control worry about multiple issues,** often despite insight that the anxiety is more intense than warranted.[32]
- Unlike other anxiety disorders, worry in GAD is **not limited to a specific trigger or social situation** (i.e., phobias). GAD patients may experience discrete panic attacks but their anxiousness is **persistent, pervasive, and focused on multiple components** of normal daily living.
- In addition to excessive worry, patients may exhibit **other nonspecific signs** including[34] irritability or fatigue, difficulty concentrating, increased startle responses, and/or sleep disturbances, including insomnia.
- Patients with GAD frequently have associated **somatic symptoms** including[31,32,34] headaches, muscle tension and myalgias, difficulty swallowing (i.e., globus hystericus), nausea, tremor or tics, sweating, lightheadedness or dyspnea, frequent urination, and/or hot flashes.
- Symptom severity fluctuates over time and is often worse during periods of increased stress.[32]
- GAD patients often seek medical care for their somatic symptoms but do not necessarily volunteer concerns about their psychological ones.[31,32]
- Screening can be performed using the 7-item Anxiety Scale (GAD-7), which has reasonable reliability, sensitivity, and specificity.[35]
- Further assessment should be made through a validated quantitative measure such as the Generalized Anxiety Disorder Questionnaire IV (GAD-Q-IV).[36]
- Initial evaluation should include the following:
  - Screening for suicidality or self-harm.
  - Assessment of anxiety severity and impact.
  - Screening for concurrent psychiatric issues including substance abuse.
- Appropriate laboratory and radiographic testing should be performed if there are potentially treatable medical conditions contributing to the patient's symptomatology.

Differential Diagnosis

- Many medical conditions are associated with or contribute to anxiety disorders including cardiac, endocrine infectious, metabolic neoplastic, neurological disorders, as well as effects due to medications, diet, toxins, and illicit substances.
- GAD must be distinguished from other psychiatric conditions (Table 4).[5,8]

Treatment

- Both medications and nonpharmacological treatments benefit GAD, but it is uncertain which is more effective. It is also unclear whether combined therapy with both modalities is more effective than either option alone.[31]
- Strongly consider **psychiatrist or mental health specialist referral** if there are[34] severe symptoms or functional impairment, signs of psychosis or suicidal ideation, comorbid medical, psychiatric, or substance abuse disorders, plans for psychotherapy, need for frequent or close follow-up, and/or patient requests for specialist treatment.

Medications

- The **SSRIs** escitalopram, paroxetine, and sertraline have all shown benefit over placebo in treating GAD and should be considered first-line agents (Table 3).[31,33,37]
  - Although data are limited, there appears to be minimal efficacy and tolerability differences amongst these medications.[33]
  - **Patients typically require at least 4 to 6 weeks of therapy with SSRIs before symptoms improve.**
- The **SNRIs** venlafaxine and duloxetine may also be efficacious in treating GAD, though trial data are mixed and limited.[31,33]
- **Imipramine** has demonstrated benefit for GAD; other TCAs are less well-studied.[31,33,37] However, the side effect profile of imipramine suggests that it should be considered a second-line agent.
- **Buspirone** improves GAD anxiety symptoms compared with placebo when studied in short-term clinical trials.[33,38]
  - It is unclear whether the efficacy of buspirone is significantly different than other antidepressants or benzodiazepines.[33,38]
  - Buspirone must be taken consistently for at least 2 weeks to achieve an anxiolytic effect.[34]
- **Benzodiazepines** have proven utility in the temporary mitigation of GAD (Table 6).[33,39]
  - However, trials have *not* shown benefit over other agents when used for long-term anxiety control.[33]
  - The prolonged use of benzodiazepines in GAD also increases risk for dependence, sedation, and traffic accidents.[33]
  - These agents should be limited to use for breakthrough anxiety.
  - There does not appear to be significant within-class efficacy differences among the long-acting benzodiazepines.[33]
- Abecarnil is a novel nonbenzodiazepine β-carboline agent with gamma-aminobutyric acid (GABA)-mediated anxiolytic effects. Clinical trials have not yet convincingly shown its benefit for GAD.[33]
- Hydroxyzine (a first-generation antihistamine) has been successfully used as an anxiolytic in GAD.[33] Data regarding its efficacy have been mixed, however, and sedating side effects may limit its usefulness.
- Gabapentin and pregabalin have shown some benefit in improving GAD symptoms but their role is yet to be defined.[40]
- Antipsychotics, including trifluoperazine and olanzapine, have yielded mixed results when used for treatment-resistant GAD.[33] The potential for serious adverse effects limits the routine use of such agents.
- Kava and valerian are herbal compounds with potential GABA-mediated anxiolytic benefits.[25] However, heterogeneity in commercially available preparations and limited clinical study caution against their use.

Nonpharmacologic Therapies

- Psychotherapy is an effective treatment for control of the GAD.
- **Cognitive-behavioral therapy (CBT)** focused on insight, education, and coping strategies reduces anxiety symptoms and is beneficial as both short- and long-term treatment.[31–33,41]
  - It is uncertain, however, whether CBT is more effective than other psychological therapies.[41]
  - It is also unclear whether ongoing CBT is more effective than supportive psychotherapy in the long-term management of GAD.[33]

TABLE 6 — Frequently Used Benzodiazepines

Drug	Onset of Action	Half-Life	Relative Potency	Usual Total Dose (mg/day)	Usual Dosing Frequency	Notes
Alprazolam (Xanax)	Medium	Interm.	4	0.75–6	tid	High-potency: increased risk withdrawal
Alprazolam XR (Xanax XR)	Varies	Long	4	0.5–6	Once daily	Absorption rate affected by food, time of day of administration
Chlordiazepoxide (Librium)	Medium	Interm.	0.1	15–30	tid	Active metabolites with long half-life of elimination
Clonazepam (Klonopin)	Rapid	Long	2	0.5–2	bid	Total doses >1 mg/day not shown to be more effective for symptom control.
Clorazepate (Gen-Xene)	Rapid	Short	0.1	15–60	bid to qid	
Diazepam (Valium)	Rapid	Long	0.2	4–20	bid to qid	
Estazolam (ProSom)	Rapid	Interm.	3	1–2	hs	High-potency. Usually used to treat insomnia.
Flurazepam (Dalmane)	Rapid	Short	0.2	15–30	hs	Usually used to treat insomnia.
Lorazepam (Ativan)	Medium	Interm.	1	0.5–6	bid to tid	
Midazolam (Versed)	Rapid	Short	0.8	5–50	tid to qid	
Oxazepam (Serax)	Slow	Interm.	0.7	30–120	tid to qid	
Quazepam (Doral)	Rapid	Long	0.2	7.5–15	hs	Usually used to treat insomnia.
Temazepam (Restoril)	Medium	Interm.	0.2	7.5–30	hs	Usually used to treat insomnia.
Triazolam (Halcion)	Rapid	Short	3.3	0.125–0.25	hs	Usually used to treat insomnia.

Higher relative potency designates more potent agents (i.e., inverse of dose-equivalents).

All benzodiazepines have longer-lasting and more potent effects in patients with hepatic impairment. CYP-450 interactions change the metabolism of many benzodiazepines.

Patients with panic disorder may need higher total doses than those with generalized anxiety disorder for symptom relief.

Short, <6 hours; Interm., 6–20 hours; Long, >20 hours; bid, twice daily; tid, three times daily; qid, four times daily; hs, at bedtime; XR, extended release.

Modified from Sadock BJ, Sadock VA. Concise Textbook of Clinical Psychiatry. 3rd Ed. Philadelphia, PA: Lippincott Williams & Wilkins, 2008.

- CBT should be administered by a skilled therapist. Data suggest that the success of psychotherapy is linked to the experience level of practitioners, though some patients may benefit from nonspecialist delivered supportive psychotherapy alone.[31]
- Relaxation training has historically been used in treating GAD but has not been well-studied in clinical trials.[31] Related methods such as "applied relaxation" and "mindful meditation" appear to have efficacy similar to other psychotherapy techniques.[33]
- Aerobic exercise and exercise training likely have general anxiety-lowering benefits but have not been well-studied in the treatment of GAD.[26]

PANIC DISORDER AND AGORAPHOBIA

General Principles

- Panic attacks are discrete sudden periods of intensive apprehension or terror, often accompanied by physiological symptoms and feelings of impending doom (Table 7).[8]
- Panic disorder is diagnosed, however, only when recurrent unpredictable panic attacks are followed by at least 1 month of persistent concern about having another panic attack or significant behavioral changes related to the attacks.[5,8]
- Agoraphobia (an irrational fear of public places, crowds, or being outside the home) may also develop in the setting of recurrent panic attacks.

Epidemiology

- Approximately 3% of American adults have panic disorder; of these, one in three develops agoraphobia. Panic disorder is twice more common in women than in men, and moderately heritable.[3,42]
- Panic disorder typically first manifests in late adolescence or early adulthood, but the age of onset extends throughout adulthood.[3,34,42]

TABLE 7	Abridged DSM-IV-TR Criteria for Panic Attack

A discrete period of intense fear or discomfort, in which four or more of the following symptoms developed abruptly and reached a peak within 10 minutes:
1. Sweating
2. Trembling or shaking
3. Chills or hot flushes
4. Shortness of breath, or sensations of smothering
5. Feeling of choking
6. Palpitations, heart-pounding, or accelerated heart rate
7. Chest pain or discomfort
8. Nausea or abdominal distress
9. Feeling dizzy, unsteady, lightheaded, or faint
10. Derealization (feelings of unreality) or depersonalization (being detached from oneself)
11. Fear of losing control or going crazy
12. Fear of dying
13. Paresthesias (numbness or tingling sensations)

Modified from American Psychiatric Association. Diagnostic and Statistical Manual of Mental Disorders (DSM-IV-TR). Text Revision. 4th Ed. Arlington, VA: American Psychiatric Publishing, Inc., 2000.

Etiology/Pathophysiology

- The underpinnings of panic disorder and agoraphobia are multifactorial and incompletely understood. Dysfunction of serotonin-, norepinephrine-, and GABA-mediated central nervous system pathways are implicated. In addition, patients may have idiosyncratic changes in autonomic system regulation.
- Panic disorder also appears to have an important cognitive-behavioral aspect, and its onset is often preceded by stressful life events.[31,34,42]
- Predisposition to develop panic attacks appears to be inheritable.[34]

Associated Conditions

- Patients with panic disorder may exhibit worsening job performance, changes in interpersonal relationships, multiple unexplained symptoms or frequent medical visits, concentration difficulties, sleep disturbances or chronic fatigue, and/or increasing alcohol/tobacco use.
- Patients with panic disorder are at high risk for developing another anxiety disorder, depression, or substance abuse.
- The risk of suicide and attempted suicide is markedly higher in patients with panic disorder, even when compared with those with other psychiatric illnesses including depression.[42]
- Panic disorder is an independent risk factor for coronary heart disease.[31]
- If untreated, panic disorder chronically recurs with an unpredictable waxing-and-waning course. Patients may experience residual symptoms, including agoraphobia and somatization, even during periods when actual panic attacks are quiescent.
- **Panic disorder is highly treatable** and the majority of patients receive benefit with appropriate therapy.[34]

Diagnosis

Clinical Presentation

- Not all patients who experience panic attacks will develop panic disorder.[34] The impact of panic disorder stems mainly from worry about future panic attacks or the possible implications of physical symptoms.
- Panic attacks may feel truly life-threatening. Patients are often consumed by recurrent "what if?" worries related to the perceived dangerousness of panic attacks and may persistently seek medical consultations despite reassurance.
- Patients with panic disorder **typically first present to emergency or primary care settings with unexplained symptoms** rather than direct concerns about panic attacks. Complaints commonly include the following[31,34]:
  - Noncardiac chest pain.
  - Palpitations.
  - Unexplained faintness.
  - Unexplained vertigo and dizziness.
  - Irritable bowel symptoms.
  - Dyspnea or tachypnea.
  - Feelings of impending doom or depersonalization.
  - Nocturnal awakenings from panic attacks.
- **Agoraphobia** sufferers typically have more severe impairment and panic symptomatology but are more likely to seek treatment than other panic disorder patients.[31]

- Screening with two questions from the Anxiety and Depression Detector yields a high sensitivity and moderate specificity for panic disorder[31,43]:
  - In the past 3 months, did you ever have a spell or an attack when all of a sudden you felt frightened, anxious, or very uneasy?
  - In the past 3 months, would you say that you have been bothered by "nerves" or feeling anxious or on edge?
  - If the patient answers "yes" to either screening question, further evaluation should be performed using a quantitative standardized instrument.
- Initial evaluation should include the following:
  - Screening for suicidality or self-harm.
  - Assessment of panic disorder severity.
  - Screening for concurrent psychiatric issues including substance abuse.
- Appropriate laboratory and radiographic testing should be performed if there are potentially treatable medical conditions contributing to the patient's symptomatology.

Differential Diagnosis

- As noted above, many medical conditions are associated with or contribute to anxiety disorders.
- Panic disorder must be distinguished from other psychiatric conditions (Table 4).[5,8]

Treatment

Strongly consider **psychiatrist or mental health specialist referral** if there is[34] severe symptoms or functional impairment; agoraphobia; recurrent panic attacks despite treatment; signs of psychosis or suicidal ideation; comorbid medical, psychiatric, or substance abuse disorders, plans for psychotherapy; need for frequent or close follow-up; and/or patient requests for specialist treatment.

Medications

- Medications improve anxiety and decrease the frequency of panic attacks, though it is unclear whether pharmacotherapy is more effective than nonpharmacological treatments.[31,34,42]
- **SSRIs** are considered the drugs of choice in treating panic disorder (Table 3). Efficacy appears similar among the SSRIs. Data also suggest comparable efficacy for extended-release venlafaxine.[31,42]
- **Benzodiazepines** are beneficial in acutely reducing the symptoms of panic attacks but have a high potential for abuse, dependence, and tolerance (Table 6).[31,34,42] Short-term adjuvant therapy with long-acting benzodiazepines may benefit some patients during the initial phase of other therapies.
- **TCAs** appear to be as effective in preventing panic attacks as SSRIs. However, they are significantly less well-tolerated by panic disorder patients and should be considered second-line agents.[31,34,42]
- **MAOIs and buspirone** have shown mixed results in the treatment of panic disorder.[31,42] Side effect and interaction profiles limit their use.
- Bupropion has not been adequately studied to support its use for panic disorder, especially as many patients report that its "activating" effects actually worsen panic symptoms.[31]
- β-blockers may help some patients control physical symptoms, though they have not shown effectiveness for panic disorder in controlled trials.[31,34]

- Gabapentin may exhibit anxiolytic benefit in panic disorder, though data are mixed.[40]
- Kava and valerian are herbal compounds with potential GABA-mediated anxiolytic benefits.[25] However, heterogeneity in commercially available preparations and limited clinical study caution against their use.
- **Side effects that mimic panic attack symptoms may occur during either initiation or discontinuation of medications.** Antidepressants should be started at half the usual initial dose and gradually titrated when increased or withdrawn. Frequent reassurance may aid patient compliance.

Nonpharmacologic Therapies

- **CBT** has an efficacy for treating panic disorder clearly supported by robust clinical trial data.
  - It is unclear whether CBT is superior to pharmacotherapy but some data suggest that the benefits of CBT may be long lasting.[31,42]
  - Combined treatment with CBT and antidepressants may be more beneficial than with either modality alone in short-term symptom reduction.[42]
  - More than one third of patients with panic disorder either cannot tolerate or do not respond to appropriate SSRI or venlafaxine therapy. Many patients who do not respond to medication will, however, respond to CBT.
  - Combination therapy with both SSRIs and CBT appears to increase the therapeutic response rate during the first few months of treatment but it is uncertain whether benefits persist after this.
  - It is also unclear whether CBT "maintenance" therapy improves remission rates after the discontinuation of medications.
  - The addition of medications may increase the dropout rate compared with CBT alone.
  - CBT should be administered by a skilled therapist. Data suggest that the success of psychotherapy is linked to the experience level of practitioners.
- Other forms of psychotherapy (including self-help treatments) have not been as well studied but may also be beneficial in treating panic disorder symptoms.[34,42]
- Aerobic exercise, breathing techniques, and relaxation/biofeedback exercises may indirectly improve panic disorder through lowering hyperreactivity to bodily sensations, though few studies have evaluated their use.[26,31,42] Similarly, yoga and meditation have theoretical benefit but have been formally evaluated only on a limited basis.[44] Although the adverse effects of such therapies are minimal, dropout rates appear to be relatively high.

PSYCHOSIS AND SCHIZOPHRENIA

General Principles

- Psychosis denotes a **disturbed perception of reality** including hallucination, delusion, or thought disorganization.
- Psychotic states are associated with increased agitation, aggression, impulsivity, and behavioral dysfunction.
- Psychosis may be due to:
  - Underlying psychiatric illness (i.e., schizophrenia, mania).
  - Substance abuse (i.e., cocaine intoxication, alcohol withdrawal).
  - Medication side effects (i.e., corticosteroids).
  - Medical illnesses (i.e., delirium, encephalitis).

- Patients have variable insight into their psychosis and may or may not recognize the derangements in their thought processes.[5,45]
- Types of psychotic symptoms include the following:
  - **Hallucinations** are false perceptions in one of the sensory modalities (i.e., auditory, visual, tactile, olfactory, gustatory). Auditory hallucinations are more common in psychoses due to a primary psychiatric disorder such as schizophrenia. However, the hallucination modality is not pathognomonic.
  - **Delusions** are false beliefs that are firmly held despite obvious evidence to the contrary. Delusions are distinct from ideas typical of the patient's background cultural, religious, or familial belief system. Common delusions include thoughts of persecution, thoughts of grandiosity or superhuman abilities, and thoughts of hyperreligiosity. Delusions are characterized as "bizarre" or "nonbizarre" on the basis of their degree of plausibility.
  - **Ideas of reference** are a common type of delusion in which a patient believes that neutral information refers specifically to him or her. Patients may believe in the receipt of "special messages" transmitted from the television, radio, newspaper, or "psychic communications."
  - **Illogical thought processes** are evidenced by nonsensical speech and loose associations, with accompanying functional impairment, bizarre behaviors, and agitation or aggression.
  - **Agitation** can manifest as both heightened emotional arousal and increased motor activity. Agitation is not exclusive to psychosis but frequently accompanies it.
- **Schizophrenia** is a severe, chronic disorder characterized by periods of active psychosis and an insidious deterioration of social, occupational, and personal functioning. Symptoms are typically subcategorized as follows:
  - **Positive symptoms,** including psychosis with hallucinations, delusions, and thought disorganization.
  - **Negative symptoms,** including blunted affect, loss of social interest, decreased motivation, anhedonia, and decreased verbal communication.
  - **Cognitive symptoms,** including deficits in memory, attention, verbal processing, and executive function.
  - **Affective symptoms,** such as bizarre or inappropriate affect and predisposition for major depression.

Epidemiology

- Approximately 1% of the American adult population has schizophrenia.
- Schizophrenia is equally frequent in men and women.
- Schizophrenia typically first manifests in men during their late teens or early twenties; women usually first exhibit symptoms in their twenties or early thirties.[3]
- Schizoaffective and mood disorder–associated psychosis may be more common in women.
- Approximately 80% of untreated manic patients develop psychotic symptoms. Psychotic symptoms in the context of mania or depression are often congruent with mood, such as grandiose delusions, but may not be.

Etiology/Pathophysiology

- The pathophysiology of schizophrenia is poorly understood.
- Studies demonstrate abnormally elevated dopaminergic activity, altered neural network activation patterns, and anatomic atrophy in the central nervous system of patients with schizophrenia.[46,47]

- These changes likely result from complex interactions between multiple genes and environmental factors.[46]
- Conditions which increase the risk of developing schizophrenia include personal history of a pervasive developmental disorder, autistic disorder, Down syndrome, and a family history of schizophrenia.

Associated Conditions

- A total of 40% to 50% of patients with schizophrenia suffer from substance abuse issues with tobacco, alcohol, or illicit drugs.[4]
- Schizophrenic patients are also predisposed to suicide, depression, homelessness, and unemployment.

Diagnosis

Clinical Presentation

- Psychotic patients should undergo a complete mental status examination.
- Patients should be specifically questioned about hearing voices, seeing things others do not see, sensations of things touching or crawling on the skin, experiencing odd smells or tastes, fears that others are following, spying on, or wish to cause them harm, thought reading, special messages from television or radio, unusual religious experiences, and special powers or abilities.

Diagnostic Criteria/Differential Diagnosis

- Criteria for the diagnosis of schizophrenia are presented in Table 8.[8]
- Schizophrenia must be distinguished from other psychotic conditions (Table 9).[5,8]
- Medical illnesses and pharmacological syndromes are associated with psychotic symptoms.

Treatment

- The treatment of psychosis and schizophrenia is complex and should be done in conjunction with a psychiatrist or similarly qualified healthcare professional.
- Treatment for psychosis should be voluntary whenever possible, but the nature of the illness may lead patients to fear or avoid treatment. Such patients may benefit from involuntary treatment, especially if they exhibit a high risk for harm to self or others.
- Symptomatic treatment of psychosis is appropriate, even if diagnostic evaluation is still in progress.
- **Goals for the acute treatment** of schizophrenia include the following[45,47,48]:
  - Preventing self-harm.
  - Controlling disturbed behavior.
  - Reducing the severity of psychosis and associated symptoms (e.g., agitation, aggression, negative symptoms, affective symptoms).
  - Addressing factors which precipitated the acute psychotic episode.
  - Connecting the patient and family with appropriate aftercare.
- **Assess the patient for risk factors for suicide or self-harm including** prior self-harm attempts, depressed mood, hopelessness, anxiety, suicidal ideation, presence of command hallucinations, extrapyramidal side effects, and alcohol or other substance use.
- Schizophrenic patients have a significantly higher prevalence of diseases including diabetes mellitus, the metabolic syndrome, coronary heart diseases, and chronic

| TABLE 8 | DSM-IV-TR Criteria for Schizophrenia |

A. Characteristic symptoms:
Two (or more) of the following, each present for a significant portion of time during a 1-month period (or less if successfully treated):
1. Delusions
2. Hallucinations
3. Disorganized speech (i.e., frequent derailment or incoherence)
4. Grossly disorganized or catatonic behavior
5. Negative symptoms (i.e., affective flattening, alogia, avolition)

Only one criterion A symptom is required if delusions are bizarre or hallucinations consist of a voice keeping up a running commentary on the person's behavior or thoughts, or two or more voices conversing with each other.

B. Social/occupational dysfunction:
For a significant portion of the time since the onset of the disturbance, one or more major areas of functioning such as work, interpersonal relations, or self-care are markedly below the level achieved prior to the onset.

C. Duration:
Continuous signs of the disturbance persist for at least 6 months. This 6-month period must include at least 1 month of symptoms (or less if successfully treated) that meet criterion A (i.e., active-phase symptoms) and may include periods of prodromal or residual symptoms manifested by only negative symptoms or attenuated form of positive symptoms (i.e., odd beliefs, unusual perceptual experiences).

Modified from American Psychiatric Association. Diagnostic and Statistical Manual of Mental Disorders (DSM-IV-TR). Text Revision. 4th Ed. Arlington, VA: American Psychiatric Publishing, Inc., 2000.

obstructive pulmonary disease than the general population.[49] Both antipsychotic medication side effects and sequelae of the primary disease seem to contribute. Such patients should undergo actively routine screening for such illnesses, with emphasis on early interventions and preventative measures.

Medications

- Antipsychotic medications are useful in the treatment of psychotic symptoms.
- In schizophrenia, antipsychotic medications are **primarily effective for control of positive symptoms.** Negative symptoms show a modest response to antipsychotics, affective symptoms respond in about half of patients, and cognitive symptoms respond minimally.[45,47,48]
- Antipsychotic medications are often classified as first-generation (a.k.a., conventional, typical) or second-generation (a.k.a., atypical). All work via dopamine-receptor antagonism. The nonspecific effect on agitation begins early; **antipsychotic effect takes 3 to 6 weeks.** Common antipsychotics are presented in Table 10.[45]
- Atypical antipsychotics are a heterogeneous class in respect to efficacy and side effect profile (Table 11).[45,50]
  - It is uncertain whether atypical antipsychotics are significantly more beneficial for the control of symptoms than first-generation agents.[45,47,50]

TABLE 9	Psychiatric Differential Diagnosis of Psychosis[5,8]	
	Defining Characteristics	**Additional Features**
Schizophrenia	• Combination of positive and negative symptoms, social withdrawal, and psychosis • Psychotic symptoms last for 1 month or longer.	• May occur in conjunction with mania or depression but mood symptoms are brief relative to the total duration of the illness
Brief psychotic disorder	• Is characterized by a total duration of <1 month.	• May be associated with borderline personality disorder (if so, symptoms usually last <1 day)
Schizoaffective disorder	• Features of both schizophrenia and mood disorder • Mood symptoms present for a substantial portion of the total duration of illness	• Psychosis persists even after mood improvements
Mood disorder with psychotic features	• Psychotic symptoms that occur exclusively during a manic or depressive episode (i.e., in unipolar or bipolar depression)	• Delusions, often mood congruent (i.e., grandiosity in mania, somatic illness in depression) • Psychosis remits when mood improves
Delusional disorder	• Nonbizarre delusions occurring in the absence of other significant psychiatric symptoms	• Common delusions include thoughts of erotomania, grandiosity, jealousy, persecution, or somatic illness
Delirium-associated	• Characterized by impaired judgment, orientation, memory, affect, and concentration, in association with a known medical illness	• Possible medical illnesses include trauma, infection, tumor, metabolic, endocrine, intoxication • Psychoactive substance use, epilepsy, withdrawal state
Substance-induced psychosis	• Because of substance abuse or withdrawal • May persist beyond acute intoxication (a.k.a., "flashbacks"). • May signal life-threatening withdrawal syndromes (i.e., delirium tremens)	
Medication-induced psychosis	• Symptoms directly attributable to known medication side effects	• Commonly seen with corticosteroids, L-DOPA
Dementia-associated psychosis	• Dementia (with decline in cognitive function) typically presents before psychosis	• Prominent in Lewy body and end-stage dementia
Ethnic/familial/societal belief system	• May contain ideas or concepts that are acceptable in the cultural context • Not considered psychosis	

TABLE 10	Commonly Used Antipsychotic Medications		
	Typical Dose Range (mg/day)	Chlorpromazine Equivalents (mg/day)	Half-Life (hours)
First-generation agents (conventional antipsychotics)			
Phenothiazines			
Chlorpromazine	300–1000	100	6
Fluphenazine	5–20	2	33
Mesoridazine	150–400	50	36
Perphenazine	16–64	10	10
Thioridazine	300–800	100	24
Trifluoperazine	15–50	5	24
Butyrophenone			
Haloperidol	5–20	2	21
Others			
Loxapine	30–100	10	4
Molindone	30–100	10	24
Thiothixene	15–50	5	34
Second-generation agents (atypical antipsychotics)			
Aripiprazole	10–30	—	75
Clozapine	150–600	—	12
Olanzapine	10–30	—	33
Quetiapine	300–800	—	6
Risperidone	2–8	—	24
Ziprasidone	120–200	—	7

Modified from American Psychiatric Association. Practice guideline for the treatment of patients with schizophrenia, second edition. *Am J Psychiatry* 2004;161:1–56.

- Atypical agents may be less likely to induce extrapyramidal side effects than high-potency conventional medications but have an increased risk for other adverse effects including weight gain.[50]
- Antipsychotic medications should be chosen on the basis of side effect profile and patient comorbidities.
- Expert opinion recommends low-dose risperidone, quetiapine, olanzapine, or aripiprazole for psychosis in elderly patients.[51]
- Adverse effects from antipsychotic medications include the following:
  - Prolactinemia (galactorrhea, amenorrhea, loss of libido).
  - Weight gain, dyslipidemia, hyperglycemia.
  - QTc prolongation (arrhythmia, sudden cardiac death).
  - Acute dystonia (acute muscular rigidity, laryngospasm).
  - Parkinsonism (masked facies, stooped posture, tremor, rigidity).
  - Akathisia (intense restlessness, restlessness).
  - Tardive dyskinesia (involuntary movements).
  - Neuroleptic malignant syndrome (rigidity, tremor, autonomic instability, mental status changes, potential for death).
- Diphenhydramine or benztropine may be helpful in treating extrapyramidal effects (i.e., dystonia, akathisia, Parkinsonism).[48]

TABLE 11   Qualitative Frequency of Antipsychotic Side Effects

Drug	EPS, Tardive Dyskinesia	Prolactin Elevation	Weight Gain	Glucose Abnormalities	Lipid Abnormalities	QTc Prolongation	Sedation
Aripiprazole	–	–	–	–	–	–	+
Clozapine	–	–	+++	+++	+++	–	+++
Haloperidol	+++	+++	+	–	–	–	++
Olanzapine	–	–	+++	+++	+++	–	+
Perphenazine	++	++	+	+	+	–	+
Quetiapine	–	–	++	++	++	–	++
Risperidone	+	+++	++	++	++	+	+
Thioridazine	+	++	+	+	+	+++	++
Ziprasidone	–	+	–	–	–	++	–

EPS, extrapyramidal side effects (akathisia, Parkinsonism, dystonia); –, rare; +, seldom; ++, common; +++, frequent.
Modified from American Psychiatric Association. Practice guideline for the treatment of patients with schizophrenia, second edition. *Am J Psychiatry* 2004;161:1–56.

- A sizable minority of schizophrenic patients do not achieve complete symptom remission despite appropriate antipsychotic medications.
- Adjuvant treatments including lithium, carbamazepine, benzodiazepines, β-blockers, valproate, and ECT have been used in schizophrenics whose psychoses did not respond to traditional therapy.[52,53]
- Associated conditions, including depression, should be addressed in psychotic patients. However, antidepressants which inhibit catecholamine reuptake can potentially sustain or exacerbate psychosis.

Nonpharmacologic Therapies

- ECT may be useful for the treatment of psychosis refractory to antipsychotic medications, those with prominent catatonic features, or those with comorbid depression or suicidality.[45,47,48]
- Psychological therapy techniques may be effective adjuvants for psychosis, though data are limited.
- Multiple psychosocial interventions, including vocational training programs and case managers, seem to be beneficial in assisting those with schizophrenia.[45,48]

Outcome/Prognosis

- Schizophrenic patients have a **chronic illness with fluctuating course.**
- >70% of first-episode patients achieve a full remission of psychotic signs and symptoms within 3 to 4 months and >80% achieve stable remission at the end of 1 year.[45]
- Predictors of poor treatment response include male gender, pre- or perinatal injury, more severe hallucinations and delusions, attentional impairments, poor premorbid function, longer duration of untreated psychosis, development of extrapyramidal side effects, and distressing emotional climate (i.e., hostile and critical attitudes and overprotection by others in one's living situation or high levels of expressed emotion).[45]
- There is significant unexplained heterogeneity in the long-term outcomes of schizophrenic patients. Poor outcome occurs in <50% of patients but, frustratingly, good outcome also occurs in <50% of patients.[47] Importantly, 20% to 40% attempt suicide and 7% will die of it.[45]

SPECIAL CONSIDERATIONS IN GERIATRIC PATIENTS

General Principles

- Depression and anxiety are **not part of the normal aging process.** These illnesses have considerable negative influence on elderly patients' quality of life.
- Older adults who require recurrent hospitalizations or long-term nursing home care have increased rates of mental health illnesses compared with their peers.
- Mental health disorders in geriatric patients seem to derive from pathophysiology dissimilar to younger adults and may involve subacute neurological degeneration or ischemia.[3,6,20,54]
- **Underlying medical conditions** (such as advanced cardiac, pulmonary, or neurological illness) predispose to depression and anxiety. The causality of such associations is complex and likely involves both physiological changes as well as psychosocial stressors.
- Medical diseases common in the geriatric population may present with psychiatric symptoms. Older adults with psychiatric symptoms should be screened for conditions including thyroid and adrenal dysfunction; diabetes mellitus; cardiac arrhythmia or

ischemia; nutritional deficiencies; malignancy, including pancreatic cancer; stroke, Parkinsonism, or neurological disorders; chronic pain; sleep disorders; occult infections; and medication side effects.

- Elderly patients with mental health disorders **often present atypically,** emphasizing somatic manifestations of their illness rather than psychiatric ones. Practitioners should exercise high levels of vigilance when evaluating older patients and avoid the mistake of simply treating symptoms without addressing possible underlying mental health issues.
- Geriatric patients are **prone to medication side effects and drug-drug interactions.** Medications should be initiated at lower doses than in younger patients and titrated slowly. Medical comorbidities should be considered when selecting therapeutic modalities and medications.
- Referral to a psychiatrist or other mental health professional should be considered for all elderly adults with mental health disorders given the complexity of care in this population.

Depression in Older Adults

- Depression can be subtle in older adults. Rather than endorsing "sadness" or "feeling depressed," older patients will often manifest depression as[43,55]:
  - Apathy or decreased interest in previous hobbies.
  - Feelings of ill health with vague somatic symptoms.
  - Lack of energy.
  - Psychomotor slowing or agitation.
  - Worsening control of comorbid medical illnesses and medical noncompliance.
  - Sleep disturbances or early morning awakenings.
  - Cognitive impairment including memory deficits and slowed information/visuospatial processing.
  - Delusions of guilt and worthlessness.
  - Auditory/visual hallucinations.
- Geriatric patients are at **increased risk for successful suicide** compared with younger adults.[3]
- Patients with symptoms of depression or a positive "Two Question Screen" should be evaluated using a **geriatric-specific metric** such as the Geriatric Depression Scale.[56,57]
- Even "minor" depression is associated with worsened function, increased mortality, and increased risk of suicide in older adults.
- Treatment should strongly be considered in such cases given the favorable response rate and benefit of intervention.
- Antidepressant medications should be considered for all geriatric patients with depression.[6]
- Skilled psychotherapy augments rates of response to medications and may alone be sufficient in mild depression if pharmacological therapy is contraindicated.[13,54,58,59]
- Data support the efficacy and tolerance of multiple classes of antidepressants in the elderly.[6,13,58]
- **SSRIs or nonselective serotonin agonists (i.e., mirtazapine, bupropion, and SNRIs) should be used as first-line agents** for geriatric depression given a more benign side effect profile compared with TCAs (Table 3).[6,13,20,58] However, these agents may cause Parkinsonism, sleep disturbances, anorexia, sinus bradycardia, and hyponatremia in the elderly.
- **Highly anticholinergic mediations,** including amitriptyline and imipramine, are **relatively contraindicated** in older adults because of risk of arrhythmia, narrow angle glaucoma, urinary retention, delirium, and orthostasis.

- Older adults also have an increased risk for cardiovascular complications from TCAs and antipsychotics.[55]
- ECT is generally safe in geriatric patients and may be especially useful for those with severe symptoms including suicidality, catatonia, and psychosis.[6,55,60]
- Remission of depression progresses more slowly in the elderly. More than half of geriatric patients treated with antidepressants eventually experience treatment response within 2 months.[6,58] If symptoms persist after 6 to 8 weeks, additional or alternative treatment options should be considered.
- Assessing therapeutic response should include evaluation of overall quality of life, performance of activities of daily living, and control of comorbid illnesses.[59]
- Maintenance treatment with antidepressants or ECT should continue for at least 12 months in older adults with moderate or severe depression to reduce the risk of recurrence. Continuance for even longer durations may be worthwhile in such patients.[6,61,62] Skilled psychotherapy is a helpful adjuvant in preventing recurrence of moderate or severe geriatric depression, but should not be used alone.[58,61,62]

Anxiety in Older Adults

- Anxiety problems, including GAD, are common in geriatric populations.[58,63,64]
- Practitioners must differentiate whether an older patient's symptoms are due to a primary anxiety disorder or secondary to other causes. Cardiac diseases, respiratory illnesses, and medication side effects disproportionately affect older adults compared with younger adults and are significantly anxiogenic if not well-controlled.
- Agitation (the physical manifestations of hyperactivity) subtly differs from anxiety but should be distinguished as it may require alternate treatment. Elderly adults with agitation do not typically experience the sense of dread or impending doom characteristic of anxiety. Agitation without clear anxiety is also frequent in patients with dementia or delirium.
- Rather than endorsing worry, geriatric patients with anxiety disorders are more likely to present with nonspecific complaints including the following[63,64]:
  - Concentration or memory difficulties.
  - Restlessness or irritability.
  - Muscle tension.
  - Vague visceral discomfort.
  - Recurrent cardiovascular or gastrointestinal symptoms without clear medical explanations.
  - Continued medical complaints despite negative workup.
  - Fatigue.
  - Decreased physical activity and functional independence.
  - Low mood or depression.
  - Increased feelings of loneliness.
  - Avoidance of certain situations, tasks, or locations.
- Anxiety prominently affects sleep in older adults; data suggest that 90% of older adults with GAD report dissatisfaction with sleep.[65]
- Anxiety disorders are frequently associated with depression in older populations.[63,64] The co-occurrence of both disorders increases the risk for suicidality and substance abuse.
- It is unclear which metrics are best to screen older adults for anxiety disorders. The Generalized Anxiety Disorder Severity Scale (GADSS) may help in evaluating for either GAD or panic disorder in elderly patients.[66,67]

- Despite the prevalence of anxiety disorders in geriatric populations, few potential treatment options have been rigorously studied.[58,63,64]
- **SSRIs** appear useful for treating geriatric anxiety disorders (Table 3). Both citalopram and escitalopram have shown benefit in the treatment of GAD and panic disorder in small trials.[68,69] Minor side effects are relatively frequent in older patients using SSRIs for anxiety and include fatigue, sleep disturbances, and urinary symptoms. More serious adverse reactions, including hyponatremia, may also occur.
- **Extended-release venlafaxine** also seems useful in treating older adults with GAD, with an efficacy, safety, and tolerability similar to that in younger patients.[70]
- **Benzodiazepines** are the most frequently prescribed anxiolytics for older patients (Table 6).[58,63,71] Compared with placebo, these medicines seem to decrease anxiety symptoms.[63] However, benzodiazepines **increase the risk for falls and cognitive impairment** in the elderly and should be used cautiously. Geriatric patients have decreased rates of drug metabolism and may tolerate intermediate-acting agents better than long-acting ones. Trials have not yet directly compared benzodiazepines with other treatments for geriatric anxiety.
- **CBT** has consistently shown promise for the management of geriatric anxiety disorders.[58,63,72,73] The benign side effects of CBT suggest that it should be considered in all elderly anxiety patients. Other psychological techniques may also be effective but have not yet been adequately evaluated.[58,63,72]
- The complementary medicine techniques of acupressure and mind-body interventions may improve the sleep symptoms of older adults with anxiety disorders, though the paucity of available data precludes definitive assessment.[74]

Psychosis in Older Adults

- Psychotic symptoms are widespread in the elderly, with prevalence estimates ranging from approximately 1% to 5% in community-based cohorts to as high as 10% to 63% in nursing home populations.[60]
- Psychosis in the elderly patients may be due to:
  - Schizophrenia/schizoaffective disorder.
  - Mood disorders (i.e., depression or mania).
  - Dementia (i.e., Alzheimer disease, Lewy body dementia).
  - Delirium.
  - Delusional disorders.
  - Substance-induced disorders.
  - Parkinson disease.
  - Medication side effects.
- **The most statistically frequent causes of geriatric psychosis are Alzheimer's dementia, depression, and delirium;** these conditions should be considered when evaluating any geriatric patient with psychosis.[60] Treatment choices should consider the etiology of the patients' psychosis.
- Up to 40% of hospitalized geriatric patients with depression manifest psychosis.[60] **All elderly adults with psychosis should be assessed for depression.** Hallucinations and delusions in patients with depression or mania are often (but not necessarily) mood congruent.
- Schizophrenia is a less frequent but important etiology of psychosis in the elderly. The majority of geriatric schizophrenic patients first developed symptoms at a younger age. **"Late-onset" schizophrenia** may, however, also occur.

- Roughly 24% of older schizophrenia patients initially manifest their illness after the age of 40 and about 4% initially manifest after the age of 60.[60] "Late-onset" schizophrenia more commonly affects women than men.
- Compared with younger schizophrenics, adults with "late-onset" schizophrenia are more likely to suffer from:
  - Visual, tactile, and olfactory hallucinations.
  - Abusive or accusatory auditory hallucinations.
  - A third-person "running commentary".
  - Persecutory delusions.
- "Late-onset" schizophrenics are less likely to display formal thought disorders or affective blunting than do younger patients.
- Unlike other forms of psychosis in geriatric patients, those with schizophrenia typically display complex, bizarre delusions and auditory hallucinations. Suicidal ideation is common in geriatric schizophrenia.[60]
- **Both ECT and antipsychotics** appear to be useful adjuvants for treating depression with psychotic features in older adults who do not respond to antidepressant medications alone.[6,51,55,60]
- Consensus statements support multidisciplinary psychosocial interventions for both older patients with chronic psychotic illnesses and their families.[58] Useful interventions include vocational/social skills training and community support programs.
- Expert opinion, consensus statements, and the few available studies all concur that antipsychotic medications are effective for psychosis or late-life schizophrenia in older patients.[51,58,60] **Atypical antipsychotics are generally preferred** for most geriatric psychotic disorders and typically used at lower doses than in younger patients.[51] Commonly used antipsychotics are presented in Table 10.
- Pharmacological treatment of psychosis in the elderly should be managed in conjunction with a psychiatrist or similarly qualified mental health specialist. Special attention should be given to patients' age-related issues including pharmacokinetics, comorbid illnesses, and polypharmacy.
- **Older patients are particularly susceptible to adverse reactions from antipsychotic medications** including (Table 11)[58,60]:
  - Parkinsonism (i.e., bradykinesia, tremor, cogwheeling rigidity, masked facies).
  - Dystonia (involuntary muscle spasms that may be painful).
  - Akathisia (feelings of increased agitation and restlessness).
  - Tardive dyskinesia (repetitive purposeless, involuntary movements).
  - Weight gain, dyslipidemia, or hyperglycemia.
  - Cardiac arrhythmias.
  - QTc prolongation.
  - Sudden death.
- In younger patients, extrapyramidal side effects (including Parkinsonism, dystonia, and akathisia) are often treated with diphenhydramine or benztropine. However, these anticholinergic agents frequently cause problems such as cognitive impairment, constipation, and orthostasis in the elderly and must be used with caution.
- The development of extrapyramidal symptoms or tardive dyskinesia in the elderly may be more frequent with use of conventional antipsychotics (i.e., haloperidol) than atypical ones.[67]
- **Antipsychotic medication therapy has been associated with an increased mortality in geriatric patients,** especially from cardiovascular or infectious etiologies. As such, atypical antipsychotic medicines carry an FDA "black box" warning regarding their use in

dementia-related psychosis. Mortality risk in the elderly may be higher with conventional antipsychotic agents compared with atypical antipsychotics.[60]

Additional Resources

MedLine Plus. Mental health. 2009. Last accessed: September 1, 2009. http://www.nlm.nih.gov/medlineplus/mentalhealth.html.

National Institutes of Mental Health. Mental health topics. 2009. Last accessed: September 1, 2009. http://www.nimh.nih.gov/health/topics/index.shtml.

PsychCentral. Mental health & psychology resources online. 2009. Last accessed: September 1, 2009. http://psychcentral.com/resources/.

REFERENCES

1. Stiebel V, Schwartz CE. Physicians at the medicine/psychiatric interface: what do internist/psychiatrists do? *Psychosomatics* 2001;42:377–381.
2. Thielke S, Vannoy S, Unutzer J. Integrating mental health and primary care. *Prim Care* 2007;34:571–592, vii.
3. National Institute of Mental Health. The numbers count: mental disorders in America. http://www.nimh.nih.gov/health/publications/the-numbers-count-mental-disorders-in-america/index.shtml. Published 2008. Accessed February 9, 2009
4. Institute for Clinical Systems Improvement (ICSI). Major Depression in Adults in Primary Care. Bloomington, MN: ICSI, 2008.
5. First MB, Frances A, Pincus HA. DSM-IV-TR Handbook of Differential Diagnosis. Arlington, VA: American Psychiatric Publishing, Inc., 2002.
6. Shanmugham B, Karp J, Drayer R, et al. Evidence-based pharmacologic interventions for geriatric depression. *Psychiatr Clin North Am* 2005;28:821–835, viii.
7. American Psychiatric Association. Psychiatric Evaluation of Adults. 2nd Ed. *Am J Psychiatry* 2006;163:3–36.
8. American Psychiatric Association. Diagnostic and Statistical Manual of Mental Disorders (DSM-IV-TR). Text Revision. 4th Ed. Arlington, VA: American Psychiatric Publishing, Inc., 2000.
9. Belmaker RH, Agam G. Major depressive disorder. *N Engl J Med* 2008;358:55–68.
10. Maurer D, Colt R. An evidence-based approach to the management of depression. *Prim Care* 2006;33:923–941, vii.
11. U.S. Preventive Services Task Force. Screening for depression: recommendations and rationale. *Ann Intern Med* 2002;136:760–764.
12. Egede LE. Disease-focused or integrated treatment: diabetes and depression. *Med Clin North Am* 2006;90:627–646.
13. Fochtmann IJ, Gelenberg AJ. Guideline watch: practice guideline for the treatment of patients with major depressive disorder. 2nd Ed. Arlington, VA: American Psychiatric Association, 2005.
14. Whooley MA, Avins AL, Miranda J, Browner WS. Case-finding instruments for depression: two questions are as good as many. *J Gen Intern Med* 1997;12:439–445.
15. Bostwick JM, Philbrick KL. The use of electroencephalography in psychiatry of the medically ill. *Psychiatr Clin North Am* 2002;25:17–25.
16. King V, Robinson S, Bianco T, et al. U.S. Department of Health and Human Services. Agency for Healthcare Research and Quality. Choosing Antidepressants for Adults. AHRQ Pub. No. 07-EHC007-3. Rockville, MD: 2007.
17. American Psychiatric Association. Practice guideline for the treatment of patients with major depressive disorder (revision). *Am J Psychiatry* 2000;157:1–45.
18. Barbui C, Butler R, Cipriani A, et al. Depression in adults (drug and other physical treatments). *BMJ Clin Evid* 2007;06:1003.

19. Butler R, Hatcher S, Price J, Korff MV. Depression in adults: psychological treatments and care pathways. *BMJ Clin Evid* 2007;08:1016.
20. Lawhorne L. Depression in the older adult. *Prim Care* 2005;32:777–792.
21. Cain RA. Navigating the sequenced treatment alternatives to relieve depression (STAR*D) study: Practical outcomes and implications for depression treatment in primary care. *Prim Care* 2007;34:505–519, vi.
22. Qaseem A, Snow V, Denberg TD, et al. Using second-generation antidepressants to treat depressive disorders: a clinical practice guideline from the American college of physicians. *Ann Intern Med* 2008;149:725–733.
23. Schatzberg AF, Cole JO, DeBattista C. Manual of clinical psychopharmacology. 6th Ed. Arlington, VA: American Psychiatric Publishing, Inc., 2007.
24. Gartlehner G, Hansen RA, Thieda P, et al. U.S. Department of Health and Human Services. Agency for Healthcare Research and Quality. Comparative Effectiveness of Second-Generation Antidepressants in the Pharmacologic Treatment of Adult Depression. AHRQ Publication No. 07-EHC007-EF. Bethesda, MD: 2007.
25. Crone CC, Gabriel G. Herbal and nonherbal supplements in medical-psychiatric patient populations. *Psychiatr Clin North Am* 2002;25:211–230.
26. Ströhle A. Physical activity, exercise, depression and anxiety disorders. *J Neural Transm* 2009;116:777–784.
27. Soomro GM. Deliberate self-harm (and attempted suicide). *BMJ Clin Evid* 2008;12:1012.
28. American Psychiatric Association. Practice guideline for the assessment and treatment of patients with suicidal behaviors. *Am J Psychiatry* 2003;160:1–60.
29. U.S. Food and Drug Administration. Antidepressant use in children, adolescents, and adults. http://www.fda.gov/cder/drug/antidepressants/default.htm. Published 2007. Accessed May 2, 2009
30. Hawton K, Townsend E, Arensman E, et al. Psychosocial and pharmacological treatments for deliberate self harm. *Cochrane Database Syst Rev* 2000;2:CD001764.
31. Shearer SL. Recent advances in the understanding and treatment of anxiety disorders. *Prim Care* 2007;34:475–504, v–vi.
32. National Institute of Mental Health. U.S. Department of Health and Human Services. Anxiety Disorders. NIH Publication No. 07-4677. Bethesda, MD: 2007.
33. Gale C, Millichamp J. Generalised anxiety disorder. *BMJ Clin Evid* 2007;11:1002.
34. National Institute of Mental Health. U.S. Department of Health and Human Services. Anxiety Disorders. NIH Publication No. 09-3879. Bethesda, MD: 2009.
35. Spitzer RL, Kroenke K, Williams JB, Lowe B. A brief measure for assessing generalized anxiety disorder: The gad-7. *Arch Intern Med* 2006;166:1092–1097.
36. Newman MG, Holmes M, Zuellig AR, et al. The reliability and validity of the panic disorder self-report: a new diagnostic screening measure of panic disorder. *Psychol Assess* 2006;18:49–61.
37. Kapczinski F, Lima MS, Souza JS, Schmitt R. Antidepressants for generalized anxiety disorder. *Cochrane Database Syst Rev* 2003;2:CD003592.
38. Chessick CA, Allen MH, Thase M, et al. Azapirones for generalized anxiety disorder. *Cochrane Database Syst Rev* 2006;3:CD006115.
39. Martin JL, Sainz-Pardo M, Furukawa TA, et al. Benzodiazepines in generalized anxiety disorder: heterogeneity of outcomes based on a systematic review and meta-analysis of clinical trials. *J Psychopharmacol* 2007;21:774–782.
40. Mula M, Pini S, Cassano G. The role of anticonvulsant drugs in anxiety disorders: a critical review of the evidence. *J Clin Psychopharmacol* 2007;3:263–272.
41. Hunot V, Churchill R, Silva de Lima M, Teixeira V. Psychological therapies for generalised anxiety disorder. *Cochrane Database Syst Rev* 2007;1:CD001848.
42. Kumar S, Malone D. Panic disorder. *BMJ Clin Evid* 2008;12:1010.
43. Means-Christensen AJ, Sherbourne CD, Roy-Byrne PP, et al. Using five questions to screen for five common mental disorders in primary care: Diagnostic accuracy of the anxiety and depression detector. *Gen Hosp Psychiatry* 2006;28:108–118.

44. Krisanaprakornkit T, Sriraj W, Piyavhatkul N, Laopaiboon M. Meditation therapy for anxiety disorders. *Cochrane Database Syst Rev* 2006;1:CD004998.

45. American Psychiatric Association. Practice guideline for the treatment of patients with schizophrenia, second edition. *Am J Psychiatry* 2004;161:1–56.

46. Jindal RD, Keshavan MS. Neurobiology of the early course of schizophrenia. *Expert Rev Neurother* 2008;8:1093–1100.

47. van Os J, Kapur S. Schizophrenia. *Lancet* 2009;374:635–645.

48. Lehman AF, Buchanan RW, Dickerson FB, et al. Evidence-based treatment for schizophrenia. *Psychiatr Clin North Am* 2003;26:939–954.

49. Oud MJ, Meyboom-de Jong B. Somatic diseases in patients with schizophrenia in general practice: their prevalence and health care. *BMC Fam Pract* 2009;10:32.

50. Leucht S, Corves C, Arbter D, et al. Second-generation versus first-generation antipsychotic drugs for schizophrenia: a meta-analysis. *Lancet* 2009;373:31–41.

51. Alexopoulos GS, Streim J, Carpenter D, Docherty JP. Using antipsychotic agents in older patients. *J Clin Psychiatry* 2004;65(Suppl 2):5–99.

52. Schwarz C, Volz A, Li C, Leucht S. Valproate for schizophrenia. *Cochrane Database Syst Rev* 2008;3:CD004028.

53. Volz A, Khorsand V, Gillies D, Leucht S. Benzodiazepines for schizophrenia. *Cochrane Database Syst Rev* 2007;CD006391.

54. Wilson KC, Mottram PG, Vassilas CA. Psychotherapeutic treatments for older depressed people. *Cochrane Database Syst Rev* 2008;CD004853.

55. Stek ML, Van der Wurff FB, Hoogendijk WL, Beekman AT. Electroconvulsive therapy for the depressed elderly. *Cochrane Database Syst Rev* 2003;2:CD003593.

56. Holroyd S CA. Measuring depression in the elderly: Which scale is best? *Med Gen Med* 2000;2(4). http://www.medscape.com/viewarticle/430554. Accessed December 23, 2009.

57. Sheikh JI, Yesavage JA. Geriatric depression scale (GDS): recent evidence and development of a shorter version. In: Clinical Gerontology: A Guide to Assessment and Intervention. New York, NY: The Haworth Press, 1986:165–173.

58. Bartels SJ, Dums AR, Oxman TE, et al. Evidence-based practices in geriatric mental health care: an overview of systematic reviews and meta-analyses. *Psychiatr Clin North Am* 2003; 26:971–990, x–xi.

59. Mackin RS, Arean PA. Evidence-based psychotherapeutic interventions for geriatric depression. *Psychiatr Clin North Am* 2005;28:805–820, vii–viii.

60. Broadway J, Mintzer J. The many faces of psychosis in the elderly. *Curr Opin Psychiatry* 2007;20:551–558.

61. Reynolds CF, Frank E, Perel JM, et al. Nortriptyline and interpersonal psychotherapy as maintenance therapies for recurrent major depression: a randomized controlled trial in patients >59 years. *JAMA* 1999;281:39–45.

62. Reynolds CF, Dew MA, Pollock BG, et al. Maintenance treatment of major depression in old age. *N Engl J Med* 2006;354:1130–1138.

63. Wetherell JL, Lenze EJ, Stanley MA. Evidence-based treatment of geriatric anxiety disorders. *Psychiatr Clin North Am* 2005;28:871–896, ix.

64. Blazer DG, Steffens DC. The American Psychiatric Publishing Textbook of Geriatric Psychiatry. 4th Ed. Arlington, VA: American Psychiatric Publishing, Inc., 2009.

65. Brenes GA, Miller ME, Stanley MA, et al. Insomnia in older adults with generalized anxiety disorder. *Am J Geriatr Psychiatry* 2009;17:465–472.

66. Weiss BJ, Calleo J, Rhoades HM, et al. The utility of the Generalized Anxiety Disorder Severity Scale (GADSS) with older adults in primary care. *Depress Anxiety* 2009;26:E10–E15.

67. Andreescu C, Belnap BH, Rollman BL, et al. Generalized anxiety disorder severity scale validation in older adults. *Am J Geriatr Psychiatry* 2008;16:813–818.

68. Blank S, Lenze EJ, Mulsant BH, et al. Outcomes of late-life anxiety disorders during 32 weeks of citalopram treatment. *J Clin Psychiatry* 2006;67:468–472.

69. Lenze EJ, Rollman BL, Shear MK, et al. Escitalopram for older adults with generalized anxiety disorder: a randomized controlled trial. *JAMA* 2009;301:295–303.

70. Katz IR, Reynolds CF III, Alexopoulos GS, Hackett D. Venlafaxine ER as a treatment for generalized anxiety disorder in older adults: pooled analysis of five randomized placebo-controlled clinical trials. *J Am Geriatr Soc* 2002;50:18–25.

71. Benitez CI, Smith K, Vasile RG, et al. Use of benzodiazepines and selective serotonin reuptake inhibitors in middle-aged and older adults with anxiety disorders: a longitudinal and prospective study. *Am J Geriatr Psychiatry* 2008;16:5–13.

72. Ayers CR, Sorrell JT, Thorp SR, Wetherell JL. Evidence-based psychological treatments for late-life anxiety. *Psychol Aging* 2007;22:8–17.

73. Stanley MA, Wilson NL, Novy DM, et al. Cognitive behavior therapy for generalized anxiety disorder among older adults in primary care: a randomized clinical trial. *JAMA* 2009;301:1460–1467.

74. Meeks TW, Wetherell JL, Irwin MR, et al. Complementary and alternative treatments for late-life depression, anxiety, and sleep disturbance: a review of randomized controlled trials. *J Clin Psychiatry* 2007;68:1461–1471.

41 Neurologic Disorders

Eric C. Klawiter, Brian Sommerville,
Leo Wang, and Todd J. Schwedt

HEADACHE

General Principles

- Lifetime prevalence of tension-type headache is 78% and of migraine is 16%.[1]
- The majority of patients who seek medical care for headache have migraine.[2]
- Two-thirds of patients with migraine who seek medical care do so in a primary care physician's office.[3]
- Headaches account for 20% of neurology outpatient visits.

Diagnosis

Clinical Presentation

History
- The diagnosis of headache depends upon a carefully taken medical history.
- Search for headache "red flags" which increase the suspicion for secondary headache disorders (Table 1).

Physical Examination
- Primary headache disorders should not be associated with abnormalities on physical examination.
- The presence of abnormal neurologic signs is suggestive of a secondary headache disorder.
- Examination should include the following:
  - General physical and neurologic examinations (including funduscopy).
  - Cerebrovascular examination (temporal arteries and carotid arteries).
  - Examination of the muscles of the neck and shoulders (range of motion and tension).
  - Examination of the temporomandibular joint (pain with palpation, clicking, and abnormal motion).

Diagnostic Testing

- A patient with a typical history, no "red flags," and a normal examination often will not need further diagnostic testing.
- When testing is necessary, it must be individualized but may include the following:
  - Magnetic resonance imaging (MRI) brain with and without gadolinium.
  - Angiography (magnetic resonance angiography [MRA], computed tomography angiography [CTA], carotid ultrasound, or conventional catheter).
  - Blood tests (e.g., erythrocyte sedimentation rate [ESR]).
  - Cervical spine imaging.
  - Lumbar puncture.

TABLE 1	Headache Red Flags

New Headaches
Beginning after the age of 50
Significant change in headache patterns or characteristics (e.g., increasing frequency or severity)
Worrisome associated features (e.g., impaired consciousness, focal weakness)
Systemic illness (e.g., cancer, HIV, other immunosuppression)
Systemic symptoms (e.g., fever, stiff, neck, weight loss)
Rapid onset of headache (i.e., "thunderclap headache")
Headache secondary to head trauma

Diagnostic Criteria

Migraine without Aura
Diagnostic criteria for migraine without aura (common migraine) established in 2004 by the International Classification of Headache Disorders (ICHD) are listed in Table 2.[4]

Migraine with Aura
- About one-third of patients with migraine have aura (classical migraine).
- Auras are recurrent attacks of reversible focal neurologic symptoms that develop over 5 to 20 minutes and last for <60 minutes and are associated with a migraine headache.[4]
- Visual aura is most common and can include fortification spectra and scotoma.
- Sensory symptoms are second most common and usually consist of paresthesias that typically involve the hand or face. Numbness is less common.
- Less common aura symptoms may also include weakness, gait instability, speech change, and others.

Tension-Type Headache
Diagnostic criteria for tension-type headaches established in 2004 by ICHD are listed in Table 3.[4]

TABLE 2	Migraine without Aura Diagnostic Criteria

≥5 attacks lasting 4–72 hours
≥2 of the following:
    Unilateral location
    Pulsating/throbbing
    Moderate or severe in intensity
    Made worse by routine physical activity
≥1 of the following:
    Nausea and/or vomiting
    Photophobia and phonophobia

Modified from Headache Classification Subcommittee of the International Headache Society. The International Classification of Headache Disorders: 2nd edition. *Cephalalgia* 2004; 24(Suppl 1):9–160.

TABLE 3	Tension-Type Headache Diagnostic Criteria

Headache lasting from 30 minutes to 7 days
Headache has at least 2 of the following characteristics:
    Bilateral location
    Pressing/tightening (nonpulsating) quality
    Mild or moderate intensity
    Not made worse by routine physical activity
Both of the following:
    No nausea or vomiting
    Not >1 of photophobia or phonophobia

Modified from Headache Classification Subcommittee of the International Headache Society. The International Classification of Headache Disorders: 2nd edition. *Cephalalgia* 2004;24(Suppl 1):9–160.

Cluster Headache
- The 2004 ICHD diagnostic criteria for cluster headaches are listed in Table 4.[4]
- Cluster headaches are more common in men than in women.
- Attacks may occur at the same time(s) of the day each day and the same time of the year.
- Unlike migraine, patients are often restless during cluster headaches.

Medication Overuse Headache
- The overuse of acute headache medications can result in daily headaches that are more resistant to usual preventative and abortive therapies.
- This syndrome can occur in those with tension, migraine, or cluster headaches.
- Frequently implicated are acetaminophen, aspirin, and combinations of caffeine and butalbital (e.g., Fiorinal, Fioricet, and Esgic).

TABLE 4	Cluster Headache Diagnostic Criteria

Severe, unilateral orbital, supraorbital, and/or temporal pain lasting
    15–180 minutes untreated
Headache associated with at least 1 of the following ipsilateral to the pain:
    Conjunctival injection
    Lacrimation
    Nasal congestion
    Rhinorrhea
    Forehead and facial sweating
    Miosis
    Ptosis
    Eyelid edema
Frequency of attacks from 1 every other day to 8 per day

Modified from Headache Classification Subcommittee of the International Headache Society. The International Classification of Headache Disorders: 2nd edition. *Cephalalgia* 2004;24(Suppl 1):9–160.

TABLE 5	Secondary Headache Differential Diagnosis

Vasculitis (e.g., temporal arteritis, primary central nervous system angiitis)
Infection (e.g., meningitis, encephalitis, abscess)
Cerebral venous sinus thrombosis
Intracranial hypotension (i.e., cerebrospinal fluid leak)
Hydrocephalus
Idiopathic intracranial hypertension (i.e., pseudotumor cerebri)
Hemorrhage (intracerebral, subarachnoid, subdural)
Mass lesion (e.g., tumor, infection/abscess, hematoma)
Systemic illness (e.g., fever, infection, severe hypertension)
Medication side effect
Upper cervical spine disease
Acute sinusitis
Temporomandibular joint dysfunction
Many others

Differential Diagnosis

Headache is a common manifestation of a multitude of diseases (i.e., secondary headache). The more common causes are presented in Table 5.

Treatment

Abortive Migraine Treatment

Triptans

- Triptans, which are serotonin receptor agonists, are the mainstay of acute migraine therapy.
- Multiple different triptans are available (e.g., almotriptan, eletriptan, frovatriptan, naratriptan, rizatriptan, sumatriptan, and zolmitriptan) and there are four routes of administration:
  - Subcutaneous, most rapid onset, and not dependent upon gastrointestinal (GI) absorption, but injection site reactions possible.
  - Nasal sprays, second most rapid onset, not dependent upon GI absorption.
  - Orally disintegrating tablets do not require water.
  - Oral tablets.
- **Triptans are most efficacious when taken at the onset of a severe headache.**
- Consider **contraindications** that include, but are not limited to, vascular disease and risk factors for vascular disease, basilar or hemiplegic migraine, and pregnancy and lactation.
- Coadministration of a triptan and a selective serotonin reuptake inhibitor (SSRI) or serotonin norepinephrine reuptake inhibitor (SNRI) may increase the risk of the serotonin syndrome. Potential risks and benefits of coadministration should be carefully discussed with the patient.

Other Abortive Treatments

- **Nonsteroidal anti-inflammatory drugs** (NSAIDs) may be taken alone or in combination with triptans.

- **Intravenous antiemetics** (e.g., metoclopramide and prochlorperazine) are commonly prescribed for nausea/vomiting and to treat migraine pain.
- **Dihydroergotamine (DHE):**
  - DHE is available IV, SC, or as a nasal spray. Parenteral DHE is usually given in combination with an intravenous antiemetic.
  - It is often used to break **status migrainosus.**
  - Several **contraindications** due to vasoconstricting effects including ischemic heart disease, coronary artery vasospasm, peripheral arterial disease, uncontrolled hypertension, and basilar or hemiplegic migraines.
  - Coadministration with CYP3A4 inhibitors (e.g., protease inhibitors, macrolides, and azole antifungals) is contraindicated.
- Others including acetaminophen, aspirin, combination analgesics (often containing butalbital and caffeine), and ergotamine. Frequent use of analgesics can lead to **medication overuse headaches.**

Prophylactic Migraine Treatment

- Recognition and avoidance (when possible) of **migraine triggers** including emotional stress, hormonal fluctuation, missed meals, caffeine withdrawal, weather changes, sleep disturbance, muscular tension, alcohol, heat, and certain foods depending on the individual.
- A **headache diary** may be helpful in elucidating specific triggers in individual patients.
- Nonpharmacologic therapies include physical therapy and biobehavioral therapy (biofeedback, relaxation training).
- The decision to treat with prophylactic medications is based upon the frequency of headaches, duration of headaches, amount of disability caused, and response to acute headache medicines.
- Drug classes include the following:
  - **Anticonvulsants: topiramate** (starting at 25 mg daily and increased to a maximum of 100 mg bid) and **valproic acid** (starting at 250 mg bid and increased to a maximum of 500 mg bid). Valproic acid is teratogenic. Gabapentin may also be effective.
  - **Antidepressants: Amitriptyline** (10 to 150 mg daily), and possibly venlafaxine and duloxetine.
  - **Antihypertensives: β-Blockers** (e.g., propranolol, starting at 80 mg/day divided tid/qid increased to a maximum of 160 to 240 mg divided tid/qid, or long-acting propranolol, starting at 80 mg daily increased to a maximum of 160 to 240 mg daily); **calcium channel blockers** (e.g., verapamil, starting at 120 mg divided tid increased to a maximum of 480 mg divided tid, or extended release verapamil starting at 120 mg daily increased to a maximum of 480 mg divided bid). Angiotensin-converting enzyme (ACE) inhibitors and angiotensin receptor blockers (ARB) may also have some prophylactic efficacy.
  - **Others:** Riboflavin, magnesium, long-acting NSAIDs, neuroleptics, herbal supplements, and botulinum toxin injections.

Tension-Type Headache Treatment

- Tension headaches are usually self-limited and responsive to over-the-counter analgesics such as aspirin, acetaminophen, and NSAIDs. The addition of caffeine may be beneficial (e.g., Excedrin [acetaminophen 250 mg, aspirin 250 mg, and caffeine 65 mg], two PO).
- Patients should be carefully counseled that too frequent use of analgesics can lead to **medication overuse headaches.**

- Patients with frequent tension-type headaches may require prophylactic measures, which may include biobehavioral therapies, physical therapy, and daily medications (e.g., amitriptyline).

Cluster Headache Treatment

- Prevention may include avoidance of triggers (including alcohol and nitrates), verapamil, lithium, valproate, corticosteroids, melatonin, and others.
- Abortive therapies include inhaled oxygen by mask, triptans (subcutaneous or nasal spray), and DHE.

Medication Overuse Headache Treatment

- The most effective "treatment" for medication overuse headaches is prevention. Patients should be encouraged to avoid frequent use of acute medications, and prophylactic treatments should be used when indicated.
- Actual treatment consists mostly of cessation of the offending acute medications, which can be difficult for many patients. The following can be employed in achieving the goal: patient education, slow taper off of acute medications, steroid taper, short-term use of long-acting NSAIDs, and hospitalization for detoxification with use of a rescue medication (e.g., DHE with metoclopramide) and the initiation of prophylactic medication.

DIZZINESS

General Principles

Definition

- Patients will use the term "dizziness" to describe a variety of sensations including vertigo, nonvestibular sensations such as lightheadedness or presyncope, and ataxia (unsteadiness or disequilibrium).
- Vertigo is defined as "the sensation of motion when no motion is occurring relative to earth's gravity and implicates a vestibular disturbance."[5]
- This section will primarily focus on the evaluation and treatment of vertigo, and this topic is also covered in more detail in Chapter 36.

Diagnosis

Clinical Presentation

History

- A careful history is of great importance in differentiating vertigo from nonvertiginous causes of dizziness and in differentiating peripheral versus central causes of vertigo (Table 6).
  - **Peripheral vertigo:** Sudden, elicited or worsened by movement, episodic, more severe, tinnitus/hearing loss common, and other focal central nervous system (CNS) findings absent.
  - **Central vertigo:** Insidious, constant, less severe, tinnitus/hearing loss uncommon, and other focal CNS findings sometimes present.
- Description of the spell, accompanying symptoms, accompanying auditory complaints, and general physical and emotional health questions can lead the examiner toward a diagnosis.

TABLE 6	Differentiating Central versus Peripheral Vertigo by History

Peripheral	Central
Sudden onset	Insidious onset
Elicited by or worsened by movement or positional change	Effect of movement or positional change less predictable
Episodic	Constant and protracted
More severe	Less severe
Hearing loss, tinnitus, and aural fullness common	Hearing loss, tinnitus, and aural fullness uncommon
Other neurologic signs and symptoms absent	Other neurologic symptoms and signs present

Physical Examination
- The neurologic examination in a patient with dizziness includes numerous specialized tests to help localize and identify the cause (Table 7).[6]
- Nystagmus is described in the direction of the fast phase.
- Classic nystagmus in **Dix-Hallpike maneuver** is characterized as the following:
  - Torsional nystagmus.
  - Brief latency lasting 5 to 20 seconds.
  - Duration <30 seconds.
  - Reversal upon arising.
  - Fatigability with repetition.

Diagnostic Testing

- **Electronystagmography** involves infrared technology, which is used to record eye movements. The battery of tests includes oculomotor, positional and caloric testing and may be useful in diagnosis and localization.
- **Audiography** may diagnose conductive or sensorineural hearing loss. Findings may lead toward the diagnosis of a peripheral cause of vertigo such as Ménière disease.
- **Brain MRI** is indicated if there are accompanying neurologic signs and symptoms, accompanying stroke risk factors, or presence of new severe headache.
- Vascular imaging (i.e., conventional angiogram or MRA) is not routinely recommended unless there is suspicion for vertebrobasilar ischemia.

Differential Diagnosis

Benign Paroxysmal Positional Vertigo
- Benign paroxysmal positional vertigo (BPPV) is the **most frequent cause of recurrent vertigo**.[7]
- Although the majority of cases are considered idiopathic, head trauma is the most common identifiable cause.
- BPPV is caused by free floating or fixed particulate debris within the posterior semicircular canal of the vestibular labyrinth.[8]
- Sudden onset of vertigo with changes in position (rolling over in bed, gazing upward, bending forward) are characteristic with a duration seconds to minutes.
- **Positive Dix-Hallpike maneuver is diagnostic.**

TABLE 7	Neurologic Examination for Dizziness	
Test	**Action**	**Interpretation**
Spontaneous nystagmus	Patient fixates on midline stationary target	Peripheral causes demonstrate fixed directional horizontal nystagmus Central causes demonstrate multidirectional horizontal, vertical, or torsional nystagmus
Gaze-evoked nystagmus	Patient fixates on target 20°–30° from midline	Peripheral causes demonstrate worsened nystagmus in midline direction of the fast phase of spontaneous nystagmus Central causes demonstrate directional change nystagmus with fast phase in the direction of intended gaze and are common in drug effect, alcohol intoxication, and CNS tumors
Smooth pursuit	Patient tracks object in all directions of gaze	Saccadic intrusions may indicate brainstem of cerebellar dysfunction
Saccades	Patient looks back and forth between two targets in a horizontal plane and then in a vertical plane	Overshoot localizes to the cerebellum Intranuclear ophthalmoplegia indicates a lesion in the medial vertical plane longitudinal fasciculus and is seen in multiple sclerosis Slow saccades may indicate brainstem dysfunction Delayed saccades are seen in cortical or brainstem lesions
Dix-Hallpike maneuver	Turn patient's head at 45° and have patient fixate in direction opposite of turned head and recline to supine position	Nystagmus is diagnostic for benign positional vertigo
Head thrust test	Patient fixates on a target while the examiner rapidly moves the patient's head horizontally	When eyes move with thrusted head and then refixate, it indicates decrease neural input from the ipsilateral ear to the vestibulo-ocular reflex and, therefore, peripheral dysfunction
Postheadshake test	Tilt the patient's head forward 30° and shake the patient's head horizontally for 20 seconds and then repeat in the vertical plane	Peripheral causes demonstrate nystagmus directed toward the unaffected side Central causes demonstrate prolonged, dysconjugate, and vertical nystagmus following horizontal headshake
Finger-nose-finger test	Patient rapidly alternates touching finger between examiner's finger and their nose	Dysmetria or past-pointing indicated cerebellar dysfunction
Gait and tandem gait	Patient walks briskly without assistance Tandem gait involves walking toe to toe in a straight line	In peripheral causes, patients may veer toward the side of the lesion Wide-based gait and inability to tandem walk indicates cerebellar dysfunction

Modified from Goebel JA. The ten-minute examination of the dizzy patient. *Semin Neurol* 2001;21:391–398.

Vestibular Neuronitis

- Vestibular neuronitis usually presents as a single episode that is severe for 1 to 2 days and improves over weeks.
- It is caused by inflammation of vestibular nerve of viral origin.
- Recovery occurs over weeks as a result of restoration of labyrinthine function or by central compensation.[9]

Vertiginous Migraine

- Vertiginous symptoms of variable duration precede or are accompanied by migraine headache, but vertigo may occur in headache-free interval.
- Often associated with typical migraine features such as photophobia, phonophobia, and osmophobia.

Ménière Disease

- Ménière disease is of the classic triad of vertigo, unilateral hearing loss, and tinnitus.
- Episodes are repetitive with each lasting from minutes to days.
- It is caused by endolymphatic hydrops, defined as an increase in the volume of labyrinthine endolymph.

Vertebrobasilar Ischemia

- Deficits may be brief and paroxysmal (posterior circulation transient ischemic attack [TIA]) or fixed (stroke).
- Many symptoms of systemic, vestibular, circulatory, and aural origin are incorrectly ascribed to posterior circulation ischemia.[10]
- Accompanying brainstem signs may include diplopia, gaze palsies, facial weakness, dysarthria, or dysphagia along with cerebellar signs of limb or gait ataxia.
- Brain MRI with stroke protocol sequences can aid in diagnosis.
- MRA may noninvasively diagnose posterior circulation stenosis or occlusion.

Other Causes

- Schwannomas, dermoid, epidermoid, and metastatic tumors can involve the **eighth cranial nerve.** Neurofibromatosis type II is associated with bilateral acoustic schwannomas with hearing loss and vertigo.
- **Ototoxic drugs** include, but are not limited to, aminoglycosides, loop diuretics, cytotoxic drugs, quinine, and aspirin.[11] Tapering or stopping the offending agent typically alleviates symptoms.
- Common **nonvestibular causes** of dizziness include orthostatic hypotension, cardiac arrhythmias including symptomatic bradycardia, drug induced, anxiety disorders, hyperventilation, and sensory disturbances with proprioceptive loss.
- **Ataxia** is frequently described as dizziness by patients, and common causes of ataxia include stroke, multiple sclerosis (MS), epilepsy, migraines, mass lesions, and many other causes.

Treatment

- Type of treatment depends on underlying etiology of vertigo.
- Vestibular suppressants such as **meclizine** are only prescribed after treatable causes of vertigo are ruled out and should only be used for several days during the acute severe phase.[12]
- Symptomatic therapy lessens severity of attacks but has no prophylactic effect.
- Suppressant treatment is recommended on an "as needed" schedule.

- Vestibular exercises may be helpful following the acute phase of vertigo.
- The **Epley maneuver** may be curative for BPPV with 85% to 90% success rate after first treatment session (see Chapter 36).[13]
- Up to 50% of patients have recurrence of symptoms with a proportion requiring additional repositioning therapy.
- Conservative treatment of Ménière disease includes low-salt diet with or without diuretics. If conservative measures fail, intratympanic gentamicin or dexamethasone injection or surgical intervention may provide resolution of symptoms.

NEUROPATHY

General Principles

- **Diabetes is the most common etiology** in the United States. Leprous neuritis is the most common cause in undeveloped countries.
- Pathogenesis varies based on the underlying cause.
- Neuropathy may involve sensory, motor, sensory and motor (sensorimotor), or autonomic nerves.
- May be primarily demyelinating, axonal, or a combination of both.

Diagnosis

Clinical Presentation

History
- Common complaints include paresthesias, numbness, pain, weakness, and autonomic symptoms.
- Questions should focus on duration, course, and distribution of complaints.
- Consider relationship to other medical conditions.
- Pay close attention to medications. Chemotherapeutic agents and antiretrovirals commonly cause neuropathy.
- Family history may identify hereditary neuropathies or toxin exposures.

Physical Examination
- Attempt to identify patterns of sensory loss in specific dermatomal or nerve distributions.
  - Diabetic polyneuropathy typically is symmetric in a stocking-glove distribution.
  - Large fiber involvement causes vibratory and proprioceptive loss.
  - Phalen maneuver (flexing wrists for 60 seconds) or Tinel sign (tapping the median nerve at the wrist) may elicit median nerve distribution pain or paresthesias in carpal tunnel syndrome.[14]
- Weakness may be a later finding.
  - Toe extension and ankle dorsiflexion weakness may be seen in polyneuropathy.
  - Isolated weakness is typical of mononeuropathies.
- Evaluate for patterns of muscle atrophy.
- As a rule, deep tendon reflexes are typically depressed or lost in large fiber neuropathy (ankle jerk lost first) and are a more prominent presentation in demyelinating neuropathies.
- Gait may be affected in severe neuropathy.
- Other signs of upper motor neuron disease are typically absent.

TABLE 8   Causes of Peripheral Neuropathy

Systemic disease
Diabetic neuropathy
Renal insufficiency
Hypothyroidism
Chronic liver disease
Celiac disease
Critical illness

Vasculitic
Systemic lupus erythematous
Scleroderma
Rheumatoid arthritis
Polyarteritis nodosa
Wegener granulomatosis
Churg strauss
CREST
Cryoglobulinemia
Vasculitis restricted to peripheral
  nerves

Infiltrative
Sarcoidosis
Amyloidosis
Neoplastic

Infectious
HIV
Lyme disease
Leprosy

Nutritional
Vitamin B_{12} deficiency
Vitamin B_1 deficiency
Vitamin E deficiency
Vitamin B_6 intoxication

Immune mediated
Chronic inflammatory demyelinating
  polyneuropathy
Guillain-Barré syndrome
Paraneoplastic
Multifocal motor neuropathy
Sulfatide antibody related
MAG antibody related

Hereditary
Charcot-Marie-Tooth disease
Hereditary liability to pressure palsies
Hereditary sensory autonomic

Physical
Trauma
Focal compression
Entrapment

Miscellaneous
Idiopathic
Chronic alcoholism
Drugs
Toxins and heavy metals

CREST, calcinosis, Raynaud phenomenon, esophageal motility disorders, sclerodactyly, and telangiectasia; MAG, myelin-associated glycoprotein.

- If there is evidence of upper and lower motor neuron signs on examination, amyotrophic lateral sclerosis or spinal cord disease should be suspected.

Differential Diagnosis
The differential diagnosis of peripheral neuropathies is presented in Table 8.

Diabetic Neuropathy
- Over 30% of diabetic patients have peripheral neuropathy.
- Symptoms progress over months to years.
- Nerves are affected in a length-dependent fashion.
- Electrodiagnostic studies demonstrate an axonal sensory-motor polyneuropathy that may have autonomic involvement.

Entrapment Neuropathies
- Systemic diseases like diabetes or amyloidosis increase susceptibility to entrapment neuropathies.

- **Carpal tunnel syndrome** is caused by increased pressure within the carpal tunnel (formed by the flexor retinaculum) producing median nerve ischemia.[14]
  - There is sensation loss in thumb, second and third digits, lateral half of fourth digit, and the adjacent palmar surface.
  - Thenar muscle atrophy can eventually occur.
  - Median nerve conduction delay is evident across the wrist on nerve conduction studies (NCSs).
- The **ulnar nerve** may become compressed in the retro condylar groove near the elbow.
  - Sensory loss in the medial half of the fourth digit, entire fifth digit, and the adjacent palmar surface.
  - First dorsal interosseous muscle weakness.
- **Radial nerve entrapment** in the radial groove of the forearm classically produces wrist drop.
- **Meralgia paresthetica** produces lateral thigh sensory complaints as a result of lateral femoral cutaneous compression at the pelvic brim.

Trigeminal Neuralgia
- Classic trigeminal neuralgia is generally thought to be due to trigeminal nerve root compression by an overlying blood vessel resulting in demyelination of sensory fibers.
- Patients suffer from lancinating pain in distribution of the fifth cranial nerve (third, second, and first divisions in order of most commonly affected).

Bell Palsy
- Unilateral peripheral facial nerve cranial mononeuropathy of unknown etiology.
- Unilateral upper and lower facial weakness with possible alteration of taste and hearing (hyperacusis).

Vasculitic Neuropathy
- Caused by peripheral nerve infarction secondary to vascular occlusion by inflammation and fibrinoid necrosis.[15]
- Classically presents as a mononeuritis multiplex syndrome but may also present as a symmetric polyneuropathy.
- Subacute progressive painful sensorimotor neuropathy.
- Usually associated with systemic vasculitic disorders but may be confined to the peripheral nerves.
- Electrodiagnostic studies reveal evidence of axonal loss.
- Nerve and muscle biopsy are diagnostic with evidence of epineural inflammation, vessel wall pathology, and axonal loss.

Chronic Inflammatory Demyelinating Polyneuropathy
- Chronic inflammatory demyelinating polyneuropathy (CIDP) is the most common type of acquired chronic demyelinating polyneuropathy.[16]
- It affects motor nerves more than sensory nerves.
- The course may be relapsing or progressive, evolving over ≥ 2 months.
- Electrodiagnostic studies demonstrate reduced conduction velocity and conduction block in multiple nerves indicating demyelination.
- Cerebrospinal fluid (CSF) protein is typically moderately elevated.
- Nerve biopsy may show evidence of demyelination.
- Biopsy is considered if there is a high clinical suspicion for CIDP, but electrodiagnostic testing is nondiagnostic.

Guillain-Barré Syndrome

- Guillain-Barré syndrome (GBS) presents as a rapidly progressive ascending weakness with areflexia and variable sensory involvement. Symptoms peak within 4 weeks.[17]
- *Campylobacter jejuni* or cytomegalovirus (CMV) infection may precede the neuropathy by several weeks.
- Respiratory muscles may be prominently involved, and ventilator support is required in 25% of patients.
- Electrodiagnostic studies typically show evidence of demyelination.
- Increased CSF protein is present in approximately 80% of patients.

HIV Neuropathy

- Distal sensory polyneuropathy is the most common neurologic manifestation of HIV.
- Neuropathy affects >50% of HIV patients.[18]
- Evidence for axonal sensory neuropathy demonstrated on electrodiagnostic studies.
- HIV neuropathy remains prevalent despite advent of highly active antiretroviral therapy.

Diagnostic Testing

Laboratories

- Initial laboratory work includes complete blood cell count (CBC), complete metabolic panel (CMP), vitamin B_{12}, folate, thyroid-stimulating hormone (TSH), hemoglobin A_{1c}, ESR, and serum protein electrophoresis (SPEP) with immunofixation.
- Additional laboratory work that should be considered depending upon the clinical scenario includes antinuclear antibodies, extractable nuclear antigens, rheumatoid factor, urine protein electrophoresis, cryoglobulins, quantitative immunoglobulins, HIV, copper, vitamin E, anti-GM1 ganglioside antibodies, antisulfatide antibodies, antimyelin-associated glycoprotein antibodies, and paraneoplastic neurological antineuronal antibodies (of which there are multiple types).

Diagnostic Procedures

- **Electromyography and NCSs** are recommended in most instances.
- Electrodiagnostic testing can help differentiate axonal versus demyelinating neuropathies.
- Distribution of involvement can be confirmed: mononeuropathy; polyneuropathy: many nerves affected, usually symmetrically; mononeuropathy multiplex: random, multiple nerves simultaneously or serially affected, usually with rapid progression; plexopathy (brachial or lumbar); or radiculopathy.
- If radiculopathy or myelopathy (spinal cord disease) is suspected, **MRI** of the appropriate level of the spine is recommended.
- **Nerve and muscle biopsy** may be useful in identifying immune-mediated (i.e., CIDP), inflammatory (i.e., vasculitis), or infiltrative (i.e., amyloidosis) causes of neuropathy. This invasive procedure should not be performed if the diagnosis can be elicited by other methods.
- Genetic testing is pertinent if a hereditary neuropathy is suspected.
- The cause of chronic polyneuropathy remains elusive in approximately 25% of cases.

Treatment

Treatment of Underlying Etiology

- Aggressive treatment of diabetes, hypothyroidism, vitamin B_{12} deficiency, and renal insufficiency may stabilize or improve the neuropathic symptoms.

- Treatment of **trigeminal neuralgia:**
  - Carbamazepine and oxcarbazepine are effective for pain reduction. Baclofen and lamotrigine may also be useful.[19]
  - Microvascular decompression of the nerve is sometimes required for those with refractory symptoms.
- Treatment of **Bell palsy:**
  - Corneal protection is necessary.
  - Treatment with oral steroids is beneficial, particularly if started within 3 days of symptom onset.[20,21] The addition of valacyclovir or famciclovir may be of further benefit for those with severe facial palsy.[22,23]
  - Prognosis is good with >90% of patients achieving full recovery.
  - Good prognostic indicators include incomplete paralysis, early improvement, young age, preservation of taste, and normal electrodiagnostic studies.
- Vasculitic neuropathy is treated with corticosteroids or immunosuppression.
- Intravenous immunoglobulins (IVIG), plasma exchange, and corticosteroids are treatment options for CIDP.[16]
- GBS typically requires hospital admission for IVIG or plasma exchange.[17]
- Entrapment neuropathies may be amenable to surgery.
  - Carpal tunnel release may be indicated if evidence of axonal loss or prolonged symptoms.
  - Ulnar nerve transposition may be necessary in refractory cases of compressive ulnar neuropathy.

Symptomatic Treatment of Neuropathic Pain

- **Nonopiate agents** remain the mainstay of therapy.
- **Antiepileptics** such as gabapentin and pregabalin are first-line agents.[24]
- **Antidepressants** such as tricyclic antidepressants (TCAs) (amitriptyline, nortriptyline) and SNRIs (duloxetine, venlafaxine) are other first- or second-line agents.
- Topical lidocaine may provide additional pain control.
- Although potentially required in some cases, opiates must be prescribed with caution given the potential for addiction and abuse.
- Tramadol is a partial opioid agonist that is generally well tolerated with somewhat less dependence and abuse potential.

Other Treatment Options

- Physical and occupational therapy can lessen disability.
- Wrist splinting, keeping the wrist in a neutral position, is helpful for carpal tunnel syndrome.
- Ankle foot orthotics aid ambulation in patients with foot drop.
- Weight loss and proper foot care is encouraged.
- Ambulatory aids may be required.

SEIZURES

General Principles

Definitions

- As proposed by the International League Against Epilepsy (ILAE) and the International Bureau for Epilepsy[25]:

- An **epileptic seizure** is "a transient occurrence of signs and/or symptoms due to abnormal excessive or synchronous neuronal activity in the brain."
- **Epilepsy** is "a disorder of the brain characterized by an enduring predisposition to generate epileptic seizures."
- The occurrence of a single seizure does not necessitate the diagnosis of epilepsy.
- An unprovoked seizure occurs without a proximate precipitant, thus excluding those associated with acute insult to the CNS or generalized systemic metabolic disturbance.

Classification

Focal Seizures

Focal seizures have epileptogenic foci in a localized region of one cerebral hemisphere and are further classified based upon level of consciousness[26]:

Simple Partial Seizures

- Simple partial seizures involve **no impairment of consciousness.**
- Can manifest as stereotypic:
  - Motor movements.
  - Abnormal somatosensory symptoms (e.g., paresthesias and hot or cold feelings).
  - Special sensory symptoms (e.g., visual, auditory, olfactory, gustatory, and vertiginous).
  - Psychic symptoms (e.g., emotion, memory, cognition, and perceptions).
  - Autonomic symptoms (e.g., epigastric sensation, pallor, sweating, flushing, and piloerection).
- Usually brief, lasting approximately 15 seconds to 2 minutes.

Complex Partial Seizures

- Stereotyped partial seizures **with impaired consciousness.**
- May include motionless staring, behavioral arrest, unresponsiveness, oral or limb automatisms, focal limb posturing, and clonus.
- Usually accompanied by postictal confusion.
- Usually lasts 30 seconds to 3 minutes.

Secondarily Generalized Tonic-Clonic Seizures

- Secondary generalization is caused by the spread of ictal discharge from a localized focus to involve both hemispheres symmetrically.
- Tonic and/or clonic movements are usually asymmetric.
- Often accompanied by postictal confusion.

Generalized Seizures

Generalized seizures involve widespread regions in both hemispheres with impairment of consciousness and include nonconvulsive (absence) and convulsive (myoclonic, clonic, tonic, tonic-clonic, and atopic) seizures.

Typical Absence Seizure

- Typical absence seizures are characterized by the following:
  - Sudden behavioral arrest, loss of awareness, and blank staring.
  - Brief, 5 to 30 seconds.
  - Immediate return to normal consciousness.

Generalized Tonic-Clonic Seizures

- Generalized tonic-clonic seizures are characterized by tonic stiffening of axial and limb muscles lasting 10 to 15 seconds.
- The clonic phase evolves from tremors that increase in frequency and amplitude to be clonic jerking with bilateral upper extremity flexion and bilateral lower extremity extension.

TABLE 9	Etiology of Seizures

Idiopathic
Presumed genetic origin
 	
Structural
Cerebrovascular
Congenital
Trauma
CNS neoplasm
Degenerative neurological
  disorder
CNS infection
	Nonstructural/metabolic
	Medications that lower seizure threshold
	  (β-lactams, alcohol, meperidine, neuroleptics,
	  antidepressants [including bupropion])
	Drug withdrawal (benzodiazepines, alcohol,
	  antiepileptic drugs)
	Electrolyte abnormalities (hyper/hyponatremia,
	  hyper/hypocalcemia, hyper/hypoglycemia,
	  hypomagnesemia, hypophosphatemia)
	Uremia
	Hypoxia/anoxia
	Acute febrile illnesses
	Drug intoxication (cocaine, phencyclidine,
	  theophylline)

- Tonic and/or clonic movements are usually symmetric.
- Typical duration of 1 to 2 minutes.
- Consciousness recovers in minutes, but postictal confusion and somnolence may last for hours.

Epidemiology
- Seizures affect almost 2 million Americans.
- The cumulative incidence of epilepsy is 3.1%, and the age-adjusted prevalence is 6.8/1,000 population.[27,28]
- The cumulative incidence of a first unprovoked seizure is 4.1%, higher than that of epilepsy.[28]

Etiology
Table 9 presents a list of the more common causes of seizures.

Diagnosis

Clinical Presentation
History
- The goal is to distinguish seizures from other paroxysmal events such as syncope, convulsive syncope, episodic movement disorders, psychological abnormalities, narcolepsy/cataplexy, and TIAs.
- A reliable description of the seizure (especially from a bystander when consciousness is impaired) should be obtained. But bystander report of seizure duration is typically unreliable.

Physical Examination
The purpose of a detailed neurological examination is to elicit focal findings suggestive of a structural lesion.

Diagnostic Testing
- The purpose of diagnostic tests is to distinguish provoked seizure from unprovoked seizure, and to determine the risk of recurrence.

- **Electroencephalogram** (EEG):
  - Thirty to forty percent of first EEGs show abnormalities.
  - Early EEGs within 24 hours have a higher yield (51%) than after 24 hours (34%).[29]
  - Epileptiform abnormalities may confirm a diagnosis of epileptic seizures and distinguish partial seizure from generalized seizure.
  - An abnormal EEG approximately doubles the risk of seizure recurrence.[30]
- **Brain MRI** evaluates for structural lesions and mesial temporal sclerosis.
- **Lumbar puncture** can rule out CNS infections if there is clinical suspicion for infection.

Treatment

General Concepts of Treatment

- **First time unprovoked seizures generally do not require antiepileptic drug (AED) treatment.**
  - Recurrence risk for second unprovoked seizure is 34% at 5 years.
  - Treatment only minimally decreases risk of second seizure.
  - The probability of achieving seizure control with AED treatment is the same for those treated immediately versus those treated after the second seizure.[31]
- The goal for the management of epilepsy is to minimize seizure frequency and medication side effects.
- **Monotherapy is optimal.**
- Medication titration should be slow using the lowest dose necessary to control seizures and stopping if toxicity is reached.
- Decrease modifiable triggers such as sleep deprivation, alcohol intake, and stress.
- Implement seizure calendars to monitor seizure frequency.
- Patients with intractable epilepsy after sufficient trials of multiple AEDs may be candidates for resective epilepsy surgery.
  - Typical workup includes a combination of long-term continuous EEG monitoring, advanced brain imaging, neuropsychological testing, and multidisciplinary team conferences at a tertiary epilepsy center.
  - Further presurgical workup may include intracranial EEG monitoring.

Antiepileptic Drugs

- **First-generation** AEDs include phenytoin, carbamazepine, phenobarbital, and valproic acid (see Table 10).
  - Advantages of use include ease of assessing therapeutic serum levels.
  - Drug-drug interactions of **enzyme-inducing** first generation AEDs (carbamazepine, phenytoin, and phenobarbital) are common and can result in as follows:
    - ○ Increased metabolism of oral contraceptive pills and reduced hormone levels.
    - ○ Increased metabolism of warfarin and reduced anticoagulant activity.
    - ○ Increased TCA levels while TCAs increase AED levels.
  - Enzyme-inducing first-generation agents cause **vitamin D deficiency.** Supplementation with calcium with vitamin D helps prevent osteopenia and osteoporosis.
- **Second-generation** AEDs include levetiracetam, topiramate, zonisamide, lamotrigine, oxcarbazepine, gabapentin, and pregabalin (Table 10).
  - Second-generation AEDs generally have the advantage of a better side-effect profile, little to no need for serum monitoring, less frequent dosing, and fewer drug interactions.
- **Rashes** encountered during AED treatment are usually diffusely erythematous, maculopapular, or pruritic.

TABLE 10 Antiepileptic Drugs

Drug	Indication	Dosing	Therapeutic Range	Side Effects	Notes
Phenytoin	Partial epilepsy SGTC	300 mg/day or 5–6 mg/kg/day in divided doses	10–20 µg/mL	Gingival hyperplasia, vitamin D and folate deficiency	Zero-order kinetics, propensity for toxicity Signs of toxicity: sedation, incoordination, nystagmus
Carbamazepine	Partial epilepsy PGTC SGTC	Start: 200 mg bid Typical dose: 800–1,200 mg/day	4–12 µg/mL	Vitamin D deficiency, leukopenia, hyponatremia	Autoinduction of metabolism Signs of toxicity: ataxia, nausea/vomiting, vision changes
Phenobarbital	Partial epilepsy PGTC SGTC	Typical dose: 60 mg bid to tid	10–40 µg/mL	Sedation, vitamin D deficiency, memory loss, depression	Signs of toxicity: sedation
Valproic acid	Partial epilepsy SGTC PG	Start: 10–15 mg/kg/day Increase by 5–10 mg/kg/day until therapeutic	50–100 µg/mL	Weight gain, tremor, hair loss	Highly teratogenic, hepatotoxic Signs of toxicity: sedation, nausea/vomiting
Levetiracetam	Partial epilepsy Adjunct for PGTC Adjunct for SGTC	Start: 500 mg bid Maximum: 3,000 mg/day		Irritability, headache, depression, psychosis	Few drug interactions, easily titrated, dose must be adjusted for reduced renal function

Drug	Indication	Dosing	Side Effects	Comments
Topiramate	Partial epilepsy PGTC SGTC	Start: 25–50 mg/day Recommended dose: 200–400 mg/day	Nephrolithiasis, paresthesias, psychomotor slowing	Improves headaches, associated with weight loss
Zonisamide	Partial epilepsy Adjunct for PGTC SGTC	Start: 100 mg/day Increase by 100 mg/week to 300–600 mg/day	Nephrolithiasis, Stevens-Johnson syndrome, dizziness	Long half-life permits daily dosing, improves headaches, associated with weight loss, contraindicated with sulfa allergy
Lamotrigine	Partial epilepsy PGTC SGTC	Start: 25 mg/day Follow titration to 250 mg bid	Rash, Stevens-Johnson syndrome, tremor	Least cognitive side effects, drug of choice if coexistent mood disorder, requires prolonged titration, drug of choice in pregnancy
Oxcarbazepine	Partial epilepsy PGTC SGTC	Start: 300 mg bid Follow titration to 1,200–2,400 mg/day	Somnolence, dizziness, headache	Less frequent side effect compared with carbamazepine
Gabapentin	Partial epilepsy SGTC	Start: 300 mg/day Maximum: 1,200 mg tid	Sedation, weight gain	Few drug interactions, dose must be adjusted for reduced renal function
Pregabalin	Adjunct for partial epilepsy	Start: 75 mg bid Increase to 300–600 mg/day	Dizziness, sedation	Few drug interactions, dose must be adjusted for reduced renal function

PG, primary generalized; PGTC, primary generalized tonic-clonic; SGTC, secondary generalized tonic-clonic.

- Most rashes subside even with continuation of AEDs.[32]
- The presence of mucosal involvement and systemic symptoms require immediate attention, as the rashes can generalize and cause fatal reactions such as toxic epidermal necrolysis or Steven-Johnson syndrome.

Benzodiazepines

- There is no role for the use of benzodiazepines for long-term management of epilepsy.
- Sometimes clonazepam is used for generalized epilepsy, particularly myoclonus.
- Disadvantages of benzodiazepines include development of tolerance necessitating escalating doses for seizure control.
- Side effects include sedation, irritability, ataxia, and depression.
- Even slow withdrawal may lead to seizures.

Discontinuation of AEDs

- The duration of active disease and of the seizure-free period influences the risk of recurrence on AED withdrawal.
- Tapering of AEDs should be slow over >2 to 3 months.
- Taper one drug at a time for patients on polytherapy.
- Currently, only the state of Maine in the United States restricts driving for patients discontinuing AEDs.
- **Unless specified by laws or guidelines, each physician needs to come to agreement with their patients on prudent seizure precautions during the withdrawal period.**

Special Considerations

Driving
- Uncontrolled loss of consciousness while operating motor vehicles can result in injury or death to patient and others.
- Longer seizure-free intervals (>6 to 12 months) are associated with reduced risk of motor vehicle accidents.
- Each state determines the seizure-free interval required, requirements for physician reporting, liability for driving recommendations, and whether mitigating factors are considered.
- State-specific rules can be found at the Epilepsy Foundation website: http://www.epilepsyfoundation.org/living/wellness/transportation/driverlicensing.cfm (last accessed December 23, 2009).

Pregnancy
- The majority of patients remain seizure-free during pregnancy.[33]
- All women of childbearing age on AEDs should be supplemented with **folic acid** 1 g daily, 4 mg/day in women taking valproate or carbamazepine.
- All AEDs are fraught with **teratogenic potential.** Valproic acid is most associated with teratogenicity in the first trimester.[34]

Alcohol Withdrawal Seizures
- Alcohol withdrawal seizures are induced by relative or absolute withdrawal of ethanol in chronic alcoholics.[35]
- Most occur between 7 and 48 hours (peak incidence between 12 and 24 hours) after cessation of drinking.
- These seizures are usually generalized tonic-clonic in type.
- >60% experience more than one seizure.

- About 33% go on to develop delirium tremens, which continues to have a relatively high in-hospital mortality.
- Treatment in the acute setting is inpatient administration of **intravenous benzodiazepines** or the resumption of libation.
- **There is no role for long-term AEDs unless there is an underlying epileptic disorder.**

DEMENTIA

General Principles

- **Dementia** is a deterioration in cognitive, reasoning, and language abilities of sufficient severity to interfere with a person's activities of daily living. This subject is also covered from the geriatrics perspective in Chapter 34.
- **Mild cognitive impairment** (MCI) is mild memory loss that may be evident on standardized testing but without significant problems in activities of daily living. Patients with MCI are at increased risk for developing dementia.
- **Delirium** is an acute impairment in awareness and orientation with disturbances of perception (i.e., hallucinations). In contrast, dementia has a more chronic steady decline with a clear sensorium in most cases.
- **Alzheimer disease** is caused by the accumulation of β-amyloid peptide, with resultant formation of neurofibrillary tangles and apoptotic cell death. Apolipoprotein E type ε4 is risk factor for accelerated amyloid deposition.

Diagnosis

Clinical Presentation

History
- Questions should focus on evaluating changes in cognition, memory, behavior, judgment, and activities of daily living. Interview both patients and their accompanying family.
- Consider prescription and nonprescription medications as possible etiologies of altered mental status.
- AD8 is a brief eight-item questionnaire that can be administered to patients and collateral sources (Table 11). Answering two questions positively provides a sensitivity of 74% and a specificity of 86% in differentiating demented from nondemented individuals.[36,37]

Physical Examination
- Mini-mental status examination is easy to administer and follow over time.
- **Cardinal features of Alzheimer disease** on mental status examination include amnestic memory loss, language deterioration, and visual-spatial impairment.[38]
- Motor, sensory, and gait deficits can be involved in later stages of Alzheimer disease.
- Primitive reflexes called frontal release signs may reemerge (e.g., palmomental, glabellar, grasp, snout, and suck).

Diagnostic Testing

- Rule out reversible causes of dementia: check CBC, CMP, TSH, vitamin B_{12}, and brain imaging. ESR, HIV, rapid plasma regain (RPR), and heavy metal screening may be evaluated if there are historical or clinical indications.

TABLE 11	AD8 Dementia Screening Interview

- Problems with judgment (e.g., falls for scams, bad financial decisions, buys gifts inappropriate for recipients)
- Reduced interest in hobbies/activities
- Repeat questions, stories, or statements
- Trouble learning how to use a tool, appliance, or gadget (e.g., VCR, computer, microwave, remote control)
- Forgets correct month or year
- Difficulty handling complicated financial affairs (e.g., balancing checkbook, income taxes, and paying bills)
- Difficulty remembering appointments
- Consistent problems with thinking and/or memory

Modified from Galvin JE, Roe CM, Powlishta KK, et al. The AD8: a brief informant interview to detect dementia. *Neurology* 2005;65:559–564.

- The likelihood of diagnosing a reversible cause of dementia is <10%.
- In most routine presentations, brain CT with contrast is adequate for ruling out structural causes.
- Brain MRI may provide more sensitivity in differentiating subtypes of dementia.
- If the clinical scenario is suggestive, indolent CSF infection should be evaluated with a lumbar puncture.

Differential Diagnosis
- Table 12 presents the differential diagnosis of dementia.

TABLE 12	Causes of Dementia

Alzheimer disease
Parkinsonian dementias
   Parkinson disease with dementia
   Dementia with Lewy bodies
   Progressive supranuclear palsy (PSP)
   Corticobasal degeneration
Frontotemporal dementia
Vascular dementia
Creutzfeldt-Jakob disease (CJD)
HIV dementia complex
Other infectious causes (e.g., neurosyphilis)
Alcoholic dementia
Posttraumatic dementia
Depression presenting as dementia (pseudodementia)
Multiple sclerosis
Normal pressure hydrocephalus (NPH)
Neoplasms
Paraneoplastic limbic encephalitis
Metabolic causes of dementia
Medication effects

- **Alzheimer disease** is a progressive neurodegenerative disorder with prominent memory, cognitive, and visual-spatial deficits.
- **Dementia with Lewy bodies** has a clinical and pathologic overlap with Alzheimer disease and Parkinson disease. In addition to memory and cognitive difficulties, patients exhibit signs of parkinsonism with rigidity, bradykinesia, and intention more than resting tremor. Visual hallucinations may be prevalent.
- **Frontotemporal dementia** is commonly misdiagnosed as Alzheimer disease. It tends to present with prominent behavioral (e.g., disinhibition, impulsivity, apathy, and loss of insight) or language abnormalities (e.g., nonfluent or fluent aphasias).[39]
- **Vascular dementia** is suggested by a step-like progression of symptoms. There will be evidence of multiple strokes on brain MRI with subcortical white matter lesions (leukoaraiosis).
- **Creutzfeldt-Jakob disease** is a rapidly progressive dementing disease often accompanied by myoclonus. It is a prion disease with familial and sporadic forms. Definitive diagnosis can only be made by brain biopsy or at autopsy, but MRI and EEG findings can be suggestive.

Treatment

Medications

Cholinesterase Inhibitors
- Donepezil, rivastigmine, galantamine, and tacrine work by reversibly binding and inactivating acetylcholinesterase (cholinesterase inhibitors).
- Starting dose of donepezil is 5 mg daily and can be titrated up to 10 mg daily.
- Use has demonstrated small improvements in cognitive and global assessments, but cost-effectiveness has been debated.[40]
- Transdermal preparations of rivastigmine may provide equitable efficacy in a preferred mode of delivery.[41]
- Common side effects include nausea, vomiting, and diarrhea.
- Possible indications for withdrawing or substituting cholinesterase inhibitors include allergic reactions, unmanageable side effects, continued cognitive decline despite a 6-month trial of the medication, and family choice.[38]

N-Methyl-D-Aspartate Receptor Antagonists
- Memantine is a low-moderate affinity N-methyl-D-aspartate receptor antagonist.
- Starting dose is 5 mg daily and can be titrated up by 5 mg per week to 10 mg bid.
- In a randomized controlled trial, combination therapy of memantine added to donepezil benefited cognition, behavior, and functional outcomes in moderate-severe Alzheimer disease.[42]

Antipsychotics
- Psychosis, aggression, and agitation have been treated with atypical antipsychotics.
- In a randomized controlled trial, the overall effectiveness of antipsychotic medications in patients with Alzheimer disease was limited by side effects and intolerability.[43]
- Extended antipsychotic use in demented patients should be reserved for those who exhibit clinically appreciable benefits with minimal side effects.

Other Nonpharmacologic Therapies
- Maintaining general health care, exercise, proper nutrition, and social interaction are vital to overall well-being.
- Caregivers and families are shouldered with many responsibilities including administering medications and promoting nonpharmacologic treatments.

- They must make decisions regarding finances and safety issues, such as driving and adequacy of living situations.[38]
- Organizations such as the Alzheimer's Association may provide family support and respite care services to caregivers.

COMMON MOVEMENT DISORDERS

- Movement disorders encompass a wide variety of conditions consisting of abnormal involuntary movements (hyperkinesis) and/or nonparetic hypokinesis.
- Disorders of movement are common, and the primary care physician is usually the first physician to identify and attempt treatment of these conditions.
- Early referral to a neurologist should be considered whenever a first attempt at treatment fails or if there is any doubt about the exact diagnosis and proper management.

TREMOR

General Principles

- Tremor is the most common movement disorder seen in the outpatient setting.
- It is defined as any involuntary, rhythmic, oscillatory movement of one or more body regions. Tremor may involve any of the extremities as well as the head, jaw, voice, or trunk.
- **Rest tremor** is a tremor in any body region that has no voluntary muscle activation and is fully supported against gravity (e.g., the patient's hand when resting in the lap).
  - This type of tremor is typically seen in Parkinson disease (PD) and related conditions, though it may also be medication induced.
- **Action tremor** is a tremor present only during voluntary activation of the affected body part (i.e., during movement or sustained posture against gravity).
  - It is seen in a variety of conditions such as essential tremor and cerebellar disease but may also be medication induced.
  - Any patient <40 years with an action tremor should be screened for Wilson disease.

Diagnosis

The initial evaluation of tremor involves screening for common endocrine and toxic causes including hyperthyroidism, hypoglycemia, caffeine consumption, nicotine use, chronic alcohol consumption, and medications.

Differential Diagnosis

Essential Tremor
- Essential tremor is a common form of postural/action tremor typically affecting the hands first and may spread to the head and/or voice later.[44] Involvement of the legs is unusual.
- It tends to run in families and typically develops in adulthood but may begin in adolescence.
- Essential tremor may begin on one side but eventually becomes bilateral/symmetrical.
- It is exacerbated by stress, fatigue, emotion, caffeine, and some medications but often improves acutely with alcohol consumption.
- It commonly causes embarrassment in social situations such as dining and may significantly impair handwriting and other essential activities of daily living.

- Severe essential tremor may have a rest component, and some patients with PD may have a postural/action tremor. Clinically significant bradykinesia and rigidity are not due to essential tremor.

Medication-Induced Tremor
- Many commonly used medications may cause tremor, both rest and action tremors, including antidepressants, anticonvulsants, antipsychotics, bronchodilators, metoclopramide, cimetidine, and levothyroxine.
- These medications may also exacerbate any underlying tremor disorder.
- Risk factors for drug-induced tremor include old age and polypharmacy.[45]
- Typical characteristics of medication-induced tremor include symmetric involvement, onset following a change in medications, and dose-related worsening.

Other Tremors
- Action and truncal tremors can be a prominent and debilitating feature of other neurological conditions affecting the cerebellum and its tracts, such as MS, stroke, neoplasm, and degenerative disease.
- These tremors are typically resistant to medical treatment, and management is generally based on occupational therapy and external modification of the patient's environment.

Treatment

- Indications for treatment of **essential tremor** are reduction in embarrassment and disability. The first-line agents are propranolol and primidone.
  - **Propranolol** (immediate or sustained release) is titrated carefully to effect, with the therapeutic dose usually falling between 160 and 320 mg daily.[44]
    - Common side effects include hypotension and bradycardia.
    - Relative contraindications include asthma, diabetes mellitus, heart failure, and heart block.
  - **Primidone** is begun at 62.5 mg daily and titrated carefully to effect, usually between 62.5 and 1,000 mg daily.[44]
    - Common side effects include sedation, nausea, and ataxia, especially upon starting the medication.
    - Long-term tolerability of primidone, however, may be superior to that of propranolol.[44]
  - Second-line medications include gabapentin and topiramate.
  - Severe or medically refractory cases may be considered for deep brain stimulator implantation. Referral to an experienced movement disorder clinic is appropriate for such patients.
- Treatment of medication-induced tremors consists of eliminating or reducing the dosage of the offending agent whenever possible.

PARKINSON DISEASE AND RELATED CONDITIONS

General Principles

Parkinson Disease
- PD is a common neurodegenerative disease caused by progressive loss of dopaminergic neurons in the substantia nigra of the brainstem, leading to dysfunction of basal ganglia circuits regulating movement.

- Lifetime risk is 2%, which increases to 4% when there is a positive family history. A small percentage of cases are associated with mutations in one of several identified genes.
- Typical age of onset is around 60, but there is considerable variability. Three percent of people >65 years have PD, and incidence increases exponentially between ages 65 and 90.[46]
- Apparent environmental risk factors include rural living, exposure to pesticides, and welding.
- A history of cigarette smoking is associated with reduced risk of developing PD.

Other Forms of Parkinsonism

- Secondary parkinsonism may be a byproduct of treatment with agents that have dopamine-blocking properties, such as antipsychotics (e.g., haloperidol, risperidone) and antiemetics (e.g., prochlorperazine, metoclopramide).
  - Ninety percent of cases begin within 3 months of starting the offending agent.[47]
  - Offending agents should be withdrawn gradually to avoid re-emergent dyskinesias.
- Other neurodegenerative forms of parkinsonism ("Parkinson-plus" syndromes) are rarer and less likely to respond to dopaminergic drugs.[48] These include dementia with Lewy bodies, progressive supranuclear palsy, multiple system atrophy, and corticobasal degeneration among others.
- Normal pressure hydrocephalus may also mimic parkinsonism. Its classic clinical triad consists of dementia, urinary incontinence, and a "magnetic" gait resembling shuffling gait of parkinsonism.

Diagnosis

- The primary clinical features of PD are tremor (initially asymmetric), bradykinesia, rigidity (sometimes with a jerky or "cogwheel" quality), and postural instability (often leading to falls).
- Other common motor findings include shuffling gait, stooped posture, loss of facial expression, decreased blinking, decreased arm swing, and occasional freezing of gait.
- Additional common nonmotor symptoms include depression and anxiety, dementia (40%), sensory complaints including pain and burning sensation in affected limbs, autonomic dysfunction, seborrhea, restless leg syndrome (RLS), and sleep disorders.[49]

Treatment

- Medical management of PD largely revolves around restoration of dopamine function in the brain via dopamine precursors such as **carbidopa/levodopa, dopamine agonists, and MAO inhibitors.**[50]
- Early treatment of PD does not accelerate the course of the disease and may even slow it down.[51]
- Typically, PD is progressive, requiring gradual increases in medication over time.
- **Levodopa,** a dopamine precursor, is generally considered to be the most effective symptomatic treatment, particularly for improving motor disability.[52,53]
  - Motor complications of treatment (e.g., dyskinesia and motor fluctuations) are more common than with dopamine agonists.
  - Other common side effects of carbidopa/levodopa include somnolence, orthostatic hypotension, dizziness, hallucinations, psychosis, anorexia, and nausea.

- Levodopa is usually given in combination with carbidopa (a peripheral decarboxylase inhibitor) in a fixed ratio (e.g., Sinemet, carbidopa/levodopa 25/100 mg). Treatment begins with low doses (e.g., half tablet tid) and is slowly increased as tolerated to effect or a maximal dosage. Usual dosage is 1 to 2 tablets tid.[53]
- **Dopamine agonists** (e.g., pramipexole, ropinirole) are also reasonable first-line therapy, particularly for those with less disability.[52,53]
  - They are slightly less effective but are significantly less likely to cause motor side effects.
  - Adverse effects are similar to those of levodopa. Peripheral edema, somnolence, constipation, dizziness, hallucinations, and nausea are more common with dopamine agonists.
  - Dopamine agonists have been associated with pathological gambling and other hedonic activities.[54]
  - Pergolide (now removed from the U.S. market) and cabergoline, both ergot derivatives, are no longer recommended treatments due to the risk of valvular heart disease and other fibrotic complications.
- Careful consideration prior to use of antiemetics or antipsychotic medications is necessary, as they may provoke an acute exacerbation of parkinsonism.
- Medically refractory cases of PD may be treated with deep brain stimulation.[55]

RESTLESS LEG SYNDROME

- RLS affects 2.5% of the population and is characterized by irresistible urge to move one's legs in response to an unpleasant, "creepy-crawly" sensation.[56]
- The symptoms are worse at night and with relaxation, leading to lost sleep. RLS may be mistaken for leg cramps and vice versa.
- Periodic leg movements (e.g., kicking, jerking) occur during sleep and tend to interrupt the sleep of the patient's bed partner.
- The etiology of RLS is unknown but is likely related to a dopamine deficit. There does appear to be a genetic component.
- Associated conditions include peripheral neuropathy, iron deficiency, renal failure requiring dialysis, pregnancy, rheumatoid arthritis, hypertension, heart disease, fibromyalgia, depression, anxiety, attention deficit hyperactivity disorder, and use of antihistamine and antipsychotic agents.
- When treatment is necessary, **dopamine agonists and analogues** dosed in the evening are first-line therapy (e.g., pramipexole, ropinirole).
- Alternative therapies include opioids, gabapentin, and benzodiazepines.
- If serum ferritin is <50 μg/L, **iron supplementation** is recommended and has been shown to improve symptoms.[56]

DYSTONIA

- Dystonias are characterized by involuntary, sustained muscle contractions leading to "repetitive twisting movements and abnormal postures of the trunk, neck, face, or arms and legs."[57]
- Early-onset (<25 years) forms of dystonia typically begin focally and gradually spread to involve other body regions, becoming progressively debilitating.
- Adult-onset (>25 years) forms usually begin within craniofacial or cervical musculature and do not migrate or progress significantly over time. Nonetheless, they may cause significant impairment in quality of life.

- Dystonias be triggered by certain actions and relieved by unusual "sensory tricks" (e.g., touching the side of one's face), leading to the erroneous impression that the disorder is psychogenic.
- Common focal dystonias include blepharospasm, task-specific limb dystonias (e.g., writer's cramp), cervical dystonia (i.e., spasmodic torticollis), vocal cord dystonia (i.e., spasmodic dysphonia), and oromandibular dystonia.[57]
- Botulinum toxin injection to affected muscles is the treatment of choice for focal dystonias.[55] Referral to a neurologist or other specialist experienced in botulinum toxin administration is recommended.

STROKE

General Principles

- Stroke is defined as a sudden-onset, focal deficit in neurological function due to ischemic infarction or intracerebral hemorrhage.
- Stroke is subdivided into several types based on presumed mechanism and associated risk factors (Fig. 1).
- Eighty-five percent of strokes are ischemic and 15% are hemorrhagic.
- Among those who survive acute stroke, the timing and degree of functional recovery is variable but most improvement occurs within the first 6 months.
- The task of secondary stroke prevention, in the form of long-term management of stroke risk factors, often falls largely to the primary care physician.
- When ischemic deficits resolve completely within 24 hours, the patient meets clinical criteria for TIA, or "mini stroke."
  - The significance of the stroke/TIA distinction is dubious, as MRI may show infarcts in patients who clinically have had a TIA.
  - Patients with TIAs are at high risk for stroke and thus should not be given less priority simply because they have no lasting deficits.
- Stroke risk is highest in the few weeks following a TIA.[58]
- Similar management principles apply to stroke and TIA patients.

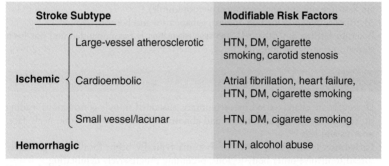

Stroke Subtype		Modifiable Risk Factors
Ischemic	Large-vessel atherosclerotic	HTN, DM, cigarette smoking, carotid stenosis
	Cardioembolic	Atrial fibrillation, heart failure, HTN, DM, cigarette smoking
	Small vessel/lacunar	HTN, DM, cigarette smoking
Hemorrhagic		HTN, alcohol abuse

Figure 1. **Stroke subtypes and associated modifiable risk factors.** DM, diabetes mellitus; HTN, hypertension.

Diagnosis

Clinical Presentation

History
- Specific stroke symptoms are referable to the brain region and vascular territory involved and are relatively sudden in onset.
- Typical stroke symptoms include hemiparesis, dysarthria, aphasia, diplopia, vertigo, numbness, and ataxia.
- **Abrupt loss of consciousness is a relatively infrequent presentation of stroke** and is far more likely to be secondary to syncope, seizure, or toxic/metabolic conditions.

Physical Examination
The examination should focus on the detection of focal neurologic deficits, such as focal weakness, deep tendon reflexes, clonus, Babinski sign, aphasia, dysarthria, ataxia, Romberg sign, diplopia, and focal sensory abnormalities.

Differential Diagnosis

- Complex migraine generally features a severe headache preceded or accompanied by a focal neurological deficit.
- Seizure can be followed by a focal neurological deficit for up to 36 hours (e.g. Todd paralysis).
- Brain tumors may occasionally present with an acute focal deficit resembling stroke.

Diagnostic Testing

- For patients with suspected ischemic stroke, **MRI** with diffusion sequences is the gold standard confirmatory test, as CT undervisualizes the posterior fossa structures (cerebellum and brainstem). **CT is excellent, however, to rule out hemorrhage in the acute setting, even for posterior fossa hemorrhage.**
- For patients with a stroke or TIA potentially attributable to carotid disease, a prompt evaluation with **carotid duplex ultrasound** is indicated to assess for carotid stenosis (see later).
- **Electrocardiography** (ECG) is indicated to evaluate for atrial fibrillation. Longer-term monitoring may be required if intermittent atrial fibrillation is suspected.
- **Echocardiography** is useful to identify mural thrombus or valvular lesions in patients with a cardiac history or abnormal ECG or who otherwise are at risk for endocarditis.
- Conventional angiography remains the gold standard for evaluation of intra- and extracranial vasculature and is generally necessary prior to endarterectomy or stenting procedures. MR and CT angiography are noninvasive imaging modalities that can be helpful in identifying stroke/TIA etiology.

Treatment

Secondary Stroke Prevention

Antihypertensive Therapy
- Hypertension is a risk factor for all strokes subtypes, and blood pressure reduction reduces recurrent stroke risk by as much as 40%.[59]
- In the immediate post-stroke setting, it is advisable to allow some degree of "permissive hypertension" to promote cerebral perfusion.

- There are **insufficient data thus far to universally recommend any one class** of antihypertensive medications for stroke risk reduction.[59]
  - An individualized approach is recommended, taking into account a given patient's particular medical problems and other circumstances.
  - The degree of blood pressure lowering seems to be the most important determinant of stroke risk reduction.

Antiplatelet Therapy
- Antiplatelet therapy reduces the risk of recurrent stroke in patients with **noncardioembolic** stroke or TIA.
- **Aspirin** (81 to 325 mg/day), **clopidogrel** (75 mg/day), or **aspirin with extended-release dipyridamole** are considered acceptable first-line therapy.
  - Aspirin is currently far less expensive than the other two options and thus is preferable for most patients.
  - There is currently no consensus about the optimal dosage of aspirin, although the risk of GI bleeding increases with higher doses.
  - Clopidogrel (75 mg/day) is an acceptable alternative for patients allergic to aspirin.
  - The combination of aspirin and clopidogrel provides no additional stroke benefit and increases the risk of hemorrhage.[60]
- Anticoagulation with warfarin has not been shown to provide superior protection against noncardioembolic stroke and is associated with an increased hemorrhage risk.[61] Anticoagulation is generally indicated for cardioembolic stroke.

Atrial Fibrillation
- **Anticoagulation with warfarin** (goal INR 2 to 3) has been shown to reduce relative stroke risk by up to 70% in patients with paroxysmal or persistent atrial fibrillation. The major complication with this therapy is increased bleeding risk.
- Any history of nontraumatic intracranial hemorrhage is generally considered a strict contraindication to anticoagulation. A history of recent or recurrent hemorrhage from other sites (e.g., GI hemorrhage) is a relative contraindication to anticoagulation, and cautious, individualized therapy is needed in such situations.
- For patients unable to take warfarin either because of unacceptable hemorrhage risk or allergy, aspirin (325 mg/day) is recommended, though it achieves only one-half the reduction in stroke risk that is afforded by warfarin.

Carotid Stenosis
- Patients with symptomatic carotid stenosis of >70% and who have a life expectancy of at least 2 years will experience a reduction in stroke risk from **carotid endarterectomy** that is superior to medical management.[62]
- Some patients with 50% to 69% stenosis will also benefit depending upon age, gender, and other risk factors.
  - Prompt referral to an experienced neurologist or vascular surgeon is mandatory for all patients with symptomatic carotid stenosis of ≥50%.
  - Cerebral angiography is usually required to confirm and precisely quantify the degree of stenosis prior to surgery.
- When carotid endarterectomy is indicated, surgery within 2 weeks is favored in patients with TIA. Larger strokes require longer interval between symptom onset and surgical intervention.
- Carotid artery stenting has yet to be as rigorously investigated as endarterectomy and is generally reserved for patients who are deemed to be high-risk surgical candidates.

Smoking Cessation
- Smoking cessation is universally recommended in patients surviving stroke.[59]
- Cigarette smoking doubles the risk of ischemic stroke.
- This increased risk disappears within 5 years of smoking cessation.

Diabetes Mellitus
- Numerous studies have shown a reduction in primary stroke risk with tighter glycemic control.[59]
- While the data for secondary stroke prevention are less abundant, improved glycemic control has such extensive health benefits that it should be the goal for all diabetic patients whether they have had a stroke or not.

Lipid-Lowering Therapy
- Observational studies suggest that hyperlipidemia is less of a risk factor for stroke than for ischemic heart disease. Patients with ischemic heart disease, however, do experience a reduction in primary stroke risk when taking either pravastatin or simvastatin.
- Patients with noncardioembolic stroke or TIA and a baseline low-density lipoprotein of 100 to 190 mg/dL but no history of ischemic heart disease have reduced risk of recurrent stroke risk after starting atorvastatin, though they have a slightly increased risk of hemorrhagic stroke.[63]
- In clinical practice, the majority of patients who have had a stroke will have one or more identifiable vascular risk factors and thus will benefit overall from the use of a statin or other lipid-lowering agent (see Chapter 8).

Valvular Heart Disease and Prosthetic Heart Valves
- A history of valvular heart disease places a patient at increased risk of embolic stroke.
- Management of valvular disease is discussed in Chapter 6.

MULTIPLE SCLEROSIS

General Principles

- Incidence of MS varies widely depending on geographical location. This variability may be influenced by environmental and genetic factors. Prevalence in the United States is approximately 1 case per 1,000.
- Typically diagnosed in early adulthood (third and fourth decade of life) and predominately affects women (2:1).
- The disease is characterized by demyelinating plaques with predilection for periventricular white matter, corpus callosum, optic nerves, brainstem, cerebellum, and cervical spinal cord white matter.[64] Immune-mediated response is initiated by both T lymphocytes and B lymphocytes with breakdown of the blood brain barrier.[65]
- Eighty percent of MS patients have the relapsing-remitting MS (RRMS) form where deficits return to baseline following relapse.
- MS may transform to a secondary progressive MS stage where deficits gradually worsen in-between relapses in addition to stepwise deteriorations.
- Primary progressive MS patients have a gradual progressive disease course from onset with no specific relapses.

Diagnosis

Clinical Presentation

History
- Attacks typically evolve over a period of days, plateau, and then improve over weeks.
- Patients may present with a myriad of symptoms and signs including focal weakness, focal sensory complaints, Lhermitte sign (electric shock sensation down trunk and limbs induced by neck flexion), unilateral loss of vision, diplopia, clumsiness, gait ataxia, and bowel or bladder complaints.

Physical Examination
The purpose of a detailed neurological examination is to elicit focal findings suggestive of a structural lesion.

Diagnostic Testing
- McDonald diagnostic criteria was first developed in 2001 and updated in 2005.[66]
- Brain MRI is the foundation of diagnosing MS.
- Cervical spinal MRI may be indicated if symptoms refer to the spinal cord or if more evidence of disease is required for diagnosis.
- CSF can be helpful in sealing the diagnosis (a concurrent serum sample is also needed).
  - Excessive oligoclonal bands represent the most specific CSF marker for MS, identified in >95% of MS patients.
  - IgG index and IgG synthesis rate may be elevated.
- Visual evoked potentials may elicit abnormal optic nerve conduction of visual stimuli as demonstrated by a prolonged P100.
- To help distinguish MS from other entities on the differential diagnosis, checking vitamin B_{12}, TSH, serum RPR, and HIV is recommended. Depending on other associated sign and symptoms, checking antinuclear antibodies and extractable nuclear antigens may be pertinent.

Treatment

Acute Treatment
- Rule out systemic causes of pseudoexacerbation such as infections or metabolic disturbances.
- Intravenous **methylprednisolone** has been shown to hasten return to neurological baseline. Typical dosing is 1 g IV/day (which can be divided into 250 mg every 6 hours) for 3 to 5 days. Intravenous steroids can be followed by a slow oral prednisone taper over 4 weeks.
- Plasma exchange can be considered if unresponsive to steroids.
- Physical therapy and occupational therapy evaluation can address rehabilitation needs.

Disease-Modifying Therapy
- Consider referral to neurologist or dedicated MS center for long-term management.
- **Immunomodulatory treatments** can reduce the inflammatory cascade that leads to demyelination and axonal damage.
  - FDA-approved treatments for RRMS include interferon-β, glatiramer acetate, and natalizumab.
  - Natalizumab is a monoclonal antibody administered as a monthly infusion and has been associated with progressive multifocal leukoencephalopathy. At this time,

it should be reserved for RRMS patients in whom alternative injectable therapies have been ineffective or not well tolerated.[67]

- Treatment of clinically isolated syndrome, or a single monophasic attack, with immunomodulatory therapy may delay progression to clinically definite MS and may delay progression of disability, but the optimal timing of treatment initiation is still being debated.[68,69]
- There are no FDA-approved treatments for primary progressive MS. Although, some clinician elect to use immunosuppressive agents.

Treatment of Related Symptoms

- Depression is common and is responsive to SSRIs or bupropion.
- Bladder spasticity and incontinence may be improved with anticholinergic drugs such as oxybutynin.
- Fatigue may be responsive to amantadine or modafinil.
- Flu-like symptoms from interferon therapy can be mitigated with pretreatment with an NSAID.

CONCUSSION

General Principles

- Concussion is defined as an alteration in consciousness secondary to traumatic brain injury.
- Primary care physicians are often responsible for providing the initial and long-term management of concussions.
- Most frequent causes in children are sports and bicycle accidents.
- Most frequent causes in adults are falls and motor vehicle accidents.
- Loss of consciousness may be the result of rotational forces at the junction of the upper midbrain and thalamus causing transient disruption of the reticular activating system.[70]

Diagnosis

Clinical Presentation

History

- Concussion may or may not be associated with loss of consciousness.
- Anterograde amnesia (inability to retain new information) and retrograde amnesia (loss of memory immediately preceding event) may be present. Anterograde amnesia typically resolves more rapidly.
- Concussion may be associated with a single brief seizure. This does not predispose to epilepsy and does not require anticonvulsant treatment.[70]
- Postconcussive syndrome includes headache, dizziness, and impairment of concentration. It lasts days to months following the concussive event.

Physical Examination

- Mental status examination to evaluate level of consciousness and memory.
- Evaluate for signs of basilar skull fracture including hemotympanum, CSF otorrhea or rhinorrhea, raccoon eyes (periorbital ecchymosis), and Battle sign (mastoid ecchymosis).
- Evaluate for accompanying neurologic signs including aphasia, weakness, sensory deficits, and ataxia.

TABLE 13	Indications for Head CT with Concussion

New Orleans Criteria[71]
Head CT is required in patients with minor head injury, GCS 15, and any of the following:
- Headaches
- Vomiting
- Age >60
- Drug or alcohol intoxication
- Persistent anterograde amnesia
- Evidence of traumatic soft tissue or bony injury
- Seizure

Canadian Head CT Rule[72]
Head CT is required in patients with minor head injury, GSC of 13–15, and any of the following:
- GCS <15 within 2 hours of injury
- Suspected skull fracture
- Signs of basilar skull fracture
- ≥2 episodes of vomiting
- Age >65
- Persistent retrograde amnesia for >30 minutes
- Dangerous mechanism of injury defined as:
  ○ Pedestrian struck by a motor vehicle
  ○ Occupant ejected from a motor vehicle
  ○ Fall from an elevation of ≥3 feet or 5 stairs

GCS, Glasgow Coma Scale.

Diagnostic Testing
- Two independently developed decision rules help select patients most appropriate for brain imaging with head CT (Table 13).[71,72]
- In prospective trials, presence of one clinical feature in either decision rule identified patients in need of immediate neurosurgical intervention and detected clinically important brain injury with 100% sensitivity.
- The Canadian Head CT Rule has increased specificity for predicting need for neurosurgical intervention when compared to New Orleans Criteria (76.3% vs. 12.1%).[73]

Treatment

- Nonopioid analgesics may benefit headaches.
- Vestibular suppressants may be indicated if vertigo is present (see the "Dizziness" section).
- Bed rest is recommended and may have palliative effects in the first two weeks following event. The strength of this recommendation is uncertain, as at least one randomized study demonstrated no effect of bed rest on outcomes at 3 months.[74]
- Cognitive rehabilitation may be beneficial.
- Several international organizations have developed consensus statements on management of concussion in athletes, specifically addressing the question of when athletes are able to return to play.[75]

- The second impact syndrome, a second concussion occurring before resolution of symptoms from the first, may be associated with cerebral edema and catastrophic effects.
- The long-term effects of multiple concussions include cognitive decline, as well documented in boxers.

REFERENCES

1. Rasmussen BK, Jensen R, Schroll M, Olesen J. Epidemiology of headache in a general population—a prevalence study. *J Clin Epidemiol* 1991;44:1147–1157.
2. Lipton RB, Dodick D, Sadovsky R, et al. ID Migraine validation study. A self-administered screener for migraine in primary care: The ID Migraine validation study. *Neurology* 2003;61:375–382.
3. Lipton RB, Stewart WF, Simon D. Medical consultation for migraine: results from the American Migraine Study. *Headache* 1998;38:87–96.
4. Headache Classification Subcommittee of the International Headache Society. The International Classification of Headache Disorders: 2nd edition. *Cephalalgia* 2004;24(Suppl 1): 9–160.
5. Committee on Hearing and Equilibrium. Committee on Hearing and Equilibrium guidelines for the diagnosis and evaluation of therapy in Ménière's disease. *Otolaryngol Head Neck Surg* 1995;113:181–185.
6. Goebel JA. The ten-minute examination of the dizzy patient. *Semin Neurol* 2001;21: 391–398.
7. Neuhauser HK. Epidemiology of vertigo. *Curr Opin Neurol* 2007;20:40–46.
8. Furman JM, Cass SP. Benign paroxysmal positional vertigo. *N Engl J Med* 1999;341: 1590–1596.
9. Baloh RW. Clinical practice. Vestibular neuritis. *N Engl J Med* 2003;348:1027–1032.
10. Savitz SI, Caplan LR. Vertebrobasilar disease. *N Engl J Med* 2005;352:2618–2626.
11. Agrup C, Gleeson M, Rudge P. The inner ear and the neurologist. *J Neurol Neurosurg Psychiatry* 2007;78:114–122.
12. Hotson JR, Baloh RW. Acute vestibular syndrome. *N Engl J Med* 1998;339:680–685.
13. Lynn S, Pool A, Rose D, et al. Randomized trial of the canalith repositioning procedure. *Otolaryngol Head Neck Surg* 1995;113:712–720.
14. Katz JN, Simmons BP. Clinical practice. Carpal tunnel syndrome. *N Engl J Med* 2002;346:1807–1812.
15. Gorson KC. Vasculitic neuropathies: an update. *Neurologist* 2007;13:12–19.
16. Köller H, Kieseier BC, Jander S, et al. Chronic inflammatory demyelinating polyneuropathy. *N Engl J Med* 2005;352:1343–1356.
17. Hughes RA, Cornblath DR. Guillain-Barré syndrome. *Lancet* 2005;366:1653–1666.
18. Simpson DM, Kitch D, Evans SR, et al.; ACTG A5117 Study Group. HIV neuropathy natural history cohort study: assessment measures and risk factors. *Neurology* 2006;66: 1679–1687.
19. Gronseth G, Cruccu G, Alksne J, et al. Practice parameter: the diagnostic evaluation and treatment of trigeminal neuralgia (an evidence-based review): report of the Quality Standards Subcommittee of the American Academy of Neurology and the European Federation of Neurological Societies. *Neurology* 2008;71:1183–1190.
20. Sullivan FM, Swan IR, Donnan PT, et al. Early treatment with prednisolone or acyclovir in Bell's palsy. *N Engl J Med* 2007;357:1598–1607.
21. Engström M, Berg T, Stjernquist-Desatnik A, et al. Prednisolone and valaciclovir in Bell's palsy: a randomised, double-blind, placebo-controlled, multicentre trial. *Lancet Neurol* 2008;7:993–1000.
22. Hato N, Yamada H, Kohno H, et al. Valacyclovir and prednisolone treatment for Bell's palsy: a multicenter, randomized, placebo-controlled study. *Otol Neurotol* 2007;28: 408–413.

23. Minnerop M, Herbst M, Fimmers R, et al. Bell's palsy: combined treatment of famciclovir and prednisone is superior to prednisone alone. *J Neurol* 2008;255:1726–1730.

24. Mendell JR, Sahenk Z. Clinical practice. Painful sensory neuropathy. *N Engl J Med* 2003;348:1243–1255.

25. Fisher RS, van Emde Boas W, Blume W, et al. Epileptic seizures and epilepsy: definitions proposed by the International League Against Epilepsy (ILAE) and the International Bureau for Epilepsy (IBE). *Epilepsia* 2005;46:470–472.

26. Commission on Classification and Terminology of the ILAE. Proposal for revised clinical and electroencephalographic classification of epileptic seizures. *Epilepsia* 1981;22:489–501.

27. Hauser WA, Annegers JF, Kurland LT. Prevalence of epilepsy in Rochester, Minnesota: 1940–1980. *Epilepsia* 1991;32:429–445.

28. Hauser WA, Annegers JF, Kurland LT. Incidence of epilepsy and unprovoked seizures in Rochester, Minnesota: 1935–1984. *Epilepsia* 1993;34:453–468.

29. King MA, Newton MR, Jackson GD, et al. Epileptology of the first-seizure presentation: a clinical, electroencephalographic, and magnetic resonance imaging study of 300 consecutive patients. *Lancet* 1998;352:1007–1011.

30. van Donselaar CA, Schimsheimer RJ, Geerts AT, Declerck AC. Value of the electroencephalogram in adult patients with untreated idiopathic first seizures. *Arch Neuro* 1992;49:231–237.

31. Musicco M, Beghi E, Solari A, Viani F. Treatment of first tonic-clonic seizure does not improve the prognosis of epilepsy. First Seizure Trial Group (FIRST Group). *Neurology* 1997;49:991–998.

32. Roujeau JC, Stern RS. Severe adverse cutaneous reactions to drugs. *N Engl J Med* 1994;331: 1272–1285.

33. Kalviainen R, Tomson T. Optimizing treatment of epilepsy during pregnancy. *Neurology* 2006;67:S59–S63.

34. Wyszynski DF, Nambisan M, Surve T, et al. Increased rate of major malformations in offspring exposed to valproate during pregnancy. *Neurology* 2005;64:961–965.

35. Victor M, Brausch C. The role of abstinence in the genesis of alcoholic epilepsy. *Epilepsia* 1967;8:1–20.

36. Galvin JE, Roe CM, Powlishta KK, et al. The AD8: a brief informant interview to detect dementia. *Neurology* 2005;65:559–564.

37. Galvin JE, Roe CM, Xiong C, Morris JC. Validity and reliability of the AD8 informant interview in dementia. *Neurology* 2006;67:1942–1948.

38. Cummings JL. Alzheimer's disease. *N Engl J Med* 2004;351:56–67.

39. Liscic RM, Storandt M, Cairns NJ, Morris JC. Clinical and psychometric distinction of frontotemporal and Alzheimer dementias. *Arch Neurol* 2007;64:535–540.

40. Crome P, Lendon C, Shaw H, Bentham P; AD2000 Collaborative Group. Long-term donepezil treatment in 565 patients with Alzheimer's disease (AD2000): randomised double-blind trial. *Lancet* 2004;363:2105–2115.

41. Winblad B, Grossberg G, Frölich L, et al. IDEAL: a 6-month, double-blind, placebo-controlled study of the first skin patch for Alzheimer disease. *Neurology* 2007;69:S14–S22.

42. Tariot PN, Farlow MR, Grossberg GT, et al. Memantine Study Group. Memantine treatment in patients with moderate to severe Alzheimer disease already receiving donepezil: a randomized controlled trial. *JAMA* 2004;291:317–324.

43. Schneider LS, Tariot PN, Dagerman KS, et al.; CATIE-AD Study Group. Effectiveness of atypical antipsychotic drugs in patients with Alzheimer's disease. *N Engl J Med* 2006;355: 1525–1538.

44. Louis, E. Essential tremor. *Lancet Neurol* 2005;4:100–110.

45. Morgan JC, Sethi KD. Drug-induced tremors. *Lancet Neurol* 2005;4:866–876.

46. Lang AE, Lozano AM. Parkinson's disease: first of two parts. *N Engl J Med* 1998;339: 1044–1053.

47. van Gerpen JA. Drug-induced parkinsonism. *Neurologist* 2002;8:363–370.

48. Poewe W, Wenning G. The differential diagnosis of Parkinson's disease. 2002; 9(Suppl 3): 23–30.

49. Fahn S. Description of Parkinson's disease as a clinical syndrome. *Ann N Y Acad Sci* 2003;991:1–14.

50. Zesiewicz TA, Hauser RA. Medical treatment of motor and nonmotor features of Parkinson's disease. *Continuum* 2007;13:12–38.

51. Fahn S, Oakes D, Shoulson I, et al.; The Parkinson Study Group. Levodopa and the progression of Parkinson's disease. *N Engl J Med* 2004;351:2498–2508.

52. Miyasaki JM, Martin W, Suchowersky O, et al. Practice parameter: initiation of treatment for Parkinson's disease: an evidence-based review: report of the Quality Standards Subcommittee of the American Academy of Neurology. *Neurology* 2002;58(1):11–17.

53. Nutt JG, Wooten, GF. Clinical practice. Diagnosis and initial management of Parkinson's disease. *N Engl J Med* 2005;353:1021–1027.

54. Dodd ML, Klos KJ, Bower JH, et al. Pathological gambling caused by drugs used to treat Parkinson disease. *Arch Neurol* 2005;62:1377–1381.

55. Siddiqui MS, Okun MS. Deep brain stimulation in Parkinson's disease. *Continuum* 2007;13:39–57.

56. Walters AS. Restless legs syndrome and periodic limb movements in sleep. *Continuum* 2007;13:115–138.

57. Tarsy D, Simon DK. Dystonia. *N Engl J Med* 2006;355:818–829.

58. Giles MF, Rothwell PM. Prognosis and management in the first few days after a transient ischemic attack or minor ischaemic stroke. *Int J Stroke* 2006;1:65–73.

59. Sacco RL, Adams R, Albers G, et al.; American Heart Association/American Stroke Association Council on Stroke; Council on Cardiovascular Radiology and Intervention; American Academy of Neurology. Guidelines for prevention of stroke in patients with ischemic stroke or transient ischemic attack: A statement for healthcare professionals from the American Heart Association/American Stroke Association Council on Stroke. *Stroke* 2006;37(2): 577–617.

60. Diener HC, Bogousslavsky J, Brass LM, et al.; MATCH investigators. Aspirin and clopidogrel compared with clopidogrel alone after recent ischaemic stroke or transient ischaemic attack in high-risk patients (MATCH): randomised, double-blind, placebo-controlled trial. *Lancet* 2004;364:331–337.

61. Chimowitz MI, Lynn MJ, Howlett-Smith H, et al.; Warfarin-Aspirin Symptomatic Intracranial Disease Trial Investigators. Comparison of warfarin and aspirin for symptomatic intracranial arterial stenosis. *N Engl J Med* 2005;352:1305–1316.

62. North American Symptomatic Carotid Endarterectomy Trial (NASCET) Collaborators. Beneficial effect of carotid endarterectomy in symptomatic patients with high-grade carotid stenosis. *N Engl J Med* 1991;325:445–453.

63. Amarenco P, Bogousslavsky J, Callahan A III, et al.; Stroke Prevention by Aggressive Reduction in Cholesterol Levels (SPARCL) Investigators. High-dose atorvastatin after stroke or transient ischemic attack. *N Engl J Med* 2006;355:549–559.

64. Noseworthy JH, Lucchinetti C, Rodriguez M, Weinshenker BG. Multiple sclerosis. *N Engl J Med* 2000;343:938–952.

65. Klawiter EC, Cross AH. B cells: no longer the nondominant arm of multiple sclerosis. *Curr Neurol Neurosci Rep* 2007;7:231–238.

66. Polman CH, Reingold SC, Edan G, et al. Diagnostic criteria for multiple sclerosis: 2005 revisions to the "McDonald Criteria". *Ann Neurol* 2005;58:840–846.

67. Ransohoff RM. Natalizumab for multiple sclerosis. *N Engl J Med* 2007;356:2622–2629.

68. Kappos L, Freedman MS, Polman CH, et al.; BENEFIT Study Group. Effect of early versus delayed interferon beta-1b treatment on disability after a first clinical event suggestive of multiple sclerosis: a 3-year follow-up analysis of the BENEFIT study. *Lancet* 2007;370: 389–397.

69. Pittock SJ, Weinshenker BG, Noseworthy JH, et al. Not every patient with multiple sclerosis should be treated at time of diagnosis. *Arch Neurol* 2006;63:611–614.

70. Ropper AH, Gorson KC. Clinical practice. Concussion. *N Engl J Med* 2007;356:166–172.

71. Haydel MJ, Preston CA, Mills TJ, et al. Indications for computed tomography in patients with minor head injury. *N Engl J Med* 2000;343:100–105.

72. Stiell IG, Wells GA, Vandemheen K, et al. The Canadian CT Head Rule for patients with minor head injury. *Lancet* 2001;357:1391–1396.
73. Stiell IG, Clement CM, Rowe BH, et al. Comparison of the Canadian CT Head Rule and the New Orleans Criteria in patients with minor head injury. *JAMA* 2005;294:1511–1518.
74. de Kruijk JR, Leffers P, Meerhoff S, et al. Effectiveness of bed rest after mild traumatic brain injury: a randomised trial of no versus six days of bed rest. *J Neurol Neurosurg Psychiatry* 2002;73:167–172.
75. Cantu RC, Aubry M, Dvorak J, et al. Overview of concussion consensus statements since 2000 *Neurosurg Focus* 2006;21(4):E3.

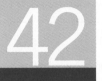

Ophthalmology

Stephen A. Kamenetzky, Michael D. Straiko, and Linda M. Tsai

- Careful history and examination are essential for correct diagnosis and treatment.
- Initial evaluation:
  - Determine the need and appropriate timing for referral to an ophthalmologist.
  - Categorize the ocular problem as acute, subacute, or chronic (Table 1).

Elements of the Clinical Ophthalmologic History

These are presented in Table 2.

Medical History

- Very important for determining relative risk of various ophthalmologic conditions and treatments.
- The severity, degree of control, and duration of the following illnesses:
  - Hypertension (HTN).
  - Diabetes mellitus (DM).
  - Vascular disease.
  - Autoimmune disease.
  - Thyroid disease.
  - Temporal arteritis/polymyalgia rheumatica.
  - Neurologic disorders.
  - Asthma.
  - Chronic obstructive pulmonary disease.

Medications

Anticoagulants, systemic steroids, and thyroid supplementation should be noted.

Family History

Glaucoma, cataracts (early or late onset), age-related macular degeneration (ARMD), ocular cancers, HTN, DM, and vascular disease should be noted.

Social History

Alcohol, tobacco, IV drug use, and living conditions are especially important.

Occupational History

Exposure to chemical substances, foreign bodies, and sunlight can be contributory.

TABLE 1	Ophthalmology Referral Guide

See immediately or send to emergency room (EMERGENCY)
Chemical burns
Acute decrease of visual acuity to ≤20/100, with suspicion of central retinal artery occlusion or temporal arteritis
Severe pain
Evidence of orbital cellulitis
Evidence or suspicion of penetrating injury to the globe, eyelid laceration, and orbital fractures

See ophthalmologist within 24 hours (ACUTE)
Corneal abrasion/contact lens
Acute decrease in vision
Mild-to-moderate pain
Preseptal (periorbital) cellulitis
Conjunctival or corneal foreign body
Hyphema
Acute visual field loss
Flashes of light or floaters

See ophthalmologist within 1 week (SUBACUTE)
Red eye with no vision loss
Red eye with no pain

TABLE 2	Elements of the Ophthalmologic History

Subjective ocular complaints
Differentiate between eyelid and eyeball complaints if possible
Change in vision
Pain
Diplopia
Flashes or floaters
Crusting
Discharge
Tearing
Redness
Photophobia

Timing
Acute (hours)
Subacute (days)
Chronic (weeks to months)

Severity
Transient versus constant
Monocular versus binocular
Subjective rating of discomfort
"Wakes me up from sleep"

Constitutional symptoms
Nausea
Vomiting
Headache
Weakness
Numbness
Dizziness

Prior ocular history
Prior trauma
Previous eye surgery
Amblyopia (lazy eye)
Cataract
Glaucoma
Age-related macular degeneration (ARMD)
High myopia
Dry eye
Blepharitis (eyelid disease)

Physical Examination

Visual Acuity

- Determination of visual acuity is the most important assessment of visual function.
- Ideally tested in each eye with a distance chart and glasses if the patient needs them.
- Near visual acuity, using reading glasses if needed, can also be checked if a distance chart is not available.
- If patients do not have their glasses with them, their visual acuity when looking through a pinhole can be checked. **Pinholing** may resolve refractive error and is useful in the patient who is not optimally corrected. This works for near vision and distance vision, but it generally does not resolve vision to better than 20/25.
- If patients are unable to see the eye chart, they should be checked to see if they can count fingers, see hand motion, or see light.
- No light perception is **absolute blindness.**
- **Legal blindness** is defined as best-corrected visual acuity of <20/200 in the better eye.
- **Driver's license requirements** vary from state to state but generally require best-corrected binocular visual acuity to be 20/70 or better for daytime driving and 20/40 or better for nighttime driving. Visual field requirements are approximately 140° binocularly.
- **Reading** is generally difficult below the 20/40 acuity range.
- **Accommodation** is the ability of the ciliary muscle to contract to make the lens shape more convex to focus at near.
  - In younger patients, **near card vision** is generally equivalent to distance visual acuity due to high accommodative ability.
  - **Decreased accommodation** (presbyopia) in patients who are >40 years leads to the need for additional convergence power for near vision (reading glasses).

Pupil Evaluation

- Compare the size and shape of pupils in light and dark conditions.
- Constriction to light and with accommodation should be noted.
- **Afferent pupillary defect (APD) (Marcus-Gunn pupil)** is evidence of optic nerve disease or significant retinal damage and should be carefully evaluated in every patient with decreased visual acuity.

External Examination of Eyelids

- Examine for evidence of erythema, edema, trauma, or eyelid lesions.
- **Ptosis** can be congenital or due to trauma, cranial nerve (CN) involvement, or senile involution.
- **Proptosis** can be seen with thyroid eye disease and orbital tumors.
- **Enophthalmos** (recession of eyeball within the orbit) can be seen after orbital trauma and rarely in breast cancer metastasis.
- **Lymphadenopathy,** especially preauricular, should be checked for, especially in conjunctivitis, orbital tumors, and infections.
- **Blepharitis and meibomianitis** are difficult to evaluate without a slit lamp examination but may be a significant cause of burning, itching, and eyelid crusting.

Ocular Motility

- May uncover deficits cause by CN palsies, gaze palsies from supranuclear etiologies, restrictive disorders after trauma, thyroid eye disease, and underlying strabismus from childhood disease.

TABLE 3	Selected Basic Ophthalmological Examination Techniques

Upper eyelid eversion
Have the patient look down. While using a cotton swab on the upper two-thirds of the upper eyelid as a fulcrum, flip eyelid over using eyelashes. To flip the eyelid back over, continue having the patient look downward and pull eyelashes back down.

Confrontation visual fields
Have the patient cover one eye. Make eye contact with the patient and explain that you want him/her to stare at your nose while you check the peripheral vision. Hold various fingers in the four main quadrants, making sure not to hold the fingers out too far into the periphery or behind the nose. *Note*: You are looking for a *large* peripheral defect such as quadrantanopias, hemianopsias, and significant visual field constriction. Minor field defects should be quantified with Goldmann or Humphrey visual field testing in the office.

Amsler grid
This checks the central 10° of vision only. Have the patient look at the center dot of the grid monocularly. While looking at the dot, have the patient note if the grid lines are straight. Have the patient mark areas where lines are distorted, broken, or missing. Make sure that the patient's fixation is not moving while attempting to delineate defects.

Fluorescein staining
Uses fluorescein strip to stain corneal epithelium. Have the patient look up, put stain on the medial portion of the bottom eyelid, and have the patient blink. Under a cobalt blue or Wood light, abrasions and ulcers will appear green.

Evaluate for afferent pupillary defect (APD)
Uses the "swinging flashlight test." When a light is directed form one eye to the other while the patient focuses on a distant target, the pupils should remain symmetrically constricted owing to the consensual light response. If the pupils dilate when the light is moved from the right to the left eye, then there is an APD of the left eye.

- Diplopia is generally not seen in chronic congenital misalignments. It can often differentiate acute, new-onset disease from chronic congenital disease.
- Nystagmus may also be noted, and patients should be sent for subspecialty evaluation unless it is long standing.

Visual Fields

- Evaluate to detect major visual field defects such as a hemianopsia or quadrantanopias (Table 3).
- **Confrontation visual fields** are standard in the primary care office and will detect gross defects.
- A **Humphrey** (computer generated) or a **Goldmann visual field** can be obtained to quantify visual field loss, especially in diseases such as glaucoma, anterior ischemic optic neuropathy, and optic neuritis.

Anterior Segment Examination

Although preferably performed with slit lamp, examination of the anterior segment of the eye can be accomplished with a penlight.

Conjunctiva

- The clear vascular epithelial covering over the sclera.
- Evaluate for foreign body and laceration in trauma.
- Generalized injection in viral and bacterial **conjunctivitis** is also associated with discharge.
- Uncomplicated conjunctivitis rarely causes pain.
- Perilimbal injection (area of sclera and conjunctiva next to the cornea) is common with **iritis.** Usually with associated symptoms of photophobia, pain, and blurred vision.
- Occasionally, **pterygia** and **pinguecula** can be seen. These are degenerations associated with sun and wind exposure. Most commonly on the nasal conjunctiva.

Cornea

- The cornea is the transparent anterior outer wall of the eye.
- Usually clear but can be cloudy and opaque in situations such as high eye pressure, decompensated corneal endothelium, scars from previous infection and trauma, and infiltrates from current infections.
- Foreign bodies and corneal abrasions may be noted under slit lamp examination.
- Any involvement of the cornea often leads to symptoms of **photophobia, pain,** and **foreign body sensation.**
- Immediate relief of pain after instillation of topical anesthetic suggests a corneal etiology.

Anterior Chamber

- The anterior chamber consists of the space between the iris and cornea and containing aqueous humor.
- Pathology is difficult to assess without a slit lamp. Suspicion of blood **(hyphema)** and inflammation **(iritis)** after trauma or spontaneously should be referred for evaluation.
- **Hypopyon,** a layering of white blood cells, is extremely suggestive of intraocular infection (endophthalmitis) or severe inflammation and needs prompt referral as well.

Iris

- Shape may be irregular after surgery or trauma.
- Pigmented lesions may be melanoma and should be referred for specialty evaluation, especially if changing in size or color.

Lens

- The lens is located just posterior to the iris.
- It is usually clear but may have a whitish or yellowish appearance with cataracts.
- After cataract surgery, the pupil may have a reflective quality from the lens implant.

Intraocular Pressure

- Quantified with tonometry or qualitatively checked with palpation.
- It varies diurnally and tends to be highest in the morning. It is not directly related to blood pressure (BP) or environmental factors such as stress or pain.
- Although **glaucoma** is multifactorial in nature, it is believed that most open-angle glaucoma can be treated by either decreasing inflow of aqueous humor (medications) or increasing outflow from the anterior chamber (medications, laser, or surgery).

- An acute severe rise in intraocular pressure (IOP) will result in corneal edema, decreased vision, pain, and usually nausea and headaches. The patient may also perceive halos or rainbows around lights from corneal edema.

Fundoscopic Examination

- **Most examinations in the office setting do not require dilation.** They are performed to assess retinal vascular health and to rule out papilledema and retinal or vitreous hemorrhage.
- Pharmacologic dilation is usually performed with phenylephrine hydrochloride 2.5% or tropicamide 1%, or both, and causes decreased accommodation for approximately 4 to 6 hours.
- For children, cyclopentolate 1% is often used in place of tropicamide and may last for 1 to 3 days.
- In the following circumstances, the patient should not be dilated without the direction of an ophthalmologist.
  - Suggestion of a shallow anterior chamber (may induce angle-closure glaucoma).
  - Patient is undergoing neurologic observation.
  - Any question of an APD.

PRESCRIBING OPHTHALMIC MEDICATIONS

Oral Antibiotics

- Oral antibiotics are not frequently used but are indicated in certain situations. In preseptal (periorbital) cellulitis or complicated chalazion with no evidence of **orbital (postseptal) cellulitis** (suggested by diplopia, pain with eye movement, decreased vision), a 10-day course of cephalexin or amoxicillin/clavulanate is used.
- Progression to orbital cellulitis is an emergency and should be referred immediately. It often requires hospitalization and parenteral antibiotics.
- For eyelid disease such as **blepharitis** and **meibomianitis,** often in association with **rosacea,** a course of minocycline, 100 mg qd, or tetracycline, 250 mg tid, for 2 to 6 weeks may be helpful.

Topical Antibiotics

- Topical antibiotics are often used for abrasions and conjunctivitis (although most is viral).
- Trimethoprim-polymyxin B (Polytrim, 1 drop tid for 5 days) and tobramycin (1 drop qid for 5 days) are used most often. Allergic reactions are possible. Drops should be discontinued if local irritation occurs. Topical sensitivity is very common with neomycin, and it should be avoided.

Artificial Tears

- Artificial tears are available over the counter.
- They are very useful for symptoms of dry eyes (foreign body sensation, redness, tearing with exposure, variable vision).
- They provide symptomatic improvement in viral conjunctivitis.
- If the patient has a history of sensitivity or is using drops more than four times per day, preservative-free artificial tears should be considered.

- Ointments and gels are very effective but will cloud vision and, as such, are best applied before sleep only.

Topical Steroids

- Topical steroids are useful in the treatment of many ocular conditions.
- Can lead to increased IOP (in up to one-third of patients), as well as glaucoma, cataracts, infection, and possible worsening and/or masking of clinical symptoms.
- **They should not be used without consultation with an ophthalmologist.**
- Antibiotic/steroid combinations should also be considered in this class.

Topical Antihistamines/Decongestants

- Topical antihistamines and decongestants are readily available over the counter as well as by prescription.
- Over-the-counter medicines such as Ocuhist and Visine should only be used for a few days at a time to avoid "rebound effect" and chronic irritation.
- Prescription antihistamines, such as olopatadine hydrochloride (Patanol, 1 drop bid), levocabastine hydrochloride (Livostin, 1 drop bid), azelastine hydrochloride (Optivar, 1 drop bid) and ketotifen (Zaditor, 1 drop bid), are available for daily use but are quite expensive.

OPHTHALMOLOGIC EMERGENCIES

Chemical Burn

General Principles

- One of the rare **true ophthalmologic emergencies** and can cause rapid, severe, and permanent eye damage.
- Alkaline substances penetrate and saponify tissues and cause more severe injury—these include ammonia, sodium hydroxide (lye), calcium hydroxide (lime), magnesium hydroxide, potassium hydroxide, and cement.
- Acids coagulate the conjunctival surface and, therefore, penetrate the eye much less. Causative acids include hydrochloric, hydrofluoric, acetic, nitrous, sulfuric, and sulfurous.

Diagnosis

- This diagnosis is made largely by history.
- On examination, eye may be red, photophobic, painful, and have epithelial defects detectable with fluorescein and a cobalt blue light/Woods lamp.

Treatment

- **Irrigate, irrigate, and irrigate![1]**
- Immediate flushing of the eye with water or normal saline for at least 10 minutes. This can be performed while the history is taken.
  - Begin flushing with any neutral fluid that is available.
  - If a Morgan lens is not available, an IV bag connected to nasal cannula placed over the bridge of the nose is effective.

- Be sure to irrigate the fornices (under the lids) to wash out any particles. Evert the eyelids if necessary.
- Do not attempt to "neutralize" the chemical with acidic or basic fluids.
- If possible, the active ingredients of the chemicals should be noted.
- pH paper should be used to measure the pH of the eye; the pH should be taken a few minutes after the eye has been flushed, before instilling any ophthalmic drops, and it should be 7.0 (if pH paper is not available, the pH square of a urinalysis strip works well).
  - pH should be checked twice 2 to 3 minutes apart. If the pH is not 7.0, the eye must be flushed again and pH rechecked.
  - Check the pH by pulling the lower lid on your own and checking the tears in the lower fornix.
  - Rarely, a retained foreign body causes continued release of the chemical and needs to be removed. This is particularly common with alkali burns.
- **Referral** to an ophthalmologist when the patient's condition is stable is required for evaluation and treatment of chemical damage.
- **Acid burns** often leave the eye red and irritated but usually do not result in serious injury.
- **Alkali burns** are especially dangerous because the eye may appear white and quiet, while deeper damage is done due to greater intraocular penetration of alkaline solution.
- A completely white eye with no hyperemia following an alkali burn is particularly ominous, as it signifies that many of the surface vessels have been destroyed.

Angle-Closure Glaucoma

- Angle-closure glaucoma is a rare disorder that occurs when the anterior chamber is anatomically narrow and the dilated iris closes off the outflow of aqueous humor, causing an acute rise in IOP.[2]
- Symptoms include severe pain, decreased vision, colored halos, corneal edema, and headache. Nausea, vomiting, and abdominal pain may also occur.
- Extremely high IOP results (possibly up to the 70s), and patients are at risk for vascular occlusions and glaucomatous damage to the optic nerve.
- An ophthalmologist manages the IOP initially with medications, but the definitive treatment is a laser peripheral iridotomy, which should be performed as soon as possible[3]; it is also done on the unaffected eye for prophylaxis.

Retinal Detachment

- Typically presents with constant photopsia (flashing lights), floaters, and a shade over the part of the vision in one eye.
- Partial detachments may not affect central visual acuity dramatically, but those that involve the central macular area with significant decreased visual acuity can be associated with an APD.
- Similar symptoms of acute onset of floaters and occasional flashes but no vision loss may be seen with acute **posterior vitreous detachment.**
- These patients need an extensive dilated retinal examination by an ophthalmologist to evaluate the status of the retina carefully and to rule out a small retinal hole, tear, or peripheral detachment.

Acute Vision Loss

- Acute vision loss (within 24 hours) with or without pain should be evaluated immediately.
- Occasionally, patients do not notice vision loss in an eye until the other eye is covered (sudden realization of chronic vision loss).
- Vision loss that is transient and returns to baseline vision may also be confused with acute vision loss (see the "Transient Vision Loss" section).

Optic Neuritis

Associated with pain on eye movement and APD (see the "Neuro-Ophthalmology" section).

Vascular Occlusion

- Ocular vascular occlusion may lead to devastating, painless vision loss.
- Often seen in people with previously diagnosed vascular disease, it may also occur in younger patients and requires evaluation for embolic (for arterial occlusion) or thrombotic (for venous occlusion) disease.

Central Retinal Artery Occlusion

- Central retinal artery occlusion causes severe painless vision loss.
- On fundoscopic examination, there may be evidence of pallor, vascular **"boxcarring,"** and a **"cherry-red spot."**
- Irreversible damage has been shown to occur after 90 minutes of occlusion, and therefore patients should be sent to the emergency room or for referral immediately.
- As an emergency measure in the primary care office, the physician can attempt to compress the eye with the heel of the hand, pressing firmly for 5 seconds, then releasing for 5 seconds over a period of 5 minutes.
  - This is designed to cause rapid changes in IOP and dislodge the embolus before irreversible retinal damage occurs.
  - An ophthalmologist can use more invasive techniques such as anterior chamber paracentesis.
  - If the patient is diagnosed quickly enough, interventional radiologists may be able to treat the patient with catheterization of the ophthalmic artery and injection with thrombolytics.[4]
- After the acute event, the patient requires a workup for embolic disease and follow-up for late ocular complications including neovascularization and its resultant complications.

Central Retinal Vein Occlusion

- Central retinal vein occlusion presents with a painless ophthalmoscopic picture of optic nerve swelling, venous engorgement, retinal hemorrhage, and cotton-wool spots, often described as **blood and thunder.**
- Although visual prognosis is poor, follow-up ophthalmologic care is imperative, as there is a high incidence of neovascularization of the retina and iris, which may lead to neovascular glaucoma and intractable pain. This may require treatment with laser photocoagulation.

Branch Artery and Vein Occlusions

- Occlusions of arterial and venous branches vary in their effect on visual acuity and should also be referred.

- Painless and frequently present with loss of a portion of the visual field.
- Branch vein occlusions may cause secondary macular edema, which can be treated with laser photocoagulation.

Ischemic Optic Neuropathies
Ischemic optic neuropathies are often associated with HTN, DM, vascular disease, and temporal arteritis (rare) and are discussed in the "Neuro-Ophthalmology" section.

Medical Evaluation
- The necessary evaluation for vascular disease varies according to etiology.
- Retinal vessel occlusions occur most commonly in patients with HTN and DM.
  - **Retinal arterial disease** may require carotid Doppler and cardiac echocardiography.
  - **Retinal venous disease** may be associated with thrombotic disease and hypercoagulable states, such as cryoglobulinemia, multiple myeloma, sickle cell disease, polycythemia vera, and lymphoma-leukemia. Complete blood cell count, proteins C and S, anticardiolipin, and evaluation for polyproteinemia may be required.

Media Opacities in Acute Vision Loss

Cataracts
The most common cause of media opacity but are usually gradual in onset (see the "Chronic Vision Loss" section).

Corneal Edema
- Corneal edema is usually associated with pain.
- There is a hazy appearance of the cornea and decreased vision.
- If gradual, it may be due to underlying corneal disease.
- Acutely, it may be secondary to increased IOP as in angle-closure glaucoma or rubeosis irides. Inflammation, infection, or opacity of the cornea may be difficult to differentiate from corneal edema with penlight examination.

Vitreous Hemorrhage
- Vitreous hemorrhage may occur after trauma or with any condition that may cause abnormal retinal neovascularization.
- It is often seen in those with diabetes, vein occlusions, retinal holes or breaks, and occasionally ARMD.
- Vitreous hemorrhage should be evaluated and followed by an ophthalmologist. Laser treatment may be needed after the blood has resorbed.
- Unresolved hemorrhage may eventually require surgical removal.
- **Terson syndrome** (vitreous and retinal hemorrhage in association with subarachnoid hemorrhage) is rare.

Retinal Detachment
Should be included in the differential diagnosis (see the "Retinal Detachment" section above).

CHRONIC VISION LOSS

Cataract

- Cataracts are the most common cause of media opacity and are usually gradual in onset (over months to years).

- Changes in the lens thickness occur with cataract development and initially can be corrected by a change in glasses.
- Cataracts are a normal part of aging; they may not interfere with visual function and may not require surgical removal.
- **Symptoms** that occur as the lens opacifies may include decreased night vision, difficulty with glare, difficulty with reading, and decreased distance acuity. Rarely, patients complain of double vision and decreased color vision and brightness in the affected eye.
- The **indication for elective surgical cataract removal** is that it affects activities of daily living.
  - Rarely, the cataract may need to be removed if it causes a secondary glaucoma or if it interferes with monitoring other ocular diseases such as macular degeneration, diabetes, or glaucoma.
  - Elective cataract surgery is performed under local or topical anesthetic as an outpatient and can be offered to any patient who is visually impaired and in stable medical health.
  - Anticoagulants required for medical care may not need to be discontinued. A recent history and physical examination are required but excessive laboratory testing is not generally indicated.[5]

Age-Related Macular Degeneration

- ARMD is a chronic, often progressive disease that affects central vision. It is often bilateral but may be asymmetric.
- ARMD may be "dry" (atrophic) or "wet" (exudative or neovascular).
- **Risk factors** include age,[6] smoking,[7] family history, (potentially related to complement factor H gene polymorphism and other genetic factors),[8,9] and race (white).
- The Age-Related Eye Disease Study demonstrated that in patients with moderate-to-severe ARMD treatment with vitamins and antioxidants reduced the rate of progression to severe vision loss.[10]
- Progression is usually slow, but sudden profound vision loss can occur if a subretinal neovascular membrane develops with hemorrhage and scarring.
- Home monitoring with an **Amsler grid** (Table 3) is recommended for early detection of central distortion.
- Relatively new treatments with injections of anti-VEGF (vascular endothelial growth factor) agents for exudative or "wet-type" macular degeneration have improved the outcome for this ocular disease.[11]

Glaucoma

General Principles

- Glaucoma is the second most important cause of blindness in the United States (after cataracts) and is the single most important cause of blindness in African-Americans.
- It is typified by increased IOP.
- **Risk factors** for open-angle glaucoma include HTN, DM, age, race (African-American), and family history.

Diagnosis

- Most patients with glaucoma are asymptomatic. Many lose significant peripheral vision before having any visual symptoms.

- IOP is determined by the rate of production of aqueous humor by the ciliary body and the outflow of this fluid through the trabecular meshwork.
  - Most normal eyes have an IOP of approximately 20 mm Hg or lower.
  - Gradual increases of IOP are tolerated well without visual complaints or pain.
  - Acute rises of IOP, as in acute-angle closure, are associated with corneal edema, pain, injection, tearing, and a mid-dilated pupil.
- The optic nerve has a depression in the center that is called the **cup of the optic disc.** The ratio of the size of the cup to total nerve head diameter is the cup disc ratio (CDR).
  - Normal CDR is up to approximately 0.4 but may vary between individuals.
  - Monitoring of optic cup enlargement, especially with concomitant IOP monitoring, is a way to quantify the severity of the progression of glaucoma.
- Frequency of visits is dictated by the IOP control and the severity of disease. General follow-up is usually every 6 months, with visual field testing every year.

Treatment

- **Medical management**[12]: Glaucoma medications either decrease aqueous humor production, facilitate outflow of fluid, or both.
  - Aqueous humor suppressants include β-blockers (timolol, levobunolol, carteolol, betaxolol hydrochloride [Betoptic]), α_2-agonists (apraclonidine, iopidine), and carbonic anhydrase inhibitors (dorzolamide, oral acetazolamide).
  - Those that facilitate outflow include prostaglandin analogs (latanoprost ophthalmic solution [Xalatan], travoprost [Travatan], bimatoprost [Lumigan]), miotics (pilocarpine), and epinephrine derivatives dipivefrin.
  - They all can have significant systemic side effects, and inquiries regarding their usage should be part of a careful medical history.
- **Laser trabeculoplasty** is usually performed with an argon laser and is done as an office procedure. It works by increasing aqueous humor outflow. It can be done a maximum of two times to each eye, and its result may be transient.
- **Surgical intervention** for glaucoma is primarily a trabeculectomy (a glaucoma "filter" surgery) and is performed on an outpatient basis. It creates a new outflow passage from the eye, which is covered by conjunctiva, bypassing the trabecular meshwork.

TRANSIENT VISION LOSS

Amaurosis Fugax

- Amaurosis fugax is transient monocular vision loss due to transient retinal arterial occlusion. The occlusion is usually caused by a cholesterol or platelet embolus but can result from vasospasm.
- Often described as a **"shade or curtain coming over the vision"** that lasts a few minutes, it is most common in patients >50 years or those with a history of vascular disease. A full ophthalmologic examination must be performed by an ophthalmologist to rule out impending vascular occlusion.
- The **most common site of an atheroma** is from the **carotids** or the **heart.** Evidence of a **Hollenhorst plaque** (refractile cholesterol plaque visible in the retinal vasculature) may be seen on physical examination.
- Medical evaluation, including carotid Dopplers, cardiac echocardiography, and basic hematologic workup, should be performed to rule out systemic disease, even in the absence of Hollenhorst plaques.

Ophthalmic Migraines

- Ophthalmic migraines cause transient episodes that usually cause at least 5 to 15 minutes of obscuration of vision.
- **Fortification** (jagged "lightning bolts") and **scintillating scotomas** (blind spot centrally with hazy edges) are characteristic. Colored lights and other visual symptoms can occur.
- Visual acuity should return to baseline after the episode, but headache or mild nausea may follow.
- A history of migraine may or may not be present. Often ophthalmic migraines develop in patients who previously had migraine headaches.
- Careful history should be taken to rule out concomitant neurologic symptoms.
- Both eyes are usually affected, although it may be sufficiently asymmetric as to appear to be monocular. Ophthalmologic evaluation is important to rule out retinal diseases.

OCULAR MANIFESTATIONS OF SYSTEMIC DISEASE

Diabetes Mellitus

- Diabetes is the leading cause of new cases of blindness in working-age Americans.
- The likelihood of developing retinopathy is directly related to the length of time a person has the disease.
  - Approximately 5 years after the diagnosis, 23% of patients have diabetic retinopathy; after 15 years, 80% have retinopathy. These statistics are similar for type 1 and type 2, with a slightly lower incidence in type 2.
- **Preventive care** is the cornerstone for decreasing visual morbidity. Stricter glucose control has been shown to decrease the rate of development and severity of diabetic retinopathy.[13]
- Diabetic retinopathy often develops without producing visual symptoms. Therefore, **yearly ophthalmologic follow-up is required once diabetes has been diagnosed.**
  - If retinopathy develops, more frequent visits may be indicated.
- Clinical trials by the National Eye Institute have shown that with early detection and treatment, the incidence of severe vision loss can be decreased by 50%.[13]
- **Panretinal and focal argon laser photocoagulation** are treatments for diabetic retinopathy that may be recommended to decrease the progression of retinopathy.[13]
- Surgical vitrectomy is occasionally required for nonclearing vitreous hemorrhages.
- **Decrease in visual acuity** due to diabetic retinopathy may not be directly related to the severity of the underlying systemic disease. Patients with mild non–insulin-dependent DM may have significant retinopathy.
  - If present, reduced acuity may be due to macular edema, macular ischemia, vitreous hemorrhage from neovascularization, optic neuropathy, optic nerve damage from neovascular glaucoma secondary to rubeosis, or retinal detachment from neovascularization and retinal membrane formation.
  - At this stage, visual acuity is not often recoverable, but laser treatment, surgical vitrectomy, or both are recommended to stabilize the process.

Hypertension

- Hypertensive changes in the retina can be chronic or acute.

- **Chronic changes** are more common and are characterized by arteriolar sclerosis and arterial/venous nicking.
- An **acute rise in BP** (usually diastolic >120 mm Hg) may cause exudates, cotton-wool spots, flame-shaped hemorrhage, and, rarely, retinal edema.
- **Malignant hypertensive retinopathy** is rare but presents with optic disc swelling and is usually bilateral. Management includes control of systemic BP.

Hypotension

A sudden decrease in BP may cause decreased perfusion of retinal and choroidal circulation, as well as optic nerve infarction. This is postulated to occur overnight. Systemic BP medication is best taken in the morning to prevent these transient hypotensive events.

Thyroid Disease/Graves Disease

- Graves disease is an autoimmune disease associated with hyperthyroidism. However, it may appear or progress in patients who are clinically euthyroid or hypothyroid.
- Tobacco usage has been associated with higher incidence of ocular complications.
- The most common manifestations include **eyelid retraction, proptosis, and corneal dryness.**
  - Serious involvement of extraocular muscles causes restrictive myopathy with **diplopia.**
  - Rarely, **compression of the optic nerve** within the orbit causes decreased vision with an APD and may require parenteral steroid therapy, radiation treatments, or surgical decompression. These patients should be referred for ophthalmologic consultation.

Sarcoidosis

- Sarcoidosis is a chronic disease of unknown etiology most common in African-American women aged 20 to 40 years.
- Focal noncaseating granulomas are histologically characteristic and can be found in affected conjunctiva and the lacrimal gland.
- Other symptoms due to sarcoidosis include anterior or posterior uveitis, retinal inflammatory disease, and even optic nerve and motility disease.
- Dry eye is common, especially in those >40 years.
- **Conjunctival biopsy** performed under topical anesthesia can give a positive tissue diagnosis but only has a high yield if a discrete granuloma is present.

AIDS

- Depression of the immune system can lead to opportunistic ocular infections.
- Common ocular manifestations include cotton-wool spots, cytomegalovirus retinitis, and Kaposi sarcoma of the eyelids. Also common are herpes zoster (shingles) ophthalmicus, herpes simplex keratitis, conjunctival microangiopathy, toxoplasmic uveitis, and central nervous system involvement.
- Yearly examination after diagnosis of AIDS is recommended, and patients should be closely monitored when CD4 counts drop below 500. Cytomegalovirus retinitis is rare in patients with CD4 counts of >50.

OCULAR TRAUMA

Corneal Abrasions

- Corneal abrasions are common and often present with significant redness, pain, photophobia, lid swelling, and a fitting history.[1]
- Pain may be alleviated with topical anesthetic.
  - **Topical anesthetics** aid greatly in examination of the eye but **should never be used for treatment,** as they may cause epithelial toxicity, decreased healing, and a neurotrophic ulcer.
- Evaluation can be aided with fluorescein staining and observation with cobalt blue-filtered light.
- Careful documentation of mechanism of injury, vision, and size of abrasion should be made.
- Treatment should include antibiotic eye drops (usually sulfacetamide 10%, 1 drop qid for 1 week, or tobramycin 0.3%, 1 drop qid for 1 week) or antibiotic ointment (polymyxin B sulfate [Polysporin Ophthalmic], 1/8-in strip bid, or erythromycin, 1/8-in strip bid).
- Ketorolac (1 drop qid for 1 week) may be used with antibiotics to decrease pain.
- If it is certain that the injury has recently occurred (within a few hours), there is no evidence of infection, there is no retained foreign body, and the patient is not a contact lens wearer, the eye may be patched.
- Any corneal haze or evidence of nonhealing abrasion should be re-evaluated by an ophthalmologist.

Foreign Body/Rust Ring

- Foreign bodies can be carefully removed either with a wet cotton tip or needle under direct visualization using a slit lamp.[1] A burr drill is occasionally used to remove rust rings.
- After the foreign body is removed, the eye should be treated with topical antibiotic (see the "Corneal Abrasions" section).
- Eversion of the eyelid should be performed to rule out retained foreign bodies under the eyelid (see Table 3).

Laceration of the Cornea, Conjunctiva, and Eyelid

- Lacerations are common after penetrating and blunt trauma.[1]
- A thorough eye examination including dilation must be performed by an ophthalmologist to rule out concurrent ruptured globe or other trauma.

Traumatic Iritis

- Traumatic iritis is common 2 to 3 days after blunt trauma and may present with decreased vision, photophobia, and dull pain.
- Patients should usually be referred to an ophthalmologist, as they may need to be treated with topical steroids. Traumatic iritis must be differentiated from bleeding (microhyphema) and infection.

Hyphema

- Hyphema is blood in the anterior eye chamber and may lead to decreased vision, photophobia, and a dull achiness around the eye.[1]
- Usually it is a result of direct trauma to the eye, but it can be caused by abnormal blood vessels (secondary to tumors, diabetes, chronic inflammation, intraocular surgery, etc.).
- It should be evaluated and followed by an ophthalmologist to rule out additional ocular involvement and manage possible complications such as re-bleeding in the eye, increased IOP, and corneal blood staining.
- Hyphema is often treated with dilation, light activity, rigid shield, and topical steroid medication but may require surgical washout if medical management is insufficient.
- The status of sickle cell disease/trait should be noted, as it affects the clearance of red blood cells from the anterior chamber through the trabecular meshwork and may lead to complications.

Orbital Fractures

- Orbital fractures are often seen due to blunt trauma.
- A thorough eye examination must be performed to rule out ruptured globe or other ocular trauma. Secondary ocular injuries should be highly suspected when motility is abnormal or vision is markedly decreased.
- Fractures should be treated with cephalexin 250 mg PO qid for 10 days. Emphasis on no nose blowing and oxymetazoline tid for 3 days aids in decreasing the risk of extension of sinus disease into the orbit and limits orbital emphysema.
- Fractures are usually re-evaluated 1 week after initial trauma.
- Many fractures are treated conservatively and are never surgically repaired.
- Indications for fracture repair from an ophthalmologic standpoint are as follows:
  - Diplopia in primary gaze.
  - Significant enophthalmos (recession of the eyeball into the orbit).
  - Unstable orbit.

Ruptured Globe

- Ruptured globe is the most serious complication of ocular trauma. **Early recognition is critical.**
- If there is any indication of prolapsed uvea, full-thickness laceration of the cornea or sclera, or distortion of the globe, the eye should be covered with a rigid shield and the patient sent for immediate ophthalmologic evaluation.
- Treat patient with antiemetics to prevent extrusion of ocular contents due to Valsalva maneuvers while awaiting definitive treatment.
- Evaluation is usually done in the emergency department, and adjunctive radiologic studies such as CT of the orbit may be helpful to evaluate the globe and rule out an intraocular foreign body.
- If ruptured globe is suspected, no eye drops should be given but systemic antibiotics are typically given.
- Definitive treatment is surgical.

Contact Lens

- Contact lens use often leads to minor trauma to the cornea.
- Contact lens wearers should be evaluated yearly to assess the health of the eye. Abrasions are common but should be evaluated because a higher incidence of infection/ulceration is associated with contact lens use.
- Contact lens wear should always be discontinued if the eye is red until a full evaluation can be done.

NEURO-OPHTHALMOLOGY

- Optic nerve disease is often detectable on careful pupillary examination by finding an APD.
- Loss of color vision and "red desaturation" or decreased perception of brightness in one eye compared to the other may also indicate optic nerve pathology.
- **Papillitis or optic disc edema** is a general term that describes acute inflammation of the optic nerve with disc elevation, edema of the nerve fiber layer, distortion of the retinal vasculature, and an APD.
- **Papilledema** is a more specific term that refers specifically to optic nerve edema caused by elevated intracranial pressures.

Optic Neuritis

- Optic neuritis is a disease of younger patients, often idiopathic, but may be associated with multiple sclerosis.
- It is an inflammation of the optic nerve.
  - May involve the optic disc (with hyperemia and optic disc swelling).
  - May be retrobulbar (with no apparent optic disc changes but more pain on extraocular motions).
- Vision may be reduced to bare light perception and it is often associated with pain with ocular movement.
- Treatment consists of either parenteral steroids or supportive care. Oral steroids have not been shown to be effective and may even be deleterious.
- Visual prognosis after a single event is good. Additional diagnostic tests include visual field testing and color vision testing.
- These patients should be followed by an ophthalmologist and referred to a neurologist for imaging to look for demyelinating disease. If the MRI reveals two or more characteristic demyelinating lesions, the patient may benefit from treatment with IV interferon-β within 28 days of symptom onset to decrease the rate of progression to clinically definite **multiple sclerosis**.[14,15]

Ischemic Optic Neuritis

- Ischemic optic neuritis is a common etiology for papillitis and vision loss in older adults.
- It is due to underlying vascular disease and often leaves a permanent altitudinal visual field loss.
- There is no effective proven treatment. It is accepted practice to start daily aspirin therapy and maximize treatment of comorbidities for vascular disease.

- Lowering the IOP with topical medications usually reserved for treatment of glaucoma may also help forward flow through compromised ocular vessels.

Giant Cell Arteritis or Temporal Arteritis

- This potentially life-threatening disease should always be considered when ION develops, especially in a patient >50 years.[16]
- Concomitant symptoms of malaise, weight loss, anorexia, scalp tenderness, jaw claudication, or shoulder/limb girdle weakness should be documented.
- Because this is a systemic disease that may lead to bilateral blindness within a few days, **early diagnosis and a high level of suspicion are required.**
- In any patient with ION, retinal arteritic occlusion, or even ophthalmoplegia, an erythrocyte sedimentation rate (ESR) should be obtained immediately.
  - If it is elevated to >40 mm/hr (or if there is a high suspicion of disease), treatment with systemic steroids (60 mg prednisone PO qd) should be initiated.
  - **A temporal artery biopsy should be performed within one week of starting steroids for histologic diagnosis.**

Papilledema

- Papilledema is optic nerve swelling from increased intracranial pressure, often seen in hydrocephalus, tumors, and pseudotumor cerebri.
- Both optic nerves normally are involved.
- Visual acuity and pupillary reflexes occasionally are normal.
- Patients may complain of transient obscurations in their vision.
- Diagnosis must involve measurement of elevated opening on lumbar puncture to confirm that the disc edema is secondary to increased intracranial pressure.

Pseudotumor Cerebri

- **Symptoms** of pseudotumor cerebri include headache, transient visual obscurations often associated with changes in posture, diplopia, tinnitus, dizziness, and nausea.
- It usually occurs in overweight young women and is more common in pregnancy.
- It is usually idiopathic but may be caused by vitamin A toxicity (>100,000 U/day), cyclosporine, tetracycline, oral contraceptives, or systemic steroid withdrawal.
- **Diagnosis** requires elevated ICP with papilledema, negative MRI and MR venography, and elevated opening pressure on lumbar puncture but with normal CSF composition.
- A full outpatient ophthalmologic examination including color vision testing and formal visual field testing is appropriate.
- **Treatment** consists of the following:
  - Weight loss if overweight.
  - Medical treatment with acetazolamide 250 mg PO qid initially, increasing to 500 mg PO qid if tolerated and necessary.
  - Discontinue any causative medications (see above).
  - Surgical treatment if medical options fail:
    - Lumboperitoneal shunt placement treats headache and prevents visual loss.
    - Optic nerve sheath fenestration prevents visual loss but usually has no effect on other disease symptoms.

Pupillary Disorders

- In the absence of trauma, pupillary disorders are often localizing symptoms of neurologic disease.
- Asymmetry of pupil size in dark or light, dilated pupils, and tonic pupils (unreactive pupils) should be evaluated.
- An APD (see Table 3) is never normal and needs to be referred for further evaluation.

Abnormal Motility

- Abnormalities of eye motility may suggest an acute or chronic CN palsy (III, IV, or VI) or extraocular muscle disorder.
- Acute changes are usually accompanied by complaints of diplopia, which may be horizontal or vertical in nature.
- Chronic changes may be asymptomatic.
- Medical conditions such as thyroid eye disease, (especially **Graves disease**), idiopathic inflammatory pseudotumor (ocular myositis), myasthenia gravis, demyelinating disease (multiple sclerosis), and cerebellar dysfunction may manifest with abnormal eye movements.

Visual Field Defects

- Visual field defects may occur from retinal and optic nerve disease but may also reflect intracranial disease.
- Lesions anterior to the optic chiasm (e.g., retina, glaucoma, and optic neuritis) produce lesions in one eye only.
- Pituitary adenomas at the optic chiasm may produce bitemporal field loss.
- Retrochiasmal (e.g., damage to the optic tracts, radiations, or the occipital cortex) lesions produce homonymous hemianopsias or other homonymous defects. Stroke is the most common cause of homonymous hemianopsia.

Intracranial Aneurysm

- Rarely intracranial aneurysms may present with ocular CN defects.
- Involvement of CN III, IV, V, and VI should suggest cavernous sinus pathology.
- Pupil-involving CN III defects can be seen in posterior communicating artery aneurysms, and MR angiography may be helpful in diagnosis.
- Diabetic or microvascular ischemic third nerve palsy usually spares the pupil and recovers spontaneously.

RED EYE

Referring to hyperemia or bleeding of the superficial vessels of the conjunctiva, episclera, or sclera, the red eye may or may not be associated with pain. However, it does not usually cause significantly decreased visual acuity.

Infections

- Infections are a common cause of the red eye. **Viral and bacterial conjunctivitis** are associated with redness, mattering, mucous discharge, and tearing.[2]

- Although topical antibiotics are useful, topical corticosteroids should **not** be used without consultation by an ophthalmologist.
- **Blepharitis** is caused by a mild eyelid infection, which can lead to a foreign body sensation (especially in the morning) and dry eye.[2]
- **Herpes simplex keratitis** can lead to corneal ulceration and scarring and should be referred to an ophthalmologist.

Keratoconjunctivitis Sicca

- Keratoconjunctivitis sicca is also known as "tear film dysfunction" or simply "dry eyes."
- Dry eyes are very common, especially in cases of lagophthalmos (incomplete closure) with Bell palsy, thyroid disease, rheumatologic diseases, contact lens wear, and age.
- Often a decrease in the protein or oil component of the tears due to eyelid disease (rosacea, blepharitis, or meibomianitis) leads to a decrease in the quality, not quantity, of tears.
- Patients may even complain of overflow tearing with extreme sensitivity to air, light, and prolonged usage of eyes, especially with near vision.
- A trial of **artificial tears** with carboxymethylcellulose along with eyelid scrubs is often recommended.
- Symptoms of dryness may be worsened by some systemic medications (antihistamines, antidepressants, or hormone replacement).

Subconjunctival Hemorrhage

- A subconjunctival hemorrhage consists of blood over the white sclera and under the clear conjunctiva.[2]
- It may be seen after inadvertent trauma or straining.
- Although these can be quite dramatic in appearance and alarming to the patient, they are self-limited, do not affect vision, and are generally painless.
- Patients may have mild eye irritation due to increased corneal dryness. Treatment involves cool compresses and artificial tears as needed.
- The patient should be questioned about other bleeding episodes or bruising, use of anticoagulants and aspirin, and HTN.
- Anticoagulants do not need to be discontinued for an isolated subconjunctival hemorrhage. If multiple episodes occur or if other systemic symptoms are present, a hematologic workup may be indicated.

Traumatic Abrasions and Laceration of the Cornea or Conjunctiva

- Traumatic abrasions and laceration of the cornea or conjunctiva may lead to redness of the eye.[1] See the "Corneal Abrasions" section above.
- The history is important in these cases and referral may be needed for treatment and follow-up especially if penetrating trauma is suspected.
- Minor abrasions can be treated with topical antibiotics, but referral is indicated if symptoms do not resolve within 24 hours.

Iritis or Iridocyclitis

- Inflammation of the iris, ciliary body, or both.
- A perilimbal distribution of redness is often present.
- This pattern is most common after trauma or with anterior uveitis and should be evaluated by an ophthalmologist.

Seasonal Allergies

- Seasonal allergies are a very common cause of red eyes.[2]
- For occasional use, over-the-counter antihistamines are reasonable, but for chronic use, new prescription medications are more effective (see the "Prescribing Ophthalmic Medications" section).

Episcleritis

- Usually localized inflammation of the episclera.[2]
- May be associated with mild pain and often resolves with topical steroid treatment.
- Episcleral redness blanches with phenylephrine. Redness from scleritis does not.

Scleritis

- Scleritis is a more serious inflammatory disorder of deeper sclera.[2]
- It may indicate a serious systemic disease such as a collagen vascular disorder or other autoimmune disease.
- Patients need to be monitored carefully for the development of scleral thinning and possible perforation.
- Scleritis is typically treated with systemic steroids.

Acute Angle-Closure Glaucoma

- Acute angle-closure glaucoma is an uncommon form of glaucoma due to the sudden and complete occlusion of the trabecular meshwork with iris.
- It is associated with corneal edema, mid-dilated pupil, and pain.
- This is a serious condition and should be **referred to an ophthalmologist immediately.**
- See the "Acute Angle-Closure Glaucoma" subsection in the "Ophthalmologic Emergencies" section.

Injected Pterygium/Pinguecula

- These are two types of conjunctival degeneration/abnormal growth on the conjunctiva that can become inflamed. They can contribute to corneal dryness as well.[2]
- Treatment is initially with artificial tears, surgical treatment is needed in some cases.

TEARING

- Tearing is a common complaint. It is often a nonspecific symptom of various underlying disorders.

- Subjective complaints are often enough to warrant an ocular evaluation.
- Quantitative measure of basal and reflex tearing is made by Schirmer testing.
- **Reflex tearing** is a common etiology.
  - This may be due to environmental and occupational irritants, pain, corneal foreign body or abnormality (infection, abrasion), and irritation caused by underlying tear film disorder.
  - Poor blink reflexes due to diseases such as Bell palsy and Parkinson disease leads to underlying corneal keratopathy with tearing.

Tear Duct Disorders

- Tear duct disorders can lead to overflow tearing due to inadequate drainage.
- In younger patients, blockage from nasal mucosal swelling, infections, and anatomic defects is common.
- In the older population, eyelid malpositions such as ectropion and entropion keep the puncta from its correct position against the globe.
- Patients with poor and infrequent blink have decreased muscle tone to force drainage of tears toward the puncta.

Conjunctivitis

- A common cause of tearing often associated with itching, discharge, and redness.[2]
- **Viral conjunctivitis** is more common, often self-limiting, and may be associated with other viral systemic symptoms.
- Treatment with topical antibiotics for **bacterial conjunctivitis** (usually more purulent) and to cover for superinfections in viral conjunctivitis is reasonable.
- The patient should be instructed to call if there is any loss of vision or symptoms do not resolve in a few days.

Anterior Uveitis

- Anterior uveitis consists of inflammation in the anterior chamber.
- Often associated with significant tearing, perilimbal injection, and photophobia.
- It is occasionally associated with systemic disease. As such, recurrent episodes require a medical evaluation guided by the patient's history and presentation which may include complete blood cell count, antinuclear antibodies, rheumatoid factor, syphilis testing, antineutrophilic cytoplasmic antibodies, human leukocyte antigen-B27, tuberculosis testing, angiotensin-converting enzyme level, and/or chest radiography.

EXTERNAL EYE AND EYELID PROBLEMS

Blepharitis

- Blepharitis is chronic inflammation and indolent infection around the eyelashes. Intermittent acute exacerbations of inflammation may also occur.[2]
- Usual organisms involved are common skin pathogens (*Staphylococcus* spp. and *Streptococcus* spp.). Blepharitis may also be more seborrheic in nature and not directly related to infection.

- Patients complain of symptoms of burning, foreign body sensation, and blurring of vision in the morning. Eye redness may also be reported.
- **Eyelid hygiene** is the most important treatment and includes warm washcloth compresses/soaks, gentle lid scrubs (with warm water and/or very dilute baby shampoo), and lid massage.
- Topical antibiotics are usually of little value.

Meibomianitis

- Meibomianitis (sometimes referred to as posterior blepharitis) is inflammation and infection around the oil glands in the eyelids proximate to the eyelid margin that may lead to burning, irritation, and sometimes a chalazion.
- Meibomianitis or blepharitis associated with rosacea may require additional treatment with oral antibiotics such as minocin or tetracycline.

Chalazion

- A chalazion is a chronic lipogranulomatous inflammatory lesion due to an obstructed meibomian gland in the eyelid. It may initially present with acute inflammatory signs and then develops into a relatively painless nodule.
- **Mainstays of treatment are hot compresses with gentle massage along with topical or oral antibiotics if indicated.**
- Conservative treatment should be carried out for 2 to 3 weeks.
- If the lesion has not completely resolved and is no longer actively inflamed, surgical incision and drainage or injection of chalazion with intralesional steroids may be recommended.
- A chalazion may be mistaken for a malignant lesion and vice versa.

Hordeolum

- A hordeolum, or stye, is an acute, painful inflammatory lesion of eyelid glands and is typically caused by a staphylococcal infection.
- Over time, a hordeolum may develop into a chalazion.
- **Warm compresses are the usual treatment.**

Potentially Malignant Eyelid Lesions

- Malignant eyelid lesions include basal cell, sebaceous cell, and sebaceous cell carcinomas.
- The length of time that a lesion has been present plus any history of recent change in size or shape should be determined.
- Any lesions of concern should be referred for further evaluation and possible biopsy for histopathologic diagnosis.
- It is important to note that sebaceous cell carcinoma can be mistaken for recurrent chalazia or refractory unilateral blepharitis.

Ptosis

- Ptosis is a common condition that may occur from congenital disease, neurologic disease, or involutional changes with aging.

• If the upper eyelid appears to interfere with the superior field of vision, or if the patient is symptomatic, surgical intervention is possible.

Dermatochalasis

• Excess eyelid skin that may cause symptoms similar to those of ptosis.
• Blepharoplasty is the treatment for symptomatic dermatochalasis.

Ectropion and Entropion

• Malpositions of the eyelid on the globe that can lead to tearing and exposure keratitis.[2]
  • Ectropion: Eyelid turned **outward.**
  • Entropion: Eyelid turned **inward.** The inward-directed eyelashes may cause keratopathy and corneal abrasions/ulcerations due to direct trauma.
• These can be repaired surgically.

Dacryocystitis

• Dacryocystitis is an infection of the tear sac from inadequate drainage of tear.
• It presents with redness, pain, and swelling in the inferomedial part of the lower eyelid.
• Acutely, oral antibiotics are necessary (cephalexin, 250 mg PO qid for 10 days).
• Surgical **dacryocystorhinostomy** is usually required after the inflammation has resolved because recurrences are likely. In a dacryocystorhinostomy, a new drainage passage is created from the tear sac to the nose.

REFERENCES

1. Khaw PT, Shah P, Elkington AR. Injury to the eye. *BMJ* 2004;328:36–38.
2. Leibowitz HM. The red eye. *N Engl J Med* 2000;343:345–351.
3. Lam DS, Tham CC, Lai JS, Leung DY. Current approaches to the management of acute primary angle closure. *Curr Opin Ophthalmol* 2007;18:146–151.
4. Biousse V, Calvetti O, Bruce BB, Newman NJ. Thrombolysis for central retinal artery occlusion. *J Neuroophthalmol* 2007;27:215–230.
5. Schein OD, Katz J, Bass EB, et al. The value of routine preoperative medical testing before cataract surgery. Study of Medical Testing for Cataract Surgery. *N Engl J Med* 2000;342:168–175.
6. Weih LM, VanNewkirk MR, McCarty CA, Taylor HR. Age-specific causes of bilateral visual impairment. *Arch Ophthalmol* 2000;118:264–269.
7. Klein R, Klein BE, Moss SE. Relation of smoking to the incidence of age-related maculopathy. The Beaver Dam Eye Study. *Am J Epidemiol* 1998;147:103–110.
8. Gehrs KM, Anderson DH, Johnson LV, Hageman GS. Age-related macular degeneration—emerging pathogenetic and therapeutic concepts. *Ann Med* 2006;38:450–471.
9. de Jong PT. Age-related macular degeneration. *N Engl J Med* 2006;355:1474–1485.
10. Age-Related Eye Disease Study Research Group. A randomized, placebo-controlled, clinical trial of high-dose supplementation with vitamins C and E, beta carotene, and zinc for age-related macular degeneration and vision loss: AREDS report no. 8. *Arch Ophthalmol* 2001;119:1417–1436.
11. Andreoli CM, Miller JW. Anti-vascular endothelial growth factor therapy for ocular neovascular disease. *Curr Opin Ophthalmol* 2007;18:502–508.

12. Maier PC, Funk J, Schwarzer G, et al. Treatment of ocular hypertension and open angle glaucoma: meta-analysis of randomised controlled trials. *BMJ* 2005;331:134–139.
13. Mohamed Q, Gillies MC, Wong TY. Management of diabetic retinopathy: a systematic review. *JAMA* 2007;298:902–916.
14. CHAMPS Study Group. Interferon beta-1a for optic neuritis patients at high risk for multiple sclerosis. *Am J Ophthalmol* 2001;132:463–471.
15. Kinkel RP, Kollman C, O'Connor P, et al; CHAMPIONS Study Group. IM interferon beta-1a delays definite multiple sclerosis 5 years after a first demyelinating event. *Neurology* 2006;66:678–684.
16. Weyand CM, Goronzy JJ. Giant-cell arteritis and polymyalgia rheumatica. *Ann Intern Med* 2003;139:505–515.

43

Screening and Adult Immunizations

Megan E. Wren

SCREENING FOR DISEASE

General Principles

- The benefit of screening depends on the prevalence of the disease, the sensitivity and specificity of the screening test, the acceptability of the test to the patient, and, most important, the ability to change the natural course of disease with treatment.
- For many diseases, there is a lack of definitive research evidence regarding the effect of screening on morbidity and mortality.
- Studies of the benefits of screening are susceptible to several forms of bias: lead time, length time, overdiagnosis, and volunteer biases.
- Many areas of controversy exist, including ages to start and stop screening, which tests to use, or whether to screen at all.
- Various professional organizations have made recommendations regarding screening for disease; **these guidelines apply only to asymptomatic patients at average risk, and they must be individualized.** Some of the most widely cited organizations include the following:
  - The American Cancer Society (ACS, http://www.cancer.org).
  - The United States Preventive Services Task Force (USPSTF, http://www.ahrq.gov/clinic/uspstfix.htm).
  - The American College of Physicians (ACP, http://www.acponline.org/clinical/guidelines/?hp).
  - The National Cancer Institute (NCI, http://www.nci.nih.gov).
  - The American College of Obstetrics and Gynecology (ACOG, http://www.acog.org).
- Table 1 presents a simplified screening schedule.

Cancer Screening

Research evidence has often been inadequate to reach definitive conclusions regarding how, when, whom, and whether to screen for various cancers. The guidelines below are a synthesis of the recommendations of the major organizations.

Breast Cancer Screening
- In 2002, a United States Preventive Services Task Force (USPSTF) review found the following[1]:
  - The relative risk (RR) of breast cancer death with mammography screening versus no screening:
    - All women, RR = 0.84, credible interval (CrI) = 0.77 to 0.91 (i.e., 16% reduction in mortality).

TABLE 1	Simplified Screening Schedule			
		Screening Recommendations		
Condition	Source			
Breast cancer	ACS	**Ages 20–39:** CBE q3 yr BSE "an option"	**Ages 40–49:** CBE q1 yr + mamms q1 yr BSE "an option"	**Ages ≥50:** CBE q1 yr + mamms q1 yr BSE "an option"
	ACOG	CBE q1 yr BSE "can be recommended"	CBE q1 yr + mamms q1–2 yr BSE "can be recommended"	CBE q1 yr + mamms q1 yr BSE "can be recommended" Mamms q2 yr until age 74
	USPSTF			
Colorectal cancer	ACS/MSTF 2008		Starting at age 50 yr: high sensitivity FOBT q1 yr OR flex sig q5 yr OR fecal DNA (interval unknown) OR DCBE q5 yr OR CT colonography q5 yr OR colonoscopy q10 yr	
	USPSTF		Age 50–75: FOBT q1 yr OR flex sig q5 yr + hi-sens FOBT q3 yr OR colonoscopy q10 yr (insufficient evidence: CT colonography or fecal DNA) Age 76–85: no routine screening Age >85: no screening	
Prostate cancer	ACS		Starting at age 50: "offer" PSA and DRE q1 yr if life expectancy >10 yr (start at 45 if FHx or if African American)	
	USPSTF		Insufficient evidence to recommend for or against screening	
Cervical cancer	ACS	**Ages 21–29:** Start 3 yr after first intercourse or by 21 yr: Pap q1 yr (if using liquid Pap q2 yr)	**Ages ≥30:** IF 3 consecutive normal Paps, then q2–3 yrs OR, Pap + HPV-DNA q3 or more yr	**Consider stopping at age:** If ≥3 normal Paps in a row and no abnormal Pap results in the last 10 yr, can stop at 70 yr
	ACOG	Pap q2 yr	IF 3 consecutive normal Paps, then q3 yr	If ≥3 normal Paps in a row and no abnormal Pap results in the last 10 yr, can stop at 65–70 yr

(continued)

TABLE 1	Simplified Screening Schedule (*Continued*)	
Condition	**Source**	**Screening Recommendations**
	USPSTF	Start 3 yr after first intercourse or by 21 yr: Pap q1–3 yr	Pap q1–3 yr	If ≥3 normal Paps in a row and no abnormal Pap results in the last 10 yr, can stop at 65 yr
Ovarian cancer	ACS	"Periodic health exams . . . might include examinations for cancer of the . . . ovaries" "Although a pelvic exam is recommended because it can find some reproductive system cancers at an early stage, most early ovarian tumors are difficult or impossible for even the most skilled examiner to feel."
	ACOG	"Data suggest that currently available screening tests do not appear to be beneficial for screening low-risk, asymptomatic women. An annual gynecologic examination with an annual pelvic examination is recommended for preventive health care."
	USPSTF	" . . . recommends against routine screening" . . . "concluded that the potential harms outweigh the potential benefits"
Lung cancer	ACS	"Informed individual decision-making . . ." "So far there is not any lung cancer screening test that has been shown to prevent people from dying of this disease"
Skin cancer	USPSTF	Insufficient evidence to recommend for or against screening
	ACS	"Periodic health exams . . . might include examinations for cancer of the . . . skin . . ."
Testicular cancer	USPSTF	Insufficient evidence to recommend for or against screening
	ACS	"Periodic health exams . . . might include examinations for cancer of the . . . testes"
	USPSTF	" . . . recommends against routine screening"

Hypertension	JNC 7	Measure BP q2 yrs (1 yr if "prehypertension" 120–139/80–89)
	USPSTF	Measure BP (interval not specified)
Hyperlipidemia	NCEP	Starting at age 20: fasting lipid profile q 5 yrs
	USPSTF	Screen men age ≥35, women age ≥45 (screen younger persons with risk factors)
Diabetes mellitus	ADA	>45 yr: consider screening with fasting plasma glucose q 3 yrs (Earlier or more frequent if obese, FHx, sedentary, Asian/Hispanic/African-American, HTN, low HDL, PCO, etc)
	USPSTF	Insufficient evidence to recommend for or against screening except in persons with HTN or hyperlipidemia
AAA	USPSTF	One-time screening for AAA by ultrasonography in men aged 65 to 75 who have ever smoked (not women)
Osteoporosis	USPSTF	Screen women aged 65+ (age 60+ if risk factors)
STDs	USPSTF	Routinely screen women ≤24 for chlamydia and gonorrhea
		Screen pregnant women for Hepatitis B, HIV, and syphilis
		Otherwise, screen according to risk factors

These are general guidelines that apply only to asymptomatic individuals at average risk for the disease; individuals with risk factors may need more aggressive screening. Screening in the elderly should be an individualized decision based on patient preference, estimated life expectancy, and comorbid conditions.

AAA, abdominal aortic aneurysm; ACOG, American College of Obstetrics and Gynecology; ACS, American Cancer Society; ADA, American Diabetes Association; BP, blood pressure; BSE, breast self-exam; CBE, clinical breast exam; CT, computed tomography; DCBE, double contrast barium enema; DRE, digital rectal exam; flex sig, flexible sigmoidoscopy; FHx, family history; FLP, fasting lipid panel; FPG, fasting plasma glucose; FOBT, fecal occult blood test; HDL, high-density lipoprotein; IFG, impaired fasting glucose; JNC 7, Seventh Report of the Joint National Committee on Prevention, Detection, Evaluation, and Treatment of High Blood Pressure; mamms, mammograms; MSTF, multisociety task force; NCEP, National Cholesterol Education Program; PCO, polycystic ovarian syndrome; PSA, prostate-specific antigen; STD, sexually transmitted disease; USPSTF, United States Preventive Services Task Force; yr, year(s).

- o Women aged 40 to 49 years, RR = 0.85 (CrI = 0.73 to 0.99) (i.e., 15% reduction in mortality).
  - o Women aged ≥50 years, RR = 0.78 (CrI 0.70 to 0.87).
- Estimates of the sensitivity of mammography were variable, 77% to 95% (i.e., 5% to 23% false negatives); sensitivity was lower among women who were <50 years, had denser breasts, or were taking hormone replacement therapy.
- In screening trials, the false-positive rate of the initial round of mammography was 3% to 6% (i.e., specificity 94% to 97%).
- The sensitivity of clinical breast examination (CBE) ranged from 40% to 69%, specificity from 86% to 99%.
- In studies, the practice of breast self-examination (BSE) was not associated with a reduction in mortality.
- In late 2009, the USPSTF published a reassessment of the available data (including additional data, relative risks being very similar to those above) stating, "For biennial screening mammography in women aged 40 to 49 years, there is moderate certainty that the net benefit is small." It emphasized the lower incidence in this group and the adverse consequences of screening.[2,3]
- Breast cancer screening includes, at a minimum, annual CBE and mammography every 1 to 2 years for women who are 50 to 74 years old.
- Data regarding those women 75 years and older are lacking.
- **USPSTF** most currently recommends the following[2]:
  - Screening mammography every 2 years for **women aged 50 to 74 years.**
  - Routine screening mammography in **women aged 40 to 49 years not at increased risk for breast cancer** is *not* recommended.
    - o Women in this age group at increased risk (e.g., deleterious genetic mutations) are more likely to benefit from mammography.
    - o The USPSTF "encourages individualized, informed decision making about when to start mammography screening."
  - The evidence is insufficient to recommend for or against screening mammography in **women aged 75 years and older.**
  - The evidence is insufficient to recommend for or against CBE in addition to screening mammography in women aged ≥40 years.
  - BSE is *not* recommended.
- The **ACS** recommends the following[4]:
  - The CBE should be part of a periodic health examination, about every 3 years for women in their 20s and 30s and every year for women aged 40 years and older.
  - BSE is an option for women starting in their 20s.
  - Yearly mammography is recommended starting at age 40 years and continuing for as long as a woman is in good health.
  - Women at very high risk (>20% lifetime risk) should undergo magnetic resonance imaging (MRI) screening and mammography every year. Women at moderately increased risk (15% to 20% lifetime risk) should talk to their physicians about the benefits and limitations of MRI screening in addition to yearly mammography.
- **ACOG** recommends CBE annually starting at age 20 years, with mammography every 1 to 2 years in the 40s and annually starting at age 50 years. BSE "can be recommended."[5]

Cervical Cancer Screening

- Cervical cancer screening with the Pap smear is recommended for all women who have ever been sexually active and who have a cervix. The ACS, USPSTF, and ACOG have fairly similar but not identical recommendations.

- Begin screening by approximately 3 years after first sexual intercourse or by age 21 years, whichever comes first (ACS and USPSTF). In November 2009, ACOG amended its guidelines recommending that screening should begin at age 21 years regardless of sexual history.[6]
- Testing interval recommendations vary:
  - **USPSTF** recommends the following:
    - Screening at least every 3 years.
    - The evidence is insufficient to recommend for or against the routine use of liquid-based cytology or the routine use of human papillomavirus (HPV) testing as a primary screening test for cervical cancer.
  - **ACS** recommends the following[4]:
    - Screening should be done every year with the regular Pap test or every 2 years using the newer liquid-based Pap test.
    - Beginning at age 30, women who have had three normal Pap test results in a row may get screened every 2 to 3 years.
    - Another reasonable option for women >30 years is to get screened every 3 years (but not more frequently) with either the conventional or liquid-based Pap test, plus the DNA test for HPV.
  - **ACOG** most recently recommends the following[6]:
    - For women aged 21 to 29 years cervical cytology screening is recommended every 2 years.
    - If a woman aged 30 years and older has had negative results on three consecutive cervical cytology tests, then she may be rescreened with cervical cytology alone every 3 years.
    - Combined cytology and HPV DNA testing is an appropriate screening test for women >30 years. The combined testing is not appropriate for women <30 years, since they frequently test positive for HPV that will clear up on its own.
- **High-risk patients** should continue annual testing (ACS, ACOG). Risk factors include the following:
  - A history of abnormal Pap smears or cervical cancer.
  - A history of exposure to diethylstilbestrol (DES) in utero.
  - HIV infection, any stage.
  - Immunocompromise, including organ transplant, chemotherapy, or chronic steroid use.
- Women who have had a **total hysterectomy** (removal of the uterus and cervix) may stop having cervical cancer screening, unless the surgery is done as a treatment of cervical cancer or precancer (ACS, USPSTF, ACOG).
- **Older women** who have had three or more normal Pap tests in a row and no abnormal Pap test results in the last 10 years may choose to stop having cervical cancer screening after age 65 (USPSTF), 70 (ACS), or 65 to 70 years (ACOG). Women with a history of cervical cancer, DES exposure before birth, HIV infection, or a weakened immune system should continue to have screening as long as they are in good health. ACOG suggests that the decision to stop screening be individualized.

Colorectal Cancer Screening

- Colorectal cancer screening should be offered to all patients aged 50 and older. Widely accepted options include the following:
  - Annual fecal occult blood testing (FOBT) with three mail-in guaiac cards and/or flexible sigmoidoscopy every 5 years; the combination is preferred over either option alone.

- Air contrast barium enema every 5 years.
- Colonoscopy every 10 years.
- Any abnormalities on FOBT, flexible sigmoidoscopy, or barium enema must be followed up with a full colonoscopy.
- High-risk persons need earlier and/or more frequent screening. These include those with the following:
  - A personal history of colorectal cancer or adenomatous polyps.
  - A personal history of inflammatory bowel disease.
  - A family history of a hereditary colorectal cancer syndrome (familial adenomatous polyposis or hereditary nonpolyposis colon cancer).
  - Women with a history of endometrial or ovarian cancer diagnosed before age 50.
  - A strong family history of colorectal cancer or polyps (cancer or polyps in a first-degree relative <60 years or in two first-degree relatives of any age). Screening should begin at age 40, or 10 years before the youngest case in the immediate family, whichever is earlier.

Lung Cancer Screening

- Lung cancer screening is not currently recommended by any major organization.
- In 2007, the American College of Chest Physicians issued updated guidelines[7]:
  - "We do not recommend that low-dose helical CT be used to screen for lung cancer except in the context of a well-designed clinical trial."
  - They also recommend against the use of serial chest radiographs, or single or serial cytologic evaluation to screen for lung cancer.
- All patients should be counseled about smoking cessation.
- Promising results have been obtained from pilot projects using low-dose spiral CT scans for lung cancer screening, but mortality data from randomized trials is not yet available.

Prostate Cancer Screening

- Available screening techniques include serum prostate-specific antigen (PSA) testing or digital rectal examination (DRE).
- Prostate cancer screening is controversial.
  - There are no randomized, controlled trials demonstrating a mortality benefit.
  - PSA screening leads to a significant number of false-positive and false-negative results.
  - The natural history of untreated prostate cancer is variable.
  - Treatment for prostate cancer may have adverse effects that decrease quality of life.
- USPSTF finds that evidence is insufficient to recommend for or against routine screening for prostate cancer using PSA or DRE.
- The ACS recommends the following:
  - *Offering* the PSA blood test and digital rectal examination yearly, beginning at age 50, to men who have at least a 10-year life expectancy.
  - Testing should begin at age 45 for **high-risk** men: African-Americans and men who have a first-degree relative diagnosed with prostate cancer at an early age (<65).
  - Men at **even higher risk** (because they have several first-degree relatives who had prostate cancer at an early age) could begin testing at age 40.
  - Health care professionals should give men the chance to openly discuss the benefits and limitations of testing at yearly checkups. Men should actively take part in

the decision by learning about prostate cancer and the pros and cons of early detection and treatment of prostate cancer.

Ovarian Cancer Screening

- USPSTF recommends *against* routine screening for ovarian cancer.
  - There is no existing evidence that any screening test, including CA-125, ultrasound, or pelvic examination, reduces mortality from ovarian cancer.
  - There is a low incidence of ovarian cancer in the general population. In women at average risk, the positive predictive value of an abnormal screening test is about 2% (i.e., 98% of positive test results are false positives).
  - Because of the low prevalence of ovarian cancer and the invasive nature of diagnostic testing after a positive screening test, there is fair evidence that screening could likely lead to important harms. The USPSTF concluded that the potential harms outweigh the potential benefits.
- ACOG and ACS do not recommend routine screening for ovarian cancer.
- Clinicians should be vigilant for early symptoms of ovarian cancer such as recent (3 to 6 months) onset of abdominal or pelvic pain, abdominal bloating, constipation or urinary urgency. Symptoms should be evaluated by pelvic examination, CA-125, and/or transvaginal ultrasound.

Screening for Other Cancers

Routine population screening is not recommended for the following cancers: endometrial, testicular, bladder, thyroid, oral cavity, or skin. Clinicians should be vigilant for early symptoms of possible cancer in those sites.

Screening for Other Conditions

Hypertension

- All patients should have their blood pressure (BP) measured every 2 years (see Chapter 3).
- Classification of BP, according to The Seventh Report of the Joint National Committee on Prevention, Detection, Evaluation, and Treatment of High Blood Pressure (JNC 7),[8] is presented in Table 2.
- Lifestyle modification includes counseling on weight loss, aerobic exercise, limiting alcohol intake, and reduction in sodium intake.
- The decision as to whether to start drug therapy should depend on the severity of hypertension, the presence of other disease, and evidence of end-organ damage.

Dyslipidemia

- The National Cholesterol Education Program Adult Treatment Panel III (ATP III)[9] recommends cholesterol screening every 5 years for all adults >20 years. Those with hyperlipidemia need more frequent follow-up. Details are available at http:// www.nhlbi.nih.gov/guidelines/cholesterol/ (see Chapter 8).
- The American Heart Association also recommends screening every 5 years, starting at age 20.
- The USPSTF recommends routine screening starting at age 35 in men and age 45 in women. Younger adults should be screened if they have other risk factors for coronary artery disease.

| TABLE 2 | Classification, Follow-Up, and Treatment of Hypertension | | |

Blood Pressure (mm Hg)	Classification	Follow-up	Treatment
<120/80	Normal	Recheck in 2 years	
120–139/80–89	Prehypertension	Recheck in 1 year	Recommend lifestyle modification Consider drugs if diabetes or chronic kidney disease (goal of <130/80 mm Hg)
140–159/90–99	Stage 1 hypertension	Confirm within 2 months	Lifestyle modification and medications
≥160/100	Stage 2 hypertension	Start treatment	Lifestyle modification and medications

Modified from Lenfant C, Cjpbamoam AV, Jones DW, et al. Seventh report of the Joint National Committee on the Prevention, Detection, Evaluation, and Treatment of High Blood Pressure (JNC 7): resetting the hypertension sails. *Hypertension* 2003;41:1178–1179.

Diabetes Mellitus

- Screen all adults with hypertension, hyperlipidemia, or cardiovascular disease.
- Routine screening in asymptomatic adults is not recommended.
- Screening of high-risk individuals should be considered at 3-year intervals.[10] **Risk factors** include the following:
  - Age >45 years.
  - Overweight (body mass index [BMI] >27 kg/m^2).
  - Impaired glucose tolerance.
  - History of gestational diabetes mellitus (DM) or delivery of an infant over 9 pounds.
  - Family history of DM.
  - Certain ethnic groups (e.g., African-Americans, Hispanic Americans, Native Americans, Asian Americans, Pacific Islanders).
- Currently, the test of choice is the fasting plasma glucose (FPG).
  - The normal FPG level is <100 mg/dL.
  - FPG level of 100 to 125 mg/dL indicates impairment of glucose tolerance.
  - FPG level of ≥126 mg/dL on two occasions is diagnostic of DM.
- A random glucose level of >200 mg/dL is considered a positive screening test and requires follow-up testing.
- In the near future, hemoglobin A1c may become the screening test of choice (see Chapter 16).

Abdominal Aortic Aneurysm

- The USPSTF recommends one-time screening for abdominal aortic aneurysm (AAA) by ultrasonography in men aged 65 to 75 years who have ever smoked.[11]
- The USPSTF recommends against routine screening for AAA in women and makes no recommendation for or against screening for AAA in men aged 65 to 75 years who have never smoked.

Coronary Heart Disease

- The USPSTF recommends against routine screening with resting electrocardiography, exercise treadmill test, or electron-beam computerized tomography for coronary calcium for the prediction of coronary heart disease (CHD) in adults at low risk for CHD events.
- The USPSTF found insufficient evidence to recommend for or against routine screening with these tests in adults at increased risk for CHD events.
- The American Heart Association recommends[12] that risk factor assessment should begin at age 20, with assessment of family history of CHD, smoking status, diet, alcohol intake, physical activity, BP, BMI, waist circumference, and pulse. Fasting serum lipoprotein profile and fasting blood glucose level should be measured according to patient's risk for hyperlipidemia and diabetes, respectively (at least every 5 years; if risk factors are present, every 2 years).

Peripheral Arterial Disease

The USPSTF recommends against routine screening for peripheral arterial disease (PAD) because there is little evidence that treatment of PAD at this asymptomatic stage of disease, beyond treatment based on standard cardiovascular risk assessment, improves health outcomes.

Thyroid Disease

Screening for thyroid disease is not routinely recommended, but clinicians should keep a low threshold for measurement of thyroid-stimulating hormone for subtle or nonspecific symptoms, especially in older women (see Chapter 17).

Obesity

Periodic height and weight measurements are recommended for all patients. The BMI is calculated by dividing the body weight in kilograms by the square of the height in meters. A BMI of >25 kg/m^2 is considered overweight, >30 kg/m^2 is considered obese, and >40 kg/m^2 is considered severely obese. Morbid obesity is obesity accompanied by medical complications.

Osteoporosis

- Women aged 65 and older should be screened routinely for osteoporosis with bone density measurement (see Chapter 37).
- The dual energy X-ray absorptiometry is the best validated test.
- Screen younger women who have risk factors: Caucasian women, Asian American women, women with low body weight, and women who have had a bilateral oophorectomy before menopause.
- All women should receive counseling regarding dietary calcium, vitamin D, weight-bearing exercise, and smoking cessation.

Sexually Transmitted Diseases

- Screen all sexually active adolescents and women aged 24 and younger (pregnant or not) for *Chlamydia* and gonorrhea (see Chapter 23).
- Screen older women (pregnant or not) for *Chlamydia* and gonorrhea only if they are at increased risk.
- Consider screening men if they are at increased risk for gonorrhea.
- Screen pregnant women for hepatitis B virus (HBV), HIV, and syphilis.

- Screen all persons at increased risk for syphilis infection.
- **Screening for HIV infection:**
  - Screen all pregnant women.
  - The USPSTF recommends screening adolescents and adults at increased risk for HIV infection.
  - The Centers for Disease Control and Prevention (CDC) recommends[13] screening all individuals between 13 and 64 years of age regardless of recognized risk factors.
- Risk factors for STDs include the following:
  - Persons with a history of sexually transmitted infections, new or multiple sexual partners, inconsistent condom use, and exchanging sex for money or drugs (or having sex partners who do) are at risk for all STDs.
  - Past or present injection drug users are also at risk for HBV and HIV.
  - Men who have sex with men are also at risk for HBV, HIV, and syphilis.
  - Household contacts of persons chronically infected with HBV are also at risk of acquiring HBV.
  - Individuals whose past or present sex partners were HIV infected, bisexual, or injection drug users, and persons with a history of blood transfusion between 1978 and 1985 are also at risk for HIV.

Alcohol Abuse and Dependence

- Screening for alcohol abuse and dependence is an important part of the routine checkup (see Chapter 45).
- Definitions (from the National Institute on Alcohol Abuse and Alcoholism at http://www.niaaa.nih.gov):
  - **Heavy or "at-risk" drinking** is diagnosed in the following group:
    - Men who consume >14 drinks per week or >4 drinks per occasion.
    - Women who consume more than seven drinks per week or more than three drinks per occasion.
    - Elderly who consume more than seven drinks per week or more than three drinks per occasion.
  - **One "drink"** is 12 g ethanol, as in 12 oz of beer, 5 oz of wine, or 1.5 oz of distilled spirits.
  - **Alcohol abuse** is a maladaptive pattern of use; manifest by continued or recurrent use despite failure in major role obligations at work, school, or home; use in physically hazardous situations; or use despite alcohol-related legal, social, or interpersonal problems.
  - **Alcohol dependence** is marked by tolerance, the presence of withdrawal symptoms on cessation, impaired control (drinking more/longer than intended), persistent desire, and continued use despite physical or psychological problems related to alcohol.
- The "CAGE" questions are a useful screening tool for alcohol dependence. Two positive responses are considered a positive test and indicate further assessment is warranted.
  - Have you ever felt that you should **Cut down** on drinking?
  - Have people **Annoyed** you by criticizing your drinking?
  - Have you ever felt bad or **Guilty** about your drinking?
  - **Eye-opener:** Have you ever had a drink first thing in the morning to steady your nerves or to get rid of a hangover?

ADULT IMMUNIZATIONS

General Principles

- Guidelines are subject to change over time and according to local public health conditions.
- Each patient's clinical context should be considered and risks and benefits weighed.
- These are general guidelines, and manufacturer's information should be consulted regarding individual products.
- Various professional organizations make recommendations regarding immunization practices. The official national policy is determined by the following:
  - The Department of Health and Human Services (HHS).
  - The Centers for Disease Control and Prevention.
  - The Advisory Committee on Immunization Practices (ACIP).
- The ACIP makes recommendations which are then reviewed by the Director of CDC and the HHS. They become official policy when published in CDC's Morbidity and Mortality Weekly Report.

Resources for Information

- Immunization guidelines are quite detailed and are periodically updated. Useful resources for accessible, up-to-date information include the following:
  - The CDC vaccine information website (http://www.cdc.gov/vaccines) has extensive information including official ACIP recommendations.
  - The Immunization Action Coalition (IAC) website has educational materials, camera ready and copyright free, at http://www.immunize.org. They have many translated documents for non-English speaking patients. The IAC also has comprehensive information about vaccines and vaccine-preventable diseases at http://www.vaccineinformation.org.

Legal Responsibilities of the Provider

- Serious or unusual adverse events must be reported to the Vaccine Adverse Events Reporting System (VAERS), whether or not the provider thinks they are causally associated. Forms are available from the Food and Drug Administration (FDA) at http://www.fda.gov/cber/vaers/vaers.htm.
- Federally approved "Vaccine Information Statements" must be given to all patients prior to administering vaccines. Copies are available from the CDC or the IAC.
- Permanent vaccination records must be maintained by all vaccine providers.

Timing of Administration

- Specified times are minimum intervals.
- Doses that are administered at shorter intervals may not result in adequate antibody response and should not be counted as part of a primary series.
- Delay or interruption in the immunization schedule does not require starting over or extra doses.
- Simultaneous administration of multiple vaccines improves compliance. In general, inactivated (killed) and most live vaccines can be administered at the same time at separate anatomic sites; exceptions include cholera, parenteral typhoid, plague, and yellow fever vaccines.

- Immunoglobulin preparations can interfere with the response to live virus vaccines.
- Tuberculin test response can be inhibited by live virus vaccines. Tuberculin skin testing can be done on the same day as the vaccination or 4 to 6 weeks later.

Hypersensitivity to Vaccine Components

- Persons with a history of anaphylactic reactions to any vaccine component generally should not receive that vaccine, except under the supervision of an experienced allergist. Vaccines may have traces of egg protein or antibiotics; the manufacturer's insert should be carefully checked.
- Contact dermatitis to neomycin is a delayed-type (cell-mediated) immune response, not anaphylaxis, and is therefore not a contraindication to vaccine use.
- Hypersensitivity to thimerosal is usually a local delayed-type or an irritant effect.
- Many vaccines may cause mild to moderate local or systemic adverse effects such as low grade fever or injection site swelling, redness, or soreness. These are not a contraindication to future doses of the vaccine.

Specific Patient Groups

Table 3 provides an overview of vaccination doses, schedules, and contraindications.

Checklists by Age

Young Adults (About 18 to 26 Years)
- Were adequate childhood vaccinations received?
  - Three doses of tetanus (DPT or DTaP, see "Tetanus, Diphtheria and Pertussis Vaccines" later) and 1 dose of measles, mumps, and rubella (MMR).
- Tetanus booster (tetanus and diphtheria toxoids [Td]) every 10 years; substitute Tdap (adult formulation with tetanus toxoid and lesser quantities of diphtheria toxoid and acellular pertussis) for 1 dose of Td.
- Students and health care workers need to have received 2 doses of measles vaccine.
- Offer varicella vaccine to those who are susceptible (never had chickenpox or vaccine).
- Offer meningococcal vaccine to those aged ≤18 and to those aged ≥19 with risk factors.
- Consider HPV vaccine (Gardisil) for women up to age 26.
- Assess risk factors that indicate the need for other vaccines: hepatitis A, hepatitis B, influenza, or pneumococcal vaccines.

Mid-Life Adults (About 27 to 49 Years)
- Were adequate childhood vaccinations received?
  - Three doses of tetanus (DPT or DTaP, see "Tetanus, Diphtheria and Pertussis Vaccines" later) and 1 dose of MMR.
- Td every 10 years; substitute Tdap for 1 dose of Td.
- Students and health care workers need documentation of 2 doses of measles vaccine.
- Offer varicella vaccine to those who are susceptible (never had chickenpox or vaccine).
- Assess risk factors that indicate the need for other vaccines: hepatitis A, hepatitis B, meningococcal, influenza, or pneumococcal vaccines.

Adults Ages 50 Years and Older
- Were adequate childhood vaccinations received?
  - Three doses of tetanus (DPT or DTaP, see "Tetanus, Diphtheria and Pertussis Vaccines" later) and 1 dose MMR.

TABLE 3 Adult Immunizations

Vaccine	Live?	Dosages[a] (For Adults Only)	Schedule[b] Number of Doses and Minimum Intervals Between Doses					Contraindications
			First Dose	Minimum Interval	Second Dose	Minimum Interval	Third Dose	
Haemophilus	No	0.5 mL IM	X					Anaphylaxis to vaccine components
Hepatitis A	No	1.0 mL IM	X	≥6 months	X			Anaphylaxis to vaccine components
Hepatitis B[c]	No	1.0 mL IM (deltoid only)	X	≥4 weeks	X	≥5 months	X	Anaphylaxis to vaccine components Administer in deltoid area only
HPV	No	0.5 mL IM	X	>2 months	X	>6 months	X	Anaphylaxis to vaccine components Pregnancy
Influenza	No	0.5 mL IM	X	Annual				Anaphylaxis to eggs or vaccine components Caution if history Guillain-Barré syndrome
Influenza, intranasal	Yes	0.2 mL intranasal	X	Annual				Anaphylaxis to eggs or vaccine components Pregnancy; immune compromise Lung disease, other chronic medical conditions Caution if history of Guillain-Barré syndrome
Measles, MMR	Yes	0.5 mL SC	X	≥4 weeks	(X)			Anaphylaxis to vaccine components Pregnancy; immune compromise

(continued)

TABLE 3   Adult Immunizations (*Continued*)

Vaccine	Live?	Dosages[a] (For Adults Only)	First Dose	Minimum Interval	Second Dose	Minimum Interval	Third Dose	Contraindications
					Schedule[b] Number of Doses and Minimum Intervals Between Doses			
Meningococcus, conjugated	No	0.5 mL IM	X					Anaphylaxis to vaccine components Caution if history of Guillain-Barré syndrome
Pneumococcus	No	0.5 mL IM or SC	X	(5 years)	(X)			Anaphylaxis to vaccine components
Polio, IPV	No	0.5 mL SC	X	≥4–8 weeks	X	≥6–12 months	X	Anaphylaxis to vaccine components
Tetanus, Td or Tdap	No	0.5 mL IM	X	≥4 weeks	X	≥6–12 months	X	Anaphylaxis to vaccine components Caution if history of Guillain-Barré syndrome Caution if history of Arthus reaction with tetanus vaccine
Varicella	Yes	0.5 mL SC[d]	X	≥4–8 weeks	X			Anaphylaxis to vaccine components Pregnancy; immune compromise
Zoster	Yes	0.65 mL SC	X					

HPV, human papillomavirus; IM, intramuscularly; IPV, inactivated poliovirus vaccine; MMR, measles, mumps, and rubella; SC, subcutaneously; Tdap, tetanus/diphtheria toxoid with acellular pertussis vaccine; Td, tetanus and diphtheria toxoids.

[a]See text for further details.
[b]Intervals are minimums to achieve adequate antibody response; longer intervals do *not* necessitate any additional doses.
[c]See text for schedule for hemodialysis patients.
[d]Keep frozen and use <30 minutes after reconstitution.

- Tetanus vaccine was first widely used in the 1940s; many older adults are not immune.
- Adults born before 1957 (i.e., age 53 in 2010) can be assumed to be immune to measles.
- Td every 10 years; substitute Tdap for 1 dose of Td for those <65 years.
- Students and health care workers need documentation of 2 doses of measles vaccine.
- All adults aged 50 and older should receive annual influenza vaccination, even if healthy.
- A single dose of pneumococcal vaccine should be given at age 65 (see "Pneumococcal Vaccine" later for other indications and revaccination schedule).
- Offer varicella vaccine to those who are susceptible (never had chickenpox or vaccine).
- Offer one-time zoster (shingles) vaccination to those aged 60 and older.
- Assess risk factors that indicate the need for other vaccines: hepatitis A, hepatitis B, meningococcal, or pneumococcal vaccines.

Documentation of Vaccinations

- If records cannot be located, the age-appropriate schedule of primary immunizations should be started. Persons who have served in the military have been vaccinated against measles, rubella, tetanus, diphtheria, and polio.
- Vaccines received outside the United States are usually of adequate potency; foreign records are acceptable if they include written documentation of the date of vaccination and the schedule (age and interval) was comparable with that recommended in the United States.

Pregnancy and Breastfeeding

- Breastfeeding is not a contraindication for any vaccine for infant or mother (except smallpox).
- **Pregnancy is a contraindication for live virus vaccines,** such as MMR or varicella, but these vaccines can safely be administered to the children of a pregnant woman.
- Influenza vaccine is recommended for all women who will be pregnant during influenza season.
- Pregnant women who are not fully immunized against tetanus should begin the primary series.
- Vaccines against hepatitis B, hepatitis A, and pneumococcus are indicated for pregnant women who are at high risk for these infections or their complications.
- All pregnant women should be tested for rubella antibodies; women who are susceptible to rubella should be vaccinated immediately after delivery.

Immunosuppressed Patients

- **Live vaccines are generally contraindicated in immunosuppressed patients,** such as those with congenital immunodeficiency, HIV infection, leukemia, lymphoma, generalized malignancy or therapy with alkylating agents, antimetabolites, radiation, or supraphysiologic doses of corticosteroids.
- Killed (inactivated) vaccines can be safely administered, but the response may be suboptimal. Vaccination during (or within 2 weeks before) chemotherapy or radiation therapy results in a poor antibody response and therefore should be delayed or repeated 3 months after therapy is discontinued.
- Because measles infection may cause serious illness in persons with HIV infection, the CDC recommends MMR vaccination for asymptomatic HIV-infected persons. Because of the theoretical risk, and one reported fatal case of vaccine-type measles

pneumonitis 1 year after vaccination,[14] the CDC believes it prudent to withhold MMR in severely immunocompromised HIV-infected patients.

- Symptomatic or severely immunocompromised HIV-infected patients who are exposed to measles should receive immunoglobulin (0.25 mL/kg; maximum dose 15 mL), regardless of prior vaccination status.

Persons with Chronic Illness

- **Hemophilia and bleeding disorders:** Many patients tolerate IM injections well if a 23-gauge needle is used and firm pressure is applied to the site for at least 2 minutes without rubbing. If the patient receives factor replacement therapy, IM vaccination can be scheduled shortly after such therapy.
- **Persons with liver disease** are at increased risk of suffering complications from many vaccine-preventable diseases. One should ensure immunity to hepatitis A, hepatitis B, pneumococcus, influenza, tetanus, MMR, and varicella.
- **Persons with chronic renal disease and renal transplant recipients** should receive influenza and pneumococcal vaccines. Hemodialysis patients should be screened for hepatitis B, and susceptible patients should receive a primary series of HBV vaccine (see the "Hepatitis B Virus Vaccine and Immunoglobulin" section for special schedules and precautions).
- **Persons with splenic dysfunction,** including sickle cell disease, or anatomic asplenia are at increased risk of contracting fatal pneumococcal and meningococcal bacteremia and should receive the vaccines. The *Haemophilus influenzae* type b (Hib) vaccine should be considered. Persons who are scheduled for elective splenectomy should receive these vaccines at least 2 weeks before the operation.

Health Care Workers

- Health care workers and first responders are at risk for exposure to and possible transmission of vaccine-preventable diseases.
- Hepatitis B is an occupational hazard for any worker with possible exposure to blood or bloody fluids.
- Influenza vaccine is recommended annually for all health care workers and can also be considered for those who provide essential community services.
- All health care workers should document immunity to measles and rubella.
- Additional vaccines are indicated for veterinarians, laboratory technicians, animal handlers, and others who may have occupational exposure to rabies, poliovirus, smallpox virus, *Yersinia pestis* (plague), or *Bacillus anthracis* (anthrax).

Travelers

- The risk of acquiring illness during international travel depends on the areas to be visited and the extent to which the traveler is likely to be exposed to diseases.
- Influenza is present in the Southern Hemisphere from April through September and year-round in the tropics.
- Travelers should be counseled about safe sex practices.
- Selected travelers may need immunization against yellow fever, cholera, typhoid, plague, meningococcus, rabies, hepatitis B, or hepatitis A.
- Resources for up-to-date information for travelers include the CDC website (http://wwwn.cdc.gov/travel/default.aspx), which has detailed information about worldwide destinations, and the CDC's toll-free 24-hour Travelers' Health Automated Information Line, 877-394-8747 (877-FYI-TRIP).

Specific Vaccines and Immunobiological Agents

Measles, Mumps, and Rubella

Indications

- Ensure that all adults are immune to measles. Adequate evidence of immunity can include any of the following:
  - A vaccination record with at least 1 dose of live measles vaccine on or after the first birthday.
  - Documentation of physician-diagnosed disease.
  - Serologic evidence of immunity (presence of measles antibodies).
  - Persons born before 1957 can be considered immune.
- Susceptible adults should receive 1 dose of MMR.
- A second dose of MMR (>1 month after first dose) is recommended for the following individuals:
  - Prior recipients of the killed measles vaccine or an unknown type in the period 1963–1967.
  - Health care workers (unless serologic evidence of immunity).
  - All students (unless serologic evidence of immunity).

Contraindications, Side Effects, and Precautions

- MMR is a live-attenuated virus; it is **contraindicated in pregnancy and is generally contraindicated in immunocompromised hosts.**[14]
- Persons with a history of anaphylactic hypersensitivity to eggs or neomycin should be given MMR only with extreme caution and under special protocols by an allergist.
- In a minority of vaccine recipients, fever (5% to 15%), rash (5%), or arthralgias (up to 25% of adult females) may develop.
- Because blood products can interfere with the antibody response, MMR administration should be delayed (consult manufacturer's information for exact intervals). However, rubella-susceptible women should be vaccinated immediately postpartum even if anti-Rho(D) (RhoGAM, WinRho, etc.) or other blood products were administered in pregnancy or at delivery. Antibody levels should be measured 3 months later to assess response.
- Tuberculin test response can be inhibited by live virus vaccines; tuberculosis skin testing can be done on the same day as the vaccination or 4 to 6 weeks later.

Polio

Indications

- Wild-type polio has been eradicated from the entire Western Hemisphere.
- U.S. adults do not need polio vaccination unless they plan to travel to endemic areas or have occupational exposure to poliovirus.

Contraindications, Side Effects, and Precautions

- Anaphylactic hypersensitivity to streptomycin, polymyxin B, or neomycin is a contraindication to inactivated polio vaccine.
- The oral polio vaccine (OPV) is a live-attenuated virus and can cause vaccine-associated paralytic poliomyelitis (approximate rate: 1 in 6 million). It is now recommended that oral polio vaccine should not be used in the United States, even in healthy children. **Only inactivated polio vaccine should be used.**

Tetanus, Diphtheria, and Pertussis Vaccines

The vaccine terminology can be confusing; all contain a full dose of tetanus toxoid.

- **DPT:** No longer available in the U.S. but still used in some parts of the world, pediatric use, full dose of diphtheria toxoid plus whole killed pertussis.
- **DTaP** (Daptacel, Infanrix, and Tripedia brands): Pediatric use only, full dose of diphtheria toxoid plus full dose acellular pertussis; take care to avoid confusion with Tdap.
- **DT:** Pediatric use, full dose of diphtheria toxoid.
- **Td:** Adult use, reduced dose of diphtheria toxoid.
- **Tdap** (Adacel and Boostrix brands): Adult use only, reduced dose of diphtheria toxoid plus reduced dose of acellular pertussis; take care to avoid confusion with DTaP.

Indications

- All adults of any age should complete a primary series of 3 doses of Td if they have not done so during childhood or the history is uncertain.
  - Tetanus vaccine was first widely used in the 1940s so elderly persons may have never received a primary series.
  - Doses that are given as part of wound management may count toward the 3 doses needed.
- **A tetanus booster (Td) is recommended every 10 years, lifelong. Many adults are overdue for boosters.**
- Only about one-third of tetanus cases result from puncture wounds; other sources include minor wounds, burns, frostbite, bullet wounds, crush injuries, and chronic wounds such as abscesses and chronic ulcers (14% of cases). Approximately 4% of patients with tetanus can recall no antecedent wound.
- Because infection does not confer complete immunity, tetanus patients should be immunized after recovery.
- See Figure 1 for guidelines for postexposure prophylaxis.

Tetanus/Diphtheria Toxoid with Acellular Pertussis

- In 2005, a Tdap vaccine was approved for use in ages 11 to 64 years.
- **Many adults are susceptible to pertussis** so the new vaccine should help to reduce pertussis morbidity among adults and reduce the transmission of pertussis to infants and in health care settings.
- The ACIP recommends a single dose of Tdap in the following circumstances:
  - To replace one Td booster in adults ages 19 to 64 years (if last dose of Td is >10 years earlier and no previous Tdap).
  - Adults who anticipate having close contact with an infant, to reduce the risk for transmitting pertussis (includes parents, grandparents aged <65 years, child-care providers, and health care personnel).
  - When possible, women should receive Tdap before becoming pregnant, otherwise immunize in the immediate postpartum period.
  - For wound management, Tdap is preferred to Td if they have not previously received Tdap.
  - Health care personnel with direct patient contact should receive a single dose of Tdap.
  - An interval of at least 2 years from the last dose of Td is suggested to reduce the risk for local and systemic reactions after vaccination, but shorter intervals may be used to protect against pertussis.

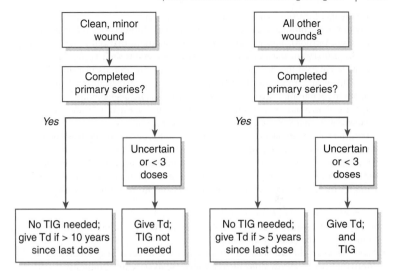

Figure 1. Guidelines for postexposure prophylaxis to prevent tetanus. [a]Tetanus-producing wounds are often not the classic puncture wounds but can include minor wounds, burns, frostbite, bullet wounds, crush injuries, and chronic wounds such as abscesses and chronic ulcers. TIG, tetanus immunoglobulin; Td, tetanus and diphtheria toxoids, adsorbed.

Contraindications, Side Effects, and Precautions
- Local reactions are common and consist of erythema, induration, or tenderness.
- Too frequent administration can produce increased rates of local or systemic reactions due to antigen-antibody complexes (Arthus-type reaction).
- Urticarial or anaphylactic reactions can occur but are rare. If such a history exists, then serologic testing to determine immunity to tetanus can be performed to evaluate the need for a booster dose. If additional doses are needed to ensure immunity, referral to an allergist is indicated.

Influenza
- Annually, many deaths occur among the elderly and chronically ill, who are at high risk for complications of influenza infection (>10,000 excess deaths in the United States in many years).
- Antibodies from previous infections or vaccinations are not fully protective against new strains because the virus undergoes constant antigenic drift (point mutations) and occasional antigenic shift (change in subtype).
- Those who are at highest risk of the disease and its complications are also the least able to respond to vaccination. Overall the vaccine is about 70% to 80% effective against vaccine-type viruses.

Indications
- Annual influenza vaccination is recommended for the following adults:
  - All healthy persons aged ≥50 years.
  - All women who will be pregnant during flu season.

- Residents of nursing homes or chronic care facilities.
- Persons with chronic cardiovascular or pulmonary disorders (including asthma, but not hypertension). This includes those with conditions that can compromise respiratory function or the handling of respiratory secretions such as cognitive dysfunction, spinal cord injuries, seizure disorders, or other neuromuscular disorders.
- Persons with chronic metabolic diseases (including diabetes), renal dysfunction, nephrotic syndrome, alcoholism, cirrhosis, asplenia, hemoglobinopathies (including sickle cell anemia), or immunodeficiency (including organ transplantation, HIV infection, hematologic malignancies, or corticosteroid use).
- Health care personnel, caregivers, and household contacts of high-risk patients (to reduce transmission to patients).
- Vaccination can also be offered to anyone in the general public who wishes to reduce the chance of influenza infection, especially those who provide essential community services and students or other persons in institutional settings.

Contraindications, Side Effects, and Precautions
- A history of anaphylactic hypersensitivity to eggs is a contraindication to the influenza vaccine (shot or intranasal).
- Side effects of the flu shot are usually limited to mild arm soreness. Placebo-controlled trials have demonstrated no increase in systemic symptoms.
- The flu shot is not a live virus and cannot cause the flu.
- The live-attenuated intranasal vaccine may cause rhinorrhea, nasal congestion, headache, or sore throat.
- Guillain-Barré syndrome has not been associated with the influenza vaccine since the 1976 to 1977 swine flu vaccine (which was associated with approximately 5 to 10 excess cases of Guillain-Barré syndrome/million vaccines).

Live-Attenuated Influenza Vaccine
- The intranasal live-attenuated influenza vaccine (LAIV) (brand name FluMist) is an option for vaccination of healthy, nonpregnant persons aged 2 to 49 years.
  - Health care workers should avoid contact with severely immunocompromised patients for 7 days after vaccine receipt.
- Possible advantages of LAIV include its potential to induce a broad mucosal and systemic immune response, its ease of administration, and the acceptability of an intranasal rather than intramuscular route of administration.
- **The intranasal LAIV should not be used in the following:**
  - Those <2 or >50 years.
  - Pregnant women.
  - Persons with chronic health problems.
  - Persons with a history of Guillain-Barré syndrome.
  - Persons with a history of hypersensitivity, including anaphylaxis, to any of the components of LAIV or to eggs.
  - Children or adolescents receiving aspirin or other salicylates (because of the association of Reye syndrome with wild-type influenza virus infection).
  - Health care workers and others who have close contact with severely immunocompromised persons during those periods in which the immunocompromised person requires care in a protective environment, such as patients with stem cell transplants.

Pneumococcal Vaccine
- Pneumococcal disease causes approximately 40,000 deaths annually in the United States.
- The vaccine contains purified capsular materials of 23 serotypes.

- Adults should receive the 23-valent polysaccharide vaccine, not the pediatric 7-valent conjugated vaccine.
- Efficacy is controversial and is estimated at 40% to 70%. Because polysaccharide vaccines do not induce T-cell–dependent responses associated with immunologic memory, there is no true anamnestic response to additional doses of vaccine (although antibody levels will rise).

Indications
- All healthy persons aged ≥65 years who were not previously vaccinated or with unknown vaccination status.
- All healthy persons aged ≥65 years who were vaccinated ≥5 years ago and were <65 years at first vaccination.
- Persons aged 2 to 64 years with chronic health conditions, including chronic cardiovascular or pulmonary disease, diabetes, alcoholism, chronic liver disease or cirrhosis, cerebrospinal fluid leaks, and functional or anatomic asplenia, including sickle cell disease.
- Nursing home residents.
- Alaskan natives and certain American Indian populations.
- Immunocompromised persons, including those with HIV infection; leukemia, lymphoma, Hodgkin disease, multiple myeloma, or generalized malignancy; chronic kidney disease or nephrotic syndrome; organ or bone marrow transplant; and immunosuppressive chemotherapy, including corticosteroids.
- The interval between vaccination and initiation of immunosuppressive therapy should be at least 2 weeks; do not vaccinate during chemotherapy or radiation therapy.

Revaccination
Revaccination is not routinely recommended and is contraindicated if the patient had a severe reaction to the first dose (Arthus or anaphylactic). A single revaccination should be considered after 5 years for those who are likely to have a rapid decline in antibody levels. Persons at highest risk include those with anatomic or functional asplenia (sickle cell disease), HIV infection, hematologic or generalized malignancy, chronic renal failure, nephrotic syndrome, or other conditions associated with immunosuppression (organ transplant, chemotherapy, corticosteroids, or other immunosuppressive medications).

Contraindications, Side Effects, and Precautions
Approximately half of patients experience injection site soreness, redness, or swelling; systemic symptoms are rare. Pneumococcal vaccine is contraindicated in those with a severe reaction to a previous dose (anaphylaxis or local Arthus-type reaction).

Hepatitis A Virus Vaccine and Immunoglobulin
The levels of antibody following hepatitis A virus (HAV) vaccine or immunoglobulin are much lower than those following natural infection and are usually below the level of detection of most commercial assays but are protective against infection (>90% effective by 1 month).

Indications for Vaccination for Preexposure Prophylaxis
- In high-prevalence populations, it may be reasonable (but not necessary) to check serology before offering HAV vaccine.
- Target groups for vaccination include the following:
  - Persons traveling to/working in countries in which HAV is endemic.
  - Men who have sex with men.

- Illicit drug users.
- Persons with chronic liver disease or liver transplant recipients (no increased risk of acquiring infection, but complications would be more likely).
- Persons with an occupational risk (e.g., laboratory workers).
- Persons who receive clotting factor concentrates.
- Vaccination can also be considered for food handlers to reduce potential transmission.

Travelers
- Travelers to Canada, Western Europe, Australia, New Zealand, and Japan are at no greater risk for infection than in the United States.
- Elsewhere, there is increased risk even if travelers observe precautions against enteric infection or stay in urban areas or luxury hotels.
- Ideally, travelers should receive HAV at least 4 weeks before travel. A second dose 6 to 12 months later is necessary for long-term protection.
- Persons who travel to a high-risk area <4 weeks after the initial dose also should receive immunoglobulin (0.02 mL/kg) at a different anatomic site.
- Travelers who do not receive the vaccine should be administered a single dose of immunoglobulin (0.02 mL/kg), which will provide protection for up to 3 months. For travel periods that exceed 2 months, the dose should be 0.06 mL/kg; administration must be repeated if the travel period exceeds 5 months.

Contraindications, Side Effects, and Precautions
- Contraindications include hypersensitivity to alum or the preservative 2-phenoxyethanol.
- The most frequent side effects are injection site soreness and headache.
- The vaccine and immunoglobulin can be given at the same time at separate anatomic sites.

Postexposure Prophylaxis
- In high-prevalence populations, it may be reasonable (but not necessary) to check serology before offering immunoglobulin.
- The immunoglobulin (0.02 mL/kg) should be given as soon as possible, but no later than 10 days to 2 weeks after exposure.
- Persons who received HAV vaccine at least 1 month before exposure do not need immunoglobulin.
- Postexposure prophylaxis is indicated for household and sexual contacts of confirmed cases (but not casual contacts).
- Day care center staff and attendees need prophylaxis if one or more cases are confirmed.
- If a food handler is diagnosed with hepatitis A, other food handlers at the same location need immunoglobulin (and should consider vaccine). Transmission to patrons is unlikely, but prophylaxis can be considered if an infectious worker directly handled uncooked or previously cooked foods and had diarrhea or poor hygienic practices and patrons can be contacted and treated within 2 weeks.

Hepatitis B Virus Vaccine and Immunoglobulin
Efficacy and Postvaccination Testing
- In immunocompetent adults, the vaccine is 80% to 95% effective in preventing disease.
- Protection is essentially complete for those with an adequate antibody response ($\geq$10 mIU/mL measured 1 to 6 months after immunization).

- Antibody levels decline over time, but protection against disease appears to persist despite undetectable antibody.
- Routine booster doses of vaccine are not recommended for immunocompetent children or adults.
- Efficacy is lower in hemodialysis patients. See below for special schedules.
- Postvaccination testing for serologic response (1 to 6 months after completion of the vaccine series) is advised only for persons whose subsequent clinical management depends on knowledge of their immune status (e.g., infants born to hepatitis B surface antigen [HBsAg]-positive mothers, dialysis patients and staff, and persons with HIV infection) or those who are expected to have a suboptimal response (age >50, renal disease, and HIV infection). Postvaccination testing should also be considered for persons at occupational risk.
- When nonresponders are revaccinated, 15% to 25% produce an adequate antibody response after one additional dose and 30% to 50% after three additional doses.

Indications

- Serologic testing may be reasonable in high-risk patients, but there is no harm in vaccinating persons who are already immune.
- The vaccine is indicated for susceptible persons in the following groups:
  - All newborns and all previously unimmunized adolescents.
  - Those at occupational risk, including health care workers and morticians.
  - Residents and staff of institutions for the developmentally disabled.
  - Hemodialysis patients, hemophiliacs, and other recipients of blood products.
  - High-risk lifestyles, including homosexual men, men and women with multiple sex partners who are seen for STDs, and intravenous drug users.
  - Household and sexual contacts with known hepatitis B carriers.
  - Immigrants from Eastern Asia or sub-Saharan Africa, native Alaskans, and native Pacific Islanders.
  - Travelers to endemic areas who will have close contact with the local population.
- Patients on hemodialysis require larger or increased number of doses, or both, to achieve adequate antibody levels.
  - Measure titers 1 to 6 months after immunization.
  - Antibody levels should be tested annually and a booster dose administered when antibody level decline to <10 mIU/mL.
  - For adult dialysis patients, use 3 doses of the special 40 µg/mL formulation of Recombivax-B (1.0 mL IM at 0, 1, and 6 months), or use 4 double doses of the regular 20 µg/mL formulation of Engerix-B (2.0 mL IM at 0, 1, 2, and 6 months).

Contraindications, Side Effects, and Precautions

The vaccine is well tolerated. Pregnancy is not a contraindication.

Postexposure Prophylaxis

- Hepatitis B immunoglobulin (HBIG) is used for postexposure prophylaxis in susceptible individuals (no vaccine or known nonresponder).
- Vaccine and HBIG can be administered at the same time, but at separate sites.
- Sexual partners of patients with acute HBV infection or who are HBsAg positive should begin prophylaxis within 14 days of the last sexual contact or if ongoing sexual contact will occur. Administer a single dose of HBIG (0.06 mL/kg) and begin the vaccine series.
- Household contacts of patients with acute HBV infection do not need prophylaxis except infants and those with identifiable blood exposure (shared toothbrush

TABLE 4	Hepatitis B Prophylaxis Following Percutaneous Exposure to Blood		

	Treatment When Source Patient is:		
Exposed Person is:	HBsAg Positive	HBsAg Negative	Status Unknown
Unvaccinated	HBIG × 1; initiate HB vaccine	Initiate HB vaccine	Initiate HB vaccine
Previously vaccinated, known responder	Recheck anti-HBs level; if adequate, no treatment; if inadequate, HB vaccine booster dose[a]	No treatment	No treatment
Previously vaccinated, known nonresponder	HBIG ×2 (1 month apart) *or* HBIG × 1 + 1 HB vaccine	No treatment	If known high-risk source patient, can treat as if HBsAg positive
Previously vaccinated, response unknown	Check anti-HBs level; if adequate, no treatment; if inadequate, HBIG plus HB vaccine booster dose	No treatment	Check anti-HBs level; if adequate, no treatment; if inadequate, HB vaccine booster dose

HB, hepatitis B; HBIG, hepatitis B immunoglobulin; HBsAg, hepatitis B surface antigen.
[a]Adequate anti-HBsAg level is 10 SRU by radioimmunoassay or positive by enzyme immunoassay.

or razor). Administer a single dose of HBIG (0.06 mL/kg) and begin the vaccine series.
• If the index patient becomes a chronic carrier, all household contacts should be given the hepatitis B vaccine.
• After any percutaneous exposure to blood, the source patient and the exposed person should be checked for HBsAg status. See Table 4 for treatment algorithm.

Varicella (Chickenpox)
• Approximately 10% of U.S. adults are susceptible to the varicella-zoster virus and its complications.
• Prior to routine immunization, approximately 100 deaths occurred annually, over half in adults. Even healthy young adults can succumb to acute respiratory distress syndrome after varicella infection.
• A reliable history of varicella is considered a valid measure of immunity; most adults with negative or uncertain histories had mild or subclinical disease and are actually immune.

Efficacy
• In adolescents and adults, the seroconversion rate is 99% after 2 doses.

- Pediatric studies show an efficacy of 70% to 90% in preventing infection and 95% protection against severe disease for 7 to 10 years.
- Cases that do occur in vaccinated persons are usually mild, with fewer than 50 lesions.
- It is unknown whether booster doses will be needed in the future.
- The incidence of herpes zoster may be less after vaccination than after the natural disease.

Indications

Two doses of varicella vaccine are indicated for all susceptible adolescents and adults, with emphasis on the following groups:
- Susceptible adolescents.
- Adults who live with young children.
- All nonpregnant women of childbearing age.
- Household contacts of immunocompromised persons.
- Health care workers.
- Workers in schools and day care centers.
- Those who live in closed populations such as colleges or the military.
- International travelers.

Contraindications, Side Effects, and Precautions

- The varicella vaccine is a live-attenuated virus vaccine.
- **Varicella vaccine is contraindicated in pregnancy** (defer pregnancy 1 month after vaccination), in individuals with compromised cellular immune function, or in adults who receive >20 mg/day prednisone.
- Approximately 25% to 33% of recipients had injection site soreness, swelling, erythema, or rash.
- In <1%, a diffuse rash developed with a median of five lesions, most caused by a coincidental wild-type virus.
- Vaccine-type virus from the varicella-like rash after immunization can infrequently be transmitted to susceptible contacts, but the secondary cases are subclinical or mild.

Herpes Zoster (Shingles)

- Latent varicella zoster virus can cause herpes zoster, as known as shingles.
- About one in five cases of zoster leads to postherpetic neuralgia (increased incidence with aging).
- Rare complications include pneumonia, cranial nerve damage, or encephalitis.
- There are an estimated 1 million cases of shingles each year in the United States.
- A live-attenuated zoster vaccine was FDA approved in 2007.
- Although both are made from live-attenuated varicella zoster virus, the varicella vaccine (Varivax) and the zoster vaccine (Zostavax) are not interchangeable—**the zoster vaccine is a much higher dosage.**

Efficacy

- Studies submitted to the FDA showed an efficacy of about 50% in preventing the occurrence of herpes zoster, ranging from 64% people in their 60s to 18% for those >80 years.[15]
- Vaccine recipients who did develop shingles had a slight decrease in pain duration (22 vs. 20 days).
- The duration of protection is unknown, but probably >4 years.

Indications

The ACIP has issued provisional recommendations.
- The vaccine is administered as a single dose.
- They recommend the shingles vaccine for adults aged ≥60 years, whether or not they report a prior episode of herpes zoster.
- Persons with chronic medical conditions may be vaccinated unless a contraindication or precaution exists for their condition.

Contraindications, Side Effects, and Precautions
- The zoster vaccine is a live-attenuated virus vaccine.
- **Zoster vaccine is contraindicated in pregnancy or in immunocompromised patients.**
- Other contraindications include a history of severe allergic reaction to gelatin, neomycin, or any component of the vaccine.
- The most common side effects are redness, pain and swelling at the site of injection of the vaccine, and headache.
- No serious problems with shingles vaccine have been identified so far.

Haemophilus influenzae Type B Conjugated Vaccine
- Most invasive Hib disease occurs in very young children but can also occur in adults with chronic pulmonary disease and conditions that predispose to infections with encapsulated organisms (e.g., splenic dysfunction, hematologic malignancies).
- Most *H. influenzae* disease in adults is due to nontypeable strains, but *Haemophilus influenzae* type B conjugated vaccine (HibCV) can be considered for adults with functional or anatomic asplenia or HIV infection (although of unproven benefit).
- Side effects of injection site such as swelling, redness, and/or pain have been reported in 5% to 30% of children; systemic reactions are infrequent.

Meningococcal Vaccine
- The meningococcal vaccine is available in two forms:
  - An older tetravalent polysaccharide vaccine (brand name Menomune).
  - The newer tetravalent meningococcal conjugate vaccine (MCV4, brand name Menactra) is now preferred because of enhanced immunogenicity.
- Both vaccines contain serogroups A, C, Y, and W135, but not serogroup B, which causes half of U.S. cases.
  - Serogroup A is the most common cause of epidemics worldwide.
  - Serogroup B is not included because the group B polysaccharide is a very poor immunogen in humans and is structurally similar to the glycosyl modification of human cell surface proteins, raising concerns of immunopathology.
- Vaccine-induced immunity is of unknown duration, and the need for revaccination is unknown.

Indications
- A single dose of MCV4 is recommended for routine vaccination of all persons aged 11 to 18 years.
- Vaccination is also recommended for persons aged 19 to 55 years who are at increased risk for meningococcal disease:
  - College freshmen living in dormitories.
  - Military recruits.
  - Microbiologists routinely exposed to isolates of *Neisseria meningitidis*.
  - Travelers to or residents of countries in which *N. meningitidis* meningitis is hyperendemic or epidemic (e.g., pilgrimage to Mecca).

- Persons with terminal complement component deficiencies.
- Persons with anatomic or functional asplenia.
- The vaccine is an option for others who wish to decrease their risk for meningococcal disease:
  - Other college students.
  - Persons infected with HIV.
- The vaccine is also used for controlling outbreaks.

Contraindications, Side Effects, and Precautions
- Adverse reactions are mild and infrequent.
- MCV4 is contraindicated in cases of sensitivity to thimerosal or other vaccine components.
- Safety in pregnancy is unknown.
- Guillain-Barré syndrome has been associated with receipt of MCV4; therefore, a history of Guillain-Barré syndrome is a relative contraindication to receiving MCV4. The nonconjugated polysaccharide vaccine (MPSV4) is an acceptable alternative for short-term protection against meningococcal disease (3 to 5 years).

Human Papillomavirus Vaccine

- This quadrivalent vaccine contains major capsid proteins of HPV 6, 11, 16, and 18 in noninfectious virus-like particles. It was FDA approved in 2006 (brand name Gardisil).
- Clinical trials indicate that the vaccine has high efficacy in preventing persistent HPV infection, cervical cancer precursor lesions, vaginal and vulvar cancer precursor lesions, and genital warts caused by HPV types 6, 11, 16, or 18 among females who have not already been infected with the respective HPV type.
- Females infected with one or more vaccine HPV types before vaccination would be protected against disease caused by the other vaccine HPV types.
- The vaccine is administered as a 3-dose series.
- The vaccine is recommended for girls at the 11- to 12-year-old checkup but can be administered to girls as young as age 9 years.
- Catch-up vaccination is recommended for females aged 13 to 26 years who have not been previously vaccinated.
- **Vaccination is not a substitute for routine cervical cancer screening** (Pap smears), and vaccinated women should have cervical cancer screening as recommended.

Rabies Vaccine and Immunoglobulin

- Most reported cases of animal rabies in the United States are in wild raccoons, skunks, foxes, and bats.
- Worldwide, wild dogs account for most cases; some U.S. cases of rabies originate from dog bites sustained abroad, even years earlier. Rabies prophylaxis in foreign countries may be inadequate.
- Vaccine side effects include injection site soreness and erythema. Mild systemic symptoms (such as headache, nausea, and myalgias) are common.
- Preexposure prophylaxis is indicated in persons whose jobs or hobbies bring them into contact with potentially rabid animals, such as veterinarians or animal handlers. Those at continuing risk should have a booster (or check serology) every 2 years.

Postexposure Prophylaxis
- The most important element of postexposure prophylaxis is immediate and thorough washing of all wounds with copious soap and water, not just antiseptics. Tetanus prophylaxis should be considered.

- Previously immunized patients should receive 2 doses of vaccine: 1 mL IM in the deltoid on days 0 and 3.
- Persons not previously immunized should be treated with the following:
  - A single 20 IU/kg dose of human rabies immunoglobulin (HRIG), up to half infiltrated in the area of the wound and half IM.
  - HRIG should be given immediately but can be administered up to the eighth day after vaccine was started.
  - Five doses of vaccine (1 mL IM in the deltoid on days 0, 3, 7, 14, and 28).
- Immunocompromised persons should be tested for adequacy of antibody response.
- The local department of health should be notified.
- The decision to initiate postexposure prophylaxis should include the following considerations:
  - Because bites to the head or neck can result in rabies in <1 week, immediate prophylaxis is indicated.
  - A healthy domestic dog, cat, or ferret should be held for observation for 10 days; if signs of rabies develop in the animal, the human contact should be immediately treated with HRIG and vaccine while the animal is tested.
  - Bites from a suspected rabid dog or cat require immediate prophylaxis. Casual contact (petting) does not require prophylaxis.
  - Bats and wild carnivores should be regarded as rabid unless proved negative by laboratory tests.
  - Bites by some animals, such as bats, can inflict very minor injury and thus be undetected.
  - **A bat found in a room with a sleeping person is considered an exposure.**
  - Small rodents (e.g., squirrels, hamsters, guinea pigs, gerbils, chipmunks, rats, and mice) and lagomorphs (including rabbits and hares) are almost never found to be infected with rabies and have not been known to transmit rabies to humans.

REFERENCES

1. Humphrey LL, Helfand M, Chan BK, Woolf SH. Breast cancer screening: a summary of the evidence for the U.S. Preventive Services Task Force. *Ann Intern Med* 2002;137:347–360.
2. U.S. Preventive Services Task Force. Screening for breast cancer: U.S. Preventive Services Task Force recommendation statement. *Ann Intern Med* 2009;151:716–726.
3. Nelson HD, Tyne K, Naik A, et al; U.S. Preventive Services Task Force. Screening for breast cancer: an update for the U.S. Preventive Services Task Force. *Ann Intern Med* 2009;151:727–737.
4. Smith RA, Cokkinides V, Eyre HJ. American Cancer Society guidelines for the early detection of cancer, 2006. *CA Cancer J Clin* 2006;56:11–25.
5. ACOG Committee on Gynecologic Practice. ACOG Committee Opinion No. 357: Primary and preventive care: periodic assessments. *Obstet Gynecol* 2006;108:1615–1622.
6. ACOG Practice Bulletin No. 109: Cervical Cytology Screening. *Obstet Gynecol* 2009;114:1409–1420.
7. Alberts WM, American College of Chest Physicians. Diagnosis and management of lung cancer executive summary: ACCP evidence-based clinical practice guidelines (2nd Edition). *Chest* 2007;132:1S–19S.
8. Lenfant C, Chobanian AV, Jones DW, et al. Seventh report of the Joint National Committee on the Prevention, Detection, Evaluation, and Treatment of High Blood Pressure (JNC 7): resetting the hypertension sails. *Hypertension* 2003;41:1178–1179.
9. National Cholesterol Education Program (NCEP) Expert Panel on Detection, Evaluation, and Treatment of High Blood Cholesterol in Adults (Adult Treatment Panel III). Third

Report of the National Cholesterol Education Program (NCEP) Expert Panel on Detection, Evaluation, and Treatment of High Blood Cholesterol in Adults (Adult Treatment Panel III) final report. *Circulation* 2002;106:3143–3421.

10. American Diabetes Association. Standards of medical care in diabetes—2007. *Diabetes Care* 2007;30:S4–S41.

11. U.S. Preventive Services Task Force. Screening for abdominal aortic aneurysm: recommendation statement. *Ann Intern Med* 2005;143:198–202.

12. Pearson TA, Blair SN, Daniels SR, et al. AHA Guidelines for Primary Prevention of Cardiovascular Disease and Stroke: 2002 Update: Consensus Panel Guide to Comprehensive Risk Reduction for Adult Patients Without Coronary or Other Atherosclerotic Vascular Diseases. American Heart Association Science Advisory and Coordinating Committee. *Circulation* 2002;106:388–391.

13. Branson BM, Handsfield HH, Lampe MA, et al. Revised recommendations for HIV testing of adults, adolescents, and pregnant women in health-care settings. *MMWR Recomm Rep* 2006;55:1–17.

14. Angel JB, Walpita P, Lerch RA, et al. Vaccine-associated measles pneumonitis in adults with AIDS. *Ann Intern Med* 1998;129:104–106.

15. Oxman MN, Levin MJ, Johnson GR, et al. A vaccine to prevent herpes zoster and postherpetic neuralgia in older adults. *N Engl J Med* 2005;352:2271–2284.

44

Smoking Cessation
Megan E. Wren

General Principles

Smokers Can Quit

- Since the publication of the first Surgeon General's Report on Smoking and Health in 1965, the rate of smoking among adult Americans has gradually decreased from 42% down to 20.9%.[1]
- Among current smokers, 70% report they want to quit.[2]
- Although individual quit attempts have a low success rate, many people can be successful with repeated attempts. In fact, **of all Americans who have smoked, half have successfully quit.**[1]
- The clinician should recognize tobacco dependence as a *chronic disease*, subject to periods of remission and relapse, and requiring ongoing counseling. Fortunately, effective interventions are now available that may be able to increase long-term quit rates to 15% to 30%.

Guidelines

- A widely accepted approach to brief office-based counseling and pharmacotherapy was published as a U.S. Public Health Service (PHS) Report and was summarized in *JAMA*.[3,4] It provides practical advice on treating tobacco addiction.
- This evidence-based guideline was sponsored and supported by many organizations, including the National Cancer Institute and the Centers for Disease Control and Prevention.
- The full Guideline is available for free at http://www.surgeongeneral.gov/tobacco (last accessed December 21, 2009), as well as a Quick Reference Guide and a Clinician's Packet.

Key Recommendations

- Tobacco dependence is a chronic condition that often requires repeated intervention.
- Effective treatments exist that can produce long-term or even permanent abstinence; every patient who uses tobacco should be offered at least one of these treatments.
- There is a strong dose-response relationship between the intensity of tobacco-dependence counseling and its effectiveness. Treatments involving person-to-person contact (via individual, group, or proactive telephone counseling) are consistently effective, and their effectiveness increases with treatment intensity (e.g., minutes of contact).
- Numerous effective pharmacotherapies for smoking cessation now exist. Except in the presence of contraindications, these should be used with all patients attempting to quit smoking.

Counseling for Behavior Change

- Brief counseling should be provided to all smokers at every visit. Interventions as short as 3 minutes can increase quit rate significantly.
- **The "Five As"** technique for brief office counseling of smokers is familiar to many clinicians. A brief summary is provided below; more detail is available in the PHS Guideline.

The 5 As

Ask

- Ask about smoking. Every patient. Every visit.
- Make it one of the vital signs so that it is not forgotten.

Advise

- Advise all smokers to quit. Physicians' advice is a strong incentive to attempt smoking cessation. Be empathetic, not confrontational.
- Use a clear, strong message such as **"Quitting smoking is the most important thing you can do to protect your health now and in the future. I can help you."**
- Personalize the message by stressing the relevance to the patient's current medical problems and symptoms. Most smokers are unaware of smoking's connection with a wide array of problems from acid reflux to osteoporosis to macular degeneration.

Assess

- Assess the smoker's willingness to make a serious quit attempt in the next 30 days (see the "Readiness for Change" section).

Assist

- Assist in the quit attempt. If the patient is ready to make a serious attempt to quit, then make smoking cessation the focus of the visit.
- Help the patient set a specific **quit date** in the next couple of weeks. Write it in the chart and on a prescription blank to make it official.
- Discuss **anticipated triggers and challenges,** and strategies to cope with them.
- The patient should enlist the aid of family and friends. Before the quit date he/she should start to break the habit by avoiding smoking in the usual places.
- Provide **educational materials.** Offer referrals to classes, websites such as http://www.smokefree.gov (last accessed December 21, 2009), or a telephone Quitline (1-800-QUITNOW) for additional counseling.
- Recommend **pharmacotherapy,** except in special circumstances.

Arrange

- Arrange follow-up in person or by phone within the first week and again **within the first month.**
- Successful quitters should be congratulated and reminded to be on guard against tempting situations and cravings, which can persist for months to years.
- Those who did not try to quit should be assessed for willingness to change and encouraged to again set a quit date when ready.
- Those who quit and have relapsed should be encouraged to learn from the experience. The physician should focus on the positive (congratulate for the days or weeks of abstinence) and help the patient feel empowered to try again by discussing strategies to cope with challenging situations.

Readiness for Change

- The Prochaska model of stages of change provides a useful framework for targeting interventions to the smoker's willingness to attempt to quit. Knowing the patient's readiness for change can guide the physician's time allotment to counseling in each visit.
- The stages form a predictable cycle:
  - **Precontemplation stage:** The smoker is unaware or underaware of the problem and has no intention of changing the behavior. The physician's role is to educate, to reinforce the need to quit smoking, and to encourage the patient to at least *think* about smoking cessation. The counseling can be quite brief, just a minute or two, but should be repeated at every visit.
  - **Contemplation stage:** The patient is aware that a problem exists but is not yet ready to make a commitment to take action. This stage may last for long periods of time. The physician's role is to strengthen the patients' self-confidence in their ability to make the change and to offer assistance in helping the patient to quit.
  - **Preparation stage:** The patient intends to take action in the next few months; this may be a brief stage. The physician should increase the intensity and specificity of counseling and help the patient determine a course of action. When a patient is really ready to commit to change, this should be the main focus of the office visit.
  - **Action stage:** This is the most visible stage, in which the addictive behavior is actually altered (for 1 day to 6 months). The physician should recommend nicotine replacement therapy (NRT) and monitor the efficacy.
  - **Maintenance stage:** The patient maintains the change (smoking cessation) and works to prevent relapse. This stage extends beyond 6 months and may last a lifetime. The physician should provide follow-up and continued support.
  - **Relapse stage:** This can also be termed **recycle** because the patient again moves through the cycle and may achieve long-term success on subsequent cycles. The physician should assist the patient in renewing the process.
- The same stages apply to any behavior change: quitting smoking or drinking, starting to exercise or follow a diet, etc. and can guide the physician's approach to counseling.

Medications to Aid Smoking Cessation

Recommendations

- **Pharmacologic therapy can approximately double the quit rate** (as compared with placebo) and should be offered to all patients except in the presence of limited special circumstances (see later).
- Established first-line treatments include sustained-release (SR) bupropion and NRT.
- Medications for smoking cessation are presented in Table 1.

Nicotine Replacement Therapy

- NRT provides an alternative source of nicotine to ease withdrawal symptoms while the patient learns new nonsmoking behaviors.
- Many studies have documented that the use of NRT can double the long-term success rate.[5]

TABLE 1	Medications to Aid Smoking Cessation			
Products and Brands (Availability)	Dosage	Side Effects and Precautions	Approximate Cost/Month	
First-line pharmacotherapies				
Nicotine gum Nicorette (OTC)	2 mg/piece (smoke <1 ppd) 4 mg/piece (smoke >1 ppd) Use at least 9 pieces/day; max 24 pieces	Mouth soreness, dyspepsia	$100–150 (10 doses/day)	
Nicotine lozenge Commit (OTC)	2 mg/piece (smoke >30 minutes after awakening) 4 mg/piece (smoke <30 minutes after awakening) Use at least 9 pieces/day; max 24 pieces	Mouth soreness, dyspepsia, and hiccups	$160–190 (10 doses/day)	
Nicotine inhaler Nicotrol Inhaler (Rx)	6–16 cartridges/day	Local irritation of mouth and throat	$250 (8 doses/day)	
Nicotine nasal spray Nicotrol NS (Rx)	8–40 doses/day	Nasal irritation	$100 (10 doses/day)	
Nicotine patch NicoDerm CQ (OTC) Nicotrol (OTC) Habitrol (OTC) ProStep (OTC) generics (OTC)	21, 14, or 7 mg/24 hours; 15, 10, or 5 mg/16 hours Use each strength for 2–4 weeks	Local skin reaction, insomnia	$80–120	

(continued)

TABLE 1 Medications to Aid Smoking Cessation (*Continued*)

Products and Brands (Availability)	Dosage	Side Effects and Precautions	Approximate Cost/Month
Bupropion SR Zyban (Rx) Wellbutrin SR (Rx) generic (Rx)	150 mg every morning × 3 days, then 150 mg bid Start 1 week before quit date; continue 3–6 months	Insomnia, dry mouth, and nausea CONTRAINDICATED if history of seizures or eating disorders	$80–190
Varenicline Chantix (Rx)	0.5 mg every morning × 3 days, then 0.5 mg bid × 4 days, then 1 mg bid Start 1 week before quit date; continue 3–6 months	Nausea, insomnia, and headache	$120–130
Second-line pharmacotherapies (NOT approved for use for smoking cessation by the FDA)			
Clonidine Catapres (Rx) Catapres-TTS (Rx) generic (Rx)	0.1–0.2 mg bid	Sedation, constipation, hypotension, and risk of rebound hypertension	$9 (generic) $120 (brand name)
Nortriptyline Pamelor (Rx) generic (Rx)	75–100 mg/day	Sedation, dry mouth, and constipation	$15 (generic) $400 (brand name)

FDA, Food and Drug Administration; OTC, over the counter; ppd, pack per day; Rx, by prescription only.

- NRT is even more effective when combined with counseling. The effectiveness of counseling increases with the intensity of treatment, but even brief interventions are of benefit.
- Studies have documented the long-term safety of NRT. Some experts advocate "harm reduction"—the use of NRT for as long as it takes to keep patients from smoking.

Safety of Nicotine Replacement Therapy

- Smokers smoke in order to get nicotine, but essentially all of the adverse health effects of smoking stem from other constituents in tobacco and its smoke. Thus, a cigarette is a contaminated drug delivery device.
- Cigarette smoke contains over 4,000 chemical compounds (the "tar"), ranging from carbon monoxide to hydrogen cyanide and 69 known carcinogens, including arsenic, benzene, and polonium-210.[6]
- Many in the public falsely believe that NRT is just as harmful as cigarettes, and they even think that NRT can cause heart attacks, lung cancer, and asthma.[7]
- The most common side effect of nicotine is local irritation, such as a rash under a nicotine patch or throat irritation from inhaled nicotine.
- NRT is unlikely to cause an addiction because of the low level of nicotine (half that of smoking) and the slow delivery to the brain.

Safety of NRT in Patients with Cardiovascular Disease

- The dose-response relationship for nicotine is flat, so the effects of smoking plus NRT are similar to smoking alone. Importantly, NRT has no "tar" or carbon monoxide. Numerous studies have documented the safety of NRT, especially as compared with continued smoking.
- Unlike cigarette smoking, NRT does not worsen endothelial dysfunction[8] nor does it cause platelet aggregation and smoking's thrombotic effects.[9]
- Transdermal nicotine in smokers with known coronary artery disease (CAD) has been shown to cause no significant differences in heart rate, blood pressure, or in duration or frequency of ischemic episodes on ambulatory electrocardiogram monitoring.[9]
- The use of nicotine gum did not increase cardiovascular deaths or hospitalizations, even in patients who smoked while using NRT and/or used NRT for more than a year.[10]
- Stress testing in smokers with CAD showed that addition of a nicotine patch improved exercise tolerance and decreased ischemia, despite continued smoking and increased serum nicotine levels. The reduction in ischemia correlated with reduced exhaled carbon monoxide levels, as the subjects spontaneously reduced their smoking while wearing the nicotine patches.[11,12] This clearly shows that **smoking while wearing a nicotine patch is not dangerous.**
- The American Heart Association supports the use of NRT to aid in smoking cessation.[13]

Specific Products
Nicotine Gum

- Nicotine gum (polacrilex) is available over the counter in 2- and 4-mg strengths; the 4-mg strength is recommended for those who smoke more than a pack a day.
- The nicotine is absorbed only through the buccal mucosa and absorption is decreased by acidic beverages, so the patient should be instructed not to eat or drink while chewing the gum or 15 minutes before. Rapid chewing, eating, or drinking will cause the nicotine to be swallowed and it will cause heartburn, hiccups, or dyspepsia.
- The gum should be chewed slowly until a peppery taste emerges, then parked between cheek and gum for buccal absorption. The gum should be chewed slowly and intermittently for approximately 30 minutes or until the taste dissipates.

- It takes several minutes for the nicotine to reach the bloodstream, so there will not be the immediate "satisfaction" of smoking.
- Patients will be more successful if they use at least nine pieces a day. They should use it on a fixed schedule: one piece every 1 to 2 hours for at least 1 to 3 months, then start to slowly taper the number of pieces per day (one piece per day every 4 to 7 days).
- The maximum daily dose is 24 pieces. Side effects include mouth soreness, dyspepsia, and hiccups.

Nicotine Lozenges
- Nicotine lozenges are available over the counter in 2- and 4-mg strengths; the 4-mg strength is recommended for those who smoke within 30 minutes of awakening.
- Similar to the nicotine gum, it is absorbed through the buccal mucosa, so patients must not eat or drink while using it.
- Patients will be more successful if they use at least nine pieces a day: one piece every 1 to 2 hours for at least 1 to 3 months, then taper off. The maximum daily dose is 24 pieces. Side effects include mouth soreness, dyspepsia, and hiccups.

Nicotine Patches
- Nicotine patches are available over the counter in several strengths.
- Each morning a patch should be placed on a relatively hairless location on the trunk or upper arm; locations should be rotated to minimize skin irritation. Hands should be washed after handling patches. The used patch should be folded in half and thrown away out of reach of children and pets.
- Any brand of patch may either be used overnight to minimize morning cravings or may be taken off at bedtime to minimize insomnia.
- A typical dosage schedule is to use the strongest patch for 2 to 4 weeks, then the intermediate strength for 2 weeks, and then the weakest strength for 2 weeks (e.g., 21, then 14, then 7 mg/day strengths).
- The most common side effects include insomnia and skin irritation. It is common to feel tingling under the patch for the first hour.

Nicotine Nasal Spray
- Nicotine nasal spray is available by prescription only and is less popular with patients (expensive and awkward to use).
- Patients should use one spray in each nostril (for a total dose of 1 mg) and should use 1 to 2 doses/hour with a maximum of 40 doses/day.
- The spray has a faster onset of action than the gum or patch and therefore has greater potential for dependence.
- The most common side effect is nasal irritation, which can be minimized by avoiding sniffing or inhaling while administering.
- The combination of the spray and patch may be more effective than the patch alone.[14]

Nicotine Inhaler
- The nicotine inhaler is available by prescription only and is less popular with patients (expensive and awkward to use).
- Each cartridge delivers 4 mg nicotine over 80 inhalations. Patients should use 6 to 16 cartridges daily for up to 6 months. The vapor is absorbed in the mouth and throat. The inhaler is puffed frequently for 20 minutes (much more frequently than a cigarette).
- Because the nicotine is absorbed only through the buccal mucosa and absorption is decreased by acidic beverages, the patient should be instructed not to eat or drink while using the inhaler or 15 minutes before.

- The most common side effects are irritation of the mouth and throat, coughing, dyspepsia, and rhinitis.

Combination Therapy

- The nicotine patch can be used for basal delivery and the gum, nasal spray, or inhaler added for "breakthrough" cravings. This is especially important if the patch must be removed at night to prevent insomnia.
- The patient should use the gum, spray, or inhaler on awakening because it will take several hours for transdermal absorption from the new patch.

Nonnicotine Medications

Bupropion

- Sustained-release bupropion (bupropion SR, marketed as Zyban, Wellbutrin, and others) is thought to work by enhancing dopaminergic activity in the central nervous system.
- Bupropion SR should be started 1 to 2 weeks before the quit date at 150 mg each morning for 3 days, then 150 mg bid for 7 to 12 weeks. Evening dosing may lead to insomnia.
- In randomized controlled trials, subjects treated with bupropion SR had **abstinence rates of about twice that in the placebo group.**[15]
- Efficacy is independent of a history of depression.
- In direct comparison studies, **bupropion SR was more effective than nicotine patches and the combination of bupropion plus nicotine patch was only slightly more effective than bupropion SR alone.**[16,17]
- The most common side effects are insomnia (about 20%), dry mouth, and nausea.
- Contraindications include a history of a seizure disorder, eating disorder, or use of a monoamine oxidase inhibitor within 14 days. Because of a 1 in 1,000 **risk of seizures,** bupropion SR should not be used in patients with a history of seizure, head trauma, brain tumor, or in those with anorexia/bulimia, hepatic failure, or those using drugs that may increase the risk of seizures (theophylline, systemic steroids, antipsychotics, antidepressants, hypoglycemic/insulin, or abuse of alcohol or stimulants). Bupropion SR is contraindicated in patients with use of a monoamine oxidase inhibitor within 14 days.

Varenicline

- The newest medication approved for smoking cessation is varenicline, a partial nicotine agonist (marketed as Chantix). It binds to the $\alpha_4\beta_2$ nicotinic acetylcholine receptors, stimulating dopamine release to reduce craving and withdrawal symptoms, while also blocking binding of nicotine to reduce the reinforcing effects of smoking (satisfaction).
- Varenicline has been shown to **more than double the placebo quit rate and is more effective than bupropion.** After 12 weeks of therapy, the 1 year quit rates were placebo 8%, bupropion SR 16%, and varenicline 22%.[18,19]
- Varenicline should be started 1 week prior to the patient's quit date at 0.5 mg once daily for 3 days, then 0.5 mg twice daily for 4 days, and then 1 mg twice daily for 12 to 24 weeks.
- The most common adverse effects of varenicline were nausea (in more than one-fourth of patients), headache, vomiting, flatulence, insomnia, abnormal dreams, and dysgeusia.

Other Medications
- **Nortriptyline** is considered a second-line agent.
  - **It is not FDA approved for smoking cessation,** but there have been several published reports that demonstrate that its efficacy in smoking cessation is better than that of placebo but less than that of bupropion SR.[20]
  - As with other tricyclic antidepressants, nortriptyline often causes dry mouth, constipation, and sedation.
  - An advantage of nortriptyline is its affordability.
- **Clonidine** is also considered a second-line agent.
  - Clonidine can approximately double the quit rate and is inexpensive, but it is rarely used for smoking cessation due to **troublesome side effects** including dry mouth, sedation, and orthostatic hypotension.
  - Abrupt cessation of high-dose clonidine can cause rebound hypertension.
  - It may be used at 0.1 to 0.2 mg twice daily.
- Benzodiazepines and selective serotonin reuptake inhibitors are **NOT** effective for smoking cessation.

Special Circumstances

Pregnancy and Lactation
- Clinicians should provide **intensive nonpharmacologic efforts** to help pregnant and lactating women quit smoking.
- **Nicotine gum is rated category C and the patches are rated category D,** but the circulating nicotine levels are only about half of those seen in pack-a-day smokers and there is no carbon monoxide.
- The American College of Obstetrics and Gynecology says that NRT can be considered if prior attempts to quit have been unsuccessful and the patient continues to smoke >10 to 15 cigarettes per day. Each patient should be informed about the presumed risks and benefits.[21]
- **Bupropion is rated as category C.**
  - A prospective study of women who used bupropion during pregnancy showed higher rates of spontaneous abortions (similar to other studies examining the safety of antidepressants during pregnancy) but no increase in the rates of major malformations.[22]
- **Varenicline is rated as category C.** There are no studies of its use in pregnancy.

Coronary Artery Disease
- NRT has been extensively studied and has been found to be **safe for patients with stable CAD** and can actually decrease myocardial ischemia (see the "Safety of NRT in Patients with Cardiovascular Disease" section).
- Bupropion overdose can cause tachycardia, conduction delays, and arrhythmias.
- Varenicline has not been reported to cause cardiac toxicity but was not marketed until 2006; studies and clinical experience are limited.

Weight Gain
- Weight gain is a significant concern for many would-be quitters.
- The average weight gain is only about 2 to 3 kg, but a minority (about 10%) may gain >12 kg.[23]
- The use of NRT or bupropion may delay or attenuate the weight gain, permitting time for the patient to focus on smoking cessation.
- Exercise will reduce the weight gain. Patients should follow a prudent healthy diet, but the period of smoking cessation is not a good time for a stringent diet.

REFERENCES

1. Centers for Disease Control and Prevention (CDC). Cigarette smoking among adults—United States, 2004. *MMWR Morb Mortal Wkly Rep* 2005;54:1121–1124.
2. Centers for Disease Control and Prevention (CDC). Cigarette smoking among adults-United States, 2000. *MMWR Morb Mortal Wkly Rep* 2002;51:642–645.
3. Fiore MC, Bailey BW, Cohen SJ, et al. Treating Tobacco Use and Dependence: Clinical Practice Guidelines. Rockville, MD: P.H.S., U.S. Department of Health and Human Services, 2000.
4. A clinical practice guideline for treating tobacco use and dependence: A US Public Health Service report. The Tobacco Use and Dependence Clinical Practice Guideline Panel, Staff, and Consortium Representatives. *JAMA* 2000;283:3244–3254.
5. Silagy C, Lancaster T, Stead L, Mant D, Fowler G. Nicotine replacement therapy for smoking cessation. *Cochrane Database Syst Rev* 2002:CD000146.
6. U.S. Department of Health and Human Services. The Health Consequences of Involuntary Exposure to Tobacco Smoke: A Report of the Surgeon General. Atlanta, GA: U.S. Department of Health and Human Services, Centers for Disease Control and Prevention, Coordinating Center for Health Promotion, National Center for Chronic Disease Prevention and Health Promotion, Office on Smoking and Health, 2006.
7. UK National Smoking Cessation Conference 2005. Available at: http://www.uknscc.org/2005_UKNSCC/speakers/alex_bobak.html. Last accessed December 21, 2009.
8. Blann AD, Steele C, McCollum CN. The influence of smoking and of oral and transdermal nicotine on blood pressure, and haematology and coagulation indices. *Thromb Haemost* 1997;78:1093–1096.
9. Tzivoni D, Keren A, Meyler S, et al. Cardiovascular safety of transdermal nicotine patches in patients with coronary artery disease who try to quit smoking. *Cardiovasc Drugs Ther* 1998;12:239–244.
10. Murray RP, Bailey WC, Daniels K, et al. Safety of nicotine polacrilex gum used by 3,094 participants in the Lung Health Study. Lung Health Study Research Group. *Chest* 1996; 109:438–445.
11. Mahmarian JJ, Moye LA, Nasser GA, et al. Nicotine patch therapy in smoking cessation reduces the extent of exercise-induced myocardial ischemia. *J Am Coll Cardiol* 1997;30: 125–130.
12. Leja M. Nicotine patches are safe to use in patients with coronary artery disease and stress induced myocardial ischemia in American College of Cardiology's 56th Annual Scientific Session. New Orleans, LA, 2007.
13. Ockene IS, Miller NH. Cigarette smoking, cardiovascular disease, and stroke: a statement for healthcare professionals from the American Heart Association. American Heart Association Task Force on Risk Reduction. *Circulation* 1997;96:3243–3247.
14. Blondal T, Gudmundson LJ, Olafsdottir I, et al. Nicotine nasal spray with nicotine patch for smoking cessation: randomised trial with six year follow up. Commentary: Progress on nicotine replacement therapy for smokers. *BMJ* 1999;318:285–288.
15. Hughes JR., Stead LF, Lancaster T. Antidepressants for smoking cessation. *Cochrane Database Syst Rev* 2003:CD000031.
16. Gold PB, Rubey RN, Harvey RT. Naturalistic, self-assignment comparative trial of bupropion SR, a nicotine patch, or both for smoking cessation treatment in primary care. *Am J Addict* 2002;11:315–331.
17. Jorenby DE, Leischow SJ, Nides MA, et al. A controlled trial of sustained-release bupropion, a nicotine patch, or both for smoking cessation. *N Engl J Med* 1999;340: 685–691.
18. Gonzales D, Rennard SI, Nides M, et al. Varenicline, an alpha4beta2 nicotinic acetylcholine receptor partial agonist, vs. sustained-release bupropion and placebo for smoking cessation: a randomized controlled trial. *JAMA* 2006;296:47–55.
19. Jorenby DE, Hayes JT, Rigotti NA, et al. Efficacy of varenicline, an alpha4beta2 nicotinic acetylcholine receptor partial agonist, vs. placebo or sustained-release bupropion for smoking cessation: a randomized controlled trial. *JAMA* 2006;296:56–63.

20. Hughes JR, Stead LF, Lancaster T. Nortriptyline for smoking cessation: a review. *Nicotine Tob Res* 2005;7:491–499.

21. Benowitz N, Dempsey D. Pharmacotherapy for smoking cessation during pregnancy. *Nicotine Tob Res* 2004;6:S189–S202.

22. Chun-Fai-Chan B, Koren G, Fayez I, et al. Pregnancy outcome of women exposed to bupropion during pregnancy: a prospective comparative study. *Am J Obstet Gynecol* 2005;192:932–936.

23. Executive summary of the clinical guidelines on the identification, evaluation, and treatment of overweight and obesity in adults. *Arch Intern Med* 1998;158:1855–1867.

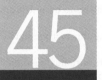

45 Alcohol Abuse
Mohsen Nasir and Thomas M. De Fer

General Principles

Alcohol use disorders are commonly encountered in primary care. Although modest alcohol use has proven cardioprotective benefits, abuse of alcohol can have detrimental physical, mental, emotional, and social effects. Alcohol-related health problems are numerous, including hepatic cirrhosis, pancreatitis, hypertension, cardiomyopathy, numerous cancers, dementia, and gastrointestinal bleeding. Fetal alcohol syndrome is the number one known cause of intellectual disability. Alcohol abuse and dependence have a heavy burden on society as a whole, as alcohol has been cited in half of all homicides and traffic fatalities. Patients of all ages, races, and socioeconomic status can suffer from alcoholism, and physicians should screen patients for alcohol use and abuse in each patient encounter.

Definitions
* **Alcohol abuse** is defined by the Diagnostic and Statistical Manual (DSM) IV as a maladaptive pattern of use associated with one or more of the following:
  * Failure to fulfill work, school, or social obligations.
  * Recurrent substance use in physically hazardous situations.
  * Recurrent legal problems related to substance use.
  * Continued use despite alcohol-related social or interpersonal problems.
* **Alcohol dependence** is a maladaptive pattern of use associated with three of the following seven behaviors over a 12-month interval:
  * Tolerance.
  * Evidence of withdrawal.
  * Alcohol is taken in larger quantity than intended.
  * Time is spent obtaining or using alcohol.
  * Persistent desire to cut back or discontinue alcohol use.
  * Alcohol use continues despite physical and psychological distress.
  * Social or occupational tasks are harmed.
* Of note, while 50% of patients with alcohol abuse will persistently have alcohol problems, only 10% will actually go on to develop dependence.
* The National Institute of Alcohol Abuse and Alcoholism defines **"at-risk" drinking** as follows:
  * Men, >14 drinks per week or >4 drinks per occasion.
  * Women, more than seven drinks per week or more than three drinks per occasion.
  * Those who habitually drink above these levels are at risk for alcoholism and alcohol-related problems.

Epidemiology
* At some point in their lifetime, over 90% of the U.S. population has had an alcoholic drink, and 80% of all high school seniors have had a drink by graduation.

- A recent study showed that lifetime prevalence of alcohol abuse to be 17.8% and the lifetime prevalence of alcohol dependence to be 12.5%.[1]
- After smoking and obesity, alcoholism is the third leading cause of preventable death in the United States.
- Approximately 85,000 deaths a year in the United States are attributed to alcohol, and the estimated costs attributed to alcohol are $185 billion yearly.[2]
- Binge drinking, defined as more than five drinks in a sitting for men and more than four drinks in a sitting for women, is prevalent among teens and college students. It contributes to high levels of risky sexual behavior, drunk driving, and poor academic performance in this patient population.
- It should be noted that patients with alcohol use disorders come from all walks of life. Physicians should not refrain from asking patients about alcohol use because they do not "fit" the stereotype of a "typical" alcoholic. Highly functional patients and the homeless, religious figureheads, educated, the young and old, poor and wealthy, and all patients should be screened for possible alcohol use.

Risk Factors
- Rates of alcohol abuse are higher in young males, single patients, those with lower income, and those from Native American or Caucasian descent. The prevalence of alcoholism is twice as high in men as in women.
- Studies have shown that those who begin drinking at an earlier age are much more likely to develop alcoholism than those who start after age 21.
- Recent evidence has shown that genetic factors can play a role in the development of alcoholism in certain people. Identical twins have been found to have a higher concordance of alcohol use than fraternal twins.

Associated Conditions
- Alcohol use disorders are associated with numerous conditions, including depression, anxiety, and other substance use disorders.
- Patients who present with alcohol use disorders should be screened for coexisting substance abuse or psychiatric disorders.
- Data from 1998 show that 30% of smokers are alcoholics and 80% of alcoholics are smokers.[3]

Diagnosis

- See the "Definitions" section for definitions of alcohol abuse and dependence.
- In this context, **screening** may be a more appropriate term.
- It should be noted in the definitions of alcohol abuse and dependence that the **amount** of alcohol consumed is not important. Although the consumption of higher amounts of alcohol may put someone at an elevated risk for an alcohol use disorder, the amount itself does not diagnose someone as having a disorder.

Clinical Presentation
- As alcoholism can affect patients of all walks of life, physicians must maintain a high index of suspicion and should question patients about alcohol consumption at each encounter.
- Screening should be done with validated tests such as the CAGE or AUDIT (Alcohol Use Disorder Identification Test) questionnaires (see the "Diagnostic Testing" section).

History

- A detailed history regarding alcohol abuse and other substances abuse should be taken at each patient visit.
- Physicians should be nonconfrontational and use nonjudgmental language when questioning patients about alcohol use.
- Patients frequently deny alcohol problems for a variety of reasons, including refusing to acknowledge the disease, shame or embarrassment, social stigma of being an alcoholic, and fear of being reported to employers or family members.
- Although physicians should be firm in discussing alcohol abuse with patients, they must also be empathic and should listen to what patients have to say about their disease.

Physical Examination

- Unless patients are intoxicated at the time of examination, the physical exam is not of great help in diagnosing alcohol disorders.
- Signs of chronic alcohol use include testicular atrophy, gynecomastia, spider angiomata, enlarged spleen, and shrunken or enlarged liver.

Differential Diagnosis

Conditions which may be associated, or confused, with alcohol disorders include depression, anxiety disorder, bipolar disorder, insomnia, and dysthymic disorder.

Diagnostic Testing

- The older **CAGE questionnaire** is the best-studied screening test for alcohol use disorders and is presented in Table 1.[4]
  - Patients who answer yes to any of the CAGE questions require further assessment and intervention. Patients who answer yes to two out of the four questions are seven times more likely to have alcohol dependence than the general population.
  - While initial studies have shown the CAGE questionnaire to be 75% sensitive, recent reports have shown it to be lower.[5] Critics point out that it **fails to identify binge drinkers and that it does not distinguish current from past alcohol use.** Although it may have its flaws, it remains a reasonable tool in screening patients in that it is quick, easy to use, and easy to remember.
- Another screening test is the **AUDIT** (Table 2).[6–9]
  - Studies have shown the AUDIT to be superior to the CAGE questionnaire in patients with active alcohol abuse or dependence.[10] It has also been found to have a higher sensitivity in populations with low rates of alcohol use.
  - The abbreviated three-item **AUDIT-C** questionnaire may also be an effective screening tool in primary care settings (Table 3).[8,11–14]
- **Perhaps, easiest of all in primary care is single question screening:** "How many times in the past year have you had five (four for women) or more drinks containing alcohol?" One or more heavy drinking days constitutes a positive screen.[8,15]

TABLE 1	CAGE Questionnaire

Have you ever felt the need to **CUT** down your drinking?
Have people **ANNOYED** you by criticizing your drinking?
Have you ever felt **GUILTY** about your drinking?
Have you ever had an **EYE-OPENER** to steady your nerves or to rid yourself of a hangover in the morning?

TABLE 2	Alcohol Use Disorders Identification Test

1. How often do you have a drink containing alcohol?
   (0) Never [skip   (1) ≤Monthly   (2) 2–4 times/   (3) 2–3 times/ (4) ≥4 times/
       to questions   month   week   week
       9 and 10]

2. How many drinks containing alcohol do you have on a typical day when you are drinking?
   (0) 1–2   (1) 3–4   (2) 5–6   (3) 7–9   (4) ≥10

3. How often do you have six or more drinks on one occasion?
   (0) Never   (1) <Monthly   (2) Monthly   (3) 2–3 times/ (4) ≥4 times/
                                                            week   week

Skip to questions 9 and 10 if total for questions 2 and 3 = 0

4. How often during the last year have you found that you were not able to stop drinking once you had started?
   (0) Never   (1) <Monthly   (2) Monthly   (3) 2–3 times/ (4) ≥4 times/
                                                            week   week

5. How often during the last year have you failed to do what was normally expected from you because of drinking?
   (0) Never   (1) <Monthly   (2) Monthly   (3) 2–3 times/ (4) ≥4 times/
                                                            week   week

6. How often during the last year have you needed a first drink in the morning to get yourself going after a heavy drinking session?
   (0) Never   (1) <Monthly   (2) Monthly   (3) 2–3 times/ (4) ≥4 times/
                                                            week   week

7. How often during the last year have you had a feeling of guilt or remorse after drinking?
   (0) Never   (1) <Monthly   (2) Monthly   (3) 2–3 times/ (4) ≥4 times/
                                                            week   week

8. How often during the last year have you been unable to remember what happened the night before because you had been drinking?
   (0) Never   (1) <Monthly   (2) Monthly   (3) 2–3 times/ (4) ≥4 times/
                                                            week   week

9. Have you or someone else been injured as a result of your drinking?
   (0) No   (2) Yes, but not in   (4) Yes, during
                                       the last year   the last year

10. Has a relative or friend or a doctor or other health worker been concerned about your drinking or suggested you cut down?
    (0) No   (2) Yes, but not in   (4) Yes, during
                                       the last year   the last year

Total score ≥8 indicates hazardous and harmful alcohol use, as well as possible alcohol dependence (≥7 for women and men >65 years).
Modified from Babor TF, Higgins-Biddle JC, Saunders JB, Monteiro MG. AUDIT. The Alcohol Use Disorders Identification Test: Guidelines for Use in Primary Care. 2nd Ed. Geneva: World Health Organization Department of Mental Health and Substance Dependence, 2001.

Laboratories
- Laboratory testing does not have a prominent role in diagnosing alcohol use disorders.
- Although tests such as γ-glutamyltransferase (GGT), liver function tests, and mean corpuscular volume can be abnormal in patients with chronic alcohol use, their sensitivity does not approach 50% and they should not be used as screening laboratories.

TABLE 3	AUDIT-C Questionnaire

1. How often do you have a drink containing alcohol?
   (0) Never (1) ≤Monthly (2) 2–4 times/ month (3) 2–3 times/ week (4) ≥4 times/ week
2. How many drinks containing alcohol do you have on a typical day when you are drinking?
   (0) 1–2 (1) 3–4 (2) 5–6 (3) 7–9 (4) ≥10
3. How often do you have six or more drinks on one occasion?
   (0) Never (1) <Monthly (2) Monthly (3) Weekly (4) Daily or almost daily

Scoring: ≥4 points for men or ≥3 points for women constitutes a positive screen.

They can be checked, however, when evaluating patients with chronic alcohol use to help manage patients.
- Blood alcohol levels may be useful in patients who appear to be intoxicated.

Treatment

- The first step in treating patients with alcohol abuse and dependence is making the patient aware that they have a disease. This should be done in an empathic and non-judgmental manner.
- Patients must be willing to change. The physician must listen to the patient and assess their readiness and willingness to change.
- Involving family members and friends is a good strategy to ensure that the patient has a strong support network when they leave the office. This should not be done, obviously, without approval of the patient.
- Brief interventions have been shown to reduce alcohol consumption.[16]
- Physicians should remember the **"Five As"** when conducting a brief intervention[8,17]:
  - **Ask:** Ask about alcohol use (see the "Diagnosis" section).
  - **Advise:** Advise the patients that their drinking puts them at high risk for alcoholism and alcohol-related problems. The specific effects of high-risk drinking should be explained.
  - **Assess:** Assess the patient's readiness to change and tailor advise accordingly (see later).
  - **Assist:** Provide specific self-help information.
  - **Arrange:** Arrange follow-up.
- Although not without critics,[18,19] the Prochaska **transtheoretical model of stages of change** is relatively well known to many clinicians and may serve to provide some very general guidelines regarding how much and what type of effort to invest. To some extent, the dividing lines between stages are arbitrary, individuals may not progress in a sequential manner between the stages, and the stages may not be mutually exclusive.
  - **Precontemplation stage:** The person is unaware or underaware of the problem and has no intention of changing the behavior. The physician's role is to advise the patient about the need to reduce alcohol consumption and the hazards of drinking. The counseling can be quite brief, just a minute or two, but should be repeated at every visit.
  - **Contemplation stage:** The patient is aware that a problem exists but is not yet ready to make a full commitment to take action. This stage may last for long periods of

time. The physician's role is to continue stressing the hazards of drinking and the benefits of behavior change. How to choose a goal can also be discussed.

- **Preparation stage:** The patient intends to take action in the next few months; this may be a brief stage. The physician should increase the intensity and specificity of counseling and help the patient choose a goal and give advice and encouragement. When a patient is really ready to commit to change, this should be the main focus of the office visit.

- **Action stage:** This is the most visible stage in which the addictive behavior is actually altered (for 1 day to 6 months). Review specific advice and continue to provide encouragement.

- **Maintenance stage:** The patient maintains the change and works to prevent relapse. This stage extends beyond 6 months and may last a lifetime. The physician should provide follow-up and continued encouragement.

- **Relapse stage:** This can also be termed **recycle** because the patient again moves through the cycle and may achieve long-term success on subsequent cycles. The physician should assist the patient in renewing the process.

- Patients should be encouraged to avoid bars and social gathering which may strongly encourage the patient to drink, and to seek help when relapse is near. Patients must learn how to cope with stress and anxiety once they abstain from alcohol.

- Constant follow-up is an integral part of treating patients. **<25% of patients will stay abstinent after a year.** Given this high relapse rate, physicians and patients may find treatment difficult and frustrating. Nevertheless, continued and consistent interaction with the patient is key to successful recovery.

Medications

- **Disulfiram,** an inhibitor of the enzyme aldehyde dehydrogenase, has been used to treat patients with alcohol use disorders once they become abstinent. Consumption of alcohol results in the accumulation of acetaldehyde and the development of symptoms including tachycardia, dyspnea, flushing, nausea, vomiting, headache, hypotension, and dizziness. Data supporting the use of disulfiram is equivocal.[20,21] It may be more effective when compliance is monitored.[8]

- **Naltrexone,** an opiate antagonist, has been used in alcoholics to decrease use. Several reviews have generally supported the use of naltrexone.[8,22–25] Recently, the COMBINE Study found better outcomes with the addition of naltrexone to medical management.[26]

- **Acamprosate,** a structural analog of γ-amino butyric acid but its mechanism of action is not fully understood. Reviews also support its use.[8,22,24,27] However, in the COMBINE Study, acamprosate was not more effective than placebo.[26]

- Benzodiazepines, β-blockers, clonidine, and anticonvulsants have all been used to treat alcohol withdrawal.

Other Nonpharmacological Therapies

- Brief interventions are 10 to 15 minutes patient encounters where counseling, feedback, goal setting, and follow-up are discussed. Numerous trials have shown these encounters to be effective in reducing drinking and increasing abstinence.[16]

- The COMBINE Study also demonstrated that cognitive behavior therapy was a helpful addition to medical management.[26]

- Alcoholics Anonymous and other support groups are wonderful community resources for patients. Physicians should have information about these resources in their office for patients who are willing to use them.

Lifestyle/Risk Modification

- Patients should be educated that abstinence is the most effective method of preventing relapse. Patients should adjust their lifestyle as much as possible to optimize their chance of remaining abstinent.
- This includes avoiding bars and other social gathering where the pressure to drink may be significant.
- In addition, patients should be aware of relapse triggers and should have numbers to call if they are in a situation where they may falter.

Diet

Patients with alcohol use disorders are prone to poor nutrition. Many may benefit from vitamin supplementation, especially folic acid.

Activity

Patients with alcohol abuse and dependence should be warned against driving and operating machinery when intoxicated.

Special Considerations

Patients who are withdrawing from alcohol, have delirium tremens or hallucinations, or have significant psychiatric comorbidity should be considered for inpatient treatment. Detailed discussion of these disorders is beyond the scope of this chapter.

Complications

- Patients who continue to abuse alcohol are predisposed to numerous health conditions. These include cirrhosis, dementia, Wernicke-Korsakoff syndrome, heart disease, malnutrition, pancreatitis, and numerous cancers.
- Women should especially be cautious when pregnant, as even small amounts of alcohol use have been shown to have negative effects on the growing fetus.

Referral

Referrals to a psychiatrist can be helpful in patients with comorbid psychiatric disease such as depression or bipolar disorder.

REFERENCES

1. Hasin DS, Stinson FS, Ogburn E, Grant BF. Prevalence, correlates, disability, and comorbidity of DSM-IV alcohol abuse and dependence in the United States: results from the National Epidemiologic Survey on Alcohol and Related Conditions. *Arch Gen Psychiatry* 2007;64:830–842.
2. Saitz R. Clinical practice. Unhealthy alcohol use. *N Engl J Med* 2005;352:596–607.
3. Miller NS, Gold MS. Comorbid cigarette and alcohol addiction: epidemiology and treatment. *J Addict Dis* 1998;17:55–66.
4. Mayfield D, McLeod G, Hall P. *Am J Psychiatry* 1974;131:1121–1123.
5. Buchsbaum DG, Buchanan RG, Centor RM, et al. *Ann Intern Med* 1991;115:774–777.
6. Saunders JB, Aasland OG, Babor TF, et al. Development of the Alcohol Use Disorders Identification Test (AUDIT): WHO Collaborative Project on Early Detection of Persons with Harmful Alcohol Consumption—II. *Addiction* 1993;88:791–804.

7. Babor TF, Higgins-Biddle JC, Saunders JB, Monteiro MG. AUDIT. The Alcohol Use Disorders Identification Test: Guidelines for Use in Primary Care. 2nd Ed. Geneva: World Health Organization Department of Mental Health and Substance Dependence, 2001.

8. Helping patients who drink too much: a clinician's guide. Updated 2005 edition. NIH Publication No. 07-3769. Washington, DC: National Institute on Alcohol Abuse and Alcoholism, 2007.

9. Berner MM, Kriston L, Bentele M, Härter M. The alcohol use disorders identification test for detecting at-risk drinking: a systematic review and meta-analysis. *J Stud Alcohol Drugs* 2007;68:461–473.

10. Bradley KA, Bush KR, McDonell MB, et al.; The Ambulatory Care Quality Improvement Project (ACQUIP). Screening for problem drinking: Comparison of CAGE and AUDIT, *J Gen Intern Med* 1998;13:379–388.

11. Taj N, Devera-Sales A, Vinson DC. Screening for problem drinking: does a single question work? *J Fam Pract* 1998;46:328–335.

12. Williams R, Vinson DC. Validation of a single screening question for problem drinking. *J Fam Pract* 2001;50:307–312.

13. Seale JP, Boltri JM, Shellenberger S, et al. Primary care validation of a single screening question for drinkers. *J Stud Alcohol* 2006;67:778–784.

14. Kriston L, Hölzel L, Weiser AK, et al. Meta-analysis: are 3 questions enough to detect unhealthy alcohol use? *Ann Intern Med* 2008;149:879–888.

15. Smith PC, Schmidt SM, Allensworth-Davies D, Saitz R. Primary care validation of a single-question alcohol screening test. *J Gen Intern Med* 2009;24:783–788.

16. Kaner EF, Beyer F, Dickinson HO, et al. Effectiveness of brief alcohol interventions in primary care populations. *Cochrane Database Syst Rev* 2007 April 18;(2):CD004148.

17. Babor TF, Higgins-Biddle JC. Brief Intervention for Hazardous and Harmful Drinking: A Manual for Use in Primary Care. Geneva: World Health Organization Department of Mental Health and Substance Dependence, 2001.

18. Riemsma RP, Pattenden J, Bridle C, et al. Systematic review of the effectiveness of stage based interventions to promote smoking cessation. *BMJ* 2003;326:1175–1177.

19. Bridle C, Piemsma RP, Pattenden J, et al. Systematic review of the effectiveness of health behavior interventions based on the transtheoretical mode. *Psychol Health* 2005;20:283–301.

20. Hughes JC, Cook CC. The efficacy of disulfiram: a review of outcome studies. *Addiction* 1997;92:381–395.

21. West SL, Garbutt JC, Carey, TS, et al. Pharmacotherapy for alcohol dependence. Evidence report number 3. (Contract 290-97-0011 to Research Triangle Institute, University of North Carolina, Chapel Hill). AHCPR publication no. 99-E004. Rockville, MD: Agency for Health Care Policy and Research, January 1999.

22. Bouza C, Angeles M, Munoz A, Amate JM. Efficacy and safety of naltrexone and acamprosate in the treatment of alcohol dependence: a systematic review. *Addiction* 2004;99: 811–828.

23. Srisurapanont M, Jarusuraisin N. Opioid antagonists for alcohol dependence. *Cochrane Database Syst Rev* 2005 Jan 25;(1):CD001867.

24. Buonopane A, Petrakis IL. Pharmacotherapy of alcohol use disorders. *Subst Use Misuse* 2005;40:2001–2020, 2043–2048.

25. Pettinati HM, O'Brien CP, Rabinowitz AR, et al. The status of naltrexone in the treatment of alcohol dependence: specific effects on heavy drinking. *J Clin Psychopharmacol* 2006;26: 610–625.

26. Anton RF, O'Malley SS, Ciraulo DA, et al. Combined pharmacotherapies and behavioral interventions for alcohol dependence: the COMBINE study: a randomized controlled trial. *JAMA* 2006;295:2003–2017.

27. Overman GP, Teter CJ, Guthrie SK. Acamprosate for the adjunctive treatment of alcohol dependence. *Ann Pharmacother* 2003;37:1090–1099.

Index

Note: Italicized *f* and *t* refer to figures and tables